Soldner / Stellmann

Individual Paediatrics

Soldner / Stellmann

Individual Paediatrics

Physical, emotional and spiritual aspects of diagnosis and counselling

Anthroposophic-homoeopathic therapy

Georg Soldner, Munich
H. Michael Stellmann†, Bad Aibling

CRC Press
Taylor & Francis Group

MedPharm
Scientific Publishers

CRC Press
Taylor & Francis Group
6000 Broken Sound Parkway NW, Suite 300
Boca Raton, FL 33487-2742

Version Date: 20140829

ISBN: 978-1-4822-0729-3 (hbk)
ISBN: 978-1-4987-1564-5 (eBook - PDF)

Visit the Taylor & Francis Web site at
http://www.taylorandfrancis.com

and the CRC Press Web site at
http://www.crcpress.com

Foreword

> The ideal of complete health is only of interest from a scientific perspective. Illness is part of being an individual.
> Novalis

The positive response to the first three editions of this book was gratifying and encouraged the authors to produce a thoroughly updated and enhanced new edition. For many colleagues this book has become a consultative resource, both for the treatment of children and the support of parents. An individualized approach to paediatrics is dependent on dialogue between parents and physician, with the child at the centre. In this way the child and, later, the adolescent can be recognized in his or her developmental potential as a unique individuality. In encountering both physical illness and psychological crises, this potential is particularly challenged; however, overcoming illness may also support the development of the child's individualization.

For this reason, it is of considerable consequence whether one approaches paediatric medicine in purely technological terms, aiming to restore complete and permanent health, or whether children are encouraged to actively overcome their health crises through providing them with sustained support in their capacity for self-regulation. The latter approach, combined with accompanying paediatric expertise, enables the child and parents to experience that they themselves can contribute to achieving the condition of health. In this process their skills are strengthened and their trust in – and familiarity with – their own capacity to overcome crises is enhanced. Health, particularly during childhood, is not a given state that only needs to be protected and maintained by means of medical intervention: health has to be permanently striven for and stabilized – even the success of an operation relies on the body's inherent capacity to self-heal. Research in recent years has shown that childrens' experiences and initiative in early childhood make a significant contribution to the development of health, on both physical and on psychological levels. Against this background, anthroposophic medicines and homoeopathic remedies can be understood as offering regulating impulses that encourage the child to overcome the pathological one-sidedness of the disease, thereby utilizing their own strength, and establishing a new, healthy equilibrium. It is evident that if this form of treatment is to be successfully practiced, it does not only require familiarity with the pathology but also a willingness to assess each patient on an individual basis with respect to their available bodily and psychological resources. Such an approach certainly does not ignore the general contributions and specific medical interventions of conventional medicine, as and when these are considered to be necessary by the physician and parents. Indeed, the doctor-parent-child relationship is supported and encouraged as and when the therapeutic approach is jointly affirmed and reviewed at suitable intervals in the light of all the available options.

The present new edition of this book has been thoroughly updated. All new material is based, as before, on the clinical experience of the authors. Parents and children feel a growing need to be acknowledged as individuals, enter a dialogue, and to be understood and involved themselves in decisions on prophylaxis and treatment. The present volume attempts to outline the foundations that can support and facilitate such a dialogue in daily practice, based on current knowledge and experience. Medical prescribing is supported by a comprehensive index and detailed table of contents, enabling quick access to specific themes and treatment options. However, to appreciate the context of individual therapeutic interventions, reading a whole chapter or subject area remains indispensible. In this respect, the book can be used both as a practical guide that can quickly be consulted, and also as a resource for a more in depth study and discussion among colleagues.

The authors would like to thank Dr. Tim Kersebohm for the agreement of the Wissenschaftliche Verlagsgesellschaft Stuttgart to publish a thoroughly revised new edition and Ms. Luise Keller for her careful editing. Many suggestions were incorporated, arising from various discussions with colleagues. The authors are indebted to René Madeleyn, Jan Vagedes, Matthias Girke, Markus Sommer and Friedwart Husemann for valuable suggestion regarding the text as a whole, and to Thomas Fuchs (Introduction), Martin Hirte (Vaccination), Till Reckert (Vitamin D), Franziska Roemer (Allergic diseases, Atopic dermatitis, Acne), Bernd Ulrich, Dieter Ecker and Bernhard Wingeier (Bronchial asthma), Karl-Reinhard Kummer, Lüder Jachens and Christoph Schempp (Atopic dermatitis, Allergies), Reinhard Schwarz (Anthroposophic medicines), and Johannes Lorentz (Rheumatology) with regard to individual chapters. We would also like to use this opportunity to thank the many other colleagues, not mentioned specifically by name, for their suggestions and critiques.

The present book has grown out of dialogue between the authors. In this context the "leading thought", expressed in the words of Novalis, have stood before us like a guiding star. The death of Michael Stellmann on 2 April 2010 represented a profound caesura, although in my experience, this dialogue continues to provide the foundation from which the form of this book derives. Very warm thanks are due to Michael Stellmann's family for allowing full access to his medical estate. This new edition is accordingly dedicated to the memory of H. Michael Stellmann, one of the great pioneers of anthroposophic and homoeopathic paediatrics.

Georg Soldner

Foreword to the first German language edition

The original stimulus for writing this book arose in response to conversations with colleagues. Nowadays, many paediatritians have the desire to extend the paradigms of their practice beyond treatment protocols that are based exclusively on conventional guidelines, derived from a so-called evidence-based science. Although, substantial and detailed documentation also exists concerning the empirical efficacy of medicines used in both homoeopathic and naturopathic practice, in the absence of an extension of corresponding disease-specific diagnostic paradigms, suggestions for possible therapeutic interventions in these fields of practice remain unsatisfactory. Such an extension, moreover, would require an integrative understanding of both physical and soul-spiritual aspects of child development. When assessed within this broader context, the potential treatment options and their associated risk factors for a specific disease thereby acquire a different perspective. A re-evaluation of risks and treatment options then becomes possible, which also takes the particular character and possible developmental role of the illness under consideration. Such a comprehensive diagnostic evaluation then provides a sound basis for assessing which therapeutic direction would be appropriate for a specific illness, and in a particular situation.

In the author's experience, descriptions of the human being and of outer nature that underlie the practice of anthroposophic medicine offer a highly differentiated lens, through which physical, soul and spiritual aspects of child development may be perceived and interpreted and possible pathologies in each of these spheres integrated into a comprehensive diagnostic picture. Not only will the rationale underlying a proposed therapeutic intervention then be evidence-based in the empirical sense, but it will also include such an individualized assessment. In the clinical setting, a comprehensive approach of this kind to diagnosis encourages the creation of a correspondingly differentiated treatment plan, in which the child can be fully honoured in every aspect of his or her individuality. Such an approach does not replace conventional paediatric training, nor will it underestimate the value of conventional scientific research and its resultant 'state of the art' treatment protocols; it rather seeks to extend the depth and scope of physicians' perceptual diagnostic ability and to enhance their capacity to differentiate between the several components or levels through which human individuality is manifests at a bodily level.

This book aims to offer suggestions for such an individualized therapeutic approach, based on the practical experience gained by the authors in their clinical practice. The path towards this goal begins during the clinical consultation with the direct perception of the child and its environment, enhanced through attentive and unprejudiced listening. The essential aspects of the pathological process under consideration will then reveal themselves. To this end, suggestions are included at the beginning of each chapter. Their aim is to extend the general diagnostic concepts in use today (e. g. pneumonia, sinusitis, asthma) so that the individual background relevant to each case of illness is included; for example, why has this particular child developed pneumonia or asthma at this particular time? In their suggestions for treatment, the authors can only – and only intend to – indicate possible interventions, even when a particular treatment has indeed shown itself to have general validity. The authors intend no more than to help prepare and offer support to paediatritians, when deciding which potential therapeutic option may be appropriate in the given case. Their intention is essentially to stimulate therapeutic skills rather than to advocate particular therapeutic measures or to offer universally valid prescriptions.

The respective limits and risks of the specified treatment proposals are indicated. The authors have consciously decided to refrain from discussing pathological conditions of which they have no personal experience or where additional therapeutic interventions cannot be suggested (e. g. as in bacterial meningitis).

This book makes use of established paediatric classifications and terminology. In so far as these were considered too restrictive, the attempt has been made to extend the boundaries of the familiar terminology in such a way that medically trained readers will find the author's thinking comprehensible. By engaging with this text, readers may simply gain a broader perspective, relevance for daily practice, of their patients and their families; their relational and communication skills may thereby be extended. They will also encounter descriptions of the art of extending medicine, based on the content and methodology of homoeopathic and anthroposophic practice. We would invite the reader to engage further in this dialogue, which will inevitably take on a different character for each individual. In this connection, the authors consider a living interest in the enhancement of skill within paediatric diagnosis and therapy to be the most important prerequisite, rather than the reader's level of previous knowledge. By approaching the text in this spirit, it should be possible to test its contents in practice. With respect to epistemological questions, we refer the reader to the established cognitive methodologies underlying the respective disciplines of natural science, humanities and anthroposophy. Homoeopathy itself arises from the spirit of the Enlightenment[1] and in that respect it embodies a clear methodology, albeit one that is restricted to an empirical approach. Anthroposophy needs to be understood as a spiritual scientific approach, whose epistemological foundations have been published, and whose relevant literature is generally available for consultation. In the final analysis, however, the contents of this book should be evaluated in the context the reader's encounter with the individual patient; their relevance and effectiveness can only be meaningfully assessed on the touchstone of clinical practice. In this spirit, the authors welcome criticism and suggestions from colleagues.

First and foremost, we would like to thank our patients who, through placing their confidence in us, have made this work possible. We would also like to extend thanks all teachers and colleagues who educated and supported us, listened to us and debated with us. The warmth engendered through such reciprocal giving and receiving has greatly strengthened our confidence.

We would also like to express particular thanks to two colleagues; to Markus Sommer, who has always made his extensive knowledge freely available to us and to Andreas Korselt. Without their committed support, it would not have been possible to write this book.

Particularly thanks are extended to Dr. Muth from the Wissenschaftliche Verlagsgesellschaft Stuttgart, who, with understanding and generosity translated our ideas and intentions into reality.

1 "Enlightenment was a desire for human affairs to be guided by rationality rather than by faith, superstition, or revelation; a belief in the power of human reason to change society and liberate the individual from the restraints of custom or arbitrary authority; all backed up by a world view increasingly validated by science rather than by religion or tradition." Dorinda Outram: The Enlightenment. Cambridge University Press, Cambridge 1995, Page 3.

In conclusion, our gratitude extends not the least to our wives for their willingness to engage with our thoughts and ideas in a warm and creative dialogue, and for the enthusiasm they have shown in doing this.

Munich/Bad Aibling, March 2001	Georg Soldner H. Michael Stellmann

Translator's notes and welcome to the English edition

A personal note about the author

Georg Soldner began treating patients under the late H. Michael Stellmann's mentorship as a medical student. He continued doing so throughout his eight years of paediatric hospital work in Munich, including three years of neonatal and intensive care. He is an anthroposophic doctor with a strong connection to homoeopathic and anthroposophic preparations, hence these aspects are emphasized in this book. I have experienced him as a highly dedicated, powerful person with encyclopaedic knowledge – not only of medicine. He really takes on responsibility for his patients, enabling them and their parents to feel secure in his care. I was surprised to hear that many of them have his mobile phone number and can call him at any time, night or day. He guides them so well that they rarely need to call him out of office hours: "This should work in such and such a way by such time, please call me at such time to tell me how the treatment is working." By demanding brief feedback from his patients, Georg continually assesses how his prescriptions are working, which is why his book is growing and changing from one edition to the next. Anyone acquainted with the complexities of everyday paediatrics knows that decades of such individual experience supported by a sound memory and digested by a keen mind can only partially be substituted by the results of scientific studies. In fact, our present reliance on guidelines and study data, together with the costs and hurdles of clinical studies, have slowed down the pace of relevant drug discoveries and undermine our art of practicing individualized medicine. Kienle and Kiene have portrayed this as follows:

> "After the golden ages between 1930 and 1965, when seminal discoveries irrevocably changed medicine, the rate of remedial innovation has continuously declined despite billions of dollars invested. The great discoveries were made by ingenious pioneering individuals who combined basic science and passionate clinical work: driven by the desire to cure patients, guided by scientific thinking; open to the unexpected, and little hampered by bureaucracy and costs. For their discoveries, clinical judgement was indispensable. Relying on small sample sizes and discarding therapies unless there were obvious effects in 10–20 patients, they found spectacular results and thus expedited innovation. Effects that could only be seen in large trials were regarded as not worth bothering about. The spectacular, ground-breaking discoveries such as sulphonamides, penicillin, cephalosporins, neuroleptics, antidepressants, steroids, etc. would possibly not have been made within the requirements of modern research bureaucracy.
> [...] As long as the doctors are, in principle, considered incapable of judging whether they help their individual patient or not, they will need strict external guidance. Clinical judgement, and its further development, is therefore a key issue for the future destiny of the medical profession. An advancement of clinical judgement could grant a renewed cognitive basis for medical expertise and medical professionalism, and could increase both the intellectual and practical autonomy of the doctor."[1]

Georg was sharpening his clinical skills and developing his habits of gathering feedback and forming clinical judgments at a transition phase, experiencing the benefits of the new developments (e.g. surfactant and 3rd generation cephalosporins) while guidelines and so-called evidence-based medicine were in the making. And while he always strives to

1 Kienle GS, Kiene H. Clinical Judgement and the Medical Profession. J Eval Clin Pract 2010;17(4):621–7

speak out of personal experience, the hundreds of references at the end of each chapter provide testimony to his appreciation for what other scientists and clinicians have contributed to modern medicine.

Georg is also the initiator of the Vademecum of Anthroposophic Medicines, a large compendium built on the experience reports of doctors around the world. So if you experience any of the indications in this book as helpful (or not helpful), please take 5 minutes to fill in this feedback form: www.merkurstab.de/Dateien/Vademecum/EN-Form-Feedback.pdf.

Useful Addresses, links and resources for Anthroposophic Medicine

- **Medical Section, School for Spiritual Science, Goetheanum:**
  www.goetheanum-medizin.ch
  The international centre for anthroposophic medicine.
- **International Federation of Anthroposophic Medical Associations:**
  www.ivaa.info
  English-language website. To find the Anthroposophic medical associations in your country, see: www.ivaa.info/about-ivaa/ivaa-member-organizations
- **Anthromed Library:** www.anthromed.org
  Offers many articles and resources in English also includes many links to suppliers etc. on www.anthromed.org/Links.aspx
- The Journal of Anthroposophic Medicine: www.merkurstab.de
- The Vademecum of Anthroposophic Medicine: www.vademecum.org

Note on vocabulary

Anthroposophy differentiates four main levels of human existence: physical, life (etheric body, which plants and animals also have), soul (with its astral body, which animals also have) and spirit (I, or Ego). When dealing with anthroposophic terminology, it is important to be aware that that words and ideas are invitations to pursue an experiential path, not substitutes for experience. This will help to avoid confusion and difficulties with words. The word ego (also referred to as Ego, I or spirit), for example, is used in anthroposophy in a manner that sometimes differs to its use in some other branches of spirituality or psychology. The term ego here refers to the self as a spiritual, creative entity, which has evolved throughout world history together with the evolving human body, thus creating bodies capable of manifesting individual spirits (hence, human bodies have an Ego-organization – also called I-organization – that lifts the astral, etheric and physical to a "higher" organizational level).

To develop a living and useful relationship to these concepts and be able to use them to extend and differentiate perception in everyday life and in relation to modern-day thinking and medicine, reading the first chapter of this book (1. Introduction) is recommendable, as well as Rudolf Steiner's basic works (e. g. "Theosophy") – where further differentiations can be found. Anthroposophically oriented doctors and therapists strive to pay attention to these four levels of being, thereby making use of modern diagnostic and therapeutic technology as well as working towards deeper insights through various meditative and observational practices and study of sources of higher wisdom.

Body, soul and spirit each have a lower and a higher aspect to themselves. Thus, our everyday thoughts and intellect are related to our spirit, but rather like a shadow is related to the form that casts it. Our feelings and emotions are related to our soul in a similar way.

Notes on the Medicines

Medicine names

1. Generally, the **German registered medicine names** and formulations have been kept in the translation because different countries use different names. Many medicines available in other countries carry the same name as the German medicines e. g. Anaemodoron, Aconitum Napellus etc, and that which is available may differ strongly per region/ country.
2. Some medicines have a different corresponding English name (e. g. Onopordon comp.). Many English names can be quickly accessed through the general **Index of Medicines** of the Vademecum of Anthroposophic Medicine (www.merkurstab.de/ index.php5?page=123). This Index of Medicines can also be used to find anthroposophic medicines carrying different names in other countries such as Great Britain (GB), Switzerland (CH) and Austria (AT) or to source similar medicinal compositions which have different manufacturers and different names.
3. The Country of manufacture is Germany unless otherwise specified. Information regarding availability of a medicine outside of the country of manufacture is not included. See manufacturer contact information below.

Procuring medicines

1. International pharmacies
   Medicines from an international pharmacy can be ordered in the country of manufacture or through a pharmacy willing to dispatch products internationally. Manufacturers and the international professional pharmaceutical associations, the IAAP and its member organizations can be consulted for further information in this regard (see Appendix I for a list of addresses).
   The situation on organ preparations is particularly difficult: Weleda UK, for example, has ceased trading most of these (mainly Wala) preparations. Especially all central nervous system ones are only obtainable through the German 'international pharmacies'
2. Special preparations
   Not all the medicines included in this book are available in 'ready-to-use' form and may need to be specially prepared (see also "prescribing medicines" below). In such cases, the basic formula is given and where relevant, the particular pharmacy experienced in preparing the medicine at the reported level of quality. The Gesellschaft Anthroposophischer Pharmazeuten in Deutschland (GAPiD, www.gapid.de) [Association of Anthroposophic Pharmacists] is actively involved in further education and certification in the field of anthroposophic pharmacy and could be of valuable assistance in this regard.

Prescribing medicines

In this book two kinds of prescriptions are used: **noncompounded** and **compounded**.

A **noncompounded** (or precompounded) order consists of a drug or a mixture of drugs supplied by a pharmaceutical company by its official or proprietary name and, if it contains more than one substance, the specific ingredients do not have to be listed.

A **compounded prescription**, also called *formula magistralis* (from Latin word magister – teacher) or *extemporaneous prescription* is an order that requires mixing of one or more ingredients (active medicaments) with one or more pharmaceutical necessities (vehicle, suspending agent). The physician selects the drugs, doses, and pharmaceutical form that he or she desires and the pharmacist prepares the medication accordingly. The name of each drug is placed on a separate line under the preceding one. The order of ingredients is as follows:

Remedium cardinale (basis). The basis is the principal drug and gives the prescription its chief action.

Remedium adjuvans (adjuvant). As the name suggests, the adjuvant is a drug that aids or increases the action of the principal ingredient.

Remedium corrigens (corrective). The corrective modifies or corrects undesirable effects of the basic or adjuvant.

Remedium constituens (vehicle). The vehicle is the agent used as a solvent in the solution, to increase the size and volume, or to dilute the mixture. The most potent or principal drug is written first, the other ingredient second, and the vehicle last, as shown in the example.

Example: Rp./

Spanish fly (pulvis)	1.57 g
Yellow wax	3.07 g
Peanut oil	0.77 g
Turpentine	0.77 g

Mix and put on textile (misce fiat emplastrum) 9 x 12 cm

There is a long list of (mainly latin) abbreviations used for compound prescriptions (see the list below and en.wikipedia.org/wiki/List_of_abbreviations_used_in_medical_prescriptions). However, such abbreviations are increasingly discouraged since they can lead to confusion (see also "conventions for avoiding ambiguity in en.wikipedia.org/wiki/Medical_prescription).

Side effects and contraindications

Manufacturer prescribing and patient information concerning side effects and contraindications is not included and is only mentioned if considered particularly relevant. This vast subject cannot be explored here at any depth. Suffice to say that the obligatory prescribing and patient information fulfils official requirements and partly reflects an inadequate level of knowledge (e. g. absence of child studies) and is therefore of varying significance for practicing physicians. Much of the information provided is more the result of a lack of knowledge rather than positively confirmed knowledge.

The official prescribing information should be consulted regarding pharmaceutical additives such as wheat starch in tablets or cetylstearyl alcohol and lanolin in ointment vehicles. The field of medicine production is continually developing and therefore changes in the medicine ranges, names, additives, and dosage forms are unavoidable. Please refer to the official prescribing information.

Note on homoeopathic potency symbols

The commonly used German symbols denoting potency strengths have been kept throughout the text, rather than using English (or other) conventions. Below is a guide to equivalency.

Potency Ratio (dilution)	German usage	German example	English usage	English example
1 to 10	D	D5	x	5x
1 to 100	C	C6	c	6c
1 to 1000	M	M7	M	7M
1 to 50,000	LM or Q	LM8 or Q8	LM	8LM

Thank you notes

My co-translators (Christian von Arnim, Susan Nurmi-Schomers, David McGregor, Jonathan Bruton, Anna Meus and Paul Motley) and the following people and institutions are warmly thanked for their involvement in this translation project: The Mahle Stiftung, Vidarstiftelsen, Hausserstiftung, the Medizinisches Seminar Bad Boll, the Medical Section at the Goetheanum, Physicians' Association for Anthroposophic Medicine (USA), New Zealand Anthroposophic Medical Association, Anthroposophic Medical Association (United Kingdom), Läkarförening För Anthroposofiskt Orienterad Medicin (Sweden), Canadian Anthroposophic Medical Association, Alicia Landman-Reiner MD, Frank Mulder MD, Stefan Geider MD, Simon Bednarek MD, Ursula Flatters MD, Nedi Eckler MD, Kenneth McAlister MD, Renee Meyer MD, Nancy Spates MD, Steven Johnson MD, Mark Kamsler MD, Michael Allen MD, Nicole Shorrock MD, David Gershan MD, James Dyson MD, Judith Klahre-Parker, Judith Soleil and Elia Gilbert from Rudolf Steiner Library, New York, and last but definitely not least the team at the Wissenschaftliche Verlagsgesellschaft Stuttgart (above all Dr. Tim Kersebohm). Please address any comments regarding the translation to Priv.-Doz. Dr. med. David Martin, Die Filderklinik, Im Haberschlai 7, 70794 Filderstadt, Germany.

Tübingen, Spring 2014 David Martin

Table of contents

Note for the reader

The present book is divided into chapters that can each be read independently. The reader will find introductory perspectives in each chapter, which support the understanding of the text as a whole. That applies above all to chapters 1, 5, 7, 6 and 3. If the book is read in that order, the methodology inherent in the volume will more easily become accessible to the reader. This applies above all to those readers who have not yet made closer contact with anthroposophic medicine. The authors focus on paediatric practice as this is reflected in the consulting room, a well as on diagnosis and therapy. However, this cannot replace the need for independent study of the methodological foundations of both homoeopathy and anthroposophic medicine.

Abbreviations

Abbreviation	Term
/d	per day
/h	per hour
/m	per month
/wk	per week
’or gtt.	drops
1 x/h	once per hour
1-2 x/d	one to two times per day
15 ml	tablespoon
1-5 x/wk	one to five times per week
5 ml	teaspoon
aa	ana = equal parts
a.c.	ante cibum (before meals)
ADD	attention deficit disorder
ADHD	attention deficit hyperactivity disorder
ALL	acute lymphatic leukaemia
AML	acute myeloic leukaemia
amp.	ampoule
cap./caps.	capsule/s
ccm	cubic centimetre (=ml)
CFS	chronic fatigue syndrome
CH	Switzerland
cm	centimetre
CNS	central nervous system
comp.	compositum
DE	Germany
DHU	Deutsche Homöopathie-Union
DGPI	German Society of Paediatric Infectiology
dil.	dilution
e. g.	for example
EPH gestosis	oedema-proteinuria-hypertension syndrome
esp.	especially
ext.	external application
g	gram
glob.	globuli
gtt. or ’	drops
gtt. a.c.	drops before meals
hr/hrs	hour(s)
hrly	hourly
i.c.	intracutaneous
i. e.	that is
i.m.	intramuscular
i.v.	intravenous
incl.	including

inj.	injection(s)
ITP	Idiopathic Thrombocytopenic Purpura.
l	litre
mg	milligram
mins.	minutes
ml	millilitre
mo.	month(s)
MRI	magnetic resonance tomography
neg.	negative
NSAID	non steroidal anti-inflammatory drug
Ø	mother tincture
p.c.	post cibum (after meals)
PCO	polycystic ovary syndrome
per os	orally
pill.	pillules
pos.	positive
p.r.n.	pro re nata (as needed)
Rh	rhythmically treated plant preparation
RSV-infection	respiratory syncytial virus infection
Rx	prescription
s.c.	subcutaneous
s.m.	submucosal
saltsp.	salt spoon = 1/8 of a tea spoon
sec.	seconds
SIDS	Sudden Infant Death Syndrome
supp.	suppositories
tab./tabs	tablet/s
trit.	trituration
wk/wks	week(s)
yr/yrs	year(s)

Selected German-English vocabulary

German	English
Apotheke	pharmacy
Augentropfen	eye drops
Eisen	iron
Essenz	essence
Fieber	fever
Flechte(n)	lichen
Honig	honey
Kreislauf	circulation
Meteoreisen	meteoric iron
Nahrung	nourishment, food
Nase	nose
Nasensalbe	nasal ointment
Nerven	nerve
Öl	oil
Puder	powder
pur	pure
quaddeln	Multiple small intracutaneous injections leading to vesicles
Quark	curd cheese
Salbe	ointment
Salbengrundlage	ointment base
Schnupfen	sniffles, head cold
Tablette(n)	tablets
Zahnung	teething
Zäpfchen	suppository

1 Introduction

(Edited and revised by James A. Dyson, MD)

Who are you? This question often lives, almost unnoticed, in the initial encounter with the newborn child. In every consultation with a patient, asking this question can help the physician to pause and, for a brief moment to observe with awe the human individual beside him or her. This feeling of reverent wonder is particularly intense when observing the newborn child. A self-reflective attitude of soul can reveal that the child is already an individual human being, i. e., the child's individuality is already present even before it unfolds and reveals itself (a feeling that also pervades encounters with seriously disabled children).

A child's life is permeated by an intentionality to bring its individuality to expression. With its birth, the newborn child takes the most incisive step on this path. It may bring the child close to death and the mother to the brink of what she can deal with and endure. The impulse that triggers the birth process, at least under normal circumstances, comes from the child itself: he or she wants to be born! Is it possible to fathom why human birth takes place so dramatically; can we discern the underlying reasons behind this?

The way this question is answered will have far-reaching consequences for how illness and death are to be understood and confronted in paediatrics. When reflecting on the deeper reality that underlies birth, it becomes evident how theoretical it would be to imagine that every illness, every crisis along the way, should be avoided; such an apparent ideal appears meaningless. Human development clearly follows a different path; only through meeting profound crisis does a new and incisive developmental step take place, Moreover, it is the individualized intentionality underlying the incarnation process that can so clearly be sensed, particularly during the physical birth and later in the presence of the newborn child. Similar developmental steps can also be experienced in older children who have come through a serious illness or maturation crisis; these steps may witness the deepening connection of the spiritual and soul individuality to the child's body.

In periods when a child is in crisis, the question "Who are you?" may often arise. One is then reconnected to that moment when it was posed for the first time. "What did you feel, what thoughts did you have, when you gave birth to your child, when you saw and held him or her for the first time in your arms?" Many mothers can, if prompted and after some hesitation, express their original feelings; and when entering subsequent periods of childhood crises, memories from the first stages of life, for example, pregnancy, birth and breast-feeding, turn out to be of key significance. An understanding for the inner necessity underlying the process of birth makes it possible to recognize the meaning, to experience the developmental moment for the child during a subsequent illness. The natural wish to avoid illnesses and crises and to suppress them finds its counterbalance in silently asking the question of the child: "Where is your intentionality leading you now? What medical or educational support do you need to proceed on your way and overcome this crisis? What are your capacities for self-regulation and what are its boundaries? What are you capable of achieving yourself and where might you need to be relieved of a task for a time?"

When physician and parents jointly adopt such an attitude and are prepared to sound these questions together, answers may be forthcoming that, in the given situation, would influence the practice of paediatric medicine.

1.1 The individualized human body

In the initial stages of life, the child's body changes from day to day. One questions whether the child is drinking enough, growing well enough, whether the rate of growth is appropriate for his or her age, and so on. The paediatrician encounters these questions on a daily basis. Acute diarrhoea with major fluid loss can quickly place a small child's life in danger. How quickly the body can change under such circumstances, losing its roundness, its healthy colour, giving a limp and wilted impression! During the twentieth century, medicine has developed the knowledge and skills to help children in such emergency situations in a way that is historically without precedent. Physicians experience deep satisfaction if a life can be saved through an intervention as minor as an infusion. But such success hides an important question: what is the nature of this life that we are called to serve as physicians, and for which we are fighting? What differentiates the living body from the body that has become lifeless?

Medical training projects a picture of the body that gives the impression of a highly complicated technical apparatus, one in which all the processes are causally dependent on one another; it refers to "information", "signals", "messenger substances" "control organs", all of which do things. On the basis of such thinking, the human body is perceived, studied and therapeutically approached as if it were an intricate physical object. In the first instance, therapeutic success may seemingly confirm this perspective, which clearly does address some aspects of the physical reality. Paediatrics undoubtedly owes a great deal, both diagnostically and therapeutically, to this rational, scientific methodology and paediatritians need to understand its therapeutic possibilities and need to be able to avail themselves of them. They are based on a scientific understanding of the laws of nature, as elaborated in terms of physics and chemistry. What science has discovered and applied in this respect relates to the "physical body".

One may ask, however, whether this picture is sufficient to comprehend the growing child. Consider, for example, the phenomenon of growth; it can cause amazement in everyone who truly observes it. It is evident that:

- growth has its original driving force within itself;
- growing organisms behave like single entities, coherent within themselves, which strive towards maturity, achieving, within qualitatively determined limits, their own particular (individual) form, structure and size;

- gowth unfolds in a time-context; an overview of living beings is only attained when all the forms they assume over time are taken into account; i. e., living beings manifest a "shape in time";
- growing organisms have an identity in space and time that spans a whole lifetime and points beyond the form that the body manifests at any particular time;
- growth is connected with regeneration; when growing organisms are injured, for example, they endeavour spontaneously to restore their form;
- the less an organism is "fully grown", the more vital is its regenerative capacity;
- with maturation, living organisms "reproduce" themselves; as their own growth dynamic reaches completion, it is transferred to their descendants and thereby renewed.

Can such characteristics be found in the domain of technology? Can the body of a "highly intelligent machine" really grow? Can it die, i. e. embrace dissolution as a whole entity when its functions expire?

In order to deepen a relationship to the principle of life, as will be outlined in this book, the reader is encouraged to take the phenomenon of the child's growth seriously, to reflect on it quietly and repeatedly. In contemplating this phenomenon, the physician encounters life in its original form, in its ability to create and maintain a body in which every process simultaneously interacts meaningfully with every other process. Throughout its entire life, a child's growth unfolds as a whole, a unity that strives to achieve a specific shape and does so only within a certain time frame. This reality cannot be grasped by the mere notion of a machine, a mechanism, be it ever so intelligent; its fundamentally character is quite other. The term "body" implies an inner coherence and an openness to the wider context in which it is embedded. In health, no part of the body works independently from the whole, nor in isolation from the living world in which it was formed – not even the human brain. The consistent internal coherence and reciprocal resonance manifesting in all living beings and life processes has been impressively and convincingly set out by Thomas Fuchs [Fuchs 2008 a, 2008 b], a philosopher and psychiatrist from Heidelberg. His ideas have a great deal to offer when developing an understanding of the physical dimension of the maturing child. Drawing from a wide range of disciplines, particularly from research in the field of infant attachment disorders, Fuchs shows that the child's organism engenders a living resonance with its environment; moreover that this has a decisive influence throughout the child's subsequent life; the greatest influence is laid down during pregnancy and the early years. He refers to an "embodied socialization", implying that the body, "the medium through which a human being exists in the world" [2008 b, 295], develops on the basis of such a relationship; neither is the human brain a genetically controlled computer but is formed as a living "relationship organ", whose fine structures and function develop in connection with and dependent upon the whole body and its surrounding world as "lived experience", (i. e., not as mere sensory data – Ed).

Recent publications in the field of epigenetics, are equally enlightening. They demonstrate that the function of DNA as stable genetic material is dependent on a living combination with proteins (mainly histones) such as chromatin. The organism restricts the "readability" of available genetic information with increasing intensity during the course of physical development and cell differentiation, thereby modifying its expression in organs and cell clusters, by influencing its action on the metabolism, through, for example, methylation of gene sequences. The important point to be noted here is the finding that "lived experiences", based on resonance of a living being with its environment, particularly apparent in the early growth phase, can affect these metabolic processes and thus epigenetically, i. e. from the outer world, modify the physical genetic material. This finding has great significance for paediatrics, for example in the field of the development of allergies [Vercelli 2004]. In relation to this, animal experiments were able to show that stressful life experiences in early childhood changed epigenetic imprinting (above all via methylation) of the genetic material in such a way that the animal's physiological ability to regulate stress was reduced throughout life [Murgatroyd et al. 2009]. This capacity is neither psychologically predetermined nor genetically inherited but is acquired as a result of epigenetic imprinting on the physical components of the genetic make-up in a living context. The work quoted from the Max Planck Institute for Psychiatry in Munich sought to investigate early influences affecting the body, which later create a disposition for depressive illnesses. The model used was a prospective comparison between laboratory animals that were allowed to remain with their mothers without interruption and animals that were separated from their mothers for three hours per day in a cage ("maternal separation stress"). This example highlights the relevance of a child's environment, including the behaviour and presence of the parents, within child development. Medical intervention in this early period can also have far-reaching physical consequences (▸Chap. 6.1).

As long ago as 1906 Rudolf Steiner (1861–1925) spoke about how experiences in early childhood can influence, even intervene in organ formation: "Everything that takes place in the child's environment, also in its moral aspect, and which the child perceives, acts on the formation of the organs, is important with regard to the physical organs ... because joy and happiness form the basis for a healthy constitution, form healthy organs; other influences can lead to illness" [Steiner 1907, 124f]. Such statements were for a long time deemed to be "esoteric" and unscientific; one hundred years later, Steiner's words have been shown to be true by animal experiments.

Moreover, epigenetic imprinting of the genetic material – and this is the second significant finding of epigenetics – can in turn be transmitted to the next generation. "The sensational element lies precisely in such a transgenerational transfer that only a few years ago was still considered to be impossible" [Kegel 2009, 82]. It has been shown, for example, that the administration of hormones to pregnant laboratory animals led to males from the affected germ line being avoided by females over several generations. [Anway et al. 2005]. Eva Jablonka, a leading researcher in this field since the mid-1990's, has referred to "epigenetic heredity and evolution", more recently extending her horizon even further to embrace the "four dimensions of evolution": "Genetic, Epigenetic, Behavioural and Symbolic Variation in the History of Life" [Jablonka 2005]. In this description, all relevant factors for evaluating human evolution are beginning to shine through.

On the basis of anthroposophic medicine and homoeopathy, the present book advocates that the human body must indeed be seen as including a distinct living entity. Such an entity needs to be conceived so specifically that each organism is understood as incorporating an underlying, individuated, species-specific "life-organization", manifesting in its growth, vitality, and physicality. Such a conception implies far more than an undifferentiated, generalized idea of life.

This life organization is not directly accessible to the senses; however, its activity becomes recognizable in the moment when natural substances – in dissolved form – are actively brought into new relationships in which they assume new structures and characteristics. Then life appears in the formation of new substances, which neither previously existed in that form in the lifeless context, nor arise in this context spontaneously, at least not in any organized way. The simplest example of this is represented by the activity of the plant leaf through which sugar-like substances, carbohydrates, are created. The formative activity of life is indivisibly linked with this substance-creating action. In this respect, the flat leaf of a plant expresses the archetypal form of a living organism. "Living entities can initially be understood … as systems that preserve their form and structure over time while their substance keeps changing. In this context such preservation should be understood as active self-organization or autopoiesis. In this process a substance acquires new, emergent characteristics, which it only obtains in the systemic context of the organism. Thus iron joined to haemoglobin behaves in a fundamentally different way from iron which occurs as a mineral …" [Fuchs 2008 b, 111].

Nutrition, i. e., the assimilation of foreign substance and energy by the living organism, is a prerequisite for growth. Moreover, plants embody life in its original form; they incorporate an organization that can metamorphose and transform salts, water, air and sun from outer nature into new substances and forms. They are not created simply through combining their constituents! In this process, the plant actively assimilates salts in soluble form (whereby it can contribute to their dissolution), separates and combines water and gases from the air by receiving the sunlight through chlorophyll; and it simultaneously transforms its environment through the resulting formation of new substance, affecting the soil, the water cycle of the earth, the earth's atmosphere and the absorption of sunlight by the earth (the green rain forest absorbs more than 80 % of incident light, the ice caps of the polar regions only 10 %). Since all living beings, including humans, always influence these relationships through their activity, we can say in this respect that all living beings on the earth constitute a unified ecological system. Within this single wholeness, they reveal, in turn, mutual inter-dependency with respect to their life activity and their life opportunities; in short, all living beings influence each other through their reciprocal and interactive relationships.

To understand the nature of the living world, it is mandatory to move beyond the established idea that the only causative principle is a (binary) sequence of happenings, such as is seen in the sequential relationship between, say, a hammer and nail. (Initially the hammer blow is taken to be the cause, and then the nail going in is the effect.) Samuel Beckett reduced this notion to absurdity in his drama "Endgame". In it, the central figure, Hamm, tries to communicate with his fellow actors Clov, Nagg and Nell – three names, each of which resembles the concept 'nail' in French, German and English respectively – and he totally fails. In living organisms and beings, all processes work simultaneously and reciprocally on one another – indeed the whole earth is a nexus of life that meteorologists already describe as an organism! The healthy interplay of physiological processes in a living organism – like two people in a productive conversation – is defined by simultaneous interaction and reciprocal resonance as opposed to causal succession. The principle of coherence, i. e., the meaningfully structured simultaneous interaction of processes, is integral to life. This concept is qualitatively different from that of causality, which has assumed such a central focus within natural sciences in the modern age. The "sense of coherence" was seen by Aaron Antonovsky (1923–1994) as a key aspect of "salutogenesis", i. e., achieving and maintaining health. The coherence of the living body and the feeling engendered by this, namely that life is meaningfully embedded in a greater context of order and destiny, form the basis of a viable concept of health.

It is no esoteric fantasy to state that coherence in living organisms encompasses both the earth and the cosmos; this is, in fact, the actual reality! Every plant actively combines the sunlit cosmic environment with the substances of the earth. The cause of plant life does not lie either in the earth or cosmos but its activity arises between both realms through correspondence, interrelationship and interaction. This life-principle is fundamentally distinct from the passively causal principle that determines interactions between inanimate objects; the living responds, whereas dead objects are determined by causal laws.

At death, the body loses the coherence that gives living form to all its processes. Bodily substances then submit to the physical and chemical laws of outer nature and their subsequent cause follows these paths. The physical body only becomes the governing reality at death; what happens in the living body, in contrast, follows a higher order, which cannot be understood in terms of the lifeless. These basic principles, this reality of the living world, also form the background against which homoeopathy and anthroposophic medicine have developed.

Samuel Hahnemann (1755–1843) referred vaguely to an organism's "life force". Anthroposophic medicine calls the individual life-organization of a living being the "etheric body" – a term which indicates that life cannot exist without inclusion of the "ether", i. e., the surrounding space, filled with sunlight. Following Goethe's scientific approach, anthroposophic research endeavours to comprehend the phenomena of life in their own terms, to penetrate the laws that govern what is alive [cf. e. g. Schad 1982, 1985].

Rudolf Steiner, moreover, perceived the activity of the life-organization, the etheric body, directly and aimed to describe such perception in appropriate terms – just like the chemist, for example, tries to frame his laboratory observations in words. Steiner's elaboration of the concept of a life-organization is based on such descriptions. He also outlined a method that enables anyone to acquire the capacity for such perception [cf. Steiner 1975].

Every science, including, for example, genetics, requires a long path of training before students begin to "see" for themselves what their lecturer has presented to them [cf. Fleck 1980]. In this respect anthroposophic medicine attempts to forge a new path, specifically when relating to the phenomenon of life. This path does not contradict the descriptions of natural science, as guided by causal analysis, but extends them through offering an enhanced understanding of the laws pertaining to living entities, including the realms of both substance transformation and of form. The essential point to grasp is that the resultant findings turn out to be productive in practice and are based on a scientific methodology that is open to scrutiny [Heusser 2010] – as also applies to all genuinely scientific methodologies.

Every encounter with a child can reawaken an interest in what is alive. Indeed what touches and moves many parents, sometimes raising their concern, is primarily the quality of life of their child. They frequently come to realize the extent to which technology has brought about conditions in which the quality of life is threatened; consider, for example, food additives which trigger allergies, car exhaust fumes which precipitate a croupy cough – many other examples could be found. Against this background of concern, acupuncture, naturopathy, homoeopathy and anthroposophic medicine are viewed in a positive light because they take account of the life of the organism as an independent force. Mainstream medicine, in contrast, is often viewed with sceptisism due to the frequent side effects of synthetically produced chemical medicines.

Anthroposophic medicine can offer a positive contribution by helping to avoid this fruitless polarization, one, that may even on occasion put the child at risk – for in reality every form of medical intervention is dependent on the living entity's inherent healing activity; a surgical procedure is in itself doomed to failure; an antibiotic relies on the active regeneration of the intestinal flora, and the same principle holds good when considering the effects of cytostatic agents in oncology, whose doses are determined to ensure that the limits of the regenerative capacity of the organism are as far as possible not exceeded. Even every "allopathic" medicine, in the last analysis, becomes subject to metabolic breakdown or detoxification and is excreted. Without encountering opposing processes, the medicine would ultimately and irrevocably poison the body. The ideal notion of a "poison-free medicine" is illusionary; situations will always arise where only a radical intervention can save life (e. g. in an emergency operation).

It is, in fact, a general principle that in embarking on any medical or therapeutic intervention, the physician must choose between one or other of two different therapeutic paths:

- On the first path, the aim is to fight, and ultimately destroy the alien process that threatens the coherence of the organism, e. g., by eliminating the pathogens in bacterial meningitis. Injuries can be surgically corrected, missing substances can be replaced, certain pathological processes suppressed or "halted". When following this path, the pathogenically causative incident or situation stands in the foreground; it is countered by an "anti" measure or a replacement, (i. e., [contraria contrariis]] "contraria contrariis").
  This method reaches its ultimate limits in those situations where the "pathogen" is the organism itself, e. g. an impaired immune regulation in allergies (atopic dermatitis, bronchial asthma) and autoimmune diseases (coeliac disease and diabetes mellitus), both of which are dramatically on the increase. The "contraria contrariis" principle has the obvious limitation that it cannot actively support vital learning processes in the organism; furthermore, albeit unintentionally, it can also cause sustained weakening of vital functions (e. g. damage to the intestinal flora by antibiotics).
- When the second therapeutic path is followed, the aim is to stimulate and enhance the organism's own activity, offering stimulus and support to strengthen its capacity for self-regulation, to modify disturbed physiological processes and restore those which promote health (salutogenesis). This principle reaches its limits where the pathological process itself exceeds the organism's capacity to overcome it in the available time. Determining these limits in each specific clinical case is a key skill of the physician, which can only mature through practice and experience.

Paediatrics will always need to make use of both therapeutic paths. In emergency medicine, the first path ("contraria contrariis") has rightly become the primary form of treatment. In situations that are amenable to the second path, assuming that it is taken up and thoroughly followed, therapeutic outcomes are often much more effective and well maintained, showing fewer side effects. Overall, they show a strengthening of the child's vitality, on which sustained health largely depends. These benefits may be attributed to the fact that the body has undergone (physiological) learning processes. By following such a path, preventive benefits will already be conferred, even during the actual treatment of the illness itself. The experience of self-regulation that children (and parents) gain through following this second path contributes to making the practice of homoeopathically and anthroposophically extended paediatrics, which is the subject of this book, deeply satisfying and rewarding.

Parents looking for an "alternative approach" would be well advised to begin by themselves taking up the path of "veneration of life" (Albert Schweitzer). Such seemingly simple practices as the quiet observation of a plant, or taking the time to calmly and unhurriedly observe an infant, can, if consciously undertaken, already reveal the basic preconditions for a living organism to develop. Particularly during pregnancy and in the first years of life, calmness is required. The embryo is suspended in a fluid envelope, in weightlessness, in which all external movement is compensated by a fine counter-movement. It is unusual for plants to change their habitat during their life. Many regulatory disorders of childhood have their origin in a lack of calmness during this first, extremely sensitive phase of life.

Other essential requirements of life include light, clean air and, above all, good quality water, a natural resource that has always been and still is in short supply. Life also depends on an appropriate, but not excessive quantity of nutritional substances that stimulate but do not replace the organism's inherent metabolic activity. Anyone assuming that a calcium tablet is incorporated directly into bony matter has failed to appreciate the most fundamental elements underlying a living entity's metabolism. Broder von Laue has described this process very convincingly [von Laue 2004]. Drinking cola and lemonade can, for example, undermine metabolic processes to such an extent that the body loses far more calcium from the bones than it can replenish, no matter how much is supplied. Young people who consume such soft drinks in excess break their bones three to five times more frequently than those who do not – even when intake of calcium is the same in each group! Conversely, osteoporosis is almost unknown in regions where people rely mainly on outdoor walking (e. g. West Africa), even if milk or other sources of calcium are not part of their diet; through their lifestyle they strengthen the activity of their life organization!

It follows from this that conversation with parents around the subject of life must assume a central position in any consultation, if an "alternative path" is even to be considered. It is almost inevitable that if parents are to pursue such a path nowadays, this step will need to be associated with a change in their habitual lifestyle. In the absence of such a change, it is illusory to imagine that either bringing up children or paediatric practice in a way that honours the true nature of life is at all possible – in fact the very notion is implausible. To ignore the laws of life, for example with respect to nutrition, already radically reduces success with homoeopathic and anthroposophic medicine. Medicine and lifestyle are indivisibly linked. This has now been confirmed in relation to studies of childhood allergies [cf. Alm and Swartz 1999, Flöistrup et al. 2006]. Respect for life can remind parents and paediatritians that in nurturing the child, it is their main responsibility to perceive, stimulate and support its own growth and vitality, and to place their trust in this process. When we have reached the stage in ourselves of perceiving, of having acquired an awareness of life and if we consider the developing body of the child as a living reality, it then becomes possible to nurture the principle of life in the child with a personal authenticity.

1.2 Stimulating self-regulation

Every disease, every injury challenges a child's life-organization; every healing process is dependent on it. To this end, the body requires an incentive, an impulse, to "change direction", to help the organism counter the momentum of the disease process (to the extent is possible). On the other hand, the organism needs support, because this "change in direction" requires strength that would otherwise be needed for growth and nutrition. "The remedies must therefore be so constituted as not only to reverse the process of the disease but also to support the decreasing vitality. The latter activity will have to be undertaken in part by diet during the illness." [R. Steiner, I. Wegman 1991, 98].

"Diet" here may be interpreted in a wider context than just food, suitable beverages and hydration, etc., which require little digestive power. The concept embraces the wider context of care, including containment provided by a calm environment, and the consciousness of adults who recognize the consequences of the child's need for a healing change in direction. In many illnesses, suitable remedies can initially be found in the field of external applications: an enema of lukewarm camomile tea can frequently relax the body when there is a high temperature; a professionally applied mustard compress can offer powerful support during a congested inflammatory process such as pneumonia, for example, if the therapeutic aim is to counter the disease by stimulating the organism's own immunological activity, avoiding the use of antibiotics.

1.2.1 Homoeopathic medicines

Homoeopathy as a treatment concept focuses wholly on the question of how the human organism can be stimulated through medicinal treatment to enable its own vital activity to bring about healing. The starting point for the homoeopathic physician is a precise phenomenological recording of the disease symptoms in the patient; not just the typical signs of the disease pathology (e. g., crepitations in the lungs) but also the accompanying symptoms specific to the individual (e. g., times when they get worse, relationship to warmth or coldness, etc.). The specific physical constitution (e. g., a thin child with a tendency to get cold, or a plump, sweating child) will also be taken into consideration. Homoeopathy can thereby stimulate and train the physician's perceptual capacity – and patients are aware when they are being perceived and taken into account as individuals.

The symptoms of disease (e. g. fever, rash, secretions, etc.) provide an image of how the organism's own activity has been transformed by the disease process. A one-sided increase in this activity comes to expression in the patient's symptoms, which, by their nature, aim to heal and eliminate foreign processes and restore wholeness. On the other hand, the organism may fail in this aim without external support and guidance; certain symptoms can, indeed, cause further damage to the organism, for example, by dissolution processes, exacerbated during inflammation). Therapeutic skill lies in addressing the self-regulation of the vital processes and giving them the right impulses and support, for example by stimulating the circulatory function, and, in the case of pneumonia, by containing the catabolic effects of an excessive or threatening acute inflammatory episode by diverting them to the periphery of the organism. Healing should be encouraged to progress from centre to periphery, from head to extremities ("Hering's law" named after Constantine Hering, the eminent pupil of Hahnemann).

Homoeopathy adopts a sceptical attitude towards the suppression of symptoms, e. g. through the use of antipyretics in a fever. Fever is an expression of the organism's own restorative activity. It is possible, for example, to observe increased mortality in measles when antipyretics are given [cf. Witsenburg 1991]. It has subsequently also been demonstrated that the use of antipyretics in early childhood promotes the development of allergies [cf. Flöistrup 2006, Beasley 2008]. A temporary exacerbation of the symptoms – i. e., an "initial aggravation" – may even be desirable in order to make way for a "swing of the pendulum back to the centre", as may happen when giving supportive treatment for a viral disease such as measles through stimulating a fever and skin rash. In the case of chronic illness, a shift of emphasis within the life organization is frequently helpful, for example, by encouraging eczema to heal through strengthening catabolic digestive processes. In such cases, a temporary modification of diet is often required, although this does not replace medicinal treatment.

The homoeopath matches the clinical picture of the illness with the drug picture (i. e., a picture of symptoms evoked by the medicine) to which it qualitatively corresponds to the greatest possible extent. The drug picture is obtained through observing the body's reaction to ingesting, as a rule, a minute dosage of a natural substance, e. g., a preparation made from belladonna or a snake poison. This reaction is a reflection of a response from the life-organization. The substance is administered to healthy test-persons as part of a drug proving; the reaction of the organism (in the various testers) is then documented. This method leads to a considerably more differentiated picture than is obtained in normal toxicological descriptions, which, in contrast, focus on the changes (often comparatively uniform) that are produced causally in the organism when the substance has been ingested in poisonous dosages.

In homoeopathic drug provings, the dosage chosen is already so minute that the reactive possibilities of the body are not toxically constrained, let alone ultimately paralyzed; they are, in fact, stimulated. In this way, the correspondence principle, in which the resulting effects arise from both sides, is demonstrated. It is therefore necessary to use a group of healthy testers, since only by considering the several reactions together can a sound drug picture be compiled. By observing the character of any further reactions that the medicine may trigger when administered in routine clinical practice, the drug picture may subsequently be significantly extended. Helpful contributions, describing differentiated homoeopathic medicinal pictures for the different life phase of the child, can be found in the Materia Medica [2007 – with numerous references] and also in the notes on differential therapy by Hirte [2008]. Grandgeorge [2004] provides additional original suggestions for paediatric homoeopathy, which have often been confirmed in practice.

The drug picture indicates the direction in which a natural substance in an attenuated dosage can influence the human organism's own activity. This knowledge is used therapeutically in homoeopathy in accordance with the "similar principle" ("similia similibus curantur"). Here the medicine, which in the healthy person triggers a specific set of symptoms similar to those of a particular illness, can produce a therapeutic reversal in the activity of corresponding symptoms in the diseased life-organization. This paradoxical action of homoeopathic medicines is not based on the strict principle of causality but on the organism's individual response to a potentized medicine, relating to its own constitution (correspondence principle). A comparable example at a psychological level is the technique of "paradox intention" (Frankl); i. e., a message which may trigger profound distress in a healthy person may liberate a healing response in an ill person. Whereas homoeopathic medicines are of little or no use for producing reliable, dose-dependent effects, they are intended to trigger responses that constitute a "reorientation" of the life-organism. These responses "correspond" to processes in the living organism and aim to generate a "resonance", as opposed to engendering direct, causally imposed effects, as intended by allopathic pharmaceuticals.

In current homoeopathic literature, classification of raw materials according to their origins within the different kingdoms of nature is gaining ground. Inspiring contributions, including paediatric indications, by Scholten in his book Homoeopathy and minerals [Scholten 1993] was followed by a speculative magnum opus by the same Dutch homoeopath, Scholten, "Homoeopathy and the Elements" [Scholten 1997], which the authors view with the greatest scepticism. In recent years, Sankaran has developed a clear system divided into mineral, herbal and animal medicines [Sankaran 2003, 2006, 2008, 2010]. In contrast to the formal catagorization, which can already be found in the large textbook by O. Leeser [Stübler, Krug 1987], Sankaran sees a deep connection between his categories and the indication and efficacy of the medicine concerned. As long ago as 1924, a systematic division into medicines derived from the mineral, herbal and animal realms, together with a qualitative differentiation of their effect on the human organism, was given by Rudolf Steiner [Steiner 1994, 227–229]. It appeared early on in the anthroposophic medical literature and anthroposophic medicines are systematically organized according to this classification. [Husemann 1956, 310–418]. Ludger Simon gives an contemporary explanation of this principle in the Vademecum of Anthroposophic Medicines [Simon 2010, 859–864, 879–899].

The raw materials for homoeopathic medicines are prepared in accordance with the principle of potentization. The aim of this process is to bring the natural substance closer to the life-organism, to subject it pharmaceutically to a kind of "digestive" process (such as maceration, trituration, dissolving and rhythmic shaking). Solvents used can include lactose (for trituration), water and water-alcohol mixtures (for dilutions); the latter can be "re-coagulated" into a solid form and stabilized by coating on pillules. The ratio of substance to solvent is fixed in degrees of, either

- 1:10 (D potencies),
- 1:100 (C potencies),
- or a combination of 1:100 and 1:500 per potentizing stage (LM potencies).

The latter range often stimulate a gentle and sustained effect without inducing a pronounced initial aggravation, which may be particularly desirable in those medicines which are more inclined to promote a strong reaction (e. g. phosphorus and sulphur).

Those who have acquired genuine, personal experience in this field of medical practice will not dispute the efficacy of homoeopathic medicines. The sensational study by Shang and Egger [2005], published in "The Lancet" proclaiming the "end the homoeopathy" [Lancet 2005], has been shown to be based on improper assumptions and scientifically untenable statistics. These errors were systematically exposed by, among others, Albonico and Ferroni in the Schweizerische Ärztezeitung [2006] [cf. also Lüdtke 2008]. In 2010, the public "dispute about homoeopathy" intensified significantly on a worldwide scale. Many newspapers like to quote a critique of homoeopathy by Edzard Ernst, formerly professor of complementary medicine in Exeter; interesting information about his career path and qualifications have been published in an interview [2010]. The authors of this book remain unconcerned by this scientific dispute.

Empirical scientific research into the efficacy of homoeopathic potencies began, remarkably, at the suggestion of Rudolf Steiner in about 1920. Righetti [1988] and Husemann [1992; 2001; 2009, 137f.] offer summaries of the history of research into potencies and the current state of such research. The effect of homoeopathic medicines cannot be deduced from the concentration of the raw material as this can be extraordinarily low, indeed sometimes to the point of being absent altogether. Hahnemann already focused much more on the solvent. Lactose and water, for example, do not represent "empty matter" but show a high degree of order within themselves. In the course of potentization, the surfaces of the raw material (e. g., iron phosphate, Ferrum phosphoricum) are initially intensively "unlocked". This enables interaction to occur between the substance itself and solvent medium. The more the process of potentization progresses, the more intensive becomes such "resonance", which the raw materials trigger in the potentizing medium. Clinically it can be observed that some so-called "high potencies" can trigger particularly strong and sustained reactions in the organism. Homoeopathic medicines can only be understood if this transition from substance to a substance-specific change in the solvent at the level of its inner organization and its resultant interaction with the organism are researched and observed in greater detail.

In many respects the living organism itself shows more of the characteristics of an interconnected, colloidally structured fluid system than of a firmly contoured mechanism. This applies above all with regard to the extracellular matrix which plays a significant role in mediating living interconnections within the organism as a whole. This matrix is of overarching importance in regulating the form and function of the cellular activity of organs themselves [cf. Hinrichsen 1990, 19f.; Vogel 1997, 117f.]. The organism itself "potentizes" the substances from outer nature as soon as they are ingested by developing colloidally organized, life-bearing fluid systems [cf. von Laue 2004]! In a colloidally dissolved form, iron, for example, as transferrin or in its function in the granulocytes (i. e., the release of oxygen radicals) acquires completely new characteristics within the organism, in contrast to its highly poisonous effect as free iron. It is remarkable that potentized iron phosphate, for example, can stimulate immune reactions which the organism otherwise carries out with the help of the most finely distributed iron, for instance, in combating a bronchopulmonary infection. In the extracellular matrix the quantitative aspect of a substance, which can be weighed and chemically analyzed, recedes completely when considered in relation to how infinitesimal quantities of the substance are subject to the life-organization and become active in the wealth of living interactions that are taking place within the matrix. The process of homoeopathic potentization may thereby be understood to correspond qualitatively to an archetypal process that also manifests in the organism itself.

1.2.2 Anthroposophic medicines

In *anthroposophic pharmacy*, as in homoeopathy, central importance is placed on the active response of the organism to the medicine. While an allopathic medicine remains active in the organism only until the latter has succeeded in breaking it down and excreting it, the anthroposophic medicine gains its efficacy through the process with which the organism reacts to it. The therapeutic aim is to stimulate or challenge the organism's own activity or, in certain functional progressions, to relieve, support and harmonize it [Simon 2010, 867–878]. Every medicine presents the organism with a specific "digestive task"; the process that the organism unfolds to meet this task is the determining factor with regard to the effect of the medicine. The anthroposophic mistletoe preparations provide a well-known example of this. They can be injected intratumorally in high concentrations where they exercise a direct cytotoxic and apoptosis-triggering effect on tumour cells [cf. Schad 1999, Stumpf 1998], similar to an allopathic agent. As a rule, however, they are not injected into the tumour but into healthy tissue or administered sublingually. Dosage regimes vary considerably, ranging from substantial material concentrations to higher homoeopathic potencies. In response to significant material concentrations, responses frequently include pronounced febrile reactions. The immunological processes that are triggered as a result can simultaneously stimulate defensive processes against tumourous diseases [cf. Kienle/Kiene 2003 for details]. Not infrequently, higher homoeopathic potencies of mistletoe have a more sustained effect on bringing the regulatory activities of the organism as a whole into order, e. g., stabilizing the warmth rhythm and the immune balance of the patient. These factors are also highly relevant in influencing both the course of the tumourous disease and the general wellbeing of the patient; they also have a role in autoimmune diseases (▸Chap. 10.9). The efficacy of the dose will vary in individual cases depending on the patient's condition and ability to respond.

Anthroposophic medicines challenge the organism's own activity in a very differentiated way. Their production and application follows the model of the human organism, which "dynamizes" all ingested substances by constantly dissolving and reforming them. The typical characteristics belonging to the substances in the external world are thereby lost; the same substances then manifest new qualities that are essential for the functioning of the organism. The calcium contained in a tablet has quite different qualitative characteristics from the protein-bound "hidden" calcium in blood serum, from which continuous small pH value-dependent quantities of ionic calcium are released. The calcium flowing into the muscle and nerve cells has a quite different effect yet again, as also does the "calcium melody" in the intracellular matrix [cf. von Laue 2004]. Anthroposophic medicine endeavours to acquire a clear understanding of how the life-organism deals with natural substances. It takes this understanding to be an actual model for pharmaceutical intentions in realizing the principle of " potentization", i. e., transforming substances from the natural world in such a way that they can release and engender formerly latent therapeutic qualities, in the context of the life-organism.

Anthroposophic medicine is also characterized by a *differentiation in the route of application of the medicine* [Simon 2010, 901–905]:

- Generally, anthroposophic medicines are used orally in dilution, trituration (trit.), or as pillules or tablets when an effect on the digestion and metabolism is required.
- Medicines are used parenterally as injections or inhalation when a direct effect on the respiration and circulatory system is intended. This application is also suitable for influencing highly inflammatory processes quickly and effectively. A convincing example of anthroposophic medicines being significantly more effective when injected than when administered orally is in the treatment of pneumonia (▸Chap. 5.1). Physicians with experience consistently confirm this finding through personal observation.
- An important modality that is specific to anthroposophic practice is the use of medicinal applications on the skin. This is not confined to measures to generate heat or reduce swellings but also includes those that aim at stimulating a subtle but substance-specific and sustained reaction in the organism. Examples of this include oxalis compresses to the abdomen after shock, metal ointment applications and ginger compresses, which exert a sustained effect on the warmth organization. Since the epidermis is ectodermal in origin, i.e, derived from the embryonic germ layer from which the nervous system

also develops, it is possible to appreciate how external applications can influence the nervous system via direct contact and "dialogue" with the skin. They may also address the soul and spiritual individuality, which, in turn, also has a decisive formative influence on processes within the life-organism. When considered as a whole, a broad and differentiated spectrum of responses can be stimulated through this modality.

Homoeopathy addresses the life-organization in purely empirical terms. In contrast, it is the aim of anthroposophic medicine to form an understanding, specific to each disease type, of the underlying pathology by describing corresponding disturbances of integration within the body's several life processes, for example, in hay fever or pneumonia. With respect to hay fever, the medicinal therapy then aims to set the body "learning tasks", which, by solving them, strengthen and regulate the life-organization with respect to its hypersensitivity to pollen. The life-organism of the child needs to counteract the tendency, inherited or acquired, to imitate outer nature, "blossoming" when nature is blossoming, as it were. In hay fever, a composition of lemon juice and quince extract is used medicinally. Lemon is a fruit in which "formative forces working from the outside to the inside are particularly strongly at work" [Steiner and Wegman 1991, 133f.]. To enhance the efficacy of this preparation, the quince has specific abilities to bind and organize fluids through the particular character of its mucilage, i. e., it specifically counteracts exudation of mucous membranes in patients with pollen hypersensitivity. The organism responds to the provocation of this slightly acidic preparation by developing a constringent ability, which enhances the integrity of mucous membranes in the nose, eyes and airways (▸Chap. 6.6). It may be administered either by subcutaneous injection, inhalation (via a nebulizer), or topically (as a nasal spray), usually in substantially measurable concentrations. The strength and frequency of dosage must be assessed according to the individual case; effectiveness may also be enhanced by increasing the strength of the preparation during the course of treatment. This method of challenging the life-organization through gradually increasing the substantial dosage, as just described in this example, may also be adopted in anthroposophic mistletoe therapy, and in the treatment of adult patients with polyarthritis [Simon 2005]. This principle illustrates a particular kind of therapeutic thinking. Homoeopathy, in contrast, often aims to achieve an enhancement in efficacy through increasing the potency, i. e., reducing the concentration of measurable content.

The original concept of "typical medicines" for typical disease processes (e. g. pollinosis, tumourous diseases, but also functional disorders of the cardiovascular system), originated with Rudolf Steiner. This category of medicines, whose varied formulations of natural substances often go back to Steiner's own indications, constitute, in the main, original pharmaceutical creations, each formulation being unique to anthroposophical pharmacy. Mistletoe preparations, in so far as they are produced from a synthesis of winter and summer sap, as suggested by Steiner, illustrate this same concept or principle. By integrating the separate substances found in mistletoe at different times of the year, the processes of synthesis capture the "time-body" of the mistletoe plant. These pharmaceutical processes, which are executed in different ways depending on the manufacturer, each imprint their own specific character on their respective preparations, so that the body reacts differently, depending on which is administered. This can be turned to therapeutic effect, in addition to the choice of the host tree and their related types of mistletoe, each of which is indicated for different types of tumour and constitution [cf. Sommer and Soldner 2000, Wilkens 2006].

Homoeopathy takes a somewhat critical view of anthroposophic pharmacy, in so much as it combines various substances in its composite, "typical" medicines, (Each mistletoe preparation is, in effect, actually already a composite medicine consisting of both mistletoe and the host tree; this becomes evident when the substances found in the mistletoe are analysed). Classic homoeopathy takes as its starting point strictly chemically defined minerals or such substances as are produced by an animal or a plant (so-called "individual preparations"). Of course the arnica plant cannot be likened to a simple individual preparation such as sodium chloride but is a complex combination of substances produced by Arnica which cannot be reduced to a single chemically active principle (as is attempted in conventional pharmacy with a poisonous plant like Digitalis). In this respect no plant can be considered to be an individual preparation when viewed from a chemical perspective. Hahnemann himself, however, also dared to produce synthetic new remedies from among the mineral preparations, e. g. Causticum Hahnemanni, which is the result of complicated chemical processes involving marble, potash and sulphuric acid as basic ingredients, which finally constitute a distillate. Being an "individual preparation", it is equally determined by the pharmaceutical process (even today, each manufacturer has its own different method of preparation!) as by the starting substances.

1

Anthroposophic pharmacy has developed a broad range of pharmaceutical processes; for example, certain plants are "synthesized" from minerals according to their natural composition, in order thereby to obtain an interrelationship of substances more specific to the disease process (as Hahnemann did with Causticum). Anthroposophic medicinal compositions (composite medicines) are not mixtures of "proven individual ingredients" but primarily new pharmaceutical products that have a rational basis and can be broadly applied in typical illnesses. In order to experience the full efficacy of these medicines, it is often necessary to administer them for a significant period of time. They have a kind of "training effect" on the organism, which often only becomes clearly apparent after several weeks but is then all the more sustained. (This applies, for example, to the application of Gencydo in pollinosis (▸Chap. 6.6) and to Cardiodoron in regulatory disorders of the cardiovascular system (cf. case histories in ▸Chap. 10.1)).

A further example can illustrate the principle that in anthroposophic medicine the pharmaceutical process by which the natural substance is brought closer to the life-organization becomes a mediator, and is just as important for the efficacy of the preparation as the natural substance itself [cf. Simon 2010]! In this context, the various preparations of the common horsetail may be considered. Equisetum arvense (cf. details in ▸Chap. 6.3.3.3) is one of the three oldest land plants on earth. It produces an enhanced concentration of silicic acid in the form of opal and has a relatively high sulphur content:

- As a *fresh decoction* Equisetum arvense can strengthen boundaries and be used as a cream to alleviate itching in atopic dermatitis.
- As an *Rh preparation* or *Wala* preparation, Equisetum is subjected to a pharmaceutical process in an aqueous environment, utilizing a rhythmic alternation of temperature and a corresponding rhythmic exposure to light and air. Through this process, the harvested plant undergoes a kind of digestion, giving rise to lactic acid fermentation. A new and inherently stable compound results from this biological reaction, which, following decanting and several steps of potentization, is available for use as an oral application or injection. These preparations maintain biological stability without the use of alcohol.

Rhythmically ordered, biologically managed pharmaceutical process of this kind, facilitating a metamorphosis of plant substance, have particular value in paediatric medicine. This is not only because they to not contain alcohol, but also because their method of production addresses the child's life-organization, mediating its independent activity. This organization gradually emancipates itself from the mother and stabilizes in the first years of life. Hypersensitivity, weeping inflammation and related dissolving processes of the skin can be reversed through its internal administration in cases of atopic dermatitis occurring in early childhood. At the same time, it addresses both the excretory and formative metabolic activity of the kidneys, in order to contain and regulate possible secondary allergic inflammation.

- If the common horsetail is cultivated on soil fertilized with silicic acid, following harvesting, an extract forms the basis for a pharmaceutical preparation (Equisetum Silicea cultum) in which the processes leading to the formation of silicic acid are strengthened. Thereby, the formative and structuring effects of the plant are significantly enhanced. This preparation is valuable, for example, in treating weeping and dyshidrotic eczema (▸Chap. 6.3.3) Through processes similar to those just described with respect to silicic acid, anthroposophic pharmacy also "vegetabolizes" metals, "potentizing" them through specific medicinal plants that have been fertilized with appropriate metallic substances. These plant extracts are then used in 1 percent (D2) or 0.1 percent (D3) concentrations. Their effects resemble those of a highly attenuated metalic potency. (Reference: Vegetabilisierte Metalle, Vademecum 2010, 914f.)
- If Equisetum arvense is "roasted" with a small quantity of sulphur, both the action of roasting and the addition of the sulphur can enhance kidney activity in chronic-inflammatory kidney diseases to a greater extent than can be achieved using a standard Equisetum preparation (▸Chap. 5.5.4, ▸Chap. 5.5.5, ▸Chap. 6.3.3) (E. cum Sulfure tostum [Vademecum 2009, 344f]).
- If horsetail is carbonized, a medicine can be obtained – Carbo Equiseti – which, when injected as a D15 potency in adults, may lead to a fall in retention values (after 2–3 days) in acute kidney failure (observations have so far been insufficient to confirm this finding in children). Equisetum tea, in contrast, can have a detrimental effect in the same situation! [von Lorenz 2007]
- Finally, a preparation obtained from the ash of the horsetail (Cinis Equiseti, D6 trit.) can have a positive effect on wakefullness and residual excretion in patients in kidney failure requiring dialysis [Wilkens 2007]. As with other Cinis preparations, its action also extends to the lungs, where it is indicated in obstructive respiratory diseases; it may also be used in treating phobic anxiety states and obsessive thoughts [Vademecum 2009, 271f].

All the above-listed indications have been derived empirically from the practice of colleagues. The reader will come across these and additional preparations of Equisetum arvense in the following chapters. For those wishing to gain a deeper understanding of this still young, living and differentiated approach to pharmacy, reference should be made to the Vademecum of Anthroposophic Medicines [2nd edition, 2010; English translation] and the loose-leaf collection edited by Michaela Glöckler "Anthroposophische Arzneitherapie" [Glöckler 2010], both of which are recommended. Whenever possible, however, the authors would strongly encourage interested physicians to participate directly in laboratory demonstrations of these pharmaceutical processes. "Hands on" personal experience has contributed very significantly to the authors' medical practice, providing it with an essential and vital foundation, and informing and inspiring their use of anthroposophic medicines. By experiencing how the medicines are produced, the physician's clinical judgment, for example recognizing their precise indication for treatment and the optimal moment to prescribe in the clinical situation, is greatly enhanced.

In summary, anthroposophic and homoeopathic medicines primarily address the organism's self-regulatory capacity, stimulating the life-organization's inherent healing possibilities. This approach is directed toward strengthening the patient's capacities to overcome, rather than to suppress, illness. The prescriber relies on the sensitivity of the organism to respond to them. In this context, paediatric medicine therefore takes on the character of a dialogue with the child's organism, its living, individually responding counterpart. This approach to treatment requires a high degree of attentiveness and thereby supports a culture of sensitive perception and listening in the interface between physician, child and parent [Girke 2007]. The patient's medical diagnosis and constitutional possibilities assume equal importance in the physician's mind. Deciding upon the right medicine and dosage, in addition to making an assessment of their efficacy, is only possible with any degree of certainty in the presence of an empathic mood of soul. To stimulate self-regulation, anthroposophic medical practice favours the use of generalized, diagnosis-related, "typical" preparations, especially at the onset of treatment, as well as medicines whose indications are specifically related to constitutional considerations. "Typical" or composite preparations owe their general diagnosis-related application to specific pharmaceutical processes. In contrast, potentized mono-preparations have greater relevance for treatment composed to support a particular individual constitution. In the experience of the authors, both composite and mono-preparations are therapeutically justified and their actions are synergistic.

An overview of the current state of clinical research in anthroposophic medicine can be found in the hta (health technology assessment) report by Kienle, Kiene and Albonico [2006, update planned for 2011], commissioned by the Swiss government, which also lists and assesses all paediatrically relevant publications.

In the present book the authors usually specify the form of administration, dosage and the manufacturer of the medicines that they use. This makes the text easier to follow, but is not intended to deter any reader from using other medicines, forms of administration or products from other manufacturers according to his or her own medical experience and views. It should be clearly stated that neither author has any conflict of interests in this respect.

1.2.3 Chronic illness and unresolved self-regulation disorders

When considered in the context of basic homoeopathy [cf. Hahnemann 1985] and its pharmacy [cf. Daems 1993], Hahnemann's understanding of chronic diseases is without doubt as relevant at the present time as in former times. At the risk of oversimplification, he identified as a significant cause of chronic diseases the repeated suppression of acute disease symptoms (e. g. a skin rash), for example, through medical measures that suppress the activity of the life-organization. When viewed in the longer term, this can lead to a fundamental change in the reactivity of the life-organism, frequently manifesting a depletion of its own activity (anergy), combined with an increasing hypersensitivity and reactivity to external stresses (atmospheric and environmental factors, pathogens, etc.). The consequences of such a weakening of the life-organism, which Hahnemann refers to in general as "psora", may be transmitted over several generations, indicating that the normal (healthy) response of the organism to a medicine, as outlined, for example, in the "similia principle", has been modified. In such cases commencing treatment with potentized sulphur and other "anti-psoric" medicines aims to reactivate the organism's ability to respond in an appropriate way. Hahnemann's theory, which for a long time was considered to be scientifically abstruse, has gained renewed relevance through the findings of epigenetics and immunological research, particularly when related to early childhood illnesses. It has, for example, been demonstrated in animal experiments that early adverse life events have deep physical effects, manifesting even on an epigenetic level, and thereby possibly influencing heredity (▸Chap. 1.1, ▸Chap. 6.1).

Paediatricians will typically encounter this problem in everyday practice in the guise of so-called atopic diseases (the term "atopic syndrome" is, in fact, just as vague as the concept of psora!). Recent studies [Alm and Swartz 1999; Gassner-Bachmann 2000] indicate that significantly fewer children present with atopic phenomena in the context of a lifestyle that optimally challenges the life-organization's activity (e. g., among children living on farms), and where this activity is less subject to suppression (e. g. through fewer vaccinations, reduced antibiotic and antipyretic prescribing). A significant correlation has been identified between a lifestyle of this kind, which, incidentally, also confers positive consequences on subsequent generations, and those families having some familiarity with anthroposophy (▸Chap. 6).

Hahnemann was an experienced physician in his own right, quite apart from being designated a "classical homoeopath". He acknowledged the importance of dietetics and gave advice about lifestyle to his patients, for example, with regard to arranging living space and balancing out physical and mental activity. Moreover, he drew attention to a further dimension of illness, as important for understanding health and illness as the life-organization itself; "But the most frequent agitation of the slumbering psora" – in the sense of being chronically ill – "as well as the most frequent aggravation of existing chronic diseases in human life arises from grief and vexation. Uninterrupted sorrow or irritation increases even the smallest traces of still slumbering psora … indeed, an innocent person may spend ten years in the Bastille or on a galley in physical agony with fewer consequences than may arise from a few months in an unhappy marriage or with a nagging conscience, irrespective of physical comforts" [Hahnemann 1983, 139f.]. Hahnemann's words resonate with current theory and understanding, for example, regarding the effect of parental stress and separation in triggering the development of allergic predispositions in the child.

Hahnemann's profound insight highlights a further dimension of the human being that needs to be identified as discrete and distinct from the physical aspect. This is the field of emotions, which embraces the entire psychological impact of interpersonal relationships.

1.3 The soul-spiritual nature of the child

"For the physical body as such, outside the context of the soul and spirit, cannot be understood at all; only the latter give it the character of meaningful reality"

Friedrich Husemann

"Not neuronal assemblies, not the brain but only *people* feel, think, perceive and act."

Thomas Fuchs

In asking the question "who are you?", the visible aspect of the person, i. e., the body, is not really being addressed. Essentially, the question refers to the nature of individuality, per se, i. e., the person, who as such remains invisible and yet embodied, "sounding through" (personare [Lat.]: resound) the personality. "Embodied mind", "embodied emotion", the process of incarnation (i. e., embodiment) of the soul and spirit are not unfamiliar concepts in current scientific discourse. By extending the concept of body as a mere physical object to include the life-organization into which individuality incarnates, the concept of "resonances between body and soul" [Verres 2005] begins to assume meaning. For the physician, this step of awareness holds a key to establishing an authentic, empathic parent-child relationship, characterized by such resonance; it expresses the ultimate and inevitable conviction that a child's body is the bearer of a soul and spiritual being.

1

In the first breath, in every movement, in every sound, the presence of the child's soul is revealed to the mother. Above all, it is in the very act of hearing that the soul element in the human being is experienced with absolute certainty. Simply to hear the sound of a bird call, ponder the experience and allow its impression to deepen inwardly is already to approach the reality of the soul. With practice, every bird species can be distinguished by this means (like the botanist can distinguish various plants by eye). In a similar way, a mother learns to understand the sounds of her child in the first few weeks of life: hunger, pain, repletion, wellbeing, unrest and tiredness become as tangible to her as if they were her own inner feelings. Frequently it is the screaming, the restlessness, the changed movements of their child that take parents to the paediatrician. Medical practice is inconceivable without acknowledging the reality of the soul; a physician with sound clinical judgment knows how to perceive its expression in the face and the movement of the child; above all, a good physician knows how to listen to the child, even to penetrate the auscultation of respiration and heartbeat with empathic awareness [Appenzeller 1989]).

Medicine refers in general terms to "the ability to express changes in emotion". With every movement, the soul reveals its essential character of fluctuation, oscillation between polarities:

- in the *movement* between tension and relaxation,
- in the *feeling* between wellbeing and discontent, sympathy and antipathy, joy and sorrow,
- in *perception*, which takes place most clearly between contrasts,
- in the rhythm of waking and sleeping.

Whereas growth takes place at rest "as in sleep", the soul element comes into its own in movement, in the social sphere, in play and interchange: in the course of evolution, ensouled beings increasingly rely on encountering others for their development, sometimes even for their very survival. What is being revealed through these phenomena, what do they conceal? Can medicine really allow itself the possibility to attribute a primary reality to the soul element?

1.3.1 The concept of the human being in medicine

It may nowadays be assumed that most paediatricians will have received at least a basic training in developmental psychology, the behavioural sciences and psychosomatic medicine, all disciplines that address the psychological dimension. These disciplines provide an indispensable basis for any serious attempt to extend conventional medical practice, including anthroposophic medicine. The paradox has to be admitted, however, that the reductionist perspective of traditional natural science does not attribute any independent reality whatsoever to the psychological aspect of the human being! To those who rigorously interpret all medical knowledge from this traditional perspective, consciousness can only be conceived as if it were "somehow invented by matter", produced by the human brain; for example, thinking must be produced by the cerebral cortex, emotions by the limbic system, will impulses related to the autonomic nervous system, hormonal influences, etc. There are few paediatricians who would be prepared to admit to holding this viewpoint, at least not in so many words, directly to a mother; but this implicit assumption pervades much of contemporary practice. Ronald Grossarth-Maticek, for example, expresses this viewpoint explicitly: "The seat of our intelligence, creativity and personal responsibility is in the cerebral cortex, which is much better developed in human beings than in the animal world. *Complicated thought processes are controlled from the cerebral cortex*" [Grossarth-Maticek 1998, 20; our emphasis]. This statement appears all the more absurd as Grossarth-Maticek himself was able to convincingly demonstrate how the soul element influences human beings' long-term health; the most significant positive factor that he identified in this respect, far ahead of exercise, nutrition, etc., was a patient's " spontaneous, emotional relationship with God" [Grossarth-Maticek 1998, 110]. However, once the concept of spirit has been excluded, a spontaneous relationship with God cannot be taken seriously in itself! Rather must it be interpreted as if it were merely the product of the cerebral cortex, i. e., derived from the machinery of the human body! If we allow these conflicting assumptions to dialogue with each other, it becomes evident that thoughts and feelings, spirit and soul, simply cannot be equated with the brain as a physical organ. Not only human experience but also philosophical analysis argues against such neurobiological reductionism [Fuchs 2008b, 26–92]

Medicine is again confronted, but now in a new guise, with the deeper question relating to its image of the human being [Girke 2010, 1–5]:

- Neurobiological research has identified neuronal correlates of consciousness down to the finest details. However, were human actions to be considered as merely the result of cerebral processes, as understood on a material level, then the dimension of moral responsibility for human action, i. e., discerning between good and evil, would become entirely virtual, as would any claim to freedom in research and teaching. To the extent that the conventional, reductionist idea or picture of what it means to be human is absorbed within medical practice, an existential contradiction arises. This becomes most evident when acknowledging the fact that in its foundations, medicine is an "applied science", originally dedicated to upholding an ethical conscience in relationship to illness and death. Against this background, the significance of recent experimental research in this field becomes all the more remarkable. It has been demonstrated that an individual's conscious intentions have greater significance with regard to the activity of individual neurons than the power of external sensory impressions [Cerf et al. 2010]. Moran Cerf's research team succeeded in recording the dynamic between conscious intentional activity and neuronal activity and were able to show that when a picture is generated as a conscious inner activity, the neuronal correlates respond more strongly than when subjected to a synchronously perceived sensory image; the former displaced the latter from consciousness. Cerf concludes "...that humans can regulate the activity of their neurons in the medial temporal lobe ... thought can override the reality of the sensory input".

- Furthermore, if conventional medicine were to take its epistemological foundations at all seriously, it would confront the fact that the very concept of " illness", when examined fundamentally, is founded not on defined scientific criteria but on ethical considerations (i. e., it is understood as a condition that "should not be") [Wieland 2006]. The difference between health and illness cannot be defined as if it were a given fact, existing objectively in the natural world; rather, it is based on culturally established judgments that vary as human consciousness and culture change. The concept of illness is not determined on the basis of isolated physical and chemical processes, but in relation to the integrity of the human organism, when viewed as a holistically functional system; i. e., health and illness can only be meaningfully distinguished in relation to a breakdown of coherence within such a system. Furthermore, health and illness can ultimately only be evaluated in their relation to the incarnating individuality, since only then is medicinal judgment able to distinction between what "should and what should not be", as the determining factor for medical action.
- In meeting the multitude of approaches within complementary and intercultural medicine, conventional medical practice is faced with a diversity of opinions regarding the image of the human being. This has corresponding consequences for diagnosis and therapeutic action; in Germany, for example, where complementary modalities are appreciated and used by many people, diverse assumptions co-exist in parallel with those of conventional medicine. Every type of medical therapy, including conventional medicine, is based upon an image of what a human being is: "That medicine depends on its understanding of the human being is therefore not to be interpreted in an arbitrary way..., on the contrary, it depends on which areas of the human being are to be focused on, when establishing the basis for treatment" [Girke 2010, 2].

Against the background of this diversity, an important event took place when, in 2004, leading representatives from conventional medicine, homoeopathy, anthroposophic medicine, naturopathy, traditional Chinese medicine and Ayurvedic medicine, as well as from cognitive science met together on the premises of the German council for medical governance under its president, J. D. Hoppe. The purpose of the gathering was to discuss the question of the image of the human being in medicine. We refer the reader at this point to the very readable volume documenting the proceedings of this conference [Girke and Hoppe et al. 2006]. This meeting was instigated by the "Dialogue Forum for Pluralism in Medicine", an organization established in 2000 at the suggestion of J. D. Hoppe. (This body has since celebrated its tenth anniversary, having meanwhile become formally established within the German governing body.

1.3.2 Presence of the soul-spiritual individuality during childhood development

> "If, alongside the physical, we grant the living, soul and spiritual elements in the human being their own reality, thereby endowing medicine with a comprehensive image of the human being which takes account of all these dimensions, we have reached the place from which anthroposophic medicine starts."
>
> Matthias Girke

Anthroposophic paediatrics regards the spiritual individuality of the child as both an ontological and functional reality, participating and exerting a potentially determining influence from the beginning of life on the development of the child's body and soul. Against this background, the physician endeavours to perceive and comprehend the physical body of the child, its life-organization, its soul and finally its spiritual individuality as distinct and equally real entities in and of themselves. While undoubtedly they all collaborate as a cohesive unified system, yet each constitutes a different level of reality: none can "create" the other, and each one is equally real The speculative notion that living organisms can spontaneously arise from dead matter and finally create a soul and spirit is alien to anthroposophic medicine. Observation of reality will confirm that ensouled living beings, from their very inception, manifest differences, even at a very basic physical level, from purely vegetative, plant life. Unprejudiced observation rather than arbitrary prejudice will reveal that it is the soul element itself that is responsible for the obvious differences between plants and animals. (Furthermore, it has yet to be proven that matter existed prior to the soul and spirit).

A central challenge of anthroposophic medicine is therefore to perceive and understand the soul element, not only in the way it unfolds at a conscious level but also in terms of its formative role within the entire bodily organization. This method of approach is essential if psychosomatic medicine is to develop into a rational and comprehensive discipline that is able to be witness to the full reality of the soul and to strengthen empathic understanding of the patient's suffering.

All ensouled organisms bear the following characteristic features:

- they form interior cavities within which organs differentiate to an increasing degree, corresponding to their stage within phylogenetic development.
- they develop organs with an independent activity: the digestive system (enabling the assimilation of solid substances); the cardiovascular system (enabling fluid circulation); the respiratory system and vocalic organs (enabling gaseous exchange) and the musculo-skeletal system (enabling independent movement and voluntary activity, capable of transforming outer nature.
- they develop sense organs for perception of the environment and a centralized nervous system, which, to an increasing degree, facilitates regulation of both the inner world of metabolism and reflective awareness of the external world.

These organic differentiations, characteristic of ensouled life, do not just appear spontaneously in the higher plants any more than they do in inanimate nature; on the contrary, their functions clearly correlate with the evolving soul element, whose functional needs they serve. It is logical, therefore, to infer that both function and individual organic form share the same derivation, namely the soul element.

In their metabolic functions, ensouled organisms manifest profound differences from the purely vegetative metabolism of plant life: mental activity, perception and movement are associated physiologically with breakdown (catabolic) processes of metabolism while growth and regeneration involve upbuilding (anabolic) processes. Typical acute inflammations, being the predominant disease-type during childhood, are connected in their initial ("day") phase with increased catabolism. This corresponds to an increased intervention of the soul and spiritual element in the physical body, i. e., it signifies an individualization of the body. The success of this process is determined by whether it passes over into the second ("night") phase, characterized by healing, upbuilding (anabolic) processes, or whether it passes into a chronic inflammatory process, i. e., into a gradually progressive breakdown (catabolic) process [cf. Girke (2010), 116–120].

Understanding this relationship, as outlined above, enables many aspects of a paediatrician's routine work to become more comprehensible. Let us consider, for example, the rhythm of sleeping and waking. In the young infant, it is already possible to observe the extent to which waking up, and the associated activities of both feeding and moving, deplete the body's vitality and cause fatigue, as if the child were in pain (which is why many parents confuse their child's fatigue with illness). The child's activity of soul, with its accompanying catabolic processes, needs to be balanced, particularly in phases of intensive growth, with frequent and long periods of sleep. During deep sleep, organic rhythms are maintained (respiration, circulation, etc.) but consciousness, discrete movements, and emotional life recede. Growth occurs mainly in sleep. A rhythmic balance between organic life and soul life is achieved in this way. During the day the soul is immersed more deeply in the body; this evokes catabolic processes. During sleep, the soul is not so engaged and the life-organization reverts to a considerable extent to its original activity, namely growth and regeneration.

In general, each rhythmic cycle expresses the balance between "up-building" and "breaking down" processes, phases during which, on the one hand, vital processes that sustain life predominate, such as inspiration and expiration, systole and diastole, contraction and relaxation of the muscles, and, on the other hand, phases in which organic activity influenced by the soul predominates. These circadian rhythms are accompanied by an increase in the levels of circulating growth hormone during sleep, and corresponding increases in adrenal hormones on waking. For health to be maintained, it is essential that this cyclic activity retains its age appropriate rhythmic balance; many illnesses originate with a disorder of this "rhythmic system".

One of the central tenets of anthroposophic paediatrics and educational practice is to recognize the importance of this age-appropriate equilibrium between up-building and breakdown processes and thereby to guide the healthy development of the rhythmical system from this perspective. In this respect, establishing regular rhythmic cycles during a child's upbringing with reference to waking, sleeping, movement and rest, eating and digesting, etc. constitutes the most important element within (preventive) "medicine". The earlier children develop stable rhythms, the more stable will be their general long-term health – and establishing this practice depends pre-eminently on the parents' approach and attitude to their child's life and environment. ▸Chap. 7 will deal with this topic in greater detail. Additional therapeutic support for these processes may also be required.

The importance of recognizing somatic expressions of the soul element becomes even clearer during times of illness. Psychological events (shock, grief, etc.) can, in their own right, lead directly to diseases in physical organs. Not only every physician, but every patient is aware of this possibility. The full implications of this insight can only be recognized, however, if the soul is granted the status of an entity in its own right and its effects on the body are given equal credibility to the reciprocal effects, i. e., to the influences of the body on the soul. Just as a cut can cause feelings of pain, so a shock can specifically effect renal functions, grief bring about disturbances in the gastric mucosa, mental and intellectual strain contribute to chronic congestion of the nasal mucosa, etc. The explanation of these organic effects is to be sought in a disruption of the structural processes within the affected organ, due to an outward "diversion" in the direction of their underlying formative activity towards the periphery of the body. This may happen, for instance, as a result of intense soul-experiences or conversely as a result of their repression. Either of these influences will tend to induce excessive catabolic activity in the vulnerable organ, or organ system.

When considering the soul organization, anthroposophic medicine refers to the "astral body" (literally, star body). The use of this term dates back to Paracelsus among others. In the context of this book, it is sufficient to point out that this term refers to the cosmic origins of the soul entity. Just as natural science relates the ultimate origin of matter to evolutionary processes in the stars, the findings of spiritual science reveal that the soul entity does not originally come from the earth but from the cosmos (in fact all human cultures share this picture). Smaller children refer to "heaven" in this context. The "spontaneous trust in God", which Ronald Grossarth-Maticek considered so essential for the human soul in maintaining health, contains at its core nothing other than a deep inner certainty of the existence of a divine creator and protector of the soul.

Artistic therapies, e. g. therapeutic painting, clay modelling and music therapy, make a significant contribution within anthroposophic medical practice and are deeply effective. Although their impact on the soul is immediate, their effects in time also penetrate the body. This has been confirmed in a longitudinal study of patients with chronic illness, financed by a statutory health insurance fund, which has demonstrated their effectiveness [Hamre 2007]. Eurythmy therapy, a unique modality within anthroposophic medical practice, enables particular disease processes to be addressed. This is achieved by engaging the patient in specific sequences of subtle but powerful bodily movements and gestures that resonate with particular soul experiences. The authors have found this therapy especially helpful in those situations where the dynamic interplay between body and soul, i. e., the interactions of the astral body and etheric body, need to be supported. The wide spectrum of conditions related to this field ranges from breathing disorders, including bronchial asthma, to behavioural disorders, including attention deficit hyperactivity disorder. The reader will find the relevant corresponding references in the appropriate chapters and also in the final section of this book. A comprehensive bibliography [Hachtel, Gäch 2007] provides details regarding therapeutic indications as well as listing relevant literature, regarding this form of therapy. Both artistic therapy and eurythmy therapy are able to achieve sustained therapeutic responses since their effects derive from the patient's own activity. Rhythmical massage therapy and external applications administered by rhythmical Einreibung, can stimulate the child's metabolic and upbuilding processes, warmth generation and distribution, and also harmonize the rhythmic interplay between soul and body, between breakdown and upbuilding processes.

"Who are you?" This question is ultimately addressed to the "I" or self, which, in the child, remains deeply concealed. What do the parents, the physician know about the being who will someday emerge from this shell, when the body has fully grown, the soul developed and incarnated, when parents have been bidden farewell and at length a person sets out on a unique path, never to be replicated?

Initially, every aspect of a child's development is held back: the newborn baby is naked; his or her warmth must be carefully protected for a considerable time. With regard to nutrition and locomotor skills, the child is continuously dependent on parents and others. "At the foundation of the most important differences between humans and animals lies the principle of retardation". At the same time the infant looks to his or her mother (anthropos [Gr.] means "one who looks up", i. e., the human being) and a process begins which lies at the core of the human condition, namely dialogue in sound and expression, word and gesture. [Verhulst 1999, 371]. Retardation in human development is to be understood in relation to the concept of learning. From the beginning, the human individuality transcends the limitation, which, in animal development, is both confined by and fulfilled within the defined limits of the species. Each animal manifests a "repetition of the same". The human individuality, in contrast, opens both physical and soul development to a new quality, namely lifelong learning. Transformative processes are evident, which are not the result of heredity or adaptation to an ecological niche, but arise from a developing inner relationship to other human beings, to the social and cultural environment. Empirical research into early childhood development has been able to show the extent to which children are physically, psychologically and spiritually dependent for the maturation of their learning processes on positive affirmation from – and the relationship with – their fellow human beings. Children, in fact, actively seeks out relationship. The value, the meaning of childhood, becomes understood, when the faculty to learn is recognized as being the central quality of the human individuality, the "I". The innermost nature of the human "I" is revealed in the child in a way that an adult is never quite able to express. Moreover, the young child's susceptibility to illness, particularly to acute inflammation, acquires its meaning against the background of the incorporation of the "I" into the soul and body, i. e., acute inflammation expresses the individualization of the body.

The "I" does not easily reveal itself in a medical consultation. An experienced physician will comprehend the body, the evolving body, and also a patient's emotions and feelings, as if these were natural phenomena. In confronting the "I" of the other person, however, something of a quite different character will be encountered; a being with memories, with a unique history in which the child's being has become embedded; a being that has not yet gelled into something "typical" or fixed, but whose future is still open, an being which develops a free space within itself, whose thoughts and impulses can always take an unexpected direction, ultimately transcending the power of prediction. Moments in which this being, this "I" is truly experienced are precious and sacred. Undivided interest, inner equilibrium, relaxed and trusting attention all contribute to such an encounter with the core human individuality. When such empathic moments translate into the clarity of cognitive awareness, and if this then becomes the leitmotif for an inner activity of will, the presence of a real being may be inwardly witnessed, an intuitive revelation of the being or the "I" may arise, i. e., "intuition". Anthroposophic medicine offers the physician a path of inner training that can support the development of such a conscious capacity for encountering the “I” of the patient [Steiner 1993, Girke 2010, 891–905, Husemann 2009, 199–220].

It is not only in the adult that human individuality can be perceived; in fact, this is already possible both in the newborn infant and in the disabled child; it is the true substance of human dignity. Individuality will be perceived in a different way, however, at the very outset of its path of development, when body and soul are still evolving their specific, individual form. In the first instance, parents and paediatricians encounter the effect of the childhood “I” primarily in its physical manifestation. Soul and spiritual aspects only gradually differentiate themselves from bodily aspects of development; the “I”, however, is always present at every level.

By the end of the first year, children wrestle to establish a new equilibrium, one that only humans are able to accomplish; the child starts to “carry its head upright”. “The fundamental difference between the upright human posture and the bearing of higher animals lies in the fact that humans are able to free themselves from the constraints of gravity. The way that human uprightness is acquired also differs from that of the animals. Whereas in animals the ability to walk is innate and often well developed from birth, in humans that is not at all the case. A blind child never spontaneously attempts to stand up or walk but has to be carefully taught how to do so. It is impossible to watch a child’s first attempts to stand up, when he or she holds on to the edge of a chair or clings to the supporting fingers of his or her parents, without having the feeling that this process resembles one of pure experimentation rather than the maturing of innate reflexes [Verhulst 1999, 169].

Not only do human beings show specifically human traits in the cerebral cortex; such traits are also present in their feet. The earliest historical evidence of human morphology was thought for a long time to be footprints (e. g., of a mother and child walking through fresh volcanic ash in Africa. These markings evidenced an ability to maintain balance and walk upright on two legs. The primates, in contrast, move along the ground using their legs and arms. Human posture itself is something unique, singular, set apart from the animal realm. It reveals a coherent, functional integration of feet, spinal column, sense of balance and brain; it manifests an overarching, transcendent principle, encompassing every functional component.

With the acquisition of upright posture, human beings simultaneously free their hands. While, at least in its potential, this functional freedom is shared with the more developmentally advanced mammals – e. g., the five digital rays of the embryonic hand in both a wild boar and human being are initially almost indistinguishable – almost all animals go on to lose this universal hand shape even before birth, in favour of acquiring a specialized, irrevocably fixed form such as a claw. And while the child learns the precision grip of thumb and index finger at the end of the first year, even primates, which are the least specialized of mammals and closest to humans, lose this functional possibility since their thumb regresses. According to Heisenberg, “Humans are unique in so much as they have retained their hand”. This example illustrates that the task of being human is much more than an intellectual or moral one; before signs of intellectual awakening appear, a child’s morphological development already reveals specifically human characteristics [cf. Portmann 1973, 36]. Morphological and functional development will always prefigure (at an unconscious level) the expression of (conscious) soul and spiritual capacities. The presence of a physically effective, human-specific and overarching organizational principle may be inferred from this. It is characteristic of predispositions that are specific to humans that, "in order to mature into acquired individual abilities", they depend to a high degree neurobioligically on "open loops that require supplementary stimulation of complementary emotional, social and intellectual competences" (i.e., of the child in relation to its caregivers) [Fuchs 2008 b, 214f.]. A wealth of developmental bodily traits could be cited, all of which illustrate comparably significant outcomes, specific to human cognitive and functional capacity [cf. Rohen 2000, 408–416]. The underlying and specifically human organizational principle that may be inferred from the above descriptions is included as part of diagnosis and therapy in anthroposophical medicine, where it is termed the "I-organization" [Steiner, Wegman 1991, 38ff.]. Its activity can be clearly identified by the observant paediatrician as the "precursor of the I".

Two basic tendencies characterize this specifically human formative principle. Firstly retention of the primary, universal (embryonic) form principle and secondly prolongation of both organic and psycho-behavioural development. Retention of an open fontanel provides the brain with more time to develop; naked skin allows for unmatched flexibility in warmth regulation and relieves respiration of this task; active prevention of snout formation, facilitated through the enclosure of the intermaxillary bone by the upper jaw, allows for the development of specifically human facial features that are absent in adult animals. Finally, the unique shape of the human head, balanced freely over the spinal column, confers on the brain its special position above rather than behind the mouth. Many other examples could be included. Their common denominator with respect to the human form is to be seen in that it retains an unspecialized, original shape. This is also the foundational morphological principle for all higher animals but through their accelerated development and specialization of function, the original form becomes distorted. This distortion may be interpreted through contrasting the nature of the astral body with that of the "I" organization. The latter serves the individualization process; the former, i.e., the astral body, manifests the formative power that leads towards differentiation in the realm of both the organs of the body and the life of feelings but which, at the same time, propels both towards the expression of contrasting extremes (as may also be experienced by humans in their instinctual drives and emotions). This tendency typically leads to the appearance of highly specialized but one-sided structures, which, at the same time, curtail further developmental possibilities. This specialized and accelerated development restricts the individualization process (i.e., of the "I" organization), on both physical and psychological levels, which, in contrast, strives to achieve equilibrium, openness, and universality. Moreover, the "I" organization has the capacity to contain and regulate the dynamism of the astral body, of the soul element, as this rushes ahead; its influence can be seen accordingly in healthy physical and psychological development. Whereas the instinctive behaviour of animals reaches a culmination with sexual maturity, in humans, development is able to continues beyond this stage. Education and paediatrics should therefore complement each other in guiding the continual maturation of the child's individuality. To this end, it is necessary to establish age-appropriate developmental goals and uphold health through encouraging equilibrium and self-regulation on the basis of the "I" organization.

Warmth and its regulation assume paramount importance when supporting the "I" organization. A stable, self-generating and regulated warmth-homoeostasis signifies the highest physiological achievement in the human organism; in fact, the capacity of human beings to regulate warmth places their development ahead of the whole of the animal kingdom. It has recently been demonstrated that the regulation of circadian rhythms in homoeothermic organisms is mediated by modulating body heat [Buhr et al. 2010]. The rhythm of human "I" activity can on the one hand be directly ascertained by measuring the intensity and rate of increase in body heat on waking; on the other hand, by the rate of peripheric dispersion of heat on going to sleep. In febrile diseases, the activity of the "I" is increasingly focused on the body. (▸Chap. 5.1) "The human "I" is connected with warmth. Not only is there physical warmth but also warmth of soul. In the soul element, this inner warmth quality also indicates the presence of the "I" in the human being." The processes of will, which are inwardly connected with the "I" and without which an "I" is inconceivable, are, by their very nature, warmth processes" [Girke 2010, 15].

A key function common to specifically human phenomena of physical development is to provide the preconditions for the development of language. Acquiring the upright gait affects the process of respiration by freeing the pectoral girdle (it is more difficult to talk when the arms are involved in carrying a heavy weight). Consequently the metabolic load that has to be managed by respiration is significantly reduced in humans (the balanced upright posture saves energy, and warmth is given off through the skin). Synchronizing with language acquisition, the growth of the anterior mandible is permanently inhibited in humans, preventing the formation of a snout and thereby retaining the anatomical shape that is a prerequisite for the development of speech. Humans also are endowed with an even row of teeth without gaps, which is a precondition for clear articulation (and is considered to be an indication of the ability to speak, when found in fossils). Language transforms the sounds made by animals into free forms, which can further differentiate and carry meaning; at one and the same time, it represents a physical, living, soul and spiritual phenomenon. Like human beings themselves, language represents a "composite phenomenon" [Verhulst 1999, 371–379]. The "I" is, indeed, the true composer of the human body.

Language development is dependent both on listening to others speaking and, above all, on being heard. The "I" requires the other "I", the you; together they create a dynamic interplay. In order to strengthen a child's self-confidence, to enable the child to find and affirm his or her own path in life, it is essential, above all else, for parents to make their active interest visible to their child, to develop a calm attitude, presence of mind, openness, and approachability. The "I" matures slowly and only in the context of interactive relationship; the process of maturation requires reciprocity, not simply input.

To the extent that children do not experience the "I" of the adult as truly approachable, they can feel deprived of recognition and may become restless, cool and sad. The love that most parents feel towards their children can easily become obscured, like clouds over the sun. This may be due to worries about their relationship with their partner, social and family pressures, and the countless small details of daily life. Not least, uncertainty and anxiety about how to engage fruitfully with their child, how to meet his or her needs, may exacerbate existing anxieties. Nonavailability, a lack of mindful presence, for example during a telephone call, while watching television or driving the car, can be even more painful for the child than the person's complete absence. Physicians are no less vulnerable to this indiscretion than are parents! Through engaging in a real conversation with the child, however, the strength to make a new beginning can always be re-established. The "I" is resilient, has the staying power to retain developmental possibilities; the child also has considerable capacity to forgive if the new beginning is meant sincerely.

Human beings share their substance, their body and their soul with the kingdoms of nature but through their "I", they grow beyond those shared kingdoms. The "I", however, provides them with a focus, and simultaneously gives them meaning. The "I" becomes their conductor and, when they become creative, also their composer. Such development, demonstrated nowhere more impressively than in human art, is initially made possible through the unique and extended duration of human childhood and adolescence. The path followed by the "I" is of necessity one strewn with crises.

By coming through each acute febrile inflammation successfully, the individuality achieves ever greater mastery over those processes of the body that derive from the kingdoms of nature, thereby overcoming the inherited aspects of the body through this activity.

During the crisis of puberty, unknown in the animal world, the young person breaks their psychological ties with parents, with the past, and may go through extremes of emotion, out of which he or she now has to create a unique and individual balance. In adolescence, young people become responsible for their decisions, for the consequences of their thinking and action. In doing so they experience the threshold of their freedom, including the freedom to take their own life. This ultimate possibility represents a schism, dividing humans from nature. Supporting the child as an individuality in such moments of crisis is more than a medical question, of taking appropriate measures; it is rather a question of presence of mind, of a loving attitude, of finding the right word or making a silent gesture.

The challenge of every physician, every therapist, will always be to transform medicine into an art of healing.

References for Chapter 1

(every reference marked with a ■ Bullet point indicates the English translation of the reference above it)

Albonico, H., B. Ferroni: Die Homöopathiestudie: Anatomie einer statistischen Operation. Schweiz. Ärztezeitung 87, 27–28 (2006)

Alm, J., J. Swartz: Atopy is less common in children of families with an anthroposophic lifestyle. The Lancet 353, 1485–1488 (1999)

Anway et al.: Epigenetic Transgenerational Actions of Endocrine Disruptors and Male Fertility. Science 308, 1466–1469

Appenzeller, K.: Grundlagen für eine neue Art der Herzauskultation. Zbinden, Basel 1989

Beasley, R. et al.: Association between paracetamol use in infancy and childhood, and risk of asthma, rhinoconjunctivitis and eczema in children 6–7 years: Analysis of Phase III of the ISAAC programme. The Lancet 372, 1039–1048 (2008)

Buhr, E., Seung-Hee, Y., Takahashi, J.: Temperature as a Universal Resetting Cue for Mammalian Circadian Oscilllators. Science, 330, 379–385 (2010).

Cerf, M. et al.: Voluntary control of human temporal lobe neurons. Nature, published online doi: 10.1038/nature09510 (2010).

Daems, W. F.: Was sind potenzierte Heilmittel? Verlag Freies Geistesleben, Stuttgart 1993

Ernst, E.: Interview, in: Homöopathische Nachrichten, April 2010, www.welt-der-homoeopathie.de, 1–3.

Fleck, L.: Entstehung und Entwicklung einer wissenschaftlichen Tatsache. Suhrkamp, Frankfurt/M. 1980

Flöistrup, H., J. Swartz et al.: Allergic disease and sensitization in Steiner school children. J. of Allergy and Clinical Immunology 117, 59–66 (2006)

Fuchts, T.: Leib und Lebenswelt. Die Graue Edition, Kusterdingen 2008 (a).

Fuchs T.: Das Gehirn – ein Beziehungsorgan. Kohlhammer, Stuttgart 2008 (b).
Gassner-Bachmann, M.: Bauernkinder leiden selten an Heuschnupfen und Asthma. Deutsch. Med. Wochenschr. 125, 924–931 (2000)
Girke, M., J. D. Hoppe, P. F. Matthiessen, S. N. Willich: Medizin und Menschenbild. Deutscher Ärzte-Verlag, Köln 2006
Girke, M.: Patient-Arzt-Beziehung. Bundesgesundheitsblatt, online publiziert DOI 10.1007/s00103-007-0312-9 (2007)
Girke, M.: Innere Medizin. Salumed, Berlin 2010.
- English translation in progress at this time – Ed.
Glöckler, M. (Hrsg.): Anthroposophische Arzneitherapie. Wissenschaftliche Verlagsgesellschaft, 1.Aufl., 3.Ergänzungslieferung Stuttgart 2010
Grandgeorge, D.: Homöopathische Arzneimittelbilder in der Kinderheilkunde. 2. Aufl. Sonntag Verlag, Regensburg 2004
Grossarth-Maticek, R.: Systemische Epidemiologie und präventive Verhaltensmedizin chronischer Erkrankungen. de Gruyter, Berlin – New York 1998
Hachtel, B., Gäch, A.: Bibliographie Heileurythmie. Veröffentlichungen 1920–2005. Natur-Mensch-Medizin Verlag, Bad Boll 2007.
Hahnemann, S.: Organon der Heilkunst. Organon Verlag, Berg 1985
Hahnemann, S.: Chronische Krankheiten, Theoretischer Teil. Organon Verlag, Berg 1983
Hamre, H. et al.: Anthroposophic art therapy in chronic desease: a four-year prospective cohort study. Explore published online, doi: 10.1016/j.explore.2007.04.008 (2007)
Heusser, P.: Anthroposophische Medizin und Wissenschaft. Schattauer, Stuttgart 2010.
Hinrichsen, K. V.: Humanembryologie. Springer, Berlin, New York 1990.
Hirte, M.: Materia medica. In: H.Pfeiffer, M.Drescher, M.Hirte (Hg.): Homöopathie in der Kinder- und Jugendmedizin. 2.Aufl. Urban & Fischer, München 2007.
Hirte, M.: Differenzierung homöopathischer Kindermittel. Urban & Fischer, München 2008.
Husemann, F.: Das Bild des Menschen als Grundlage der Heilkunst. Verlag Freies Geistesleben, Stuttgart 1956.
Husemann, F., O. Wolff: Das Bild des Menschen als Grundlage der Heilkunst, Bd. 1, 10. Aufl., S. 16. Verlag Freies Geistesleben, Stuttgart 1991.
- Huseman, F. Wolff, O.: The Anthroposophical approach to medicine: v. 1, 2. Steiner Books, Great Barrington, M. A. 1983, v.3 Mercury Press, Spring Valley, N. Y. 2003.
Husemann, F.: Rhythmusphänomene beim Wirksamkeitsnachweis potenzierter Heilmittel. Der Merkurstab 45, 73–91 (1992).
Husemann, F.: Rehabilitation von Benvenistes Forschungen über homöopathische Hochpotenzen, Der Merkurstab 54, 335–336 (2001).
Husemann, F: Anthroposophische Medizin. Verlag am Goetheanum, Dornach 2009.
Jablonka, E., Lamb, M.: Evolution in Four Dimensions. Genetic, Epigenetic, Behavioural and Symbolic Variation in the History of Life. MIT Press, Cambridge 2005.
Kegel, B.: Epigenetik, 2.Aufl. Dumont, Köln 2009.
Kienle, G., H. Kiene: Die Mistel in der Onkologie. Schattauer, Stuttgart 2003.
Kienle, G., H. Kiene, H. Albonico: Anthroposophische Medizin in der klinischen Forschung. Schattauer, Stuttgart 2006.
- Kienle GS, Kiene H., Albonico HU. Anthroposophic medicine: effectiveness, utility, costs, safety. Schattauer, Stuttgart, New York 2006.
Lancet Editorial. Lancet 366, 690 (2005).
Laue, H. B. von: Kalzium als Substanz und Prozess im Menschen. Der Merkurstab 57, 78–95 (2004).

Stübler, M., Krug,E.(Hrsg.): Leesers Lehrbuch der Homöopathie, 5 Bde. 2. bzw. 3. Aufl. Haug Verlag, Heidelberg 1987.

Lorenz, S. von: Carbo Equiseti, Indikation bei akuter Niereninsuffizienz. In: Indikationen anthroposophischer Arzneimittel aus gesichteter ärztlicher Erfahrung. Gesellschaft Anthroposophischer Ärzte in Deutschland (Hrsg.). Der Merkurstab 61, 1, Supplement (2008).

Lüdtke, R., Rutten, A. L. B., The conclusions on the effectiveness of homeopathy highly depend on the set of analyzed trials. J.Clin.Epidemiology, published online doi: 10.1016/j.jclinepi.2008.06.015 (2008).

McCarthy, M.: Critics slam draft WHO report on homoeopathy. Lancet 366, 705–706 (2005).

Murgatroyd, C. et al.: Dynamic DNA methylation programs persistent adverse effects of earla-life stress. Nature neuroscience, published online doi:10.1038/nn.2436 (2009).

Portmann, A.: Biologie und Geist. Suhrkamp, Frankfurt/M. 1973.

Righetti M.: Forschung in der Homöopathie. Grundlagen, Problematik und Ergebnisse. U. Burgdorf Verlag, Göttingen, 1988.

Rohen, J. W.: Morphologie des menschlichen Organismus. Verlag Freies Geistesleben, Stuttgart 2000.

▪ Rohen, J. W.: Functional morphology : the dynamic wholeness of the human organism. Adonis Press, Hillsdale, N. Y. 2007.

Sankaran, R.: Einblicke ins Pflanzenreich,2 Bde. Homoeopathic Medical Publishers, Mumbai 2003.

Sankaran, R.: Survival – The Mollusc. Homoeopathic Medical Publishers, Mumbai 2008.

Sankaran, R.: Struktur. Erfahrungen mit dem Mineralreich. 2 Bde. Homoepathic Medical Publishers, Mumbai 2010.

Sankaran, R.: Sankarans Tabellen. Homoeopathic Medical Publishers, Mumbai 2006.

Schad, F., B. Matthes, H. Matthes: Intraläsionale Viscumtherapie bei hepatocellulärem Karzinom. Der Merkurstab 52, 120–122 (1999).

Schad, W. (Hrsg.): Goetheanistische Naturwissenschaft, Bd. 1, Allgemeine Biologie. Verlag Freies Geistesleben, Stuttgart 1982.

Schad, W. (Hrsg.): Goetheanistische Naturwissenschaft, Bd. 4, Anthropologie. Verlag Freies Geistesleben, Stuttgart 1985.

Scholten, J.: Homöopathie und Minerale. Stichting Alonissos, Utrecht 1993.

Scholten, J.: Homöopathie und die Elemente. Stichting Alonissos, Utrecht 1997.

Shang, A., M. Egger et al.: Are the clinical effects of homoeopathy placebo effects? Comparative study of placebo-controlled clinical trials of homoeopathy and allopathy. Lancet 366, 726–732 (2005).

Simon, L.: Arzneimittelfindung am Beispiel chronische Polyarthritis. In: M. Glöckler, Anthroposophische Arzneitherapie, 3–1–3–27. Wissenschaftliche Verlagsgesellschaft, Stuttgart 2005.

Simon, L: Grundlagen anthroposophischer Arzneitherapie. In: Vademecum Anthroposophische Arzneimittel. 2.Aufl. Der Merkurstab 63, Supplement (2010), 842–909.

Sommer, M., G. Soldner: Die Mistel und ihre Wirtsbäume. Differenzierung zur Optimierung der Therapie. Der Merkurstab 53, 29–43 (2000).

Steiner, R.: Wie erlangt man Erkenntnisse der höheren Welten, 24. Aufl. R. Steiner Verlag, Dornach 1993.

▪ Steiner, R.: Knowledge of the higher worlds : how is it achieved? GA (complete works) 010. Rudolf Steiner Press, London 2004.

Steiner, R., I. Wegman: Grundlegendes zu einer Erweiterung der Heilkunst, 7. Aufl. R. Steiner Verlag, Dornach 1991.

▪ Steiner, R., I. Wegman: Fundamentals of therapy : an extension of the art of healing through spiritual-scientific knowledge. GA (complete works) 027. Mercury Press, Spring Valley, N. Y. 1999. Also available as: Extending practical medicine: fundamental principles based on the science of the spirit. Rudolf Steiner Press, London 1996.

Steiner, R.: Die Erziehung des Kindes vom Standpunkt der Geisteswissenschaft, Vortrag Köln 1.12.1906. GA 55, 2.Auflage, 118–132, R.Steiner Verlag Dornach 1983.

- Steiner, R.: The education of the child and early lectures on education. GA (complete works) 034. Anthroposophic Press, Hudson, N. Y. 1996.

Steiner, R.: Die Kunst des Heilens vom Gesichtspunkte der Geisteswissenschaft, Vortrag London 29.8.1924. GA 319. 3.Aufl., 226–247, R.Steiner Verlag Dornach 1994.

- Steiner, R.: An outline of anthroposophical medical research : abridged report of two lectures, London [28 Aug 1924 & 29 Aug 1924]. GA (complete works) 319. Anthroposophical Publishing, London 1926. Also published as: "Art of healing from the perspective of spiritual science" in the book: The healing process, Anthroposophic Press, Hudson, NY 2000.

Stumpf, C. et al.: Intratumorale Mistelapplikation bei stenosierendem Rezidiv eines Cardia-Carcinoms. Der Merkurstab 51, 85–88 (1998).

Vercelli, D.: Genetics, epigenetics, and the environment: switching, buffering, releasing. J Allergy Clin Immunol 113, 381–386 (2004).

Verhulst, J.: Der Erstgeborene. Mensch und Tier in der höheren Evolution. Verlag Freies Geistesleben, Stuttgart 1999.

Verres, R.: Was uns gesund macht. 2.Aufl. Herder, Freiburg 2005.

Vogel, H. H.: Zur Krankheitsdisposition. Verlag Natur-Mensch-Medizin, Bad Boll 1997.

Wieland, W.: Medizin als praktische Wissenschaft – Die Frage nach ihrem Menschenbild. In: Girke et al., Medizin und Menschenbild, 9–28. Deutscher Ärzte-Verlag, Köln 2006.

Wilkens, J.: Misteltherapie. Differenzierte Anwendung der Mistel nach Wirtsbäumen. Sonntag Verlag, Stuttgart 2006.

Wilkens, J.: Cinis Equiseti, Indikation bei dialysepflichtiger Niereninsuffizienz. In: Indikationen anthroposophischer Arzneimittel aus gesichteter ärztlicher Erfahrung. Gesellschaft Anthroposophischer Ärzte in Deutschland (Hrsg.). Der Merkurstab 61, 1, Supplement (2008) – in print –

Witsenburg, B. C.: Masern-Sterblichkeit und Therapie. Der Merkurstab 45, 177–178 (1992).

2 Disorders following abnormal birth

Later, as I was looking at these pictures, I saw something which I had missed in the rush. No trace of the cute face we expect in a baby. The brow furrowed, the mouth contorted in pain. An old man with large, knowing eyes was looking at me. Who was this being? Where did he come from? What did he feel? What did he know? I became curious.

Walter Schels, *Das offene Geheimnis*

2.1 Anamnesis and diagnosis

The drama of giving birth involves the close interaction between the child's and the mother's organism. Any disruption of this interaction can place the development of the child at risk both directly and in the long-term. Hence it is important to be *aware of and scrutinize any divergence from the natural course of delivery not just in neonatology but in every paediatric anamnesis.*

- Was the birth spontaneous or was it induced?

Every induced birth represents an encroachment for the child. Because under normal circumstances the foetus triggers the birth itself – mediated by the action of its adrenal gland – while at the same time preparing its metabolism for the forthcoming stress of birth: it wants to be born! The time of birth is co-determined by the expected child, something that is manifested at the hormonal level. Although the maternal oestrogens determine the contractions, they are stimulated by cortisol which comes from the child. How does the child know that the time for birth has arrived? One thing is certain: a dialogue about the right time for the birth develops between mother and child in which the child has a significant input and "choice" [Martinius 1997]. *If the birth is induced from the outside, this can mean a shock for the child,* disrupt the normal interaction between the child's and mother's organism and impair the child's stress tolerance. This example clarifies the difference between a process being induced by the action of the child's individuality or through a medical intervention. In the former case the soul and spiritual individuality unites in a positive way with the physical event whereas in the latter case the consequence can be a connection between the soul and physical entities which is not quite right and labile. The perception, diagnosis and treatment of such shock experiences are very important because it can prevent a long-term disposition for disease.

- Did birth occur naturally or by caesarean section?

> The face of this mother giving birth touched me deeply. I had never before seen such an expression – with so much pain, but also energy and resolution – in a face. (...) I was spellbound by the change in her face. A moment ago still contorted with effort – now relaxed, beautiful, satisfied.
>
> Walter Schels

The expulsive phase through the maternal birth canal is of fundamental significance for the child's and mother's experience of the birth. In contrast to a caesarean section, the child itself breaks out of its cover in that the head, which normally goes first, moves down through the lesser pelvis in a cross-like rotating movement [cf. Husemann 2009, 245–254]:

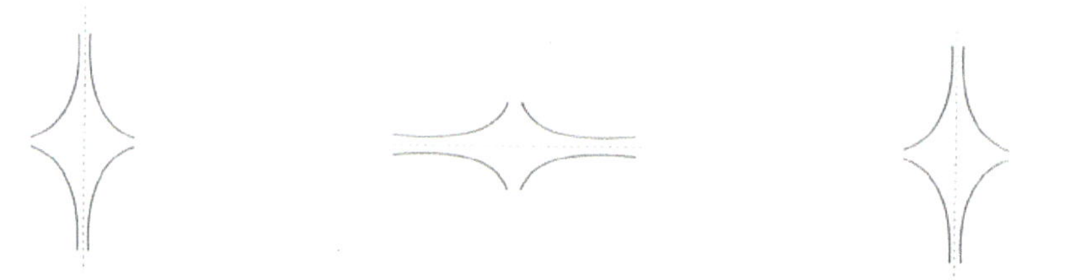

Fig. 2.1 Anterior fontanelle at the in height of the pelvic inlet, pelvic cavity and pelvic outlet.

On amniorrhexis (i.e. when "the waters break"), clear amniotic fluid and blood initially flow from the birth canal. While the child's compressed thorax largely empties its fluid-filled lungs and the umbilical circulation is increasingly prevented, the child comes close to a physiological state of asphyxia. With the emergence of the limbs, the decisive counter-movement of the child is initiated: the first breath, which is prepared and called for by the preceding event.

A child which is delivered by caesarean section awakens quite differently during birth. The sequelae often manifest physically in the sphere of the respiration e.g. in "wet lungs" syndrome. The psychological sequelae are less frequently taken into account. Depending on whether it is a planned or emergency section, the consequences for the child can vary considerably. The experience of the mother is also fundamentally different depending on whether she was able to give birth to her child by herself. Her confidence in her own body is often reduced by a section – particularly with regard to further births; the connection with the child is placed under stress during the confinement period through the sequelae of the operation and anaesthetic. A general anaesthetic or the administration of strong analgesics during birth is of considerable significance for the child and should be therapeutically compensated.

- Was delivery rushed or delayed? Were aids (forceps, vacuum extraction) or obstetric interventions (e.g. Kristeller's method) required?

A rushed delivery can traumatize the child as much as the use of forceps or vacuum extraction. While external injuries and fractures are more easily recognized, a possible lesion of the spinal column is considered less frequently. The atlanto-occipital junction and the cervical spine can be affected (e.g. atlas dislocation) [Deeg et al. 1998, 597–602; Upledger and Vredevoogd 2000, 304–309].

They do not have any directly visible sequelae and are therefore difficult to diagnose. But experience in practice shows that in some children displaying

- pronounced trimenon colics,
- gastroesophageal reflux disease,
- delayed development of motor functions,
- expressive speech development disorders,
- activity and attention disorders (ADHD)

such mainly *birth-related disorders of the craniocervical junction* are of causal significance. That applies in increased measure to newborn and premature babies who underwent nasotracheal intubation. Therapeutically, early *craniosacral therapy/osteopathic treatment* by an experienced, certified therapist is often manifestly effective (significant improvement can occur already after 1–3 treatments). The principle of this therapy and the start of its use for infants is described vividly in Upledger's autobiographical account [Upledger 2002, 48ff.]. The comprehensive physiological importance of the cervico-occipital junction – the intramural nervous system of the whole gastro-intestinal tract, among other things, starts here in the embryo, revealing the importance of this region in reflux and abdominal colics – is set out in B. Christ's account which culminates in the statement that "the region of the cervico-occipital junction must be seen as a 'vital centre' of the human being" [Christ 1990, 831). This can draw our attention to the fact that the head displays fundamentally different formative principles from the rest of the body – it is created wholly from the outer germ layer, the ectoderm [Rohen 2000, 350] – and that the undisturbed *junction between the head and the body* is of vital anatomical and functional importance (e.g. for the coordination of all movement processes) in early childhood. The *indication* for craniosacral therapy arises from the above anamnesis and the examination results in which asymmetries (e.g. subtle side differences in the region of the upper cervical spine; torticollis), irregularities of tone (above all in the trunk musculature), and disorders of the movement flow are of importance (to understand the craniosacral movement cf. Upledger and Vredevoogd 2000, 49–62). They must be distinguished from neurologically defined clinical conditions.

Generally familiar sequelae of a difficult delivery are asphyxia and – above all in neonates – intracranial haemorrhage.

- Was the birth significantly premature or was the child overdue?
- What was the birth weight?

If we understand the formation of bodily substance as the work of the child's life organization over time, then these anamnesis questions acquire fundamental importance for an understanding of the child's constitution. The response in the first instance reflects the intrauterine growth conditions (feeding through the mother): What time, what opportunity did the child's life organization have for its primary development? Thus early and sustained placental malnutrition over a long period (before the 34th week of pregnancy) can reduce the total number of cells throughout life, lower growth potential and later intelligence [for references cf. Wollmann 2004] and mean an increased risk of cardio-vascular diseases and type 2 diabetes [Beinder 2007].

Birth weight i. a. reflects the activity of the child's life or formative forces, the etheric body, during the foetal period [for the concept of the etheric body ▸Chap. 1.1. as well as Steiner and Wegman 1991, 12, 98]. If we consider that a quarter of children who are too light during the gestation period display disorders as early as the perinatal period [Keller and Wiskott 1991, 176], it becomes clear that small-for-date births can often have more serious consequences than a purely premature birth (after the 32nd–34th week of pregnancy). Significant therapeutic help can be provided here by homoeopathy and anthroposophic medicine.

Children who are born truly *overdue* can give rise to the question whether they themselves hesitated before birth or whether a manifest pathology paralyzed the initiation of birth. Many years of practical experience teach us to pay particular attention to this initial situation of an overdue birth: what is concealed behind such hesitancy? It happens not infrequently that an illness or crisis affects these children at a later date which they can only manage with difficulty (a quasi second birth). If overdue children are initially seen frequently during the nursing period in order to observe and examine them carefully, it may be possible, in good time, to give them the help they require on their path of incarnation.

2.2 Treatment

Neonatological first care generally observes the following sequence:

1. Warmth,
2. Respiration,
3. Circulation,
4. Nutrition, substance substitution.

This sequence is based in the first instance on therapeutic experience. But it can also lead to a deeper understanding of the components of the child's being.

2.2.1 Maintaining warmth

The preservation of a stable body temperature is physiologically the primary (and most complex) task of the human organism. That is also reflected in its position in neonatological first care. It directly makes clear the extent to which all bodily processes are dependent on homoiothermy, the preservation and regulation of warmth. The circadian day-night rhythm of the organism is also regulated through the warmth organization [Buhr 2010]. Before birth, the unborn child lives in the maternal warmth cover and the placenta is the central organ of foetal temperature regulation [Kaufmann 1990, 202]. It is remarkable in this connection that Rudolf Steiner in 1924 refers to the placenta (chorion) as "the physical correlate of the I-organization" in the foetal period [Steiner 1989, 308]. The relationship between the human individuality and warmth was already addressed above (▸Chap. 1.3). The temperature regulating centre, the most important source of warmth for the unborn child, still lies at the periphery – just like the sun acts as a source of heat from the environment for all poikilothermic and plant organisms. With birth and the dying off of the placenta, the "lost half of the human being" [Schad 2008], the child's individuality, and with it body temperature, enter the body: the healthy newborn almost doubles his or her own warmth generation in comparison to the foetus. This great increase in the development of body temperature at birth, but also every time the child wakes up, in febrile diseases and physical activity corresponds directly to the incarnation of the individuality in the body and the development of its will activity. And only homoiothermy makes it possible to develop will activity at any moment, whereas snakes, for example, lose any possibility of independent activity merely through the cooling of the environment.

The human warmth organization is superior to all other living beings with regard to its performance and regulatory ability [Aschoff 1971, 43–113; Husemann and Wolff 1991, 102]. This freedom is realized in human beings above all through their naked skin without fur, feathers or scales: it is no longer protein structures such as hair or feathers but the subcutaneous fat which protects people against loss of heat; and the large number of sweat glands and the regulation of cutaneous perfusion allow them the unique freedom to dissipate and regulate heat. Some of these central functions of the human skin only mature late in pregnancy and in the first year of life: a premature child has little subcutaneous fat to fall back on, his or her sweat glands are not yet functioning in the first days of life and the subcutaneous fat doubles in the first year of life. Furthermore, the loss of heat in the region of the head and face cannot be significantly regulated – but these areas comprise a large part of the body surface in infants while the limbs, in which human beings can vary heat dissipation to an extraordinary degree, are still hardly developed. This makes the cultural and therapeutic task very clear; the newborn infant must be observed particularly attentively as to his or her warmth situation and appropriately covered.

The human individuality also lives and acts in the self-generated warmth perceived by others, and the importance of warmth in establishing a relationship between the self and another becomes directly perceptible in the newborn: when it is first placed at the mother's breast, it is not only the maternal breast which warms up but in this moment the infant also experiences a warming impulse right into the periphery, and the same applies to the father who also experiences this moment! It has been shown that the experience of such a moment after birth reciprocally deepens the bond between child and parents.[1]

Hence the careful observation of the child's warmth situation and its therapeutic support is fundamentally of the greatest importance – not just in neonatology. The quiet, careful handling of the newborn which reduces medical diagnosis to the necessary minimum without rigid routine, is a prerequisite for warmth protection. The physical proximity to the mother, pre-warmed cloths, woollen (!) baby clothes including head covering (20 % of the body surface) provide the child with the necessary warmth cover. Parents are always surprised how much more stably infants can maintain their temperature when they are wearing a woollen bodysuit! Research into sudden infant death syndrome (SIDS) has made the vital importance of body temperature and heat regulation clear, for example through the risk of hyperthermia or also hypothermia (!) of the infant during sleep [Poets 2003, 163]. Above all, inhibiting the necessary heat loss in the head and facial region can have fatal consequences [Kinney 2009, 800]. Poets advises feeling the temperature between the shoulder blades during sleep: the skin should be warm without sweating. During the day the temperature in the limbs should additionally be checked: with the possible exception of the time before feeding, the hands and feet should be warm. But if a

1 A strong parallel rise in oxytocin can be measured in the mother [Uvnäs-Moberg 2005]. The authors are grateful to Markus Sommer for the reference to the corresponding results in attachment research.

weakness and lability of the child's warmth organization becomes apparent – wherein observing the periphery is as important as the core temperature – therapeutic measures are indicated. This is the case especially with premature and small-for-date babies; but antibiotic treatment can also frequently (measurably) disrupt the warmth organization.

An effective way of warming is a regular all-body oil rub (torso and limbs)

- 1–2 x/d, e. g. with **mallow oil** Wala.

This oil composition contains extracts of elder, linden and sloe blossom as well as St John's wort oil, among other things.

In premature babies and newborns, it can be gentler to avoid all plant extracts in the oil to begin with and to do the rub with warmed olive or almond oil [Ulrich 2002, 69]. The warming effect is noticeable particularly in the limbs as they grow and remain warm. As long ago as the end of the nineteenth century, the well-known British homoeopath Burnett [1993, 11] observed and publicized the therapeutic and preventive effect of regular all-body oil rubs in infants. It was noticeable that they thrived better and there was a reduction in the seriousness and frequency of infectious diseases – e. g. in a comparison of twins.

2.2.2 Asphyxia, respiratory regulation disorders and SIDS

The peri- and postpartum asphyxia of the child has today become a domain of neonatal intensive care medicine with regard to first care. But even with the full deployment of the methods of intensive care medicine the effect of potentized medicines can be repeatedly experienced.

The following is specifically effective

- **Tartarus stibiatus D6 trit.** Weleda/**C6–30 pillules** (various manufacturers)

initially e. g. 2 pillules/1 small saltsp. sublingually every 5 min., with onset of effect half-hrly to hrly, maintenance dose one dose 3–5 x/d.

Case history

A paediatric colleague was able to observe the action of Tartarus stibiatus while a doctor with the helicopter emergency service. He was called to an infant who had been born extremely prematurely with consecutive tracheomalacia following long-term ventilation. The intubation of this child was highly risky, even under hospital conditions, because of the level of difficulty. He therefore accompanied the cyanotic and hypercapnic child to the hospital without intubation in the first instance and instead administered Tartarus stibiatus as set out above. On arrival at hospital the child had practically normalized blood gases and intubation was no longer necessary

Tartarus stibiatus is made from a compound of antimony trioxide with the potassium salt from tartaric acid ("wine stone") [Stübler and Krug 1987, 435]. This becomes soluble in the antimony compound – which is also highly poisonous. In homoeopathic potency we can observe that the constriction of the lower airways is relieved and mucous congestion is dislodged from them as well as respiratory activity as a whole being stimulated and stabilized. Indications for Tartarus stibiatus in newborns and infants are all states of threatening asphyxia, obstruction of the airways with a mucous rattle and circulatory insufficiency, pale skin colour and threatening respiratory regulation weakness (cf. also pneumonia, bronchiolitis, pertussis and severe reactions to vaccination [Vademecum 2010, 795]). Tartarus stibiatus is one of the most important medicines in paediatrics and should always be promptly available in the medical bag and office.

If – above all in premature babies – there is immaturity of the respiratory centre (cumulative phases of periodic respiration, cumulatively longer apnoeas), the administration of

- **Tartarus stibiatus D6 trit.** Weleda
  1 saltsp. 3–5 x/d

over a longer period is also indicated. Here the action can be intensified through the simultaneous administration of

- **Carbo Betulae D12 trit.** Weleda
  1 saltsp. 2 x/d

Carbo Betulae, birch charcoal, is made by heating wood under air-restriction: release of heat with simultaneous disruption of the oxygen supply and release of carbon dioxide forms the "physiology" of the charcoal kiln – but also characterizes the pathophysiology of asphyxia and probably also SIDS [Kinney 2009, 798]. In potentized form, Carbo Betulae has the effect of intensifying the respiratory activity of the organism, and in particular exhalation, thus also relieving the circulation (stasis in the microcirculation and blockage in the venous circulation). Central respiratory paralysis is countered and the function of the respiratory centre is stimulated, which is, after all, meant to adjust the breathing (out) activity with regard to the formation of heat (and the release of carbon dioxide) in the organism.

The question arises here as to whether the administration of Tartarus stibiatus and Carbo Betulae can act to prevent *possible sudden infant death syndrome (SIDS)*. Great progress has been achieved in the prevention of SIDS through

- avoiding the accumulation of heat and hypothermia,
- avoiding the prone position,
- breast feeding,
- the child sleeping in the parental bedroom but in a separate bed,
- avoiding soft mattresses and underlays for the sleeping infant,
- avoiding/restricting smoking [Poets 2003, 161],
- a regular rhythm of life as far as possible, including at weekends/public holidays.

Here it is noticeable that the *balance* of closeness and distance as expressed for example in the rhythm of breast feeding and letting sleep, sleeping in the parental bedroom but in his or her own cot, is of material importance. The *individual perception of the needs of the child* has a protective effect while SIDS is facilitated above all if the parents smoke. The toxic effect of Nicotiana tabacum can lead to a *deformation of the rhythmical system* – and in potentized form can, in turn, be used as a valuable medicine for disorders in this sphere [Wilkens 2002, 396].

Affected infants with nicotine withdrawal syndrome and respiratory regulation disorder following nicotine exposure in pregnancy can be given Carbo Betulae in the form of a composite medicines with potentized Nicotiana tabacum:

- **Nicotiana comp. pillules** Wala
  2 pillules 2–4 x/d.

SIDS is a failure of the respiratory regulation in the child. Respiration corresponds directly with the experience of the soul in the body (e.g. pleasure, pain) and is the result of the activity of the soul organization (the astral body) (▸Chap. 1.3). The respiratory activity which starts with birth only stabilizes gradually; it is fundamentally more labile during sleep when the soul and spiritual individuality and the vital processes of the body partially separate [Steiner and Wegman 1991, 16] and the waking presence of the soul entity recedes. It is clear that the "entry" of the soul into the body is connected with the respiration, takes place in respiration. Waking up intensifies the respiratory processes; it was possible to show in prospective studies that children who died from SIDS were subject to cumulative phases of incomplete awakening [Schechtman et al. 1992].

SIDS research has shown the high degree to which this event is dependent on attentiveness, the lifestyle habits of the parents, on cultural conventions, rhythm and balance in living with the baby, and that risk arises above all through addictive behaviour by the parents, loss of a partner and poverty. Addiction is the result of one-sided fixation arising from psychological needs which become dominant over the I and exercise a one-sided catabolic effect on the body. If the carer consciously wants to act on the breathing processes in the child's soul and support them, this is dependent on the presence of his or her I, and particularly the preservation of the balance between the child and the parents [cf. on this parent-child connection in general Rudolf Steiner 1995, 33]. States of exhaustion, relationship problems, money worries and unresolved dependencies can interfere with parental attentiveness and freedom of action. The example of SIDS shows that *detailed parent counselling* has saved the lives of more infants than technically elaborate interventions (polysomnography, monitors, etc.). The *preventive medicinal approach is of supplementary* importance in this respect. The authors recommend treatment with Carbo Betulae D12 and Tartarus stibiatus D6 in the above dosage for children with a known immaturity of the respiratory regulation (apnoea tendency) and children who are deemed to be at risk as the result of affected siblings or following an apparent life-threatening event (ALTE [cf. Erler 2003]). If these children are monitored with a home monitor, this allows the success of the treatment to be controlled. In the practice of the authors, it was possible to repeatedly observe a significant and rapid fall in apnoea frequency and a stabilization of the respiratory rhythm. Information with regard to the SIDS risk can, in contrast, only be provided through studies. Beyond that, all the therapeutic perspectives described in this chapter (heat regulation, shock treatment, attention to the craniocervical junction, etc.) are of preventive importance.

2.2.3 Shock sequelae

Each state of shock places the connection between soul and body, the incarnation of the individuality, at risk and makes it more labile. Psychologically, a shock primarily produces anxiety and restlessness; but it can also have sequelae which persist for a long time, such as sleep disturbance.

A severe shock physically places vital functions at risk particularly in the sphere of the circulation and kidney/adrenal gland activity. Shock treatment can be of relevance for all the disorders discussed in this chapter. Anthroposophic and homoeopathic treatment is also pertinent if history reveals that an earlier shock experience is the probable cause of clinical disorders (see case history below).

The most important potentized medicine for shock and shock sequelae is

- **Aconitum D10–30 pillules** Wala/**C200** pillules (various manufacturers)
  - acutely 1 × 2 pillules D30 (newborns and infants) or 3 × 2 pillules D10,
  - for shock sequelae depending on the age of the child 1 × 2–5 pillules D20 in the evening,
  - for shock sequelae in the distant past with severe anxiety 3 × 2–3 pillules C200 at 12-hourly intervals each

Aconitum napellus, aconite, forms aconitin, "probably the most poisonous of all alkaloids; 3 mg are enough to kill a horse" [Madaus 1999, Vol. 1, 395]. This strong mountain plant which can be found up in regions up to a height of 3000 m, prefers nitrogen-rich soils fertilized by animal excrement. Its flower is bilaterally symmetrical (like the face, for example), dark blue and turns away from the sky (in contrast to radially symmetrical composite flowers like arnica or calendula, which are never associated with strong toxicity).

Aconite produces attack-like symptoms of poisoning with existential fear, circulatory insufficiency (cardiotoxic) and acute anuresis. "It opens the sodium channels and leads to uncontrolled persistent excitation up to the complete exhaustion of cell function. The poisoned person freezes into a 'pillar of salt'" [Vademecum 2010, 41]. The indication for Aconitum in treatment of shock is given if the child has suddenly got into a situation which has triggered severe tension and anxiety and in which he or she is at the mercy of external forces – even if these may be people who medically want to save his or her life. A sign of such an acute state of shock can be delayed or suspended diuresis (conversely the positive effect of potentized Aconitum can be seen, among other things, in the restoration of diuresis). The initial administration of Aconitum improves the response to Tartarus stibiatus, for example, in acute asphyxia if this was triggered by shock-like circumstances of birth. Aconitum is also effective in peripartal shock events lying a long time in the past.

Case history

In a five-year-old boy with serious bronchial asthma who had been treated largely unsuccessfully for years, a thoroughly retaken anamnesis revealed a postpartum asphyxia. This led the mother of the child, a doctor's assistant, to feel an anxious *certainty that the child would die.* It subsequently turned out that the mother herself had suffered from asthmatic disorders since that time. On the basis of the continuing complaints following an event which lay a long time in the past, Aconitum in higher potencies was administered both to the mother and the child: first in D30 and then in D200. The mother's complaints disappeared almost completely as a result; the child's asthma, which before the start of this treatment could only be managed with inhaled steroids, could be decisively improved; it became possible to discontinue the inhaled steroids altogether (now three years of follow-up). Undoubtedly the early administration of Aconitum, indeed, directly after the birth, would have been significantly more effective – with the result that perhaps no one would have detected the effect.

2

Tab. 2.1 Comparison of Aconitum and Opium

Aconitum	Opium
Toxic root node	Dried latex of the seed pod with narcotic effect
Anxiety, tension	Sopor, atony
Neuralgiform pain	Painless state
Acute anuresis	Paralytic ileus, atonic obstipation
Over-wakeful, excessively strong inhalation	Sleepy, stertorous respiration

The state of shock which requires Aconitum as a medicine primarily provokes excessively strong and (anxiously) self-perpetuating inhalation (cf. the relationship with bronchial asthma in above case history). A polar shock effect can occur e. g. through a *general anaesthetic*. The soul entity is detached (too much) from the physical body and cannot afterwards find its way back to its normal activity in the body. The child is not tensed up but primarily atonic, the respiration stuporous (strong tendency for apnoea!), the facial features appear limp and painless. A key sign of this state is the inactivity of the intestinal musculature to the extent of paralytic ileus.

This state of shock, which often involves opiate-related anaesthetics, has its medicinal equivalent in potentized

- **Opium C30 pillules** (various manufacturers)
  3 × 2 pillules at an interval of 6–12 h each.

This medicine should be considered particularly after a section under general anaesthetic or after the administration of opiates during birth. But Opium can show a dramatic effect also in other comparable situations.

Case history

A two-year old girl undergoes an operation for retrocession and reimplantation of the right ureter into the bladder. Postoperative complications require two emergency operations within five days. The child subsequently develops paralytic ileus; all measures to evacuate the intestine fail. The child is in a bad general state of health, apathetic and indifferent; she just wants to be left in peace. Opium C30 is prescribed by telephone in the dose set out above. Bowel movement starts six hours after the first administration; the child starts to take some food again and recovers in a few days following this administration

Aconitum and Opium correspond to two *polar states of shock* (Tab. 2.1): In one case the soul activity in the body, and thus respiration, anxiety, pain, is elevated – in the other case there is a partial excarnation of the soul and spiritual individuality which leaves the life organization to its own devices (regression into an almost plant-like state). All the symptoms set out can only be helpful in identifying this basic shift in the soul and physical integration of the child.

The following is suitable for external application following shock

- **Oxalis ointment 10 %** Weleda
  massage in pea-sized quantity in a clockwise direction between the sternum and navel 1–2 x/d.

The delicate, thin, sour-tasting leaves of common wood sorrel (Oxalis acetosella) "flourish even at 1/70 of full daylight whereas they perish in strong sunlight as a result of the destruction of the chlorophyll." [Madaus, Vol. 3, 2049]. The leaves display sensitivity (e.g. to touch) and mobility (they fold up and down together like an umbrella e.g. when touched or if it rains, and they do so within a few minutes) in a way which is otherwise only typical for a flower. Even the roots of Oxalis are contractile, which helps the plant to avoid being covered on the forest floor.

Physiologically it is the *gastro-intestinal tract* in its vital regenerative power and its independent movement on the one hand, and its pronounced "innervation" on the other which corresponds to some of the characteristics of Oxalis. The "enteric nervous system" (ENS), whose mass is comparable with that of the brain, develops in the intestinal wall in parallel with the development of the central nervous system; the gastro-intestinal tract is the organ in the human body with the most nerves outside the CNS! This ENS, like the CNS, is permanently influenced by the early experiences of the child. A gentle rhythmical Einreibung with Oxalis ointment is indicated if shock experiences have led to a regulatory disorder of this system, a state of *vegetative hypersensitivity* has occurred (e.g. intestinal colic, meteorism, stool irregularities). The soul and neuronally mediated activity is not immersed unconsciously in the function of the digestive tract but irritates the child's perception of its body – we can refer to this as *hypersensitivity of the sense of life* [Soesmann 1995, 29], a frequent consequence of shock, but which can also occur at particular ages in the form of so-called umbilical colic at around the age of three to five.

An Oxalis rhythmical Einreibung can balance such a state of inner hypersensitivity. It can also be used in the kidney region if shock experiences have caused a disorder of this organ area (cf. the impressive case history from M. Sommer in the Vademecum of Anthroposophic Medicines [Vademecum 2010, 638]).

Treatment with *potentized silver* has a very broad balancing effect in the event of shock, continuing the above shock treatment with herbal medicines and rounding off and consolidating their action. Here the action of silver is – organically related – primarily aimed at the *nervous and sensory system*. The characteristics of silver display an affinity with all ectodermal organs in the human organism. It has the greatest conductivity of all metals, corresponding to the nerve fibres which achieve their full conductivity by the age of seven. Nerve fibres are argyrophilic, i.e. they can be histologically selectively stained (Golgi staining). Silver can be used to make perfect mirrors just as the sensory and nervous system reflects the environment and the inner world of the organism. Shock experiences can disrupt the development and function of this system and weaken its vital foundations. This applies particularly if the etheric body, the life organization of the child, is still very immature or weak as is often the case in premature or small-for-date babies.

Silver is the metal which is the most supportive of life and least toxic for humans. Whereas microorganisms can be killed even by finely distributed traces of silver (oligodynamic effect), water sterilized with silver is completely harmless for humans. Silver wires and plates are common surgical instruments and are tolerated by the human organism without a problem. Potentized silver has a fundamentally *supportive action on the life organization* and can balance the too deep penetration of the conscious soul life which has a catabolic and paralyzing effect on the life processes. Therapeutically potentized silver reduces the sensory hypersensitivity of the child, his or her nervosity and anxiety, in treating the effects of shock. The rhythmical alternation of waking and sleeping, the replacement of mental consciousness processes, associated with catabolic physical processes, by physical anabolic processes is supported. Potentized silver is particularly important for premature and small-for-date babies (see below).

Various silver preparations are used medicinally in anthroposophic medicine:

- **Argentum met. praep. D6 trit.** Weleda
  1 saltsp. in the evening–1 saltsp. 3 x/d
- **Argentum/Rohrzucker pillules** Wala
  3 pillules in the evening (neonates)–7 pillules (infants)/d

In this medicine developed by H. H. Vogel [1994, Vol. 1, 137] silver (Argentum met. D5) is potentized together with cane sugar D9 [Beiblätter Natura 2000, 41–50]; it is specifically suitable for the treatment of shock sequelae.

- **Bryophyllum Argento cultum Rh D3 dil.** Weleda (alcohol-free – cf. ▸Chap. 1.2.2)
  3 gtt. 3 x/d – infants 3 × 5–7 gtt.

The starting substance in the latter preparation is a Bryophyllum (life plant, "Goethe Plant") specially cultivated with a silver-containing fertilizer over several years. In this way the plant "potentizes" traces of the metal; this process of the "vegetabilization of metals" goes back to a suggestion from Rudolf Steiner. Bryophyllum, an extraordinarily vital succulent plant with smooth, meaty leaves, grows in dry and warm regions of the earth in which the strong sunlight threatens the vitality of the plant through dehydration. Bryophyllum counters that by closing its stomata during the day, thus separating the process of photosynthesis from the respiratory process. At night it inhales the carbon dioxide required for carbohydrate synthesis from the air and binds it in the form of crassulacean malate so that Bryophyllum becomes increasingly acid towards the morning and then converts the carbon dioxide in the air into carbohydrates through photosynthesis. As "brood leaves", Bryophyllum primarily propagates vegetatively by growing small plantlets on the edges of the leaves which then drop off and grow into new plants. Bryophyllum displays a clear moon and silver affinity as understood by anthroposophic medicine through its night-time activity, unusual for plants, and its productive abundance. The pharmaceutical process of the "vegetabilization" of silver in this way brings the action of the silver pharmaceutically closer to the organism and its life organization: shock-related sleep disturbance and hysteriform states of agitation provide an important indication for this medicine [cf. Schneider 2001]. The nightly "poisoning" through acid accumulation in Bryophyllum corresponds to the nightly states of unrest, the vegetative hyperexcitability in children which can be treated with Bryophyllum Argento cultum [Schramm 2009, 331–333].

If the original shock experience was accompanied by toxic burdens (e.g. anaesthesia, antibiotics), the sulphur compound of silver, silver sulphide, can be administered:

- **Argentit D6 trit.** Weleda
  1 saltsp. 3 x/d [Vademecum 2010, 107]

2.2.4 Birth trauma

The most serious birth traumas relate to the circulation: cerebral hypoxaemia and ischaemia. If there is any reasonable suspicion of hypoxic, ischaemic or haemorrhagic brain damage (e.g. after a protracted birth which had to be ended with a section) the attempt can be made with potentized medicines to prevent or reduce the long-term consequences.

Potentized copper has a broad compensating effect in this situation:

- **Cuprum met. D30 pillules** (various manufacturers), **Cuprum met. praep. D30 amp.** Weleda
  1–2 pillules 1–3 × in 24 h, 0.3 ml per os or 0.5 ml i.v.

This is the most important potentized medicine for *vasospasms;* other indications for the administration of copper are: hypoxaemia (cyanosis), bad peripheral circulation (delayed refill reaction, cool extremities), epileptic attacks with cerebral blood flow disorders or following asphyxial brain damage, stuporous depression of consciousness and a tendency for muscle spasms (both of the smooth and cross-striated muscles).

Underlying these symptoms is the difficulty of the soul organization, the astral body, to combine with the life organization through *respiration*: it remains "stuck halfway", exhalation and respiratory rhythm cannot get going, the child threatens to sink into the night of hypoxia. The tendency for vasospasms, for cramps reflects an astral body which has become "stuck" and cannot therefore give the life organization any impulses. The soul entity is fighting for incarnation but does not succeed in creating the required conditions: specifically in the sphere of respiration, the gas tensions, the child threatens to regress to intrauterine physiological conditions which are now totally inadequate for the growing independence of respiration and warmth generation.

The embodiment of this pathology is the *unsuccessful separation from the mother.* Physiologically, the phenomenon is relevant in this connection that the maternal serum copper level rises two to three fold during pregnancy which is mirrored in the child at birth by maximum corpuscular iron concentrations in the blood: the ratio of child haemoglobin to maternal haemoglobin is between 3:2 and 2:1. The child needs the iron to break out of the maternal cover and be able to incarnate while the mother uses the substantial qualities of copper, among other things, to envelop, hold and nourish the unborn child (while her Hb is physiologically falling). We have here, in archetypal form, the *polar and complementary relationship between iron and copper* which is of fundamental importance for the treatment of respiratory disorders (cf. ▸Chap. 6.5). In this context iron stands for inhalation, the development of independent movement and body temperature, copper for exhalation, relaxation and separation, for physical catabolic processes stimulated by the soul entity.

Copper in higher potencies is indicated if these qualities are at risk: in paediatrics it is often indicated for a *tendency to go into spasm* (airways, vessels, musculature) and a *maternal bond which is too close.* Serious cerebral ischaemia can be prevented or its effects mitigated in neonatology through its spasmolytic effect. In our own experience stressed newborns recover considerably faster with the administration of Cuprum D30.

The authors have had positive experiences with it in recent years when undertaking follow-up treatment after birth trauma with

- **Chamomilla Cupro culta, Radix eth. Dec. Rh D3 dil.** Weleda (alcohol-free)
  3–5 gtt. 2–3 x/d.
  In epilepsies in infancy D2 can be more effective (1–2 gtt. 2–3 x/d, contains alcohol, diluted in a little water).

In this specific anthroposophic medicine, traces of copper are taken in through the roots of the camomile plant and "potentized" in the plant's metabolism (cf. the explanation above on the vegetabilization of metal in Bryophyllum Argento cultum, ▸Chap. 2.2.3). In this way the copper acts finely on the child's sentient organization, above all with an antispasmodic effect, combined with the calming action of the camomile root which is particularly pronounced and therapeutically valuable in infancy. In this way the copper therapy can be deepened following birth trauma.

The positive effect of Arnica montana in blunt traumas, haematomas and haemorrhagic insults is well known.

At the slightest suspicion of an intracranial brain haemorrhage

- **Arnica e pl. tota D30 pillules/amp.** Wala
  1–3 × 1 pillule within 24 h, 0.3 ml i.v.

can be administered immediately together with Cuprum D30; such bleeding almost always occurs on the basis of hypoxaemia and fluctuations in perfusion. Manifest brain haemorrhages (ultrasound grading ICH II–IV) require Arnica in ascending order of potency:

- **Arnica e pl. tota D6 pillules** Wala
  1 pillule 3–5 x/d for 1 week, then D12, 1 pillule 2 x/d for 1 week and finally D30 1 pillule 1 x/d for 3 days (follow-up treatment ▸Chap. 8.2.1.2).

In cephalohaematoma:

- **Arnica e pl. tota D4 pillules** Wala
  1 pillule 3–5 x/d, then
- **Arnica 10 % ointment** Weleda
  applied externally 2 x/d.

In general, the *joint administration of Arnica and Cuprum in D30*, 3 × within 24 h, is to be recommended, alongside any treatment for shock and asphyxia if there is any suspicion of peripartum cerebral damage.

A *cerebrospinal fluid circulation disorder* (hydrocephalus) can be the consequence of extensive intracranial bleeding. The implantation of a shunt is not always required.

In our own practice we could repeatedly observe that the administration of

- **Stannum met. praep. D20–30 trit.** Weleda
  1 saltsp. 2 × or 1 x/d

was able to reduce the extent of the hydrocephalus and the pressure of the cerebrospinal fluid.

Stannum met., zinc, is used as a metallic medicine in homoeopathy and anthroposophic medicine; in paediatrics above all for the stasis of fluids in the connective tissue which can be caused, among other things, by inflammations or circulatory disorders [cf. Husemann and Wolff 1986, 443–445]. Cerebrospinal fluid circulation disorders are best treated with higher potencies (D20–30); fluid congestion of the lungs, especially in pneumonia, with medium-high potencies (D10–15), while e.g. in a testicular hydrocele external application (0.4% ointment Weleda [Vademecum 2010, 768] is possible.

Case history

A baby born prematurely in the thirtieth week of pregnancy is suffering from grade III intracranial bleeding with progressive enlargement of the subarachnoid spaces. Shunt implantation appears unavoidable. At the request of the mother, treatment with Arnica e pl. tota D6 and Stannum met. praep. D20 according to the above doses is initiated approx. seven days postpartum. There is no further increase in the hydrocephalus; on the contrary, a slow but continuous improvement is determined. Fourteen years after birth the developmental neurological findings are normal and there is only moderate enlargement of the interior subarachnoid spaces.

2

The initial treatment with Stannum and Arnica should be subsequently continued with

- **Hypophysis/Stannum glob.** Wala
  2–5 pillules 1–2 x/d for 3–9 months or longer.

A serious clinical picture in neonatology which requires intensive treatment is *hypoxic-ischaemic encephalopathy* following asphyxia, which above all in premature babies results in cerebral tissue damage (leukomalacia). Circulatory and kidney function is labile or considerably impaired; cerebral seizures can occur. The incarnation of the soul and spiritual individuality is seriously impaired; the body threatens to fall into a vegetative state. The children often appear stuporous, hypotonic; if they are not intubated, a shrill crying or whining with little modulation is noticeable, among other things.

Treatment with

- **Helleborus niger D12** Wala
  1–2 pillules 2–3 x/d

can be tried here to supplement the other therapeutic perspective set out above

The reader can find a comprehensive account of Helleborus niger, the Christmas rose, as a true polycrest of homoeopathically and anthroposophically extended paediatrics, in the references [Swoboda 2005, Merkurstab 6/2010]

The treatment of seriously ill newborns in hospital with *external applications* should not fundamentally be neglected either. In this situation of abrupt separation from the mother and unavoidable invasively painful treatment, the importance of the skin as a sensory organ should not be overlooked (particularly with regard to neurological disorders!). Loving attention and touch of the skin acquires its importance and justification also from the perspective of today's neonatal intensive care. *Massaging oil into the back* in a craniocaudal direction, for example alternating between rose oil and sloe oil (▸Chap. 2.2.1) is advisable.

If there is the clinical suspicion of a *peripartum-related lesion of the cervical spine/craniocervical junction* (Chap. 2.1) the child should be examined and, as necessary, manually treated by an experienced osteopathic therapist. Many complications can be avoided in this way!

In the event of positive findings, medicinal treatment is possible with

- **Hypericum D12 pillules** (various manufacturers)
  3 pillules 1 x/d e.g. in the afternoon and
- **Disci comp. c. Stanno pillules** Wala
  2 pillules 2 x/d e.g. in the morning and evening.

In paralysis related to birth trauma, e.g. Erb's palsy or facial paresis, the healing process can be improved through the administration of

- **Hypericum ex herba D6 pillules** Wala
  2 pillules 3 x/d together with
- **Arnica e plans tota D6 pillules** Wala
  2 pillules 3 x/d.

In cases resistant to therapy, additional treatment with potentized homologous organ preparations can be recommended e.g. in facial paresis related to birth trauma.

- **Nervus facialis GI Serienpackung III (=D5–30) amp.** Wala
  0.3–0.5 ml (per os!) 1 x/d (or each 2nd day), starting with D5 in ascending order of potentization.

In paediatric practice, *potentized organ preparations* administered in the form of *potency series* (series packages) have repeatedly shown themselves to be effective if vital regenerative processes are to be stimulated in particular (homologous) organ-specific areas. In primary abnormal vitality or damage lying further in the past, the authors administer the potency series in ascending order; in acute damage and inflammatory components they do so in descending order. The ampoules are administered *per os* by drawing the contents of a whole ampoule into a syringe and then dispensing the required quantity from that. Cf. the specific treatment chapters on the application of potentized organ preparations in acute or chronic inflammations.

2.3 Counselling and treatment in cases of premature birth, birth defects and prolonged pregnancy

2.3.1 Treatment goals for babies born prematurely and with birth defects

Neonatology today enables premature babies from the 32nd week of pregnancy or earlier to have a largely normal prognosis with regard to survival and permanent disability. But if we pose the questions that were formulated in ▸Chap. 2.1 (birth anamnesis), it becomes clear that these children and their parents – above all the mothers – have quite a different birth experience from most full-term neonates.

> The event mostly happens quickly and without preparation. Women prepare themselves for a normal pregnancy and the birth of a healthy child so that they are unprepared and taken negatively by surprise by a premature birth. ... Mothers feel totally caught off guard in this situation. .... The parents are suspended between joy (about progress) and depression (about setbacks), indeed, in extreme cases between life and death. They do not know what to prepare for and that is the greatest stress of all."
>
> [Markovich and de Jong 2008, 16, 32]

The mother feels pain about the fact that she was not able to carry her child to term, which for her can mean owing the child something and not having provided the baby with something he or she needs for life. Sustained traumatization occurs in many mothers in this connection [Jotzo and Poets 2006]. Often the course of delivery has to be manipulated, not infrequently through tocolysis in the first instance, possibly the administration of steroids ("lung maturity"), and the birth itself is rarely a spontaneous event and is accompanied by a great deal of anxiety and nervousness. In such a situation the pregnancy should always be enquired about and any – often abrupt – trigger for the premature birth sought (▸Chap. 2.4, Pregnancy anamnesis, and ▸Chap. 2.2.3, Shock sequelae). At the same time paediatricians can ask themselves how all of this was experienced by the child and which sequelae can still be perceived.

As a rule, a prematurely born baby is paediatrically cared for and hospitalized. Helpless and hypersensitive, the neonate – depending on the circumstances which led to the premature birth and which are necessary for his or her care – is missing the natural *correspondence of the mother*: as living warmth envelope, as perceptive and responding soul entity, as a nourishing human reference. This happens with increased frequency and intensity the more premature the child is: incubator care, stomach probe, unavoidable injury through blood taking and infusions, intubation and artificial respiration, and, finally, not infrequent occurrences of reanimation lead to fundamentally different circumstances to those of a normal birth in which the soul awakens to life.

Case history

A nine-year-old boy is presented in practice for short stature. The blood sample necessary for diagnosis cannot be taken: even three adults cannot hold the fearfully struggling child! The child was delivered in the 28th week of pregnancy by emergency section when a routine gynaecological check surprisingly revealed a pathological CTG. Apgar 0 directly after birth, primary reanimation. This experience in practice gives us an idea of the depth to which such a birth experience can be inscribed on a person's constitution. The child suffered serious mixed asthma at the age of nine, pronounced difficulties in falling and staying asleep, pronounced anxieties and contact disorders. Alongside the short stature, the medical findings revealed overgrowth of the intestinal flora with Candida albicans – appropriate diet and therapy led to a sustained improvement in his subjective feeling of health – as well as considerable intervertebral blockades in the region of the craniocervical junction and thoracic spine. By means of treatment in accordance with the principles set out here, absolutely with the inclusion of topical steroids in aerosol form to begin with, for example, but beyond that with the use of potentized medicines (internal and inhalation), a temporary antimycotically effective diet, rhythmical massage therapy, osteopathic treatment, supported by advisory consultations with the parents, it was possible largely to remedy all the problems described within three years with the exception of the short stature. In the follow-up phase (17 years) after conclusion of the treatment, statural height also normalized. The effectiveness of the osteopathic treatment impressed the boy to such an extent that he decided to become a physiotherapist and today works very successfully in this profession.

Modern neonatology has recognized the irreplaceable nature of the *conscious development of the mother-child relationship* ("kangarooing"), the sensory care of the child through touch of the skin, the perception of maternal warmth and the mother's scent, the taste of breast milk, the experience of the sense of equilibrium through gentle rocking on the mother's stomach [Jotzo and Poets 2006]. It is remarkable that Rudolf Steiner's differentiated account of sensory development and its importance in child development has been fully confirmed by neonatology today [Ulrich 2002; Einführung in die Sinneslehre: Soesman 1995]. The importance of the *father* also comes into focus much more clearly: "The father plays a crucial role in this first period after the [premature] birth." [Markovic and de Jong 2008, 30]. This aspect cannot be highlighted enough in present-day paediatric practice. "The drama of paternal deprivation" [Petri 2009] can have lifelong consequences and it is also a task of doctors and nurses to ensure the "inclusion of the father" in caring for the premature baby and that a lasting bond can be established between the child and his or her parents.

On the other hand a premature birth need not only have negative consequences, as is shown, for example, in the biography of Elisabeth Kübler-Ross: as an underweight triplet, something of her later empathy, her perceptual capacity and energy may perhaps also be due to that. Because premature babies clearly undergo an existential test in the first weeks of life which challenges their will to live to a much greater extent than a normal birth. And anyone who has worked in neonatology and has attentively followed the life of his or her former patients will also begin to ask about the nature of the spiritual individuality he or she has encountered and the meaning of the destiny of a premature birth for the child and its parents. In this context a lot depends on the way in which the child and his or her parents were supported by physicians and nurses during their extreme human experience.

Modern neonatology confronts the paediatrician with new kinds of diagnostic and therapeutic problems, above all in extremely premature and small-for-date babies. Many of them display lasting disabilities which do not, however, limit a clearly defined ability to a greater or lesser extent as is the case with full-term neonates, but diffusely relate to a number of so-called partial functions in the sphere of perception and motor development, a general impairment of the ability to concentrate, but also to the sleeping-waking rhythm, eating behaviour, growth, etc. Many of these things do not subsequently mature – and the scope of such impairments can only fully be seen at kindergarten and with early school age. The child and his or her environment often suffer in that the spiritual and creative potential of the child is contradicted by his or her soul and psychosocial as well as physical difficulties with which both sides have to struggle. A great deal of *patience* is required here in the support of these children who frequently do not master their difficulties and show their strengths until the latter half of childhood and adolescence.

Diagnostically, it is not just the physical immaturity evident after birth which is decisive but above all the continuing impairment of the living potential of the child, its life and growth forces in time. This aspect is generally termed "life force" in homoeopathy, and in anthroposophic medicine with greater differentiation as "life body" or "body of formative forces" [Steiner and Wegman 1991, 25] This is manifested physically among other things in the growth processes, in the metamorphosis of form as well as in every process of physical regeneration. The connection between reduced general growth potential and reduced intelligence in extremely premature or small-for-date newborn is generally familiar [Saigal 2003]. From an anthroposophical perspective this is interpreted as relating to the same life forces which initially produce growth as well as physical organ development. After they have fulfilled these tasks, they are released for functional tasks – whereby there are some organ areas (e. g. in the intestinal mucosa, bone marrow) in which these forces always remain strongly linked to their body-forming tasks and others in which they are liberated to a much greater extent. That applies in particular to the nervous and sensory system which has largely been developed physically by the age of approx. 7 or 8 and has little regenerative potential.

The *metamorphosis of the life forces* referred to here is also of crucial importance for so called "*school readiness*" – alongside the development of psychological maturity. It is very important not to start premature children at school until they are ready for this metamorphosis – otherwise the early entry to school deprives them of life forces which they urgently need to finish the development of their organs. Many extremely premature and small-for-date children display partial hypotrophic organ development, clearly lagging growth (here treatment with growth hormone can definitely have a helpful effect), and hypothrophy of their life organization, their etheric body. Accordingly, they have difficulties in releasing their etheric life forces and using them for their own soul and spiritual organization. On the other hand the life organization, the etheric body, develops in time and the most effective therapeutic measure is frequently to delay putting the child's life forces "in the service" of cognitive performance by a year. Thus ADHD research has in the meantime been able to show in general (not specifically related to neonates) that the probability of stimulant treatment, i. e. hyperactivity and attention deficit disorder in school, falls by half at age 10–14 if enrolment in school lies one year later than in the comparison group [Elder 2010]. This finding is of particular significance for premature and small-for-date children and a clear scientific argument in the question of the *right school enrolment time.*

On the basis of these preliminary remarks we can now formulate the goals which we pursue diagnostically, therapeutically and in parent counselling *in addition to established neonatology:*

- stimulating the child's own growth forces and guiding them in their activity where necessary (e.g. through potentized medicine, but also i.a. through external applications)
- supporting the soul and spiritual individuality of the child such that he or she can achieve as far as possible a harmonious connection with his or her own body, compensation of psychologically damaging experiences and the normal development of perception and activity [cf. Ulrich 2002]
- supporting the parents through counselling such that they feel themselves understood in their psychological situation and, on the other hand, receive the necessary help in understanding their child's situation and, on that basis, learn to handle him or her properly.

2.3.2 Premature birth

In order to implement the therapeutic goals described, the therapeutic approaches outlined above under ▸Chap. 2.2 are fundamental for the following ▸Chap. 2.3.2.1 and ▸Chap. 2.3.2.2: warmth protection, support of respiratory activity and regulation, treatment for shock sequelae and birth traumas. *Supplementary perspectives* will be set out below. They are described in their order in terms of the *functional threefold organization of the organism* (nervous and sensory system, rhythmical system, metabolic and limb system), which represents a fundamental perspective for anthroposophic medicine [Girke 2010, 20–36]. It not only enables a clearly structured understanding of the human corporeality [Rohen 2000], but is also of help in understanding the different actions and relationships of the soul entity with regard to these three systems [Steiner 1983, 150–163].

2.3.2.1 Nervous and sensory system disorders

The nervous and sensory system stands in the foreground in human foetal and infant development. But it is not only the brain, nervous system and sensitive parts of the sense organs which are formed from the ectoderm, the outermost germ layer, but also the epidermis (as well as the mammary glands and dental enamel). At the beginning, the ectodermal germ layer of the embryo develops the clear and transparent *amnion,* within which the foetus floats almost weightlessly in the amniotic fluid. The amniotic fluid is biochemically almost identical in composition to the cerebrospinal fluid. According to the Archimedes principle, the brain, too, in vivo weighs only about 30 g through the buoyancy of the cerebrospinal fluid (in adults) [cf. Rohen 2000, 152, and Steiner 1980, 35] and thus subsequently floats at rest for the whole of life in the same weightlessness as the complete foetus during pregnancy.

A premature birth in the first instance always means a *premature loss of the amnion as a foetal organ, as a buoyant space, as the central organ of the embryonic life organization*: "We have to know the following: the amnion is the physical correlate of the etheric body" [in pregnancy – Steiner 1989, 308]. The spherical shape of the head, the maturation of the sensory and nervous system is directly connected with the amnion (just like the brain throughout life can only function adequately in the specific milieu of the subarachnoid space). Through the premature birth the senses and the skin are prematurely exposed to the external world (it is indicative that the clinician determines the degree of prematurity from the skin and the skin appendages) and the pathology, with its long-term consequences which results from premature birth, is focused on the nervous and sensory system. So a therapeutic balance is of particular importance here.

An initial, directly active and, in principle, long-known therapeutic possibility is external applications on the skin; the epidermis is itself an original derivative of ectodermal development. The fundamental importance of the experience of touch with regard to the development of the nervous system in early childhood is generally accepted. *Every external application through the skin has a direct effect on the nervous and sensory system.* At the same time it is possible to influence the activity of the visceral organs in a rhythmical, stimulating or, indeed, calming way through the skin. *Rhythmical Einreibungen and rhythmical massage therapy as indicated by Wegman and Hauschka* have proved themselves to be particularly effective in the follow-up care of premature and small-for-date babies [Ulrich 2002]. As early as intensive care, and even more so afterwards, we can pay heed to the following alongside "kangarooing":

- Protection against bright light, attention to a day-night rhythm (the amnion is protected against daylight, retinopathy of prematurity (ROP) is promoted by too early vision). Exercising restraint with regard to photo flashes!
- Cradling movement (mother's stomach, "kangarooing", "hammock" – tried and tested in long-term neonatal patients) to stimulate the child's life organization and sense of balance. The latter is closely related to the I. Such cradling movements are an archetypal function of the amnion; e. g. in chicken embryos, which develop outside the mother's body, there is an active generation of rocking movements (recalling the sea as the source of life) [Scarf 2000]
- Speaking, quiet singing with the child: the newborn can already distinguish language from every other acoustic event [Lutzger 1996, 184]. CD or MP3 players are particularly alien to the child in this phase of life.
- Good taste experiences above all of breast milk to prevent eating disorders and loss of "inner appetite" (▸Chap. 6.5).
- Warm touch (with the palms of the hand, not the finger tips), providing security, carefully supporting the head, carefully observing and protecting the warmth of the child.
- Clear shapes and colours (e. g. yellow-orange walls/blue-violet veil above the bed), a few simple objects, at the beginning without sharp contours (simplest Waldorf doll, woollen bird).

A *home visit* is valuable in this context when the child is discharged from neonatal hospital care (it is frequently the case that at the beginning these children can only receive adequate medical care through home visits).

The development of the nervous and sensory system is positively influenced by *whole-body rhythmical Einreibungen of the skin*, initially with almond or olive oil, then – alternating with **mallow oil** Wala (warmth cover) as already mentioned – with

- 10 % rose oil (e. g. **Rosa e flora 10 % oleum** Wala)

The child grows calmer, more relaxed and often also sleeps better after this application.
A pronounced calming and sleep-promoting action is supported by rhythmical Einreibungen, above all of the back and legs with

- **Lavandula, Ol. aeth. 10 %** Wala

which in the first weeks/months of life can be diluted with olive oil to contain 2–5 % of etheric lavender oil.
As a potentized medicine administered per os (!), the following organ preparation corresponds particularly to rose oil in its universal action on all ectodermal organs

- **Amnion Gl amp.** Wala

It can be administered in the first weeks of life daily in the evening in D8 (0.2 ml per os); if the patient first comes for treatment some time after the premature birth, higher potencies (D12–30) are indicated (e. g. 0.3 ml per os in the evening every second day).

A reduction in hypersensitivity as well as of restlessness and sleep disturbance can be observed; on the other hand the vitality of the ectodermal organs is positively influenced. The administration of amnion can also ameliorate illnesses and psychological disorders beyond the neonatal period which have developed as the result of the traumatic loss of sheathing in early childhood [Vademecum 2010, 65] and/or are connected with primary reduced vitality and hypersensitivity e. g. of the skin (important medicine in atopic dermatitis ▸Chap. 6.4.3.6.1).

Case history

An approx. eight-week-old infant is presented in the practice for treatment of obstructive bronchitis. The treatment with Tartarus stibiatus D6 and other medicine shows an unexpected lack of success. The repeat anamnesis makes clear that the premature birth of the child in the 36th–37th week of pregnancy (i. e. relatively close to the due date) and the resulting hypersensitivity of the child are of pathogenic significance in this case. The administration of Amnion Gl D8 leads to the cure of the symptoms, which had previously been resistant to treatment, within a short period of time.

States of restlessness in hospitalized premature babies following interventions with anaesthesia, the use of (refractory or addictive) sedatives and opiates, as well as in premature babies following discharge from hospital, respond well to

- **Aurum/Valeriana inject/glob. velati** Wala
  0.5 ml per os/5 pillules per os 1–4 x/d

This composite medicine acts above all to stabilize the vegetative nervous system of the child. In this context we refer specifically once more to the medicines Oxalis and Argentum as already discussed (▸Chap. 2.2.3).

One specific lesion of extremely premature children in the region of the sensory and nervous system is *retinopathy of prematurity (ROP).*

In addition to and continuation of the normal ophthalmological diagnosis and treatment, limited improvement can be achieved – also at a later time still – with the administration of

- **Hypericum D10–12 pillules** (various manufacturers)
  2–5 pillules 1 x/d in the morning,
- **Chrysolith D6 trit.** Weleda [cf. Leitgedanken zu Chrysolith in: Vademecum 2010, 311]
  1 saltsp. 1 x/d in the afternoon
- **Cerebrum comp. A pillules** Wala
  2–5 pillules 1 x/d in the evening

In the experience of the authors, this treatment must be continued for a sufficiently long period of time – approx. 6 to 9 months. In children older than 6 months Hypericum can be replaced with phosphorus (same potency and dosage) and thus be administered in alternation.

2

2.3.2.2 Respiratory disorders: bronchopulmonary dysplasia and recurrent lower respiratory tract infections

The immaturity of the barrier organs of the skin and lungs limits the successes of neonatology in extremely premature children. Here the focus is often on acute lung immaturity. The following suggested treatments relate to children whose respiratory organs have been damaged and compromised in their development to such an extent through the consequences of artificial respiration, oxygen toxicity and similar things, that an – individually different – mixed picture of interstitial chronic inflammation of the lungs, damage to the respiratory epithelium and bronchial hypersensitivity (hyperresponsiveness), inflammation and mucous congestion develops: the consequences can be restrictions of the respiratory volumes with dyspnoea and (in greatly varying measure) oxygen demand, failure to thrive and gastroesophageal reflux, chronic relapsing, more or less obstructive bronchitis and relapsing pneumonia [Thomas and Speer 2005]. If in practice we see milder forms of bronchopulmonary dysplasia (BPD) today, they can nevertheless impair the development of the child's respiratory organs in a sustained way. Infections with RSV viruses during infancy have a particularly serious effect on the affected children, which is why the authors support RSV prevention with Palivizumab recommended for this patient group and have so far not observed any serious side-effects.

Some anthroposophic treatments have shown themselves to be therapeutically so effective in this context that savings could be achieved in allopathic medicines. That is also of importance in so far as, for example, systemically administered corticosteroids in the early postnatal phase can cause cerebral damage [cf. Thomas and Speer 2005, 218], topical (inhaled) steroids can, among other things, negatively influence growth and bone density and beta-sympathomimetics can increase any already existing restlessness in the children affected. In general the long-term value of the steroid inhalations widely used today for this clinical picture is controversial so that the reduction and – if possible – careful tapering off of the steroid treatment is a legitimate therapeutic goal. Diagnostically we should think in neurologically impaired premature babies of *gastroesophageal reflux* which occurs cumulatively with BPD and can to a considerable degree bring about, maintain and worsen pulmonary inflammations and requires very careful investigation and treatment.

A base medicine suitable for the children concerned is

- **Tartarus stibiatus comp. trit.** Weleda.
  3 × 1 saltsp./d, then 1–2 x/d

administered over several months.

Here Tartarus stibiatus (▸Chap. 2.2.2) in D6 has been processed together with Quarz D12. Potentized rock crystal has the effect here of making the chronic inflammation recede and inhibiting scarring; it promotes the regeneration and restoration of the physiological function and form in the region of the airways. For many premature babies quartz is a central medicine in a very general sense as it also stimulates the warmth organization and counters a general sensory hypersensitivity. In this way it promotes the thriving of these often delicate and sensitive children with their tendency to become too cold (cf. also the homoeopathic medicinal picture of Silicea [Hahnemann 1983, Vol. 5, 240–292; Hirte 2007, 962–965], anthroposophical substance observations on quartz [Husemann and Wolff 1986, Vol. 2, 402–407] and the current account in the Vademecum of Anthroposophic Medicines which provides comprehensive references [Vademecum 2010, 700–707].).

This medicine is supported by the administration of

- **Prunus spinosa e flora. et summit. D3 pillules** Wala
  1–3 pillules 3 x/d.

Prunus spinosa is made from the flowers and shoots of blackthorn. It is indicated if there is a weakness of the life forces and a danger of the organism becoming too physical. That is often precisely the case in relapsing bronchopulmonary inflammation of premature babies. Blackthorn as a bush forms one of the hardest woods of indigenous woody plants (= extreme physicality of a living organism). On the other hand its toughness, its active tendency to propagate and its early, intensive flowers in early April show great vitality. By processing the flowers and shoots and administering them in a stimulating, low potency, precisely this vital pole of the plant is highlighted pharmaceutically. This blackthorn preparation significantly strengthens the life organization particularly in the region of the rhythmical system, of heart and lungs.

This medicine was also given, among others, to the nine-year-old patient described in the case history above (▸Chap. 2.3.1) in whom the weakness of the life forces manifested in the form of chronic mixed asthma, lack of appetite, underweight and short stature following a premature birth in the 28th week of pregnancy. The etherically strengthening action of blackthorn can clarify the function of the lungs in the formation of physical substance: *in the inner vitalization of the nutritional substances catabolized and assimilated in the digestive tract, the build up of own life-supporting substances is crucially dependent on intact lung function.* On the one hand the health of the lungs is to a high degree dependent on adequate nutrition (as shown by the example of cystic fibrosis, the course of which is strongly dependent on a sufficient intake of food, but also by the example of tuberculosis which is associated with hunger and lack of light). On the other hand premature babies with chronic pulmonary disease in particular show that the growth of the organism is limited by lung function. Rudolf Steiner explicitly referred to this connection in a fundamental lecture of 1922 [Steiner 1989, 99–118]. It is helpful for the doctor to keep the following in mind: hunger for food comes in particular measure from the lungs and is often restricted when this organ is diseased. Conversely, adequate nutrition is a basis for the recovery of the lungs – something which also applies to children with bronchopulmonary dysplasia.

Ginger wrap

The ginger wrap is particularly suitable as an external application for children with bronchopulmonary dysplasia in acute febrile bronchitides which mostly show an obstructive component but which can also display a transition to bronchial pneumonia:

- Put two teaspoons of Pulvis Zingiberis in 250 ml of water heated to approx. 70 °C.
- Cover and allow to draw for 5–10 minutes, then immerse cloth for wrap and squeeze out.
- When warm (not too hot, but do not allow to cool either) place on chest and immediately wrap with a molton [molton is a soft cotton hush cloth] and wool cloth/scarf.
- Let the child lie for approx. 20 minutes (small children 10 minutes at the beginning, then increase to 20 minutes) in the wrap.
- It is essential to ensure that the feet are warm before applying the wrap. If necessary, carry out a foot bath, or massage the legs with oil.

The slow but sustained effect of this wrap stimulates the inner heat formation of these often thin and easily hypothermic children and at the same time has a deeply reassuring and anxiety-removing effect which is particularly valuable in formerly premature babies. While mustard as a rough, yellow flowering plant (with sulphur characteristics) accumulates its allyl mustard oil in the seeds and has a directly stimulating effect on the metabolism and blood circulation as a mustard wrap (▸Chap. 5.1.1.4.2), ginger concentrates its essential oils in the rhizome. In this signature the plant reveals a strong relationship to the nervous system which is also expressed in its action on the central nervous system (e.g. central antiemetic effect). The action of the ginger can be understood as relieving the one-sidedly excessive activity of the astral body in the head pole so that it can engage in the digestion and metabolism as a toning and secretolytic effect. That relieves the respiration.

In the last few years, the authors have had impressive positive experiences with this accompanying treatment for children with serious bronchopulmonary dysplasia; both in the clinical phase and in the out-patient continuation of the treatment. Infections (e.g. RSV) and other *complications had considerably worsened the pulmonary situation, leading to a vital risk to the children and which was difficult to manage.*

Here potentized phosphorus turned out to be a crucial medicine – initially administered individually, then in combination with other medicines – best given in infancy as

- **Phosphorus C12 pillules** Gudjons
  3 pillules 1–2 x/d (administered per os in the morning and possibly afternoon).

This treatment can be effectively supplemented through the administration of

- **Echinacea/Argentum pillules** Wala
  3 pillules 1–2 x/d (administered in the afternoon and evening)

The children concerned were seriously physically impaired but psychologically and mentally alert (apart from clinical sedation) and – as soon as the illness allowed – interested; despite their situational disorders (sleep disturbance, states of restlessness, anxiety, eating disorders, etc.) they radiated an intense relationship with their closest reference persons. Phosphorus in medium potentization contributes to the child's organism damping down excessive inflammatory processes and, on the other hand, the soul and spiritual entity of the child better uniting with the body (▸Chap. 5.1.1.4). Potentized phosphorus is the *most important homoeopathic/anthroposophic medicine during and after corticosteroid treatment* (together with Apis mell.) and can be used to continue it in a regulatory and non-suppressive way (▸Chap. 1.2). After early infancy the authors use phosphorus in pulmonary diseases, above all in the form of LM (=Q) potency as LM6.

The combined treatment of phosphorus in a lower to middle potency and Argentum metallicum in a higher potency (D30) has often proved its worth in anthroposophic medicine in infections which have been difficult to treat. For the parenteral (i.v.) application of

- **Argentum met. praep. D30 amp.** Weleda
  0.3–1.0 ml i.v.

for infections with CRP elevation there are positive experiences also in clinical neonatology. "According to experience so far, the alternation of phosphorus and Argentum (e.g. as a phosphorus injection in the morning and Argentum injection in the evening) can be considered to be a kind of "basic therapy" for serious infectious diseases." [Girke 2010, 126]

The authors also had very good experiences in the parenteral application of

- **Argentum D30/Echinacea D6 amp.** Weleda [Vademecum 2010, 112f]

In addition to phosphorus, particularly with *relapsing pneumonia*, the longer term use of following composite medicine

- **Pulmo/Vivianit comp. amp.** Wala
  preventively 0.5 ml/d per os or 1 ml with 1–2 ml NaCl 0.9 % as inhalation
  acutely 3–4 × 0.3–0.5 ml/d per os or possibly 1 x/d 1 ml s.c. or as inhalation

has shown itself to be very effective (▸Chap. 5.1.1.4).

Once the child has reached the age of 4 to 6 months, the longer term administration of

- **Phosphorus LM6** (= Q6) (various manufacturers)
  1–2 gtt. in a little spring water in the morning intensifies the action of Pulmo/Vivianit comp. particularly in the winter when there is little light.

For severe anxiety and restlessness a compress with

- **Lavandula, oleum 10 %**
  on the chest

or gently massaging this oil into the back in a craniocaudal direction has a relaxing and calming effect.

Particular care should be taken with regard to the *prevention of rickets* in these children (▸Chap. 3.2) – for the early stages of rickets frequently appear clinically, in the first instance, in the form of relapsing and unusually serious inflammation of the airways. A check of the (25OH) vitamin D level is helpful.

Nutrition is of material importance, something which was already referred to previously. On the one hand, many premature babies have a clear *vitamin and trace element deficiency* – iron deficiency, which increases the susceptibility for infections, is probably the most familiar but there is frequently also a selenium deficiency, etc. In premature babies with chronic inflammation there should, without fail, be sufficiently comprehensive lab controls and, as necessary, substitution. Furthermore, children with problems of the airways who are fed *cow's milk/derivatives* in the first 18 months of life frequently display an *elevated level of mucous congestion* and a tougher mucous consistency. Here, changing over to a diet without cow's milk is to be recommended, at least on a trial basis – the effect occurs, if it occurs, after a few days. On the other hand these children are particularly dependent on adequate nutrition.

As far as diet is concerned, mare's milk [Bühlbäcker 1996] is, in the experience of the authors, of particular importance for premature babies (and also full-term neonates) with chronic relapsing and above all inflammatory disorders of the airways. The best experience was with high fat content mare's milk. It was introduced into anthroposophical child nutrition by Madeleyn [1997, 270], initially at the Gemeinschaftskrankenhaus Herdecke and currently in the paediatric department led by him at the Filderklinik in Stuttgart. He was able to show that this milk represents a possible alternative for premature babies down to 1,800 g. Mare's milk is offered in Demeter quality (frozen or powdered, e. g. Kurgestüt High Odenwald, tel. 06274–242, D-62429 Waldbrunn, delivers throughout Germany). Due to its great hygienic quality, is does not necessarily have to be pasteurized. As a natural food it is therefore, by a long way, most similar to human breast milk if breast milk is not available or only available in insufficient quantities – which is often the case in premature babies with chronic pulmonary disease. The 2.5 % to 3.5 % addition of germ oil is required for calorific balance, supplemented by starch additive (2.5 % to 4 %, e. g. cornflour), which can also be used for thickening (in gastroesophageal reflux). It is noticeable when feeding with mare's milk that *the tendency to develop infections is reliably reduced in children* together with the benefits of very good gastrointestinal tolerance and low allergenicity in these patient groups (in the experience of the authors this can present a problem only in children with already very pronounced atopic diseases). Historically [cf. Bühlbäcker], mare's milk was considered also in times past to be a medicine for inflammatory respiratory diseases which are difficult to treat. Also in the experience of the authors, it cannot just be described as a food but also as a *medicine for children with chronic relapsing respiratory diseases*. The development of the sense to taste is also supported and not damaged as is the case with conventional hydrolysate formulas which have no proactive immunological effect. Mare's milk has also proved its worth for tube feeding children in intensive care.

2

2.3.2.3 Bowel disorders and metabolic disorders

Premature birth means that the three great barrier organs of the skin, lungs/airways and gastro-intestinal tract are unavoidably overwhelmed and subject to an unphysiological situation (in relationship to their level of maturity). It is often insufficiently considered that *intensive perceptual processes* take place at these barriers which are of far greater importance at this age than later on: thus the taste of the first food, for example, fundamentally shapes the relationship of the child to food, his or her appetite behaviour, etc. When dealing with premature babies it is therefore not just the substance and material aspect (e. g. composition of the food) which is important, but also the aspect *of the shaping sensory experience which is associated with it for the child.* Anyone who, for example, compares the taste of hydrolysate formula with the taste of human breast milk or also fresh animal milk (e.g. mare's milk) will have to admit that the child will grow up in two separate worlds depending on what he or she is fed in this sensitive phase of life.

Developing a taste for different foods per os continues to be a decisive challenge in neonatology: it would be quite possible, as such, to offer enough human breast milk for all newborns if (as was commonly the case in the former East Germany until 1989) "surrogate donation" were permitted and promoted. Breast milk optimizes thriving, contributes significantly to reducing the risk of infection (above all also with regard to the hazardous necrotising enterocolitis) and best supports normal intestinal flora. If breast milk is not available, mare's milk (see above, section 2.3.2.2) is a possible alternative, above all in children with cystic fibrosis (mucoviscidosis), but also for short bowel syndrome and children with intractable diarrhoea [Madeleyn 1997, 270].

For the *medicinal treatment of the intestine and metabolism*, the anthroposophic and homoeopathic approach to therapy offers numerous therapeutic possibilities – in contrast to allopathy (▸Chap. 4). A small selection is listed below which has proved its worth for treating premature babies in the practice of the authors

If the patient is or was exposed to a toxic medicinal burden after birth (e.g. parenteral antibiotic/antimycotic treatment) and if there is a need to stimulate the detoxifying excretory processes of the child,

- **Equisetum cum Sulfure tostum D4 trit.** Weleda
  1 small saltsp. 3–4 × per os

can be administered.

This particularly stimulates elimination via the kidneys (mild diuretic effect without disruption of the electrolyte balance) and is also effective for oedemas e.g. as the result of hypoproteinaemia or various renal disorders.

This medicine is based on a pharmaceutical indication from Rudolf Steiner. The horsetail (Equisetum arvense) – generally known for its stimulating action on the kidneys – is roasted together with 1 % (by weight) of sulphur and then potentized by trituration (in this respect the medicine corresponds approximately to Equisetum D4/Sulphur "D6"). As a result the – clinically replicable – excretion-supporting effect of Equisetum clearly increases; the potentized sulphur also activates detoxifying excretory processes in the liver/gall bladder region. This can indicate the comprehensive effect of Equisetum c. Sulfure tostum in toxic metabolic burdens.

In *hyperexcitability* (the infant often overflexes), irritability, tendency for hiccups, hypersensitivity to all sensory stimuli, tendency to develop rhinitis, tendency for obstipation and development of inguinal and umbilical hernias after the toxic action of medicines and anaesthetics,

- **Nux vomica D6–C30 pillules** (various manufacturers)
  3 pillules (D6) 3 x/d–1 x/d to 2 x/wk (C30)

is a very effective, detoxifying medicine. Nux vomica and Sulphur/Equisetum c. Sulfure tostum are particularly suitable for introducing the treatment.

If it is primarily an *intestinal problem* with changing stools, obstipation or diarrhoea, shifts in the intestinal flora (mycosis, bacterial abnormal colonization), the administration of low potentized fern preparations [Sommer and Soldner 1990, 289–296] has proved successful.

- **Aquilinum comp. amp./pillules** Wala
  0.2–0.3 ml 3 x/d per os/3 × 2–3 pillules

in combination with symbiotic control, e.g. with

- **Colibiogen®** for children: ¼–½–1 tsp./d (▸Chap. 4.6).

If there are painful symptoms with colics, meteorism and possibly stool irregularities – this can facilitate the tendency of premature babies to develop inguinal hernias but can also be reinforced by the latter – the administration of the following has proved its worth

- **Oxalis Rh D4/dil.** Weleda
  in combination with
- **Belladonna Rh D6-4 dil.** Weleda (alcohol-free)
  3 gtt. before each breast feed or before a meal (▸Chap. 4.4.4).

The more delicate and younger the child, the more preferable a higher potency.

2

This medication achieves vitalization, and at the same time a reduction of hypersensitivity in the region of the gastro-intestinal tract.

Toxically-related functional liver damage with medicinally-related icterus, biliary excretion disorder and the corresponding intestinal symptoms can be treated phytotherapeutically with the administration of *greater celandine preparations.*

Greater celandine, Chelidonium majus, displays an interesting signature in its plant form: the rounded lobed green leaves have lactiferous ducts (poppy family) running through them which contain a deep yellow, sharp tasting, alkaloid containing latex. Phytopharmaceutical research has shown that a greater celandine extract has a *choleretic and spasmolytic* effect on the bile ducts and the intestine as a whole. Thus this plant – used since time immemorial for liver/gall bladder disorders [Madaus 1999, Vol. 2, 919–927] – represents one of our most effective and universal medicines for stimulating bile production and elimination, as reflected in research and practice [Daems 1992, Vol. 1, 9–42; Wolff 1990, 121].

Concentrated – often standardized – preparations are not suitable for premature babies; lower potencies are better tolerated, e.g.

- **Chelidonium (e rad.) D2-6 pillules** (various manufacturers)
  2–5 pillules 3 x/d

One preparation specifically aimed at bile production is the aqueous potentized

- **Chelidonium Ferro cultum Rh D3 dil.** Weleda
  3–5 gtt. 2–4 x/d (alcohol-free).

It is complemented by

- **Taraxacum e pl. tota D3 pillules** Wala
  1–3 pillules 2–3 x/d

Sulphur is combined with these herbal medicines as a basic mineral reactivation and detoxification medicine for the metabolism in homoeopathically potentized form:

- **Sulphur D6–30 trit.** Weleda
  1 saltsp. daily or weekly

or, with particular effect on bile flow (also proven in status post choledocal cyst),

- **Natrium sulfuricum D6 pillules/D8 dil.** (various manufacturers)
  3 pillules or gtt. 2 x/d

In all parenchymal changes of the liver, particularly fibrotization processes following total long-term parenteral nutrition in combination with hepatotoxic medicines, the composition of lady's thistle, liver organ preparation and apple mistletoe can be recommend on the basis of many years of experience by the authors:

- **Carduus marianus/Viscum comp. pillules** Wala
  3–5 pillules 1–3 x/d.

2.3.2.4 Consultation with parents

It is important to find out at the beginning what is really going on in the parents psychologically: not just the rational questions they ask but also their feelings, which many do not dare to express immediately. It can be helpful to point out that many mothers of premature babies have feelings of anxiety as well as questions about being at fault etc. The task regarding the child and its situation should be carefully broached only once the psychological situation of the parents has been heard and accepted, as far as possible in correspondence with the questions of the parents themselves. Emphasis should be placed on the extent to which the newborn, and particularly the premature baby, develops on the basis of its *sensory experience* and the importance which accrues to parents and the opportunities they have (▸Chap. 2.3.2.1) even on an intensive care ward. The concrete suggestion that they should touch the child, to cradle and talk quietly to him or her, possibly giving a rub and gently massaging of the back can help the parents to build a bridge to their child and give him or her support. Another important piece of information is that these children are often very uncertain in their instinctual behaviour so that e. g. the sleeping-waking rhythm has really to be learnt by them through the behaviour of the parents. *They not only require more parental empathy but also parental guidance* in the field of rhythm and nutrition. Finally, particularly with premature babies who are disabled or have been seriously ill for a longer period of time, it is necessary to ensure that the child does not cause the relationship between the parents to grind to a halt but that they quite deliberately once a week, for example, set aside some time for themselves. There is, above all, often a risk in this situation that the mother becomes isolated with her ill child which can have serious consequences for both.

2.3.3 Birth defects and growth disorders related to premature birth and birth defects

Diagnostically, underweight at birth can indicate a number of things: not just intrauterine malnutrition but also e. g. genetic disorders or also a familial constitutional moment (family, pregnancy anamnesis). Whatever the case may be, it is important to see underweight children frequently at the beginning in order to observe their development oneself and to intervene diagnostically and therapeutically at an early stage if there is unsatisfactory progress.

Alongside nutritional anamnesis and advice, the following organ preparation has proved its worth in the event of failure to thrive and in s/p intrauterine malnutrition

- **Organum quadruplex amp.** Wala
  0.2–0.3 ml per os in the evening.

The same applies with regard to failure to thrive in hypoproteinaemia as occurs e.g. in serious, generalized atopic dermatitis in infancy or with regard to failure to thrive with serious toxic medicinal burden.

Silver sulphide works in the same way in the field of potentized mineral medicine,

- **Argentit D6 trit.** Weleda [Vademecum 2010, 107]
  1 saltsp. 1 × nocte–3 x/d per os.

In addition, the *whole-body massage with mallow oil* is of particular importance for these children (▸Chap. 2.2.1)

If there is the impression that the infant stops drinking after a short period although still feeling hungry, has a distended stomach and fails to thrive – as if his or her metabolism were rejecting the food or were unable to process it –

- **Lycopodium clavatum C30 pillules** Gudjons
  3 pillules in the afternoon or evening or per day as appropriate for up to 2 weeks

is a constitutionally effective medicine (▸Chap. 4.7.4).

A central medicine for growth and form-giving disorders in anthroposophic medicine is

- **Hypophysis/Stannum pillules** Wala
  3 pillules 1 x (–3 x)/d. for 3–9 months.

It stimulates the activity of the pituitary gland which plays a central role in the regulation of the growth processes. Stannum in medium potency, on the other hand, supports form-giving processes (▸Chap. 2.2.4). In general, we can say that Hypophysis/Stannum strengthens the growth and form-giving impulses coming from the head pole (cf. the physiology of the pituitary gland) while e.g. Organum quadruplex stimulates the metabolism in the large visceral organs.

In principle the pregnancy anamnesis (▸Chap. 2.4) is important for discovering any stressful events or toxic influences. In our experience, failure to thrive in alcohol embryopathy is very resistant to treatment but these children too benefit in the medium term from the medication indicated above.

2.3.4 Prolonged pregnancy

Under normal circumstances, birth is triggered by the child. This is preceded by the conditions surrounding the child in utero becoming scarce not just in terms of space but also with regard to nutrition through the placenta – as is the case physiologically towards the end of the normal gestation period. If the child feels “too content” it becomes overdue.

Thus it makes sense that a short *fast by the mother* in this situation can speed up the triggering of the birth: the nourishing maternal cover is reduced a little and the child's initiative to get born encouraged.

This can be supported medicinally if the mother takes a **stinging nettle preparation** which is strengthened still further in its effect through special iron fertilization of the plant:

- **Urtica Ferro culta D2 dil.** Weleda
  3 × 10–15 gtt.

This medicine has generally proved its value in anthroposophical obstetrics as a help in preparing the birth in the final weeks of pregnancy (supplemented by **Cuprum met. 0.4 % ointment** Weleda or **Kupfer-Salbe rot** Wala 1–2 x/d massaged into the mother's perineum in order to help prevent an episiotomy).

Constitutionally, an overdue baby can indicate a reluctance in the incarnation process, a kind of "laziness" to master life's tasks oneself. It can repeatedly be observed in the course of development of overdue babies that part of the drama of birth is made up later in a critical illness during infancy or as a small child. Here the doctor can ask himself or herself whether a constitutional treatment is appropriated (e. g. the administration of Calcium carbonicum LM6) with the aim of stimulating the child's own activity. Thus the administration of medium-high and LM potencies of Calcium carbonicum (=Conchae) has the effect, among other things, of speeding up dental eruption, reducing excessive head sweating, stimulating intestinal activity and thus generally supporting the infant to mature. In any event, it is advisable to see these children regularly every 4 to 6 weeks in the first six months of life.

2.4 Pregnancy anamnesis

The circumstances of the pregnancy, the birth, the marital situation of the parents at the time, the life situation (rural/urban) etc. together produce a picture of the 'initial conditions' of a person's life which often already indicate with surprising clarity what will later emerge as life themes ... These initial situations indicate the issues. They indicate the meaning of an event before it has even developed.

Matthias Wais

Doctors rarely learn anything of substance when they ask "whether something special occurred during pregnancy". On the other hand it can often be seen in children with chronic problems such as e. g. bronchial asthma (▸Chap. 6.5) that there were often serious disorders in this period or even before (!) which throw their shadow into the present – but which can be handled productively once they are known. Pregnancy anamnesis belongs to the intimate sphere of paediatric anamnesis; we must not act like a bull in a china shop; collecting the information requires an appropriate setting but on the other hand also open and targeted questions.

Case history

Both parents of a four-year-old boy always accompany the child and make a sober impression. The boy enters the consulting room like a clown, a little rascal. If he does not want to do something and starts screaming extremely loudly, the father has to hold him. The mother remains very restrained in her gestures. The boys appears hyperactive, without distance. Large eyes quickly seize up all the interesting objects in the room. The first time he comes he is limping but then immediately whizzes through the room.

The written anamnesis which was requested beforehand reads as follows with regard to the pregnancy: "Vaginal mycosis in 15th week of pregnancy, course of pregnancy normal, pregnancy without complaints, birth 38th week of pregnancy very fast, episiotomy + vaginal tear." On further questioning it emerges that the older brother of the patient was meant to be born by section but came too fast and with considerable injuries to the mother. This already throws a different light on the words of the written anamnesis which does not mention this previous, defining experience of the mother.

The boy is presented because of a rheumatic oligoarthritis (complete case report ▸Chap. 10.9). The diagnosis makes the doctor think that there is more hidden under the smooth surface of the pregnancy anamnesis. After careful further enquiries in the parent consultation, the following emerges: the father's brother's dog bit the first son, the brother of our patient, in the head when the mother was six months pregnant. It happened before her eyes. Since then, contact with her brother-in-law has broken off. The boy's father reports: "My brother is very dominating and it only works if I go along with him like a dog (!)." The father's brother lives near the family. He did not get in touch when the pat. was born.

A year later the father is treated psychotherapeutically for panic attacks. Now we again ask about the life story of the father. The result: "I have been accompanied by anxiety for all of my life. As a child I suffered from nightmares for eight years and was treated with barbiturates during this period (age 1–8). My father was an alcoholic and was himself seriously abused as a child. My mother comes from East Germany and in turn grew up in West Germany separately from her father. She did not get to know her father until 15 years after the fall of the East German regime. It turned out that for years she had lived two kilometres away from her father.

During the consultation it is often helpful to ask the questions in reverse order – backwards from birth, from external factors (job, moves) to the personal and relationship circumstances. Some questions can only be asked in the parent consultation without the child. The following outline is set out systematically for the sake of clarity.

Did pregnancy occur

- spontaneously?
- as an unwanted "accident"?
- "planned", possibly with medical intervention?
- was it preceded by a longer period of contraception?
- "Pill": liver strain, hormonal disorders of the mother?
- were there previous terminations of pregnancy or miscarriage?

- was conception and the period when the pregnancy was determined experienced as trauma, happiness or with ambivalence?
- what is the attitude of the father, the mother to the pregnancy?
- was the relationship shaken, dissolved or strengthened?

The basis for a successful pregnancy is the *interaction of the child's and mother's organism.* This interaction assumes openness towards one another and a certain equilibrium. It is very strongly co-determined by the *soul and bodily interaction in the maternal organism* – and this in turn is influenced by the mother's present and past psychological experiences.

That is also what underlies the above questions: was procreation experienced by the mother as "conception" – meaning that she experiences herself in a certain equilibrium with the father on the one hand and the child on the other and is open for both – or does she have ambivalent or hostile feelings (e. g. because the father does not want the pregnancy or because she is mentally focused on another e. g. professional goal)? Or is she anxious – e. g. with in vitro fertilization – about a failure of the pregnancy or complications? Does she feel guilty about a previous termination of pregnancy? Is there an exaggerated wish for a child whereas previously a pregnancy was rejected for a long time? In any case, the equilibrium which is required by the child's interaction with the mother may in many ways be placed at risk and consequently these problems do not end with birth.

Without wishing to impose a particular perspective on the reader, the authors hold the view that in the act of procreation a body is created by the parents in which an independent soul and spiritual individuality gradually incarnates. Depending on the responses to the questions above, this individuality encounters different conditions for incarnation: the maternal physical and soul sheathes are ready to receive it to different degrees.

Unwanted children often have to fight for their incarnation; there is a greater accumulation of premature and small-for-date births among them; they mostly require enhanced help from us. Inwardly we can sometimes observe a strong dynamic on the part of these children of wanting to go beyond the parents and distance themselves from inherited traits – on the other hand they may make great demands on their parents after birth, for example through recurring illnesses.

Wanted children have it "easier" by comparison, they mostly grow up more harmoniously. That means we have to be all the more alert when they do fall ill – after all, it was so easy before! The ability to overcome an acute illness, which coincides with the ability to break down the body inherited from the parents, to a certain extent in fever, for example, and – starting with this "model" – to build it up again in a new individualized form, can still be underdeveloped in these children to begin with. Particularly after weaning, when the borrowed immunity from the breast milk gradually begins to recede, these children can undergo a dramatic acute illness. This can be understood as a challenge to now also start developing the combative side physically and psychologically, as, for example, can come to expression in fever and associated metabolic activities.

We find today that the mother/parents can indeed have a positive attitude to the pregnancy but that in the subsequent period – subjectively quite unconsciously in part – the mother does not adjust physically and psychologically to the pregnancy but is constantly distracted from the child in her activity and experience, e. g. as part of a stressful occupation. Not infrequently, only the occurrence of complications leads to a change of direction, e. g. premature bleeding, early contractions, which force the mother to sign off work and take more rest.

Calmness, trust, attentive behaviour which includes the attentive perception of the unborn child, care for one's own body and own needs and those of the partner, support the development of the child in a particularly sustained way. Epigenetic (▸Chap. 1.1) and immunological research (▸Chap. 6.1 to ▸Chap. 6.3) confirms the far-reaching influence of the pregnancy on the developing body of the child – quite apart from the well-known harmful effects of alcohol and nicotine. Stress and anxiety during pregnancy have a negative effect – at all levels, be it the regulation of the genetic material, the future ability for self-regulation, placental perfusion, the psychological ties with the child or the risk of early contractions. From a paediatric perspective it is important to align the medical checkups for the pregnant woman with these objectives in order to stabilize the parent-child relationship and support the attentive behaviour of the mother. Unfortunately the practice in such checkups is not evaluated at all in this respect and there is frequently no communication between the gynaecologists and the paediatricians. The authors were able to observe that establishing regular cooperation between paediatricians and gynaecologists can have a positive effect – many gynaecologists have never asked themselves whether, for example, behavioural problems in the infant might be dependent on the type and nature of care during pregnancy (and how that might be prevented).

If the medical checkup during pregnancy is aimed primarily at the early discovery of deficits and anomalies in the unborn child, without pursuing as an equal goal the stabilization of the relationship between the mother (and father!) and the child, the checkup itself can turn into a source of anxiety and stress in pregnancy. The ever earlier and more perfect ultrasound diagnosis, for example, which is carried out in Germany in particularly great numbers, can not infrequently put the mother and father in an unintended situation which initially puts great psychological stress on them and triggers shock experiences.

Case history

A 26-year-old student phones the paediatric practice. She fell ill with leukaemia (ALL) when she was ten years old. Now she is twelve weeks pregnant. She has just returned from a gynaecological checkup. Blood analysis and ultrasound, she was told, show a statistical risk of 1:168 that her unborn child could develop Down's syndrome. Without any further discussion she was advised to undergo further diagnosis. But the risk of a miscarriage caused by amniocentesis or a chorionic villus biopsy lies at 0.5–1 % and thus within the same probability range as the trisomy risk.

In order to contain the situation and get it under control, a longer conversation with the mother and father is held in the practice that same day. Only now do the parents become fully aware of the risk entailed by the proposed diagnostic investigation in relation to the assumed risk, only now do they have the opportunity to make a considered judgement, only now can they jointly reflect on their own attitude to a possible disability in their child and come to a decision.

Such occurrences have become increasingly common in our own practice in the last ten years. No matter whether this wish for perfection, for the earliest possible certainty, for the exclusion of all risk comes from the frequently inexperienced parents or from the doctor, the consequences of anxiety and stress fall back on the unborn child. The great benefit provided by ultrasound in the planning of the birth, in identifying a disparity between the child's head and the mother's pelvis, etc. is globally overshadowed by forms of medical care and diagnosis in pregnancy which are not primarily guided by the life of the child but by the ideas of others: be it the desire to have a child of a particular gender among Chinese or Indian parents, be it the wish for the perfect child which is so common in Germany. Whatever the decision and behaviour of the parents and doctor, the important thing is to take decisions regarding preventive diagnostic investigations with an awareness of the possible consequences and to balance them with a consideration of the possibility of non-intervention. For every diagnostic investigation *is already a breach of the envelope* which surrounds the human foetus, every diagnostic measure can have far-reaching consequences for the mother-(father-)child relationship. That is why it is so important that everyone involved should resist the systemic pressures and take the time for dialogue.

In the paediatric practice and clinic, a detailed enquiry about events which have placed a burden on and unsettled the mother-child relationship during pregnancy is very important:

- *Relationship conflicts, difficult relationship with parents,* excessive demands from the already existing family have a particularly strong effect on the unborn child.
- *Occupational stress* (above all in first-time pregnancies), e. g. long time spent working at a screen, frequent driving, high levels of responsibility and time pressures draw the mother's strength outwards and facilitate placental undernourishment and (postnatal) childhood restlessness. What women (and men) consider to be normal today is very remote, particularly in this respect, from what would be appropriate. The same applies to the – so frequent – change of house during pregnancy.
- Another important question is the one relating to *stimulants* such as nicotine and coffee which in turn indicate that the mother is in part physically and psychologically distracted from the child; they negatively affect the child's nervous system (and respiratory system) and can, for example, lead to sustained post partum sleep disturbance. In such cases this information helps in giving targeted homoeopathic treatments to the child (▸Chap. 7.1).
- *Early contractions and preeclampsia* have, in the final instance, as their unconscious goal the rejection and premature birth of the child. They can be triggered by an infection in the child, for example, as a means for saving both mother and child; miscarriages are frequently caused by a child's deformities. They can also be an expression of a weakness in the mother's life forces or physical constitution and which are insufficient to carry the pregnancy to term. Finally, they can also be a manifestation of an unconscious antipathy or ambivalence towards the pregnancy. Here there is a risk that this is not identified and continues to work as a pathological factor in the family for a long time after the birth.

Two polar opposite medicines are used preferentially for complications in the second half of pregnancy, as mentioned above: beta-sympathomimetics (e. g. Partusisten®) and magnesium sulphate. The former elevate the stress levels of the organism such that a specific "stress profile" is enforced: bronchial dilatation, tachycardia, immobilization of the smooth muscles in favour of the maximum active readiness of the cross-striated muscles. The heart has to cope with this contrast and enable it: the most dangerous side-effect of this medicine is acute cardiac failure through a collapse of the rhythmical order of the heartbeat. Beta-sympathomimetics thus produce a slackening of the uterine muscles; but at the same time both the mother's and child's organism is placed in a state of stress which had as its original purpose to ward off an external threat. A tachycardia can be observed in the mother and child as a stress symptom which is also used as a measure for determining the dose of the medicine (and as a dosage limit). Beta-sympathomimetics essentially correspond to substances which the animal (and human) organism produces for stress regulation (e. g. adrenalin).

In contrast, magnesium plays a central role in the plant metabolism. The effect of magnesium sulphate aims to make the organism more "vegetable-like", to paralyse the agitation of the soul entity in the body: accordingly, magnesium intoxication leads to a hypothermal sleep state; the substance is fundamentally very much less toxic than beta-sympathomimetics.

Newborns whose mothers were given a lot of magnesium before birth can stand out due to subnormal temperature, muscle hypotonia and drowsiness. There has been some discussion [Mittendorf et al. 1997, 1517] as to whether the administration of magnesium sulphate post partum is associated with elevated mortality (through SIDS). On the other hand, after tocolysis resulting from beta-sympathomimetics children often stand out after birth due to restlessness and, in the observation of the authors, show a greater tendency for bronchial asthma. This can be due to the kind of situations which trigger premature contractions – e. g. shock experiences of the mother – having a harmful effect on the child's growing organism e. g. in the respiratory tract [Steiner 1989, 204]; but perhaps tocolysis also underlies the observed phenomenon as a direct effect. It is, in any event, remarkable that an illness now occurs in the child which medicine once again treats (suppressively) with beta-sympathomimetics.

Therapeutically, a thorough and empathetic discussion with the mother or parents is in itself often already a significant help: guilt feelings and anxieties can be dismantled, and the perception of all those involved can also be sensitized, for example with regard to another pregnancy. What is achieved in this situation is obviously very dependent on the attending doctor.

Medicinally, potentized copper,

- **Cuprum met. praep. D6–20 trit.** Weleda
  1 saltsp./d in the evening

is the most important medicine (▸Chap. 2.2.4) for abnormal pregnancy anamnesis.

It is indicated when the interaction between the mother's and child's organism was impaired such as to cause *placental vasospasms, premature contractions,* perhaps also *extreme nausea* and *weight loss* in the early stages of pregnancy. If there is a diagnostic indication that such disorders represent a significant trigger of the child's pathology needing treatment, and, above all, if there is an apparent resistance to treatment of this pathology, Cuprum can be administered, preferably in the evening. The further the pregnancy lies in the past and the more intense the psychosomatic problem is in the child itself, often characterized by an ambivalent relationship with the mother, the higher is the potency chosen. The treatment duration is 3 to 6 weeks.

A therapeutic problem is represented today not only by the increase in premature births, but also the *increase in diagnostic interventions during pregnancy which, as* mentioned above, are often willing to tolerate the possibility of a miscarriage which may be triggered as a result. They also often imply the question as to whether the pregnancy should be carried to term at all. Thus an *amniocentesis,* for example, involves not just an injury to the child's sheathing but also a profound ambivalence towards the pregnancy. It is naive to assume that there will be no consequences.

Therapeutically

- **Amnion Gl D8–12–30 amp.** Wala
  0.3–0.5 ml/d nocte per os

can be of help (▸Chap. 2.3.2.1), e. g. in increased states of restlessness and sleep disturbance after birth. There are also positive experiences in administering 1 amp. Amnion D8 to the mother s.c. after amniocentesis [Vademecum 2010, 66].

Shock experiences in pregnancy, particularly if they have led to complications or even premature birth, can be treated with Aconitum, Opium, Argentum/Rohrzucker, Oxalis ointment (▸Chap. 2.2.3).

Toxic burdens can also be of importance: *Exposure to amalgam,* but also its removal, can be of pathogenic importance in infant eczema and states of restlessness, for example; here the administration of

- **Hepar sulfuris D6 trit.** Weleda
  1 saltsp./d

may have a cleansing effect as well as the administration of

- **Silberamalgam D30 pillules** Staufen
  5 pillules 1 × wkly.

Finally,

- **Natrium muriaticum LM/Q6** (various manufacturers)

should be mentioned as an important and extensive medicine. It represents the most important medicine, especially for girls, if due to exposure during pregnancy and in the neonatal period *there was depressive inhibited development of the child.* It is noteworthy that a fondness for a salty taste (keynote for Natrium muriaticum) correlates with low birth weight! [Stein et al. 2005]

Case history

A former premature baby of the 27th week of pregnancy is presented in practice at the age of 2½ years because of lack of appetite, obstipation, short stature and chronic-obstructive bronchitis. Delayed walking at 18 months (corrected age). The mother is a secretary, French; the father is her former boss who, although he visits the mother and child several times a month, has his own family and hides his paternity. The mother wanted the pregnancy and does not verbally blame the father, but a sad expression is apparent in the mother and child; furthermore, the mother does not find it easy in the current situation to find her bearings in a German city. In reality she continues to find it very painful that the father does not acknowledge her and his child. As a result, Natrium muriaticum LM6, 5 gtt./d in the morning is prescribed: the first thing to happen is that the girl's mood lightens significantly, her appetite increases and, above all, the bronchopulmonary symptoms which had previously been resistant to treatment for more than nine months heal completely and permanently within 3 weeks (follow-up observation period:

two years). The obstipation (no bowel movement for up to 7 days!) normalizes. In the follow-up at the age of 18 – the child did not come to the practice in the interim period – a 152 cm tall girl in stable health (the mother is also small in height) presents who in the meantime lives with her mother back in France where she successfully graduated from secondary school, having jumped a class as a result of her school performance. Her behaviour is reserved and inhibited, the relationships with people of her own age not as deep as the girl would like.

Natrium muriaticum, potentized table salt, is indicated above all in situations where a severe psychological experience cannot be overcome through grieving and causes emotional responsiveness to permanently freeze. We might think of Lot's wife who looked back and turned into a pillar of salt: by looking back she cannot let go and this prevents her from going into the future at the right time [Coulter 1989, 433].

References for Chapter 2

(every reference marked with a ■ Bullet point indicates the English translation of the reference above it)

Aschoff, J.: In: Physiologie des Menschen, Bd. 2, 43–113. Gauer, Kramer, Jung (Hrsg.). München 1971.

Beiblätter der Zeitschrift Natura 1926–1936. Natura Verlag Dornach, 2000.

Beinder, E.: Fetalzeit und spätere Gesundheit. Dtsch Ärztebl **104**, A 644–650 (2007).

Bühlbäcker, A.: Zur Verwendbarkeit von Stutenmilch, Kumyss und Eselsmilch als Diätetika und Heilmittel unter besonderer Berücksichtigung der Bedürfnisse des Säuglings und des Frühgeborenen. Deutsche Hochschulschriften 1104. Verlag Hänsel-Hohenhausen 1996.

Buhr, E., Seung-Hee, Y., Takahashi, J.: Temperature as a Universal Resetting Cue for Mammalian Circadian Oscilllators. Science, **330**, 379–385 (2010).

Burnett, J. C.: Zarte, zurückgebliebene, schwächliche und im Wachstum behinderte Kinder. Müller & Steinicke, München 1993.

Christ, B.: Entwicklung der cervico-occipitalen Übergangsregion. In: Humanembryologie, 831–834. Hinrichsen, K. V. (Hrsg.). Springer, Berlin, New York 1990.

Coulter, C.: Porträts homöopathischer Arzneimittel, Bd. 1, 2. Aufl. Haug Verlag, Heidelberg 1989.

Daems, W. F.: Chelidonium/Curcuma comp. – Eine Heilmittelstudie. Persephone Bd. 1, 9–42, Dornach 1992.

■ Daems, W. F.: Chelidonium Curcuma Comp. A Medicament Study. Persephone 1, Mercury Press, Spring Valley, N. Y. 1998.

Deeg et al.: Ist der plötzliche Kindstod Folge einer lageabhängigen Minderperfusion des Hirnstammes? Schr. f. Kinderheilk. **6**, 597–602 (1998).

Elder, T: The importance of relative standards in ADHD diagnoses: Evidence based on exact birth dates. J.of Health Economics **29**, 641–656 (2010).

Erler, T., A. Grunske: Scheinbar lebensbedrohliche Ereignisse im Säuglingsalter. Mschr. Kinderheilk. **151**, 520–526 (2003).

Hahnemann, S.: Chronische Krankheiten, Bd. 5. Hüthig-Medizinverlage, Heidelberg 1999.

Hahnemann, S.: Chronische Krankheiten, Bd. 5, 240–292. Organon-Verlag, Starnberg 1983.

Hirte, M.: Materia medica. In: Homöopathie in der Kinder- und Jugendmedizin. 2.Aufl. Urban & Fischer, München 2007.

Husemann, F., O. Wolff: Das Bild des Menschen als Grundlage der Heilkunst, Bd. 1, 10. Aufl. Verlag Freies Geistesleben, Stuttgart 1991; Bd. 2, 4. Aufl., 1986.

- Huseman, F. Wolff, O.: The Anthroposophical approach to medicine: v. 1, 2. Steiner Books, Great Barrington, M. A. 1983, v.3 Mercury Press, Spring Valley, N. Y. 2003.

Husemann,F.: Anthroposophische Medizin. Verlag am Goetheanum, Dornach, 2009, 245–254Verlag Freies Geistesleben, Stuttgart 1996.

Madaus: Lehrbuch der biologischen Heilmittel, Bd. 1, Bd. 2, Bd. 3. Olms Verlag, Hildesheim 1999.

Madeleyn, R.: Anthroposophische Kinderheilkunde. Der Merkurstab **5**, 270 (1997).

Marcovich, M., de Jong,M.: Frühgeborene – zu klein zum Leben? Kösel, München 2008.

Martinius, J.: Süddeutsche Zeitung **246**, 6 (1997).

Merkurstab **63**, 6, Sonderheft Helleborus niger (2010).

Mittendorf et al.: Is tocolytic magnesium sulphate associated with increased total paediatric mortality? Lancet **350**, 1517 (1997).

Poets, C. F.: Der plötzliche Kindstod. In: Pädiatrie. Lentze, Schaub, Schulte, Spranger (Hrsg.). 2. Aufl. Springer.

Jotzo, M., C. F. Poets: Wenn Leben mit Leid beginnt. Mschr. Kinderheilk. **154**, 630–638 (2006).

Kaufmann, P.: Placentation und Placenta. In: Hinrichsen,V. (Hrsg.): Humanembryologie. Berlin, Springer, 1990.

Keller, W., A. Wiskott: Lehrbuch der Kinderheilkunde, 6. Aufl. Thieme Verlag, Stuttgart 1991.

Kinney, H., Bradley,T.: The Sudden Infant Death Syndrome. N Engl J Med **361**, 795–805 (2009).

Lutzker, P.: Der Sprachsinn., Berlin – New York 2003.

Petri, H.: Das Drama der Vaterentbehrung. Reinhardt Verlag, München 2009.

Rohen, J. W.: Morphologie des menschlichen Organismus. Verlag Freies Geistesleben, Stuttgart 2000.

- Rohen, J. W.: Functional morphology: The dymanic wholeness of the human organism. Adonis Press, Hillsdale, N. Y. 2007.

Saigal, S. et al.: School-age outcomes in children who were extremely low birth weight from four international population-based cohorts. Pediatrics **112**, 943–950 (2003).

Schad, W.: Das Amnionschaukeln bei den Sauropsiden. Der Merkurstab **53**, 297–304 (2000).

Schad, W.: Die verlorene Hälfte des Menschen. Verlag Freies Geistesleben, Stuttgart 2008.

Schechtman VL. et al., Sleep state organization in normal infants and victims of the sudden infant death syndrome. Pediatrics **89**, 865–870 (1992).

Schneider, C.: Bryophyllum Argento cultum bei kindlicher Hysterie. Der Merkurstab **54**, 327–330 (2001).

Schramm, H.: Heilmittel der anthroposophischen Medizin. Urban & Fischer, München 2009.

Simon, L.: Schmerztherapie mit homöopathischen Heilmitteln. Haug Verlag, Heidelberg 1987.

Soesman, A.: Die zwölf Sinne. Verlag Freies Geistesleben, Stuttgart 1995.

- Soesman, A.: The twelve senses. Hawthorn Press, Stroud, U. K.1990.

Sommer, M., G. Soldner: Die Farne. Der Merkurstab **43**, 289–296 (1990).

Stein, L. J., B. J. Cowarth, G. K. Beaucamp: Salty taste acceptance by infants and young children is related to birth weight. Longitudinal analysis of infants within the normal birth weight range. Eur. Journal of Clinical Nutrition, 1–8 (2005).

Steiner, R.: Meditative Betrachtungen und Anleitungen zur Vertiefung der Heilkunst. Gesamtausgabe Bd. 316, 2. Aufl. Rudolf Steiner Verlag, Dornach 1980.

- Steiner, R.: Course for young doctors: meditative contemplations and instructions for deepening the art of healing: lectures for physicians and medical students. GA (complete works) 316. Mercury Press, Spring Valley, N. Y. 1994.

Steiner, R.: Von Seelenrätseln. 5. Aufl. R.Steiner Verlag, Dornach 1983.

- Steiner, R.: Riddles of the soul. GA (complete works) 21. Mercury Press, Spring Valley, N. Y. 1996.

Steiner, R.: Physiologisch-Therapeutisches auf Grundlage der Geisteswissenschaften. Gesamtausgabe Bd. 314, 3. Aufl. Rudolf Steiner Verlag, Dornach 1989.

- Steiner, R.: Physiology and therapeutics: four lectures, Dornach, October 7–9, 1920. GA (complete works) 314. Mercury Press, Spring Valley, N. Y. 1986.

Steiner, R., I. Wegman: Grundlegendes zu einer Erweiterung der Heilkunst nach geisteswissenschaftlichen Erkenntnissen. Rudolf Steiner Verlag, Dornach 1991.

- Steiner, R., Wegman, I.: Fundamentals of therapy: an extension of the art of healing through spiritual-scientific knowledge. GA (complete works) 27. Mercury Press, Spring Valley, N. Y. 1999. Also available as: Extending practical medicine: fundamental principles based on the science of the spirit. Rudolf Steiner Press, London 1996.

Steiner, R.: Heilpädagogischer Kurs. Gesamtausgabe Bd. 317, 8. Aufl. Rudolf Steiner Verlag, Dornach 1995.

- Steiner, R.: Education for special needs: the curative education course; twelve lectures for doctors and teachers given at Dornach between 25 June and 7 July 1924. GA (complete works) 317. Rudolf Steiner Press, London 1998.

Stübler, M., E. Krug (Hrsg.): Leesers Lehrbuch der Homöopathie, 3. Aufl. Haug Verlag, Heidelberg 1987.

Swoboda, F. (Hrsg.): Documenta Homöopathica Bd.25, Maudrich Verlag, Wien 2005.

Thomas, W., C. P. Speer: Bronchopulmonale Dysplasie Frühgeborener. Mschr. Kinderheilk. **153**, 211–219 (2005).

Ulrich, B.: Menschenkundliche Überlegungen zur Behandlung von Frühgeborenen. Der Merkurstab **55**, Sonderheft Pädiatrie, 68–71 (2002).

Upledger, J. E., J. D. Vredevoogd: Lehrbuch der CranioSacralen Therapie, 4. Aufl., 304–309. Haug Verlag, Heidelberg 2000.

Upledger, J.: Auf den inneren Arzt hören, 4. Aufl. Heyne, München 2002.

Uvnäs-Moberg, K.: The Role of Oxytocin in the Development of Attachment and Maternal Adaptions during the postpartum Period. Vortragsabstract. Internationales Symposium am 2./3.12.2005 in München anlässlich der Verleihung des Arnold-Lucius-Gesell-Preises 2005 an Prof. J. Kennell, Prof. M. Klaus und P. Klaus.

Vademecum Anthroposophische Arzneimittel. 2.Aufl. Der Merkurstab **63**, Supplement (2010).

- Vademecum of anthroposophic medicines, CD format. Medical Section of the School of Spiritual Science, Dornach, Switzerland 2009

Vogel H.-H.: Wege der Heilmittelfindung, Bd. 1. Natur Mensch Medizin Verlag, 1994.

- Vogel, H.-H.: Finding remedies: spiritual knowledge of man and naure; a contribution toward understanding anthroposophic remedies, based on the example of the Wala remedy compositions. V 1, 2 Natur-Mensch-Medizin, Bad Boll 1994.

Wilkens, J.: Nicotiana tabacum in homöopathischer Potenzierung in seinen praktischen Möglichkeiten. Der Merkurstab **55**, 393–403 (2002).

Wolff, O.: Choleodoron. Weleda. Korr.bl. f. Ärzte 128, 121 (1990).

Wollmann, H. A.: Zu klein bei Geburt (SGA). Mschr. Kinderheilk. **152**, 528–535 (2004).

3 Disease prevention

"Meaning cannot be given but must be found."

V. Frankl [1992, 22]

"That it is worth investing energy in, committing oneself to and championing at least some of the problems and demands of life, that they are a welcome challenge rather than a burden one would like to be rid of."

A. Antonovsky [1997, 36]

With these words A. Antonovsky describes the feeling of meaningfulness and significance which, associated with the feeling of comprehensibility and manageability of the world, gives rise to the "sense of coherence" in a person. What are the factors which determine whether or not a person develops healthily in the course of his or her life? We are familiar with the possibly disease-causing and pathogenic relevance of social and hygienic conditions, the infectious and genetic causes of disease and similar things. But that is countered by the observation that the healthy development of the individual is not dependent solely on his or her circumstances but on the inner ability to maintain one's own health. This has a physical, mental and individually spiritual dimension.

Authors such as Frankl or Antonovsky recognized in people who had remained healthy or returned to health despite extremely adverse circumstances that the ability to give "*meaning* to life" (Frankl) was of crucial importance. The sense of coherence, the trust in one's ability to understand and manage the world – that there is possibly a meaningful context in life, destiny and the development of one's own biography – can play a stronger role than the sum of disease-causing influences: the forces of *salutogenesis* cannot be understood on the basis of purely pathogenically-oriented thinking and action.

The ability to maintain human health is clearly linked with the spiritual individuality, the I of a person. The challenge [Antonovsky 1997, 36] of giving meaning to life, of recognising and oneself creating meaningful connections, is not a feature of any other living being in nature but a specifically human one [Frankl 1992a, 56ff.]. The full capacity to meet that challenge is not developed until adulthood. But the abilities in that respect are formed to a crucial degree in childhood and each individuality brings its own prerequisites.

A positive development is promoted in childhood on the one hand through the affection towards and trust in the child, through a positive attitude that there is meaning in things, and on the other hand through the availability of resistance which the child can learn to manage. The absence of such resistance and challenges can lastingly weaken the development of the health-preserving, inner coherence of the individuality [Bundeszentrale für gesundheitliche Aufklärung, *Was erhält den Mensch gesund?* 1998, 31]

The development of the child takes place in the context of the development of the body, the physical, vital and psychological context of life, contexts which are clearly differentiated in anthroposophic medicine [Steiner and Wegman 1977, 7–19]. At all these levels the child can learn to overcome resistance and thereby acquire necessary, individual abilities. This process becomes particularly clear in the act of adopting an upright posture, in the active overcoming of gravity, the achievement of walking upright, which is acquired through the body-related activity of the human I [Steiner and Wegman 1991, 29]. In this context it also becomes noticeable that each child takes this step *at a different time*; a quality lies therein which characterizes his or her individuality as much as do his or her physical traits. In moments of crisis, in acute fever for example, the activity of the individuality as it affects the body, which finds its direct expression in the human warmth organization, can rise far above the normal measure; and this correspondingly intensifies not just the elimination of pathogens but also transforms the physical body inherited from the parents, gives it new characteristics and wrests new abilities from it. It happens not infrequently that this own activity – including the crisis of puberty – is perceived by adults as itself being the problem which needs to be resolved, as being meaningless and superfluous. Parents and doctors are much too little aware of this dimension of fever, for example. The same applies to the fact that only humans go through the crisis of puberty and that this is meaningful and necessary for real, inner independence to be achieved from the parents. In contrast, animals reenact the life of their parents once they reach sexual maturity. The singular importance and length of human childhood [Kipp 1980] only becomes comprehensible when the reciprocal penetration of the soul and spiritual aspect with the physical body is understood. *The "sense of coherence", which Antonovsky refers to in connection with salutogenesis and which decisively develops in childhood and adolescence, does not correspond to a purely intellectual but to a soul and physical reality. The child actively individualizes himself or herself to the extent that he or she succeeds in making his or her body into an expression of his or her individuality down as far as the immunological events, as the shape of hands and face.* The body inherited from the parents offers the possibility for this and at the same time represents an obstacle, as does the family at a psychological level. Human development is not based on conserving what has been inherited; on the contrary, the child must be given sufficient opportunity to transform and newly shape the inherited prerequisites of his or her existence. This process of detachment and reorganization cannot succeed without moments of crisis; illness and crisis are necessary companions of human individualization.

The human immune system illustrates *the connection between individuation and health in a specific way. This is a learning* system which increasinly moves beyond what is genetically inherited in its development. The organism actively intervenes in the genetic material with the development of the T- and B-lymphocytes ["Rearrangement", Wahn et al. 2005, 52], thus developing the necessary diversity of antibodies and lymphocyte surfaces on the one hand and their coherence in the form of the immunological individuality and identity of the organism on the other [Hinrichsen 1990, 351f]. The quality of the "I-organization" is clearly expressed in this process. The immune system represents a context of physical coherence which includes and penetrates all the organs. Differentiating what belongs to the "self" and what is foreign represents a central quality and competence of the healthy human immune system. At the same time it illustrates that this individualization process is only possible on the basis of radical catabolic processes – not just (as in the digestive system, which is also the main field of activity of the immune system) with regard to external nature but also with regard to the substance inherited from the parents. Epigenetics has researched this aspect increasingly extensively in recent years and shown the extent to which the child's organism reshapes the "inherited body" during pregnancy and early childhood and also how much the later capacity of human beings to self-regulate the organism – and thus their health – is dependent on these early learning processes. The question about disease prevention must primarily focus on this dimension of human development and paediatrics has to ask itself: is the number of children who possess good self-regulatory ability (psychological and physical) at school age increasing or decreasing – and how is this connected with the practised form of disease prevention and treatment?

We find equilibria of opposing processes at all levels of the human immune system. The *immune regulation* as "orchestrator" of these processes is therefore of overriding importance with regard to the issue of health and illness; it represents an independent, active process of the individual. *The pathology of many children in countries with a western lifestyle is today characterized by increasing disorders in the development of immune regulation: Chronic inflammatory, allergic diseases and autoimmune diseases such as childhood diabetes mellitus arise from a disorder of individuation at a physical level, an insecure, labile identity, in which the secure differentiation between "self" and "foreign" is not managed.* Foreign substance from the environment, e. g. certain proteins, can penetrate the barriers of the organism, appear inside the organism in the "wrong place" and cause irritations; at the same time the organism starts to attack and dissolve its own structures immunologically, e. g. its own barriers or also vitally necessary inner organs such as the islet cells of the pancreas.

Human beings are hardwired to individualize immunologically to the same extent as they do, for example, in their thinking. This process, like learning to think, requires a chronological order, requires *the right challenge at the right time.* Acute inflammatory diseases in infancy, undergoing and actively overcoming intestinal parasitosis (e. g. worms) can promote immunological learning; the absence of such challenges favours e. g. allergy development or chronic-inflammatory bowel diseases. When acute inflammatory diseases occur, the immune system is adequately activated: nonspecific and specific immune system, cellular and humoural response, become equally active and that is clearly how the organism can best learn to regulate the event. Protective immunization in infancy for example only activates the humoural immune response whereas the cellular one is not "trained" correspondingly and thus has a one-sided effect on the specific immune system although the proper order of the learning process would require the prior activation of the nonspecific immune system.

Individual development is characterized by each person requiring different challenges to develop their individuality; and medical experience teaches us that children can fall ill both epidemically, on the one hand, and quite individually, each in his or her own time, on the other. The same applies to crises of psychological maturation. – *Collective disease prevention* is linked with a tendency to blank out the perception of the child's individuality and to lose the respect for its development and chronological laws.

Vaccination e. g. against mumps at twelve months, combined with manipulated measles, rubella and chickenpox viruses and preservatives, provokes a different learning process from actively undergoing mumps which in the observation of the authors, for example, has a positively detaching effect in a pre-existing excessively close mother-child relationship (▸Chap. 5). Studies have shown that for example *undergoing mumps in childhood in contrast to having the mumps vaccination reduces the risk in girls of developing an ovarian carcinoma in later life by approx. 20 %.* This link has been known since one of the first case-control studies on ovarian carcinoma [West 1966] and has been confirmed in six further studies [incl. Newhouse et al. 1977]. In 2010 researchers established why undergoing mumps, but not the mumps vaccination, can protect against ovarian carcinoma [Cramer et al. 2010]. In children mumps is usually experienced as a mild disease [Speer and Gahr 2009, 372], there is no danger to life and extremely rare risks such as labyrinthine hearing loss in no way offset the risk of an ovarian carcinoma. It is indeed difficult to justify the mumps vaccination in childhood. It has shifted the typical age of onset of disease today into the group of 16–24-year-olds in which 30 % of the affected men develop orchitis which does not exist in childhood. Ovarian carcinomas are a relatively frequent malignancy; in Germany alone more than 8000 women fall ill with the disease per year and their prognosis is bad: two thirds of those affected die within five years. Omission of the mumps vaccination could save up to 20 % of these patients from developing an ovarian carcinoma, yet this information is not included on websites and in the standard medical works.

The fear of another malignant neoplasm, the malignant melanoma is something of which in contrast all parents and already many children are aware. Mortality from malignant melanomas among women in Germany is approx. 20 % of mortality from ovarian carcinomas.[1] But this means that the possible protection if all women underwent mumps as children could arithmetically prevent almost as many fatal ovarian carcinomas as fatal melanomas occur in total in women each year. All the media carry reports that children should no longer be allowed to play outside without sunscreen as sunburn drastically increases the risk of later malignant melanoma. That sunscreen with sun protection factor 10 reduces the production of vitamin D in small children through sunlight by 95 % (in SPF 15 this is 99 %) is never mentioned. It is, incidentally, precisely the ovarian carcinoma, for which the lack of sunlight and vitamin D probably represents a considerable further risk factor: "Women between the ages of 45 and 54 die five times more frequently in the north of the USA of ovarian cancer than women in the southern states" [Small 2007, 152]. But also for the malignant melanoma itself Tremezaytues and Reichrath note in *Der Hautarzt*: "More recent data in the literature indicate a less favourable clinical course of the melanoma disease if there are low 25(OH) vitamin D serum levels. ... Epidemiological studies show that with increasing distance of the dwelling place from the equator the risk rises of dying from various malignant tumours (incl. mammary, ovarian, colonic and prostate carcinoma)." [Tremezaygues and Reichrath 2010, 484]. Whereas sunlight is currently described by dermatologists as the "complete carcinogen" [Krutmann 2001], it must be emphasized from the aspect of disease prevention that *sunlight (which can really be absorbed) and the vitamin D synthesis dependent on it are of irreplaceable importance for humans and particularly for children, e. g. for an intact resistance against infections and very probably as a protective factor against many different carcinomas. This is confirmed by a review in the German Ärzteblatt* [Zeeb and Greinert 2010] on "The importance of vitamin D in the prevention of cancer". The relationships set out here are an example of how short-sighted disease prevention can be if it works with negative images. As with medical check-ups during pregnancy (▸Chap. 2.4.), we have a purely pathogenically fixated attitude here which is fine for treating acute meningitis but not for helping people achieve a healthy lifestyle. Instead anxieties are deliberately stoked.

1 The Epidemiological Divison of the German Cancer Register Heidelberg in 2008 [dkfz Krebsatlas für die 20 häufigsten Krebstodesursachen in Deutschland, 2010] showed a proportion for ovarian carcinomas of 5.9 % in women dying from cancer in Germany, malignant melanomas 1.3 %. The proportion of women who died from uterine cancer was 2.2 % in the same year.

To close the circle, we can look at the prognosis of melanoma patients in contrast to the prognosis of women with an ovarian carcinoma: the result is "that in a statistical comparison with the general population patients with a tumour depth of < 1.5 mm have the same *or indeed better (tumour depth < 0.75 mm) life expectancy*" [Braun-Falco 2009, 1320]. *Every second person diagnosed with a melanoma in Germany has a tumour depth of < 0.75 mm!*[1] This means that for the majority of melanoma patients life expectancy is not reduced. That is not as a rule communicated to patients in this form either.

If we look at these facts, we begin to wonder:

- Why is a vaccination like the mumps vaccination in childhood recommended uncritically as necessary disease prevention if the disease is not life threatening, complications rarely occur and it has been shown for more than 40 years that mumps in childhood can protect against later mumps in men with the risk of inflammation of the testicles and, above all, can protect many women against an ovarian carcinoma?
- Why is the protection against ovarian cancer through a childhood disease, which does not bring in a great deal of money, worth so much less than the protection against the much rarer and prognostically more favourable malignant melanoma? What is the relationship between the fact that more women in Germany die of ovarian carcinomas than cervical carcinomas and the public awareness of the HPV vaccination in childhood, on the one hand, and the possible protection against ovarian carcinomas through the *omission of a vaccination in childhood*, on the other? Normally only the pill is named as prophylaxis for ovarian carcinomas, once again a product of the pharmaceutical industry.
- Why are sunscreens with high sun protection factors recommended uncritically when leading dermatologists have to admit at the same time that the proof that sunscreens protect against malignant melanomas is "still outstanding" [Wolf 2009, 292] and evidence is growing that vitamin D deficiency is already widespread during adolescence [Reckert 2009, 583] – an observation which we can confirm through the many blood levels we have determined in adolescents ourselves.

In summary it is hard to avoid the impression that

- *narrow, purely specialist perspectives* (e. g. of dermatology or the German Standing Vaccination Commission STIKO) *quickly lose the view of the overall context*, for example with regard to the benefit to the organism of absorbing sunlight or the long-term consequences of suppressing childhood diseases;
- *commercial interests* (in the sale of vaccines, sunscreen, etc.) *are involved in highlighting or suppressing scientific* findings (in terms of Evidence-Based Medicine, the connection between mumps and ovarian carcinomas backed by better evidence than the effectiveness of sunscreens in melanoma prophylaxis, which is not to say that the authors consider sunburn in children to be harmless).

1 The reasons for this are unknown. It is suspected for example that these patients on average have a healthier lifestyle before or at the latest following diagnosis than the average population. Malignant melanoma for example more frequently affects people in positions of social responsibility and relatively rarely people in occupations involving heavy physical work, even if the latter work a lot in the sun.

The term "evidence" should not push aside the judgement of the individual doctor. In so far as the doctor can base his or her actions on scientific arguments and his or her own observations, he or she is entitled and obliged to place them alongside the current evidence-based medical guidelines as an equal source of knowledge [Kienle/Kiene 2010] and to conduct the dialogue on disease prevention with the patients or their parents in an unbiased and open-minded way. Individual medical judgement belongs just as much to the necessary foundations of "shared decision making" as the "best available evidence" within the meaning of the respective established medical standard.

Seen from a medical perspective, fewer and fewer children are today achieving satisfactory immunological maturity in Europe and the USA. Prevention in medicine should respond to this new challenge today and thereby also self-critically ask the question whether the action of paediatrics in developed western countries is not itself part of a wrong "immunological curriculum". The role played by affluence combined with a one-sided scientific thinking has already been recognized in the example of infant food: the replacement of breast milk, which continually adjusts to the needs of the infant in a living way, with standardized, industrial ready-to-use foods which allegedly "contains everything" has serious repercussions for the maturation of the child. Measurable losses of cognitive development potential (▸Chap. 4.1) and the loss of psychological warmth in the experience of breast feeding correlate with the known disadvantages for the development of the child's metabolism, the risk of obesity and much else. It has been known for some time that acute infections such as bacterial meningitis and otitis media occur with far greater frequency in the absence of breast feeding. That breast feeding performs a valuable function in the healthy maturation of the immune system's "early programming" in early infancy can be seen in Crohn's disease for example: "Children who had never been breast fed had more than three times the risk of developing Crohn's disease than children who had received breast milk" [Koletzko 2010, 760]. It gives pause for thought if in a country like Canada chronic-inflammatory bowel diseases increased between 1993 and 2005 by 33 % in the under nine age group [Benchimol 2009]. Koletzko refers to the "other side of the coin of our culture"; yet the question of nutrition, dealing with worm infections (whose rigorous elimination probably correlates with an increase in chronic inflammatory bowel diseases, while the administration of worm eggs (Trichuris suis) was able to improve the course of ulcerative colitis and Crohn's disease [Summers 2005a, b]), the effect on intestinal flora of antibiotics and sugar consumption, etc. also concern paediatric practice and not just our culture (therefore putting them beyond influence) as a whole. Although the suspicion is growing that precisely the frequent use of antipyretics and antibiotics in treatment as well as the density and early timing of protective vaccinations can negatively influence the development and individuation of the immune system, while on the other hand the positive effect on the incidence of allergies of an anthroposophical lifestyle (including much greater restraint in the use of the above medical measures) can be scientifically shown [Alm and Swartz 1999, Flöistrup et al. 2006], the mainstream in paediatrics is still oriented towards substituting more and more physical abilities of the child or manipulating them in their development. Here the benefit of these measures for the individual child is increasingly questionable while the manufacturers of vaccinations and infant food increasingly influence medical research and development as their sales rise.

Perfected disease control cannot replace health development. The lifelong development and preservation of health is an active process which in the long term depends on the individual himself or herself, his or her physical and psychological learning processes. These should happen at the right time: on an immunological level the *own activity of the child's immune system in the first years of life, the acquisition of the ability to balance and regulate this immune system, are of crucial importance. The preventive horizon encompasses not just childhood but the whole of life.*

For today's children the carcinoma will top the list of causes of death in adulthood. In terms of prevention, there is empirically backed proof of the value of acute febrile diseases in carcinoma prophylaxis [up-to-date overview in Girke 2010, 423f; Albonico 1996a]. The mumps-ovarian carcinoma example set out above underlines this connection.

Disease prevention must not be equated with isolated, specific and expensive measures for individual diseases (cf. the "Wuppertal Manifesto" [Hirte et al. 2010]). On the contrary, every medical intervention should be examined from the perspective of salutogenesis: what does it mean in the long term for the ability of the organism to actively maintain its health? A great gap has opened up in this field between treatment and prophylaxis. The administration of antipyretics, antibiotics and similar things, for example, *has been shown to weaken* the ability of the organism to regulate itself and maintain its own health and leads to an increased allergy risk [Flöistrup 2006] (▸Chap. 6.1). In many cases such medicines can be replaced by a procedure which primarily observes, stimulates, guides and supports the organism's own activity. Direct "mandatory" allopathic intervention is thus restricted to those cases where own regulation is not possible or has become highly problematic.

The therapeutic approach of anthroposophic medicine and homoeopathy as represented here is guided throughout by the principle that in treatment the own activity of the organism *should be primarily supported.* This means that treatment of the disease and prevention directly pass over into one another; accordingly the reader will find *in all chapters of this book perspectives on disease prevention.* Under the living conditions of western industrialized states, long-term successful health promotion will be able to get by less and less with technically standardized, manipulative disease prevention. This procedure is based on an outdated negative image (acute inflammation as enemy of the child), the one-sidedness of which itself contributes to new diseases occurring on a large scale which themselves can no longer be satisfactorily manipulated and managed. Alongside the suppression, manipulation and substitution of the organism, medicine must learn the skill to stimulate and support the living organism and give it the necessary impulses; this requires an understanding of the living individuality, the ability to identify the right time and what is necessary in each individual case. Against this background the doctor and parents will have to keep answering questions in paediatric practice as to which method of disease prevention is the most appropriate for the child individually.

3.1 Providing medical advice regarding disease prevention and parents' individual decisions

> Health promotion is the process of enabling people to increase control over, and to improve, their health. To reach a state of complete physical, mental and social well-being, an individual or group must be able to identify and to realize aspirations, to satisfy needs, and to change or cope with the environment.
>
> WHO [1986]

The authors do not take the view that the administration of vitamin K or D, of fluoride or that vaccination should be generally rejected. Such an attitude fails to take the step to individual freedom and responsibility and adopts a similarly simplifying and authoritarian position with regard to the child and parents as the attitude which says that the same (standardized), general vitamin, trace element and vaccination prophylaxis is *incumbent on* the doctor and family. Indeed, many parents and fellow doctors today believe that they are fundamentally obliged to carry out the measures mentioned. What is at stake here is the defence of the right of parents to care for their children on the basis of the freedom of the human being and his or her right to life and physical integrity (*Basic Law of the Federal Republic of Germany*, Articles 1 and 2), including the free self-determination of preventive measures. The free and democratic constitutional order is related to the *principle of the free choice of therapy* and that applies in particular in the field of *disease prevention*; above all if it includes medical intervention in a healthy patient. The duty of care of parents and doctors in exercising their responsibility has to be based on their freedom of choice. But this freedom remains abstract if it is or has to be exercised by one of the parties alone. In reality young parents, often barely familiar with their new responsibilities, are lacking the necessary basis for making a decision – here they are dependent on a fair and appropriately timed dialogue with the doctor and written information which leaves them free in their decision. The necessary decisions should be taken by both parents *after an interval* following the meeting with the doctor. On the other hand the doctor himself or herself is normally not entitled to take and implement a decision in the field of disease prevention. There is a binding requirement under law to enter a dialogue in which the current preventive recommendations and risks are set out in order thereby to enable the parents to make an individual judgement as to the way which is correct, appropriate and adequate for the child. The aim of what follows is to clarify by means of selected topics of paediatric disease prevention how the *basis can be created on which the necessary decisions can be judged.* The authors undertake these advisory discussions above all in the context of the second to sixth preventive medical checkups in the first year of life (in Germany there are 6 standardized paediatric examinations of a child in the first year). However, the topics of vaccination and vitamin D/sunlight remain of relevance throughout childhood and adolescence. In this context it is vital to include the mother *and* father in this process (in so far as the legal prerequisites exist for both parents) and of course the young person himself or herself. Only a decision to which all those involved can agree is sustainable in the long term! As a result, such an approach in the practice of the authors leads to *various, individualized ways of prevention.*

3.2 Vitamin D, rickets prevention, sun exposure and sun protection

... the healthy development of form-giving processes can only occur in the field of the I-organization

Rudolf Steiner, Ita Wegman

Vitamin D Deficiency is largely also due to our culture which invented glass, the bulb and sunscreen and which shuts itself off from sunlight and creates interior spaces ...

T. Reckert

We were recently able to show that rigorous UV protection can lead to vitamin D deficiency

L. Tremezaygues, J. Reichrath

We studied breast milk in recent years and were able to show that it contains six of a total of eight analyzed UV filters, some of them with oestrogen-like effects

Margret Schlumpf

"We need outside light for life. Not just as light which has already been captured in matter in nature through food (e. g. in the form of the carbohydrates resulting from photosynthesis); we also need it directly. If we do not have it in the doses well adjusted by the earth's atmosphere, we become ill. In extreme cases, a child will get rickets" [Reckert 2009, 578]. With these words the anthroposophical paediatrician Till Reckert begins his thorough work *Sonnenlicht, Vitamin D, Inkarnation* which has provided this chapter with important stimuli. With this introduction Reckert takes his starting point at the level of life: life on earth is based on its coordinated coherence with sunlight (▸Chap. 1.1). "Sense of coherence" (Antonovsky) as an expression of health is based on the reality that every living organism is dependent on harmonious coherence with its earthly and cosmic environment, that the physical life organization, the etheric body, lives in this coherence. If we see the ray of light as the archetypal phenomenon of the straight line in nature – just as we can see the archetypal phenomenon of the sphere in the water drop – it is very easy to understand intuitively that the development of crystalline substance in the services of our own upright posture, the development of the skeleton, is particularly dependent on sunlight. It also separates water and salt in nature and enables those processes in nature which are opposed to earthly gravity. Rudolf Steiner described the "absorption of sun forces" as central for the development of the child's body in the first years of life [Steiner 1994, 55f.]

What a difference to the way this subject is presented in public opinion: the fear of sunlight and the ubiquitous recommendation to use sunscreen (particularly with regard to UV-B which provides a necessary basis for the development of vitamin D in the skin) stands in contrast to the current recommendation to administer high doses of vitamin D in food supplements and the renewed practice of administering loading doses of vitamin D e. g. to the residents in homes for the elderly. In the latter case "the risk of a hip fracture [in 2 independent studies] under the active treatment even rises significantly ... The reasons for this paradoxical effect are unclear. It may be caused by the treatment regime with a single high dose per year" [*arznei-telegramm* 12/2010]. Clearly a purely substance-oriented and a real life view cannot be reconciled: because there is neither the time nor opportunity for these "elderly women" and men "living in a home" to spend adequate time in the sunlight, the idea is to give them an intramuscular injection of the "finished product" once per year. The consequences show that a person's exposure to light and unphysiologically high substitution doses can have different effects – which can in general cause us to be more cautious about administering ultra-high doses of vitamins. The same practice of vitamin D loading doses in infants was criticized in the early 1950 s by the anthroposophical paediatrician zur Linden for its sometimes devastating effects (hypercalcaemia and atherosclerosis); vitamin D substitution was avoided as far as possible in anthroposophical paediatrics with the consequence that cases of rickets did occur now and again in the children cared for in that way.

3.2.1 Sun exposure anamnesis

If as paediatricians we become aware of this subject, and if – analogously to a nutritional anamnesis – we obtain from all our patients a *sunlight anamnesis*, the experience can be increasingly unsettling:

- Particularly in the winter months, many mothers hardly find the time to spend a sufficient period outside in the daylight with their small children in the midday hours.
- Children with disabilities who are looked after in institutions during the day and are often restricted in their own movement, frequently spend insufficient time in daylight due to staff shortages or staff absent on sick leave (the rules for prisoners are stricter).

3

Case study

A 15-year-old patient with a serious visual impairment attends an all-day school for blind and visually impaired children. On most days, the children do not go outside into the playground. When the paediatrician requested that the school should ensure that this does happen, the school management replied through the mother that the paediatrician should explain why it was necessary for the pupils to go outside during the day, something that the school could not currently do due to staff shortages.

- Pupils in secondary all-day schools only spend short periods outside in daylight during the week in the winter months and have little opportunity for vigorous exercise. At the same time football training for boys in the autumn and spring frequently takes place at dusk with floodlights. The vitamin D levels of young people measured in our own practice correlate with scientific data which for Parisian adolescents in late winter produced an average 25-OH vitamin D level of 8.2 ng/ml [Grant and Hollick 2005], whereby all the experts agree that values below 10 ng/ml are pathological and associated with the risk of rickets or osteomalacia at every age. If we bear in mind that adolescence forms a crucial phase in the development of the skeleton for the whole of life, it gives us a measure of the significance of these findings. But cardiovascular diseases also increase with such low levels; a study [Pilz 2008] showed that the risk of sudden cardiac death increased by six to seven times at a level of 10 ng/ml in comparison to levels above 30 ng/ml. It is worth noting that specifically the cardiovascular system is crucially dependent on exercise and the absorption of sunlight!
- Pregnant women are frequently under great stress and often cannot find any opportunity to spend adequate time outside in daylight during the week. The situation is particularly difficult for mothers with a migrant background from Islamic countries: "It

was possible to show that the mothers of infants with rickets frequently themselves suffered from a clear vitamin D deficiency and needed treatment [Dawodu and Wagner, 2007]. On the other hand newborns of mothers with risk factors are already at risk: in Rotterdam 63 % of newborns of veiled or dark-skinned mothers had a 25-OH vitamin D level under 10 ng/ml compared to 16 % of newborns of mothers without these risk factors" [Dijkstra et al. 2007, quoted from Reckert 2009, 584].

- It is to be recommended that each doctor should obtain a picture through anamnesis of the really lived *coherence with sunlight* and at the same time to direct the attention of the patient or the parents to the subject by this means.

3.2.2 Vitamin D deficiency and sun protection during pregnancy and breast feeding

Foetal development during pregnancy and in the first year of life is characterized by *anabolism*. Transformed, physically absorbed sunlight forms a basic condition of human incarnation. On 29 August 1924 – before the description of vitamin D by Windaus in 1927 – Rudolf Steiner characterized the connection between sunlight and the function of the uterus in the following terms, which was no doubt difficult for his listeners to understand: "Then we come to study how in the embryonic period the human being enters the physical world from the spiritual world, and there we find that there is a special relationship between the forces which are present in phosphorus and the phosphorus compounds and the forces which exist in the uterus. If these forces did not exist in the uterus, rickets would simply occur in every person. The uterus constantly acts as a doctor against rickets." [Steiner 1994, 242]. "Phosphorus" means bearer of light, and the inner sun of the human body, its warmth and dynamism, essentially rests on the metabolism of high-energy phosphates. The connection between the uterus, pregnancy and vitamin D has only recently been scientifically established [Evans 2006]: for the active metabolic vitamin D_3–1.25(OH) is not produced and regulated only in the kidneys but also "locally" in individual organs. "One of the first tissues after the kidneys in which the vitamin D receptor and 1-alpha-hydroxylase could be shown to exist was the placenta. … Mice which cannot produce 1-alpha-hydroxylase are infertile (even if the consequences for the calcium metabolism are compensated for). It is assumed today that vitamin D_3 produced locally in the placenta is important for a local immune tolerance and the nidation of the foetus." [Reckert 2009, 586]

What Rudolf Steiner expressed intuitively in the words: "Then rickets would occur in every human being", can today be physiologically confirmed. Without autonomous vitamin D_3 production in the uterus human pregnancy would probably not occur. As the *regulatory action of the vitamin D metabolism is linked with the activation of vitamin D3–25(OH) into vitamin D3–1.25(OH), this discovery means that the placenta itself (always assuming a sufficient supply of vitamin D!) regulates the active vitamin D3–25(OH) level of the foetus.*

Research has been able to show that a vitamin D deficiency in pregnant woman can compromise the build up of the body of the unborn child in a sustained way: intrauterine growth retardation, small gestational age births, arterial hypertension in the mother, premature contractions, an increase in amniotic infection syndromes, elevated section rates and an increase in Th1-related autoimmune diseases such as type 1 diabetes mellitus correlate with vitamin D deficiency in the mother. The newborn can develop rickets with hypocalcaemia. In a globalized world it is therefore particularly important to observe as a doctor:

- does the mother have a dark skin type which makes vitamin D synthesis in the skin up to ten times slower than in a so-called "Celtic skin type" with light skin and reddish hair?
- does the mother mostly wear a veil in daylight for cultural reasons or does she only rarely go outside during pregnancy e. g. for occupational reasons or reasons of lifestyle?
- is there maternal obesity which increases the risk of a vitamin D deficiency for lifestyle reasons and due to the changed metabolism for liposoluble substances?

With regard to child health, the most important and particularly sustainable preventive measure for rickets is the sufficient absorption by and "storage of sunlight" in the mother's body. Vitamin D_3 formed in the skin is stored in a simple hydroxylated form in the liver (this storage vitamin D_3–25(OH) is used to measure the vitamin level). Human beings can quite easily store enough for a period of three to four months and thus survive the "vitamin D winter" (correlating in southern Germany with the time from 1 November-1 February and thus with the old Celtic calendar which celebrated the start of winter and spring on these dates). Here there are indications that self-produced vitamin D is stored to a greater extent than vitamin D taken per os as a substitute.

We would absolutely recommend measuring the mother's blood level if there is any indication of a vitamin D deficiency. The most important "substitution" for a vitamin D deficiency is the recommendation – vigorously presented – for the mother to spend sufficient time outside, for her to do so daily (except extremely light-skinned women), *not to use any sunscreen as long as she is at home but to adapt to the sun over the course of the year, expose the skin to it in sufficient measure and to judge the time spent in the sun such that no erythema occurs* [cf. the recommendation of Zeeb and Greinert 2010]. The link between vitamin D deficiency and the use of sunscreen with a higher sun protection factor has been scientifically shown [Querings and Reichrath 2004; Tremezaytues and Reichrath 2010]. In summer, midday should of course be avoided whereas in the transitional periods in October and March only the hours around noon allow the sufficient development of vitamin D. The skin can adapt to the sunlight at the home location through daily exposure to the sun (except in the "Celtic" skin type 1 which only makes up 2 % of the German population) and thereby build up strong natural light protection without losing the ability of vitamin D synthesis through sunlight. If the mother practices such "light nutrition" she will also ensure that the right amount of sunlight is absorbed by her child. There is not just a physiological difference in producing vitamin D in this way rather than eating a tablet (because exercise has a complementary effect to sunlight/vitamin D on the physiology of the skeleton, the musculature and the cardiovascular system), but the psychological and spiritual experience is also fundamentally different. It is a remarkable fact which correlates with observations in practice that vitamin D deficiency can also reinforce seasonal winter depression whereas conversely exercise and a sufficient vitamin D level is associated with enhanced psychological wellbeing. The relationship with the sun represents a central question for every human culture and the symbol of the point and circle represents the sun worldwide. Vitamin D deficiency poses the question, expressed positively, as to our relationship with the sun.

We have referred several times already to *skin type*: the different skin types I-VI distinguished by dermatology [Höger 2005, 393] represent adaptations of the skin to exposure to the sun in particular regions of the earth. They indicate that the time for sufficient vitamin D production and the pigmentary protection of the skin against sunburn are balanced for each skin type in accordance with the local light conditions under which each skin type has formed through adaptation. At a time of globalization in which Irish immigrants celebrate barbecue parties on Australian beaches and black African couples experience the polar nights on the Norwegian Lofoten, in which outside work has been largely replaced by factory halls and offices with computer screens, and medical students sit in lecture theatres without natural light, this natural adaptation of the human skin to sunlight (which is estimated to have taken place over approx. 10,000 years) requires cultural and medical support: in the form of *light protection and sunlight substitution.* Light protection through sunscreen can become necessary above all through travel and the associated, sudden exposure to more intense sunlight. Substitution measures are indicated above all where the home location/life circumstances do not permit sufficient sunlight to be absorbed in relation to the skin type and the intake through natural sources (fish from cold oceans, avocados, eggs from free-range chickens) is limited.

Light protection through sunscreens with higher sun protection factors is a problem for pregnant women and breast feeding mothers and for children to the extent that chemical UV filters are absorbed and can be eliminated through breast milk for example, sometimes with hormone-(oestrogen-)like effects. In animal experiments the effect of the corresponding substances on male and female genitalia have been shown, for example [Schlumpf et al. 2008]. That is why the authors categorically advise pregnant and breast feeding women against the use of sunscreens with chemical (higher) sun protection factors (apart from exceptional cases of extremely sensitive skin and unavoidably high UV exposure). Children, if they require sunscreen, should accordingly be given products based on zinc oxide and, as appropriate, titanium dioxide – if the skin is unbroken (they contain nano particles).

How can the skin be protected naturally against excessively strong radiation from the sun?

- Choice of time of day to spend outside.
- Appropriate clothing ("textile protection") in strong sunlight.
- Adaptation through regular exposure: there is a strong indication that *(mobility-related) sudden exposure to unusually strong sunlight* is particularly damaging for skin up to and including oncogenesis. On the other hand the skin can develop a considerable "sun protection factor" through regular exposure [Jachens 2006, 48].
- Antioxidants such as vitamins A and E in natural foods (e. g. sandthorn) and sunscreen agents, flavonoids, polyphenols, e. g. in green tea, "actives" in cosmetic products [Krutmann 2009].
- Sunscreen with physically acting sun protection factors (zinc oxide, titanium dioxide).
- The question of *vitamin D substitution in pregnancy and the nursing period* – if the natural absorption of vitamin D cannot be increased because of the time of year or for reasons of locality or lifestyle and the deficiency has been shown to exist – is handled pragmatically by the authors. In each case it appears more effective and less risky to ensure a sufficient maternal vitamin D supply than to start with postpartum paediatric compensatory treatment when it is actually too late. The substitution of vitamin D in the mother, if undertaken, should be done daily in doses of between 500 and 1,000, max. 2,000 IU/day. A range above 20 ng/ml vitamin D_3–25(OH) should be aimed for;

the oft-quoted significantly higher serum concentrations require careful monitoring and themselves contain risks in the event of a massive substitution [*arznei-telegramm* 2010; Shroff et al. 2010]. The aim should always remain to return to natural forms of vitamin D absorption as soon as possible.

3.2.3 Rickets

Rickets poses a risk to the child's development in a characteristic way:

- In *craniotabes*, the first clinical manifestation of rickets, the ossification of the skull remains at an embryonic stage, as it were; the fontanelles remain wide open, the membrane bone is so soft it can be compressed, above all parietally; the strong sweating of the child is typical, particularly on the head. The child *cannot maintain the spherical shape of the head in the face of gravity*; an angular deformation threatens.
- In *rickets complicated with tetany*, the most acutely threatening manifestation of rickets, the drop of the available calcium in the blood leads to muscle failure up to and including laryngospasm and thus to the threat of respiratory paralysis. In the same period (most frequently at about the sixth month of life) a *deformation in the region of the rib cage* (rachitic rosary, Harrison's curve) can be observed in the skeleton.
- Finally, rickets becomes manifest in a *failure of limb development*: the children do not become erect, epiphyseal wear and a pathological atrophy of the long tubular bones already mark the third stages of rickets development.

We can at a very early stage observe – mostly sour smelling – sweating on the head, clearly increased restlessness during sleep and poor feeding above all in the evening. These important general clinical symptoms often precede skeletal findings. In parallel to the second phase of rickets, in which the latter can spread from the head to the rib cage and particularly the respiration, we can observe *greater susceptibility to infection and a very much more serious course of infectious diseases* above all of the airways. A characteristic example of this is infant bronchiolitis (▸Chap. 5.1.5). Thus rickets is a disease in which both the vital functions of the immune system and the physical crystallization and development of the skeleton are at risk of remaining immature and entering into a pathological process of disintegration which endangers body shape, respiration, free upright posture and movement. Something of the nature of rickets becomes particularly clear in its consequences for *dentition*; there can be a delay not just in the eruption of the first teeth and thus the attainment of independence from (breast) milk but the development of the second, permanent teeth can be seriously damaged particularly in the crown. Yet nothing symbolizes the ability to mineralize more clearly than the teeth which represent the hardest and most durable substance which our body can produce; at the same time nothing embodies more clearly our ability to separate ourselves from the external world, the ability to destroy and dissolve everything invasive. And thus we can indeed observe that after the teeth have erupted the healthy small child is immunologically significantly more stable than previously, and above all while the teeth are erupting. *When all these things are taken together, rickets represents the inability of the child to give its body the necessary form.*

The vitamin D prophylaxis which is generally practised throughout the first year of life is equivalent to *hormonal substitution treatment*. For looked at from the perspective of its effect on the metabolism – and also in terms of structure and synthesis – active vitamin D is a hormonally active substance (steroid hormone). Even if the substance as administered is not yet the active form of the hormone – in contrast to vitamin D_3–1.25(OH) substitution for children with kidney failure – and the organism can thus regulate the vitamin D activation itself, vitamin D substitution in infants does nevertheless intervene in their metabolism and can lead to problematic consequences. That is shown by current studies [Bäck et al. 2009, Gale et al. 2008, Hyppönen 2004] which show *that vitamin D substitution in infants can raise the rate of allergic rhinitis, atopic allergies and bronchial asthma in later life* (follow-up observation periods of 9 years and more) (so-called Th2-mediated chronic-inflammatory diseases – in contrast to the Th1-mediated diseases, type 1 diabetes mellitus or Crohn's disease for example). These data show that the concerns raised by anthroposophic medicine about a *general, untargeted vitamin D prophylaxis in infancy* is not without a scientific basis. In view of a globalized world, completely different skin types and very different light conditions in central Europe in summer and winter, it makes sense also to individualize *vitamin D prophylaxis in infancy.* The aims of such preventive treatment should, if possible, not be framed purely in negative terms:

- "Never administer vitamin D": illusory in view of premature babies, children from migrant families, children who are constitutionally (see below) prone to rickets and chronic diseases.
- Give everyone the same dose "so that nothing happens": something always happens. Studies on allergy risk in particular show that in the field of collective hormone substitution there is no such thing as no consequences. What may be barely adequate for one child is superfluous for another – and thus a risk without benefit.

The gold standard in this (as in other) fields should rather be the question, related to rickets:

- Can the child develop and mineralize his or her skeleton and teeth sufficiently from out of his or her own forces? Does he or she have sufficient light reserves to strengthen, individualize and regulate his or her form physically and immunologically? How can I fundamentally support this process, how can I stimulate it if necessary (e.g. with anthroposophical or homoeopathic medicines) and when do I have to support it through substitution?

If we ask ourselves this question, we become more attentive towards the child and his or her parents. Anyone who wishes not just to avoid illness but support incarnation will attempt, to begin with, to perceive the child's incarnation process individually. Thus the constitutional circumstances of the body and soul are of great importance (▸Chap. 3.2.5.). It is further important to be aware that the ontogenesis of the human being is designed to extend the course of events, to maintain *physical development in a fluid or developing state for a long time and* to prolong its completion for as long as possible" [Kipp 1980, 28f.]. We *first need to understand human physiology* – we might call it a physiology of freedom – before we intervene. The founders of anthroposophic medicine, Rudolf Steiner and Ita Wegman, expressly emphasize in their remarks on this subject that the bones of the human being are formed "by the I-organization" [Steiner and Wegman 1953, 68]. This means that the same principle is at work in *human* skeletal development as in upright gait, speaking and thinking – something which animals do not have. We can now ask: is general vitamin D prophylaxis a help or hindrance with regard to the individual success of bone development? For it can really only be a matter of enabling the child to build up his or her body himself or herself and only to use substitution when it has become clear that he or she cannot do so out of his or her own strength. That is certainly not the case for every child.

3.2.4 Practical implementation of individualized rickets prevention

When as part of the second preventive medical checkup the parents and doctor decide whether a general or an individual vitamin D prophylaxis should be undertaken, it is important to inform the parents about the commitment which is involved in the latter way.

- It is responsible to undertake individual rickets prevention only if the child is *presented at the practice every four weeks* in the first six months of life and, as necessary, beyond that in the first winter six months – thereafter every six weeks to completion of the first year of life or in the second winter six months.

The *careful observation* of the child and his or her development – *before* any medical intervention – is the basis for doing the child full medical justice. The things which have to be taken into account in this context have already been described. The second element is the *anamnesis*. That can highlight those children who are *particularly at risk* from rickets [Madeleyn 1995, 560]:

- *Premature and small gestational age babies* (SGA): here there is an increased risk of rickets above all if the child cannot be taken outside as a result, for example, of a greater susceptibility to infection. No general recommendation can be made here because the individual conditions can vary greatly [Madeleyn 1995, 560].
- Children who are not breast fed or who are weaned early are very much at risk of rickets if they are not given the normal (vitaminized) powdered milk. Feeding infants in cases of atopic dermatitis with pure almond milk or non-adapted soya food from the health food shop – which is in any case fraught with problems – also creates a disposition for rickets. Similar to premature and small gestational age babies, the absence of vitamin D can raise the incidence of rickets to 50 %. On the other hand all foods licensed as infant food contain vitamins; the quantities of vitamin D they contain should be included in the medical considerations. The infant food must, of course, contain sufficient calcium, but calcium absorption is, in turn, strongly vitamin D-dependent.
- Children of parents with a migration background coming from regions closer to the equator than the practice location. It should be taken into account that up to 80 % of Iranian women, for example, exhibit a vitamin D deficiency and hence more frequently tuberculosis as a result of the practice of wearing the veil. The cultural migration background is just as important as the geographical one. In general the doctor ought to try and assess whether there is already a maternal vitamin D deficiency (see above). Because it generally applies that "the content in breast milk of vitamin D-active components is scarce" [Reckert 2009, 581].

Apart from these easily identified children at risk, there is a risk of rickets which is not so easy to detect. Here the anamnesis must endeavour to discover the real living conditions of the family. The first question is of course about sufficient time spent outdoors. After the neonatal period, i. e. the first 28 days of life, the child should spend at least half an hour but preferably at least an hour per day under a blue sky. Where this is not regularly possible (e. g. mother's occupation, etc.), the child *cannot* adequately advance the mineralization of his or her skeleton – because this is essentially dependent on transforming the light into hormonally effective (chemical) substance! However, the child does require a transitional time of approx. four weeks in the neonatal period to adjust his or her heat generation and regulation as well as respiration to the extrauterine conditions. We have observed the increasing trend to expose newborns to the atmospheric conditions as early as after a few days. Apart from on mild summer days, this generally represents an excessive demand on the child. It is therefore urgently to be recommended that within this time the child is brought up in the stable and adapted environment of the home – because the child must also be able to digest the external atmosphere with all its changes, not just the food. The essential thing above all is to maintain a *stable inner warmth regime* for which the child urgently requires this transitional period.

Whereas we can react relatively easily and plausibly to the information that the child has insufficient exposure to light, wide-ranging surveys among doctors have shown that the tendency for rickets arising from the absence of a vitamin D prophylaxis was observed particularly among those children who grew up in families with problematical warmth conditions. Here the term warmth must be used in its full dual meaning: on the one hand it is important for rickets prevention carefully to observe the warmth organism of the child. The contrast of stable body heat with the relative coolness of the light-flooded atmosphere in particular promotes the intervention of the I-organization in skeletal development. From the perspective of anthroposophic medicine, the latter represents a relative cooling, a release of heat from the developing bone substance (cf. the chemistry of salification) whereas rickets can be understood precisely as an "adhesion" of warmth to the bones, something which also resonates in the Latin term for the disease, rach-itis, in so far as every inflammation (-itis) designates a location in the organism which is relatively too warm and displays a tendency to dissolve its structure [Steiner and Wegman 1991, 68f).

In contrast, there is a problematic warmth situation for the child if there is an insufficient perception of him or her and his or her warmth requirements are neglected (e. g. not dressed warmly enough). On the other hand there is a warmth problem in a metaphorical sense if the parents have anxieties or there are serious conflicts in the relationship between the parents or with the child (cf. also pregnancy, birth, nursing period). An increase in rickets should be anticipated in such a marred atmosphere.

Finally, it is self-evident that we have to take account of *diseases of the child* with regard to rickets prevention particularly if they

- make staying outside impossible for longer than a week (e. g. pneumonia in winter)
- are associated with longer-term disorders of resorption (gastrointestinal diseases, cystic fibrosis, etc.) and/or liver, gall bladder and kidney function.
- bring with them genetically an elevated infection risk and restraint of the body-related activity of the I-organization (e. g. children with Down's syndrome)

A further significant – third – element in individual rickets prevention is *to identify the constitution of the child.* The latter disposes the child quite differently to rickets disorders. Both homoeopathy and anthroposophic medicine have endeavoured to provide a differentiated description of the physical and soul constitution of the small child. We will deal with that in greater detail in the following section.

The careful consideration of all the points as set out leads to four possible consequences at each presentation. Of course these evaluations are not independent of the parental judgement but form the basis for a consultation in which the path to be taken is decided with the parents:

- The child does not require medical intervention, nutritional and lifestyle advice and regular checks are adequate.
- The child requires constitutional support with anthroposophic/homoeopathic medicines, but not vitamin substitution.
- The administration of vitamin D is indicated as there is a recognizable risk.
- The child displays manifest signs of rickets and requires immediate treatment for rickets.

If as part of *rickets prevention the decision is taken to administer vitamin D,* the authors generally administer dosages between 250 and 500 IU daily. It should be emphasized once more here that this only applies if the state of health of the child, the vitamin D supply from breast milk or through vitaminized infant food and/or the seasonal sunlight do not provide a sufficient supply. The principles of (calcium and) vitamin D treatment for rickets are generally known. *Vitamin D substitution in proven vitamin D deficiency* and seasonal or individual inability to produce vitamin D by natural means can become necessary in any age group. We will only refer here to the example of oncologically ill children and young people who frequently do not see daylight for weeks or months and are exceptionally at risk of infection.

Below we will deal with the possibilities of constitutional rickets prevention in infants and small children with potentized medicine and external applications.

3.2.5 Constitutional medication for infants

In the first six to eight weeks of life the authors do not, as a rule, yet administer potentized mineral medicines which intervene in the constitution. In an early recognizable weakness of the warmth organization (e. g. warmth distribution) and the integration of sensory impressions (both point to the I-organization), the life and I-organization can be strengthened with the administration of potentized

- **Apis mell. D12 pillules** Weleda, DHU
  2–3 pillules 1 x/d in the morning

to help incarnation as explained above. Cf. also the principle in the Vademecum of Anthroposophic Medicines [Vademecum 2010, 91–96]

The honeybee itself embodies in all of its activity, on the one hand, a consistent relationship with the sun and light by which it is guided and from out of which it creates its strictly formed and, for an insect, very temperature stable structure. All the perceptions of the individual animal are constantly integrated into the bee colony; the whole colony is focused on a single central point in the queen bee which generates a synthesizing and life promoting action in the colony. On the other hand bee venom leads to dissolution in the victim in the form of an inflammatory oedema. Administered as D12, Apis mell. can stimulate the child to stabilize its warmth regulation and start to crystallize its mineral form from out of the sunlight. In relation to the organs, Apis mell is particularly effective with regard to the *kidneys*, the inner centre of the vitamin D metabolism, as well as with regard to the periphery of the circulatory system and the *basic substance of the connective tissue* [Vogel 1994, Vol. 1, 110f., Vol. 2, 712], which is fundamental for all form-giving processes in the organism [Hinrichsen 1990, 22f.].

- A generally effective mineral medicine in rickets prevention is potentized
- **Apatit D6 trit.** Weleda

This substance is directly related to the most finely distributed, highly structured form of crystallizing mineral substance in human bones – a complex calcium compound containing phosphorus, chlorine and fluoride. In low potentized form, e. g. 1 saltsp. in the morning, Apatit stimulates the process of mineralization in the skeleton (▸Chap. 3.4.1). (The effect should not be confused with the specific constitutional effect of calcium phosphate produced in the chemical laboratory [Calcium phos.] which is described in greater detail below). Specifically in premature and small gestational age babies, potentized Apatit can be given at a very early stage.

After no later than the twelfth week of life, it is also preventively necessary to take account of the *constitution of the child*. Hence we will briefly characterize the most important constitutional types – in so far as relevant here.

3.2.5.1 Potentized oyster shell calcium (Calcium carbonicum H, Conchae)

Probably more than half of the *infants requiring preventive treatment* accord with the constitution described in the *medicinal picture of Calcium carbonicum Hahnemanni and* also clearly characterized in the anthroposophical understanding of the human being [Husemann 2009, 63–78]:

- *"Much mass without strength"*, i. e. children who quickly put on weight in the nursing period, often are above-average weight at birth and also give a calm, satisfied sympathetic and slightly lethargic impression in their behaviour; motor and skeletal development lag behind weight development.
- These children accordingly *sleep relatively much* and through the night relatively early, before teething or the start of the development of rickets makes their sleep more restless again.
- The *metabolism thus predominates*; they give the impression that the fluid predominates – in the plump forms, but also in the *relatively reduced tone* of the child and in the *comparatively strong tendency to sweat*. This appears above all in the head alongside the feet and hands; we have the impression as if the fluid is overflowing outwards and upwards. In anthroposophical terms we can say that the etheric element predominates in relation to the formative forces so that the physical element is insufficiently mineralized; also that the foreign matter from the external world is insufficiently stopped or overcome. These children accordingly have a tendency particularly to develop *infection-related catarrh*, muco-tympanum and consecutive otitis, cow's milk intolerance (in the sense of an insufficiently developed barrier in the gastro-intestinal tract) and food-related eczema, above all on the head and cheeks.
- The *warmth regime is "upside down"*: hot, sweaty head and cool, damp feet and hands characterize this constitution (acutely this would be typical for Belladonna which can be considered to be "acute Calcium carbonicum").
- The *relative weaknesses of the formative forces*, in anthroposophical terms the delayed intervention of the astral body and I-organization, are revealed on the one hand in this reversal of the warmth structure (I-organization), and on the other in the typical sour smell of the excretions (perspiration and stool). Every excretion is seen anthroposoph-

ically as the product of astral activity in the etheric; the same applies with regard to every reaction in the organism tending towards the sour. We can see these sour excretions as an attempt to control the fluid-etheric entity through pruning – just as a gardener produces form and refinement from pure growth through pruning. However the attempt to do this does not quite succeed in these children to begin with, which is why there is the strong tendency to sweat at the least effort (drinking!).

To a certain extent all these things are still physiological characteristics of the infant in the first trimester Accordingly this constitution is also encountered far more frequently at this age than later on – many infants and small children thus pass through *a constitutional change* in their development which in a certain respect is really physiological at this age; it indicates, after all, that the body inherited from the parents has been profoundly transformed by the child. Accordingly we apply oyster shell calcium, Conchae or Calcium carbonicum Hahnemanni preventively above all where the above characteristics remain very strongly dominant and/or for a conspicuously long period of time.

Children with this constitution have a phlegmatic nature; they do not like to be approached too directly or too vigorously (something which to a certain extent applies to all infants).

Accordingly mildly elevated forms of potentization which nevertheless intervene in the constitutional structure have proved themselves very effective in treatment, e. g.

- **Calcium carbonicum LM6** (later possibly LM12) Arcana
  2 gtt. diluted in some still spring water 1 x/d [Wolff 1991].

This medicine should be given daily until the one-sidedness has balanced out or there is the impression that the effectiveness stops or begins to turn into the opposite. This can either be followed by a break to observe the further development or one can move directly to LM12. Higher LM potencies are rarely of use at this age in particular.

As an alternative to an LM potency

- **Conchae D6–20 trit.** Weleda
  1 saltsp. 1–3 x/d can be administered whereby an increasingly high potency should be administered the closer the action is to be focused to the head (D20 in a tendency for craniotabes and strong sweating on the head, D12 in mucous congestion of the airways, D6 to support the incarnation in the metabolic and limb region)

A composite medicine based on potentized oyster shell with a wide application is

- **Conchae/Quercus comp. S trit.** Weleda
  1 saltsp. 1–3 x/d

which with **Calcium carb. D10** also contains **oak bark D4** and metallic **zinc D10**. This medicine has been specifically developed for rickets prevention. It also acts on susceptibility to infection [Vademecum 2010, 353] and eczema in infancy based on the constitution as set out.

In rarer cases the potentized calcium carbonate of the oyster shell can also be of relevance with regard to thin infants who tend to be underweight: here we find the tendency for sour diarrhoea connected with the typical sour (head) sweating, intolerance of milk and a strong anxiety. These children stand out above all through their *impaired assimilation*. The medicine Magnesium carbonicum (▸ Chap. 4.4.4), which is indicated for *aggressively tense* children who tend towards milk intolerance and sour diarrhoea, must be differentiated from that.

Infants with pronounced characteristics of the Calcium carbonicum constitution have a comparatively high risk of rickets; the perception of this constitution thus often indicates the same as the indication for prophylaxis with the potentized medicine. This treatment can, if required, be intensified with sulphur baths. The previously recommended Dr. Klopfer sulphur bath is no longer available. A replacement is

- Sulphur baths (**Spitzner Balneo Schwefelbad**)
  5–10 ml per 10 litres of bath water (depending on bath size), approx. twice weekly

The development of *craniotabes* which, if moderately pronounced, can be very well treated with the measures set out, is particularly characteristic of these children. At the same time the treatment specified forestalls the otitis media which occurs so frequently in these children. The application of Calc. carb. in higher potentization frequently leads to an acceleration of dentition. It has been observed that the frequent application of high potencies (D/C200) can negatively influence the amelogenesis of the teeth. For this reason we prefer medium potencies or the LM potencies referred to.

3.2.5.2 Potentized quartz crystal (Silicea, Quartz)

A quite different constitution also displays a high risk of rickets which mostly manifests only at a slightly later time and can then often be associated with severe bronchopulmonary infections (e. g. bronchiolitis, staphylococcal pneumonia, etc.). These children stand out through a generally *low vital warmth*. Their body is *thin*, they tend to be *small* and their birth weight lies below the average; we find an above average number of premature infants among these children (for Calc. carb., an overdue birth date tends to be typical). Their *growth is slow* and the metabolism displays much less activity than in the type we considered first. The infants mostly seem quiet; their fingers are noticeably *slender* and the forehead predominates in the face while the lower jaw is very delicately formed – again in contrast to the typical Calc. carb. constitution.

Both constitutional types have the tendency to sweat in common, yet these children often display a rather cool, non-smelling perspiration on the head whereas the *foot sweat* often has a foul smell. The *fontanelle* also remains *open for a long time* (and typically here *also the small fontanelle)*. The skin is *pale, delicate and diaphanous*. The facial expression is *wide awake and calmly "objective"* (not as spontaneously smiling and sympathetically inclined as in Calc. carb.), the child has a neutral and clear soul presence and often seems to be undecided for a long time about entering into the necessary, life-affirming physical activity – he or she for example drinks quite differently from the typical Calc. carb. infant.

These characteristics recall *rock crystal* from which the silicic acid medicine can be obtained following a process developed by Hahnemann (Silicea), but which can also – as customary at Wala and Weleda – be directly triturated and potentized (quartz). The transparency and beautiful form, but also the inner coolness and rigidity (combined with a complete loss of own warmth), which characterize rock crystal are also indicators of a tendency in these children. Although primarily they do not obviously tend towards formlessness, they are at risk of rickets. This is because the formative forces, the I and astral body, do not keep the body-building metabolism sufficiently supplied in these children but exhaust themselves in the region of the head: The body atrophies, too little substance is built up and too little heat is released. Therapeutically, the maintenance of the warmth organization acquires the greatest importance in the Silicea constitution (all-body oil rhythmical Einreibung daily, ▸Chap. 2.2.1). Medicinally we can consider Equisetum arvense in a low potency (D2, D3) to begin with. Here silicic acid – Equisetum species can have a silicic acid content of 40 to 70 percent in their ash – is present in the plant in highly concentrated form as opal combined with a relatively high content of *sulphur.* It is precisely the vitality of sulphur which is missing in these children, and thus we can see the *horsetail as a kind of model for combining silicic acid with sulphur.*

One possible course of action is

- **Equisetum Silicea cultum Rh D3 dil.** Weleda
  5 gtt. 3–4 x/d (alcohol-free! – cf. ▸Chap. 1.2.2) for 2–4 weeks, then
- **Quarz D6 trit.** Weleda
  1 saltsp. 3 x/d for 4–6 weeks, then
- **Quarz D20 trit.** Weleda/**D20 pillules** Wala
  1 saltsp. 1 x/d or 3 pillules 1 x/d for 4–6 weeks.

In acute infections in this early phase of life Pulsatilla is frequently the indicated medicine, not infrequently in alternation with Ferrum phosphoricum.

If the metabolism is to be supported to an even greater extent, (e. g. if there is clear underweight in s/p small gestational age birth), the following potentized organ preparation is particularly suitable

- **Organum quadruplex comp. amp.** Wala
  0.3–0.5 ml of the amp. 1 x/d–3 × weekly administered per os

and, if Quarz D20 is given in the evening, the following as a complementary medicine

- **Abrotanum D1–3 dil.** custom-made by e. g. Apotheke an der Weleda
  2–3 gtt. 1–2 x/d (relatively mild bitter tolerated by children – for mechanism of action cf. [Vademecum 2010, 869])

As the risk of rickets may not become apparent so quickly in the Silicea constitution, we emphasize that clear signs of this constitution are an indication for preventive treatment with the above medicines or another form of Silicea therapy. It is further worth noting that these children react with particular sensitivity to *vaccination* – and that Silicea D30, 3 pillules given immediately and possibly 12 h following vaccination, is the best medicine to prevent vaccination side-effects. In any event, from a constitutional perspective it is clear that the various constitutions respond with different degrees of sensitivity to vaccination. Since in the typical Silicea constitution the nervous and sensory system dominates – something which also comes to expression in the dominant forehead and eye area – and on the other hand the metabolism remains relatively weak, corresponding to the delicate lower jaw, there is a particular susceptibility for sustained irritation of the nervous system (e. g. sleep disturbance, shrill screaming during the night, restlessness following vaccination) and simultaneous further blockages of the immune system (e. g. candidiasis following vaccination, elevated frequency of infections of the airways, etc.). For the metabolic quality of the pathogen is also weakened in the vaccine while the aim is to imprint the immune system's "memory": what might be described as a perception without oneself becoming metabolically active – e. g. in the form of a fever. This character of vaccination touches on the weak point of Silicea as the substance itself has the tendency to develop insufficient metabolic activity in relationship to the perception.

3.2.5.3 Calcium phosphoricum; Calcium fluoratum (Fluorite)

Another important constitutional medicine is pure calcium phosphate

- **Calcium phosphoricum LM6** Arcana, **C12 pillules** Gudjons
  2 gtt. or 3 pillules 1 x/d in infancy and early childhood

Children who need this medicine to assist their constitution are often overlooked to begin with: frequently their problems only develop in the transition from infancy to early childhood and increase until they reach school age. The risk of rickets is considerably less. A constitutional characteristic is that these children on the one hand have a tendency for *lymphatic reactions*: large lymph nodes primarily in the neck, but a slender neck, large tonsils which can be rimous quite early on, and a clear *sensitivity to cold* like Calc. carb. in accordance with the lymphatic constitution. On the other hand the appetite is variable and there is a tendency of *frequent paroxysmal stomach pain* and later of frequent *headaches*. They sweat less, mostly on the back of the neck. The tendency for rickets tends to exist more in the thorax and particularly the limbs (which is why this medicine can be found in Kent's Repertory as typical for greatly delayed learning to walk). Psychologically these children are significantly more alert, curious and willing to explore as early as infancy than the Calcium carbonicum constitution.

The problem arises not so much from the one-sided dominance of one pole than from the difficult or unsuccessful penetration of the formative forces coming from the head and the vital metabolic dynamism resident in the body. The latter is managed much better than in Calcium carbonicum, but a constantly alternating predominance of the nervous and sensory pole on the one hand (wakefulness, intellectual development) and the metabolic processes on the other (coming to expression in lymphatism and also the headaches) can occur in these children. The appetite changes accordingly. Without constitutional treatment this conflict between the nervous and sensory and the metabolic poles can manifest later in very pronounced cases as aseptic bone necrosis in which the equilibrium of blood supply and bone formation breaks down (for example in the region of the femoral head in Perthes' disease; ▸Chap. 9.4.1). The disposition for idiopathic scoliosis is also elevated in this constitution (▸Chap. 9.3.3). This inner contradiction of these inherently active children therefore threatens specifically the areas of the skeleton associated with great mobility while craniotabes in particular, i. e. an ossification disorder in the completely immobile parts of the skeleton, is typical for Calcium carbonicum. Calcium carbonicum is obtained from the completely rigid oyster shell (exoskeleton) while phosphate is involved in the development of the skeleton in fishes; and it is precisely in the fishes that a highly segmented, flexible endoskeleton starts to develop; fish (salmon or eels, for example) turn into "curious" sea creatures who travel long distances and who are very alert in comparison to the molluscs. Calcium phosophoricum therefore comprises great mobility in relation to the human constitution but also changeability, prematurity (e. g. of intellectual development) and delay (e. g. of dentition). Great length growth with little weight gain, a slim figure with pronounced lymphatism exist simultaneously, alongside one another. The therapeutic goal is to actively support a balance of these tendencies in the first five to seven years of life; only then can the spine properly develop in school age which otherwise reflects the imbalance, the failure of the nervous and sensory and the metabolic poles to penetrate one another.

Finally, we refer to *Calcium fluoratum (fluorite)*. Premature, excessively strong mineralization, early dentition, noticeably large and dense teeth, hypermobile joints and a rather smaller head which hardens early is characteristic of these children. They are often inwardly restless and not very impressionable which can turn into a considerable social and educational problem. From a constitutional perspective they are not at risk of rickets; substitution with vitamin D or indeed fluoride can reinforce their pathological tendencies. Here it is important to revitalize the fluid vital element, the etheric body, and counteract the premature development of the body.

The administration of the following is suitable for this purpose to begin with

- **Argentit D6 trit.** Weleda
  1 saltsp. 1–3 x/d

followed by the administration of

- **Fluorit D12 trit.** Weleda
  1 × 1 saltsp./d in the morning and
- **Magnesium fluoratum D12**
  1 × 3–5 pillules in the evening.

Children with this constitution can graphically illustrate the problems which can arise from undifferentiated general preventive treatment for rickets.

3.2.6 Rickets treatment

Phosphorus as potentized medicine is located at the boundary between prevention and treatment of rickets. Phosphorus means the bearer of light. And therapeutically we can experience in a very impressive way how this substance can very strongly influence the activation of light in the child's organism – not just in a positive way! We referred above to the way that the action of sunlight in the child's metabolism promotes the mineralization of the skeleton; how the child adopting an upright posture, but also the reduction of sleep, of pure anabolism is connected with that. Phosphorus in deep – also in very subtly diluted – potencies enhances this action of the formative forces which are intimately connected with the human I. The physiology of the vitamin D metabolism up to and including its immunological importance makes the therapeutic effectiveness of phosphorus clear and comprehensible: for deep phosphorus potencies reinforce this process, promote immunological competence precisely in the region of the lung and the efferent urinary tract and support the ossification of the skeleton particularly in the region of the thorax and the extremities, the action of light in the metabolism.

This effect is particularly apparent in the season of the year with the least light. Parents several times told us that they had the impression after administering phosphorus that the eyes of their child, which were dull and matt, started to "shine" again – while medically a clearly increasing resistance against infections could be observed.

Phosphorus is certainly not just a medicine for the phosphorus constitution within the meaning of homoeopathy. On the contrary, the above action can benefit very many children whereas constitutional "phosphorus children" are rare. But with the wrong dosage the danger very quickly arises that the children become too alert, develop restlessness and sleep disturbance and can severely drop out of their harmony. Hence phosphorus should not be given without a clear indication. Slight craniotabes, in particular, *without* general signs of rickets such as sleep disturbance, greater perspiration, etc. (see above) is *not* necessarily a phosphorus indication. On the contrary, this is given if

- there is a general threat of rickets developing,
- there is the risk of a serious infection of the airways (threat of pneumonia with weak resistance, season with little light) or the tendency for urinary tract infections,
- ossification in the region of the thorax and the extremities is lagging
- the child in general gives the impression of a lack of light.

Here the LM potencies have once again proved very effective for us:

- **Phosphorus LM6** Arcana
  1 × 1–2 gtt./d in the morning in a little spring water.

The following composite medicine complements phosphorus

- **Rose Iron (Roseneisen)/Graphit pillules** Wala
  3–5 pillules 1 x/d in the afternoon (can be given up to 3 pillules 3 x/d)

This medicine often leads to a stabilization of appetite, promotes motor development and obtaining an upright posture in the first year of life as well as stabilising relapsing infections of the airways.

If the occurrence of craniotabes is observed with an increase in sweating (not every craniotabes can simply be assessed as being related to rickets – it is always essential to include the overall state), the administration of the following has proved its worth alongside the specified constitutional and general treatment possibilities

- **Cichorium Plumbo cultum Rh D3 dil.** Weleda
  3–5 gtt. 3 x/d

We prefer the aqueous potentization of chicory, Cichorium intybus, in which previously a lead salt was herbally processed and pre-potentized, as it were, within a three year period (▸Chap. 1.2.2), to the use of a lead ointment.

If there are already signs of childhood rickets the substitution of calcium (!) and vitamin D is of course the primary treatment. In additional we will briefly refer to some treatment possibilities beyond these measures here.

In addition to calcium and vitamin D, the frequent administration of

- **Conchae 5 % trit.** Weleda can have a stabilising effect.

The most important external treatment is regular **sulphur baths** every second day, best in the late afternoon (▸Chap. 3.2.5.1). This can further be supported by

- **Hypophysis/Stannum pillules** Wala
  3–5 pillules 3 x/d
- **Roseneisen (Rose Iron)/Graphit pillules** Wala
  3 × 3 pillules.

and the constitutionally most effect medicine in deep potency.

We would emphasize once again here that careful continuous preventive care, linked with the most individually tailored rickets prophylaxis based only on indications, makes such states of manifest rickets extremely unlikely. They do, however, remain a possibility. If there is uncertainty in preventive care, the indication e. g. for laboratory clarification (Ca, phosphate, AP, Vit. D_3–25(OH) etc.) should be generously set.

In closing it should still be mentioned that *regional* differences (even between northern and southern Germany) are of great importance in rickets prevention and treatment. The intensity of the sunlight but also the consistency of the soil (sandy or calcareous) and the atmosphere (e. g. many foggy days) create specific conditions which produce a risk of rickets in children which is regionally very different. This is only one example of the way in which the doctor has to know and take account of the locational qualities and for that reason alone cannot simply take on the way of working of a colleague working somewhere completely different.

3.2.7 Sun protection and vitamin D deficiency in children and teenagers

The introductory observations in ▸Chap. 3 as well as ▸Chap. 3.2.1 to ▸Chap. 3.2.3 set out the key considerations with regard to this subject which will only be briefly summarized here for practice:

- A sunlight (and exercise) anamnesis is a key part of a preventive medical checkup when there are unclear disorders, susceptibility to infection and chronic-inflammatory diseases. *Vitamin D deficiency can occur at any age, including among adolescents, and requires intervention.*
- *Advice on sun protection* should be given regularly as the recommendations made by the media, pharmaceutical industry and government can have a detrimental effect on the children and adolescents concerned (toxic hormonal side effects of chemical sun protection factors, vitamin D deficiency, etc.)
- The goal should be sufficient time spent outside in appropriate clothing, with sufficient exposure of the skin to light, avoidance of sunburn above all through textile protection, shades, choosing the right time to spend outside during the height of summer (avoidance of midday) and in the transitional months (benefit of midday), *active exercise in light, natural adaptation to the local sunshine without sunscreen* to the extent permitted by skin type and the time exposed to the sun.
- Use of sunscreen with physical sun protection factors and antioxidants in situations where the (unaccustomed, extended) exposure to the sun makes this necessary to avoid sunburn. This applies e. g. with regard to visiting high mountains, the beach in swimwear, etc.
- Eating food with high vitamin D content in seasons when there is less light (pollack, eggs from free-range chickens, avocado, veal, etc.)
- Advice adjusted for skin type: children with a Mediterranean skin type hardly ever develop sunburn but require longer in the sun while children with a Celtic skin type require careful measures to prevent sunburn but quickly develop higher vitamin D levels in sunlight.

3.3 Vitamin K prophylaxis

Vitamin K, like vitamin D, is a fat-soluble substance which has a far-reaching effect on the developmental processes in the human organism. In the plant world it serves the process of photosynthesis as phylloquinone (vitamin K_1), thereby enabling a sunlight-dependent process for the development of substance and form: we can see an initial affinity with vitamin D. In his account of vitamin K prophylaxis, Madeleyn [2005] refers to the work of Iwamato et al. [2004] which shows that during growth the production of osteocalcin, a bone matrix substance with great affinity to apatite, is dependent on vitamin K and that the administration of vitamin K can increase bone mass at this age. The direction in which vitamin K works in the animal and human organism is thus related to vitamin D. Atherocalcin is also a vitamin K-dependent protein: "Atherocalcin is probably connected with the development of atherosclerosis" [Biesalski 1997, 63]. Vitamin K was present in the cord blood of 156 newborns only in extremely low levels or not measurably at all and maternal vitamin K levels do not correlate with the content in cord blood. It is clear that the placenta ensures extremely low vitamin K levels in the foetus [Greer 2010, incl. review of the literature]. The importance of vitamin K for a sufficient measure of blood clotting clearly starts with the birth, the "landing", of the human being and is held back in the weightlessness of the "cosmic" foetal world. The problem area of vitamin K prophylaxis thus presents itself before the transition between these two so different phases of human development.

Bile acids are involved in the absorption of vitamin K. Vitamin K is hydroxylated to its biologically active form in the liver and then enables the carboxylation of the vitamin K-dependent clotting proteins (factor II, VII, IX, X, C and S proteins); in vitamin K deficiency "they appear as inactive clotting proteins in the blood" [Biesalski 1997] and display a vitamin D deficiency as "PIVKA-II". There is not yet a secure method to diagnose a vitamin K deficiency in newborns by determining PIVKA II [Greer 2010, 546].

Vitamin K prophylaxis in breast fed infants is motivated in that

- breast milk contains very low vitamin K levels (0.1–0.2 µg/100 ml – cow's milk contains a level which is approx. seven times higher (comparable with the higher calcium and phosphate content of cow's milk). It is worth noting that human breast milk itself clots much more finely in the gastro-intestinal tract than cow's milk.
- vitamin K deficiency bleeding can occur in *purely breast fed infants* in approx. one in 10,000 children, which in a third takes the form of serious, often lethal brain haemorrhage. Here the delayed intracranial bleeding following the neonatal period is particularly feared.
- *Breast fed children with cholestasis* are particularly affected by delayed bleeding, also when given 1 mg vitamin K solution after birth and daily substitution of 25 µg of vitamin K. While 25 of 30 Dutch breast fed children with biliary atresia suffered delayed bleeding under this regime, it was only one of 88 bottle-fed children. A satisfactory screening for these children among newborns does not yet exist. They can only be protected through extremely high-dosage vitamin K prophylaxis (2 mg after birth and 12 weeks of 1 mg weekly per os or 1 × 1 mg i.m.).

Eating green vegetables (chlorophyll), olive oil, oats, fresh green salad, carrots and broccoli can raise the vitamin K level of breast milk. The following influences can promote vitamin K deficiency in breast milk (loc.cit.):

- nutritional deficiency and malnutrition, e.g. lack of green vegetables,
- hepatotoxic medicines, above all anticonvulsants, tuberculostatics, thyrostatics,
- laxatives,
- diseases of the liver and bile ducts, coeliac disease, chronic inflammatory bowel diseases
- antibiotics. [Biesalski 1997, 63ff.].

The hepatobiliary system and intestinal digestion and absorption are thus also of relevance in the mother and must be investigated through anamnesis.

The issue is why the vitamin K level of breast milk is regulated so low in the correspondence between mother and child. The newborn's blood clotting system which, although functionally equivalent, displays considerable differences to the adult, undergoes a thorough transformation in the first weeks of life and only then is there an adaptation to the situation (and factor concentrations in the blood) with which we are familiar in the adult. This transition is partially controlled by the breast milk in the slow and, in comparison to animals, deferred way characteristic of humans: the form-giving processes of the human being in infancy are thereby without doubt held open for longer than in animal physiology which also gives rise to the possibility of vitamin K deficiency bleeding in rare single cases. Toxicity through the vitamin K solutions used today is not known [Greer 2010, 546]. The question as to whether the parenteral administration of high doses of vitamin K in the neonatal period is associated with an elevated incidence of leukaemia in childhood has not been proved, but neither has it been disproved [Golding et al. 1992, Klebanoff et al. 1993].

The research of Rudolf Steiner and Ita Wegman [Steiner and Wegman 1991, 87] on blood clotting can provide an important reference with regard to a deeper understanding of this issue: "The *development* of the organism is essentially a transformation of the protein substance so that the latter is able to work together with the mineralizing forces. These are contained in calcium, for example." But that precisely is the function of vitamin K in blood clotting, to enable the interaction of clotting factors with calcium through decarboxylation processes, thus allowing stable (red) thrombus formation. In the same passage Steiner and Wegman point out that the process of blood clotting in humans is regulated under the influence of the I-organization. In this connection it is also worth looking at the physiological development of humans in its specific chronological character, referred to above, its "retardation" in comparison to animals, which is also an expression of the action of the human I-organization [Verhulst 1999]. We can see the motif that the form-giving and fixing processes, which are linked to the substance of calcium, are retarded in the human organism both in bone development (low vitamin D level in breast milk) and in blood clotting *in order to allow for the greatest individualization in the development of the body.* That precisely is where the problem emerges with regard to the current paediatrically favoured general preventive measures in childhood: vitamin D, vitamin K and fluoride as a joint collective measure one-sidedly promote the early solidification of the child's organism, and they do so by means of a substitution which overrules the individual regulation of the organism. On the other hand vitamin K deficiency bleeding, which can end terminally in its intractability, is a serious complication which today can be largely prevented.

The doctor and parents must decide what course to take. The corresponding parent guide [Vagedes and Soldner 2010, 40–42] and information sheet [cf. Leitlinie und Merkblatt zum Thema Vitamin-K-Prophylaxe 2009] offer basic information which can help to prepare a decision in consultation with the doctor. The following applies with regard to healthy full-term neonates:

- The oral prophylaxis recommended in Germany with the triple oral administration of 2 mg vitamin K, and particularly the Danish/Dutch pattern of 2 mg administered postnatally and the weekly administration of 1 mg per os for 12 weeks (see above), work with unphysiological doses which are far removed from the model of human physiology. They are reasonable above all if there is an elevated risk of a vitamin K deficiency, be it because of *maternal disorders* (e. g. antibiotics, taking anticonvulsants etc.), or because of disorders in the child (in so far as the latter do not require parenteral administration). Furthermore, the Danish/Dutch pattern is the safest one if delayed bleeding in children with cholestasis is also to be avoided. In order to recognize children with cholestasis at the earliest possible stage, determining the direct bilirubin is recommended in breast fed children with icterus at the age of 2 weeks [Benchimol 2009]. As there are indications, and it also corresponds to the physiological ratio of vitamin K resorption, that (also subclinical) restrictions of gall function (with elevated AP values) foster a vitamin K deficiency (in the sense of reduced resorption of fat-soluble substances), vitamin K prophylaxis is indicated above all in instances in which restrictions or stresses on gall function may be assumed in the neonatal period. More severe or prolonged icterus or the administration of hepatotoxic medicines may already point in this direction.
- Very much more physiological is the procedure, also previously practised in Holland, with the administration of 1 mg vitamin K after birth and a daily prophylaxis with the administration of 25 µg (= 2 drops) of a formulation prepared in the pharmacy:

Vit. K1 – oily solution	*12.5 g/gtt.*
Phytomenadione (Ph. Eur.)	6.26 mg
Ol. Amygdalarum	ad 20.00 g

  which remains usable for twelve weeks when stored in a cool, dark place. Further details on its production and a possible source of supply with experience in producing it is offered by the See-Apotheke Bodolz (www.seeapotheke.de) pharmacy [Massag 2005]. The administration of 1 mg post partum serves to prevent early bleeding.
- Finally, the parents of healthy newborns also have the possibility of rejecting such preventive treatment and avoiding the early administration of substances other than breast milk. Their argument might be that the correspondence between the breast feeding mother and infant, developed over long evolutionary periods, is probably optimally adjusted for the interaction between the physical and soul-spiritual individuality of the human being and that risks such as foetal vitamin K deficiency bleeding lie in a probability range which applies to almost every action in everyday life (way to school, travelling in a car, etc.) as a background risk and dimension of human destiny. Neither has the safety question yet been resolved through long-term comparative studies. If it should turn out, for example, that early high doses of vitamin K entail serious long-term consequences for the infant thus treated, and be it in small percentages, a risk of side-effects of one in a thousand or less might nevertheless be of high relevance given an NNT (number needed to treat) of 1:10,000 for this measure. If parents decide to proceed along this path – after being thoroughly informed about the risks – such a preventive decision should as a rule be accepted by the doctor. In this context the doc-

tor should particularly refer to vitamin K-rich foods (see above), which have been shown to increase the vitamin K content in the mother, as well as determining and observing known and possible risk factors for the heightened incidence of vitamin K deficiency with particular care.
- Separate preventive recommendations apply with regard to premature babies and children with an early diagnosis of chronic diseases which go beyond the present framework.

Prevention from the perspective of anthroposophic medicine must above all take the activity of the I-organization into account (▸Chap. 3.2). The I-organization works not just in the development of consciousness but in the whole of the human organism. The action of the I-organization in the metabolic sphere, which is relevant for human will development ("cholerics"!), is set out in greater detail in ▸Chap. 4. Here the intervention of the I-organization in the hepatobiliary sphere is of particular importance: "The development of the liver and gall bladder proceeds wholly in parallel with the strength of the I-organization received by the human being" [Steiner 1989, 114]. At this point Rudolf Steiner refers to "lethal pathological states in childhood" which are connected with biliary secretions. A risk is clearly contained in the insufficient intervention of the I-organization in this sphere (shock experiences associated with birth might also play a role here). The infant's vitamin K resorption is just as much dependent on the healthy maturation of the infant's hepatobiliary function as on the corresponding situation in the gastro-intestinal tract of the maternal organism.

3

The following is suitable to stimulate the maturation of the hepatobiliary function in newborns with regard to the I-organization
- **Chelidonium Ferro cultum Rh D3** Weleda
  2–3 gtt. 3 x/d before breast feeding (alcohol-free).

This medicine may be indicated particularly in protractedly icteric breast fed infants (for details on this aspect cf. ▸Chap. 4.3.3). The possible diagnosis of these children were referred to above. This medication represents a complementary perspective in diagnosis and treatment which should not be understood as a replacement for the administration of vitamin K but as a look at the individualized developmental process which is implicit in this topic.

3.4 Questions concerning general fluoride prophylaxis – tooth delay prevention and dental disorders

It is normal paediatric practice today to hand parents a prescription, unasked, as part of the second preventive medical checkup (U 2) which provides for the daily administration of a combination of 500 IU vitamin D and 0.25 mg fluoride. In parallel there is normally the second oral administration of vitamin K (2 mg), corresponding to approx. 600–700 times the dosage which the infant takes in per day at this point physiologically through breast milk. There is no information about the fluoride content of breast milk in the standard works of paediatrics [Lentze and Schaub et al. 2003, Speer and Gahr 2009]. New studies [Yamur et al. 2007] show a fluoride content in breast milk of 0.006 to 0.017 ppm

[Chuckpaiwong 2000]. The current paediatric guideline on the administration of fluoride to infants in Germany recommends 0.25 mg/d – 15–40 times the amount of normal fluoride concentration in breast milk – and that daily! – from the fifth day of life [DGKJ 2010, B 5–4]. This contrasts with the recommendations of the specialist group responsible for dental health: "From the perspective of dental medicine, the systemic administration of fluoride is no longer indicated today except in exceptional cases" [Speer and Gahr 2009, 912]. In the same textbook S. Koletzko emphasizes "the very effective reduction both of the number and extent of carious lesions" [loc. cit. 75] without dealing with the content or possible deficiency of fluoride in breast milk. The fluoride concentration in cord blood is controlled by the placenta, the fluoride concentration in breast milk is largely independent of food and drinking water. The scientific panel of the European Food Safety Authority EFSA notes in its opinion: "Fluoride content of the body is not under physiological control." [EFSA 2005]. This is contradicted, on the one hand, by the facts as set out and scientific studies which show that the fluoride content in the embryo and infant is precisely regulated at a low level as long as such regulation is not disrupted from outside through unphysiological doses. On the other hand we can concur with the EFSA opinion to the extent that in exogenic fluoride intake (fluoride tablets or swallowing fluoride-containing toothpaste) the resorption rate in infants (90 %) and small children is very high and the organism – as is shown by the example of dental fluorosis acquired in the first three years of life – cannot compensate for the too high intake of fluoride *because of insufficient self-regulation in this case.* The EFSA currently accepts, for example, that children in the first three years of life are given quantities of fluoride through normal prophylaxis today which trigger moderate dental fluorosis in 5 % of the affected children. In this context it must be pointed out that *it is generally agreed that caries is not a diseases arising from a fluoride deficiency* (analogously to rickets resulting from a deficiency of vitamin D for example) [Hirte 2007, 295]. On the contrary, there is a good argument to say that the low fluoride intake of the breast fed infant is an essential component of the food which Koletzko calls "the ideal food for the healthy infant in the first year of life" [loc. cit. 68]: human breast milk. Koletzko emphasizes in the same passage: "There are impressive recent study results which link food intake and growth in early childhood with the risk of illness in old age." Rudolf Steiner was the first to emphasize as long ago as the 1920 s that one would not necessarily see the difference between children brought up on breast milk or on artificial, cow's milk-based infant food immediately but that it would clearly emerge at the age of 65 [Steiner 1999b, 188] and that then sclerosis (Steiner: "calcification") would occur in those children who had not been fed breast milk. This view is confirmed today. But so far no one has undertaken a long-term study to compare infants with unphysiological vitamin K and fluoride substitution and infants fed breast milk. It is evident that the untargeted, generalized administration of fluoride to infants is a mass experiment which lacks any evidence as to its long-term effect.

The question which has to be asked here is: what path does this enormously elevated and clearly unphysiological fluoride concentration take in the developing organism? And here we can see that the majority of the fluoride with which the organism is preventively flooded travels into the skeleton (and is incorporated into the apatite there instead of hydroxyl ions). The activity of the osteoblasts is stimulated and ossification speeded up. The more fluoride the bone contains, the more brittle it becomes (something that has been shown by research on fluoride treatment for osteoporosis): "Fluoride accretion in bone increases bone density but excessive long term intake reduces bone strength and increases risk of fracture and skeletal fluorosis (stiffness of joints, skeletal deformities)." [EFSA 2005]. At the same time these bones are less accessible for osteoclasts which inhibits the catabolic and transformation processes in the skeleton of essential importance in growth.

Children who have taken fluoride tablets display dental fluorosis more frequently (paralleled by concordant skeletal changes!) than children who were only treated with toothpaste containing fluoride [Schütte 2003, 16, Hetzer 1999]. The influence of the young age of the child, in particular, on fluorosis development has been documented [Levy et al. 2010, Burt 2000]. Dental fluorosis clearly shows that the administration of fluoride causes the child to age more, that it introduces a sclerotic quality into the skeleton which is built up by the child out of his or her I-organization as he or she creates his or her form [cf. on this perspective of anthroposophic medicine Girke 2010, 41–44]. Thus the generalized administration of fluoride tends to *speed up the ossification and inhibition of skeletal* plasticity. *Here the summation effect arising from the interaction of vitamin K doses working on the skeleton* (▸Chap. 3.3) *and vitamin D substitution throughout the year should be observed, indicating a speeding up and qualitative transformation of ossification and dentition.*

At this point we can note that the development of the human form is the expression of a *retardation* in comparison to animal development. The I-organization makes itself felt in human skeletal development in that it keeps it open for longer (e.g. the fontanelles in apes close at about birth, in humans at 1–1½ years: this allows the brain to evolve in the first year of life.) This retardation is shown particularly in the development of the teeth and the change of dentition: The change of dentition starts in

- macaques at 1½ years
- gorillas, chimpanzees at 3 years
- humans at 6–7 years.

The growth of the anterior dental arch stops in human beings at the age of 2–3, their jaw does not develop into a snout and the anterior dental arch retains its shape at the time of language acquisition. This brief sketch should indicate to the reader that one should first understand the specifically human physiology of ossification and dentition before any medical intervention. What is clear in any event is that the regulation of fluoride intake through the placenta and breast milk is precisely coordinated with this slow form of ossification which is specific to humans. Looked at from this aspect, we have to reach the conclusion that the early fluoridation of the infant ignores the activity of the human I-organization in its anabolic activity. If we consider that the metabolism in the sphere of the mineralization of the skeleton works with far greater intensity in the child than in an adult, we can appreciate that the process of skeleton development and formation takes place in a different way if the fluoride content in the skeleton and the teeth rises. No research has yet taken place into the consequences for the joints.

There are references to a negative influence on the fertility of women and men in regions with high concentrations of fluoride in the drinking water [Freni 1994]. It was possible to show in animal experiments that there is an inhibition of testicle function following the long-term administration of fluoride [Chinoy 1992, 1994] and there are even references to an elevated incidence of osteosarcomas under fluoridation [Hoover et al. 1991] – osteosarcomas occur above all in the skeletal regions with the greatest dynamic growth. If this alarming information is confirmed, it would be another indication of the possible negative influences of the administration of fluoride on ossification in humans. Hirte [2007, 290–297] cites further risks.

All these things are being done without adequate information for parents: they are only told about dental caries without the systemic consequences of the administration of fluoride ever, as a rule, being mentioned. Anyone who perceives the physical form of the human being also as an expression of his or her soul being, who understands the development of the skeleton as an essential body-forming activity of the human individuality, *will also be able to see the risk of alienating the physical body from the individuality which ensouls it through the generalized, unphysiologically elevated administration of fluoride to infants; because physical solidification, undertaken from the outside and uniformly speeded up, may at the same time be compromised in its quality.*

Case study

A twelve-year-old patient at the time displayed moderate dental fluorosis on her incisors following the common vitamin D-fluoride prophylaxis in early childhood. At the age of fourteen, a devitalization in the dental root of three teeth occurs in this patient at an interval of approx. 2 months between each occasion – despite immediate dental intervention. It is suspected that the root has also been affected as part of a dental fluorosis. On consultation with our colleague Markus Sommer the latter proposes a homoeopathic treatment which has proved itself in fluoride damage:

- **Magensium fluoratum D12**
  5 pillules 1–2 x/d.

Following administration of this medicine for 6 months, there is no further root damage in the teeth of this patient. Then the medicine is discontinued. Only six weeks later the root dies off in a fourth tooth. Since then the patient has been undertaking continuous treatment with Magnesium fluoratum D12 for the last 18 months and has been free of further inflammatory and degenerative changes of the dental roots.

Ex juvantibus this case study can make clear that the tooth itself becomes sclerotic under the administration of fluoride: sometimes to the extent that it prematurely loses its living connection with the whole of the organism.

If we look at the quality of fluorine as an element, an aggressive reactivity oriented towards solidification (highest electron negativity of all elements) is revealed which produces a passivated fluoride in combination with the respective reaction partner which is very difficult to attack chemically (thus the purpose of the fluoridation of corticosteroids is also to delay their break down by the organism as much as possible). This quality of extracting the substance from a living interplay of combination and dissolution and giving it a solid form is in principle a *sclerotizing* quality. The fluoride content of breast milk is correspondingly small and is composed in such a way *that the infant remains capable of development, above all.* Physiologically the fluoride content in human bone gradually increases with age in parallel with the ageing process. *On the other hand this quality of fluorine is physiologically present in the development of dental enamel*[1]: In contrast to the osteoblasts which make the bones, the adamantoblasts which make the enamel die off

1 Cf. Steiner [1999a], 319: "Then we can see that overcoming chemical properties in this way, working towards pure mineralization, is really the same as the process which develops the teeth in the organism."

completely by the age of eight – also a fluorine quality. Thus it is no surprise that dental enamel becomes more resistant to acid and thus to caries when it absorbs fluoride. But it does so above all through saliva and the topical use of e.g. fluoride toothpaste [Stösser 2008].

The *homoeopathic* perspective is of significance as expressed in the *medicinal picture of Calcium fluoratum* (= fluorite). Here we can distinguish between two types, one which has included too little of this substance in his or her physical development and one which is governed too much by it. The latter displays strikingly large teeth which often erupt at an early stage; psychologically these children are often not very impressionable, of "singular contentment" [Borland 1961, 37–39] and not very sensitive also in respect of their own illnesses (▸Chap. 3.2.5.3). The fluoride deficiency type, on the other hand, tends towards defective enamel, early caries, severe weakness of the connective tissue and driven, jerky aimless activity. The common element between them is the *lack of animated movement and sentience*: This is a significant trait which makes the homoeopath consider potentized fluoride (Calcium fluoratum and other fluoride salts). The fluorine quality comes to expression most radically from a homoeopathic perspective in the medicinal picture of Acidum fluoricum. In his inspiring "Homöopathie und Minerale", Scholten [1993, 173f.] characterizes it in a way which has also repeatedly proved its worth in practice for the authors when arriving at an indication for prescribing a homoeopathic fluoride salt: an emphasis on materialist values, rapid movement, also driven sporting activity, "*hard, fast, urgency*". Such a characteristic can make one stop and think as a doctor about the consequences for the child of the iatrogenic adjustment of the fluoride balance. Husemann [Husemann 2010, 42–64] gives a profound account from the perspective of anthroposophic medicine of the physiological importance of fluorine for childhood development, including a case study with Acidum fluoricum.

- **Magnesium fluoratum D12** pillules DHU
  3–5 pillules 1–2 x/d
- **Argentit D6 trit.** Weleda
  1 saltsp. 1–2 x/d

have a balancing effect if we want to undertake follow-up treatment in children treated with fluoride. In addition, Argentit has particularly proved its worth in children with excess doses of vitamin D.

3.4.1 Tooth decay prevention

It is difficult to start with the individual perception of the child in the field of caries prophylaxis, as the development of the permanent crowns is hidden in the first seven years of life. On the other hand, early childhood caries possesses predictive importance with regard to the permanent teeth [Stösser 2008, incl. references]. Is the child specifically at risk of caries? Is a healthy diet and careful oral hygiene sufficient or is medicinal prophylaxis indicated?

On the basis of the practical experience of the authors, the following perspectives arise with regard to an assessment of the *caries risk*:

- Family anamnesis (caries of the parents and siblings). This aspect (of the inherited body) is very important.

- Premature and small gestational age babies.
- Early childhood rickets. Its avoidance is central to successful caries prophylaxis.
- Children who "went to sleep with the bottle for a long time"
- Physical constitution: delicate children or children who appear robust but are nevertheless easily susceptible to illness (for therapeutic possibilities cf. ▸Chap. 3.2.5).
- Psychologically, children are mainly at risk of caries who are inwardly restless and (often secretly) anxious, have a tendency to withdraw inwardly but cannot come to rest either. Typical in this respect is also, for example, the tendency to develop throat inflammations in kindergarten and at school as an expression of the psychological inability to cope in the social sphere. There is often a great addiction to sweet things in this group. But changes in the saliva, which plays a central role in the remineralization of the dental enamel, are also involved in the greater tendency of this group to develop caries. For saliva reflects the intervention of the soul entity in the physical entity.
- *Mouth breathing* represents another relevant risk factor. "If the teeth remain dry", above all during the night, the central remineralization through the saliva is missing which is only guaranteed if the child breathes through the nose.
- Intellectually, very intelligent children are often particularly affected by caries (they are also fond of sweet things). This aspect will be discussed in greater detail below (cf. indication for quartz in this chapter).
- We often find extremes among children with psychomotor retardation (large, completely caries-free teeth or very rapidly progressing tooth decay).

As early as his first medical course, Rudolf Steiner pointed to the importance of "starting to observe the dental development of the child from the first tooth onwards, whether he or she develops less enamel or has a tendency for small teeth to grow" [Steiner 1999a, 242]; and he pointed here particularly to the importance of *fluorine and Magnesium* in preventing caries. More modern research has shown independently that a certain ratio of fluorine and Magnesium is required for the optimum development of tooth enamel.[1]

In the experience of the authors over many years and after numerous experiments, certain mineral medicines in low potencies, as a rule, have proved their value in preventing caries, including in specific compounds containing Magnesium and fluorine. The first to mention is

- **Apatit D6 trit.** Weleda
  1 saltsp. 2 x/d,

a complex compound of calcium with phosphates as well as hydroxyl, chloride and fluoride ions (▸Chap. 3.2.5), a substance which we already mentioned for the prevention of rickets. It also comprehensively supports the growth of the skeleton and the teeth without driving them in a one-sided direction.

Apatite itself contains various substance qualities in balance: the quality of fluorine, which aims to harden the fluidity of chemical processes in the mineral sphere; the quality of the phosphates, which enable the buildup of a hard but, in principle, soluble, transformable mineral substance in animals and humans; and the quality of calcium as basic substance of all mineralization processes in animals and humans. Finally, it is precisely the hydroxyl

1 We are grateful to our colleague Markus Sommer for this reference, too.

ions which point to the living origin of these mineral substances which only come about with animal life. The OH^- content of the hydroxyapatite in the organism is reduced with the amount of fluorine that is administered.

In contrast to the administration of fluoride, giving Apatite D6 does not involve any material substitution; on the contrary, it controls the mineralization of the teeth and skeleton in the sense that the various essential qualities in this respect are balanced and sustained in their effect. Apatite can (▸Chap. 3.2.5) be given to children at risk from early in the first year and it can be given for a long time.

An important medicine in caries prophylaxis, particularly if there is delayed dentition, a tendency for delicate or small growth and weak biliary function (fat digestion, soft stool consistency, light stool colour) is natural magnesium sulphate

- **Kieserit D4–6 dil.** Weleda
  3–5 gtt. 2–3 x/d

It speeds up dentition and promotes the process which Rudolf Steiner [1976, 241] summarizes for Magnesium in the image that through the action of Magnesium "that which is to be given a plastic form" (i. e. essentially the fluorine) is sufficiently available. Thus Magnesium sulfuricum activates the fluorine metabolism in the same way that sulphur does in respect of the silicic acid metabolism. At the same time low potentized magnesium sulphate intensifies the digestion processes through stimulating bile secretion.

Tooth enamel mineralization means the radical release of all energy from the crystallizing substance, a separation of the imponderables from ponderable matter, of the life forces from physical bodily nature. Rudolf Steiner points out in the above context that the organism can manage this all the better the more the imponderable penetrates the ponderable in another location, namely in the sphere of the metabolism and the abdomen; that is to say, the stronger the life organization wholly penetrates the physical substance of the body in those locations and keeps it in movement. If, on the other hand, a significant part of the maternal life forces, the metabolic energy in the sphere of the abdomen, is placed at the service of the child and not the mother's own body, the teeth and jaws begin to acquire "too much vitality" and to dissolve [Steiner 1976, 317]. An important role is clearly played here by changes in the saliva during pregnancy. Saliva occupies a key overall position with regard to the remineralization of the tooth enamel and dental health.

In practice it can be observed that *caries particularly increases when there is primarily too little vitality in the digestive organization* (indication for Magnesium sulf. or Kieserit) or the digestive processes become disordered for a longer period of time (tendency for diarrhoea, intestinal dysbiosis/mycosis, etc. – cf. ▸Chap. 4). Here the consumption of sweet things plays an important role; conversely, the desire for sweet things increases the weaker the digestive ability becomes. It is therefore an important *principle of caries prophylaxis to strengthen and order the digestive and metabolic processes.* It should be emphasized here that *nutrition*, giving the child solid food in good time early on, sufficient chewing, fresh fruit instead of fruit juices which attack enamel and intestinal flora (!), and a healthy amount (no fundamental ban) of sweet things are basic. Millet and oats represent particularly valuable cereals in the diet, vegetables preserved by spontaneous fermentation can stabilize healthy bacterial flora in the digestive tract and above all also in the mouth cavity itself. Instead of disinfecting mouth washes, as often recommended today, the authors tend to recommend giving a few fork-fulls of raw sauerkraut each day in the winter months from the age of three, for example, which together with its valuable content supports the oral flora and provides the intestine with valuable so-called roughage. Raw sauerkraut is one of the cheapest and most effective possibilities of "symbiotic control". The following is suitable as an external application which stimulates the vitality of the digestive organization

- **Chlorophyllum D1 ointment**, custom-made, e.g. by Apotheke an der Weleda
  massage into the stomach 2 x/wk-1 x/d (pea-sized quantity)
  [goes back to a suggestion from Rudolf Steiner; Vademecum 2010, 45]

Whereas Kieserit, i.e. natural magnesium sulphate, intensifies the digestion in low potencies, potentized sulphur

- **Sulphur LM6** Arcana
  3–5 gtt. 1 x/d

primarily has an ordering effect on the digestion and metabolism and reduces the desire for sweet things.

Sulphur intensifies the link between the life forces and the physical organism in the metabolic sphere and at the same time counters processes and impulses from the metabolic sphere which are active "in the wrong place": physically as inflammatory dissolving tendencies in the "nervous and sensory pole" (up to and including caries), psychologically through metabolically determined impulses such as e.g. a craving for sweet things, aggressiveness when hungry, etc. Sulphur is indicated as an interim medicine for some weeks if there is a strong craving for sweet things, a tendency for dysbiosis, flatulence, changing stools, s/p antibiotics and an excessive metabolism "in the wrong place", for example in the form of purulent inflammations of the skin or recurring inflammations of the airways.

If there is insufficient digestive activity in the child, the action of sulphur can be effectively supplemented with

- **Pancreas GI D4 amp.** Wala
  0.3–0.5 ml per os 1 x/d in the afternoon.

In view of the relationship already mentioned above between Magnesium and fluorine in the development of dental enamel,

- **Magnesium fluoratum D12 pillules** DHU, Staufen
  5 pillules 1 x/d,

mentioned above in ▸Chap. 3.3 represents an ideal guiding medicine. It can be given, preferably in the evening, over a long period of time (e.g. Apatite in the morning, Magnesium fluoratum in the evening). Mezger [1999], who, among all the homoeopathic doctors, has studied the magnesium salts most intensively and introduced Magnesium fluoratum in therapy, interestingly says that this medicine has an effect on the pancreas.

If there are clear anamnestical signs of considerable problems in the development of dental enamel, the authors recommend the supplementary administration of the following medicine for specific periods in the first seven years

- **Dens Gl D6 amp.** Wala
  0.5–1 ml per os 2 x/wk, for 9 months if possible in the first 3 years.

It has been shown that organ preparations in the first years of life can support anabolic processes in the organism with particular effectiveness. There have also been impressive experiences with the Dens preparation *when there has been traumatic loosening of the milk teeth*. We had the impression on several occasions that the threatening devitalization of the tooth could be avoided by this means. In such cases the dose is 0.5–1 ml per os 1–2 x/d.

One cause of caries lies in the equilibrium of digestive and limb activity and nervous and sensory activity increasingly being displaced: refined food and the absence of physical work and movement prevent the necessary engagement in the "metabolic pole" while at the same time people today are often greatly challenged in the intellectual sphere. Studies such as of the mountain farmers in the Alpine Goms valley in the Swiss canton of Valais [Goebel and Glöckler 1984, 375], where the state of the teeth among the inhabitants radically deteriorated after the valley was opened up through the Furka road leading to change of diet, provide evidence of this. The connection between the *ectodermally* formed tooth enamel and the nervous and sensory system are also of relevance here. Too great a stress on the nervous and sensory system is just as relevant for the development of caries as a primary weakness or culturally determined underload of the metabolic and limb system.

3

Potentized rock crystal is suitable for balancing the consequences of intellectual overload,

- **Quarz D12–20 pillules/trit.** Wala, Weleda
  5 pillules or 1 saltsp. 1 x/d in the morning (▸Chap. 3.2.5.2).

Has a complementary effect to potentized fluorine compounds.

Quarz is generally indicated when intellectual stress quickly leads to the exhaustion of the child's vital forces. We point out only in general that a constitutional treatment carried out with care and caution as well as the perception and therapeutic balancing of mental unrest and anxieties can also achieve a lot with regard to the tendency to develop caries. On the other hand we must caution that, for example, the too early or too frequent administration of very high potencies – particularly with regard to Calcium carbonicum and phosphorus – can lead to mineralization disorders.

Positive results are reported by dentists and paediatricians with regard to the early onset of caries and caries prophylaxis with

- **Aesculus, Cortex D50 dil.** (custom-made by Apotheke an der Weleda)/**pillules** (See Apotheke Bodolz seeapotheke@seeapotheke.de)
  3 pillules/gtt. (under age 2), 5 pillules/gtt. (under age 7) 1 x/d–3 x/wk each for approx. 7 weeks, then a break of 3–7 weeks [Vademecum 2010, 45–47]

This was proposed by Rudolf Steiner [Steiner 1999a, 318]: the potentized extract of the bark of the horse chestnut is intended to contribute to allowing the tooth enamel to solidify enough so that the vital chemical processes can be sufficiently damped down in favour of the necessary mineralization process. With regard to the associated treatment concept, cf. the quoted information in the Vademecum of Anthroposophic Medicines, second edition, 2010. The authors alternatively refer to the medicines set out in this contribution. They prefer pure apatite to the medicine Apatit/Phosphorus comp. (Weleda).

In practice, the doctor will give medicines such as sulphur and quartz for a set period, e.g. 4 to 6 weeks, whereas medicines such as Apatit or Magnesium fluoratum may also be necessary for a long period of time. ◘ Tab. 3.1 gives an overview of the various possibilities of caries prophylaxis.

◘ **Tab. 3.1** Overview of caries prophylaxis

Nervous and sensory system	Dentition process	Digestion and metabolism
▪ Quarz D12–20	▪ Apatit D6 ▪ Magnesium fluoratum D12	▪ Kieserit D4–6 ▪ Sulphur LM6 ▪ Pancreas Gl D5–8

In summary, the following should be taken into account with regard to caries prophylaxis:

- Adequate period of breast feeding in the first year which protects against caries.
- Prevention of rickets
- Dental care from the time that the teeth erupt, if possible without toothpaste or alternatively with a non-fluoridated toothpaste suitable for children, until the child is approx. 5 years old.
- If there is a greater risk of caries/evidence of plaque on the teeth, sparing use of a reduced-fluoride toothpaste suitable for children once a day in the evening, if possible not until the age when only a small amount of it will be swallowed (age 5)
- Avoidance of longer periods of breathing through the mouth.
- Avoidance of sucking on the bottle.
- Whole food, sufficiently long periods between meals, avoidance of cariogenic foods (which as a rule also involve a high glycaemic burden and thus the risk of obesity, for example).
- Regular dental checkups, but restraint with regard to excessive paediatric dental action. Not every recommendation is mandatory! As necessary, always choose topical fluoride applications over the systemic administration.

3.4.2 Delayed teething

In delayed teething – evident not just at its late occurrence but also in a certain stagnation of development and in typical teething-related problems which do not end with the eruption of the teeth –

- **Kieserit D6 dil.** Weleda
  3–5 gtt. 3 x/d

has proved successful. Constitutionally, the single administration of Conchae or Calcium carbonicum Hahnemanni LM6 to D30 and/or Silicea D6 to D30 is helpful in the first instance.

3.4.3 Teething troubles, difficult dentition syndrome

This area has largely become a field of parental self-medication today.

Proven medicines:

- **Chamomilla e rad. D6 pillules** Wala
- **Magnesium phosphoricum D6–12 pillules** DHU
- **Belladonna/Chamomilla pillules** Wala

5 pillules 1 x/nocte to 3 x/d each, acutely (at night) 5 pillules 3 × at short intervals.

- **Viburcol supp.** (indicated if there are purely pain symptoms), or
- **fever and teething supp.** Weleda (good experiences also in the first year of life, indicated if there are simultaneously signs of inflammation)

1–2 x/d each, above all in the evening.

3.4.4 Pulpitis, parulis

Ulceration processes in the region of the dental root in damaged milk teeth tend to predominate in paediatric practice, whereby the dental root of the milk tooth is naturally subject to a catabolic process as part of the change of teeth. In these inflammations the purulent secretion often comes out through the development of a fistula. The exaggerated ambition of dentists to conserve damaged teeth as "placeholders" should be viewed critically in the case of parulis.

The following medicines are suitable for conservation:

- **Periodontium/Silicea comp. amp.** Wala
  0.5 ml per os 2–3 x/d (the most effective medicine)

possibly supplemented by

- **Conchae comp. pillules** Wala
  5 pillules 3 x/d,
- **Pulpa dentis Gl D30 amp.** Wala
  0.5 ml per os 1–2 x/d.

In acutely painful inflammations,

- **Hepar sulfuris D12 pillules**
  5 pillules 2–3 x/d

can initially be given in alternation with Silicea comp./Pulpa dentis in place of Conchae comp.

3.4.5 Teeth grinding, bruxism

Nocturnal teeth grinding (bruxism) in itself only represents a symptom; it belongs to the sphere of abnormal nocturnal spasmodic movement which is connected with the soul not being able to properly disengage from the body on going to sleep and a part of soul activity from the day persisting or being concluded during sleep.

A medicine which particularly supports the disengagement of the soul entity from the body on going to sleep and in the first half of the night is

- **Belladonna Rh D20 dil.** Weleda
  5 gtt. (alcohol-free)/d in the evening.

If the teeth grinding occurs in association with pavor nocturnus (night terrors), mostly in the second half of the night, then there is a deeper-reaching disorder.

Here

- **Kalium bromatum D12–C30 pillules** DHU

in individual dosage can produce a thorough improvement.

If the teeth grinding occurs in association with a recurring worm infection, a pale and unhealthy appearance and – above all during the worm infection – aggressive and restless behaviour which is difficult to manage paedagogically, this shows that the soul entity cannot penetrate the metabolic sphere during the day (which comes to expression in inadequate catabolism in the gastro-intestinal tract). The child displays extreme irritability which is only a reflection of his or her inability to assert himself or herself against the food and the parasites ingested with it in the metabolic sphere. As a rule, the behaviour of these children improves as soon as the worms are killed off with allopathic medicines.

Sweeping improvement can often be achieved here by giving

- **Cina D12–C30 pillules** DHU

which not only improves or cures the teeth grinding but also the irritability, susceptibility to parasites and unhealthly pale appearance.

This shows the therapeutic principle that a pathological process during the night should make us consider what process is too weak or incomplete during the day. Thus Cina has the effect of strengthening the digestive ability of the child during the day. But that also causes the other symptoms disappear.

3.5 Vaccination[1]

We have to recognize that a great deal of insecurity and uncertainty lives – I would say, has to live – in the vaccination question. That lies in the nature of vaccination itself. In view of these uncertainties, not only the decision which we reach is crucial for me in my capacity as advisor to the parents –the way in which we reach that decision is just as crucial.

H. U. Albonico

Decades of paediatric work and the exchange of experiences with others have led me to value the fundamental outlook of the parents regarding this subject and largely to respect it because they are most closely connected with the destiny of the child; and also to exercise restraint with regard to medical intervention in infancy if there is not an urgent need. Such restraint coincides with that of many parents when they sense that the body of their infant should actually be "inviolable" – and that includes a vaccination which is not strictly necessary right now.

W. Goebel

We do, however, expect that parents who are restrained with regard to vaccinations also grant their children the necessary rest, treatment and recuperation in any illness which may occur as a result.

W. Goebel, M. Glöckler

Influenza vaccination: policy versus evidence.

T. Jefferson

Successful protective vaccination against smallpox was carried out in China as long ago as the sixth century AD. The idea of preventive vaccination reached Europe at the end of the eighteenth century through the medicine practiced in the Islamic world. Edward Jenner carried out the first smallpox vaccinations in England in 1796 – but after the vaccination his own son suffered mental disability at ten months and died at the age of 21. Smallpox was eradicated in the twentieth century so that the smallpox vaccination, which was itself a risky procedure, was no longer necessary.

Such eradication is probably not globally possible for other pathogens such as the measles virus, for example. The German Standing Vaccination Commission STIKO, for instance, has expressly moved away from the goal of eradicating the measles virus (STIKO expert Jan Leidel at the 2010 Wuppertal vaccination congress). But since the measles virus can cause high mortality when it enters a population which has not previously come into contact with it and has no immunity (thus approx. 40,000 of the 148,000 inhabitants of Hawaii died from measles in 1848 when the virus reached the islands), the vaccination strategy of "global elimination" (i. e. with the aim that measles only any longer occurs in very rare instances, without the virus being eradicated) now being pursued with measles *means a long-term, sustained dependence of the global population on the early vaccination coverage of 95 % of the population*. But in places where the real diseases of the population are malnutrition, lack of drinking water, absence of medical care and frequent occurrence

1 In collaboration with Martin Hirte.

of tuberculosis – in poor, socially disorganized countries – measles claims hundreds of thousands of victims even today. Will a vaccination coverage rate of 95 % be achieved in those countries? Meanwhile each case of measles in Germany is closely monitored by the health authorities although in 2007 not a single death resulted from the 3826 cases of measles notified in the EU [Euvacnet 2008]. In countries with a "western lifestyle" it is no longer acute but chronic inflammations, above all *the enormous increase of allergies and autoimmune diseases*, which in the meantime represent the main problem for paediatrics and which in rare cases such as bronchial asthma or diabetes mellitus can also lead to death (in recent years, more children and adolescents have died of bronchial asthma than of measles in Germany; in the USA, 97 deaths resulting from type 1 diabetes mellitus under the age of 20 are assumed to have occurred in 2005 [Bartick and Reinhold 2009, e1052]).

The only *prevention for these diseases* which has so far been identified and for which there is any evidence is lifestyles which either lead to wider contact with, above all, bacterial pathogens by the pregnant mother and the infant (farm children) and/or the restrained handling of vaccination and suppression of acute diseases ("anthroposophical lifestyle" cf. ▸Chap. 6). J.-F. Bach, who cannot be accused of any affinity with anthroposophical or homoeopathic thinking, summarizes it like this: "There is a certain irony in the fact that we must now search for new ways to reproduce the infectious diseases against which we have been fighting with great success over the past three decades. The challenge is an important one because of the high morbidity of allergic and autoimmune diseases" [Bach 2002]. The question therefore arises: *in a society with a "western lifestyle" and limited resources, what medical strategy, what form of prevention and therapy make the greatest contribution today to the prevention of serious diseases that are a threat to our wellbeing and health on a long-term basis?* The "Wuppertal Manifesto", which emerged from the first national conference on differentiated vaccination in Germany on 1 and 2 October 2010, reflects the basic position of the authors on the subject of vaccination and prevention as related to Germany. We therefore reproduce it in its entirety in this section:

Wuppertal Manifesto [Ärzte für individuelle Impfentscheidung 2010]

The most effective preventive measures against infectious and life-threatening diseases worldwide are living conditions fit for human beings, health education and access to education, healthy food and clean drinking water. In contrast to these active approaches to the promotion of health, "protective" vaccination is a defensive measure. It can be useful as a supplementary measure in order to prevent certain life-threatening diseases.

The expenditure for every protective vaccination must be balanced against its individual and social benefit. In this way it has to be subject to comparison with other forms of disease prevention which, as a result of the limited funds available in national health systems, are deprived of resources because of expensive vaccination programmes.

Possible long-term consequences of vaccination programmes must be better studied and considered independently of the influence and interests of the vaccine manufacturers. In this context the following requires particular consideration:

- the negative effects on the maturation of the immune and nervous system above all of young infants,
- the increasing loss of robust immunity in the population acquired through the response to the respective pathogen; its replacement with a shorter and less competent vaccination immunity,

- the shift of diseases into age groups subject to greater complications and the spread of new pathogens or pathogen types as the consequence of extensive elimination and eradication programmes.

The dramatic increase in chronic diseases such as bronchial asthma or diabetes mellitus as early as childhood, observed in recent years and decades in countries such as Germany, makes it urgently necessary to investigate issues of disease prevention in larger contexts than has happened hitherto. Sustainable health development requires new concepts which are fundamentally different from a constantly increasing number of vaccinations, given at an ever earlier age, to eliminate individual sub-groups of pathogens.

The current practice of vaccination recommendations, which are increasingly interpreted as obligations, does not do justice in any respect to the scientific, health and economic requirements of modern, integrated preventive medicine and is an anachronism in this form:

- the Standing Vaccination Commission STIKO neither has the staff nor financial resources to undertake an independent, comprehensive and scientific evaluation of vaccination programmes,
- it furthermore formulates its vaccination recommendations independently of any necessary consideration of health economics or alternative prevention concepts,
- there is a lack of independence from particular interests such as those of the vaccine manufacturers among a majority of members of this body, an independence which is required if its formulations are to be credible.

Hence we demand that

- disease prevention and health promotion in Germany shall be supervised by a scientific institution to be newly created,
- this institute shall work with credible independence from the interests of individual groups involved in the prevention concept (e. g. the pharmaceutical industry),
- this institute shall use transparent and clear scientific criteria in the evaluation of measures for disease prevention and health promotion and shall take account of the diversity of therapeutic directions and possible service providers,
- prevention of acute and chronic diseases in childhood and adulthood shall be integrated in an overall concept and that they shall be studied in their context,
- the role which protective vaccination can play in this overall concept shall be balanced against other preventive measures in a health system with limited resources. (...)

(...)

Dr. Martin Hirte, Dr. Steffen Rabe, Georg Soldner,
Dr. Stefan Schmidt-Troschke, Dr. Christoph Tautz

3.5.1 Vaccination and prevention

> As it has not been shown that an influenza vaccination reduces the number of exacerbations and complications in children and adolescents with asthma, such a vaccination for this disease cannot in general be recommended.
>
> S2-Leitlinie Asthma im Kindesalter 2010

In recent years, the recommendations of the Standing Vaccination Commission in Germany, STIKO, and the individual federal states have kept growing; close connections between many STIKO experts and the vaccine manufacturers have been shown to exist, 14 of 16 members have conflicts of interest. The flu vaccination which since 2010 has been recommended by the federal state of Saxony from the seventh month (!) is an example which illustrates the conditions characterized by the internationally respected vaccine expert Tom Jefferson in the following words, even before the outbreak of swine flu: "The optimistic and confident tone of some predictions of viral circulation and of the impact of inactivated vaccines, which are at odds with the evidence, is striking. The reasons are probably complex and may involve a messy blend of truth conflicts and conflicts of interest" [Jefferson 2006]. In children under the age of two the efficacy lies within the placebo range [Hobermann 2003, Smith et al. 2006], in over two-year-olds no effect on severe disease courses and complications has been documented [Jefferson 2005] – ear infections can even occur more frequently among vaccinated children than ones who have not been vaccinated! "In healthy under sixty-five-year-olds, studies were not able to show any influence of vaccination on the frequency of hospital admissions and mortality from flu and flu complications" [Demicheli. 2004]. "Vaccination effects (!) could not be shown in patients suffering from bronchial asthma or cystic fibrosis either" [Smith et al. 2006]. It is, furthermore, remarkable that fundamentally the benefit of acute inflammatory diseases, for example, is not mentioned once by the STIKO – there is no oncologist on the commission either! Thus studies have shown that "*the melanoma risk falls by about 20 % in flu with temperatures under 38.5 C. If the temperature rises above that figure the risk even falls by 35 %*" [Kölmel 1999, quoted from Sommer 2009, 19]. Every sunscreen manufacturer would be overjoyed if he could show such an effect of his product on the prevention of melanomas.

If the whole of the German population were to be vaccinated against flu once a year, that would cost more than 1bn euros – as long ago as 2009, flu and swine flu vaccinations were leaders in the field of vaccination doses sold, followed by the TBE vaccination. The expenditure of the statutory health insurance funds on flu vaccinations has in the meantime risen to a multiple (two-figure range) of all homoeopathic medicines taken together. In the age of evidence-based medicine, critics like to highlight the lack of efficacy of homoeopathic medicines in scientific studies, while the evidence of the efficacy and, above all, the benefit of the flu vaccination (which changes every year, it has to be said) is still outstanding and the potential of serious side effects, for example the verified connection between Guillain-Barré syndrome and flu vaccination [Juurlink 2006], has been demonstrated. The triggering of autoimmune diseases – including in the sphere of the nervous system up to and including acute demyelinating encephalomyelitis [Nakamura 2003] – must arouse concerns. Paediatricians will look with alarm at the impressive and serious publication by Watanabe [2010], for example, in which one (!) paediatric nephrologist reports about four children aged between 5 and 7 each of whom developed acute Henoch-Schönlein purpura (HSP) one day after influenza A (H1N1) vaccination. Watanabe also reports about seven further cases reported in the literature. Five of the total of eleven affected children displayed immunologically-related diseases incl. HSP, reactions to medicines or food allergies in their history, six did not. One patient developed terminal kidney failure, one chronic glomerulonephritis. From this and other publications, the authors derive a contraindication for the flu and H1N1 vaccination for children with autoimmune diseases, particularly on the rheumatic disease spectrum. As it is known that crucial decisions in the human immune system occur in the first year of life, particularly with regard to autoimmune diseases and allergies, a recommendation such as the one on vaccination by the region of Saxony is all the more incomprehensible from a professional perspective. Hand washing (and a face mask, as appropriate) represent procedures which have fewer side effects are probably more effective for protecting oneself or one's child, as relevant, from infection (cf. ▸Chap. 5.4.)

The introduction of the *chickenpox vaccination* for children was the subject of fierce debate, both in terms of the matter itself and economically. It is indicative that before the vaccine was introduced it was suggested that it would offer sufficiently long protection. That had to be quickly corrected once it had been introduced: the recommendation to vaccinate twice against measles, mumps, rubella and chickenpox in the second year of life means the introduction of a dual vaccination; and then there are the costs which arise to the health system as a result which funds are not therefore available for other tasks. Here another problem is revealed: *the issue of mixed vaccines.* For, it turns out, the combined quadruple MMRV vaccine carries twice the risk of a seizure than the separate administration of MMR and the chickenpox vaccination! These data, collected for an American health insurance company [Kaisers Permanente 2010], expressly show that the claim that the number of components in a vaccine does not matter is untrue. That can also be seen, for example, in a comparison of the reported side effects of a pentavalent vaccine with a hexavalent one in pre-approval studies. The fact that the hexavalent vaccine Hexavac had to be withdrawn from the market after unexplained deaths [Zinka 2006, von Kries 2005] (formally for other reasons), shows that increasing the components in a mixed vaccine can produce unpredictable risks for the child to be vaccinated. On the other hand doctors are put under great pressure from the health insurance funds to make use of mixed vaccines.

It is worth noting that the information about complications arising from chickenpox in childhood (in 1996–2000 a total of four deaths, whereby it remains unclear what other health problems there were in these cases) clearly rose in 2003 and 2004: more than 1,000 hospital admissions with 10 deaths were suddenly to be deplored [epid. bull. 2005] and the STIKO revealed in 2004: "The actual figure could lie at … 25–40 deaths per year" [epid. bull. 2004] [cf. Hirte, 2011, section on chickenpox vaccination]. These figures will make every practicing paediatrician shake their head. With regard to the complications arising from chickenpox as against the complications arising from the vaccine, the summary of product characteristics for VARILVAX and VARILRIX merely notes that there are no indications that such complications were more frequent following vaccination than falling ill with wild-type VZV [arznei-telegramm 2008]. As the treatment of chickenpox does not represent a problem for the experienced doctor which would make him or her consider vaccination, the question must be asked here also: *what is the benefit* of undergoing chickenpox in childhood and of contact with children suffering from chickenpox? To begin with, paediatricians can benefit from chickenpox because the herpes zoster rate of paediatricians is the lowest in the population: the good recurring boost for paediatricians through chickenpox protects them particularly effectively against shingles. This protective effect is lost to whole societies which eliminate chickenpox in children: American experts predict that a wave of ever younger adults in the USA will fall ill with herpes zoster due to the absence of the boost through varicella [Brisson 2002, Thomas 2002]. Thus it is no surprise that the German College of General Practitioners and Family Physicians DEGAM – far removed from any suspicion of being an opponent of vaccination – published a position paper "Impfen um jeden Preis?" (Vaccination at any price?) [DEGAM 2009]. The DEGAM points out that the chickenpox vaccination "contains the risk of a shift to an older age" in which the disease (like many childhood diseases) takes a more serious and risky course. It does not see any convincing evidence of the benefit of vaccination.

In contrast, M. Wrensch found an unexpected result with regard to the question as to the benefit of going through chickenpox: she was able to show in a comparison of two independent patient groups that the risk of brain tumours, particularly of a glioblastoma multiforme, is higher in adults if they have not caught chickenpox or have a low antibody status. The odds ratio, i. e. the relative probability of the occurrence of a malignant brain tumour, was 0.59 for the group which had suffered from chickenpox [Wrensch et al. 1997, 2005]. The ESPED data also indicate that the risk of falling ill with type 1 diabetes mellitus is reduced through chickenpox [ESPED 1998]. Both of these are serious diseases. In 2010 it was possible to demonstrate the benefit of undergoing chickenpox – in contrast to vaccination! – for the prevention of atopic dermatitis in childhood [Silverberg 2010]. The current state of scientific knowledge thus argues against a chickenpox vaccination in early childhood, while in contrast the vaccination of young women without immunity can protect them against infection during pregnancy. There are further links between undergoing acute inflammatory diseases in childhood and tumorous diseases in adulthood: the benefit of mumps in the prevention of ovarian carcinomas was already mentioned in the introduction to ▸Chap. 3. Albonico [1996a] found indications in his study which support the argument that there is a reduction in the risk of developing a carcinoma by undergoing febrile childhood diseases. Further references on this subject can be found in Girke [2010, 423f.].

The pneumococcal vaccination reveals an additional problematic side of vaccination strategies: the *replacement* and "flourishing" of bacterial strains which were hardly prevalent up to that point and which in the case of sickness can cause greater problems than their original epidemiologically prevalent conspecifics. The vaccination itself originally appeared to be very successful in reducing invasive pneumococcal diseases in the USA. But soon bacterial strains which were not affected by the septavalent vaccine replaced the strains which had been displaced: "Serotype 19A, which is both resistant to antibiotics and a common cause of disease, is not affected by PCV 7 [the septavalent pneumococcal vaccine originally approved for infants] *and is increasing worldwide including in countries without PCV 7*" [Dagan, Klugman 2008, 785]. In Europe, on the other hand, no effect on acute otitis media was shown in studies with the septavalent vaccine in Holland [Le et al, 2007], the vaccine had been developed for American conditions. Yet it was declared as the recommended vaccination in Germany by the STIKO under optimistic assumptions: "With a vaccination rate of 80 %, the STIKO anticipates a reduction in invasive pneumococcal diseases in under two-year-olds of 53 %. If this also applies to serious and fatal courses, seven deaths and 15 cases of complications in this age group would be prevented under the most favourable circumstances with vaccine costs of at least 140 million euros" [arznei-telegramm 2006, 89] – others calculate 176 million euros. In northern France the incidence of pneumococcal meningitis rose twofold after the introduction of Prevenar (septavalent), in infants by 6.5 times [Alexandre and Duibos 2010]. The cause was pneumococci which were not covered by the septavalent vaccine. This example shows particularly clearly the effect of transferring a vaccination developed for US conditions to a quite different environment of mother and child. In the meantime the subject of serotype replacement has become such a problem, and the efficacy of septavalent vaccine is clearly so inadequate, that a 13-valent pneumococcal vaccine has already been introduced after the 10-valent vaccine "Synflorix" arrived in 2010. Data on the safety and efficacy of such measures are difficult to collect or, indeed, obtain. Fourteen unexplained deaths occurred among Argentinean study participants in the clinical trial of Synflorix. In the Netherlands, over 100,000 doses of Prevenar were withdrawn from the market after three unexplained deaths [Hirte 2011, Pneumokokkenimpfung, Nebenwirkungen]. Thus the pneumococcal vaccine is an example of a risky intervention in the ecology, the bacterial environment and the social world of humans – a mass experiment with an uncertain outcome in which it is difficult to obtain reliable scientific data about drug safety and efficacy due to the rapid changes in this field. An added difficulty is that most pneumococcal vaccinations are carried out in practice as an "add on" to a hexavalent vaccination, for example. In 80 % of the deaths which were reported at the same time as the pneumococcal vaccination (that does not necessarily imply any causality), other vaccinations were carried out simultaneously.

A further characteristic feature in this field, which already became evident in the information on the pneumococcal vaccine or on the duration of the protection in the varicella vaccination, is the constant *outdatedness and contentiousness of the information, including the recommendations of the STIKO:* even in the period between the completion of this manuscript and the publication of the book certain observations may no longer be relevant. A look across the border can be instructive in this context. Thus a country like Austria reaches different conclusions in its 2010 vaccination plan from its larger neighbour as to which vaccinations are publicly recommended: the HPV vaccination, for example, not at all, the hexavalent vaccination in the first year just twice instead of three times, the pneumococcal vaccination just three times instead of four times. That contrasts with the "claim of infallibility" asserted by the STIKO recommendations as a "scientific standard" in court for example. If we look further afield in Europe, it becomes even clearer that the vaccination recommendations of national authorities can vary considerably and are constantly changing. To speak of a "scientific standard" in this context is euphemistic.

The question as to whether vaccination contributes to intensifying the health problems of children in western industrial states is a matter of concern. One example from 1999/2000 is the question to what extent the introduction of the Hib mass vaccination directly contributed to a rise of diabetes mellitus in Finland. The *arznei-telegramm* [1999] calculated in November 1999 an additional case of diabetes mellitus in childhood "per 1,700 Haemophilus influenzae vaccinations carried out according to the customary pattern today ... Parents of children to be vaccinated should be informed about the possible risk." This magnitude lies significantly higher today than the rate of invasive Hib diseases leading to lasting complications or the death of the child before the introduction of the vaccination; according to Classen and Classen [1999], 58 cases of diabetes can be expected in 100,000 vaccinated children, whereas approx. seven deaths and seven to 26 cases of long-term damage through Hib diseases are prevented. R. von Kries and H. J. Schmitt [1999] immediately responded as spokesmen of the STIKO: "Informing parents that 'the Hib vaccination could cause diabetes' is to spread false information on the basis of the current data available." In contrast, the group led by Wahlberg [2003] was able to show that in Hib vaccinated children immunological risks of the development of childhood type 1 diabetes (elevated IA-2A and GADA antibodies) could be shown to exist 5.9 and 3.4 times more frequently and that the titre of the IA-2A antibodies lay significantly higher than in children who had not been Hib vaccinated. The risk should be particularly considered if a family member of the core family has already fallen ill with type 1 diabetes mellitus [cf. Hirte 2011].

This question can only really be clarified through *long-term, comparative studies of vaccinated and non-vaccinated subjects.* When, however, in the study for the HPV vaccine Cervarix the (new) adjuvant of the vaccine was also contained in the "placebo" of the comparison group (and only the antigen against HPV was not), it cannot but come as a surprise – in view of the fact that 8 % of those vaccinated with the active treatment and 10 % of those treated with the placebo (!) reported on serious events after the vaccination (e. g. diabetes mellitus or autoimmune diseases) – that the authors [Romanowski 2009] failed to see any connection between these events and the vaccination. The only way to explain it is that the word "placebo" to describe the "placebo" ampoule containing the adjuvant had such suggestive power that the authors of the study began to believe it themselves while a real control group for the HPV vaccine (e. g. NaCl ampoules for the placebo group) was lacking.

The field of protective vaccination in childhood occupies a special position in paediatrics. A real *fanaticism* exists in this area, frequently on both sides. Anyone who surfs the relevant pages on the Internet will not find a problem of children and young people today which is not related to protective vaccination by its fanatical opponents. That is evident in the literature from as long as 150 years ago. In 1924 Rudolf Steiner considered it necessary to state in a meeting with doctors: "The fanatical opposition to these things" (the reference is to the general smallpox vaccination) "is not what we are aiming for but we want to change things on a large scale through insight" [Steiner 1989, 288]. Today, too, it is the concern of the authors, like many like-minded anthroposophical and homoeopathic colleagues, to enable parents *to make a free vaccination decision based on insight* and thus to occupy an independent position between fanatical opponents and demagogic supporters of vaccination who want to replace any dialogue with compulsion.

Against the background of often confusing and contradictory data, it is essential that the advising doctor *has comprehensive and up-to-date information.* The present volume cannot do that; there is, however, excellent literature available meanwhile which seeks to introduce some calmness to the debate. Some of it is constantly updated on the Internet or is published as updated manuscripts. We expressly refer here to

- *"Impfen – pro und contra"* from the classic homoeopathic paediatrician Martin Hirte [2011]. This work is suitable as a source of information for parents while at the same time providing in a comprehensive and impressive manner the knowledge which the doctor in daily practice does not necessarily have directly to hand. This section of the book owes many key references to Martin Hirte.
- The *website* of the Verein der Ärzte für individuelle Impfentscheidung www.individuelle-impfentscheidung.de which is maintained and constantly updated by the classic homoeopathic Munich paediatrician Steffen Rabe. It offers the relevant up-to-date information to anyone interested.
- *"Schutzimpfungen selbst verantwortet"* by Wolfgang Goebel, fourth edition [2009]. This book impresses above all through the attitude of the author, an anthroposophical paediatrician and founder of the paediatric department at the Gemeinschaftskrankenhauses Herdecke hospital, which comes to expression in his account regarding vaccination advice and decision-making, as well as in the very impressive account of a measles encephalitis case from the perspective of the parents which can teach us a great deal about supporting these seriously ill children.

- The *arzneimittel-telegramm* which publishes important up-to-date information on vaccines on an ongoing basis.

In view of the controversy among the experts, *the doctor's experience regains its importance with regard to the advice he or she gives* – as long as there is also a scientific case which support that experience. There is no pressing epidemiological emergency situation in the German-speaking countries for any of the diseases under discussion. Against this background the authors argue for and practice *an individually differentiated approach to vaccination.*

3.5.2 The decision to vaccinate – general considerations

The goal is a free decision by the doctor and the parents which can stand the test of time as a personal decision of all those involved even in the event that vaccination side effects or disease complications occur. This is only possible if there is sufficient information about the benefits and risks of the vaccination; what is of equal importance, however, is that *trust should be created.* Decisions based on stirring up fear [Barth and Bengel 1998] do not provide a solid basis and can rightly be challenged.

The most important trust is the trust in the individuality of the child itself. If the child is supported educationally and medically in such a way that in crisis situations the focus is on his or her own potential to overcome a disorder, such trust can grow. ▸Chap. 5 explains such perspectives regarding our understanding of illness and therapy in acute-inflammatory diseases in greater detail, something which can also be of relevance when advising on vaccination. If parents experience the gain in independence and health which children can develop from overcoming such diseases [Kummer 1992], their anxiety arising from a desire to protect the child from the challenge to and test of its own forces often disappears. A key prerequisite along this path is that the doctor should be available in such crisis situations. (That will increasingly only be possible through the collaboration in trust among several doctors).

Trust arises when the attempt is made to ensure that as far as possible *both* parents come to a unanimous decision. The quality of the decision can be measured, among other things, in that it leads to a reduction in parental anxiety and not an increase in anxiety in one parent because his or her concerns are ignored by his or her partner and the doctor. The doctor himself or herself is obliged to explain the applicable STIKO recommendation or national vaccination recommendation as being the scientific standard, the diseases and risks against which the vaccination is supposed to protect, and the vaccinations, including their possible side effects. He or she must also explain the consequences of not vaccinating (e.g. possible exclusion from kindergarten and school in the absence of a measles vaccination or if the child falls ill with measles). That is very relevant for working single mothers, for example. If the doctor suggests a vaccine which is not recommended for the given age, he or she must also explain that the state bears no liability if vaccination damage results.

It is clear that, given the wide range of views and facts which have to be taken into account today when deciding whether or not to vaccinate, parents must have obtained some prior basic information through vaccination evenings, reading the literature suggested under 3.5.1 for example, or information sheets such as the information sheet on measles vaccination from the GAÄD *before discussing vaccination with the doctor. The advisory meeting with the doctor serves to clarify open questions and put the vaccination decision on an individual footing.* Legally, written information alone is never sufficient;

adequate time must always be provided for the parents of the child or young person to be able to ask questions and make an informed decision.

In view of the many different possible vaccinations, the meetings on this subject must be *spread out*; the number of vaccinations which can be discussed at one meeting varies individually. Hence it is important to draw up a *plan* for the vaccinations to be discussed which is determined by the STIKO vaccination plan as the standard and the chronological urgency of the vaccination decision. In this way it can be calmly decided *whether and when* a vaccination is given. The result should be transparently documented for both sides. The authors prefer to document the vaccination decision in the preventive care record (the *Gelbe Heft* in Germany), as well as placing a copy in the patient file or electronic documentation.

Contraindications (see the respective Summary of Product Characteristics for each vaccination!) must be carefully taken into account in all vaccinations discussed. The authors *do not vaccinate* if there are even slight signs of an acute – and be it a "harmless" – disease. The same applies as far as possible when other family members are suffering from acute infections, a journey or move is imminent within two weeks (or longer depending on the vaccination), or exceptional psychological or, indeed, physical stresses are likely to happen during this period. Restraint is called for with regard to all identifiable allergic and autoimmune diseases. That also concerns cases of polyarthritis occurring in early childhood, for example. H. Truckenbrodt [1997], not known as an opponent of vaccination, notes in this respect: "Many paediatric rheumatologists have furthermore observed that an outbreak or reactivation of the disease has occurred in, at minimum, a chronological connection with vaccination … The interval between vaccination and the occurrence of symptoms ranges from a few days to weeks".

Mixed vaccines offer the benefit of a reduced burden on the child of painful injections, adjuvants and preservatives. But from an immunological perspective they represent an elevated "sensory deception" [Meinecke 1999] of the immune system which can give us reason to anticipate negative consequences on the further maturation of the immune system. Side effects are more difficult to identify and treat. Pentavalent and hexavalent vaccines display particularly pronounced side effects in studies and in practice.

With regard to the question of booster vaccinations, the *determination of vaccination titres* has proved successful. Thus in 90 % of cases one measles immunization is adequate if the vaccination titre is measured (and entered in the vaccination record, if positive, in place of the second vaccination). Booster vaccinations at school age are largely superfluous if vaccination titres are measured before vaccination. Conversely, that is the only reliable way to discover gaps in vaccination. Another important use of vaccination titres is to obtain certainty about the immunity of young women before a pregnancy or of travellers before trips to countries with poor medical care and particular infection risks (e. g. polio, diphtheria). People with statutory health insurance must bear the costs themselves and taking blood can also be stressful; but on the other hand the risk of vaccination side effects can be minimized with the simultaneous optimization of patient safety as the number of refresher and booster vaccinations can be significantly reduced.

3.5.3 Aspects on timing of vaccinations

Insights into the development of the nervous system, into immunological development and the toxicity of vaccines in the first year of life place the focus ever more on *the question of the vaccination timing*. On the other hand the social pressure on the parents increases massively if access to communal facilities such as crèche and kindergarten is dependent on undertaking all the recommended protective vaccinations at the times recommended by the STIKO. That is demanded, not least, by the German Medical Assembly and already practiced by some private providers (at the time of going to press of this edition). In this increasing tension the doctor can highlight a number of key considerations:

- *Neurodevelopmentally*, almost half of all human brain growth takes place during the first year of life. The human brain is characterized by its special plasticity and adaptability in this phase of life but it is also particularly sensitive. The transition from the "germ state" of the pluripotent stem cells to the state "become image" of the differentiated nerve cells is particularly sensitive. In the course of this differentiation, methylation processes of the DNA occur (which as "bookmarks" restrict the readability of the genetic information of the cell nucleus, thus prescribing a specific text which is required for stable cell differentiation). This "epigenetic regulation" is still in full swing in the first year of life. This fact illustrates – as does the development of the immune system – the extent to which the human organism develops its living form not just through heredity but also through the development and transformation of what is inherited, something which requires a longer time than in comparable animal organisms. It was Rudolf Steiner who was the first to point out that the experience of the environment in early childhood has an "organ-forming" effect (cf. ▸Chap. 1.1). *Aluminium salts*, preservatives and other adjuvants of vaccines (we need only think of the new flu vaccines) can disrupt the differentiation of the nervous system through their inhibiting action on the nerve growth factors and the *epigenetic regulation*. If we combine the hexavalent vaccine Infanrix Hexa and the pneumococcal vaccine Synflorix, for example, the doctor is administering 1.2 mg of aluminium! Breast milk contains 4–65 µg/l, that is one twentieth of this amount at maximum (whereas soya food can contain up to 2400 µg/l and must also be considered as very problematical in this respect [Ernährungskommission DGKJ 2006]). Another factor which must be considered is that the aluminium is administered parenterally in the vaccine as a hydroxide and is not assimilated through the intestine. At the same time the blood-brain-barrier of the infant is still more permeable than that of the more mature small child. Another factor to be considered is the sensitive process of myelination of the central nervous system which is in full swing in the first year of life and which can also be disrupted in the way described above: nerves which have not yet been myelinated are more susceptible to toxins. Such toxic effects are known from animal experiments and experiments with human nerve cells [Petrik 2007]. Modern vaccines such as the hepatitis B vaccine are suspected of triggering the *demyelination process by immunological means*. The whole of the motor system can be affected (toxic effects of aluminium hydroxide were also found in motor neurons) [Shaw 2009]. The risk that vaccination in the first year of life can delay and inhibit motor development, and thus the incarnation of the child's soul and spiritual entity, should be taken seriously in view of these research results.
- Against this background the recommendation of the STIKO to administer the scheduled vaccinations to premature babies based on the date they were born and not on their calculated birth date is incomprehensible. The authors do not just see this as being associated with clearly worse tolerance and, in view of the low body weight, an even higher toxic burden, they also consider the argument that it prevents possible apnoeas in infant with whooping cough as self-contradictory. Liese and Knauf themselves write:

"With regard to the safety of vaccinations [for premature babies], special attention should be paid to the possible occurrence of apnoeas and bradycardias in very small premature babies; here monitoring is recommended above all in the context of the first vaccination [! – what about the second vaccination?]" [Liese and Knuf 2009]. That is why the authors recommend starting from the calculated birth date unless there are clear reasons for any other procedure in individual cases.

- *Immunological findings* about the development of the immune system also suggest a procedure with regard to the *timing of the vaccination* which is different from the recommendations of the STIKO. The latter are guided solely by the criterion of the earliest possible protection against infection. The *nonspecific immune system* develops primarily in the first year of life. The complex findings about this development are set out in detail in ▸Chap. 6.1. Premature penetration of the childhood barriers at this age promotes the development of allergies. At this age the ability to differentiate between "self" and "foreign" matures not just with regard to the conscious awareness of one's own body and its boundaries ("body schema") but also immunologically, particularly in the thymus-dependent maturation processes of the T cellular immune system. In this sphere the DNA of the lymphocytes is opened, changed and individualized by the child's organism ("rearrangement", ▸Chap. 6) – once again maximally during the first year of life. Comparable processes have also been demonstrated for the B cellular immune system in the first year of life. The development of the individual *immune regulatory balance* is crucial in this maturation process. Vaccinations in the first year of life stimulate Th_2 lymphocytes, the physiological dominance of which during pregnancy must be reversed in the first year of life, at the wrong time. Vaccines one-sidedly stimulate this branch of the immune response which is required for memory formation in the sense of a specific immunity mediated by the vaccine. In the normal development of the immune system in early childhood, the focus is initially on nonspecific resistance in the management of acute infections which the child has actually undergone. Such a response of the immune system – which supports the immune regulation in the first year of life – is characteristically different from the response which is triggered through vaccination, specifically in the first year of life. Using the example of the early childhood tetanus-diphtheria-whooping cough vaccination, it was possible to show that the stimulation of the child's Th_2 cells increases, the more the infant still has antibodies passed from the mother, i. e. the earlier vaccination takes place. A Canadian research group found clinically in the 11,531 children it studied that the same vaccine *was associated with only half the asthma incidence at the age of 7 (DPT) when the first vaccination was administered at least 2 months later than specified in the national vaccination plan* (which provides for the first vaccination at 2 months) [McDonald 2008]. With this study at the latest, European doctors also have scientific arguments for questioning the early recommended time for the start of vaccination.

This result expressly shows that comparative long-term studies would have to be presented in order to be able to evaluate this recommendation at all. Currently the recommendations for the early vaccination of infants are no more than "eminence-based" recommendations without scientific backup regarding their long-term benefit (or damage) for the vaccinated child. *At the same time this study makes clear that the question as to the time when vaccination should take place is just as important as the question what is vaccinated.* That is also important for parent counselling.

- Loading vaccines with aluminium hydroxide has the purpose of stimulating the reaction of the child's immune system to the administered antigen. It is worth noting that the adsorption of egg protein (ovalbumin), for example, with aluminium hydroxide and its parenteral injection is an established model for allergically sensitizing guinea pigs in asthma research! Only low antigen quantities are required to produce "IgE antibodies in addition to IgG": "The addition of an adsorbtion agent" [aluminium hydroxide] "clearly produces considerable differences in sensitization" with the declared aim of the "permanent sensitization" of the laboratory animal. Bordetella pertussis is also used as an adsorption agent for the sensitization of guinea pigs ("guinea pigs are generally used as a model for human bronchial asthma as there are many similarities between both species (sic!)" [Mahdawi 2005, 11]). "It has been shown in animal models to induce sensitization that aluminium hydroxide additives increase IgE production" [Plewig et al. 2004, 178f.]. The aluminium hydroxide content of vaccines must be seen as even more problematical against this background, particularly in the first year of life in which the immune regulatory balance develops and the child also increasingly comes into contact with foreign protein through food, for example.
- Acellular pertussis vaccination in early childhood promotes the strong release of IgE and Th2-specific cytokines. "Our data show that the cytokine profile of 6-months-old children is influenced by the composition of the whooping cough vaccine they were given at the age of 2, 3 and 4 months" [Mascart 2007, quoted from a lecture by M. Hirte in Wuppertal 2010]. The depth to which vaccination can inscribe itself in the body of the immature child cannot be expressed more clearly. R. Bernsen notes an increased risk of asthma at school age related to early whooping cough vaccination – not, however, if whooping cough itself has been suffered [Bernsen 2008]. Thus the vaccination antigens of the pertussis vaccination and aluminium hydroxide present particular risks in the first year of life. An overview of the aluminium content of various vaccines can be found in Hirte [Hirte 2011].
- But the maturation processes of the immune system as described not only mean that early vaccination can promote allergies, but also that it can weaken the *resistance against infection*. Aaby [2000] was able to demonstrate this effect dramatically in infants and small children in West Africa: children who had been vaccinated at an early stage against diphtheria, tetanus, polio and infantile paralysis (for which many more reasons exist in West Africa than in Germany) showed twice the mortality in the subsequent period than the comparison group. The causes of death were above all malaria and intestinal infections; socially these children tended to be better off and better fed than the comparison group. In our own practice, too, a clear rise in the susceptibility to infection can repeatedly be noted after protective vaccinations.
- The aim of vaccination is to manipulate the specific immunological memory formation. But the organism only develops the corresponding ability from about the age of one, while infant vaccination principally calls forth *premature specific memory formation*. "Only on conclusion of the first year of life, and thus on achieving the upright posture typical of human beings through learning to walk, does the specific immune response really get going…" [Meinecke 1999, 70]. The currently dominant vaccination strategy for infants thus does not correspond to the "physiological curriculum" of the human immune system. This plausibly explains why vaccination at this age can impair the immune regulation of the child. Yet the capacity of the immune regulation expresses a central aspect of the physical I-identity, the effectiveness of the I-organization in the body.

Against the background of these insights it becomes increasingly plausible *only to start vaccinating children as far as possible once they have started to walk independently*. The achievement of independent upright posture corresponds with the first crucial maturation of the nervous and immune system. The respiration also significantly stabilizes at that time, SIDS to all intents and purposes no longer occurs from that time onwards; thus the danger that vaccination could provoke such an event also largely disappears. Finally, the first teeth have mostly also erupted by this time and children are particularly susceptible to infection while this is happening.

On the other hand, early vaccination of the Hib vaccination and, to a certain degree, whooping cough vaccination is of significance as invasive Hib diseases are most frequent at six to seven months. This does not apply in the same way to most other vaccines. It should be noted, however, that the "herd immunity" of the Hib vaccination has in the meantime greatly reduced the infection risk of infants. On the other hand, one vaccination is sufficient after the first birthday. With whooping cough, it is not possible to immunize the infant through vaccination at the age at which whooping cough can take a threatening course, namely the first four months. The whooping cough vaccination particularly appears to promote the Th2-dominated regulatory disorders of the immune system, something which is linked with the nature of the whooping cough antigen (which, after all, is also used to sensitize animals, see above). Anyone who wants to protect infants against a whooping cough infection must ensure the perfect immunization of their environment, above all the adults. Such a strategy is not very realistic, even if that is being attempted today. In this respect parents can decide whether they want to have any older siblings of an infant vaccinated. The authors point out that undergoing whooping cough (after the age of one and before puberty) not only offers the best immunization into adulthood, but that with the homoeopathic-anthroposophical treatment of whooping cough important developmental steps and also the cure of chronic diseases such as bronchial asthma can often be observed. Here, too, then the benefits of childhood diseases must be balanced with the risks.

The timing of the vaccination plays a role in other respects in measles and mumps, for example: here the complication rate rises sharply from the age of nine and with the onset of puberty, which can be an argument for vaccination at that point, unless the organism has developed immunity by then, for parents who do not want to vaccinate their children at an earlier stage against these diseases. With regard to measles, there has been a new development in so far as the feared subacute sclerosing panencephalitis (SSPE) occurs above all following infant measles which is becoming relatively more frequent due to the lack of natural immunization of many mothers. The vaccination of infants is possible in principle from the ninth month at the earliest, so that increasing numbers of infants enter a "window" (predicted many years ago) in which they do not have any immunity of their own. Against this background there is an added consideration if there are older siblings of having them vaccinated as necessary in order to protect the infant.

By carefully considering the timing of vaccination and discussing it between the doctor and parents, we become aware of the chronological developmental dynamics of the child's own organism and thus of the child's etheric body, the life organization at work in growth and all chronologically ordered processes of organ development ("body of formative forces"). That in itself incorporates an important point of view which supports attention to and respect for the living self-development of the child and our trust in it.

3.5.4 Description of vaccines

These vaccinations are recommended for as early as the first six months and must if possible be discussed in the first two months of the child's life in order to enable a free vaccination decision without pressure of time.

3.5.4.1 Haemophilus influenzae serotype B (Hib)

The frequency of this disease peaks with regard to bacterial meningitis in the first year of life. The benefit of vaccination comes about particularly through early vaccination from the fourth month. Non-vaccinated children benefit from the vaccination coverage of the rest of the population ("herd immunity"). This is countered by immunological risks, above all the suspicion that it can promote diabetes mellitus (see above) and possibly also bronchial asthma and atopic dermatitis (several observations of our own). After the age of one, a single vaccination is sufficient for immunization. A non-aluminium-containing single vaccine (ActHib®) is available in Germany, Hib is a component in pentavalent and hexavalent vaccines.

3.5.4.2 Pertussis (whooping cough)

This disease is potentially life-threatening in the first year of life and particularly the first four months (apnoea, encephalopathy – at approximately the same time when there is a risk of SIDS). The vaccination does not yet protect children in this phase of their lives; infants are infected, increasingly with the introduction of the vaccination, by adults. The STIKO recommends that adults, above all parents (to be), have themselves vaccinated. But even vaccinated persons can transmit whooping cough. The critical arguments on whooping cough vaccination were set out in ▸Chap. 3.5.3. Whooping cough and vaccination particularly put children with prior cerebral injury at risk.

Specific indications for vaccination can be serious diseases of the rhythmical system: organic heart defects, pulmonary diseases, symptomatic serious scolioses e.g. in myopathies. On the other hand the authors have also seen serious side effects in this respect in particular (e.g. repeated pneumonia after whooping cough vaccination in a child with spinal muscular dystrophy). A single vaccine is not currently available in Germany.

3.5.4.3 Tetanus

A real risk, apart from burns, does not exist until the child starts to play outside from about the age of twelve to eighteen months (in central Europe). Most recently, the necessity of this vaccination was clearly made an issue even within STIKO (Jan Leidel, personal communication). The total number of tetanus cases in the USA has fallen to approx. 30 cases each year as opposed to ten times that number before the introduction of the vaccination. The mortality from tetanus in the case of illness lies at approx 10% among the under sixties and is even lower in childhood; the prognosis for this disease has therefore very clearly improved. Yet it should be pointed out that puncture wounds in particular continue to carry the risk of tetanus. Practical experience shows that when unvaccinated children suffer an injury with a risk of tetanus (animal bite, puncture wound, dirty wound which the child has sustained outside the house) everyone involved quickly becomes nervous and the combined active/passive vaccination carries greater risk than the active immunization alone. It should also be pointed out that when young people travel to poor countries, the risk rises considerably and the medical infrastructure there is unlikely to be able to guarantee the same cure rate as in the USA or Germany. There therefore continues to be good reason for a protective vaccination once the child is walking. The authors have observed families in which several siblings reacted hypersensitively to the vaccination, sometimes repeatedly. In each case the vaccination should be preceded by an enquiry about hypersensitivity in previous vaccinations and this should be taken seriously as appropriate.

3.5.4.4 Diphtheria
Despite largely insufficient vaccination cover among adults, only individual cases of diphtheria occur any longer among adults in Germany (approx. 1 case/2 years) and in children no case has occurred in over ten years. The vaccination continues to be relevant for travelling, diphtheria currently only occurs after journeys to risk countries. Risk countries are particularly countries which suffer acutely from social disorganization, war, malnutrition; Germany experienced major diphtheria epidemics in and after the Second World War, Russia a smaller epidemic in about 1990. There is a high lethality in individual cases, above all through too late diagnosis (approx. 20 %). As there is no single vaccine the use of which could still be justified, it should be considered in early childhood that immunity at the age when adolescents and young adults frequently travel to countries with a diphtheria risk can only be achieved through a long-term strategy. From that perspective the combination with tetanus can be recommended.

3.5.4.5 Polio
No risk of new infections in the EU; the goal of this vaccination is protection when travelling and the continued maintenance of herd immunity. It can be combined with tetanus and diphtheria, but a good single vaccine is also available.

3.5.4.6 Hepatitis B
No proven benefit in infancy which would outweigh the known vaccination risks apart from holiday trips to high risk countries or the correspondingly intensive contact with virus carriers in the family or immediate environment (vaccination for risk groups). Considerable risk of unwanted vaccination side effects; suspected of triggering autoaggressive diseases [Girard 2005]. The vaccination must be discussed in every case with young people as part of their preventive medical checkup (J1, J2), (risk of sexual and drugs-related transmission, risk for specific professional groups, e. g. in the medical field).

3.5.4.7 Pneumococci
The problem area has already been discussed in ▸Chap. 3.5.1. There can be no doubt that pneumococcal meningitis is particularly serious, but the sustained decline of this disease is not assured by the vaccine according to the current state of knowledge and the vaccine itself carries risks which cannot exclude death as a result of vaccination in individual cases. In view of the very high NNT (number needed to treat) to prevent a pneumococcal meningitis, this starting position is not very encouraging even excluding the costs. Currently one 10-valent and one 13-valent vaccine are new on the market; only insufficient information about their safety and side effects is available. There are only the manufacturers' studies, data collected over the long-term are not available. Prevenar13 has a very much reduced aluminium content compared to the 10-valente vaccine Synflorix.

Figures on invasive pneumococcal diseases from various European countries show very varying effects of the vaccine, there are many references to the danger of a serotype replacement by more adverse, antibiotic-resistant pneumococci; possible rebound effects as in northern France have been referred to in ▸Chap. 3.5.1. On the other hand, the development of resistance to antibiotics in pneumococci is alarming at an international level. A therapeutic approach as represented by homoeopathy and anthroposophic medicine, which does not use antibiotics in many cases of acute inflammations, would possibly appear to represent the safest long-term strategy to avoid falling into the trap of cumulative serious infections with antibiotic-resistant pathogens. As far as the early vaccination timing of the pneumococcal and Hib vaccination is concerned, it should be pointed out that *breast feeding and stopping smoking each reduce the risk of bacterial meningitis in infants by three to four times.*

Pneumococcal vaccinations are particularly useful when the spleen has been lost. If a pneumococcal vaccination is wanted for the infant, he or she can be vaccinated twice in accordance with the Austrian vaccination plan and once after the first birthday. If there is no vaccination until after the first birthday, one vaccination is sufficient (as for Hib). In the view of the authors, this vaccination should not be combined simultaneously with other vaccinations.

The following vaccinations should be discussed from the second year of life:

3.5.4.8 Rotaviruses

Rotavirus infections can, as a rule, be easily treated. Falling ill with the wild-type virus enables the development of a stable immunity and important learning processes of the immune system. The vaccines are contaminated with swine viruses; possible associations of the vaccination with intususception and Kawasaki disease [Oberle 2010] represent additional arguments against this vaccination.

3.5.4.9 Varicella

Medicinal therapy is available for immunosuppressed children. The vaccination is reasonable in exceptional cases or for young people without immunization (e. g. young women without immunity before a pregnancy!). Except in the neonatal period, deaths occur with varicella almost only in situations where there is immunosuppression; on the other hand, several deaths were reported in the USA following vaccination [Wise 2000] and most recently there were reports of two cases of stroke after chickenpox vaccination [Wirell 2005] (cf. also ▸Chap. 3.5.1).

3.5.4.10 Measles

There is a single vaccine for measles (Masern-Merieux®). As there are strong arguments against the early immunization for chickenpox, mumps and rubella in childhood, and girls are potentially at greater risk of developing an ovarian carcinoma in adulthood through the mumps vaccination (see the introduction to ▸Chap. 3), this vaccine should be considered. A single vaccination immunizes 92–98 % of all vaccinated children which can be shown through the titre control after 1–3 months (entry in vaccination record replaces second vaccination). The combined MMR vaccine is suitable primarily for boys of school age if the aim is to reduce the mumps risk (vaccine protection against mumps is very unreliable). Girls can be given a separate single rubella vaccination in puberty if there was no (titre control!) natural (= more sustainable) immunization in childhood.

Eight to ten percent of all patients in Germany today who have fallen ill with the disease are infants whose mother transmitted no or only weak maternal passive immunity. In other countries, e.g. Spain and the USA, the percentage of infants who have fallen ill rises to over 50%. In parents with a migration background, a possible higher infection risk in their home country should be taken into account and they should be warned about taking the infant to such countries. Mothers who still underwent wild-type measles transmit more stable (maternal passive immunity; this is, however, getting less because of the falling booster effects from wild-type measles [Hohendahl 2006]). The question of *sibling vaccination* is of particular importance here, as for whooping cough, because the absence of the booster effect means that the immunity of the infant obtained from the mother becomes increasingly unreliable in the second six months of life both in relation to vaccinated and to naturally immunized mothers, and the feared SSPE appears to occur cumulatively with infant measles. The observed cases of SSPE should in any event be a reason to keep unprotected infants strictly separated from measles patients. The trigger in all cases of SSPE is the wild-type virus even if cases of illness have repeatedly been observed in which the SSPE manifested a short time after the measles vaccination.

The risk of complications in measles clearly rises after the age of nine, particularly the risk of encephalitis. Thirty percent of all people who fell ill in Germany in recent years were adults. Measles in third world countries should also be warned against: it is neither permitted to import from/take measles to those countries nor can it be recommended to expose oneself to the risk of catching measles by travelling through such countries. Hence, given a lack of immunization, vaccination in adolescence is not just relevant from an individual medical perspective but also of great social relevance in a globalized world. The disease can take a serious course also in pregnancy, but the risk to the unborn is not elevated as is the case with rubella or chickenpox. On the other hand a pregnancy in the three months following vaccination should be avoided. As the duration of the vaccination protection is uncertain, and numerous adults were only vaccinated once, a titre control might be sensible also in adulthood. (The STIKO instead generally recommends a refresher vaccination for certain population groups (born after 1970, no wild-type measles, vaccinated only once)).

The measles vaccination is a live vaccination. Complications, e.g. seizures, tend to occur at the start of the second week following vaccination. The authors vaccinate above all when it is certain that the person will not be subject to any unusual stresses in the 14 days following the measles vaccination, will not undertake any long journeys and the doctor can be reliably reached if there is a reaction (e.g. vaccine-associated measles, which accompany a particularly reliable immunization). As set out above, the risk of a seizure doubles for MMRV vaccination. Among the possible side effects, the manifestation of epilepsy should be taken particularly seriously. Here, as in other cases (e.g. serious autoimmune hepatitis 11 days after measles vaccination), the authors have been forced to note repeatedly that such cases are rarely reported. It must therefore be assumed that the figures for the side effects of the measles vaccination are distorted by considerable underreporting. There is no reliable data on the safety of measles vaccines to date [Demicheli 2005].

A significant factor in the case of measles is *the social exclusion of non-immunized children from schools and kindergartens* when measles cases occur in these institutions. The Society of Anthroposophical Physicians in Germany has had comprehensive legal opinions prepared with this in mind [Hesse 2007]. The doctor should always aim for a calm dialogue with the health authorities in order to limit (initially exaggerated) exclusion measures to a rational level. Parents should be informed about possible consequences when taking the vaccination decision (namely having to look after their child possibly for 2–3 weeks).

Children who have undergone measles tend to suffer less from atopic allergies in comparison to vaccinated children [Rosenlund 2008, Alm and Swartz 1999], frequently display clear developmental progress after the illness [Kummer 1999] and there are suggestions of a protective effect produced by measles on the risk of developing carcinomas in adulthood [Albonico 1996a]. The least risk of complications is at kindergarten age.

3.5.4.11 Rubella (German measles)

Pregnant women are better protected through natural immunization in childhood than through vaccination immunity. A serological check is required in puberty; if there is a lack of immunity, a one-off vaccination with the single vaccine and subsequent titre control is frequently sufficient. Alternative immunization as part of the MMR vaccination.

3.5.4.12 Mumps

No relevant risks in childhood. Boys are at risk of mumps orchitis from the onset of puberty. The main age when illness occurs as a result of the vaccination is 16–24. Mumps outbreaks affect a high percentage of people who have been vaccinated twice, the protection is distinctly unreliable. If mumps immunization is wanted for boys, the MMR vaccination at about the age of nine (with prior titre control as appropriate) promises the greatest success; according to our own titre controls, relatively many boys developed no or only insufficient protection after MMR immunization. In contrast to the time before the vaccine was introduced, the seroprevalence in the US population shows an immunity of only 90 % in adulthood, insufficient for achieving "herd immunity" [Kutty et al. 2010]. This shows that the mumps vaccination probably does not make a positive contribution to the prevention of mumps complications. If the protective effect of mumps against ovarian carcinoma in women is included [Cramer et al. 2010], there is no assured indication for the mumps vaccination, at least in childhood.

3.5.4.13 Meningococcus

This vaccination reaches only approx. 30 % of the meningococci (type C) circulating in Germany; their importance was beginning to wane even before the introduction of the vaccination. In 2008, three children under the age of 15 died of group C meningococci. The duration of the vaccination protection is doubtful and thus calls into question how much the vaccination recommended for one-year-olds protects young people (elevated risk from nicotine, alcohol and s/p antibiotic treatment). In small children, the vaccination protection begins to fall as soon as after one year [Hirte 2011]. The tolerance of the currently used vaccines is equally not very good; in Great Britain there were six deaths in 2001 and 2003 alone after vaccination in early childhood [Mirror 2006]. Travel vaccination for regions where they are endemic (African "meningitis belt").

3.5.4.14 Tick-borne encephalitis

In Germany, the expenditure on TBE vaccines is the second highest after the flu vaccines – in great contrast to their proven use. The vaccination can be considered for children over the age of three who live in real natural epicentres of TBE. In Germany, there is no case of lasting TBE complications under the age of 12 [Hirte 2011]. There is no scientific evidence about the benefit of the TBE vaccination in childhood. There was not a single difficult course with permanent damage or death among 371 Slovenian children aged up to 15 [Lesnicar 2003]. On the other hand, the convalescence of the affected children can take a very long time which can indicate vaccination if there is a prolonged stay in high risk areas. The risk to adults is significantly more serious, particularly if aged over 50. As far as refreshing the vaccination protection is concerned, determining the level of protection by titre is particularly useful here in the experience of the authors, as vaccinated children mostly still show a very high titre after 3–5 years. The risk of side effects must be taken seriously, e. g. triggering an inflammatory episode in a pre-existing rheumatic disease.

3.5.4.15 Hepatitis A

Relatively frequently indicated for long-distance trips with poor food hygiene. A vaccination more than 6 weeks before start of the trip is sufficient as a rule. Should be vaccinated singly.

3.5.4.16 Influenza

Should only be considered in childhood in exceptional circumstances (▸Chap. 3.5.1).

3.5.4.17 HPV at school-going age

The introduction of the HPV vaccination for girls aged 9–13, and in any event before the first sexual encounter (cohabitarche), represents a current example of the complexity of vaccination decisions:

- Parents have to decide about vaccinating their partly already pubescent children against a sexually transmitted disease; the alternative is the conscious prevention of such diseases (which cannot be prevented through vaccination in the case of e. g. hepatitis C and AIDS) and regular gynaecological checkups (which threaten to be undermined by the vaccination).
- The vaccine was approved without a single phase III study having been published – at the time that the vaccination was made mandatory in Texas, there merely existed two Congressional abstracts of such phase III studies! [Abholz 2007] Furthermore, there is no phase III study of children under the age of 12!
- The costs of introducing the vaccine are so high that Australia, for example, has already forced a price reduction in order to be able to introduce it at all. The long-term benefit, the duration of protection and the long-term consequences of introducing the vaccine (e. g. replacement by other pathogenic HPV viruses) were unknown at the time of the introduction of the vaccine. Austria decided for that reason not to include the HPV vaccination in the national vaccination plan.
- The adjuvants of both vaccines have not so far been transparently tested for their safety (▸Chap. 3.5.1). The side effects reported in connection with the HPV vaccination, including autoimmune diseases and deaths [NVIC 2009] following vaccination, “are real and cannot simply be swept under the carpet” [Gandey 2008]. In Germany and Austria, at least four deaths were registered following HPV vaccination [Hirte 2011]. This means that several years after the introduction of the vaccination there continue to be serious concerns about the safety and harmlessness of the vaccine.

That is why the authors have decided to publish the 2007 HPV vaccination guideline of the Society of Anthroposophical Physicians in Germany here in order to make it easier for readers to reach a decision.

Guideline on HPV vaccination of the Society of Anthroposophical Physicians in Germany (Der Merkurstab 60, 2, 2007; loc. cit. also the information sheet for patients

The HPV vaccination which has now become available is highly praised by the medical societies and the media as a breakthrough in the prevention of cancer and has therefore received much publicity. Various parties are calling for the blanket introduction of the vaccination. Patient information frequently originates with the pharmaceutical companies and the demand among parents and young people is great.

A differentiated assessment of the connection between HPV infections and cervical carcinomas as well as of the effect of the HPV vaccination is not easy given the current one-sidedness of the data available but all the more necessary for the proper care of our patients.

With this in mind, we hereby, in the form of this guideline and the associated patient information sheet, present a critical help, deviating from the current recommendation, to reach a considered judgement.

Human papillomaviruses

Human papillomaviruses have a size of 55 nm and are thus very small even for viruses. The double-stranded DNA with approx. 8,000 base pairs is enclosed by an icosahedral capsid. HPV replicates in the nucleus of the affected cell. Certain differences in gene sequence makes it possible to identify more than 100 subtypes. Differences in the capsid allow bonding with specific epithelial cells. The viral replication is associated with a pronounced proliferation of the epidermal cell layers. Parakeratosis and hyperkeratosis as well as the formation of koilocytes occurs. In the event of a malignant transformation, whereby the viral DNA is integrated into the host DNA, an activation of oncogenes can be shown to occur in the host chromosome.[1] Primarily cellular and only slight humoural immune reactions mean that there is frequently a spontaneous regression.

The cutaneous HPV types cause warts in school age children. They mostly reduce in size within two years.

The genital mucosal HPV types (approx. 40) are sexually transmitted. The low-risk types 6 and 11 are the main agents of the anogenital warts (condylomata) which also often show a spontaneous regression. Approx. 13 high-risk HPV types can lead to the development of dysplasia and neoplasia mainly in the vaginal portion of the cervix. In such dysplasia, too, 50 % of the cases are no longer evident after 1–2 years. The persistence of the HPV infections of the cervix increases with the age of the woman,[2] i.e. the spontaneous regression is much more frequent in young women.

The genital HPV infection is transmitted sexually. The use of condoms does not help against HPV 6 and 11, protection through condoms against infection of the cervix with high-risk types has been proven.[3]

About 70 % of all people have been infected at least once with a genital HPV in the course of their life. The prevalence lies between three and 50 %

1 Friese, K., A. Schäfer, H. Hof: Infektionskrankheiten in Gynäkologie und Geburtshilfe, 97. Berlin 2003
2 Friese, K., A. Schäfer, H. Hof: Infektionskrankheiten in Gynäkologie und Geburtshilfe, 98. Berlin 2003
3 Winer, R. L. et al. in New Engl. J. Med. 354, 2645–2654 (2006); quoted in GebFrauenheilk. 66, 1120–1121 (2006)

Cervical neoplasia

A high-risk HPV infection is detected in 99% of women with an invasive cervical carcinoma. 70% of them are type 16 and 18. The reverse conclusion must not be drawn, namely fewer than 1% of women with a high-risk HPV infection get a carcinoma. In CIN I or II a regression takes place in 50–56%, in a further approx. 25–35% their state remains stable over many years and only 14–20% develop into CIN III.[1],[2] Even in CIN III, a regression of 10 to 33% has been described.[3] Persistence and progression are more frequent in cervical lesions, e.g. due to other infections.

As a rule it takes approx. ten years for an HPV infection to lead to an invasive carcinoma.

Following conization in CIN II or III, the further course was HPV negative in 80–90% of patients.

High-risk HPV infections appear to be a condition for the development of a cervical neoplasia. Other known co-factors are: taking the pill (resulting from substance and not just possible promiscuity), nicotine, and probably also other vaginal infections such as chlamydia, and undoubtedly many other hitherto unknown factors.

Routinely determining HPV with a Pap smear neither has therapeutic nor clear prognostic consequences and merely promotes anxious alienation and the fixation on a virus result which has probably disappeared again a few months later. In a Pap III or IIID result the differentiation between high-risk and low-risk HPV can influence the further treatment.

It is argued that the success of gynaecological cancer screening through cervical smears is shown in the reduction of the incidence from 35/1000 (1971) to 12/1000 (2001) in recent years, although participation in screening is 50% at maximum. That does not yet make clear for which part of the reduction screening is responsible. What is certain is that there has been a jump in the number of conizations based on results which can also regress spontaneously.

If dysplasia is diagnosed in a woman, it may be possible to support the possibility of spontaneous regression with an anthroposophical treatment.

HPV vaccine

The human papillomavirus vaccine consists of virus-like particles (VLP) which are produced in yeast cells with recombinant DNA. They do not contain any DNA. Gardasil®, contains VLP of HPV 6, 11, 16 and 18; Cervarix® of HPV 16 and 18. These particles trigger a humoural immune response. Aluminium is added as an adjuvant; its allergenic effects have been scientifically known for a long time (Wahn 1994, 113).

Vaccination is currently generally recommended before cohabitarche. The vaccine has been approved by the European licencing authority from the age of nine both for girls and boys. But there are no studies of children and young people of this age! Gardasil® was studied in women aged between 15 and 25 with an observation period of just 4.5 years.

1 IARC: Handbooks of cancer prevention, vol. 10. Cervix cancer screening. Lyon: IARC Press, 2005; zitiert in 2

2 Hillemanns, P., G. Mehlhorn, F. Rinnau, P. Soergel, M.W. Beckmann: HPV-Infektion: Impfung, Diagnostik und Therapie. GebFrauenheilk 67, R1–R28 (2007)

3 Kind, E., M. Kuhlmann: Zervikale intraepitheliale Neoplasien, 1477. In: Beckermann, M., F. Perl: Frauen-Heilkunde und Geburts-Hilfe. Basel 2004

The existing studies on Cervari®, only tested on 1113 young women, show that there was seroconversion in almost 100 % of the test persons, and antibodies formed against a first HPV infection with type 16 or 18 in 91 %. The follow-up examination was after 3.5 years [meanwhile 6.4 years, Romanowski 2009]. A phase III study is currently being carried out. Whether there will be any regression at all in carcinoma development is currently just speculation and cannot be demonstrated within this period either.

With Gardasil® there is a placebo-controlled study with only 552 women (aged between 16 and 23). After 2.5 years, an HPV infection was determined in four of the active treatment group and 36 women of the placebo group (89 % protected). This study does not allow us to draw any conclusions about assured protection against cancer either. No carcinoma was observed in any of the women in either group!

It must further be taken into consideration that Gardasil® only vaccinates against two, Cervarix® against four of the 13 HR types. First indications of a serotype replacement have already been observed:[1] this means that the vaccination effect can be considerably reduced in the medium term through a vaccination-induced shift in the spectrum of so-called high-risk HP viruses.

Gardasil® was approved although no phase III study was published. The premature approval of a vaccine would only make sense if it was to deal with a rapidly spreading and frequently occurring disease. The opposite is the case. Mortality and incidence of the disease are steadily decreasing, probably because of the increasing use of condoms and the deployment of early detection.

Forming a judgement

It is not easy for adolescents and their parents to form their own judgement about the vaccinations available, given the way vaccines are promoted. The first prerequisite is good information about the connection between HPV and cervical carcinomas as well as about possible effects of the vaccination. The information sheet which accompanies this guideline also refers to medical and educational aspects of the vaccination decision: what does such a vaccination communicate with regard to sexual education?

It is further worth observing that the risk of being infected with HPV is directly linked with sexual behaviour. Everyone has a choice in the matter. German AIDS Relief is already warning about the negative influence of the HPV vaccination on safe sex behaviour.

The cancer screening available today furthermore offers the possibility of diagnosing, observing and, if necessary, treating dysplasias mostly in good time.

Looked at from this perspective, cervical carcinomas are a type of cancer with optimum opportunity of prevention through sexual behaviour and early detection. The necessity of taking action against cervical carcinomas with a large-scale vaccination campaign is not, therefore, given.

Dr med. Bart Maris, Gynaecologist, Krefeld
Georg Soldner, Paediatrician, Munich
Dr med. Angela Kuck, Richterswil/Switzerland
Dr med. Gabriela Stammer, Gynaecologist, Wennigsen/Hannover

---

1 HPV vaccine Gardasil. arznei-telegramm 37, 117–119 (2006)

3.5.5 Approaches to vaccination in practice

Parents who want to discuss an individual course of action for protective vaccination with their paediatrician are often met with a primary refusal (numerous reports to the authors). It is important for parents to assert their right to make their own decision in the field of disease prevention and to inform themselves accordingly. Opinions on the constitutional position [Zuck 2006] confirm the right of parents and doctors to make an individual decision in the question of protective vaccination; there is no mandatory vaccination in Germany.

Both Wolfgang Goebel [2009, 104–109] and Martin Hirte [2011] set out possibilities for an alternative course of action to build up the child's vaccine protection. The authors point the parents to their publications before the advisory meeting is held in the practice. We can report from our own practice that the vaccination decisions of parents can vary considerably if the doctor really takes the time to provide individual advice. In view of the range of vaccinations and combined vaccinations which are meanwhile on offer, as well as the confusing and intransparent information situation, these meetings are taking increasingly longer despite the doctor becoming ever more experienced in these matters. But so much depends on a viable decision, including the legal aspects [cf. Goebel 2009, 151–162], that this is time well spent.

For central Europe, we can begin by stating in the words of Wolfgang Goebel: "Anyone who does not want to vaccinate in the first year of life, does not ... currently incur a widespread risk, but in rare cases possibly a major one" [Goebel 2009, 108]. There is much to be said for starting with the vaccinations once the child begins to walk independently. Anyone who then does not want to use the common pentavalent and hexavalent dead vaccines quickly encounters problems if they still want to use vaccines approved in Germany for this age. Fortunately a single Hib vaccines is available again. Anyone who only wants to vaccinate for whooping cough, diphtheria and tetanus, can make use of Infanrix® vaccine which is approved for use from three months. The hepatitis B vaccination cannot really be recommended for infants not in the risk groups, which is why the hexavalent vaccine is seldom used in our own practice. Single vaccines for children are available here.

Yet in all other respects the doctor and parents, if they have an individual vaccination plan which deviates from the standard, are often dependent on combination vaccines which are only approved for use from the fifth year of life (for boosters). For the latter there are no public vaccination recommendations for infants and thus no rules governing compensation if complications arise; they are only available for "off label use" at the doctor's responsibility. The authors and many colleagues have for many years practiced such a procedure; numerous vaccination titre controls have shown with regard to the proposal set out below that sufficient immunization of the children can, as a rule, be achieved by this means. On the other hand, parents can only suggest such a procedure to their doctor and not claim it as a right; in this instance a free decision is required by both sides, a conscious assumption of responsibility, because it means moving outside the recognized standard.

Most widely accepted, also by parents who are critical of vaccination, is to build up

- *tetanus protection*, for which a single vaccine not containing thiomersal is available which is vaccinated a total of three times as part of the initial immunization.

Combinations with the weakened diphtheria vaccine ("d")[1] are to be recommended as otherwise the development of diphtheria immunity is not possible until adolescence with-

1 Sitzmann [2001] confirms that the reduced "d" vaccination dose almost always achieves sufficient protection against diphtheria at this age.

out superfluous additional vaccination against tetanus. Combinations are available for this which in terms of their approval are intended as boosters but, in the experience of the authors, are also suitable for initial immunization. The polio vaccination can be combined or done at a later time. The following proposal has expressly been developed for situations in which parents wish to avoid as many as possible vaccinations for which there is no compelling evidence, so that the immunological and physical individuation of their child is disrupted as little as possible. Not all the recommended vaccinations are therefore taken account of here. Parents should, of course, also always be offered the opportunity to vaccinate their child in accordance with STIKO.

Possible alternative vaccination procedure [cf. also Hirte 2011]

- When the child reaches walking age, two Td vaccinations (best with Td-rix®) at an interval of 6–12 weeks. Third vaccination after 6–12 months.
- Alternative vaccinations are
  - only tetanus in infancy
  - the triple combination with polio (e.g. Revaxis®); alternatively the single polio vaccination three times later in childhood or adolescence
  - triple vaccination with whooping cough, e.g. if there are serious underlying diseases of the heart and airways (Infanrix®)
- Hib: vaccination three times with ActHib® from the third month, e.g. for premature babies, if the parents so wish. Alternatively a single vaccination after the first birthday.
- Pneumococci (Prevenar13®) for risk groups: vaccination three times in infancy from the third month or twice from the sixth month or single vaccination after the first birthday; for vaccinations before the first year of life booster vaccination in the second year. The age peak of pneumococcal meningitis lies in the second six months of life as with Hib. Most at risk are children with a CSF fistula, congenital immunodeficiencies or following a splenectomy.
- Measles/mumps: single measles vaccine Measles-Merieux® for girls from the ninth year; to be considered for girls and boys from kindergarten age and before the birth of younger siblings. After vaccination, titre determination at an interval of 2–3 months. Combination measles-mumps-rubella (MMR) vaccine in boys of school age with a view to the mumps immunization and renewed titre control after one vaccination.
- Rubella: for girls from puberty. Prior antibody testing can identify and verify whether natural immunization has already occurred. Otherwise titre control after the first vaccination (here, too, one vaccination is sufficient as a rule).
- Chickenpox: for girls who have not had chickenpox, before puberty to protect against chickenpox in pregnancy.
- Hepatitis B: for infants whose parents are carriers. To be considered in the case of parents with a migration background from countries in which hepatitis B is endemic (e.g. many far eastern countries) if regular visits home are planned.
- For premature babies who meet the indications for RSV prophylaxis with Palivizumab, the authors have had good experiences with this passive prophylaxis and have not so far observed any significant side effects in their own practice.
- Meningococci: primarily travel vaccination; in individual cases of diseases of the immune system. Explain the risks to young people.

For the *hepatitis B vaccination* outside the risk groups, it can be sufficient to discuss the indication with young people and until the age of 18 with their parents. From this age the infection risk increases significantly depending on sexual contacts, travel to distant countries, drug abuse and also social engagement, e. g. in the medical sphere.

In principle all parents should be made aware that they need to consult their doctor in good time regarding possible and required preventive measures before travel to remote countries. Here the precise location and, in the case of malaria prevention, also the time of year of the planned trip plays a role. The discussion should, if possible, take place before the trip has been firmly booked as it may be possible, after a thorough consideration of the risks, to reorganize some journeys or delay them for a time if this is necessitated by developing the required protection.

3.5.6 Side effects – general considerations

The observable *reactions to the vaccines* in use today are clearly different from those of classic smallpox vaccination to which the homoeopathic response was to give Thuja or mercury [Imhäuser 2000, 155f]. It is noticeable that the focus in respect of the consequences has shifted to allergic and autoimmunological disorders and damage to the central nervous system. The approach developed by H. H. Vogel [1996, 74–80] regarding allergic and hyperergic reactions can help to explain this action of vaccines. He starts from the *mesenchymal matrix* which has been shown to be of crucial importance for the embryonic differentiation of the organs: the extracellular matrix is the starting point for the morphogenesis of the organism [Hinrichsen 1990, 19f.]. The course of the epigenetic regulation of the cell nucleus during cell differentiation is probably connected with the cell surroundings, the matrix, and their action on the cell. This transparent and fluid organization combines all physically differentiated organs into a unity for the whole of life [Vogel 1996, 74]. Rudolf Steiner and Ita Wegman [1977, 77] already spoke about the importance of the "interaction of the organs" and referred to the "silicic acid organism" which penetrates the whole organism and unites it. It is indeed the case that the mesenchymal matrix contains a relatively high quantity of silicic acid and in terms of its qualitative characteristics corresponds in many respects to a colloidal solution of silicic acid.

Rudolf Steiner and Ita Wegman [1977, 76] link this silicic acid, which is organized in a living way by the organism, with two key processes:

- the inner limitation of growth in accordance with morphogenesis,
- the separation of the organism from the "pure actions of nature" so that "the former does not have to perpetuate the actions of nature but can develop its own".

They also emphasize the particular importance and dynamics of these processes during childhood (empirically the human organism contains relatively more silicic acid the younger it is).

Physiologically it is of great importance that natural substances have been completely broken down before they enter the sphere of the matrix. If a disorder of the protective epithelial barrier occurs (such as e. g. in childhood asthma at the bronchial mucosa), foreign substances can penetrate the matrix and provoke a "dislocated" inflammatory digestive process which in turn can lead to the damage or destruction of organ structures arising from the mesenchyme (cf. ▸Chap. 6).

By administering protective vaccinations parenterally, a foreign body is deliberately implanted in the sphere of the matrix which bypasses the barriers and nonspecific digestive and immune processes. This irritation is strengthened further by the use of aluminium hydroxide, facilitating an enormous, allergenic immune response (▸Chap. 3.5.3). It is known that Al-OH and whooping cough bacteria antigens are the "strongest known adjuvants for the induction of IgE antibody synthesis" [Wahn et al. 1994][1]. The local reactions to vaccines, up to and including the serious clinical picture of macrophagic myofasciitis, are triggered above all by adjuvants of the vaccines. "But if isolated shreds of perception penetrate 'undigested' into the depths, they act like disorganized developmental stimuli on the child's organism at the time when it is engaged in differentiation" [Vogel 1996, 74].

"From this perspective, vaccinations represent concealed sensory stimuli which do not penetrate the consciousness and which are equivalent to sensory deception" [Meinecke 1999, 70]. We can concur with this statement from C. Meinecke from the point of view that vaccinations circumvent the sense organs and barriers of the organism and represent a dislocated perceptual process. The relationship with the genesis of allergic diseases is thus evident. With that in mind, Rudolf Steiner's statement about the origin of carcinomas is particularly shocking: "It can also be that the dynamics, the forces which are active in a sense organ – which must be active there to a certain extent so that the sense organ can develop – are active in the wrong place. ... Then there is a great tendency for a sensory organ to develop in the wrong place. *And that manifests itself as a carcinoma, as cancer* (emphasis by the authors). Only if you have insight into the human organism will you be able to understand that *in the carcinoma you have the tendency to form sense organs which have been dislocated across all systems*" [Steiner 1982, 179].

That clearly states the basic problem associated with parenteral protective vaccination, particularly in the first year: it induces a perceptual process in the organism in the wrong place (direct access from outside to the mesenchyme) and often at the wrong time (with regard to the perceptual ability of the specific immune system). The organism *must* respond to the vaccination by "developing a sense organ in the wrong place". Meinecke [1999] rightly describes this as undermining the order in the organism, its normal sensory and intentional activity (!), and "contributing to weakening it". Such a point of view also allows for a better understanding of the possible side effects of vaccines and their treatment.

3.5.7 Complementary treatment options during and after vaccination

3.5.7.1 Supportive medicinal treatment

The previous section provides the rationale for the supporting treatment which is generally used by the authors with parenteral vaccinations, namely *the administration of silicic acid in homoeopathic potentized form*. It occupies a central place in the above descriptions by Rudolf Steiner and Ita Wegman [1991] as well as in the treatment developed by H. H. Vogel [1994, 74] for allergic and hyperergic disorders: "The high potency of quartz is intended" to stimulate "the ... I-organization" to combine "in particular with the organ connective tissue" and the warmth events occurring here (description by H. H. Vogel [Vogel 1994, 695] of the indication for Quarz/Oxalis comp. Wala). Vogel [1996] perceives a specific problem when there is a one-sided, dislocated call on the sensory organization "while the warmth organism (I-organization) relatively falls behind in its development." But therein lies the problem of vaccination: the organism is to be induced or forced to undergo a sensory and memory development without developing a corresponding activ-

1 This reference is missing in the third and fourth editions of the work!

3

ity in its warmth organization (we can also call it will activity) (e. g. a fever and rash in measles).

The administration of

- **Silicea/Quarz D20–30 pillules** (various manufacturers)
  1–3 × 5 pillules at intervals of 12 h following vaccination
  (irrespective of constitution type)

can counter this dissociation and an over-sensitivity of the organism.
From the perspective that the vaccination represents a lesion for the muscle and a risk for the nervous system, the authors give a one-off potentized dose of the "silicolous plant" [Vogel 1994, 140]

- **Arnica e planta tota D15 pillules** Wala
  1 × 5 pillules.

In homoeopathy, Silicea is considered to be one of the most important medicines for and after vaccination [Coulter 1991, 121–125]. The "fear of needles and injections" is well known; curiously, it represents a prominent mental symptom in the medicinal picture of Silicea. In the observation of the authors, children whose constitution is similar to the homoeopathic Silicea type before the vaccination are particularly prone to vaccination side effects.

In these children and for a generally very pronounced *fear of injections* treatment with Silicea before the vaccination (starting approx. four weeks beforehand) can significantly improve the tolerance of the injection, for example

- **Quarz D20 pillules** Wala or **Silicea LM6 dil.** Arcana
  3–5 pillules or 3 gtt. in water daily in the morning.

Potentized silicic acid in higher potencies also represents an important medicine in the treatment of vaccination side effects and complications.

3.5.7.2 Treating side effects

3.5.7.2.1 Apnoeas and hypotonic-hyporesponsive episodes

In the first year, particularly in premature babies (born before the thirty-seventh week of pregnancy), apnoeas can occur cumulatively following vaccination, particularly if the STIKO vaccination plan is applied in accordance with the chronological and not the corrected age [Liese and Knuf 2009]. M. Hirte [2005, 83] quotes various authors on this subject: "The younger the children are when they are vaccinated, the more likely they are to suffer states of apnoea and a dangerous drop in heart rate".

In the same period, cot (crib) death represents the most important vital threat to infants in central Europe (▸Chap. 2).

For apnoeas and preventively for infants vaccinated early, (vaccination up to the completed fourth month, corrected for age from calculated birth date), the authors prescribe

- **Tartarus stibiatus D6 trit.** Weleda
  preventively 3 × 1 saltsp., therapeutically up to 5 x/d.

This medicine can also be considered for hypotonic-hyporesponsive episodes (HHE) which represent a circulatory and consciousness disorder probably triggered by the central nervous system. Within 48 hours of vaccination they lead to reduced responsiveness, muscular hypotonia and pallor including cyanosis. Such episodes were observed most frequently after whooping cough vaccination [Hirte 2011].

In addition to Tartarus stibiatus,

- **Helleborus niger D6–12 pillules/amp.** Wala
  3 × 2–3 pillules/0.3 ml per os/d is indicated in such cases.

Helleborus acts here as an anti-shock medicine – not dissimilar to opium in its indication [Soldner 2010, 511] – with a toning effect on the renal, adrenal and central nervous system.

3.5.7.2.2 Shrill crying or screaming

This symptom occurs primarily after vaccination with whooping cough component but can occur after any vaccination, particularly in view of the mixed vaccines which are now preferred. Mansoor and Pillans [1997] report that in New Zealand shrill screaming was reported ten times more frequently after the DTP-Hib combination than after the DTP combination. This is screaming which lasts from several hours to days and can hardly be quieted (Cri encephalique). It indicates in all cases a sustained irritation of the central nervous system.

The external application of the following can be particularly effective for shrill screaming

- **Arnika-Essenz** Wala/Weleda
  1:10 dilution as a cooling compress around the head (used for a longer period of time) or also sprayed regularly on the head.
- **Apis mell. D12–30 pillules** (various manufacturers)
  3–5 pillules 3 x/d
- **Helleborus niger D12–30 amp.** Wala
  0.3 ml per os 3 x/d
- The homologous **vaccine nosode** in D30 or C30 (obtainable from Staufen-Pharma and partly from Gudjons)
  1–3 × 3–5 pillules.

The external application of Arnika-Essenz is also to be recommended as the initial treatment for older vaccinated children who develop a high temperature and serious headaches after the vaccination. The external action of Arnika on the head in these syndromes surpasses in the experience of the authors almost all internally administered medicines in its prompt reliability. Irrespective of the vaccination, K. R. Kummer has described (numerous observed cases; verbal information) the external application of diluted arnica essence three times a day as being very reliably effective for infections with a high temperature and symptoms of a starting encephalopathy.

Afterwards, or in parallel as appropriate, treatment with *potentized autologous blood* as developed by Imhäuser [2000, 187–198] (C5, 7, 9, 12 in ascending potentization, ▸Chap. 6.3) can be carried out (starting with C5 daily, subsequently higher potencies 2–3 × wk). The administration of the homologous vaccine nosode and of potentized autologous blood is generally suitable for the treatment of vaccination side effects and complications. Thus a colleague S. Rabe told the authors verbally about a child which after hepatitis B vaccination developed *cold urticaria persistently for several months* which resisted all allopathic attempts at treatment. The symptoms disappeared rapidly and on a sustained basis following administration of the hepatitis B vaccine in high homoeopathic potentization as the sole medicine!

3.5.7.2.3 Infection susceptibility and allergic reactions

An *elevated susceptibility to infections* can be noted comparatively frequently after vaccination. The slow or negative response of the symptoms to symptomatic treatment is a characteristic feature – while not infrequently treatment can be rapidly and sustainably successful if the corresponding vaccination is taken into account as a possible trigger (cf. also the above case of vaccination-associated cold urticaria).

The most important medicines in these cases are

- **Quarz D20 pillules** Wala
  3–5 pillules 1 x/d
- **Echinacea e pl. tota D3 pillules** Wala
  3 × 3 pillules/d
- **Lien comp. pillules** Wala
  3–7 pillules 1–3 x/d
- **Potentized autologous blood as developed by Imhäuser** (▸Chap. 3.5.7.2.2, shrill screaming)
- The homologous **vaccine nosode** e.g. in D30/C30 Staufen Pharma/Gudjons
  1–3 × 3 pillules as a single dose
- Care of the warmth organization through appropriate clothing and, as necessary, oil rhythmical Einreibungen e.g. with **mallow oil** Wala.

For *allergic reactions* (e.g. urticaria), the therapeutic principles set out in ▸Chap. 6 apply similarly to acute episodes of allergic diseases following vaccination alongside the use of the vaccine nosode.

3.5.7.2.4 Cerebral seizures and neurological sequelae

Here the authors are aware of a series of complications some of which were very serious. Alongside fateful circumstances, the authors consider that the way in which the vaccination decision was taken as well as consideration of contraindications and acute disorders play an important role [cf. Bütikofer 1997]. Thus a case of transverse myelitis following MMR vaccination at the age of 15 months was credibly reported to us in which the child had been vaccinated in the same meeting at which vaccination had been "discussed" despite concerns which had been voiced repeatedly by the mother.

Known neurological complications following vaccination include meningitis and encephalitis, Guillain–Barré syndrome, paralysis and epilepsy. Rare focal inflammatory brain damage has also been seen on several occasions by the authors, e.g. Rasmussen's encephalitis, Landau-Kleffner syndrome and others. These disorders are often difficult to influence therapeutically for any medical direction.

Alongside constitutionally-related prescriptions, the following medicines should be primarily considered (▸Chap. 3.5.6.2.1, ▸Chap. 3.5.6.2.2):

- **Amnion Gl D30 amp.** Wala, **Apis mell. D30, Vaccine nosode D30, pot.** autologous blood C12 in hyperergic inflammation-related disorders of the nervous system
- **Bryonia D30, Stannum met. praep. D30** particularly in inflammation of the meninges and disorders of the cerebrospinal fluid pressure, **Cuprum met. praep. D30** in vasospasms
- **Agaricus muscarius D12, Helleborus niger D12, Hypericum D12–C30,** homologous organ preparations Wala as descending potency series Gl D30 to D8 in detectable lesions of the nervous system.

In all cases consideration should be given to Silicea D30 or C30 (various manufacturers)/ Quarz D60 amp. Weleda and Arnica (=Arnica e radice) D12–30 internally, Arnika-Essenz externally diluted 1:10 as a wrap or 15 ml/bath). In conclusion, we will report about a particularly tragic case in which no medical direction has so far been able to influence the epilepsy in any pervasive way (allopathically, almost every possible anticonvulsant incl. bromides was used).

Case study

(Doctor's letter from the Kehl-Kork Epilepsy Centre, when the child was aged 2½)
Diagnosis: "Infant brain damage, presumably as the result of postvaccinal encephalopathy following second DPT combination vaccination (diphtheria component) with serious impairment of mental development, lack of speech development, considerable impairment of statomotor developmental with hypotonic infantile cerebral palsy and underlying hemiparesis on the right and symptomatic focal and generalized epilepsy with grand mal and myoclonic seizures.

Synopsis

M. is the first child of healthy parents (...). In terms of the family anamnesis, there are no indications of isolated seizures, epilepsy, physical or mental disability. Regular pregnancy and spontaneous delivery with cephalic presentation in mature child (...). Initial normal development, documented as such through to the U4 preventive medical checkup. The examination carried out 14 days before the epilepsy manifestation on 13.6.... (at 5 months) ... on occasion of the second DPT and polio vaccination showed the child to be healthy.

On 25 and 26.6.1990, a total of three grand mal seizures occurred with staring expression and rhythmical convulsive movements of the right arm and left leg. Admitted to children's hospital ... on 27.6.... The cerebrospinal fluid was slightly yellow and clouded together with an artificial admixture of blood. (...)

The CT result was judged to be normal at this point. The EEG controls repeatedly revealed specific indications of a left temporo-parieto-occipital epicentre with activation during sleep in the sense of clear generalization tendencies of the HSA. (...)

An MRT carried out in March (of the following year) found an indistinctly limited white matter lesion in the region of the posterior horn of the left lateral ventricle. After separate assessments by two independent radiologists, the lesion suggests that ischaemic damage has occurred there.

Starting from the developmental stage reached at the time that the epilepsy manifested, M.'s development stagnated almost completely thereafter.
(...)
The parents examined the question of whether the vaccination may have been responsible for the damage in detail. A legal expert consulted by them in this connection classified the event as the likely result of a whooping cough vaccination. Such an assessment is not tenable in our view, given the long interval between the vaccination and the start of the illness as well as the absence of the typical clinical picture for a diffuse vaccination encephalopathy. In contrast, the following facts support the postvaccinal hyperergic vasculitic genesis of the epilepsy caused by the diphtheria component of the mixed vaccine:

1. ... the child had developed healthily and normally up to the onset of the illness, there is no indication of a genetic disposition for epilepsy.
2. The period between vaccination and the manifestation of the illness (up to 14 days) is typical for a postvaccinal hyperergic vasculitic encephalopathy following diphtheria vaccination.
3. The illness manifested after the second diphtheria vaccination (more than one diphtheria vaccination is the prerequisite for the scientific hypothesis of a hyperergic vasculitic reaction).
4. The cerebrospinal fluid was coloured yellow when the illness manifested, indicating the transfer of red blood corpuscles and their disintegration ... hours or days before the LP.
5. There is a typical vascular ischaemic pattern of damage with neuroradiological indications of terminated focal ischaemic damage on the left, corresponding neurological unilateral symptoms on the right and epicentre signs in the EEG on the left.

This unequivocally serious epilepsy with an estimated number of approx. 400 to 550 grand mal seizures so far, must be assumed to be a principal factor in the harm caused to the further mental and motor development of the child".
The doctor's letter contains nine references to diphtheria damage, including a publication by H. Stickls [1978, 636] on the blockage of the middle cerebral artery following a diphtheria-tetanus booster vaccination in a six-year-old boy from 1978, as well as a publication by H. Mittermeiers [1959] on generalized anaphylactic toxic blood vessel wall injury with sinus thrombosis following active diphtheria vaccination.
The boy has been under the paediatric care of the authors for several years; there continue to be approx. 10 to 20 cerebral seizures (alternating between specifically focal and grand mal seizures) per month despite allopathic anticonvulsants and homoeopathic or anthroposophical medication. Clear symptomatic progress could nevertheless be achieved in recent years, to which dolphin therapy in the USA made an impressive contribution. Of the potentized medicines, Secale cornutum D12 to D30, which displays a special relationship with the vascular pathology as presented, had a beneficial effect alongside Agaricus and others (▸Chap. 8.1).
The doctor's letter from the Munich Clinic for Child and Adolescent Psychiatry from 2000 closes with the observation: "The assessment of the developmental age based on behavioural observation produced a developmental age of about 1¼ years" (biographical age 9 years). "In summary, this is a boy with difficult-to-treat epilepsy. He has only recently learned to walk ..."

When this case was briefly presented by one of the authors as part of a "Munich Vaccination Conference" at the Dr v. Hauner'schen University Paediatric Hospital, several colleagues spontaneously expressed their sadness. In conversation with colleagues, some of them admitted that they were unaware of the possibility of such complications; the authors also only learned about it specifically through dealing with this particular patient, the study of doctors' letters and the literature. A member of the STIKO who was present said spontaneously that in view of the epidemiological situation in Germany many parents would probably not agree to a diphtheria vaccination in infancy if they knew or were told about the possibility of such complications. He concluded his verbal considerations with the sentence: "But the parents aren't really that interested in the detail..." A lawyer who was also present explained the legal situation with regard to such vaccine damage – which has been recognized by the courts for some time: if a doctor has obtained knowledge of such a vaccination side effect through personal experience, even if it does occur extremely rarely, he or she is obliged to tell the parents about it in his or her practice even if such a possible consequence of vaccination has not yet been (is no longer?) mentioned in the literature. On the other hand, the authors are also aware, through reports from colleagues, of two children of kindergarten age in southern Germany who died of diphtheria at a time when M. was DPT vaccinated. The children had not been vaccinated because neither parent wanted it and were probably infected by adults who had travelled back to Germany from regions in which diphtheria is a frequent occurrence.

This example clearly illustrates the necessity of weighing up contradictory fundamental perspectives when taking a decision about vaccination. The ability to consider such things and come to an individual decision is a direct expression of the human I. It is enabled through truthful, transparent information which does not try to manipulate the act of coming to a decision from outside and force it in a predetermined direction, through a discussion in which the doctor places trust in the parents' ability to come to such a decision. Then the vaccination decision can represent an important experience, a learning process for all sides.

3

References for Chapter 3

(every reference marked with a ■ Bullet point indicates the English translation of the reference above it)

Aaby, P. et al.: Routine vaccinations and child survival: follow up study in Guinea-Bissau, West Africa. Br. Med. J. 321, 1435–1438 (2000).

Abholz, H.-H.: Impfung gegen Gebärmutterhalskrebs – Würdigung einer ungewöhnlichen Impfstoffzulassung. Z. Allg. Med. **83**, 57–60 (2007).

Albonico, H. U.: Häufigkeit fieberhafter Infektionskrankheiten im Kindesalter in der Vorgeschichte von Karzinompatienten. Der Merkurstab **1**, 1–19 (1996a).

Albonico, H. U.: Vortrag im Rahmen der Ärztetagung Individuelle Impfberatung und -entscheidung 11.5.1996. Gemeinschaftskrankenhaus Herdecke, Manuskriptdruck des Arbeitskreises für individuelle Impfentscheidungen S. 55, beziehbar über W. Goebel, ehem. Leitender Arzt der kinderheilkundlichen Abteilung am Gemeinschaftskrankenhaus Herdecke, Beckweg 4, 58313 Herdecke (1996b).

Albonico, H. U.: Krankheit – Angst – Impfung. Der Merkurstab **4**, 236 (1998).

Alexandre, C., Duibos, F.: Rebound in the incidence of pneumococcal meningitis in northern France: effect of serotype replacement. Acta Peiatr. **99**, 1686–1690 (2010).

Alm, J. S., J. Swartz: Atopy in children of families with an anthroposophic lifestyle. Lancet **353**, 1485–1488 (1999).

Antonovsky, A.: Salutogenese. Zur Entmystifizierung der Gesundheit. dgtv, Tübingen 1997.

Antonovsky, A.: Unraveling the mystery of health: how people manage stress and stay well. Jossey-Bass Publishers, N. J. 1987.

Antonovskys Modell der Salutogenese – Diskussionsstand und Stellenwert. Bundeszentrale für gesundheitliche Aufklärung (BZgA), Köln 1998

Arzneimitteltelegramm **11**, 120 (1999).

Arzneimitteltelegramm **10**, 89 (2006).

Bach, J.-F.: The Effect of Infections on Susceptibility to Autoimmune and Allergic Diseases. New Engl. J. Med. **347**, 911–920 (2002).

Barth, J., J. Bengel: Prävention durch Angst. Stand der Furchtapellforschung. Forschung und Praxis der Gesundheitsförderung, Bd. 4. Bundeszentrale für gesundheitliche Aufklärung, Köln 1998.

Bartick, M., Reinhold, A. : The Burden of Suboptimal Breastfeeding in the United States : A Pediatric Cost Analysis. published online : www.pediatrics.org/cgi/doi/10.1542/peds. 2009–1616 (2009).

Benchimol, E. et al. : Early diagnosis of neonatal cholestatic jaundice. Can Fam Physician, **55**, 1184–1192 (2009).

Bernsen, R. M. et al. : Reported pertussis infection and risk of atopy in 8–12 year-old vaccinated and nonvaccinated children. Pediatr Allergy Immunol **19**, 46–52 (2008).

Biesalski H. K. et al. (Hrsg.): Vitamine. Thieme, Stuttgart 1997

Borland: Kindertypen. Arkana Verlag, Heidelberg 1961.

Braun-Falco, O. et al.: Dermatologie und Venerologie. 5.Aufl., Springer, Berlin 2009.

Buchwald, G.: Impfen – das Geschäft mit der Angst. Knaur 1997.

Bütikofer, J.: Aufklärungspflicht aus juristischer Sicht. Dtsch. Ärzteblatt **26**, C 1324 (1997) – Wir zitieren aus der uns vorliegenden Rohfassung des Manuskripts.

Bundeszentrale für gesundheitliche Aufklärung: Was erhält den Menschen gesund? Köln 1998.

Burt et al: The effects of a break in water fluoridation on the development of dental caries and fluorosis. J Dent Res **9**, 2000, 761–769.

Chinoy, NJ et al.: Reversible Fluoride Induced Fertility Impairment in male Mice.Fluoride **25**, 71–76 (1992).

Chinoy NJ et al.: In vitro toxicity in human spermatozoa. Fluoride **27**,4 (1994).

Classen, J. B., D. C. Classen: Association between type 1 diabetes and HIB vaccine: causal relation is likely. Br. Med. J. **319**, 1133 (1999).

Chuckpaiwong S. et al: Fluorid Analyer der menschlichen Muttermilch in abgelegenen Gebieten von Thailand. J trop Med Public Health **31** 583–586 (2000).

Coulter, C.: Portraits homöopathischer Heilmittel, Bd. 2, Haug Verlag, Heidelberg 1991.

Cramer, D. et al.: Mumps and ovarian cancer: modern interpretation of an historic association. Cancer Causes Control **21**, 1193–1201 (2010).

Dagan R., Klugman, K.: Impact of conjugate pneumococcal vaccines on antibiotic resistance. Lancet **8**, 785–795 (2008).

DEGAM: Impfen um jeden Preis? Z Allg Med **85**, 94–96 (2009).

Demicheli, V. et al.: Vaccines for preventing influenza in healthy adultes. Cochrane Database Syst Rev 2004(3): CD001269.

Demicheli, V. et al.: Vaccines for measles, mumps and rubella in children. The Cochrane Database of Systematic Reviews 2005 Issue 4.

Deutsche Gesellschaft für Kinderheilkunde und Jugendmedizin: Leitlinien Kinderheilkunde und Jugendmedizin. Urban&Fischer, München 2010.

Dijkstra S. H. et al.: High prevalence of vitamin D deficiency in newborn infants of high-risk mothers. Arch Dis Child **92**, 750–753 (2007).

Ehrengut, W.: Leserbrief zu "Aktueller Stand der Keuchhustenschutzimpfung". päd. praxis **3**, 555–559 (1992).

Ehrengut, W.: Zusammenhang zwischen Polio-Impfung und Guillain-Barré-Syndrom. Pädiatrie hautnah **7**, 466–467 (1998).

Elswood, B. F. et al.: Poli vaccines and the origin of AIDS. Medical Hypotheses **42**, 347–354 (1994).

EFSA: European Food Safety Authority, Gutachten des Wissenschaftlichen Gremiums für diätetische Produkte, Ernährung und Allergien (NDA) auf Ersuchen der Kommission über den zulässigen oberen Aufnahmewert für Fluorid, EFSA-Q-2003-018 (2005).

Ernährungskommission der Deutschen Gesellschaft für Kinder- und Jugendmedizin, Ernährungskommission der Schweizerischen Gesellschaft für Pädiatrie: Stellungnahme zur Verwendung von Säuglingsnahrungen auf Sojaweissbasis. Paediatrica **17**,16–19 (2006).

ESPED-Jahresbericht 1998. www.esped.uni-duesseldorf.de/jabe1998.htm.

ESPED-Jahresbericht 2004: Invasive Infektionen durch Streptococcus pneumoniae (Pneumokokken): Geimpfte Fälle (01.01.2004–31.12.2004). www.esped.uni-duesseldorf.de/jabe2004.pdf.

Flöistrup, H., J. Swartz et al.: Allergic disease and sensitization in Steiner school children. J. Allergy Clin. Immunol. **117**, 59–66 (2006).

Frankl, V.: Ärztliche Seelsorge. 4. Aufl. Gustav Fischer Verlag, Stuttgart 1992a; 5. Auflage Urban und Fischer, München 2000.

Frankl, V.: Psychotherapie für den Alltag. 6. Aufl. Herder Verlag, Freiburg 1992b.

Freni, S. C.: Exposure to high fluoride concentrations in drinking water is associated with decreased birth rates. J. Toxicol. Environ Health **42**, 109–121 (1994).

Gandey, A.: HPV vaccine adverse events worrisome says the key investigator. Actions Traitements 26.7.2008.

Gerst, T.: Impfstatus und Prävention. – Tätigkeitsbericht vom 109. deutschen Ärztetag. In: Deutsches Ärzteblatt **103**, A 1524 (2006).

Girard, M.: Autoimmune hazards of hepatitis B vaccine. Autoimmun. Rev. **4**(2), 96–100 (2005).

Girke, M.: Innere Medizin. Salumed, Berlin 2010.

- English translation in progress at this time – Ed.

Goebel, W., M. Glöckler: Kindersprechstunde. Urachhaus, Stuttgart, 11. Aufl., 1984, 15. Aufl. 2005.

Goebel, W.: Schutzimpfungen selbst verantwortet. Verlag Freies Geistesleben & Urachhaus, Stuttgart, 4. Aufl. 2009.

Golding, J et al: Childhood cancer, intramuscular vitamin K and pethidine given during labour. BMJ **305**, 341–346 (1992).

Grant, W. B., Hollick, M. F.: Benefits and Requirements of Vitamin D for Optimal Health. Alternative Medicine Review 10 (2005)

Greer, F. R.: Vitamin K the basics – What´s new? Early Human Developmet **86**, S43–47 (2010).

Evans K. N. et al: Effects of 25-Hydroxyvitamin D and 1.25 – Dihydroxyviamin D 3 on Cytokine Production by Human Decidual Cells. Biology of Reproduction **75**, 816–822 (2006).

Griffin, M. R. et al.: Risk of seizures and encephalopathy after immunization with the Diphtheria-Tetanus-Pertussis-Vaccine. J. Am. Med. Assoc. **263**, 1641–1645 (1990).

Hesse, J. M.: Rechtsgutachten. Ausschluss nicht geimpfter Kinder vom Schul/Kindergartenbesuch und andere Maßnahmen der Gesundheitsämter bei Auftreten von Masernerkrankungen. Vereinbarkeit mit Infektionsschutz (IfSG) und Grundrechten? Merkurstab **60**,357–368 (2007).

Hetzer, G: Dentalfluorosen: Prävalenz, Risiko und Bewertung von Schmelzflecken. In: Per os prophylaxe, Sonderheft 1999, 36–39.

Hinrichsen, V.: Humanembryologie. Springer Verlag, Berlin – New York 1990.
Hirte, M.: Impfen – Pro und Contra. 2. Aufl. Knaur 2005, 3. Aufl. 2008, 4. Aufl. 2011.
Hirte, M.: Fluor. In: H. Pfeiffer, M. Drescher, M.Hirte (Hg.): Homöopathie in der Kinder- und Jugendmedizin. 2.Aufl. Urban & Fischer, München 2007.
Hirte, M., Rabe, S., Soldner, G., Schmidt-Troschke, S., Tautz, C.: Wuppertaler Manifest. www.individuelle-impfentscheidung.de (2010).
Hobermann, A. et al.: Effectiveness of inactivates influenza vaccine in preventing acute otitis media in young children: a randomized controlled trial. JAMA **290**, 1608–1616 (2003).
Höger, P, Kinderdermatologie, Schattauer, Stuttgart 2005.
Hohendahl, J. et al.: Masern- und Mumpsantikörperstatus bei Neugeborenen und ihren Müttern – Verlauf im ersten Lebensjahr. Klin. Pädiatr. **218**, 213–220 (2006).
Holt, P. G. et al.: Developmental factors associate with risk for atopic disease: implications for vaccine strategies in early childhood. Vaccine **21**, 3432–3435 (2003).
Hoover R. N. et al.: Time trends for bone and joint cancers and osteosarcomas in the Surveillance, Epidemiology and End Results (SEER) Program, National Cancer Institute. In: Review of Fluoride: Benefits and Risks. US Public Health Service, F1–F7 (1991).
Husemann, F.: Anthroposophische Medizin. Verlag am Goetheanum, Dornach 2009.
Husemann, A.: Der hörende Mensch und die Wirklichkeit der Musik. Verlag Freies Geistesleben, Stuttgart 2010.
Imhäuser, H.: Homöopathie in der Kinderheilkunde. Haug Verlag, Heidelberg, 7. Aufl. 1985, 12. Aufl. 2000.
Impfen – Routine oder Individualisation. Hrsg. von der Arbeitsgruppe für differenzierte Impfungen (1999), Postfach, CH-3000 Bern 9.
Iwamato, J. et al.: Differential Effect of Vitamin K and Vitamin D Supplementation on Bone Mass in Young Rats Fed Normal or Low Calcium Diet. Yonsei Medical Journal **45**, 314–324 (2004).
Iyengar, G. V.: Elemental composition of human and animal milk, a review. Upsala 1979 – zit. nach Goebel, W., M. Glöckler: Kindersprechstunde, 13. Aufl. Urachhaus, Stuttgart 1998.
Jachens, L.: Hautkrankheiten ganzheitlich heilen. 2.Aufl. Urachhaus, Stuttgart 2006.
Jefferson, T.: Influenza vaccination: policy versus evidence. BMJ **333**, 912–915 (2006).
Juurlink, D. N. et al.: Guillain-Barre Syndrome after Influenza Vaccination in Adults: A Population-Based Study. Arch Intern Med **166,** 2217–2221 (2006).
Kaiser Permanente (2010, June 29), Combination MMRV Vaccine linked with two-fold risk of seizures, study finds.
Kienle, G., Kiene, H.: Clinical judgement and the medical profession. J. fo Evaluation in Clinical Practice. published online doi: 101111/j.1365–2753.2010.01560.x.
Kipp, F. A.: Die Evolution des Menschen im Hinblick auf seine lange Jugendzeit. Verlag Freies Geistesleben, Stuttgart 1980.
Klein, T.: Sonnenlicht. Hygieia Verlag, Dresden 2007.
Koch, M. A.: Impfungen können und müssen besser genutzt werden (Editorial). Bundesgesundhbl. **1**, 1 (1996).
Koletzko, S., Uhlig, H. H., Hygienehypothese: Schlüssel zur Ätiologie und Pathogenese von CED? MSchr Kinderheilkd **158**, 759–765 (2010).
Koskiniemi, M., A. Vaheri: Effects of Measles, Mumps, Rubella Vaccination on Pattern of Encephalitis in Children. Lancet **343**, 31–34 (1989).
Kries, R. v., H. J. Schmitt: Diabetes mellitus nach Hib-Impfung? Kinderärztl. Praxis **8**, 589 (1999).
Kries, R. v. et al.: Sudden and unexpected deaths after the administration of hexavalent vaccines (DTPa-IPV-HBV-Hib): Is there a signal? Eur. J. Pediatr. **164**, 61–69 (2005).

Krober, M. S. et al.: Decreased measles antibody response after measles-M. R.-Vaccine in infants with colds. JAMA **265**, 2095 (1991).

Krutmann, J: Die Verwendung von topisch applizierten DNS-Reparaturenzymen zum Schutz der menschlichen Haut gegen UVB-induzierte Schäden, Bundesgesundheitsbl. **44**, 480–483 (2001) Krutmann, J.: Actives. Der Hautarzt **60**, 294–300 (2009).

Kummer, K. R.: 1001mal Masern – prospektive Untersuchung von 886 retrospektive von 115 Verläufen in der Praxis. Der Merkurstab **52**, 369–375 (1999).

Kummer, K. R.: Aktuelles zum Thema Impfungen. Der Merkurstab **55**, 57–58 (2002).

Kummer, K. R.: Aktuelles zum Impfen. Der Merkurstab **56**, 228–229 (2003).

Kummer, K. R.: Aktuelles zum Impfen. Der Merkurstab **57**, 59 (2004).

Kummer, K. R.: Impfungen im Kindesalter. Schriftenreihe "gesundheit aktiv", 5. Aufl. 2005.

Kutty P. et al.: Seroprevalence of Antibody to Mumps Virus in the US Population, 1999–2004. J Infectious deseases **202**, 667–674.

Kyle, W. S.: Simian retroviruses poliovaccine and origin of AIDS. Lancet **339**, 600–601 (1992).

Le, T. M. et al.: Effect of pneumococcal vaccination on otitis media with effusion in children older than 1 year. Eur J Periatr.**166**, 1049–1052 (2007).

Leitlinie und Merkblatt zum Thema Vitamin-K-Prophylaxe der Gesellschaft Anthroposophischer Ärzte in Deutschland (GAÄD). Der Merkurstab **60**, 62–65 (2007).

Lesnicar, G. et al.: Pediatric tick-borne encephalitis in 371 cases from an endemic region in Slovenia, 1959 to 2000. Pediatr. Infect. Dis. J. **22**, 612–617 (2003).

Levy S. et al.: Associations between fluorosis of permanent incisors and fluorid intake from infant formula, other dietary sources and dentifrice during early childhood. J Am Dent Assoc. **141**, 1190–1201.

Liese, J. G., Knuf, M.: Impfungen von Frühgeborenen. MSchr f Kinderheilk **157**, 758–766 (2009).

Mahdawi,W., Ein neues pharmakologisches Screeningverfahren für neue und bekannte Antiasthmatika und Antiallergika am ovalbuminsensibilisierten Meerschweinchen in einem Zweikammerganzkörperplethysmographen. Diss. Ludwig-Maximilians-Universität München 2005.

Mascart, F. et al.: Modulation of the infant immune responses by the first pertussis administrations. Vaccine **25**, 391–398 (2007)

Massag, B.: Niedrig dosierte Vitamin-K-Prophylaxe bei Neugeborenen. Der Merkurstab **58**, 50 (2005).

Madeleyn, R.: Rachitisprophylaxe aus der Sichtweise der anthroposophisch erweiterten Medizin. Der Merkurstab **48**, 558 (1995).

Madeleyn, R: Vitamin-K-Prophylaxe bei Neugeborenen. Der Merkurstab **58**, 49–50 (2005).

Mansoor, O., P. Pillans: Vaccine adverse events reports in New Zealand 1990–1995. New Z. Med. J. **110**, 270–272 (1997).

McDonald K. et al.: Delay in diphtheria, pertussis, tetanus vaccination is associated with a reduced risk of childhood asthma. J Allergy Clin Immunol **121**, 626–631 (2008).

Meinecke, C.: Hepatitis-B-Impfung – Gegenwärtige Indikationsstellung und Problematik eines Konzepts. Der Merkurstab **52**, Sonderheft Hepatitis, 68–77 (1999).

Mezger, J.: Gesichtete homöopathische Arzneimittellehre, Bd. 2, Haug Verlag, Heidelberg 1999.

Mirror.co.uk: 'Vaccine link' to 18 dead tots. 13. Febr. 2006. www.mirror.co.uk/news/topstories/tm_objectid=16696993 %26method=full%26siteid=94762-name_page.html.

Mittermeier, H.: Generalisierte anaphylaktisch-toxische Gefäßwandschädigung mit Sinusthrombose nach aktiver Diphtherieschutzimpfung. Mschr. Kinderheilk. **107**, 288 (1959).

Nakamura, N. et al.: Neurologic complications associated with influenza vaccination: two adult cases. Intern Med. **42**, 191–194 (2003).

Newhouse, M. et al.: A case control study of carcinoma of the ovary. Br. J. Prev. Soc. Med. **31**, 148–153 (1977).

National Vaccine Information Center (NVIC): An analysis by the National Vaccine Information Center of Gardasil & Menactra daverse event reports to the Vaccine Adverse Events Reporting System (VAERS). Februar 2009.

Plewig, G., Kaudewitz, P., Sander C. A.L Fortschritte der praktischen Dermatologie und Venerologie. Springer, Berlin 2004.

Pilz, S. et al: Association of Vitamin D deficiency with heart failure and sudden cardiac death in a large cross-sectional study of patients referred for coronary angiography. J Clin Endocrinology **93**.3927–3935 (2008).

Portmann, A.: Biologie und Geist. Burgdorf Verlag, Frankfurt/M. 2000.

Querings, K, Reichrath, J: A plea for detection and treatment of vitamin D deficiency in patients under photoprotection. Cancer Cause Control **15**, 219 (2004).

Rabe, S.: Impf-Info, 5. Aufl., Manuskriptdruck, Rathausgasse 2, 81241 München, 2002; im Internet: www.impf-info.de.

Reckert, T.: Sonnenlicht, Vitamin D, Inkarnation. Der Merkurstab **62**, 577–593 (2009).

Romanowski, B. et al.: Sustained efficacy and immungenicity of the human papillomavirus (HPV)-16/18 AS 04-adjuvanted vaccine: analysis of a randomised placebo-controlledtrial up to 6.4 years. Lancet **374,**1975–1985 (2009).

Rosenlund, H.: Allergic Disease and Atopic Sensitization in Children in Relation to Measles Vaccination and Measles Infection. Pediatrics **123**, 771–778 (2009).

Schlumpf, M., et al.: Developmental toxicity of UV filters and environmental exposure: a review. Int J Androl **31**, 144–151.

Scholten, J.: Homöopathie und Minerale. Stichting Alonissos, Utrecht 1993.

Schütte, T.: Untersuchungen über den Fluoridgehalt des Trinkwassers aus privaten Wasserversorgungsanlagen der Region östliches Münsterland. Dissertation Institut für Hygiene, Univ.klinikum Münster 1983.

Shroff, R. et al.: The virtues of vitamin D – but how much is too much? Pediatr Nephrol, published online DOI 10.1007/s00465-010-1499-9.

Siedler, A., A. Tischer: Masernerkrankungen in Deutschland. Kinderärztliche Praxis (2002), Sonderheft "Impfen 2002", 8–12.

Sitzmann, F. C.: Consilium Infectiorum 2001/43, Frage 3447.

Silverberg, J. I. : Association between varicella zoster virus infection and atopic dermatitis in early and late childhood: a case-control study. J Allergy Clin Immunol **126,** 300–305(2010).

Smith, S., Demicheli, V. et al.: Vaccines for preventing influenza in healthy children. Cochrane Database Syst Rev 2006 (1): CD004879.

Soldner, G.: Helleborus niger. Der Merkurstab **63**, 508–517 (2010).

Speer, C., Gahr, M.: Pädiatrie. 3.Aufl. Springer, Berlin 2009.

Stehr, K., U. Heininger: Aktueller Stand der Keuchhustenschutzimpfung. pädiatr. praxis **4**, 391–402 (1991).

Steiner, R.: Physiologisch-Therapeutisches auf Grundlage der Geisteswissenschaften. Gesamtausgabe Bd. 314, 3. Aufl. Rudolf Steiner Verlag, Dornach 1989.

Steiner, R.: Das Zusammenwirken von Ärzten und Seelsorgern. Pastper os medizinischer Kurs. Rudolf Steiner Verlag, Dornach 1994.

- Steiner, R.: Pastoral medicine: the collegial working of doctors and priests: eleven lectures delivered in Dornach in September of 1924. GA (complete works) 318. Anthroposophic Press, Hudson, N. Y.

1987. Also published as: Broken vessels: the spiritual structure of human frailty. Anthroposophic Press, Great Barrington, M. A. 2003.

Steiner, R.: Anthroposophische Menschenerkenntnis und Medizin, Gesamtausgabe Bd. 319. Rudolf Steiner Verlag, Dornach, 2. Aufl. 1982, 3. Aufl. 1994.

- Steiner, R.: The healing process: spirit, nature and our bodies: lectures, August 28, 1923-August 29, 1924, in various cities. GA (complete works) 319. Anthroposophic Press, Hudson, N. Y. 2000.

Steiner, R.: Mensch und Welt. Gesamtausgabe, Bd 351. Rudolf Steiner Verlag, Dornach, 1999 [b].

Steiner, R.: Geisteswissenschaft und Medizin, Gesamtausgabe, Bd. 312. 7.Auflage, Rudolf Steiner Verlag, Dornach 1999 [a].

- Steiner, R.: Introduction to anthroposophical medicine. GA (complete works) 312. SteinerBooks, Great Barrington, M. A. 1999.

Steiner, R., I. Wegman: Grundlegendes zu einer Erweiterung der Heilkunst nach geisteswissenschaftlichen Erkenntnissen. Rudolf Steiner Verlag, Arlesheim 1953, Dornach 5. Aufl. 1977, 7. Aufl. 1991.

- Steiner, R., Wegman, I.: Fundamentals of therapy: an extension of the art of healing through spiritual-scientific knowledge. GA (complete works) 27. Mercury Press, Spring Valley, N. Y. 1999. Also available as: Extending practical medicine: fundamental principles based on the science of the spirit. Rudolf Steiner Press, London 1996.

Steiner, R.: Anthroposophische Menschenerkenntnis und Medizin. Gesamtausgabe Bd. 319. Rudolf Steiner Verlag, Dornach 3. Aufl. 1994.

- Steiner, R.: The healing process: spirit, nature and our bodies: lectures, August 28, 1923-August 29, 1924, in various cities. GA (complete works) 319. Anthroposophic Press, Hudson, N. Y. 2000.

Stickl, H.: Verschluss der Arteria cerebri media nach Diphtherie-Tetanus-Auffrisch-Impfung bei einem sechs Jahre alten Jungen. Der Kinderarzt 636 (1978).

Stösser, Fluorid zur Prävention der Milchzahnkaries. Per os prophylaxe und Kinderzahnheilkunde **30**, 17–25.

Thomas, S.: Contacts with varicella or with children and protection against herpes zoser in adults: a case-control study. Lancet **360**, 678–682 (2002).

Tolzin, H. U.: impf-report Nr. 24/25. Tolzin Verlag, Augsburg 2006.

Tremezaygues, L, Reichrath,J.: Zur Bedeutung des Vitamin-D-Stoffwechsels in der humanen Haut.

Truckenbrodt, H.: Impfungen bei chronischer Arthritis. pädiatr. praxis **52**, 42–43 (1997).

Vagedes, J., Soldner, G.: Das Kindergesundheitsbuch. 3.Aufl. Gräfe und Unzer, München 2010.

Vandermeulen C. et al.: Long-term persistence of antibodies after one or two doses of MMR-vaccine. Vaccine **25**, 6672–6676 (2007).

Verhulst, J.: Der Erstgeborene. Mensch und höherer Tiere in der Evolution. Verlag Freies Geistesleben, Stuttgart 1999.

Verstraeten, T. et al.: Safety of thiomersal-containing vaccines: a two-phased study of computerized health maintainance organization databases. Pediatrics **112**, 1039–1048 (2003).

Vogel H.-H.: Wege der Heilmittelfindung, Bd. 1, Bd. 2. Natur Mensch Medizin Verlag, Bad Boll 1994.

- Vogel, H.-H.: Finding remedies: spiritual knowledge of man and naure; a contribution toward understanding anthroposophic remedies, based on the example of the Wala remedy compositions. V 1, 2 Natur-Mensch-Medizin, Bad Boll 1994.

Vogel, H. H.: Organe der Ich-Organisation. Natur Mensch Medizin Verlag, Bad Boll 1996.

Wahn, U., R. Seger, V. Wahn: Pädiatrische Allergologie und Immunologie. 2. Aufl. G. Fischer Verlag, Stuttgart 1994, 3. Aufl. Urban & Fischer, München 1999, 4. Aufl. Urban & Fischer, München 2005.

Wahlberg, J. et al.: Vaccinations May Induce Diabetes-Related Autoantibodies in One-Year-old Children. Ann. N.Y. Acad. Sci. **1005**, 404–408 (2003).

Watanabe: Henoch-Schönlein purpura folllowing influenza vaccinations during the pandemic of influenza A (H1N1). Pediatr. Nephrol published online DOI 10.1007/s00467-010-1722-8.

West, R.: Epidemiologic study of malignancies of the ovaries. Cancer **19**, 1001–1007 (1966).

Windorfer, A.: Zentralnervöse Infektionen im Kindesalter. Mschr. Kinderheilk. **143**, 605–616 (1995).

Wirrell, E. et al.: Stroke after varicella vaccination. J. Pediatr. **145**, 845–847 (2005).

Wise, R. P.: Postlicensure safety surveillance for varicella vaccine. JAMA **284**, 1271–1279 (2000).

Wolf P., UV-Filter. State of the art. Hautarzt **60**, 285–293 (2009).

Wolff, O.: LM-Potenzen und vegetabilisierte Metalle. Der Merkurstab **50**, 127 (1991).

Wrensch M. et al: History of Chickenpox and Shingles and PRevalence of Antibodies to Varicella-Zoster Virus and Three Other Herpesviruses among Adults with Glioma and Controls. Am J Epidemiol **161**, 929–938.

Wrensch M et al: Does prior infection with varicella-zoster virus influence risk of adult glioma? Am J Epidemiol **145**, 594–7 (1997).

Zinka, B. et al.: Unexplained cases of sudden infant death shortly after hexavalent vaccination. Vaccine **24**(31–32), 5779–5780 (2006).

Zuck, R.: Gutachterliche Äußerung für die GAÄD wegen Impfbeschluss des 109. DÄT zu berufsrechtlichen Sanktionen gegenüber Ärzten. Der Merkurstab **59**, 549–555 (2006).

4 Digestive tract disorders and gastrointestinal diseases

Breast feeding is a learning process of mother and child[1]

4.1 Breast feeding and early development of the digestive and immune systems

Breast feeding represents the most important act of disease prevention and healthy development in human life. The newborn is physically incapable of digesting any natural foodstuff other than breast milk – or milk made similar to it. The greatest growth spurt in postnatal life occurs during the breast feeding period in parallel to the development of a digestive tract which is capable of functioning independently: organ formation, growth and organ activity cannot be separated at this age.

The existential importance of this process is expressed in the term "suckling" which indicates both the own activity and the dependent child. – Breast milk is finely attuned to the vital needs of the child's organism, itself being living substance and not a nutritional solution. In terms of age breast milk is always "newborn" whereas powdered milk and bottled food can be significantly older than the child itself. During the whole breast feeding period and also in the course of each individual occasion that the child is breast feed [Koletzko 2009, 70] the milk changes in accordance with the needs of the child's organism in quantity and quality and is thus an expression of a sensitive regulatory organization which envelops mother and child. In this phase of life, mother and child are still directly connected at the level of the life organization, the etheric body. The child experiences in substance the interaction between perception and response in what he or she receives from his or her breast feeding mother as nutrition. That can create a "sense of coherence" in the soul. Breast feeding fulfils the need for understanding, for responsiveness and attention. The research into salutogenesis, into the resilience of children has made the importance of this quality clear.

4.1.1 Breast feeding and the human being's relationship to fats

Obesity research has shown that breast fed infants develop better self-regulation with regard to food intake and the feeling of satiety. Among 10,000 Bavarian children aged 5 to 6 the prevalence of obesity in children who were never breast fed was 4.5 %, in children who were breast fed only 2.8 %, corresponding to a reduction of more than 35 %. Beyond

1 Koletzko B. et al. [2010]

4

that there was a clear dosage-effect relationship: In the children who were breast fed for a period of six to twelve months the prevalence had fallen to 1.7 % [Zwiauer 2001, 73]. These data show that breast feeding exercises a sustained influence on the way that children deal with fats. The human fat metabolism has a central, direct relationship with the warmth organization and the ability of the skin to regulate warmth (cf. Section 6.4.2 in detail); healthy infants double their fat content in the first year of life from 14 to about 28 %. No terrestrial animal develops such a fat content; only marine mammals and hibernating animals get anywhere close to such a level. Free living mammals have an average fat content of 2 to 5 %. The question of fats, the build up and regulation of body fats, is a question of the I-organization and so it is no surprise that obese people can only regain control over their fat metabolism through individual commitment in their I. The maternal commitment through breast feeding strengthens this ability already in the infant.

Mammals and human beings have homoiothermy, the internal warmth autonomy, in common; in the universality of the human warmth organization such warmth autonomy (with the parallel possibility of remaining active under all ecological conditions, being able to develop an independent will) reaches a qualitatively new level, the level of the I-organization. After birth the newborn must double his or her warmth generation; brown adipose tissue physically enables this step. It has been shown in mammals that breast milk activates warmth generation after birth [Hondares 2010]. This makes the direct influence of breast milk on the effectiveness of the I-organization clear. It is supplemented by the research finding that the organism gives its components a uniform temporal shape through the self-regulation of warmth and that the circadian rhythm of mammals is regulated through warmth [Buhr 2010].

It can give us cause for thought that Ita Wegman and Rudolf Steiner pointed out in 1925 that the mother transfers "her own formative forces of the I-organization to the child" through the fat in breast milk and thus "add something to the formative forces which have already been transferred through heredity" [Steiner, Wegman 1991, 59]]. The relationship between the human organism and the fats is indeed something unique. Through their subcutaneous fat human beings can forgo the species-specific specialization of the skin in the form of fur, feathers and scales (all protein substances). Protective warmth and warmth generation are only connected in this radical form with fat in human beings, 98.5 % of the human warmth reserves are stored in the fatty tissue. At the same time obesity and anorexia represent characteristic ways for human beings to fall ill which are connected with the achievement, or lack, of autonomy; to the present day they cannot be cured pharmacologically but ultimately only through strengthening the I activity of the patient. As long ago as 1925, Steiner and Wegman characterized the human fat metabolism in such a way that they noted in obesity a tendency towards chronic subcutaneous inflammation triggered by excess fat ["parasitic warmth centres", l. c. 60] while on the other hand acknowledging the importance in terms of the pathology of fat deficiency (e. g. epidermal in atopic dermatitis). In doing so they were decades ahead of scientific research.

Their formulation that breast milk "added something to the formative forces which have already been transferred through heredity" indicates qualities which are today the subject of epigenetic research (▸Chap. 1.1.) and are connected with the regulation of the DNA developing in pregnancy and early childhood (breast feeding period), that is, in a time when the life organization of the child is physiologically still directly connected with the mother. It can further be related to the human shape as a whole in so far as human beings form a "fat sculpture" and, for example, the chubbiness of the cherubic infant as much as the beauty of the adult woman are directly connected with the sculpted form of the fatty tissue (female primates, for example, do not have a developed female breast outside lactation). Obesity or anorexia are reflected in the achievement or otherwise of the human form. Their incidence has increased in societies with a western lifestyle to the same extent (with anorexia, for example, eightfold in Germany since 1960) as autoimmune and chronic inflammatory disorders for example (see below), which are associated with a regulatory weakness at the level of the I-organization and for which breast feeding has in many instances shown itself to be an effective preventive. In breast feeding the incarnation of the child's individuality is supported in its embodiment (▸Chap. 1.3.2).

After fatty tissue, the human brain is the most fatty organ (40 % of dry weight). Breast feeding actively supports brain development and can have a measurably positive influence on intelligence. Here both the composition of the breast milk (long-chain omega-3 fatty acids, fat profile) and of the child's metabolism play a central role [Caspi 2007]. A longitudinal cohort study from Christchurch, New Zealand, investigated the connection between the breast feeding period and cognitive abilities as well as the exam performance from the age of 8 to 18 in 1000 children and young people. Even after correction for various cofactors, a longer breast feeding period was significantly associated with

- better performance of intelligence at the age of eight and nine,
- better reading and mathematical performance from the age of 10 to 13,
- better final exams at age 18 [Horwood 1998],
  - never breast fed: 22.2 % without school leaving exam,
  - < 4 months breast fed: 19.2 % without school leaving exam,
  - 4 months breast fed: 16.4 % without school leaving exam,
  - ≥ 8 months breast fed: 14.0 % without school leaving exam ($p < 0.05$).

The composition of the fats in human breast milk can in turn be influenced through the nutrition of the mother e. g. with biodynamic milk products [Rist et al. 2007].

4.1.2 Breast feeding, intestinal flora and immunological development of the infant

The chemical analysis which shows the (fluctuating) content of salts, fats, proteins and carbohydrates covers up *the living organization and function of breast milk as it changes over time* and thus the key difference from any artificially produced infant food which only ever represents an imitation of life at the level of what can be physically and chemically understood (and done). Breast milk possesses living enzymatic activity, e. g. through fat splitting enzymes, antimicrobially effective lactoferrin. It contains bacteria which act as "starters" of healthy intestinal flora and through its composition it controls the development of the child's intestinal flora. Through its IgA content it contributes to the development of a functioning intestinal wall; only the influence of breast milk turns the intestinal into a functioning barrier between internal and external world (▸Chap. 6, Allergic diseases). In the first 3–4 months of life breast milk contains up to 100 million leucocytes/l, the maternal nonspecific immune system (granulocytes, macrophages) initially takes care of the child's gastro-intestinal tract through breast feeding until the infant's own immunological competence has developed. Breast fed children are five times less likely to fall ill with infectious enteritis [Koletzko 2009, 71], but also approx. three times less likely to develop bacterial meningitis (Hib, pneumococci, cf. ▸Chap. 3.5), which underlines the fundamental importance of the gastrointestinal mucosa as barriers between internal and external world.

At the same time breast milk has a "probiotic" effect. The intestine of the newborn is still sterile. In the first three years human beings develop flora inside their digestive tract, above all in the mouth cavity and large intestine, which comprises about 400 different types of bacteria and which is specific to each person, showing a high level of intraindividual stability throughout life [Kummer 1998]. The colonization of the digestive tract is introduced on the one hand by the maternal vaginal flora (in vaginal births) and on the other by bacteria in breast milk. After a caesarean section there is a delay in the development of the intestinal flora. Here analyses show that the Lactobacillus flora in breast milk display clear regional differences: women living in rural areas in Japan or Sweden showed e.g. up to 50% L. reuteri in their breast milk whereas this bacterium with its valuable function with regard to intestinal flora and protection against infection was hardly present in the breast milk of women living in urban areas of Peru, Denmark or Israel [Sinkiewicz 2005]. This correlates e.g. with the fact that chronic-inflammatory bowel diseases are increasing faster in cities than in the country and that contact of mother and child with farm animals has shown itself to be a strongly protective factor in allergies and chronic inflammatory bowel diseases (reduces the risk by 50–60%!) [Koletzko, Uhlig 2010, 760]. "Probiotics" initially represents the opposing concept to "antibiotics". The facts set out above also explain why antibiotics can disrupt a healthy development more profoundly in the first year of life than later on because they disrupt the development and individualization of the intestinal flora. In summary, we can say that the development of a healthy digestive system correlates with the basic quality of the etheric: *living coherence*, which comes to expression in breast feeding, in the contact between the mother and the natural environment, in the assimilation of the maternal bacteria in the child's digestive tract. Biodynamically produced foods, the enjoyment of vegetables preserved by spontaneous fermentation (e.g. raw Sauerkraut), the avoidance of antibiotics supports the development of a healthy digestive and immune system in mother and child (▸Chap. 6.1, "anthroposophical lifestyle").

At the same time the development the child's intestinal flora points to a polar quality: human beings cannot live without cultivating death in their intestine throughout their life. The foods imbibed have to be radically broken down until their have lost any character of the organism from which they originate (that does not apply to breast milk). If we look at the development of the human digestive system over the long term, we can see in the mature human digestive system that human beings realize a *unique universality* with regard to the cosmos of possible foods: no other highly developed living being is able to digest such diverse substances – from the above perspective we might also say able to subject such diverse substances to death in its own digestion – as the human being! This aspect can illustrate the depth to which the human I-organization incarnates in the digestive tract in the course of childhood. Thus many food intolerances disappear by themselves in the course of childhood because the digestive power of the child grows and one-sided food likes or dislikes in small children often fade in the second half of childhood.

What we have said about the digestive process applies equally with regard to the defence of the organism against intestinal flora: only a fraction of this intestinal flora in the urinary passages means a serious infection; mere traces of this flora in the blood means septicaemia. The penetration of the intestinal flora through the mucous layer to the intestinal wall is a central pathogenic factor in chronic inflammatory bowel diseases. In a healthy digestive tract both sides must be kept differentiatedly apart and no alien life must penetrate the inside of the organism. This necessary polarization is effected by the higher aspects of the human being: at the "threshold" between intestinal lumen and organism, the life of external nature must "die" and integrate itself with the laws of the human organism. The intensive pervasion of the intestinal wall by the human immune and nervous system (see below), the connection between the digestive system and the physical activity of the sentient and I organization only becomes comprehensible if this threshold character between life and death is recognized. "Death resides in the intestine" and is controlled there by the higher components of the human being throughout life.

Healthy intestinal flora itself provides a healthy etheric basis for this necessary catabolic process. It enables the complete breakdown of food, eliminates dangerous microorganisms, synthesizes vital resorbable vitamins and prevents the adhesion of harmful bacteria to the intestinal wall. The human astral body also comes to essential expression in the differentiated *gas tension relationships* which are set up in the intestine with the help of the intestinal flora (anaerobic conditions in the large intestine lumen as opposed to high oxygen tension in the intestinal wall). On the other hand abnormal bacterial colonization of the small intestine or disorders of carbohydrate digestion, for example, can be shown to exist through the concentration of hydrogen in the exhaled air, and reflect a pathological release of gases in the intestinal lumen which is no longer guided by the astral body.

The human immune system takes its starting point from the digestive tract. Two thirds of this system are located in this area. It is precisely in dealing with the intestinal flora, in the management of life in the intestine, that the child's immune system develops its equilibrium of aggression, delimitation and killing of everything alien, on the one hand, and tolerance for what belongs to the body, on the other. A profound individualization and physical identification process correlates immunologically with the development of the intestinal flora. Ultimately every activity of the immune system which dissolves alien qualities in the organism and excretes them is a "par-enteral" digestive activity. Breast feeding ensures the best prerequisites in this learning process: The thymus (▸Chap. 6.3) of breast fed children also develops more strongly than the thymus of children who have not been breast fed [Koletzko 2009, 71].

The immune tolerance, *the self-regulation of the immune system* develops better on a sustained basis than in infants fed with formula food: the probability of otitis media between 6 and twelve months is reduced by half in breast fed children, the probability of an allergic inflammation of the airways is verifiably lower as late as the age of seven [Zwiauer 2001, 72, 74]. This living quality means that breast milk even has an organ-forming effect on the child's digestive tract – a quality which no artificial infant milk possesses. If the child continues to be breast fed when gluten-containing food is introduced, the risk of coeliac disease falls by half [Koletzko 2010, 682]. That is shown particularly clearly by the effect of breast milk on the epigenetic regulation ("early programming") as coeliac disease can only develop if there is a genetic predisposition but most infants develop an (epigenetic) tolerance to prolamines (alcoholic grain-based proteins) [Zimmer 2003]. Thus breast feeding also promotes learning processes for a healthy immune tolerance and immune regulation after solid food has been introduced. That is shown, finally, by chronic inflammatory bowel diseases (IBD): the risk of developing Crohn's disease rises more than threefold in children who have not been breast fed, much clearer than the risk for ulcerative colitis [Koletzko and Uhlig 2010, 760f.]. But Crohn's disease has increased by more than six times in the last 50–60 years, ulcerative colitis approx. by three times. Breast feeding has a positive salutogenetic effect in that the child's organism learns to keep the intestinal content, intestinal flora and intestinal wall apart by means of a stable "mucosal block", a living layer of mucosa which separates the intestinal content and intestinal wall and can keep the latter virtually sterile [cf. Girke 2010, 665]. In chronic-inflammatory bowel diseases, but also in coeliac disease, a living quality between the intestinal wall and intestinal content is lost which is otherwise physiologically built up after birth under the influence and with the substantial support of the breast milk.

If we add up in the way of western industrialized societies what the result would be if 90 % of US mothers were to breast feed their infants for six months, experts calculate an annual "saving" of more than 900 childhood deaths and of 13bn US dollars for the national health system when compared to the current situation [Bartick, Reinhold 2010]. At the same time this makes clear which preventive measure in western industrialized societies displays the most assured efficiency and sustainability (cf. ▸Chap. 3) and the contribution made by women who breast feed their babies for a sufficiently long period of time. Acknowledging this can also be an aspect of paediatric activity.

Breast milk also acts differently than "dead" nutrition, including every aspecific milk, on the development of the child's own bodily substance. The protein in human breast milk is used almost without loss for building up the child's bodily substance (the protein content in breast milk, in relation to resorbable protein, lies at less than 1 g/dl) and therefore places minimal burden on the kidneys through the excretion of nitrogen. Breast milk does not first have to be completely broken down by the child's organism with a great deal of effort in the way that foreign nutrition does, which invariably leads to the corresponding losses. Instead it can pass over directly into the child's anabolic processes, the child's organ formation in the whole organism.

The replacement of breast milk through artificially adapted food is only possible in that the deficiency in vital quality is compensated through a surplus of substance, above all protein. Thus infants fed with formula milk display "clearly higher insulin concentrations in their plasma … than breast fed children. High insulin levels may have a stimulating effect in the early development of adipocytes" [Zwiauer 2003, 86] and are thereby in turn connected with the development of obesity and an increase in type 2 diabetes mellitus in the population. A key aspect in any artificial infant food is that it irritates the child's gustatory sensation (and development!). There is no research yet on the long term effects of the bitter taste of hydrolyzed, hypoallergenic infant food on the later appetite behaviour of children. Artificial infant food further has an irritating effect in forcing the infant to engage in significantly stronger catabolic activity in the digestive tract and metabolism than breast milk. Gall bladder and pancreas activity are irritated and provoked through every breast milk replacement as the enzyme activity of breast milk is absent and at the same time more substance has to be broken down and digested than in breast feeding. That allows us to understand, on the other hand, why icterus neonatorum lasts longer in breast fed children than in those who have not been breast fed. The infant organism must vitalize such milk with a great deal of its own effort, something that can be seen, among other things, in that almost half the protein of powdered milk is excreted and not used for building up bodily substance – *a burden above all on the kidneys, and which can lead to an increase in restlessness in the infant.* The nitrogen burden of artificial infant food speeds up the maturation process of the kidney functions, but thereby also the mental awakening with all possible consequences. Stronger organic catabolic processes are accompanied by increased mental sensations. [Steiner and Wegman 1977, 16f.; Vogel 1995, 47–52, 69;

Portmann 1983, 225–233; Fintelmann 1994, 85] Such stimulation of the kidney activity indirectly influences intestinal activity, (tendency for colics, meteorism, change in voiding rhythm).

Breast milk itself today contains irritating factors for the child's digestive tract, e. g. in its content of harmful substances (which is not an argument against breast feeding). A considerable part of fat-soluble harmful substance which is stored in the maternal organism and is otherwise difficult to excrete occurs in breast milk. Thus every infant must today deal with irritating and indigestible components of food which undoubtedly can also contribute to disorders of the digestive tract.

4.1.3 Breast feeding and embodiment of the childhood sentient and I-organization

Breast feeding means that through the living maternal food the child becomes quiet, that he or she goes to sleep while the nutrition is resorbed and own substance is built up. In contrast, *colic* after food means that an irritation, an abnormal feeling in the soul has been triggered at the boundary of external and internal world, at the intestinal mucosa, which in turn leads to a painful reaction to the food which has been taken in. That raises the question as to the *presence of the sentient organization in the digestive tract*. Whereas the strength of the life organization comes to expression in the constantly regenerating intestinal mucosa, particularly in the fine, leaf-like villi and microvilli of the small intestine, a picture emerges in the intestinal wall which is very much determined by the astral body, the soul and animal-like organization of the human being. The gastro-intestinal tract is the organ in the human organism with the most nerves outside the CNS; the "enteric nervous system" (ENS), also called "little brain", is equal in mass to the brain. The growth of the intestinal wall also occurs parallel to growth of the brain. As early as the start of the second year of life, loss of length of the small intestine can no longer be compensated (short bowel syndrome). This not so well known fact shows particularly clearly that the intensive regeneration of the intestinal mucosa in the intestinal wall, like brain development, faces a quality which is pervaded by intensive formative and catabolic processes. An initial reason for such intensive innervation can be seen in the fact that *the whole of the digestive tract possesses the capacity of independent movement* – extending as far as the villi of the mucosa ("villi pump"): The gastro-intestinal tract moves "like a snake in the abdomen" (snakes are able to digest everything coming from outside). The invagination of an independently moving gastro-intestinal tract represents an archetypal act of animal body formation.

Self-movement is not possible without self-perception. *By far the most nervous connections between the ENS and CNS are of an afferent sensitive nature! The gastro-intestinal tract is a highly sensitively (largely unconsciously) perceived interior space*, the "*sense of life*" [Steiner 2002, 23] of human beings is intensively connected to this organ. Whether or not a person feels well is decisively dependent on the quality of his or her experience at the skin and intestine, his internal and external barriers. Breast feeding, sensitive touch can make an infant calm and satisfied. The oral cavity is the most sensitive and intimate area of the human being as such (something that underlines the soul and spiritual importance of breast feeding once again and should also be considered by every paediatrician who makes an examination in this area). Children between the ages of three and five often experience the independent movement of the intestine in a painful way. On the other hand the peristalsis in the gastro-intestinal tract also reflects soul experiences: accompanying movements of the intestinal wall can be observed in people who are dreaming.

The child appears to undergo and fix learning processes in his enteric nervous system in the same way as in the central nervous system. Both nervous systems interact intensively and are permanently marked by early relationship and environmental experiences. Against this background a "*visceral hypersensitivity*" can develop as early as the first year of life. The intestinal content is experienced – figuratively speaking – like a scratchy vest on dry skin, not like a welcome treat; antipathetically stressed hypersensitivity leads to paraesthesia and hypertonically spasmodic disorders of the motor functions with the corresponding functional digestive disorders. Hypersensitivity, hyperresponsiveness and motility disorders thus so form the beginning of a development in which the action of the sentient organization, the astral body, in the digestive tract threatens to become independent and paralyzed [Girke 2010, 657]. The abnormally increased activity of the sentient organization can lead to a chronic subacute inflammatory disorder of the intestinal wall which comes to expression in infants in strong trimester colics [Rhoads 2009]. Disorders of the intestinal flora favour such a development; neurogenically the enteric nervous system can itself cause inflammations (like ends of the vagus nerve in asthma).

In adults with irritable bowel syndrome, the beginnings of their disorder can often be traced back to early childhood. Negative biographical experiences of mother and child during pregnancy and early childhood can come to expression in such disorders. Clinical observation shows that children whose development in utero was strongly burdened by unrest, shock experiences of the mother, medical intervention, etc. have a much greater tendency for states of unrest and disorders of the digestive process than children whose pregnancy was undisturbed [Papousek 2009, 563]. The word "irritation" brings to expression that ultimately the *soul organization of the child* is irritated. Infections and food intolerances can then become the acute triggers of such a disorder. The soul entity here requires particular guidance and integration through the I. Therapeutically the attempt must be made to prevent parts of the human sentient organization from making themselves independent and splitting off, and to support their reintegration into the realm of the I-organization and its regulation. The mother, the parents play a key role in this respect. Her I exercises the strongest effect on the embodiment of the soul and spiritual individuality of the child. The corresponding therapeutic support of the parents can have a sustained positive effect on subsequent development. Against this background, the use of potentized organ preparations of the vegetative nervous system (Plexus coeliacus, Plexus gastricus – Chap. 4.7.1.2) has been shown to be helpful in medicinal treatment in recent years.

Breast feeding requires calm. Perhaps the most important thing in the process of breast feeding is that in that moment nothing and no one is more important than mother and child. *Attention and appreciation of the other promote the incarnation of the human I.* Telephone and media should not have access to the mother at that time; siblings should learn to respect the period when the mother is breast feeding. Because that precisely lays the foundation for a *feeling of self-esteem in the child*: Moments in which nothing is more important than the child himself or herself gives the child the feeling of his or her own value. For women who might have worked up to that point it is often a new experience to switch off the phone and "only" breast feed in peace. The feeling of restlessness, the need to be "networked", give way only gradually to the enjoyment and pleasure which can be experienced in breast feeding.

The mother breast feeds her child face to face – a fundamentally different relationship than can be found in the animal kingdom. The *correspondence of body and soul inherent in breast feeding* feeds the child much more comprehensively than can be understood from a purely nutritional and physiological perspective.

In delicate, breathing interplay between mother and child it is not only the composition of the breast milk which is adapted to the needs of the child; an elementary learning process in the soul takes place at the same time [Dornes 1993]. *The capacity of understanding matures* – in mother and child; both influence and transform one another significantly; *Physical and soul correspondence are indivisible here* [Fuchs 2008, 191–194]. It is noteworthy that breast feeding cuts the risk of sudden death syndrome (SIDS) by approximately half [Vennemann et al. 2009]. Breast feeding stabilizes the breathing of the child. In situations where physical breast feeding is impossible the soul aspects of the act of breast feeding are all the more important; the mother can compensate for the absence of breast milk through attention, calmness and perception of the child.

Warmth is located between these soul and food related aspects of breast feeding. Watching and maintaining the warmth of the infant meets both an elementary physical (▸Chap. 2) and soul need. Warmth transmits calmness, attention and security; Children whose warmth situation is intact behave significantly more calmly than children who have to compensate for a reduction in body temperature – even only occasionally – through breaking down their bodily substance. Breast feeding itself supports the infant to keep warm.

Every paediatrician will look after children who cannot be breast fed for various reasons. But if as physicians we observe and communicate the importance of breast feeding in its entirety, possibilities and opportunities become clear for compensating some of the loss which artificial baby food inevitably brings.

4.2 Breast feeding counselling

> You, the Big, go and rest in honour of the Small; for its hour is its world and your hour is the cosmos.
>
> J. R. Jiménez

Against this background breast feeding counselling should be given special medical attention before (!) and after birth. Thus clear information about the connections set out above can strengthen the motivation to breast feed. Suitable parental guides [Goebel and Glöckler 2008, 321–328; Vagedes and Soldner 2010, 123f] can support the mother, the advice of experienced midwives and breast feeding counsellor be very helpful. A *relaxed posture* during breast feeding is important for milk flow, prevents mastitis and helps the baby to latch on to the nipple in the right way [see Vagedes and Soldner 2010, 124]. The importance of putting the baby to the breast soon after the birth is generally known; if the father also experiences this moment, it can strengthen his ties to the child.

Unfortunately, *mixed feeding in the first days of life* continues to be widespread. The natural fact that the child only receives little food in the first three days of life, loses weight and manages with low blood sugar levels is respected too little as a *natural and in itself sensible arrangement*. The natural shortage of food and weight loss after birth appears meaningful from the perspective of the incarnation of the soul and spiritual entity: Physical catabolic processes and the awakening of the soul and spiritual entity in the body go in parallel (the incarnation of Christ in the baptism in Jordan is followed by 40 days of fasting in the desert – an archetypal image for the incarnation process referred to here). The temptation of mixed feeding should be resisted for as long as the situation is not pathological (e.g. with premature babies or small-for-date births; cave childhood hypoglycaemia with maternal diabetes!). As decisively as intervention is required in these cases, any intervention without good reason in the form of a sugar solution or, worse still, "hypoallergenic" food ("as a precaution") should be equally avoided. Any administration of sugar can lead to an unwanted reaction and irritation of the intestinal mucosa; any foreign protein in this sensitive situation of the first days of life increases the long-term risk of food intolerances and disrupts the development of the digestive tract. The information from the mother that there was mixed feeding in the first days of life is important with regard to the aspects set out above and an important point to be noted in the patient notes.

It cannot be the task of this book to add to the existing literature on maternal nutrition during breast feeding, on breast feeding itself and on nutrition for infants and toddlers [e.g. Goebel and Glöckler 2008, 321ff.] We will discuss here a number of additional aspects of importance in paediatric practice.

Mastitis of the mother occurs most frequently with the first child. The cause can often be found in the tense posture of the mother during breast feeding. In practice the principle applies: no mastitis of the mother without tension in the shoulder region (on the same side)! That is why it is important the mother *should learn the proper position for breast feeding* (e.g. through instruction from the midwife) and not be left to cope by herself. Together with frequently putting the baby to the breast or expressing milk, galactostasia can be treated with quark compresses, possibly with the addition of honey.

In acute cases the breast can be treated with

- **Mercurialis perennis, 20% tincture for external use** Weleda 1:10 dilution as a compress,

in the healing phase or at night

- **Mercurialis perennis 10% ointment** Weleda
  suitable as a massage ointment which must be carefully wiped off before the next feed [cf. Vademecum 2010, 584]

An important therapeutic measure for mastitis, as necessary, is an enema with 1 litre of approx. 30 °C warm camomile tea.
Internally we can initially administer

- **Apis Belladonna cum Mercurio pillules** Wala
  5 pillules hourly.

If there is severe sensitivity to touch, stabbing pain when breast feeding or moving, alternatively

- **Bryonia D6 pillules** (various manufacturers)
  5 pillules every two hours

or as composite medicine

- **Bryonia comp. pillules** Wala
  7–10 pillules every two hours.

With slightly less pronounced sensitivity to touch and reducing milk flow
- **Phytolacca D12 pillules** (various manufacturers) can be considered as an alternative.

With fever or progressive inflammation this treatment is intensified with injections of
- **Argentum/Quartz amp.** Wala,

supplemented as necessary in the event of severe fever/unfavourable course by
- **Lachesis D30 amp.** (various manufacturers),
- **Mamma Gl D30 amp.** Wala
- **Argentum D30/Echinacea D6 amp.** Weleda
  as mixed injection i.v.

The injections are administered s.c. (upper arms) or i.v., preferably in the late afternoon (17.00–19.00).

Women today often approach their task as a mother with a very awake consciousness and intensive intellectual preparation. But as a result they also become aware of many risks whose real extent is initially difficult for the still inexperienced mother to judge and which not infrequently lead to *great worry about the child.* Wakeful intellectuality alone does not provide calmness and support. These can only grow out of life experience – and therein also lies the task of the doctor, midwife and nurse which cannot be replaced by any book or any person who is less experienced in these questions.

If the mother is physically very *exhausted* as a result of the birth or a subsequent illness she can be supported with
- **Levico comp. amp.** Wala
  1 ampoule per os and
- **Blackthorn elixir** Weleda
  3 × 15 ml (do not take after 17.00) daily.

In the situation frequently encountered in practice today in which the mother suffers nervous exhaustion and then mostly reports restlessness and colics in her infant, the mother can be prescribed
- **Neurodoron® tab. (Kalium phosporicum comp. tab.)** Weleda
  1–2 tab. 2 x/d

If there is a strong *tendency of the mother to become tense* combined with *fears about the child* a one-off i.v. injection of
- **Cuprum met. praep. D30 amp.** Weleda

can have a relaxing and tension-relieving effect. The effect can be strengthened through the administration of magnesium in substance form.
- **Melissa Cupro culta D2 dil., Rh D3 dil.** Weleda
  5–10 gtt. (D2), 10–15 gtt. (Rh D3) 3 x/d

which warms through, relieves tension, has a calming and also a soporific effect is particularly suitable for further treatment [Girke 2010, 659]. Melissa is characterized, among other things, by a high magnesium content.

4

Strong maternal *fears*, for example after a difficult birth, can be countered with

- **Aconitum e tub. D20–30 pillules** Wala
  D30: one-off administration of 3 × 5 pillules every twelve hours
  D20: 5 pillules daily in the evening

and the treatment can be continued, above all with depressive components of fear, with

- **Hypericum ex herba D2 pillules** Wala (frequently more effective than medicines with a greater substance concentration!)
  5–10 pillules 3 x/d

or with gold in the vegetabilized form of St John's wort treated with gold fertilizer (cf. ▸Chap. 1.2.2.)

- **Hypericum Auro cultum D2 dil., Rh D3 dil.** Weleda
  5–10 gtt. (D2), 10–15 gtt. (Rh D3) 3 x/d.

Insufficient lactation is often connected with physical or nervous exhaustion as well as lack of rest and too little sleep and is rarely organic in origin. Alongside the familiar measures, drinking more, lactation teas, frequently putting the child to the breast, the possible treatments outlined above provide significant help in the case of exhaustion and tension. It is also of help if the mother lies down ¼ hour before breastfeeding and tries to calm herself outwardly and inwardly.

If all these measures have failed, the organ preparation

- **Mamma Gl D6 amp.** Wala [Vademecum 2010, 569]

as injection s.c. in the upper arm and subsequently as ampoule has proved effective in individual cases.

If in the initial breast feeding period, for example in the event of a premature birth, there has to be mixed feeding, age-adapted *mare's milk* [Madeleyn 1997] with starch and oil additive (approx. 2–3 %) might be considered as a comparatively vital and mostly well tolerated supplement to breast milk. In contrast to the guidelines currently in force the authors have had good experiences with it; in particular, mare's milk appears to strengthen the immunological competence of infants which accords with historical experience [Bühlbäcker 1996]. As the child will not normally have any further contact with such milk after weaning, the sensitization risk is significantly smaller here than for cow's milk derivatives (which, in contrast to mare's milk, have to be artificially adapted). Better than mare's milk, however, is *donated breast milk* which will surely experience a revival one day (having been common in former East Germany, for example, until as recently as 1989): for in total there is always enough breast milk available for all in the population as a whole and the infection risks as such are absolutely manageable.

Every soul relationship is significantly determined by the *rhythm* of the encounter. Rhythm can create order and limits, the rhythm of rest and movement in itself gives strength. There is no shortage of opinions on the rhythm of breast feeding today. In practice it has shown itself to work if free interplay between mother and child is initially enabled in the neonatal period in which both often find a rhythm which does not require any external guidance or correction. After the first four weeks of life the period between feeds should not be *less* than three hours (▸Chap. 4.4); during the night a free period of four hours should be endeavoured in order to prevent the mother becoming exhausted.

The rhythm of breast feeding should be organized in such a way that the mother has sufficient time and space for her day-to-day concerns and recuperation. That is all the more likely to succeed, on the other hand, the more she can devote herself to her child during breast feeding.

Nipple anomalies can be overcome with nipple shields or, if necessary, expressing the milk. The *lingual frenulum* under the infant's tongue should be observed in case it hinders breast feeding; if intervention is necessary, it should take place at an early stage in order to enable trouble-free breast feeding [Forlenza 2010].

4.3 Digestive tract disorders during the neonatal period

If in the first days after birth digestive disorders occur in the form of poor feeding or atonic vomiting, this can be the consequence of a *birth trauma* and require the corresponding causal treatment as described in ▸Chap. 2.2.4. After the required differential diagnosis has been undertaken (exclusion of infection, above all), the treatment as set out may be sufficient in individual cases for the clinical pictures described below. For pyloric spasm an extended understanding of the disorder is still worthwhile even when operational treatment is carried out.

4.3.1 Poor feeding in the newborn

Normal feeding behaviour arises from a *physical* interest. *Soul activity* is at work in the latter which comes to expression for example in the *excretion of stomach acid* (a process which still takes place very modestly in the newborn and, in a remarkable parallel with kidney function, only matures in the course of the first year of life). The ability of the child to break down the food he or she takes in, destroy its connection with nature and thus unlock it to build up his or her own body substance culminates in *gall bladder and pancreas secretion.* It is an organic expression of personal *will activity* (that has found its linguistic expression in the term "choleric" [Steiner and Wegman 1991, 54–56]). Breast milk here relieves the infant of part of this digestive work through its own content of digestive enzymes; the "physical interest" of the child must nevertheless manifest itself in sufficient excretion by the gall bladder and pancreas so that digestion, and with it feeding, can start normally.

In *poor feeding infants* these processes can be stimulated through plant bitters (non-alcoholic). Extracts of the yellow gentian root (▸Chap. 4.6.3.3),

- **Gentiana lutea Rh 5 % dil.** Weleda
  1–2 gtt. before meals, have proven their worth or
- **Gentiana Magenglobuli (Stomach remedy)** Wala
  1–2 pillules dissolved in liquid before meals,

containing extracts of gentian root, wormwood, dandelion and low potentized Nux vomica and having a slightly bitter taste.

If the main problem is an *acid deficiency in the stomach, found mostly in generally hypotonic infants* (e. g. newborn with Down's syndrome!), it is possible to stimulate the intervention of the sentient organization, the astral body in the digestive tract through the administration of

- **Acidum hydrochloricum D2 dil.** Apotheke an der Weleda [Girke 2010, 644]
  1 gtt. diluted in water before meals, possibly in combination with 2–3 pillules Gentiana comp. Wala.

A comprehensively effective homoeopathic medicine for the above disorders is potentized clubmoss,

- **Lycopodium clavatum C30 pillules** Gudjons[1]

This medicine is indicated especially for infants who initially voraciously demand the breast but stop drinking very quickly. These children give the impression as if the food lies in their stomach like a stone. They lack the necessary digestive power above all with regard to bile secretion so that they have a tendency for meteorism and constipation. The *discrepancy between a ravenous voracious appetite and digestive weakness* is a leading indication for the administration of Lycopodium. The children display a skinny, often distended body and not infrequently an impressively beautifully shaped head with an alert facial expression. The normal growth process in early childhood which starts at the head pole and descends into the body (and only later into the limbs) is retarded.

The clubmoss itself, as one of the earliest land plants at all (together with ferns and horsetail), today displays a strongly retarded vitality; the development of a new generation takes 14 to 15 years in total which is very unusual at this stage of plant development. The plant spores used are very rich in *aluminium* which also has a retarding action on living digestive and metabolic processes in animals and humans (cf. homoeopathic medicinal picture, ▸Chap. 3.5). Aluminium as a substance underlies many *antacids*. Homoeopathically potentized Lycopodium can gradually lead to the cure of a constitutional digestive weakness. The most important complementary medicines are sulphur and Carbo vegetabilis, which should be administered as an intermediate medicine if Lycopodium is to be repeated.

A "Lycopodium state" can also occur *iatrogenically if hepatotoxic medicines* (e. g. certain antibiotics) or *lengthier parenteral nutrition* were necessary. Here colleagues on neonatal intensive-care wards were able to observe impressive medicinal effects (▸Chap. 4.4.4).

4.3.2 Atonic vomiting in the newborn

The overall symptoms of the child suggest *hypotonia*; the food dribbles out of the mouth. The child fails to thrive properly (lack of weight gain). The question as to a birth trauma is particularly important here (pay attention to craniocervical junction!).

1 The Lycopodium preparation from Gudjons, which is triturated in the first stages of potency, is particularly effective in the experience of the authors. Trituration corresponds to the strongly mineral character of the clubmoss spores (high aluminium content).

Because of its regulating action, we can therapeutically administer

- **Cuprum met. praep. D30 trit.** Weleda
  as a single dose 1–3 × 1 saltsp. (possibly to be repeated after one week) which in this case counters vasospasms in the craniocervical junction and intracranially.

Another important treatment is the external application of

- **Arnica e flora 10 % Oleum** Weleda/Wala
  from the back of the head along both sides of the spinal column to kidney level (2 x/d). This aims to stimulate the necessary toning starting from the head

If atonic vomiting is accompanied by restlessness, we should consider

- **Magnesit D6 trit.** Weleda (= Magnesium carbonicum nat.)
  1 saltsp. after treatment with Cuprum 3 x/d.

4.3.3 Icterus neonatorum

Neonatal jaundice (icterus neonatorum) is a specific human phenomenon [Stockhausen 1993, 386]. Humans here develop a bile producing process which appears "unnecessarily complicated" and which only gets going gradually during breast feeding. From a purely scientific perspective it is difficult to see any sense in that. In contrast, anthroposophic observation shows that bile formation can be seen as an important act of human will activity in the human body.[1] When Stockhausen [1993] writes: *"The most important physiological cause of icterus neonatorum is therefore birth and cutting the umbilical cord"* (emphasis in the original) – i. e. the interruption of placental secretion – then this also makes clear that the glucoronidation and elimination of bilirubin is something *qualitatively new* which must be initiated at birth. If we accept that human beings have qualitatively different scope with regard to their will activity from any animal, but that internally, too, they achieve unique universality in the digestion of different foods in the course of childhood (▸Chap. 4.1.2), we can also contemplate the thought that the human individuality in the form of the I-organization "sets itself against the flow of nutrition" in bile secretion [Steiner 1991b, 161; Girke 2010, 710f.]. The connection between bile secretion and vitamin K resorption emphasizes that the will activity of the I, which is closely connected with the blood, can only maintain itself physically if it succeeds in developing sufficient bile secretion.

From the perspective of anthroposophic medicine, biliary (and pancreatic secretion is thus directly connected with the human I which only becomes fully active in the body together with the soul entity through the act of birth. This I lives as an "inner sun" in the body; it is directly connected with the singular warmth organization of human beings which forms the basis for their ongoing ability to act independently of external circumstances (▸Chap. 4.1.1). This I works functionally very strongly, excluding and overcoming all external aspects of nature within the digestive tract. Here it is remarkable that external sunlight and support partially substitute for all these I activities (▸Chap. 3.2) which ultimately also underlies light therapy[2].

1 Rudolf Steiner refers to the connection between I activity and the evolution of the liver and gallbladder system in his lecture of 27.10.1922 to physicians in Stuttgart [Steiner 1989].

2 Rudolf Steiner refers to the connection between the action of the sun and the physiology of the child in the first years of his or her life in his lecture of 11.9.1924 [Steiner 1984b, 55ff.].

Neonatal jaundice therefore challenges the child's will to actively intervene. The more icteric the child becomes the sleepier it becomes; the more active its bile production and excretion becomes, the more alert and active the infant becomes.

In order to reach a reasonable *indication* for treatment, we must first distinguish whether the child is healthy as such or whether a pathology is hidden behind the icterus (infection, serious blood group compatibility with anaemia, etc. – cf. above, enzyme defects, biliary atresia, etc.). The determination of the direct bilirubin in the second to third week of life can be of decisive importance in this respect (▸Chap. 3.3, Vitamin K deficiency). If the child is healthy, medicinal support is justified if the child becomes lethargic, begins to feed poorly, becomes too sleepy and a vicious circle thus threatens to ensue in which the bilirubin continues to rise. In a healthy newborn, values above 20 mg/dl are an indication for phototherapy. Lower thresholds apply for jaundice occurring in the first three days of life, in infants with a positive direct Coombs test, and in premature infants. Below this limit, the treatment set out below is almost always sufficient in our experience. *Hospitalization* is *rarely required* for these children. In contrast, hospitalization for *ill, dystrophic or exsiccated children* is undoubtedly important both diagnostically and therapeutically. *Therapeutically, warmth* takes a primary position. The reason for this is clear from the above explanations. In practice we can see that warmth protection (▸Chap. 2.2.1) is of central importance with regard to the progression of the jaundice.

To stimulate the activity of the gall bladder, massaging the organ (circular motion on right costal arch) with

- **Ferrum met. 0.4% ointment** Weleda 5.0
  Vaseline:Penaten aa ad 20.0,
  pea-sized quantity daily in the morning,

has proved itself as an *external application.*

Internally we can initially administer

- **Sulphur D30 pillules** (various manufacturers)
  2 pillules in the morning (possibly repeated on second and third day of treatment) followed by
- **Chelidonium Ferro cultum Rh D3 dil.** Weleda (non-alcoholic)
  3–5 gtt. before each breast feed, possibly supplemented by
- **Natrium sulfuricum D6 pillules** (various manufacturers)
  3 pillules before each breast feed.

Natrium sulfuricum has a specifically stimulating effect on bile secretion which can also be used to stimulate the detoxification processes through the liver.

For poor feeding ▸Chap. 4.3.1.

An *enema* with physiological saline solution at 37 °C has a stimulating and relieving effect.

4.3.4 Pyloric spasm

Male infants, firstborn and premature babies are more frequently affected by this clinical picture. "The maximum development of the *musculature* occurs close to the pylorus. The wall thickness of this section of the stomach is not reached anywhere else in the digestive tract" [Girke 2010, 626]. The symptoms – the rush of acidic vomiting after the meal, the typically distressed and bad tempered facial expression – clearly show that we have *hypertonicity*, i. e. a strengthened, spasmodic intervention of the soul entity. The pylorus musculature is hypertrophic and hypertonic. This illness can be easily treated today through an early sonographic diagnosis and operation. However, the operation does not solve the question as to how the soul entity of the child, which at first clearly cannot integrate properly into the physical body, can find the proper relationship. An alternative is intravenous treatment with Atropine. Conventional treatment can be usefully extended by complementary medicine; with an early diagnosis it is often possible to avoid an operation if there is the appropriate therapeutic patience.

Physiologically, the pyloric canal brings about a rise in the internal stomach pressure (resistance function) in the course of stomach peristalsis, which culminates in approx. 2 % of the chyme being "ejected" from the stomach into the duodenum [Rauber and Kopsch 1987, 327]. This, in turn, is followed by relaxation of the stomach. The pylorus thus performs an essential *rhythmical function* as guard between the acid environment of the stomach and the alkaline one of the duodenum. From an anthroposophical perspective, the processes up to and including this barrier are primarily dependent on the soul organization, the astral body, while the ultimate dissolution of food as a substance which is alien to the organism is dependent on the I activity in the gall bladder and pancreas. It then moves into the field of activity of the etheric in the small intestine (whose activity is largely independent of the sleeping-waking rhythm).

Rudolf Steiner and Ita Wegman [1977, 107–114] referred to "hypertrophy of the astral body in the stomach region" with regard to pyloric spasm in a case study. Symptomatically we can see *an exaggeration of the resistance principle* at the pylorus which no longer mediates rhythmically on coming into contact with the chyme in the stomach but reacts purely "antipathetically". There is a head-like increase in size and hardening of the musculature, a retrograde, head-oriented peristalsis, and – as always where the soul entity intervenes in the physical entity with abnormal strength – an *abnormally painful awakening* of the child (while physiologically the transfer of the chyme to the duodenum is associated with fatigue and the need for sleep). *Waking, catabolic soul activity* blocks the effectiveness of physical will activity (gall bladder, pancreas) and living anabolic processes which lead to sleep and underlie growth. If the healthy "antrum, pylorus and first part of the duodenum ... form a functional unit" [Rauber and Kopsch 1987, 327], this functional unit separated during pyloric spasm. The rhythmical system between the nervous and sensory and the metabolic parts of the human being has been disrupted. A similar basic disorder in relation to the soul entity is noted by Rudolf Steiner e. g. for bronchial asthma (symptomatically lack of appetite and nausea are typical for an asthma attack). In principle it is true of *spasmodic clinical pictures whose symptoms come to expression in attacks*, that the immersion of the soul entity in the body "gets stuck half way" and *does not find the transition to the relaxation phase.* The soul entity becomes blocked instead of rhythmically being released under the guidance of the I (e. g. in breathing out, the relaxation of the musculature).

It now becomes comprehensible why prematurely born babies more frequently suffer from pyloric spasm, since in their case the immersion of the soul entity in the body takes place prematurely and irregularly. It is also probably no accident that Rudolf Steiner and Ita Wegman [1977, 107–114] describe a premature baby born in the 34th week of pregnancy in the case study mentioned above, which subsequently fell ill with epilepsy and motor disorders after suffering pyloric spasm [cf. in detail Soldner and Sommer 2007]. The pathopsychology described clearly indicates a connection with gastroesophageal reflux disease (▸Chap. 4.6.1)

Therapeutically *copper* is fundamentally the most important medicine for this disease type (▸Chap. 2.2.4). We initially administer

- **Cuprum met. praep. D30 trit.** Weleda
  3 × 1 saltsp. at 12 hourly intervals.

Potentized copper has a *regulating effect* on the tone of the stomach musculature; it can induce the soul activity *to become rhythmical again and thus lead over into relaxation itself*, as would normally be the case. This treatment should also be carried out if the child has already been operated on and only comes for treatment subsequently.

The treatment can be continued with copper in the form of an external application of low potentized blue vitriol:

- **Cuprum sulfuricum D3 dil.** Apotheke an der Weleda
  2 x/d rub several drops into the skin in the region of the pylorus

Additionally

- **Cuprum/Nicotiana ointment** Wala
  1–2 x/d gently massage into stomach in an uncoiling spiral [Vademecum 2010, 380]

Copper carbonate provides inner relaxation in the form of

- **Malachit D4–6 trit.** Apotheke an der Weleda
  1 saltsp. 3 x/d

Malachite, deep green copper carbonate, is particularly suitable for introducing the relaxation ("breathing out") of the soul entity in the sense of a transition "into the anabolic night side" [Girke 2010, 646] (cf. also its relevance for sleep disorders, ▸Chap. 7.1)

At the level of the plant kingdom the application of the potentized form of *Belladonna* corresponds to the circumstances described above. A closer examination of this medicinal plant shows how the process of growing and fruiting associated with ensouled life penetrates the living in such a way in Belladonna which can never be found in this form in non-poisonous plants (the blossoms develop under the leaves with a violet colour). Strict organizing principles are at work in the deadly nightshade [Grohmann 1968, 156ff.]. Belladonna has its general therapeutic importance because it represents *the poisoning of living (typically plant-like) anabolic processes through soul and soul-related processes which have penetrated too deeply*. This medicine is particularly indicated when the soul entity is dammed up and cramps or just tension of some kind occur (cf. homoeopathic medicinal picture) [Husemann 2009, 15–30; Stellmann 1979].

For pyloric spasm we can use

- **Belladonna Rh D6 dil.** Weleda
  3 gtt. before each meal

supplementing the treatment with potentized copper or copper compounds.
Specifically in the case of pyloric spasm

- **Nux vomica D12 pillules** (various manufacturers)
  2–3 pillules 3 x/d is effective.

In its specific action on the gastric nervous system

- **Plexus gastricus D30 amp.** Wala
  0.3 ml per os daily–every 2 days

can be an effective help.

The homoeopathic medicine Nux vomica is made from the – strongly cupriferous! – seed of Strychnos nux vomica which contains strychnine as a significant poisonous substance [Lewin 1992, 789; Madaus 1979, 1985–1996]. The action of the poison deforms the activity of the astral body in the digestive tract into tetanoid hypersensitivity and stiffening spasms. In cases of strychnine poisoning it was still possible to obtain undigested active strychnine from the stomach of a corpse six years after death occurred: An image for something indigestible "sitting heavily on the stomach" causing profound irritation and paraesthesia. If these toxicological experiences already illustrate phenomenologically that Nux vomica represents a simile of the infant suffering from pyloric spasms, Rudolf Steiner explains [1999, 371] Nux vomica as working when "those areas of the human organism, whose real task is to dissolve, are turned into a kind of sense organ,", and that its action dampens the *hypersensitivity* above all in the region of the stomach so that a relaxation occurs.

In the conservative treatment of pyloric spasm the most can be achieved with the medicinal sequence Cuprum – Belladonna – Nux vomica supplemented by external copper applications. The general paediatric principles apply with regard to *diet* and *positioning*.

4.4 Trimester colics

Rarely is there such a gap in paediatrics between the experience of pain and helplessness in parents and child on the one hand and assurances from the doctor ("it will pass", "that is normal at this age") on the other. In medical practices, but also in the out-patient departments of paediatric clinics, *colicky pain and states of restlessness* in the first three months of life (and somtimes a lot longer than that) represent an increasingly frequent therapeutic problem. Valuable clinical research and therapeutic approaches have been undertaken by M. Papousek, N. v. Hofacker and others as part of the "Sprechstunde für Schreibabys" [Papousek 2004]. The authors owe important ideas to this research. The specific importance of the gastro-intestinal tract as the ensouled internal space of the newborn is emphasized by more recent research (▸Chap. 4.1):

- the development of the enteric nervous system (ENS) in early childhood strongly influenced by biographical events,
- the (possibly long-term) importance of *visceral hypersensitivity* (as analogous to bronchial hyperresponsiveness),
- the verification of increased calprotectin values in the stool of cry-babies as a sign of *inflammatory irritation* of the intestinal mucosa,
- the possible efficacy of *probiotics* such as Lactobacillus GG Reuteri in trimester colics

and more indicate that the digestive tract is an important organic setting for trimester colics without it being possible to reduce these events to "flatulent colics" for example.

4.4.1 Symptomatology and anamnesis

The most visible *symptom* on the first visit to the doctor is the often exasperated helplessness and desperation of the mother while the infant has finally gone to sleep during the drive to the doctor. If the father accompanies mother and child he can mostly only support his wife's descriptions: It becomes clear that the parents have become completely

4

worn down in their effort to pacify the screaming child. In many cases they report that it becomes worse in the course of the day towards evening: the child screams and demands food, drinks in a restless and hectic way, hardly calms down during the meal and then starts screaming again soon after. Although the child is worn out, he or she only sleeps for a short period, waking up again screaming. It is constantly being picked up although that is also of less and less help. Often it is said that the child suffers a lot of "flatulence"; but if we enquire more closely it is difficult to determine whether the flatulence was there already before the screaming or only occurred in the course of it, whether it is cause or consequence. If the parents are asked to keep a *sleep record* it often becomes clear that there is a pronounced *lack of sleep*: short periods of sleep with frequent waking above all in the first half of the night, difficulty in getting to sleep and an overall sleep period which is much too short in relation to the day.

Premature babies are affected to a greater extent; premature babies tend as a rule to suffer these states of restlessness for longer than full-term babies. According to studies by Papousek [2009, 563], a careful *pregnancy anamnesis* results in the following picture in persistent or excessive screaming of the infant (to be differentiated from normal trimester colics through the extent and duration): Of all affected mothers

- 7 % started the pregnancy with in vitro fertilization,
- 19 % received tocolysis, which in turn begs the question about the cause of premature labour,
- 6 % were depressive during pregnancy,
- 30 % reported conflicts with their partner during pregnancy,
- 16 % conflicts with their families of origin,
- 51 % prenatal fears and stress,
- 9 % experienced the birth as traumatic,
- 15 % were separated from their child soon after birth.

Currently 44 % report a stressful relationship with their partner and 36 % a tense relationship with their families of origin, 33 % of the women affected feel a lack of social support. The high percentage of *postpartum depression* in the affected mothers (40 %) is particularly striking, whereby more recent studies have shown that twice as many fathers are also affected in comparison to men of the same age in general. The *revival of stressful childhood experiences* (40 %) and the unmanaged loss of reference persons in the past (16 %) must also be taken into account. All of these things place a burden on the living relationship between mother (and father) and child with psychological feelings of ambivalence. Such *psychological stress* has an irritating effect on the unborn child as early as in utero, particularly on the *barrier organs*: digestive tract, respiratory tract and skin develop the tendency as a result of such influences to become *hypersensitive* with a simultaneous weakening of vitality (both things correlate very closely – ▸Chap. 6.5, Bronchial asthma). *Premature babies* display this tendency in a particularly pronounced form. Medicines (tocolytics!) and recreational drugs (nicotine, coffee) during pregnancy must be investigated in detail during anamnesis.

The consequences of shock, particularly through a *birth trauma*, are important causes of childhood states of restlessness (▸Chap. 2.2.3, ▸Chap. 2.2.4); as is *hypothermia* (▸Chap. 2.2.1). Depression disrupts the resonance between mother and child (▸Chap. 4.1.3.), conflicts with her partner or family of origin place a stress on the mother-father-child ties through the transfer of unresolved psychological conflicts. Other factors that can have an irritating effect are:

- foreign food together with or instead of breast milk,
- medicines (administration of vitamins or fluorine, antibiotics as relevant),
- lack of rhythm,
- lack of quiet.

4.4.2 Diagnosis

It is easy to diagnose "trimester colics" symptomatically; it is difficult to understand the underlying event and on that basis to develop an understanding of the child and his or her parents which leads to a well-founded therapy.

- What underlies the presented symptoms?

The decisive factor is that the *rhythm* is disrupted through which the child's soul and spiritual entity immerses itself in the body, acts in it and disengages itself again. The start of respiration and an actively catabolic digestive process in the child's intestinal tract after birth is qualitatively different from the purely anabolic life processes that can, for example, also be found in plants. According to anthroposophical understanding, the soul and I of the child start working in the body here in processes which are essentially connected with the *breakdown* of substance (food, but also own physical substance in the oxidative metabolism) and the *release of energy*, enabling the awakening of *consciousness* and the activation of own *will activity*. In healthy children these "day processes" take them out of themselves to a *tipping point* at which the pendulum swings the other way and *anabolic* "night processes" take precedence culminating in *sleep* [Girke 2010, 18–20]. The *liver*, as the central organ of the human life organization, the etheric body, shows this morphologically in that it increases by up to 20 % in volume at night. With the start of bile secretion at about 3.00 or 4.00, i. e. of catabolic digestive processes, it loses volume correspondingly again. But also in the intestine itself the acidic (soul-triggered) gastric secretion is followed by bile and pancreas secretion initiated by the activity of the I in the body. This not only concludes the breakdown of the food but at the same times turns the chyme alkaline, leading to the absorption processes in the small intestine and the subsequent anabolic processes. This happens in a place which is physiologically removed from consciousness, in which conscious sentience is pathological (e. g. intestinal colic). Thus secretion and motility of the digestive tract as far as the upper duodenum is also dependent on the waking state while the activity of the small intestine is not significantly affected by the state of wakefulness. In a healthy person the activity of the soul and I in the body by itself leads to a tipping point which in turn leads to the disengagement of these entities of the human being: breathing in – breathing out; wakefulness – fatigue – sleep – waking up. But the tensing and relaxation of muscles can also be understood in this sense. The soul and spiritual entity takes hold of the organ concerned, activates it, but then normally disengages again such that the organ in turn can build itself up again (and grow).

With birth the necessity thus arises for the infant himself or herself to develop and stabilize a rhythm between the above-mentioned polarities. This rhythm does not exist in that form before birth, *is not a given*, and means – in the sleeping-waking rhythm, for example – the *replacement* of other rhythms active during pregnancy. As little as children will learn to stand and walk if they do not have a human model *to imitate*, as little will they find their own rhythm if the human environment fails to guide and support this process through its own behaviour (▸Chap. 4.4.3).

If we take the relationship between catabolic and anabolic activity as our guiding perspective, we can interpret the symptoms set out in ▸Chap. 4.4.1 such that the therapeutic procedure directly arises from it.

4.4.2.1 Nutrition

Breast milk is easily transformed into anabolic activity and actively relieves the child's anabolic processes, e. g. pancreatic activity. Everything *indigestible*, e. g. toxic substances in breast milk and allopathic medicines, increases the child's catabolic processes and has an irritating effect.

4.4.2.2 Warmth

Keeping warm relieves the catabolic metabolism, which at rest primarily serves to maintain homoiothermy (▸Chap. 2.2.1) – hypothermia makes and keeps a person awake.

4.4.2.3 Shock sequelae

Any shock either produces a close or loose connection of the soul and spiritual entity with the body (▸Chap. 2.2.3); that prevents a normal rhythm in the sense set out above which must be returned therapeutically to its normal centre position.

4.4.2.4 Sleep deficit

This is always a catabolic process; the "sleep balance sheet" by means of a sleep record illustrates directly the *extent of the disorder*. The achievement of a healthy sleeping-waking rhythm is a key therapeutic objective.

4.4.2.5 Feeding difficulties; meteorism

These tend to be *a consequence rather than cause*. If the response to signs of tiredness is feeding, the activity of the soul and I in the upper digestive tract is called on again and held fast there – the changeover to absorption and anabolic activity is passed by and sleep is made impossible. Flatulence and painful intestinal contractions can, on the one hand, be the consequence of (e. g. artificial or toxic) nourishment which the child cannot fully digest. It acts as an irritant which calls forth abnormal sensitivity in and activity of the soul entity in the lower digestive tract. That is frequently also the case when the child is fed too frequently and therefore the catabolic process in the upper digestive tract is overwhelmed and becomes insufficient. But the nutrition (e. g. wholemeal bread which is difficult to digest, indigestible protein) or the consumption of coffee and nicotine of the mother can also be too much for the child's digestive system. But flatulence also occurs as the direct consequence of soul activity which has penetrated too deeply into the physical body: After a prolonged period of screaming many infants display spastic intestinal convolutions and a distended intestine which was previously not the case.

The time sequence of the trimester colics is now also easier to understand: the soul and spiritual entity increasingly penetrates the body in the course of the day; the maximum body temperature, which is normally reached between 17.00 and 18.00, is the direct result of the physical presence of the soul and the I. This means that the *main tipping point* in the relationship between soul and body lies at about 18.00 (in accordance with the median of the sunset). If we understand trimester colics essentially as the failure or displacement of this tipping point or the failure to reach it, it becomes comprehensible why the infant's restlessness increases from about 17.00 to 18.00. *Until school age, the evening period represents a particular challenge for parents today* because the constant activating, rousing tendency of the "western lifestyle" places in doubt our perception of the child's tiredness and the necessary release of the child from the day and the parents from the child. Thus many adults respond to signals from the child that he or she no longer feels "comfortable in his or her skin" not by slowly ceasing their activity with regard to the child and allowing peace to set in but by *increasing their activity*. That is often involuntarily reinforced if the father returns home from work between 18.00 and 20.00 and wants to spend some time with the child. A vicious circle thus ensues whose characteristics were set out at the beginning.

4.4.3 Indications for supporting parents therapeutically

A detailed *explanatory discussion* which includes the perceptions and feelings of the parents and sets out the connections (▸Chap. 4.4.2) in a comprehensible way follows anamnesis and examination. Another aspect is to train the "sense of life": perceiving when the child gets tired so that the parents then *change their behaviour to start disengaging from the child* so that the soul entity of the child can be released from being tied into the physical body. It is important to include the father in this discussion.

The period in which the child is picked up, has its nappy (diaper) changed, is fed and where the focus is on active attention should not exceed one-and-a-half hours. Then it is time to put the young infant down again and prepare him or her for sleep and then to leave him or her alone. As this can be very difficult at the beginning, it is important to discuss in each individual case how the parents can disengage themselves at that point: e. g. by means of a ritual with a defined end through *which the child's soul is handed over to the care of its true home.* Because the soul of the child was not procreated by the parents like his or her body; on going to sleep it is transferred into the care of the realm whence it originates (no matter how the parents interpret this in religious terms). The parental fear that the child might feel abandoned is countered, on the one hand, by this handover and, on the other, by the mother now undertaking some manual activity around the house which the child perceives quietly, thus providing assurance of the mother's presence – but it must be equally assured that the mother, now disengaged from the child, can turn to other things (this becomes easier with every child, and the problem of trimester colics increasingly rare). A strict *minimum gap* between meals of three to four hours prevents the upper digestive tract from being overloaded.

Keeping a sleep record makes it easier for the physician and parents to see how far there has been success in implementing these basic principles. It is important to support this development patiently; recrimination and adopting an attitude of checking up on the parents are misplaced.

If in the first weeks of life the child is not put in a romper suit but completely swaddled – e.g. in a large baby blanket – thus keeping the (still uncoordinated) limb movements under control, the small infant is given the necessary hold he or she requires. In this way the infant is still relieved of the difficult task of coordinating his or her limbs in a guided (and thus not disconcerting) movement. The swaddling clothes at the same time allow for an important experience of touch: being held and an elementary perception of self, even after the mother lays the child down out of her arms.

Ensuring that the infant stays warm, including a calming oil massage (▸Chap. 2.2.1) and relaxed breast feeding (▸Chap. 4.2), are of essential importance. The extent of activating sensory impressions for the child should be discussed; the most important thing is that quiet sets in from 18.00 (not being on the way to or from somewhere, no media, no telephone) and that the father returning home from work adapts to this mood of letting go. In extreme screaming phases between feeds the child should be comforted for a short while without feeding to communicate the presence of the adult without the latter getting into counterproductive activity. Here the father should relieve the mother during the night who herself should without fail get enough sleep.

With regard to her own food the breast feeding mother can take care to ensure that she avoids as far as possible onions, garlic, cinnamon, heavy wholemeal bread and one-sided nutritional habits. A nutritional record of the mother over three to four days avoids stressful medical (unnecessary) advice and as a rule helps quickly to identify the elements which can be changed and optimized without turning the mother's customary habits, and thus her feeling of wellbeing, upside down. If at all, coffee should be drunk in small quantities in the morning, alcohol and nicotine avoided altogether, the latter in any case throughout the house.

4.4.4 Suggestions for medicinal treatment

The prescription of

- **Belladonna Rh D4 dil.** Weleda (▸Chap. 4.3.4),
- **Oxalis Rh D4 dil.** Weleda, (▸Chap. 2.2.3)
  (both without alcohol) 2(–3) gtt. before meals,

has fundamentally proved its worth for children with trimester colics.

Belladonna as a medicinal plant corresponds to a state in which the soul activity penetrates too deeply into the child, dams up and, above all, cannot disengage itself, remains "stuck". That corresponds to the homoeopathic lead symptoms: worse in the early evening hours until midnight, waking again shortly after falling asleep with pain or active unrest and strong screaming. The child looks actively congested; during colicky pain he or she overstretches himself or herself.

In terms of differential therapy,

- **Colocynthis e fructibus D6 pillules.** Wala
  1–2 pillules before meals, possibly dissolved in liquid,

is indicated if the child doubles up with his or her colicky pain and if he or she has a tendency to diarrhoea.

The action of Belladonna is oriented towards the digestive tract in the specified deep potencies. What interpenetrates in the plant: toxin development in the (metabolically active) pole of blossom and fruit, and vegetative anabolic processes (leaves and shoots), is separated in human beings trough the homoeopathic application. Belladonna D4 *simultaneously has a cramp-releaving and vitalizing effect* on the digestive tract – in contrast to significantly higher potencies.

Oxalis D4 counters hypersensitivity and increased irritability in the sphere of the dormantly unconscious life processes in the middle and lower digestive tract as suffered by

Tab. 4.1 Copper vegetabilized through medicinal plants for trimester colics. Dosage: 2 gtt. 2–3 x/d (D2) and 3–5 gtt. 2–4 x/d (Rh D3) each

Chamomilla Cupro culta D2, Rh D3 dil. Weleda	**Tabacum Cupro cultum Rh D3 dil. Weleda**	**Melissa Cupro culta D2, Rh D3 dil. Weleda**
Irritable children, challenging aggressive, tendency to diarrhoea and flatulence. In s/p birth trauma	Periodically recurring, acutely occurring colics with nausea, strong pallor; key factor: periodicity	Children with reduced vitality, low body temperature, cold extremities; loving children

the small infant. This can be raised to pathological levels by numerous possible influences some of which have already been discussed. In wood sorrel (Oxalis), vital anabolic processes are combined with extreme light sensitivity, great irritability and mobility in the leaves which otherwise only occur in plant blossoms. In homoeopathic potencies, Oxalis tends to counter visceral hypersensitivity, Belladonna pathological soul activity in the digestive tract raised to painful spasms. The medicine can also be applied externally e. g. as an Oxalis compress on the stomach, (soak compress in **Oxalis Folium 20 %** Weleda diluted 1:50 in warm water, squeeze out and apply as warm stomach wrap)

This treatment can be supplemented during its course with the mineral medicine iron carbonate in the form of

- **Siderit D6 trit.** Weleda
  1 saltsp. 2 x/d

That (gently) intensifies the catabolic action of the gall bladder and pancreas in such a way that the digestive process in the lower intestinal sections is relieved and a one-sided hypersensitivity of the soul entity is countered.

If there is manifest maldigestion (above all with artificial infant food) including badly digested stools and foul smelling flatulence, the preparation

- **Cichorium/Pancreas comp. pillules/amp.** Wala
  3 × 3 pillules/d or 0.5 ml per os 1–2 x/d is indicated.

The organ preparation it contains in low potency has an activating effect on the pancreas; the same applies for Cichorium with regard to the gall bladder and pancreas, while Stibium represents an important metallic medicine (in D6) when life processes can maintain themselves in the small and large intestine which were not fully dissolved and destroyed in the upper digestive tract (e.g. maldigestion, but also intestinal infections – (▸Chap. 4.5.2).

The indication of potentized copper for trimester colics becomes clear from the description of pyloric spasm and *copper* as a medicine (▸Chap. 4.3.4) abnormal, painful awakening, hypertonic activity of the soul entity, turning to spasms, in the musculature of the digestive tract, impaired rhythm, the absence of the timely transition to the sleep and relaxation phase.

“Vegetabilization” (Tab. 4.1) is one possibility of using copper therapeutically in this sense. Here medicinal plants are fertilized with a copper solution in certain processes so that they absorb greater amounts of copper and integrate it into their life context. For three years the plants are harvested, composted and their residues used to fertilize the next generation so that the metal is "potentized" through the plant itself, i.e. introduced into a medium in fine distribution which here is the plant substance itself. Here medicinal plants are used which have effects related to copper which are intensified and modified through the vegetabilization of the metal[1] [Busse 1994, Madeleyn 1994].

If it is difficult to differentiate between the medicines set out in ▫Tab. 4.1, then

- **Nux vomica/Nicotiana comp. pillules** Wala
  up to 4 × 2 pillules daily

has proved itself for severe colicky pain (particularly a tendency to obstipation)[2]
If the infant is obviously not feeding well with a simultaneous voracious appetite, strong flatulent colics, above all in the period between 16.00 and 20.00, and is not thriving well, we can bear in mind

- **Lycopodium C6–30 pillules** Gudjons
  2–3 × 3 pillules daily (C6); C30 3 pillules for 3–7 days each evening

(▸Chap. 4.3.1). In acute colics and simultaneous *tendency to overstretch* Lycopodium can be supplemented with

- **Mandragora off. e rad. D6 pillules** Wala
  2 pillules as required, up to ½-hourly [Vademecum 2010, 555]

Mandragora, the mandrake, is particularly effective when there are underlying disorders or weaknesses of the liver and gall bladder system [Mezger 2005, 968]. As a toxic plant (Solanaceae), Mandragora acts in a very similar way to Belladonna for acute pain in which a tendency to overstretch backwards is noted (the opposite is the case with Colocynthis and Magnesium phosphoricum). The authors owe the reference to Mandragora for trimester colics to Reinhard Schwarz.

If spasmodic states of restlessness occur as early as the first weeks of life – typical trimester colics generally only start from the third or fourth week of life – and if anamnesis reveals that there has been drug exposure through anaesthesia (section) or other chemical medicines, a suitable initial treatment is

- **Nux vomica D30 pillules**
  1–3 × 2 pillules at 12-hourly intervals.

If there is a *disorder of the intestinal flora* – e.g. after antibiosis in the early infancy period and with artificial nutrition – the corresponding replacement and, as necessary, symbiotic control is required (▸Chap. 4.6).

If infants with a *protracted course* in whom the colics persist beyond the twelfth week of life (corrected for gestation age) come for treatment, and if previous treatments have failed to work, *potentized magnesium salts* can often play a key role (▫Tab. 4.2). That also applies if the child begins to reject breast milk or shows signs that it does not tolerate

1 The suggestion for this procedure comes from Rudolf Steiner
2 The authors have had good experiences with this medicine in the treatment of stenosing bowel diseases (e.g. not completely resectable Hirschsprung's disease) with full, distended and dilated intestinal sections and inflammatorily changed mucosa (supplemented by Carpellum Mali comp. trit. Weleda).

Tab. 4.2 Differentiation between the three most important magnesium salts in the treatment of the disorders described.

Magnesium phosphoricum D6–12 pillules (various manufacturers)	Magnesium carbonicum = Magnesium D6 trit. (Weleda)	Magnesium muriaticum D4–6 pillules (various manufacturers)
▪ Spasmodic, suddenly occurring colics which improve through warmth ▪ Neuralg. pain (teething pain) ▪ Sensitive, open ▪ Vomiting, singultus	▪ Thin, dystrophic, small stature ▪ Does not even tolerate breast milk ▪ Most violent colics, acidic, greenish diarrhoea, ▪ Angry, intense attacks of screaming, soul entity less open than Mag. phos. ▪ Tendency towards gastro-esophageal reflux (▸Chap. 4.7.1)	▪ Weak digestive activity, above all liver weakness with too little bile secretion; maldigestion; tendency towards constipation with rectal inactivity, ▪ Grumpy, fearful but not violent.

breast milk well. The life forces in these children are mostly weak with a more profound disorder in the structure of the etheric body [cf. Soldner, Wilkens and Sommer 2006].

We can understand the action of magnesium better if we take account of its central position in the anabolic metabolism of nature. Magnesium, as the central metal of chlorophyll, enables the plant to receive sunlight[1] and transform it into the energy which underlies all vegetable life processes and is directly transferred into building up living substance. In animal and human physiology the presence of magnesium is required for many processes, particularly in the more anabolic ones, although magnesium itself as a so-called "co-factor" – e.g. in bone generation – always stays in a living fluid state and does not physically crystallize and become chemically bound like for example the calcium salts.

Scholten also emphasizes using homoeopathic application of magnesium salts for tendencies to spasms and colics.. "In my experience Magnesium carbonicum and Magnesium muriaticum are the *most important medicines for children of divorced or quarrelling parents.* Here the fear of losing the parents is real" [Scholten 1993, 27]. If we compare this statement with the research of Papousek (▸Chap. 4.4.1), it immediately becomes clear that *potentized magnesium salts* have a central indication in protracted and excessively screaming infants particularly in the event of *postpartal maternal depression as well as relationship conflicts between the parents and with the families of origin*, but also following tocolysis during pregnancy (loss anxiety). We can consider magnesium when the parental sun no longer shines in the family or only a dull light reaches the child through dense cloud cover.

Breast milk itself does not only have materially nourishing but also light related aspects, for example in its content of vitamin D and immunoactive substances (▸Chap. 3.2). If the magnesium-containing chlorophyll in the plant enables the sunlight to be absorbed, the magnesium compounds described can equally strengthen the inner light, the life organi-

1 The flame of magnesium is the brightest of all the elements and is similar to sunlight: "Objects lit up by magensium throw deep shadows even in sunlight because magnesium light is more intensive on earth than even sunlight." [Hollemann-Wiberg, Lehrbuch der anorganischen Chemie, 81st-90th edition. Walter de Gruyter, Berlin 1976, 683].

zation of the child in its digestive function and ability to assimilate food. Infants requiring treatment with potentized magnesium salts are often thin, tend to be small in stature and easily excitable. They do not digest and resorb food well and tend towards food allergies. The activity of the liver, gall bladder and pancreas in particular is generally too weak or impaired. The *fear of aggression* ("pacifism", Scholten) emphasized in homoeopathy in the context of potentized magnesium salts which can, on the other hand, have as its counterpart uncontrolled *bursts of aggression*, correlates organically with a weakness in the ability to "resist" food coming from outside and to overcome it. This ability is connected with the function of the gall bladder and pancreas (▸Chap. 4.3.3) which can be stimulated by administering Magnesium carbonicum, muriaticum and fluoratum (▸Chap. 3.4). This in turn can have a healing effect on inflammatory irritations of the intestinal mucosa and visceral hypersensitivity.

Potentized magnesium salts, above all magnesium D6, are often effective for colicky pain also in connection with *gastroesophageal reflux* (▸Chap. 4.7.1) in children in the second trimenon (particularly in breast fed children).

4.5 Acute gastrointestinal illness

4.5.1 Acute gastroenteritis

This common clinical presentation in paediatric practice can be supported through the appropriate therapeutic action, potentially reducing hospital admissions.

Acute vomiting, nausea and lack of appetite as symptoms of the irritation of the gastric mucosa can be caused by a wrong diet, swallowing a lot of chlorinated swimming-pool water, as well as by a developing infection. These symptoms must be differentiated carefully from other (possibly hidden) diseases affecting other organs (e. g. otitis media, bact. meningitis) particularly when there is fever, pain and poor general state of health (beware of superficial telephone consultation!). The general state of health is the most significant general factor in the diagnosis of acute diseases in early childhood.

Alongside general dietary treatment, the following medicines are suitable for the initial therapy of acute vomiting without diarrhoea

- **Nux vomica D6 pillules** (div. manufacturers, ▸Chap. 4.3.4)

administered in alternation with

- **Ipecacuanha D6–12 pillules** Weleda
  3–5 pillules half-hourly, then less frequently

Ipecacuanha is especially indicated when vomiting is at its worst during the night. A clean tongue of the patient is also an indication for Ipecacuanha, whereas patients with a white-coated tongue as a rule respond better to treatment with

- **Antimonium crudum D12 pillules** (var. manufacturers)
  (same dosage as Ipecacuanha)

Antimonium crudum is particularly indicated in patients displaying a tendency to formlessness. Ipecacuanha, in contrast, corresponds to an active astrality and the patients may suffer at other times from coughing with the urge to gag or asthma which worsens at night and during damp weather.

Electrolytic solutions without artificial flavouring (e.g. Oralpädon® without flavouring) or chamomile tea are to be recommended in all cases of gastroenteritis. But after vomiting the child should not drink anything for at least 30 minutes if possible in order not to provoke renewed vomiting. If the condition of the child or considerable nausea do not allow the rapid administration of suitable fluids, then an *enema with the above electrolyte solution* or chamomile tea mixed with electrolyte (9 g table salt per litre) is almost as effective as an infusion. Before school age, it can be administered with a rubber bulb for infants and small children (size 4, holds 130 ml) which should also be kept in the office and the doctor's bag for acute cases. The enema is administered slowly with fluid at body temperature and repeated after two hours as necessary. As a rule, the large intestine quickly resorbs a considerable quantity of the fluid. This directly supports the circulation, and the child's nausea is calmed in a way similar to an infusion. In addition, there can be a mildly laxative effect in the event of acute vomiting which significantly relieves the digestive tract as a whole. If such a treatment is to be considered for the pre-school or school-age child, an irrigator (250–400 ml volume) is suitable [cf. Vagedes, Soldner 2010, 53f.]. By using this measure, the authors were able to prevent hospital admissions for acute gastroenteritis almost completely.

If the symptoms primarily include acute vomiting, diarrhoea and circulatory insufficiency, the most important medicine is

- **Veratrum e rad. D6 pillules Wala, Veratrum album D6 pillules** (div. manufacturers)
  5–7 pillules hourly; as the patient recovers 5 x/d.

Veratrum tones the circulation – it is also tried and tested for hypotonia of the circulation (!) – which is also important during gastroenteritis in small children so that they can overcome the illness and start taking food again.

A proven composite medicine for acute vomiting and diarrhoea, including traveller's diarrhoea, is

- **Bolus alba comp.** Wala
  1 tsp. in 100 ml water/day, administered every 30–60 mins.

Administered in smaller doses [Sommer 1999], it has also shown itself to be an effective *preventive* in this context. Some children might reject the aniseed taste of the medicine. For the first-aid kit, Veratrum album D6, Bolus alba comp. Wala and a temperature-stable symbiosis-controlling medium (e.g. Perenterol®) are generally sufficient together with an electrolyte solution.

In acute *diarrhoeal disorders*, specifically rotavirus diseases, and particularly when the child is small,

- **probiotic Lactobacillus preparations** (e.g. Infectodiarrstop® mono)

can reduce the duration of the illness [Koletzko 2009, 79]. The set combination with an electrolyte solution has proven to be less effective for the authors because if it is rejected then neither component can be used; we prescribe electrolyte solutions without flavour and then, separately, a probiotic as appropriate.

Slimy diarrhoea which increases with *every intake of food* (gastrocolic reflex) and is accompanied by *fever* may react positively to

- **Geum urbanum D1, Rh D3 dil.** Weleda
  5–10 gtt. D1 (older children), Rh D3 (without alcohol) < 2 years 3–6 x/d

This medicine was also used successfully by the authors for infants and small children in a paediatric clinic, e. g. in rotavirus infections. D1 is also efficacious for older children in the event of acute enteritis with the modalities described [Vademecum 2010, 465]. In the event of *rotavirus enteritis*, effectiveness also has been shown for

- **Tormentilla eth. Dec. (original mother tincture)** Weleda
  3 gtt. (one year old) and 5–10 gtt. (older children) 3 x/d [Subbotina 2003].

If in the course of the illness strong, colicky *abdominal cramps occur with the child doubling up,*

- **Veratrum e rad. D6 pillules.** Wala and
- **Colocynthis e fruct. D6 pillules** Wala

jointly administered hourly, then 5 pillules each 5 x/d are effective. In the event of very strong pain

- **Magnesit D6 trit.** Weleda

can be added. This combination has repeatedly proved very effective for the authors. All three medicines are simultaneously effective for diarrhoea.
For severe *exhaustion*, with severe fluid loss due to illness or with a highly febrile course, anxious restlessness and poor feeding, the administration of

- **Chininum arsenicosum D6** (var. manufacturers)
  5 × 5 pillules/d

in combination with **Veratrum album** is indicated. This medicine, which is rarely directly available at home or in pharmacies, should not be absent in the office or clinic.
If the child predominantly suffers from diarrhoea, and if the latter consists of *foul-smelling stools* which are ejected in attacks of defecation, two medicines take precedence: for *undigested stools and aggressive restlessness* in the child

- **Olivenit** (= nat. **D6 trit.** Weleda)
  1 saltsp. 3–5 x/d

as well as the efficacious herbal medicine

- **Podophyllum D4 dil./pillules** (var. manufacturers.)
  5 x/d to 5 gtt./pillules hourly.

In the convalescent phase this is positively followed by

- **Levico D3 dil.** Weleda
  5–7 gtt. 3 x/d

possibly in combination with control of symbiosis.

For the medicinal treatment of acute *gastroenteritis in older children*, two set of medicines have often proved their worth in practice in addition to the treatment described above:

- **Nux vomica olpx** Madaus
  hrly to begin with. Alternate with
- **China olpx** Madaus
  depending on age 3–10 gtt./per dose.

China olpx and **China D12 pillules** in combination with **Colibiogen® Kinder**, 1 tsp./d, are frequently indicated and successful in practice in *postenteritis syndrome* (Chap. 4.5.4.).

- **Salix/Rhus comp. pillules** Wala alternating with
- **Veratrum comp. pillules** Wala
  5–7 pillules each 3 x/d

are a pair of medicines for febrile gastroenteritis with relapsing abdominal colic (cf. ▸Chap. 4.5.2)

Suitable *teas* include blueberry tea (place 1 ml dried blueberries in 200 ml cold water, boil for 10 mins., strain), blackberry leaf tea (pour 250 ml hot water over 2 tsp. blackberry leaves, allow to brew for 15 mins., strain) and haresfoot clover tea (place 2 tsp. haresfoot clover = Trifolium arvense, Herba in 250 ml cold water, boil for 2 mins., strain) [Pahlow 1993, 96f., 155ff., 227f.].

For *control of symbiosis* following acute gastroenteritis cf. ▸Chap. 4.6.4, the *diet* should follow the general paediatric principles; breast fed children should continue to be given breast milk.

4.5.2 Acute salmonellosis and salmonella elimination

The *diagnosis of acute salmonella* should initially be made empirically. The main symptoms are of enterocolitis, frequently with an initial high fever; the general state of health of the child is often clearly impaired. Anamnestically, microbial exposure may be determined. The fever persists as a rule for three to four days. Infants under six months may have a septic course.

Two medicines should initially be considered in a *highly febrile, difficult course*: if there is severe exhaustion and hyperaesthesia with a hot, red head, almost every child will resist being examined and just wants to be left in peace

- **Arnica e pl. tota D6 pillules Wala/dil.** Weleda
  5 pillules/gtt. 5 x/d

is indicated. If the child presents as "typhoidally" (typhos, Greek: fog) dazed, apathetic, completely devitalized,

- **Baptisia D6 pillules** (var. manufacturers.)
  5 pillules 5 x/d, possibly hourly to begin with

can be a medicine of crucial importance (it is not readily available in pharmacies either and should therefore be kept at the clinic) [Emmrich 1998].

With a sustained high fever an i.v. injection of

- **Argentum met. praep. D30 amp.** Weleda
- **Baptisia D6 amp.** Staufen
- **Chininum arsenicosum D6 amp.** Staufen

intensifies the therapy in the first days of illness as a mixed injection.

A basic medicine for acute salmonellosis is potentized stibnite, antimon sulphide [Rissmann 2010, Bovelet and Bräuer 2010], in the form of

- **Antimonit D6 trit.** Weleda (= Antimonium crudum D6)
  1 saltsp. 3–5 x/d [Vademecum 2010, 71]

The action of the antimony ore, with its fine needles, in potentized form is aimed primarily at stimulating the formative forces in the sphere of the digestive tract. The salmonellosis can be seen as an indicator that these organ-forming forces in the child have been weakened in the sphere of the digestive tract – due to constitutional reasons, or because of an excess of foods which weaken the digestion. through their content of fat, sugar and proteins which are difficult to digest (ice cream, salads with mayonnaise, etc.). *Antimonite, the sulphur compound of antimony, strengthens the individualizing formative forces, the (unconscious) activity of the I in the life entity;* it does so especially where permanent vital regeneration forms the basis of organ activity and the organ must form, establish and maintain its shape within this moving, flowing balance. Such organic areas primarily include the intestine and, on the other hand, the blood and bone marrow. Here potentized antimony preparations are of universal therapeutic importance [Steiner and Wegman 1991, 85–89]. From this perspective the Salmonella infection signifies a "tendency to destroy the formative forces" [Steiner and Wegman 1991, 88] which are naturally always present in the intestine and have to be managed by the human digestive organization; that directly gives rise to the *therapeutic aim of permanently strengthening the organ-forming forces in the sphere of the small and large intestine.* The necessity to strengthen form is illustrated by the experience that treatment with antibiotics for salmonelloses causes more damage in the medium term than it produces benefit, as such treatment is linked with a weakening of these formative forces.

The weakened state of the lower digestive tract is reflected in patients through their basic apathetic and irritable mood, white coated tongue and mushy liquid stools which can be interspersed with firmer lumps; tenesmus can also occur.

The effect of antimonite can be intensified through massaging the abdomen with

- **Stibium met. praep. 0.4% ointment** Weleda
  massage in a pea-sized quantity in a clockwise direction[1].

The following composite medicine has generally proved its worth in acute salmonellosis:

- **Antimonit D6 trit.**
  in combination with
- **Salix/Rhus comp. pillules** Wala
  5–7 pillules 5 x/d

for approx. 7 days. The latter represents an anthroposophical composite medicine which is difficult to assess. But its efficacy in *highly febrile enterocolitis and salmonellosis* was repeatedly experienced by the authors to be wide-ranging both in clinical and out-patient practice, including as monotherapy [Vademecum 2010, 731].

If there is severe fluid loss and the associated emaciation, administering

- **Chininum arsenicosum D6 pillules** (var. manufacturers)
  5 pillules 5 x/d

can be of help in the course of the illness.

Control of symbiosis is to be generally recommended, e.g.

- **Colibiogen®** for children
  1 tsp./d
- **Mutaflor Suspension**
  1 ml/d

It is not unusual for symptoms of colicky pain to recur in the course of acute enterocolitis while the diarrhoea gradually subsides. Suitable treatment for this second disease phase is

- **Veratrum comp. pillules** Wala (which also contains potentized antimony)
  3–5 × 5–7 pillules/d

and if that is not sufficient, sips of

- **Bolus alba comp. Pulvis** Wala
  1 tsp./100 ml water/day.

1 We are grateful to Dr. F. Husemann for this advice.

Salmonella carriers – a problem which occurs more frequently with antibiotic treatment – always require thorough *symbiotic control* following the appropriate stool diagnosis (▸Chap. 4.6). Beyond that, the administration of the appropriate nosode in D30, 5 pillules 1 × weekly, and the continuation of the treatment set out above with antimonite D6 trit. 1 saltsp. 2 x/d, and Stibium met. praep. 0.4 % ointment, 1 x/d massaged into the abdomen, is generally successful.

4.5.3 Campylobacter jejuni enteritis

The centre of this disease in the digestive tract generally lies somewhat higher up than it does for salmonellosis. In its treatment it is important to include the upper digestive tract, above all the *stomach* and to strengthen its function.

Bitters are particularly suitable in this context; for children under the age of nine

- **Gentiana Magenglobuli (Stomach remedy)** Wala
  3 × 3–5 pillules/d,

for older children and adolescents (even more effective)

- **Enzian-Magentonikum (Gentian Stomach tonic)** Wala

The activity of the soul and spiritual entity in the upper and middle digestive tract, which is often too weak in these patients, is more strongly engaged as a result (▸Chap. 4.3)

In order to strengthen the organ-forming force in the directly affected organ area, (particularly the lower small intestine), the following should be administered [Engel 2010, Simon 2010]

- **Kalium aceticum comp. D4 trit.** Weleda
  3 × 1 saltsp./d

Alongside the basic treatment measures, which can be supplemented by the appropriate nosode as appropriate, the administration of the following has often proved itself symptomatically

- **Salix/Rhus comp.** Wala
  5–7 pillules 5 x/d
- **Bolus alba comp.** Wala
  1 tsp./100 ml water/day, administered one teaspoon at a time (▸Chap. 4.5.1 and ▸Chap. 4.5.2).

4.5.4 Post-enteritis syndrome

It is not unusual in paediatric practice to encounter the problem that prolonged diarrhoea occurs after gastroenteritis, particularly if the *diet* was carried out inconsistently or for an insufficient length of time. Irrespective of the triggering cause, damage to the mucosa occurs which in this situation leads to an inability sufficiently to split disaccharides such as lactose, or to completely dissolve the food in its natural context. Children who already display constitutional difficulties in detaching themselves from their mother and asserting themselves independently with regard to the external world are frequently affected by postenteritis syndrome.

Therapeutically, the omission of milk, sugar, fatty foods and especially fruit juices for a period of 10 to 14 days is important with a correspondingly modified diet. Medicinally, the administration of the following has proved itself

- **China D12** (var. manufacturers)
  5 pillules 3 x/d

together with

- **Colibiogen® Kinder**
  1 tsp./d for 2 to 3 weeks.
- **Stibium arsenicosum D8 dil.** Weleda
  5–7 gtt. 2 x/d

The authors owe the latter to a suggestion from H. Magerstädt; a greatly proven medicine in practice.

4.5.5 Acute acetonaemic vomiting

This rare but dramatic clinical picture, which in individual cases can frequently relapse, affects mainly girls in infancy and at pre-school age. The affected children perceive their environment very intensively; they can be very jealous and demanding and develop an "unconscious cunning" in influencing the people around them. On the other hand they are easily overwhelmed in *processing* their soul impressions and feelings, and then have a tendency for impressive, paroxysmal hysterical gestures. In that respect they are completely at the mercy of their emotions which can act infectiously on the people around them. If adults fail to succeed in maintaining a mental calm which is based in the I, by approaching the child with anxiety for example, they can exacerbate his or her symptoms (▸Chap. 7.6, Respiratory affective spasms). This is a typical hysterical clinical picture in the sense of anthroposophic medicine.

The soul entity of these children is too strongly connected with the surrounding world and too little involved with processing and digesting what is taken in by the body from the outside world. That leads to over-sensitivity in the upper digestive tract (▸Chap. 4.3.4); if an irritation occurs in this sphere, the child reacts with excessively strong vegetative agitation as if something foreign has penetrated the body and cannot be digested. The paroxysmal vomiting and change in the metabolic situation – reminiscent in its gesture of hyperventilation tetany – are the attempt psychologically to reject and get rid of what actually should be managed and digested by the body. As the connection between the soul and spiritual entities and the body becomes more and more intensive in the course of childhood, the maturation of the child itself leads to a cure in the longer term (similar to respiratory affective spasms and related clinical pictures).

In dealing with the affected patients, it is necessary to discover the circumstances which might be overexerting the child psychologically. If the clinical picture is transparently explained in a consultation, the required inner calm and security can be communicated to the parents so that they can support the child in the right way.

Medicinally the acute administration of

- **Acetone D10 dil.** Staufen
  5 gtt. 2–4 x/d

and, at an early stage, an enema with electrolyte solution in sufficient quantity are crucial. Constitutionally

- **Ignatia D30 pillules** (var. manufacturers)
  7 pillules dissolved in 50 ml water, 3 × 1 tsp./d for 3 days

is often the decisive medicine, which might have to be repeated several times.

Like Nux vomica, this medicine is strongly related to the hyperexcitability of the vegetative nervous system – also toxicologically. The ignatia plant is a creeper like Gelsemium which lacks independent uprightness. All the homoeopathic medicines obtained from creepers have the common characteristic that the patients these medicines help are vegetatively very excitable and psychologically at the mercy of their emotions (cf. stage fright with Gelsemium). Just as these plants need a tree, the patients at this phase require another person who can help them to become upright. And the more that other person exudes and embodies a strong I and sovereignty over their soul entity, the more the clinical picture recedes. Generally this means that in the affected family at least one of the parents has not yet sufficiently developed these qualities. Consultation with the parents (i. e. mother *and* father) is therefore of fundamental importance with regard to treatment.

The very experienced anthroposophical paediatrician Annegret Fauth told the authors about her oft-proven positive experience with the following:

- **Antimonit D4 trit.** Weleda
  depending on age and weight, 1 saltsp. ½ to 1-hrly for approx. 24 hours

in combination with

- **enema (retention enema) 30 ml camomile tea 1:1 with glucose electrolyte solution**
  ½-hrly to begin with.

Dr Fauth summarized the response to the therapy in the following words: "It is like giving water to a dried out flower".

4.6 Nutritional advice, thrush, intestinal mycosis and dysbiosis (dybacteriosis)

The main part of this chapter is devoted to disorders of the intestinal flora, mycosis and dysbiosis. Doctors are frequently confronted with the question as to which kind of nutrition or, as appropriate, diet is healthy for the child. Chronically relapsing infections or atopic dermatitis in infancy, for example, can often not be treated without individual nutritional advice, which may range from omitting the inevitable cocoa in the morning to the elimination of fizzy apple drinks as the basic beverage (which can be the case in poorer families). *What is the "gold standard" of healthy nutrition?* And how can individual nutritional advice succeed under the pressure of daily practice so that it respects the lifestyle of patients and yet still makes for significant changes?

In recent years, the following salutogenically-focused principles have proved their worth. We will introduce them at the start of this chapter in abbreviated form.

Nutritional record

What is currently being eaten and drunk should form the basis of any nutritional advice. The best thing is if for approx. 4 "typical days" (e.g. Thursday-Sunday of a normal week, not at Christmas or on holidays) the food and drink of the child is recorded with time of intake and sent to the doctor.

The doctor can then check the record in a quiet moment and mark for discussion those foods and drinks which are questionable or need to be changed. At the same time he gains an insight into the actual nutrition of the child which no verbal anamnesis can provide.

At the subsequent meeting, nutrition can be discussed with the parents/mother on the basis of the record – with or without the child, depending on age. The following principles have proved themselves in this context:

- Does *breakfast offer* the basis for sufficient satiety during the morning? Does the child eat breakfast at all? How early must he or she get up to have time and an appetite for breakfast? Oats (wetted the evening before), sourdough bread with butter (and a freely chosen spread, not Nutella® if possible) offer a good foundation for example. Pure "white flour preserved food" or just a drink are not sufficient. This point is particularly important specifically for children with attention deficit or concentration disorders in school or behavioural disorders in kindergarten.
- *Drinks* should be warming in the winter and may contain a delicate herbal taste (tea) as appropriate; freshly squeezed (!) fruit juices make a good "highlight". Sugary drinks are fundamentally unsuitable! Families can save a lot of money if they offer their children sensible drinks.
- Children should be given a *warm lunch* with sufficient *fresh ingredients*, e.g. raw vegetables and salad. Cooked food should, if at all possible, be *prepared by oneself.*
- The *evening meal* should not be eaten too late and be easily digestible (salad better at lunch, soup is well suited for the evening). It can be very helpful if Dad leaves the house a little bit earlier in the morning so he can be home at 18.30 in the evening, for example! The period of the evening meal and going/being brought to bed is the most precarious and important time in the whole course of the day, and can be managed a lot better if both parents are present.
- *Nutritional breaks* (i.e. times with *no* food) are indispensible for a healthy digestion. In childhood five meals (incl. in-between meals) are ideal.
- *Sweet foods are not a problem* if the family rigorously follows the principle of only eating such sweets *which have been made at home.* When we hold surgery, this principle appears to us to be the best way to prevent intestinal mycosis (and special diets!). Homemade cakes, a sweet desert, homemade Christmas biscuits have a different effect from ice cream bought at the supermarket, daily chocolate, sweets from the sweet shop and such like. This suggestion sounds harsh but also brings freedom and substantially improves (like a homemade lunch) the delivery of necessary nutrients for the child, reduces the intake of salt and the consumption of sugar, etc. At the same time it saves a lot of money which should be used to buy quality food (organic, biodynamic, good animal care).
- *High quality fats*, cold water fish if they are liked, high quality vegetable oils, butter *are not fattening* and are filling, thus preventing the excess consumption of carbohydrates/sugar. Fresh eggs from chickens which have truly been able to peck in the sunlight and ripe avocados are valuable and even contribute to the provision of vitamin D.

- *No low fat foods*, fresh whole milk. In studies, certified raw milk from the farm regularly performs best (e. g. with regard to allergy risk), but contains a residual risk of pathogenic E. coli infections.
- *If possible, avoid canned food*. Dried foods (air-dried ham, dried fruits) in contrast are valuable if eaten in appropriate quantities. Some foods are appropriately available in deep frozen form. Foods which are available fresh should be bought and eaten when they are as fresh as possible.
- The important thing is that bought foods should be *pre-processed as little as possible*. The more we prepare food ourselves, the better it is tolerated and the less there is of additives and preservatives (incl. salt). The *taste* is also better and more individual.
- *Transparent meat products* (escallop, a roast, chicken) are preferable to many sausage goods. Meat with lemon or after freshly squeezed orange juice is digested better, particularly with regard to iron intake. In vegetarians, ferritin and vitamin B12 should be checked at appropriate intervals.
- *Fermented milk products*, intestinal symbionts from raw sauerkraut, Kanne Brottrunk® or other sources should be on the menu.
- *Vegetables* should be eaten in sufficient quantities, including in soups or raw (carrots, for example), or as filling for lasagne etc.
- *Nuts* (walnuts, hazelnuts, almonds) are valuable foods and should not be absent if tolerated. Peanuts, on the other hand, are superfluous for infants (choking risk) and not very suitable for older children. Peanut allergies are hardly ever cured, in contrast to other food intolerances.

What reads like yet another list of instructions should not be presented as such. A more creative approach is to *identify those three steps* which bring child and parents closer to these principles without abandoning everything that has so far constituted the family's lifestyle. We can keep repeating this process and thereby achieve a lot more with regard to good compliance in the family than through programmatic lectures and instructions. Subsequent checks with a new record and a second consultation after an appropriate interval increases the effectiveness of such an approach considerably.

After all, *food intolerance* is a major issue today. This book deals with that in greater detail in many places (coeliac disease, atopic dermatitis, etc.). In general these rules apply:

- It must always be determined individually what food the child does not tolerate. No laboratory test can provide the sole proof here, careful observation (elimination and exposure) is crucial.
- Many food intolerances disappear as the child matures – re-exposure at reasonable intervals is often sensible and liberating.
- At children's parties or visits to other families, the food and drink which everyone else is eating and drinking should only be restricted for the child if the intolerance is absolutely certain. Anyone who practices a reasonable regime at home (see above) can cope with a lot of things as a guest.
- Food intolerances can be seasonal (e. g. in pollinosis patients) and they can be dependent on *location* (e. g. tomatoes tolerated in Mediterranean countries, not tolerated in Holland).
- *Seasonal* foods such as strawberries should not, if possible, be eaten outside the season because then the risk of intolerance is higher. The concept of *"food from the region"* is helpful here!

Finally, there should be a word during the consultation about the "how" of the meal. A healthy digestion – that is also the message of this chapter – is dependent on the engagement of the soul and spiritual individuality, on its forces which are physically active in the digestive tract. Saying grace, the taste and smell of the food, the style in which the table is set and in which we eat has a profound effect on the development of the digestive and metabolic system of the child (and thus the physical basis of its will forces). The omnipresent profusion of inferior, pre-cooked foods places such an attitude at risk. We place greater value on food we prepare ourselves. Children should be involved in that from an early age.

4.6.1 Symptoms and causes

In a thorough review of the current literature in conventional and complementary medicine, as well as through his own experiences in practice, the paediatrician K. R. Kummer [1998] reaches the conclusion that it must currently remain open as to whether intestinal mycosis "is a primary or secondary disorder". However, in general we view the growing spread of Candida albicans or Aspergillus niger as *the consequence of a digestive and immune weakness* of the child – even if fungi in turn have a negative effect on the organism as a whole.

The newborn has a primary weakness of the digestive and immune systems, and these systems can only function in an age-appropriate way together with breast milk. The lack of breast feeding, but also a cesarean delivery, pose a risk to the normal development of the intestinal flora; if there is no vaginal delivery, the initial physiological colonization of the intestine in the newborn does not happen. (▸Chap. 4.1.2) Candida albicans as such is *not* part of the initial colonization of the intestine in newborns [Tannock 1994] and the *candidiasis which frequently occurs in infancy today* is connected to a great extent with whether or not the child is artificially fed and whether there is a susceptibility to candida in the parents, particularly the *mother* (see below).

If we consider mycosis to be a consequence, and if we search for a treatment related to its cause, Pasteur's insight that the *terrain* is (almost) everything applies here. We must therefore primarily diagnose the terrain and treat it on that basis. In the best case, a purely symptomatic antimycotic treatment becomes redundant. As a first approximation, we can describe the intestinal milieu in which Candida albicans can thrive as an environment where the food in the digestive tract *takes a wrong turn:* it is not fully dissolved and then resorbed, but it *remains partially undigested* and cannot pass through the "barrier" of the intestinal wall. At the same time it is not promptly excreted, but starts to ferment in a way which is not controlled by the organism, providing the breeding ground for abnormal colonization of the intestine, e. g. through Candida albicans or Aspergillus niger. Another possibility is that mainly carbohydrates in the food have already been *broken down before they enter the organism* and can no longer be subjected to a rhythmically structured, gradual catabolic and transformative process. This leads to an *abnormally fast passage through the upper digestive tract* and to the short-term *flooding of the following parts of the intestine with broken down carbohydrates* some of which are converted by the metabolism of yeast fungi before the intestine can resorb everything. That is the case, for example, in the consumption of sweets, fruit juices and white flour products. As this produces an abnormally rapid rise in the blood sugar level, candidiasis can also easily occur at other mucosal surfaces (e. g. vaginal mycosis in adolescents). The organism always responds to such a rapid rise in the blood sugar level with a counter-regulation; thus eating sweets produces symptoms of hypoglycaemia (e.g. a rise in restlessness, concentration disorders) including a burning desire for something sweet. This can result in a vicious circle.

If we consider that all carbohydrates ultimately owe their origin to the resorption of sunlight by the plant, *the organism normally accesses light reserves for its activities* through catabolic activity, resorption and the subsequent respiration of the carbohydrates. Fats tend to have more of a character of warmth reserves, but the boundary between them is blurred. A spreading intestinal mycosis always exists by skimming off part of these absorbed light reserves for itself and depriving the organism of them.

The metabolism of fungi differs from the bacterial metabolism in that it *remains incomplete* [Kummer 1998, 68f.], thereby *creating intermediate products,* including (fusel) alcohols and histamine, which have a *toxic, beclouding effect* on the human organism. After excretion by the fungi (or also acutely after release by the fungi following antimycotic treatment) they are resorbed by the child's intestine in considerable quantities and have *a toxic effect particularly on the liver* [Friedrichsen 1990]. Thus with the increase in fungal growth in the intestine, the GGT rises to pathological levels, something which is also familiar to us from regular alcohol consumption. The *fungal metabolism poisons the child's metabolism* with consequences which can reach as far as the *sphere of volition and consciousness*!

Fungi normally prefer damp, humid (and often cool) places. In themselves they do not have a positive connection with the light. They are satisfied with an incomplete catabolic metabolism which *reflects in caricature the insufficient catabolic and digestive process of the human host underlying intestinal mycosis*. In contrast to the metabolism of the physiological intestinal flora, "fermentation which limits itself and only produces a relatively small yield of energy is one of its characteristics ... This behaviour with regard to matter, the *retardation of full digestion* in favour of partial metabolic stages, reveals an aspect of fungal pathology which has not been studied a great deal so far: fungi *prevent* the complete digestion which the human organism requires" [Kummer 1998, 69]. The primary insufficient catabolic and digestive process is further inhibited and weakened by the mycosis.

Basic *symptoms* which can be the expression or consequence of intestinal mycosis now become more comprehensible in their context:

- fermentative dyspepsia, meteorism, colicky stomach pain (▸Chap. 4.4),
- sour and foul smelling stools,
- changing appetite, halitosis, furred tongue,
- sleep disturbance, mood changes, states of restlessness,
- lack of energy, abnormal pallor, deep shadows under the eyes,
- sudden attacks of tiredness and fluctuating concentration.

It is notable that

- nocturnal enuresis

with an existing intestinal mycosis can sometimes be improved through the corresponding treatment. This indicates how important it is for the individuality of the child to master the digestive processes with regard to controlling other processes in the sphere of the "metabolic human being".

4.6.2 Diagnosis

According to the anthroposophical understanding, the catabolic activity surrounding food in the upper and lower sections of the intestine reflects the intervention of the soul and spiritual individuality in the body (▸Chap. 4.1.3.). Digestion of the food not only makes available the substances to build up the body, but above all provides the energies that are required for motility and sensitivity, for developing consciousness and free action, for the maintenance of the homoiothermic warmth organization. This action of the soul and I in the body is first expressed in secretion processes of the saliva, stomach acid, bile and of the pancreas (▸Chap. 4.3.3, cf. [Girke 2010, 725]). In the sense of the old humoural physiology they embody the qualities of "hot" and "dry" (the bitter and sour) and their actions are opposed to the development of mycosis. A central prerequisite for the activation and effectiveness of these secretions is *chewing* and the *teeth*. Thus the tendency for nappy (diaper) thrush usually heals up after the teeth have erupted. Conversely, the inflammation of the mouth and inhibited chewing during the eruption of the teeth particularly promotes mycosis. Persistent intestinal mycoses in children with severe disabilities may be connected with chewing disorders. Nothing illustrates the above more clearly than the necessity to take an active and thorough bite in order to initiate the full digestion of the food. It becomes self-evident that apple juice has precisely the opposite effect on the organism from an apple which has been eaten by the child himself or herself, and that the consumption of something sweet is different from the activity of accessing sweetness through one's own activity. Stimulating such own activity is therapeutically vital and also the real purpose of a diet.

Soul and spiritual activity is preceded – particularly in the child – by the process of *perception*. Thus the perception of the food, its sensory qualities is necessary for initiating the required digestive processes in the upper and middle digestive tract. Breast milk, self-prepared natural foods, and food which has to be thoroughly chewed develop this sphere of the senses differently from industrially prepared ready-food and very strongly broken down or processed foods. If we intensify the child's processes of perception through the corresponding diet and, for example, through bitters (as appropriate for his or her age), we can in many cases achieve a clear increase in the digestive activity of the child.

Mycosis predominates in situations in which the perception of the food, the chewing and formation of saliva as well as the secretions of stomach acid, bile and pancreatic secretions are insufficiently activated through wrong nutrition. Patients whose inner ability to fully dissolve, overcome, and utilize the external world in the form of food is organically or constitutionally impaired, are particularly susceptible to this.

This raises the question as to how the doctor can perceive the constitution of the patient and the various organ functions in order thus to individualize the diagnosis.

Many children today have the tendency to immerse themselves too strongly with their soul activity in the perception of the surrounding world while the engagement in the body of the higher components of the human being, the I and astral body, lags behind; as does the penetration of the metabolic processes by the soul and spiritual forces. Their relationship with food is often very unstable, fluctuating, psychologically shaky or one-sided. The original vital interest is absent in this sphere because it has been displaced to the sphere of the nervous and sensory pole (▸Chap. 4.5.5). "As a consequence the digestion is too weak and cannot adequately execute the processes for assimilating the foreign food. The human being is too much directed outwards with his or her attention, allows foreign processes to penetrate himself or herself too much, and has too strong a secondary reaction" [Kummer

1998, 69]. Here we can see a transition to allergic reactions (▸Chap. 6) which are often reinforced by intestinal mycoses: "The fungi, as foreign substance, may well themselves represent an allergen" [Kummer 1998, 69]. This becomes comprehensible through the basic constitutional situation described above: the organism perceives insufficiently what it internalizes as food and gives an incomplete response. The allergic reaction forces itself on this state as a secondary reaction in order to try and bring the penetrating foreign substance to perception and digestion – but now at the wrong time, in the wrong place and to the wrong degree.

The opposite of the constitution described above is represented by children with an unbridled predominance of the metabolic impulse, in which the vitality of the organic sphere gains the upper hand over the formative tendencies (▸Chap. 4.5.2). These children cannot cope with the food which they enjoy eating, possibly to excess. They have a tendency leading towards inflammation and diarrhoea, towards speeding up the metabolic processes and, in so doing, towards the loss of the necessary barrier function of the intestinal mucosa. Such a constitutional situation can lead to secondary food intolerances. This *"hysterical" constitution* has a tendency to come to expression in the metabolic field while the "*neurasthenic constitution*" [Husemann and Wolff 1986, 142–154] lives too strongly in the nervous and sensory sphere and combines itself too much with the environment. In both cases a treatment which removes the ground from under the mycoses will have a beneficial effect on the constitution and thus also the allergic tendencies of the child.

With regard to the *diagnosis of impaired organ functions* of the gall bladder, pancreas, stomach and spleen cf. ▸Chap. 6.3.

The probable *existence of mycosis requiring treatment* is supported by the symptoms and diagnostic context set out above. If the fungal infestation itself is not clinically obvious (such as for example in oral or nappy (diaper) thrush), a careful *stool examination* is necessary, repeatedly if necessary. With little (mycological) effort and suitable agars[1] this can be done in the doctors clinic, while the laboratory diagnosis of a *bacterial dysbiosis* should be made in a laboratory with experience in that field. The colony and bacterial count should be recorded semiquantitatively. The bacterial count alone will only reveal something about the necessity of treatment in the event of a very high bacterial count. If there is a low to medium bacterial count in the stool, the doctor will have to decide primarily on the basis of the symptoms and connections set out above whether or not the child is *ill* or whether there is merely a non-standard result (requiring monitoring) with which the child's organism will be able to cope.

As treatment always has very radical consequences, especially through the required diet, only careful diagnostic consideration will fulfil the doctor's responsibility towards the child. In individual cases, the diagnosis can be supplemented with swabs (tonsils, genitals if there is suspicious fluor); if a blood serum test is carried out, the liver values, particularly of GGT, the trace elements iron, magnesium, zinc and selenium, as well as vitamin B_{12} and folic acid are of specific interest, because in the event of intestinal dysbiosis cumulative deficiencies can be found which in turn negatively influence the digestive processes.

1 The use of selective agars, e.g. Nickerson Agar (suggestion by M. Sommer), is particularly simple.

4.6.3 Treatment

4.6.3.1 Oral thrush

Oral thrush in infants is generally induced through contact. In breast fed children the breast of the mother must therefore also be treated, in non-breast fed children hygiene must be observed (bottles and nipples teats should be cleaned physically and boiled).

Locally, the candidiasis can be treated by swabbing the mouth (cotton wool swabs) after the meal with

- **Tea tree oil** aqueous dilution of approx. 1:20

which, diluted approx. 1:10 with calendula oil, is also suitable for treatment of the mother's breast (dabbing the nipple with lemon juice from the seventh month of pregnancy onwards acts as a preventive).

Internally the following can be administered orally before the meal

- **Borax D6 amp.** DHU/Staufen
  5 gtt. (0.2 ml) at a time.

If necessary, Borax can be alternated with

- **Mercurius cyanatus D6 amp.** DHU/Staufen
  5 gtt. (0.2 ml) at a time before each second meal.

The liquid form is more effective than pillules; the use of ampoules avoids the toxicity of alcohol for infants.

Since with each case of oral thrush there is a threat that the yeast fungal growth will spread to the whole digestive tract, a preventive treatment should always be considered which at the same time supports local healing in the mouth.

According to our own observations the nosode

- **Monilia albicans D6** pillules Staufen
  3 pillules 2–3 x/d is effective in combination and in alternation with
- **Gentiana Magenglobuli (Stomach remedy)** Wala
  2–3 pillules 2–3 x/d

Both medicines sensitize the perception processes in the upper digestive tract and intensify its catabolic activity with regard to the invading yeast fungi; here the slightly bitter taste of Gentiana is necessary for its action.

As a rule, *nappy (diaper) thrush* is a symptom of intestinal mycosis which is symptomatically often restricted to the period before and around the time that the teeth erupt and in that case can be adequately treated locally.

Locally, the following is once again suitable

- **Tea tree oil**
  diluted 1:10–1:20 with calendula oil.

The experienced anthroposophical paediatrician H. Pechmann reports very positive experiences with

- **Rosemary ointment 10 %** Weleda
  applied several times/d [Vademecum 2010, 724], it has also frequently proved its worth for the authors.

To cleanse the skin, whey and calendula oil can be used instead of water; for acute symptoms initial treatment with

- 0.1 % aqueous **gentian violet stain solution** (= NRF 11.69 methylrosanilinium chloride solution)

is suitable. As protective ointment

- **oxyplastine ointment**

from Switzerland is suitable, among other things, or

Sulphur praep.	3.0
Kamillosan ointment	10.0
Ol. Jecoris	30.0
Zincum oxyd.	30.0
Adeps lanae	ad 100.0 [Goebel and Glöckler 2008, 699]

This ointment is suitable for various superinfections of the skin.

Case study

Even in nappy (diaper) thrush, it is worthwhile investigating the cause. A 14-month-old girl was brought to the surgery with nappy (diaper) thrush which had not responded to treatment for two weeks. As this child had never otherwise suffered from candidiasis, the question arose as to why such symptoms had suddenly arisen which were so difficult to treat. Only at this point did it emerge that the candidiasis had occurred two to three days after the first tetanus vaccination. The child was given Silicea D30 (5 pillules) once and subsequently 3 pillules 3 x/d of Echinacea e pl. tota D3 Wala. The candidiasis healed within half a week.

4.6.3.2 Nutritional advice for intestinal mycoses

If after infancy *intestinal mycosis in need of treatment* is diagnosed, the first and most important step is *individual nutritional advice* for the family. A proven method in this respect has been to prepare a written *nutritional record* (food and drink, approximate quantity and time of day, documented without any gaps) as a basis which the doctor can assess before the meeting: what are the eating and drinking habits which could promote the growth of intestinal fungi? The greatest problem regarding a specific diet is that it undermines the family all eating the same meal together – a great psychological strain on every child. That is why the whole family should, as far as possible, adapt its food correspondingly – as a rule, everyone benefits! The timing of such a change should also be considered: it should not, for example, be placed just before Christmas. Nutritional advice has various tasks:

- For many patients, it clarifies for the first time the effects of their nutritional habits.
- It explains the factors which in the concrete individual case and in general influence mycosis.
- In detail, it discusses a *strict dietary plan* which, under normal circumstances, must be adhered to for three weeks and
- the type and scope of "healthy nutrition" which has to be continued afterwards for at least the same period.

The key thing is that the doctor or nutritional adviser should explain the aim of the change in nutrition to the parents and, in so far as permitted by age, to the child. By changing nutritional habits, and *through the resulting effort of will required by the child himself or herself*, the child can be made to feel much better and in full command of his or her powers (which often makes dealing with the child a lot easier). The decision to embark on this path should be taken from a position of understanding; a voluntary diet strengthens, a passively followed diet weakens the will! In paediatrics much depends in this context on the *attitude of the parents*; if the child feels that they are following the medical advice out of insight and because they think it is right, they will appear credible.

A clear *time limit* for the diet is also important. Afterwards the family should go back to deciding freely what it eats and drinks; not many will simply return to the *status quo ante* if there has been proper advice at the beginning.

At this point it is necessary to fundamentally address the *familial environment* of a child with intestinal mycosis. Frequently, at least one of the parents himself or herself has a problem in this area. It is not easy to decide whether transmission through a contact person (given a bacterium which is ubiquitous as such) or constitutional similarities are significant – apart from those cases where the focus of the illness lies wholly with the parents (e.g. a single mother with pronounced depression and candidiasis – in such a case, which was treated by the authors, every treatment of the mycosis in the child failed to begin with). In any event, it is to be recommended that before any treatment *a stool examination is undertaken for all of the family members*. This shows, on the one hand, that constitutionally and organically healthy children are not normally susceptible to mycosis; on the other hand the child, as mentioned, is often not alone with its problem in the family, something which clearly raises the motivation to change the nutrition of the whole family at least for the period set out above. Many families experience that in a very positive way, leading to a permanent modification of their eating habits which is important for the long-term success of the treatment.

Sufficient time should be available for the nutritional consultation by the doctor or a specialist. The many questions associated with practical implementation can also be discussed, for example, as part of an evening meeting with a group of parents of patients. Copies of general lists as to what should be avoided and what is helpful should be made available and discussed (◘ Tab. 4.3).

In the medical consultation the length and scope of the "strict diet" should be defined for the individual patient as well as the duration of the diet as a whole. The corresponding entries by the parents in the nutritional record are intended for this purpose to document the necessary changes; fact sheets can supplement that. Sufficiently long breaks without calorie intake are also important (▸ Chap. 4.6.3.3 below, gall bladder activity). What the

Tab. 4.3 Dietary information with regard to the treatment of intestinal mycoses.

Dietary information	Food
The following should be generally avoided:	■ Sugar and white flour products, sugary drinks ■ Sweet fruit, compote, fruit juices, including diluted ■ Chocolate, cocoa products ■ Ready-meals, deep frozen food, tinned food ■ Ice cream ■ Yeast-containing foods, freshly baked bread ■ Pasta, white/polished rice ■ Peanuts ■ Hardened fats, deep-fried foods ■ (For young people) alcohol
Recommended within limits	■ Fresh fruit (except bananas) ■ Bread: sourdough and fermented bread are recommended
Recommended foods	■ Vegetables other than pulses (peas, soya) ■ Pickled vegetables, e. g. raw sauerkraut ■ Soups garnished with vegetables seasoned to stimulate the digestion (fibre, "ballast") ■ Salad, if possible eaten at lunch ■ Raw vegetables, well chewed, if possible eaten at lunch ■ Sour milk products of all kinds (buttermilk, yoghurt, quark, etc.) ■ Millet, oats, spelt, barley, buckwheat, pre-cooked cereals e. g. as flakes, muesli (wetten and allow to soak), fresh grain porridge ■ Meat of organic and if possible Demeter quality, e. g. combined with a little freshly squeezed lemon juice ■ Fish, also combined with a little lemon juice ■ Sour milk drinks (e. g. Kanne Brottrunk®), ■ Sesame, sunflower seeds, linseed ■ Hazelnuts, almonds

child is able to digest at all can vary considerably. An abrupt change of nourishment to whole food can have the effect of making an (above all neurasthenic) child with a weak digestion even more ill, develop more severe meteorism, thrive even less – and suffer clearly more. Under these circumstances it is better to strengthen the child in its digestive activity medicinally *before* a strict diet and gradually to move the food over to the diet.

The constitution of the child is an important aspect: children, with a *"hysterical"* constitution (▸Chap. 4.6.2), in whom the digestion and metabolism are vital as such, but are overworked because of their relative dominance, are already being treated "causally" through the implementation of a consistent diet in combination with symbiotic control (see below) and mostly improve drastically with such treatment. What they are lacking is moderation and rhythm in their nutrition; if they learn to find and keep the latter, their digestive organization is once again in a position to manage its task.

In the *"neurasthenic"* type – whom the paediatrician encounters with increasing frequency as a result of a western lifestyle, e. g. through the decline in natural physical exercise and the growth in intellectual activity – the root of the digestive disorder lies deeper, as explained above (▸Chap. 4.6.2). In these children *medicinal therapy* plays a crucial role in order to achieve the required intensification of the catabolic and digestive processes in the upper and middle digestive tract and thus to create the basis for healing.

4.6.3.3 Stimulating the digestion as long-term treatment for intestinal mycoses

The central herbal medicine for intestinal mycoses is the *root of yellow gentian, Gentiana lutea.* The shape of the plant gives a sturdy and stocky impression while its leaves are positioned crosswise in opposition (like for example the stinging nettle) and are large and elliptical with pronounced curving veins. The root can be dug out only with great difficulty and extends far into the ground in which it is firmly anchored; yellow gentian grows primarily in the chalk alps of central and southern Europe. The plant concentrates bitter substances in the hard, strong and tough-fibred root, including amarogentin which has the highest bitter value of indigenous bitters. The taste of the root extract is exceptionally intense and the aftertaste is reminiscent of iron.

The stocky, powerful shape, the crosswise opposition of the leaves, the deep connection with the earth, the taste and scope of the bitters (stomach and duodenum) give yellow gentian a quality which is related to *iron* [Steiner 1963, 116–119]. In nature, iron is most closely connected with the earth of all the metals; it gives the earth its characteristic colour, belongs to the most frequent elements in the earth's crust and in all likelihood essentially makes up the earth's core. The earth is the planet with relatively the most iron in the solar system. Iron extraction from the food and assimilation happens via processes in the stomach and duodenum. Iron is not just the respiratory metal in the blood, which may be considered the central organ of the human warmth organization and all will processes. Every act of will, every time a region of the body warms up is primarily associated with an increase in blood flow. Iron is equally indispensible for the human immune system (e. g. granulocyte function) and for the integrity of all the barrier organs; and thus also for demarcating the external world, breaking down and overcoming internalized natural processes, and for the rhythmical autonomous activity of human beings with regard to nature. Iron enables the human individuality to control nature both inside the body and externally and to recruit nature for his or her own intentions [Selawry 1985, 258–269].

It is mandatory that the treatment stimulates this body-related I-activity. In phytotherapeutic (as opposed to potentized homoeopathic) concentrations, the root of yellow gentian activates such "iron" activity in the upper digestive tract; *this is the region where the iron in food is resorbed.* Children with low ferritin levels, whose food has a lack of iron and/or who have weak iron resorption are more prone to developing mycoses. It is therapeutically important to take this aspect into account! The bitter root extract of Gentiana lutea activates iron resorption and through the experience of the bitter taste directly stimulates stomach and bile secretion in the child and thus the engagement of the soul and I in the metabolism [cf. Leitgedanken zu Gentiana lutea in: Vademecum 2010, 460]

Therapeutically, the authors primarily use

- **Gentiana Magenglobuli (Stomach remedy)** Wala
  3 × 3–7 pillules/d,

in adolescents and adults the sugar and alcohol free

- **Enzian-Magentonikum (Gentian stomach tonic)** Wala
  3 × 1 small tsp./d.

These medicines are very important in the treatment of mycoses for every constitutional type. In the event of iron deficiency and a tendency for anaemia

- **Gentiana 5 % dil.** Weleda 10.0
  Anaemodoron dil. Weleda 40.0
  ad 50.0 dil., 3 × 5–15 gtt.

and as follow-up treatment above for girls in the second septennium

- **Ferrum pomatum D1 dil.** Weleda
  3 × 5–10 gtt.

The elimination of candida fungi can be further promoted by administering

- **Myrrhinil intest. tab.**
  up to 3 × 3 tab./d.

From the perspective of anthroposophic medicine, *the process of bile production,* its concentration in the gall bladder and subsequent ejection on entry of the chyme into the duodenum (which is also "injected" by the pylorus, (▸Chap. 4.3.4) represents a significant "iron process" in the digestive event. Bile is the result of a primary catabolic process of the erythrocytes in the spleen; here the iron itself is retained by the organism. Bile is a highly active substance which is extraordinarily toxic if released into the organism. Through being retained in the gall bladder and with the subsequent ejection process into the duodenum, the bile flow is "arterialized" and thus becomes even more intensely catabolic in the intestinal lumen. (This process is weakened if we constantly snack and do not maintain a rhythm of eating and not eating). But other than with the stomach and pancreatic enzymes, the activity of the bile *directly passes over into unlocking and assimilating the warmth contained in the food* (in the form of fats; enterohepatic circulation of the bile fluid). Thus bile activity in a unique way represents the two sides of I activity with regard to nature in the same two ways that they are active in the substance-related handling of iron. Finally, bile also stains the stool – very comparable with the brown colour which iron gives the crust of the earth – and stool colour is one of the ways to assess the activity of the gall bladder. This is also one of the factors which plays a key role in the voiding rhythm. *The stimulation and rhythmization of gall bladder activity through diet and medicines is one of the cornerstones of mycosis treatment.*

Greater celandine, Chelidonium (Radix), whose familiar bile stimulating and simultaneously anticonvulsive effect can be intensified further if the plant is fertilized with iron salts during cultivation over three years, has proved itself therapeutically (Chapt. 1.2.2):

- **Chelidonium Ferro cultum** Weleda
  in smaller children administered as Rh D3 (non-alcoholic), from school age as D2 dil., 5–7 gtt. 3 x/d.

If the effect is insufficient or if the patient displays a clear lack of drive and weaknesses of the digestion, the treatment is intensified by administering

- **Vesica fellea/Ferrum D4/8 amp.** Wala
  0.5 ml 1 x/d before the main meal.

The treatment can be supported by externally massaging into the region of the gall bladder at the right costal arch

- **Ferrum met. 0.4 % ointment** Weleda
  pea-sized quantity in the morning

Finally *chicory*, Cichorium intybus, with its universally stimulating and harmonizing action on the digestion in the upper abdomen, is an important medicine for mycosis treatment. This spreading composite produces new, delicate blue flowers each morning in the summer which quickly wilt and are replaced daily by new ones. The angular rough-haired stem is hollow and the whole plant is infused with a bitter latex. Apart from the bitter and tannin substances it contains, its much finer and more differentiated thin shape strikes the eye in comparison to gentian, in accordance with the unshaded locations of the plant at waysides and on banks and waste land [cf. Diederich 2006]. The universal effect of chicory on the stomach and duodenum, on gall bladder and pancreas activity, but also on the spleen and kidneys has been known about for centuries [Madaus 1999a, 966–974]. Its effect on these organs is directed at the living etheric entity in equally stimulating and *formative* measure; Cichorium intybus has a sustained effect on the development of self-regulation of digestion and resorption in the upper sections of the intestine. The plant itself displays strongly formative forces in its growth and as a composite realizes the greatest possible order in the plant realm in the sphere of the flower. Particularly noteworthy is the repeated flowering each day at sunrise – in human beings the catabolic activity above all of the gall bladder must also start again afresh each morning in a daily rhythm; there is a special relationship between the daily rhythm and the human I [Steiner 1988, 148–160]. Therapeutically we can experience that the addition of Cichorium makes the treatment work better and deepens its effect – a herbal effect which is difficult to label but very much to be valued. A specific symptom pointing to the choice of this medicine is undigested food components in the stool [cf. Leitgedanke und leitende Indikation von Cichorium in: Vademecum 2010, 313].

- **Cichorium Rh D3 dil.** Weleda
  5–10 gtt. 3 x/d.

If – as described using the example of the *neurasthenic constitution* – the basic constitutional problem of the patient is that his or her I-organization fails to guide the activity of the soul deeply enough into the metabolism, if the soul is not active enough in the metabolism in a perceptive and catabolic capacity and thus vital organ activity is damaged and the poison of foreign life spreads, then the medicine which works most deeply and thoroughly is *phosphorus*. If we understand digestion, the tapping and respiration of carbohydrates, as tapping the *light* in the food through the I, which requires it for its activity, we can understand the action of phosphorus as *intensification of inner light formation*. Mycosis, on the other hand, deprives the organism of part of its nutritional light reserves which it continues to bind in poisonous catabolic products. Such light formation acts right down as far as stimulating the immunological perceptive and digestive processes (cf. also the action of phosphorus e. g. in the chronic infection of the urinary tract, ▸Chap. 5.5.3). The carbohydrate metabolism in the organism takes place substantially in closest interaction with the phosphate metabolism (phosphorylation of glucose, transfer of energy from the breakdown of carbohydrates to energy-rich phosphates, etc.) which absorbs the energy released through respiration e. g. in the form of ATP until it is released through human activity.

From a homoeopathic perspective the medicinal picture of phosphorus is closely connected with unstable blood sugar levels as is typical for many patients with mycosis problems (▸Chap. 4.6.2). As part of the treatment of mycosis,

- **Phosphorus LM6 dil.** Arcana
  2–5 gtt. daily each morning

can be prescribed over a longer period.

An important indication for the administration of phosphorus in the way set out here is the *prior treatment with corticosteroids*, which create a susceptibility for mycoses in the same way that antibiotic treatments do. In these patients, phosphorus can contribute to creating a counterweight to the consequences of such treatment particularly with regard to the immune system itself and to stimulating inner light formation.

With this indication, but also in general, if there is circulatory lability and weak adrenal gland function the treatment with phosphorus can be supplemented by

- **Glandulae suprarenales comp. pillules** Wala
  5–7 pillules in the morning and at midday.

Bacterial dysbiosis and intestinal mycosis frequently occur as the consequence of *antibiotic treatment* – particularly if the latter was not accompanied by measures for symbiotic control (see below).

In these cases an initially low potency of sulphur is indicated, preferably as natural silver sulphide,

- **Argentit D6 trit.** Weleda
  3 × 1 saltsp./d for 2–4 weeks.

After prior treatment with Argentit, the organism of these patients responds significantly better to the treatment set out above.

In depressive states (▸Chap. 7) which can lead to persistent symbiotic disorders and intestinal mycoses due to their paralysis of inner and outer will activity and inner light penetration, *Hypericum perforatum* in substantial or low potentized form is a very efficacious medicine also in childhood. The effect can be described in abbreviated form as one of *"plant phosphorus"* (cf. the strong connection with light and the photo sensitizing characteristics of the plant and the substances it produces). St John's wort extracts and *Ferrum sidereum* (a crystalline, noble natural form of iron which also contains phosphorus among other things) are the most important medicines which act on the metabolism in *depressive children*:

- **Hypericum Auro cultum D2 dil.** Weleda
  5–10 gtt. 3 x/d
- **Ferrum sidereum D6 trit.** Weleda
  3 × 1 saltsp./d

The infusion of the abdomen and hypothermic parts of the body with warmth is supported by massaging in

- **Mallow oil** Wala (▸Chap. 2.2.1).

For a sustained treatment of mycosis, diet and the specified medicines for stimulating the digestion and breaking down food represent a crucial measure to activate the child's organism. But it should also be taken into account that the mycosis itself leads to *consequential damage of the intestinal mucosa* and often also to measurable *nutritional deficiencies* (e. g. zinc and selenium deficiency). Here replacement therapy could be considered, as necessary, which in place of zinc and selenium tablets can also consist of resorption stimulating treatment (Zincum met. D6 trit. Weleda, D3 trit. Apotheke an der Weleda, Sulphur selenosum D4–6 trit. Weleda, ¼ tsp. 1 x/d of each) and dietary measures (e. g. wheat germ powder as a source of zinc).

A broadly based, vitalizing effect on the function of the intestinal mucosa and the excretory activity of the gall bladder and kidneys is achieved through the preparation

- **Aquilinum comp.** Wala [Sommer and Soldner 1990]
  2–3 × 5–10 pillules/d or ½–1 drink amp./d

This can treat the harmful action of the mycosis on the intestinal mucosa and the excretion of toxic burdens from the liver and kidneys via the gall bladder and urine can be stimulated. The authors also consider it to be a basic medicine for any symbiotic control. The medicine should and can be administered over a long period.

Therapeutic success in intestinal mycosis can often be recognized in that the patient feels greater vitality and strength and that health and the ability to concentrate are subject to less fluctuation; the child appears to be more present in himself or herself and has greater ability to act.

In some cases – above all in children with chronic underlying diseases – sufficient therapeutic success can only be achieved through the addition of *antifungals*. Like antibiotics, they fundamentally represent a "backup solution" in the approach advocated here if the forces which the organism can develop itself are not sufficient. In any event, it is better to act on the digestion and metabolism in an ordering and strengthening way *before* administering a Nystatin preparation, for example, to reduce the antimycotic treatment to the absolutely necessary minimum, and also to carry out after-treatment with the specified preparations in order to achieve stable success. Nystatin as an antifungal agent is taken in the first week of treatment in solution *after* each bigger meal and from the second week of treatment *before* the meal in tablet form or in solution three time daily.

Although in the practise of the authors the administration of Nystatin is rarely required, there are individual patients who have experienced a significant improvement in their health through antifungals if the above treatment concept can be followed.

4.6.4 Symbiosis control – dysbiosis (dysbacteriosis)

K. R. Kummer [1998, 71f.] refers to the *antagonism* between the physiological bacterial intestinal flora and intestinal fungal growth. Supporting the *physiological bacterial intestinal flora* acts against being overrun by yeast fungi such as Candida albicans. Every treatment which aims to change the "terrain" of the digestive tract therapeutically must also take care to ensure that a "new crop" is sown so that the growth of the physiological flora displaces pathogenic growth and the intestine can fulfil its function. But even without any mycosis, the wrong types of food or gastroenteritis can lead to an imbalance in the bacterial intestinal flora (dysbiosis) with the corresponding digestive disorders [Friedrichsen 1990].

Diagnostically, the appropriate *stool analysis* is helpful which differentiates the various types of bacteria semiquantitatively.

We must, however, refer in principle to the specialist literature with regard to this subject [cf. Kummer 1998, 2005]. Two possibilities of symbiotic control are set out generically below which are carried out by the authors in each mycosis treatment, for example, together with the therapy set out in ▸Chap. 4.6.3.

Preparations with cell-free lysates of E. coli should be administered to begin with:

- e.g. **Colibiogen® Kinder** Lösung
  1 tsp./daily in the morning in weeks 1–3,
- or **Pro-Symbioflor®**
  1st week 5–10 gtt. 3 x/d
  2nd week 3 × 7–15 gtt.
  3rd week 10–20 gtt. 3 x/d

This should be followed by preparations made of Enterococcus faecalis:

- e.g. **Symbioflor® 1**
  from 3rd week 10–20 gtt. 3 x/d
  also over a longer period if necessary

and overlapping with that or also alternatively a substitution with coli bacteria:

- e.g. **Mutaflor®** Suspension
  0.5–1 ml/d. (very well tolerated) for approx. 3 weeks
- or **Symbioflor® 2**
  in the afternoon 1 × 5 to 1 × 20 gtt.
- in older children: **Mutaflor®** mite
  1 cap. 1–2 x/d.

This can be supplemented by stimulating the acidulation flora with the administration of Lactobacillus GG acidophilus:

- e.g. **Paidoflor®** (cultured lyophilisate of Lactobacilli)
  2 × ½ to 2 × 1½ tab./d depending on age
  2–4 weeks or longer

or in gastroenteritis,

- e.g. **InfectoDiarrstop®** mono LGG powder
  1 bag/day

The acidulation flora occupy a central position in the terminal ileum, i.e. still in the region of the small intestine; their substitution and stimulation should be considered on the one hand in gastroenteritis (the stool is too "small intestine-like" in acute diarrhoea) and on the other in *chronic dysbiosis with a tendency to mycosis and susceptibility to infection* [cf. Kummer 2005, 450].

During antibiotic treatment, protecting the intestinal flora with the administration of Saccharomyces cerevisiae

- e.g. **Perenterol®**, **Perocur®** cap.
  1 cap. 1–3 x/d

has proved effective (for infants and small children open the capsule and mix the content with a little liquid).

4

4.6.5 Acute appendicitis

It is, of course, self-evident that a manifest acute appendicitis must remain the domain of the surgeon or paediatric surgeon. This condition has become rare today. It is worth noting that "it is not the (preventively undertaken) appendectomy in childhood but the appendicitis itself (with appendectomy as necessary)" which reduces the risk of ulcerative colitis to two thirds – renewed proof of the idea that acute and chronic inflammations stand in an inverse relationship to one another [Koutroubakis et al. 2002, Girke 2010, 672]. The unmistakeable symptoms of a child with acute appendicitis are the often restricted ability to walk upright (only able to walk hunched forward or not at all), sensitivity to jarring (e. g. the patient reports that being driven on an uneven road was painful), pain on the slightest percussion of the abdominal wall (muscular defence), aggravation with every movement and the sudden onset. Furred tongue, possibly nausea and vomiting, mostly blocked stool. The illness can often be suspected simply by inspection of the patient while for the experienced doctor temperature measurements and laboratory findings (urine status, CRP) tend be merely of differential diagnostic significance. Palpation can be difficult in the event of the atypical position of the appendix but often leads to a diagnostic result if carried out carefully. A little known sign is an acupuncture point under the right fibular head which is painful on pressure (whereas there is no pain at this point on the left). Examination by an experienced ultrasound examiner has decisively improved the preoperative diagnosis.

As an initial measure on suspicion of appendicitis, which might still have an inhibiting effect in the early stages (cf. the impressive experiences of Wotschke [1963]), the administration of the following is suitable

- **Belladonna D4 dil., D6 pillules** Weleda
  3–5 gtt. D4 or 5 pillules D6 ¼-hrly to begin with
- **Cichorium Rh D3 dil.** Weleda
  5–10 gtt. ¼-hrly (▸Chap. 4.6.3.3)
- **Antimonit D6 trit.** Weleda (▸Chap. 4.5.2)
  1 saltsp. hrly
- **Mercurius dulcis D6 dil.** DHU
  5–7 gtt. 3 x/d

Suitable external measures are cool compresses in the area of the appendix, possibly supplemented by a cooled lemon slice on the McBurney's point. Careful (not too high) introduction of a camomile tea enema. Fasting.

As part of taking blood (CRP, blood counts, etc.)

- **Argentum met. praep. D30 amp.** Weleda
  1 ml i.v.

can be administered.

The administration of these medicines must not delay clarification of the diagnosis (sonography) and, as necessary, surgical care!

4.7 Treatment indications for chronic gastrointestinal disease

4.7.1 Gastroesophageal reflux disease

4.7.1.1 Clinical diagnosis

While the vomiting of stomach content may be considered a physiological process in the first months of an infant's life, gastroesophageal reflux disease represents a painful disease for the child which in its severe forms can be destructive on the oesophagus (resulting in peptic stenosis, Barrett's oesophagus) and in individual cases causing life threatening (aspiration pneumonia, bleeding, and apnoea in young infants. This clinical picture is of particular significance in children with cerebral palsy (50–75 % of children with spastic quadriplegia display a pronounced and often difficult to treat pathological reflux) and in children with s/p oesophageal atresia and diaphragmatic hernia. A timely diagnosis is of great importance, on the one hand, because of the suffering it causes the little patients and, on the other hand, due to the secondary damage. We particularly refer to relapsing stridor, chronic obstructive bronchitis and relapsing pneumonia in children with cerebral palsy which not infrequently have their true cause in a reflux disease without the latter itself directly appearing clinically. The disease can manifest or recur clinically in children with cerebral disorders at any age, triggered, for example, by acute infections.

As only some of the lead symptoms are described in the literature, they are listed once more below:

- The key factor is a *worsening of the child's state when her or she lies down* and an improvement when he or she sits up, irrespective of which symptom is leading (screaming, vomiting, coughing, sour mouth odour, etc.). This symptom is often the only one which reveals the true cause of the symptoms at an early stage!
- Screaming attacks (when recumbent!), sour mouth odour and increased vomiting are typical symptoms in infants and small children. The refusal of food and weight loss can additionally occur in the course of the disease.
- Later the pain is projected nonspecifically into the stomach and then specifically into the back next to the spinal column on the left along the oesophagus.
- At night the parents can often hear the child swallowing as he or she swallows the rising stomach content (associated with that is the typical sour mouth odour particularly in the morning).
- Stridor, sustained obstructive respiratory ailments and relapsing pneumonia should always make us think of a reflux disease. Conversely, chronic pulmonary diseases can also reinforce gastroesophageal reflux!
- Stereotypical rotation and extension of the head (Sandifer's syndrome) mostly indicate a massive reflux problem.

Case study

A reddish-blond four-month-old boy has come to the surgery for investigation because for weeks he has been showing a subfebrile temperature for reasons which are not clear; all inflammatory parameters are normal also on renewed investigation. When laid down on the examination couch, the face of the child turns dark red and he screams as loudly as he can, clearly in pain. The physical examination reveals a child who is not gaining in weight (feeding the child is very difficult, the mother reports), who is very difficult to examine and has systolic blood pressure of 136 mmHg! The child shows no disability and

no malformation of the upper gastrointestinal tract. He is immediately admitted to hospital to exclude an adrenal tumour and for further diagnosis.
Hypertonicity is clinically confirmed which is initially treated with calcium channel blockers; tumour screening is negative. The very experienced developmental neurologist, who happens to be on duty when the child is admitted, immediately diagnoses gastro-esophageal reflux disease on the basis of the symptoms described above. In the further course of treating the reflux disease all the findings are normalized. But the child remains difficult in his social behaviour, his ambivalently close bond to his mother, his fussy eating habits and variable tendency to seem uncomfortable. From the perspective of the anthroposophical understanding of the human being, we can speak of an early disorder of the sense of life, from the perspective of conventional paediatrics of a regulatory disorder of the autonomic nervous system which is not healed with a cure for the reflux disease.

The diagnosis is confirmed most reliably by gastroscopy with a biopsy. But the most important thing is an early clinical diagnosis.

4.7.1.2 Treatment

The first measure is to place the child in an *inclined position*, if possible at an angle of approx. 25°. An improvement as a result of the inclined position is an important diagnostic confirmation particularly in infants; it is to be recommended in a supine position now that the prone position is obsolete. The second recommendation is *frequent small meals*, in infants and small children with *thickened food* (e. g. Nestargel® 0.5 g/100 ml or a correspondingly prepared powdered milk (AR=Antireflux)). It is important to identify any *food intolerance* at an early stage and to omit milk, for example, if it is not tolerated; this can make a crucial contribution to the improvement of the disorder.

A very effective measure in many cases – also in the above case study – is qualified *craniosacral/osteopathic treatment*. The relationship particularly between disorders of the craniocervical junction and disorders in the function of the upper gastrointestinal tract is quite close, something which is also explained embryologically through the source of the innervation of large parts of the digestive tract in the region of the craniocervical junction. An early osteopathic diagnosis and, as necessary, treatment is urgently to be recommended particularly in children with reflux disease who do not show any cerebral palsy or anatomical malformation of the oesophagus. Important indications can be found in the birth anamnesis and a careful examination of the child (▸ Chap. 2.1).

A simple and often effective measure is the administration of

- Alginat (**Gaviscon Advance® Suspension** (aluminium-free!))
  2.5–10 ml depending on age up to 3 x/d in the evening after meals,

which spreads in a protective film over the stomach content and thus reduces acid reflux episodes.

This substance can be administered as early as in infancy without problems; it is important to give it especially in the evening after meals. In less severe cases the administration of antacids (proton pump inhibitors) can be avoided in this way in combination with the treatment set out below.

On the other hand in children with cerebral palsy and with s/p oesophageal atresia the administration of

- **Antra Mups®** (Omeprazol)
  in age-appropriate dosages

can often not be avoided and is necessary to prevent the above secondary damage to the oesophagus and airways.

This medication is almost always to be preferred over operational intervention (e.g. fundoplication) and re-operations, particularly in the above children. There is still no reliable information in Germany with regard to the long-term consequences of surgical anti-reflux procedures; the experiences of the authors with surgically corrected reflux disease are overwhelmingly negative. Well-founded indications for surgical anti-reflux procedures are rare [cf. Koletzko 2004, 1031]

In his lecture cycle *Das Initiatenbewusstsein* ("Initiate Consciousness") [Steiner 1993], Rudolf Steiner provides a profound characterization of what he perceived in his spiritual research as the possible unconscious soul state in the region of the stomach: a powerful "backward movement" may be active in this region – a strong soul connection with the world of the dead as experienced by the soul before birth, an influence from this part of the soul world which is too strong. This might well manifest itself in the stomach region as illness.

In the view of the authors it seems natural to consider this aspect when a *physical* "backward movement" occurs in this region and persists pathologically beyond the third month of life after acid formation in the stomach has already set in to a considerable extent. From this perspective we can say that the child remains too strongly in a prenatal regressive state. In this context Rudolf Steiner refers to the substance of copper; a correct dosage can regulate the balance between digestion and respiration [Steiner 1993, 76]. These two areas must be polarized following birth after they were filled and flooded by amniotic fluid before birth: whereas it is a physiological part of the respiratory process to breathe in and breathe out, i.e. to reverse the direction of movement regularly, this precisely does not apply with regard to the gastro-intestinal tract.

Copper is not only the core metal for the treatment of diseases of the stomach region but it is also a far-reaching medicine in the event of a too close, regressive mother fixation and disorders arising from the birth itself and their consequences.

It is particularly notable in Steiner's account that he appears to refer casually to *Asafoetida,* a powerful Umbelliferae native to Iran and Afghanistan "which only occurs on gravelly and sandy soil with a saline subsurface" [v. Volkmann 1960, 83]. The plant forms a mighty thigh-sized root whose gum, asant, provides the source material for the homoeopathic medicine. It contains etheric oils, two thirds of them organic disulphides which give it a disgusting smell ("stinking gum"). Asafoetida was traditionally a component of the "Pillulae antihystericae" Sydenhams, for example; in anthroposophic medicine Rudolf Steiner emphasizes that the quality of the smell of asafoetida indicates a Saturn (lead) quality of the plant [cf. Steiner 2001, 84]. In the anthroposophical understanding of the human being asafoetida strengthens and regulates the intervention of the sentient organization, of the astral body in the metabolic area, thus countering regressive tendencies, a rise upwards of metabolic processes, and promotes the incarnation of the higher components of the human being in such a way that healthy, propulsive peristalsis is stimulated. We could formulate it as follows: treatment with stinking gum is intended to ensure that what belongs below the diaphragm stays there. The French homoeopath Didier Grandgeorge, as intuitive as he is practically oriented, describes the main paediatric indication of asafoetida as "the reverse peristalsis". In asafoetida the peristaltic movement from the mouth to the anus is "in reverse as if the organism was spitting everything that comes from the outside out again. Furthermore, we have to consider that the child is nourished in the uterus through the umbilical cord. After birth he or she has to come to terms with the latter being severed and has to change over to taking in food through the mouth and intestine. This changeover does not happen" [Grandgeorge 2004, 46]. From this perspective reflux disease represents an *unsuccessful postnatal polarization of digestive and respiratory pathways and a regressively oriented pathology.* It is no surprise that children with birth-related cerebral palsy and spastic quadriplegia suffer particularly from this disease. [Cf. in this connection Soldner and Sommer 2007, 33]

Against this background the following homoeopathically potentized herbal medicines have proven themselves therapeutically:

- **Asa foetida C12 pillules** Gudjons
  3–5 pillules 1–2x/d

above all for infants with reflux disease; for reflux disease in combination with relapsed obstructive respiratory diseases and pneumonia, for children with an identifiable *ambivalently close mother fixation.* The sound of the rising stomach content audible during the night is also typical.

Belladonna is also an important medicine for reflux disease, either as an individual medicine (Rh D4–10 dil. Weleda) or from the second year of life in the very reliable and effective combination

- **Pulvis stomachicus c. Belladonna trit.** Weleda[1]
  ½–1 dosage spoon 2–3 x/d

Lead symptoms are *very severe screaming attacks with reddening of the face*, above all in the evening and after being put down in the first half of the night. Children with a tendency to macrocephaly, close to the Calcium carbonicum type, even if they tend to be quite thin with gastroesophageal reflux disease.

- **Plexus coeliacus D15 amp.** Wala
  0.5 ml per os 2 x/d (alternatively **Plexus gastricus D15–30 amp.**

has grown in importance for the authors in recent years as an organ preparation (▸Chap. 4.1.3). It is effective, among other things, for gastroesophageal reflux in infancy with failure to thrive and a characteristic increase in pain when put down [Vademecum 2010, 668] and is intended to counter a chronifying disorder of the enteral nervous system.

- **Iris versicolor D4–6 pillules** DHU
  5 pillules 3 x/d after meals.

Iris is generally effective for *excess stomach acid and acid reflux* from the stomach, also familiar as a medicine for weekend migraine; from an anthroposophical perspective it therefore counters metabolic processes surging up into the nervous and sensory pole of the human being.

- **Abies nigra D6 tab.** DHU, **D4 pillules** DHU
  3 x/d before meals.

1 The authors are grateful to D. Ecker (Filderklinik) for informing them about his very positive clinical experiences which they confirmed in practice (also in cerebrally disabled children)

Wilkens [2006, 100] refers to the connection between Abies nigra and diaphragmatic hernias and disorders of the stomach meridian. In homoeopathic examination stomach symptoms, postprandial pain, reflux and foul-smelling breath as well as a *strong inner feeling of coldness* dominate. This is particularly relevant in *children with s/p oesophageal atresia* who frequently display difficulties in generating their own warmth and a susceptibility to colds. Especially in such children, almost all of whom have problems of gastroesophageal reflux disease, Abies nigra is a profoundly working medicine which can be administered for a long period of time.

Copper can be administered to start treatment – above all following birth disorders – as

- **Cuprum met. praep. D6–20 trit.** Weleda
  1 saltsp. in the evening for 3–6 weeks

In gastroesophageal reflux with its characteristic deterioration when recumbent and during the night, therapeutically potentized copper carbonate in the form of malachite is suitable in less severe forms during infancy:

- **Malachit D6 trit.** Apotheke an der Weleda
  1 saltsp. 4 x/d [Vademecum 2010, 568]

More broadly indicated is the following carbonated copper (malachite), effective for the stomach, as

- **Chamomilla/malachite comp. amp.** Weleda
  ½ ampoule orally 1–3 x/d, in older children/adolescents (e.g. with cerebral disability) also s.c. 2–3 x/wk

which has a stronger warming and harmonizing effect and also alleviates pain. It contains the copper-related medicinal plant **Tabacum** in potentized form as an important component.

The external application of copper in combination with Tabacum *in the bladder region or massaged in for the kidneys* (cf. the basic thinking in [Sommer and Soldner 2007]) is also important for simultaneously deepening and relaxing the activity of the soul organization:

- **Cuprum/Nicotiana ointment** Wala
  massage in thinly 2 x/d

As a supplement and follow-on treatment the following should be considered for gastroesophageal reflux disease in infancy (cf. a more detailed explanation under ▸Chap. 2.2.4):

- **Chamomilla Cupro culta, Radix eth. Dec. D2 dil./Rh D3 dil.** Weleda
  2–5 gtt. (D2) 3 x/d diluted with a little water/3–7 gtt. (Rh D3) 3–5 x/d,

whereby the D2 dil. acts a little more strongly but contains 18% alc./vol. while the Rh D3 dil. is alcohol free [cf. also Engelen 2005, 222f.].

- **Magnesit D6 trit.** Weleda
  1 saltsp. 3–4 x/d

is an effective medicine for milk intolerance, failure to thrive, severe pain, refusal of basic food (vegetables) and excess acid (▸Chap. 4.4.4) [Vademecum 2010, 557]

One effective possibility of using copper in therapeutic dosage with iron, traces of arsenic and sulphuric acid in long-term treatment is *Levico water*. Most effective is Levico strong water which is administered diluted with water, at maximum approx. 1 gtt./year of life in the morning for approx. 7 weeks in ascending and descending dosage (start gradually, e.g. for a five-year-old child: first week 3 gtt./d, second week 4 gtt./d, third to fifth week 5 gtt./d, week six as two and seven as one). It is suitable for older children with chronic reflux disease and has a strongly roborating effect which is very much what is wanted in these cases (▸Chap. 6.5.6.3.2). The treatment can be repeated several times per year. If Levico strong water (Starkwasser) is not available, D1 dil. Weleda can be used instead.

4.7.2 Coeliac disease

4.7.2.1 Clinical picture

Bad mood, pallor, bloated abdomen, stomach pain, diarrhoea (malabsorption), weight loss, failure to thrive and laboratory findings (above all iron and zinc deficiency, elevated transaminases, gliadin, transglutaminase and endomysial antibodies can lead to a diagnosis which is backed up by a suction biopsy of the small intestine. In our own practice the general experience has been confirmed that coeliac disease can manifest oligosymptomatically and also without specific symptoms. A corresponding diagnosis should be considered particularly in the case of

- children with autoimmune diseases (in our own practice including children with type 1 diabetes mellitus, dermatomyositis, chronic multifocalosteomyelitis, etc.),

who in the event of a coincidence with coeliac disease can experience a significant improvement in the course of the disease through a gluten-free diet. Keller [2003] describes the case of a girl who was treated with Prednisolon (with all the associated consequences) for two years for suspected autoimmune hepatitis because of a 50-fold elevation in transaminases before anyone thought of coeliac disease – cured with the corresponding diet and ten years of normal development.

Case study

An 8¾-year-old girl was referred by the ophthalmologist. She had initially been taken to see an orthopaedist six years previously with swelling and pronounced pain in the right ankle after jumping off a wall. The injury had significantly increased in the two weeks after the jump. Treatment with rest for suspected traumatic ankle distortion. Three months later with the injury persisting, MRT: syndesmosis rupture, rupture of ant. tibiofibulare lig., ant. talofibulare and calcaneofib. with evidence of synovitis and joint effusion. Four months after the occurrence of the injury she was taken to the paediatric surgery department of the university clinic, rheumatoid factor, ASL, C3, but not ANA were determined, the ESR of 29/62 was ignored, a primary lymphoedema was diagnosed. Eleven months after the injury another MRT was performed in the paediatric surgery department, extensive increase in soft tissue around the bony structures of the tarsus, the ligaments and tendons in this region. Twelve months later the girl still cannot put her weight fully on her right leg, the ankle and forefoot are hyperthermic and tender. Diagnosis: reflex dystrophy following ankle trauma. Continued physiotherapy and lymph drainage. The mother had carried the child a lot after the injury. The parents then bought a buggy and pushed the girl for a long time. She is their first and only child.

Nineteen months after the injury ophthalmic examination: Iridocyclitis of the right eye with synechia, band keratopathy and cataracta complicata with a decrease in visual acuity to 0.5; the girl had been complaining about blurred vision for a month. In the diagnosis at the German Centre for Childhood and Adolescent Rheumatology 23 months after the injury, ANA 1:1280, Hb 10.3 g/dl, slightly elevated ESR, slight thrombocytosis. The prescribed medicinal treatment was not initially followed due to scepticism about conventional medical methods. Inflammatory episodes in the eye in the following 2 years. Now the family feels secure with their new ophthalmologist and carries out his topical therapy. In the last year rapid growth of cataract. Visual acuity down to 0.25. Surgical removal of the lens was planned but could not be carried out due to continued inflammatory activity in the eyes. The ANA-positive iridocyclitis with oligoarthritis is the reason for the referral from the ophthalmologist.

We were able to collect the following information regarding the past history which is not mentioned in any doctor's letter: the mother has been ill with Crohn's disease since her youth, underwent an operation because of that 27 years ago. Since then she has by her own decision successfully followed alternative concepts and eats gluten-free, which is good for her. She looks older than she is, a close symbiosis in the family is noticeable, the girl slept in her parents' bedroom until she was four, the father has had a skin rash on his right ankle for the last two years (!). The grandmother on the mother's side also suffers from Crohn's disease. When the patient was two years old, the mother had two miscarriages and was very anxious in the period before the second miscarriage. More recently the patient has suffered from itchy eczema on the left elbow. As a small child, she never had any fever or childhood diseases. At the age of seven she had 39–40 °C fever for a week, since then has been more independent, robust, the inflammation of the ankle is very much improved, she is running and jumping again. By character the girl is alert, makes precise observations, and is orderly. But the situation with the right eye has not yet improved. During the consultation she drew a girl (far above the "ground") in the upper right half of the paper and in the middle of the sheet in the lower half a sun under an arch. The digestion of the child is normal.

The complex therapy with anthroposophic medicines, incl. Iris bovis D30, Vespa Crabro D15, Equisetum cum Sulfure tostum D15 and Solum Inject aa Oral, produced a clear calming in the eye according to the ophthalmologist (▸Chap. 10.9). Weight and height approx. seventy-fifth percentile. During the second presentation (the family lives 100 km away) two months later, endomysium AB (1:1280), transglutaminase AB (> 128 U/ml), gliadin IgA (46 U/ml) and IgG (121 U/ml) were determined for the first time in the life of the patient. Ferritin 7 ng/ml (normal 20–200), zinc normal, *ANA 1:1280 and thus at the same level as four years ago*. ESR 23/56 mm. The abdomen was judged to be clinically normal also gastroenterologically. The gastroduodenoscopy and laboratory tests ordered by the author led – to the surprise of the gastroenterologist who performed the examination – to the diagnosis of coeliac disease Marsh IIIc with highly enlarged and flattened villi, deepened crypts, increased lymphoplasmacellular infiltration of the lamina propria. Lactase activity was reduced; the other disaccharidases were normal (very surprising with Marsh III!)

Five months after the start of a gluten-free diet the *ANA have fallen to 1:320*, the inflammatory activity in the right eye has disappeared completely without steroid eye drops, there are no longer any clinical symptoms on the right ankle; the lens can be removed. The mother reports that the morning mouth odour which the girl has had since the age of three has disappeared "as if by magic". A strong ambivalence in the relationship with the mother became apparent in the last few months: on the one hand the girl expressed a fear of school, on the other hand she became aggressive towards the mother (for the first time). The proven medicine for school phobia, Ambra grisea C12, made the anxieties clearly recede (all these symptoms point to a strong mother fixation).

This is not the only case in the practice of the authors: thus a multifocal aseptic osteomyelitis in a 14-year-old patient from Italy, treated with limited success using homoeopathic-anthroposophic methods, was completely cured when doctors in Milan diagnosed coeliac disease and treated it with the corresponding diet. This patient too had a clinically normal digestion. It was noticeable that he had a close connection with his parents, was an only child, that the mother suffered from depression and the patient cried in deep empathy when the mother was feeling bad, that he was a good pupil and pianist and took little pleasure in exercise out in nature. The multifocal (aseptic and rheumatic) osteomyelitis affected the lower extremities the muscles of which were conspicuously weak.

The close mother fixation, the frequent status as an only child, a rather head-focused (slightly large-headed) constitution with a relatively weak connection between the individuality and the lower limbs (sometimes also a relatively cool stomach) was a common feature in several children with coeliac disease in our own practice. The association of coeliac disease and diabetes mellitus (approx. 5%) points to the typical constitution of type 1 diabetes mellitus patients: "Influences which either prevent the necessary incarnation of the higher components of the human being in the metabolic and limb organization or restrict the effectiveness they have already achieved in this region of the threefold organism [head – chest cavity – metabolic/limb section] create a predisposition towards type 1 diabetes mellitus" [Girke 2010, 299]. This observation can easily be transferred to children with coeliac disease and explains the clinical observation from an understanding of the whole human being. It throws a light on the case study set out above:

- The close mother fixation causes the soul and spiritual entities to incarnate more slowly (▸Chap. 1.3). The higher components of the child's being detach themselves more slowly from the maternal mantle (bond), weakening the development and emancipation of her own etheric body, life organization because the latter requires such an impulse from the soul and spirit. This is precisely what happens with regard to the digestion (▸Chap. 4.1) and movement.
- An only child often suffers particularly few febrile infections in early childhood. Febrile children's diseases strengthen individualization, the incarnation of the soul and spirit, and thereby also the emancipation from the mother. Conversely the position of being an only child can greatly strengthen the bond with the parents and particularly the mother.
- The etheric body of the child makes itself independent from the top downwards, craniocaudally. In the constellation which we have set out, the child's development is dissociated because it progresses faster in the head than in the limbs.
- Maternal anxieties and depressions reinforce the tendency above all in empathetic children to keep the I and astral body "above and outside". Rheumatic inflammation, paralysis, its connection with imitation and the position of the eye in this process is set out in ▸Chap. 10.9.
- In this case there was the additional trauma following the jump off the wall. Previously the girl liked exercise, now she became dependent on parental, and above all her mother's care. The mouth odour, which had disappeared "as if by magic" after adequate dietetic therapy, developed during this phase. The parents had largely taken over a basic function of the limbs, independent movement, again. Rudolf Steiner's concept of the "metabolic and limb system" indicates that a lack of movement or the failure of the soul and spirit to incarnate properly in the movement of the limbs can also affect the

vitality of the metabolic region which receives its impulses from the soul and spiritual entity. Clinical research, which today has recognized the central salutogenetic role of movement ("exercise") in metabolic diseases, confirms this connection.

Coeliac disease belongs pathogenically to the spectrum of (Th_1-accentuated) autoaggressive disorders in which a disorder of the child's immune regulation induces an autoaggressive inflammation. Type 1 diabetes mellitus, like rheumatoid arthritis, originates immunologically in this disease spectrum. The autoaggressive inflammation is directed in rheumatic oligoarthritis against the synovia of individual joints but also the periarticular ligaments and tendons as well as against the uvea and the associated structures, in diabetes against the pancreatic islet cells and in coeliac disease against the mucosa of the small intestine. If "cross reactions" occur in this context, these diseases can clearly reinforce one another. The autoaggressive inflammation in coeliac disease is stimulated by the gluten (prolamin) of cereals (wheat, barley, rye, oats) working together with the body's own transglutaminase. At least six months of breast feeding has a protective effect, i. e. protecting against too early contact with foreign protein, as does feeding small amounts of gliadin around the sixth or seventh month while breast feeding continues – because the organism most easily develops the necessary tolerance of gluten if breast milk is present. Breast milk turns out to be a "master in the art of tolerance", breast feeding to be a crucial support in the phase of the first contact with foreign foods.

"A meta-analysis of six case control studies showed that the risk of coeliac disease is reduced by half if gluten is introduced with the solid food *while breast feeding is still taking place*" [Koletzko et al. 2010, 682, author's emphasis]. The incidence is also increased by too late gliadin contact. It is striking that as a result of cereal breeding, wheat in particular has a far higher percentage of gluten than two generations ago thus making it more toxic for humans: to the present day the development of conventional industrialized agriculture has failed to follow sustainable objectives with regard to ecology and health, and even less so with regard to seeds. Biodynamically cultivated cereals are to be preferred. It has been proven that most people do *not* develop coeliac disease even if genetically predisposed to do so; it has not yet been clarified scientifically [Zimmer 2003] why this is so – clearly a question of the epigenetic immune regulation (▸Chap. 4.1.2). It is equally clear that the organism in many children can limit the gluten intolerance to a latent state. From the perspective of complementary medicine, the following consequences arise:

- The direction set out in this book, which consistently aims for a successful development of the child's immune regulation in terms of prophylaxis and treatment, including the use as far as possible of biodynamic or organic foods, is likely to be a protective approach with regard to coeliac disease.
- Children with manifest coeliac disease require a rigorous diet corresponding to general paediatric principles (also lactose-free at the beginning).
- The authors have experienced cases which clinically lost their gliadin intolerance again with the treatment described below. The initial diagnosis of a gliadin intolerance must not immediately be equated with irreversibility. The question as to what distinguishes transitory gluten intolerance from lifelong coeliac disease has not been scientifically clarified [Zimmer 2003]. In controlled re-exposure, oats may be considered as a cereal which has high value in terms of nutritional physiology.

- If clinical and laboratory controls (biopsy findings, as necessary, following re-exposure) show that the patient has retained his or her gliadin intolerance, uncontrolled gliadin exposure should be warned against on the basis of the significantly higher risk of developing further autoimmune diseases or the increasingly frequent long-term occurrence of malignomas of the gastrointestinal tract.

4.7.2.2 Treatment possibilities

At the time of diagnosis, *serious damage to the mucosa of the small intestine* has mostly occurred. The child cannot adequately assimilate essential substances such as e. g. iron; his or her inner metabolism is malnourished, also leading to the psychologically and physically observable signs of illness.

If at the time of diagnosis there is diarrhoea with maldigestion/malabsorption (classic coeliac disease picture), the administration of

- **Podophyllum D4, subsequently D6 dil./pillules** (various manufacturers)
  3–5 gtt./pillules 5 x/d

at the start of treatment for at least 4 to 6 weeks has proved itself; the drops seem to be even more effective than the pillules. Symptoms suggesting the choice of Podophyllum are sustained painless, copious, foul smelling, diarrhoea, which can sometimes shoot out, and which can alternate with constipation; in general there is a great deficiency of vital warmth – a symptom which can often be observed in children with coeliac disease. A central medicine to strengthen the working together of the four entities of the child's being has shown itself to be

- **Pancreas GI D4 amp.** Wala
  0.5–1.0 ml/d per os for a long period

It is indicated not only for the diarrhoea described above but for any digestive weakness. It strengthens the vitality and digestive activity of the child. By this means this organ preparation [Steiner, Wegman 1991, 116] clears the path for the physically oriented activity of the higher components (astral body, I) in the "metabolic human being". If there is also *anxiety and a weak digestion* the following is suitable

- **Pancreas/Meteoreisen amp.** Wala
  at the same dosage [Vademecum 2010, 645]

This treatment can be supplemented above all by the administration of

- **Aquilinum comp. pillules** Wala
  3–7 pillules 3 x/d (depending on age)

(▸Chap. 4.6.3.3) which supports the regeneration and redifferentiation of the mucosa [cf. Sommer and Soldner 1990], and

- **Antimonit D6 trit.** Weleda
  3 × 1 saltsp./d.

As a *tea*, a preparation with blackberry leaves and dried blueberries is suitable for diarrhoea and proven villous atrophy (▸Chap. 4.5.1). *Symbiotic control* is indispensible with this disease (▸Chap. 4.5.4) as well as controlled vitamin and trace element substitution to begin with. After the first acute phase of the disease has subsided, the medicinal administration of Podophyllum can be followed by a potentized, constitutionally active mineral medicine. Silicea (quartz) is most frequently considered (D6-20) (▸Chap. 3.2.5.2): There is generally a primary weakness of the body building metabolism and a lack of body heat in children with coeliac disease. Significantly less frequently Calcium carbonicum, Magnesium carbonicum (▸Chap. 4.4.4) and Calcium fluoratum (▸Chap. 3.2.5.3) are indicated.

In terms of diet the generally familiar dietary rules apply. If the above therapy is carried out, the attempt can be made after a year at the earliest to introduce oats into the diet in a controlled way with careful clinical and laboratory observation of the course. If there are significant co-diseases, such as the iridocyclitis in the case described above, the authors recommend the longer-term abstinence from the re-exposure to gluten. *Millet* can be positively highlighted from among the gluten-free cereals. It particularly accords with the needs of the small child in many of its characteristics. The authors have repeatedly been able to observe the way in which the trophic condition of the skin has improved rapidly and impressively with millet. It appears to represent a significant supplement in the diet of these children. Quinoa and amaranth are also very valuable foods for children with coeliac disease.

In coeliac disease, the healing process can be significantly supported by *eurythmy therapy*. In learning to cope with food and the environment, great importance obtains in this context to the infusion of the body with warmth, the equilibrium between the sensory and nervous pole and the metabolic pole, loosening the symbiosis with the parents, and the internalization of iron qualities.

4.7.3 Chronic inflammatory bowel disease – Eosinophilic colitis, ulcerative colitis and Crohn's disease

4.7.3.1 Disease types and individualized paediatrics

Case study

A four-year-old boy with *eosinophilic colitis* came to the practice for the first time. The disease started at 17 months. He is his mother's fourth child. His oldest half-brother (24 years old) has an alcohol problem. His older half-sisters (22) are healthy. The boy himself was apparently 18 days (!) overdue. Breast fed exclusively for eight months, then some solid food. At the age of 11 months, the father of his half-siblings died of cancer at the age of 47, something which was a deep shock for the mother. "I weaned him very quickly" (from a letter of the mother) and the boy "ate normally". Measles, mumps and rubella vaccination was given at 15 months. At 17 months bloody diarrhoea starts, proven allergic sensitization above all to chicken protein and less so to wheat and rye flour. None of the elimination diets incl. Neocate® lead to any stabilization, bloody diarrhoea persists. Child was admitted to kindergarten at two-and-a-half years, growth retardation (< 3rd percentile) and multiple psychosocial developmental deficits. Severe intestinal bleeding occurred a few days later. "I have noticed that [the boy] acts out strongly through his intestine," the mother says.

Currently renewed bleeding, diarrhoea, in the meantime a pollinosis has manifested. The boy has over time been given numerous homoeopathic medicines by his mother, montelukast was not successful. Steroids did not completely stop the bleeding either. A gastroscopy and colonoscopy at the age of four histologically confirmed the diagnosis of eosinophilic colitis (typically for "IBD", the pathologist did not want to exclude other chronic-inflammatory bowel diseases such as Crohn's disease altogether purely on the basis of the histology).

The boy has now been treated by the author in collaboration with a reference centre for eosinophilic colitis in northern Germany for seven years. Progress under anthroposophically homoeopathic as well as allopathic treatment (including the administration of Trichuris suis ova) remained inconsistent for three years. The intestinal bleeding also made the parenteral administration of iron necessary. Then, four years ago, as the situation grew more critical in December, the author consciously went back to consider the start of the illness once more. Clearly the mother, who had separated from the father of the half-sisters, had been shocked and overcome by the news of the death of her first husband. There was a rupture in a relationship which until that point was very symbiotically focused (overdue pregnancy, long breast feeding period, solid food too late). The experience must have aroused anxiety in the boy. He is noticeably childlike in all social situations, maladjusted, he lacks a feeling for appropriate social distance and is anxious and experiences much negativity with children of his own age. It became clear that the then rupture probably triggered great anxiety and the boy immediately reacted with panic if he was "left alone by the mother", e.g. following admission to kindergarten. Accordingly, he regularly woke up each night between one and two in the morning and slipped into his parents' bed.
Thereupon the following medicine was prescribed by telephone – the family lives 800 km away (Chap. 2.2.3): *Aconitum C200 pillules*, 3 × 3 pillules/d for three days. Directly afterwards (in the same week) the bloody diarrhoea ceased to date (4 years of follow-up). The strength of the potency reflects the assumption that the original triggering event lay several years in the past. Calprotectin and lactoferrin in stools as inflammatory markers have remained moderately high to date – a diagnosis which is not unusual also in other IBD in remission.
Since then there has been no treatment of the intestine other than a repetition of Aconitum in psychologically stressful situations. Treatment with growth hormone in view of the boy's strongly retarded growth had been started some considerable time before this therapy. The multiple developmental deficits and ADHD symptoms have represented a significant therapeutic challenge in the last few years. The boy has clearly benefited in his development from eurythmy therapy.

This case study reflects the perspectives which were developed in ▸ Chap. 4.1.

Chronic-inflammatory bowel diseases are often preceded by *an experience of loss* – e.g. a death in the family, the end of a friendship. On the other hand the patients are sensitive and dependent in heightened measure on their social relationships; normal to pronounced intelligence contrasts with remaining too childlike in their psychological experience and behaviour [Keller and Wiskott 1991, 1179].

Case study

A mother, who wants to present her 12-year-old son at the surgery writes down a brief anamnesis on three pages. The disease started six months ago when the boy weighed 37 kg and was 153 cm tall: continuous loss of weight, one month later anal abscess treated surgically, stomach pain, feeling of abdominal fullness, postprandial nausea, increasing concentration problems, feeling of coldness and cold intolerance (in summer and autumn), continuation only of surgical and homoeopathic treatment by the local paediatrician without success: six months after onset 28.5 kg BW, CRP 8.2 mg/dl, leucocytes 15,800/µl, thrombocytes 983,000/µl, Hb 10.0 g/dl, endoscopically Crohn's oesophagitis and attack of the colon, above all the rectum.

The mother wrote: "A diagnosis which initially made us parents very depressed. [Her son], in contrast, accepted the illness and informed himself about it from the doctors. They .... were pleased about his openness and thirst for knowledge. But as his mother I can also see that he "swallowed" a lot and tried to come to terms with these events by himself. .... About myself still: two years ago (1½ years before manifestation of the disease) I suffered a spinal cord infarction [cause unexplained, no known risk factors]. Arms and hands are paralysed. Intensive and specific therapies enable me to live a largely independent life again. Even writing ... It was of course a disastrous event for the family and for me. But I started immediately taking things as they are and gained control of daily life again through the therapies. During this time there were major problems with [her son]: change of school from primary to upper secondary school, *complete academic failure* (emphasis in original). Then change to intermediate secondary school with repetition of class 5 with great success. He has developed into a good student now in class 6."

Another and yet common language becomes audible here:

- The *sudden and unexpected loss of the "nurturing basis"*, the mother, the primary school world, *childhood*: the manifestation of chronic-inflammatory bowel diseases peaks at about the age of 12–14 [Buderus 2010, 747], i.e. at the threshold of puberty, of disengaging oneself [normally gradually but steadily] from the nurturing and caring basis of the family, of creating new relationships with people of one's own age, the profound changes in one's own body, the first soul and spiritual awakening of one's own individuality [cf. Keller 2010]. In the gospels, two accounts reflect this polarity: on the one hand the 12-year-old Jesus in the temple who amazes those around him and alarms his parents – Mary calls out: "My child, how could you do treat us like this (Luke 2:48) – and on the other hand the 12-year-old daughter of Jairus who is thought to be dead by all those around (Luke 8:49) and is restored to life after the healing of the woman who has been bleeding for twelve years: in Palestine, menstruation set in on average at the age of 12 (as bone finds have shown) ... If in this critical phase between 9 and 14 such a loss of support and attention in the family and at school occur at the same time, then this can be more than the young person is able to "digest", "swallow" or indeed "cast off". Pathopsychologically we might start to recognize the origin here of the dwindling of the "mucosal block", the protective living mucosal layer between the intestinal content and the intestinal mucosal barrier which plays a central pathogenic role in chronic inflammatory bowel diseases (▸Chap. 4.1.3, [Girke 2010, 665).

- We can reflect on what the adequate treatment of this shocking loss of maternal security would have meant for the patient – this case study can serve to underline once again the importance of the aspect of treatment for shock in preventive medicine!
- It is characteristic of this family (one of the boy's aunts also suffered from Crohn's disease) that everyone involved tries to "keep a cool *head*" (although they can be emotionally excitable). Psychologically they deal with a lot by themselves. "From a psychological and spiritual perspective, children with Crohn's disease tend to be more withdrawn, sceptical, unapproachable and independent in comparison to children with ulcerative colitis" [Vagedes, Soldner 2010, 156]. That is also how this patient presented in the seven years which have in the meantime passed since the first diagnosis.
- *"Crohn's disease is functionally marked by the dominance of the nervous system,* i. e. by a 'cephalic development in the wrong place'. In this connection the granuloma which characterizes Crohn's disease is a significant finding. … The 'cranial capsule' of Crohn's fibrosis with the surrounding lymphatic infiltrate shows the quality of the nervous and sensory system" [Girke 2010, 667]. This characteristic is underlined by the typical *catabolic metabolism and weight loss, by the pain (and stenoses of the intestinal passage as relevant)*: the Crohn's patient enters into a dynamic of physical catabolism in which the basis of the body's anabolic activity, the digestive and absorption process above all in the small intestine, is "walled off": the "wall" between these patients and the environment is reflected in their digestive tract, which after all should always be simultaneously perceived as original ensouled inner space (▸Chap. 4.1.3): here too "things come to a halt", forward passage and exchange come to a standstill while life threatens to dry up.

In this case it was only possible to control the acute situation to begin with by means of a conventional treatment plan: a frequent situation in chronic inflammatory bowel diseases in which the position of the complementary medical and salutogenetic approach to treatment is to be sought in the achievement and stabilization of remission rather than the management of the acute episode. It should nevertheless never be excluded that when even the standard treatment fails, an anthroposophical and homoeopathic treatment concept as set out below can enable the management of an acute disease episode (as has been experienced by the authors e. g. with florid colitis which had continued to bleed in a 2-year-old patient even with the administration of a high dosage of steroids). On the other hand the recurrence rate is high and the physician using anthroposophical and homoeopathic treatment should always examine in good time which treatment concept is appropriate for the patient at any given time. Any preliminary ideological decision should be avoided here!

Organically the *symptoms are those of powerlessness: while* the digestive tract usually represents an organ in which the "external world" in the form of the intestinal content, including the intestinal flora, is governed, formed, devitalized (to the extent of physiological water removal in the large intestine) and is brought rhythmically to excretion, something which the child can place under its conscious control from about the age of three, this order breaks down in chronic inflammatory bowel diseases. In this way the ulcerative colitis dissolves the border between inside and outside; the blood as the central inner organ of respiratory and will activity flows out, the organism thereby becomes deficient above all in iron. The disease process not infrequently also spreads to the bile ducts – just as conversely ulcerative colitis can often be observed in sclerosing cholangitis. This connection also indicates that in these diseases *the catabolic activity of the organism, which is physiologically directed against the ingested food* (▸Chap. 4.1.3, ▸Chap. 4.3.3), *loses its power and orientation* and the digestive organs of the organism themselves become subject to a pathological catabolic process.

From the perspective of anthroposophic medicine, all catabolic and excretory processes are an expression of the activity of the soul entity and the astral body in the physical body; the latter must be guided by the I-organization if the catabolic process is to run a useful course for the whole of the organism. Hence the therapy must initially address, strengthen and physically engage the individuality, the I of the patient, in order to control the one-sidedly catabolic dynamic of the astral body. This is reflected immunologically in both diseases in a *polar failure of the immune regulation* (which is a function of the I-organization): *in ulcerative colitis and eosinophilic colitis as well as in chronic allergic inflammation we find a one-sided immune reaction of the* Th_2 *lymphocytes, while Crohn's disease and coeliac disease are characterized by a dynamic dominated by* Th_1 *lymphocytes.* In ulcerative colitis the barriers dissolve, as in atopic dermatitis and bronchial asthma; in Crohn's disease the gastro-intestinal tract segmentally loses flexibility and threatens to stenose or develop wall-breaching fistula and abscesses (as individual joints threaten to lose their flexibility and become deformed through inflammation in Th_1-dominated rheumatoid arthritis).

Therapeutically the consultation with the patient is important with this goal in mind. Alongside the anamnesis (biography, experience of loss, family anamnesis) it is a matter of finding access to the individuality of the child or the adolescent and in the further course to guide them out of their powerlessness in stages. This path is significantly supported in adolescence by *artistic therapy* to the extent that the physician can prescribe it specifically and guide it through regular therapeutic discussions with the therapist. The family bond of ulcerative colitis patients in particular is high. In childhood and adolescence, it can be the goal of artistic therapy in particular gradually to loosen the inner dependence on and bond with the family which is *strongly determined by the super-I* (and often very performance-related above all in ulcerative colitis); also to aim to open up an inner soul space which the child or adolescent can move into and in which he or she can also be physically present.

The goal of the *medicinal* therapy from the perspective of anthroposophic medicine is also to anchor the soul entity and I-organization of the patient properly in the *organism.*

4.7.3.2 Complementary medicine treatment indications

To begin with, let us refer once more to the *shock, the sudden or threatening aspect of security.* The corresponding therapy has been outlined elsewhere (▸Chap. 2.2.3) but also requires creative concepts in individual cases. To this end it is necessary to uncover the source of the disease dynamic anamnestically.

Set out below are mainly typical treatment possibilities which the authors have found to be effective individually or in a treatment concept.

- In the experience of the authors, treatment with **potentized autologous blood** as indicated by Imhäuser [2000] in children with ulcerative colitis is a valuable basic treatment; it is also effective in many allergic clinical pictures (▸Chap. 6.3.3.4).
- C5, 7, 9, 12, 15 in ascending potentization 3–5 gtt. 3 x/wk in the morning for 4–6 weeks each, from C9 only 2 x, in C15 only 1 x/wk.

The universal relevance of this treatment lies in the blood being the central organ of the human individuality, the I-organization [Steiner and Wegman 1977, 40] in the organism, in so far as this I can be seen as intervening tangibly in the body *through the will.* The warmth organization of the human being is the organization of the blood flow through the organism; every will process comes to expression through a change in perfusion. Ulcerative colitis as a clinical picture shows that the individuality of the patient remains too strongly dependent on the family and external world with his or her soul entity and does not face up sufficiently to the environment through the will to conquer his or her own autonomy. "Blood ties", the blood flow of heredity, dominate individualization; on the other hand the patient threatens to lose his or her own blood to the outside (ulcerative colitis). Treatment with potentized autologous blood can be seen as an appeal to the I-organization to unite more deeply with its own central organ.

Phosphorus works in a similar direction, e.g.

- **Phosphorus LM6 dil.** Arcana
  3–5 gtt./d in the morning

In patients with ulcerative colitis (and eosinophilic colitis) it not only counters the bleeding tendency but as treatment over a longer period significantly strengthens their self-confidence, their psychological independence (▸Chap. 5.1.1.4.3). The treatment with potentized phosphorus is particularly important if the patient has previously been treated with *corticosteroids,* something which in practice is frequently the case with this disease.

In order to learn to control the inflammatory process in the lower intestinal sections, it is important for the patient to strengthen the activity of the gall bladder and pancreas which physiologically have the strongest breaking down effect on the intestinal content and in which the intervention of the astral body and I in the digestive process becomes particularly manifest. It is a matter of guiding this catabolic process in the right direction whereas it becomes increasingly autonomous in the disease and turns against the organism itself.

In therapeutic practice the following has proved particularly effective

- **Cichorium/Pancreas comp. amp./pillules** Wala
  ½ ampoule 2 x/d per os, in adolescents also 1 ml s.c. in the region of the left costal arch 1 x/d–1 x/wk or 7–10 pillules 3 x/d.

While the Pancreas organ preparation stimulates the activity of the pancreas at the level of the etheric body, Cichorium and antimony act on the astral body and I-organization in the sense set out above. Antimony can also counter the structural dissolution and bleeding tendency in the lower intestinal section.

This therapeutic intention can be supplemented by

- **Gentiana Magenglobuli (stomach remedy)** Wala
  5–10 pillules 2–3 x/d

above all for *lack of appetite, burdening through allopathic medicines, stress* – also suitable in patients with *Crohn's disease with severe weight loss* to stimulate digestion and resorption of food and thus physical anabolic processes.

Antimony takes a central position in the treatment of ulcerative colitis [cf. Principle and leading indication in Vademecum 2010, 772; Hannesen 2004, 46f]

For ulcerative colitis, eosinophilic colitis with bleeding tendency

- **Stibium met. praep. D6 amp., trit., supp.** Weleda
  acutely 10 ml i.v. 1 x-several x/d, also in infusion solution, also rectally as an enema at body temperature or supp. 2–3 x/d, for maintenance trit. 1 saltsp 1–3 x/d.
- **Marmor D6/Stibium D6 amp., trit.** Weleda
  in the same indication and dosage (no supp. available), above all for psychological lability, hysterical constitution ("hysterical" as defined in anthroposophic medicine) to give the child greater support and protective sheathing.

For slimy diarrhoea and mucous colitis, a potentized joint trituration of antimony sulphide and mercury is suitable

- **Aethiops antimonialis D6 dil./tab.** DHU
  ½–1 tab./5–7 gtt. 3–5 x/d.

Extracts of tormentil, Potentilla tormentilla speed up tissue repair phytotherapeutically and reduce the *bleeding tendency in ulcerative colitis* [Huber 2009].

- **Tormentilla eth. decoct. (original mother tincture)** Weleda
  5–20 gtt. 3 x/d depending on age

can be administered for nervously tense and greatly stressed patients, also mixed with Valeriana (valerian) original mother tincture in a ratio of 2:1 (Tormentilla:Valeriana). It should not be administered for too long after the bleeding has stopped. If food intake already triggers (gastrocolic reflex) diarrhoea, if there is *strong sensitivity in the stomach region and a tendency for diarrhoea*, a suitable herbal tincture is

- **Geum urbanum eth. decoct. (original mother tincture)** Weleda
  5–10 gtt. 3–6 x/d (in infancy Rh D3) [Vademecum 2010, 465]

In both tormentilla and avens (Geum), we are dealing with the rhizome of delicate, unobtrusive plants. Rudolf Steiner [Steiner 2001, 119f.] spoke about the efficacy of Geum urbanum in such a way that the intended action on the *enteric nervous system ENS* was directly apparent: "The nervous and sensory apparatus is stimulated specifically in the digestive organs and so that is where we have the predominating action of the I. ... We will therefore have to combat diarrhoea, we will have to combat mucous discharges from the intestine." From this perspective it becomes comprehensible how roots such as avens, containing etheric oils with the corresponding scent, or tormentilla, which already displays a relationship with the metabolic system through its red colour, can address specifically this side of the intestine which has been referred to in ▸Chap. 4.1.3. as being central to the effectiveness of the astral body and I-organization in the digestive tract, acting primarily in the intestinal wall.

A further basic medicine in anthroposophic medicine for the treatment of chronic bowel disease is **Digestodoron**® Weleda (▸Chap. 6.3.3.2; Vademecum 2010, 390f)

A universally important, if more symptomatically acting medicine in anthroposophic medicine for chronic inflammatory bowel diseases is

- **Bolus alba comp. pulvis** Wala
  1 tsp./100 ml water, of which (depending on age) and symptoms 30–150 ml/d taken by the teaspoon or in sips.

This medicine, which contains extracts of Geum urbanum, Chamomilla, Gentiana and Arsenicum album in D4 among other things, has its role in ulcerative colitis as well as in Crohn's disease. Symptomatic forms of

- diarrhoea,
- inflammatory changes of the mucosa in oesophagus, stomach, small and large intestine,
- stress

are intercepted by the use of this medicine. Many patients learn to use this medicine as needed. The aniseed taste can be an obstacle with small children but older children and adolescents accept it as a rule [Vademecum 2010, 225]

In more severe inflammatory activity and a tendency for bleeding, the application of

- **Salix/Rhus comp. pillules Wala**
  5–7 pillules 3–5 x/d

can have a very positive effect. Its indication is also relatively broad.

Studies have shown the value particularly in ulcerative colitis of *symbiotic control* with E. coli Nissle:

- **Mutaflor® Suspension, cap.**
  1 ml per os 1 x/d, in older pupils 1 cap.

is used regularly by the authors for *symbiotic control* (▸Chap. 4.6.4) in ulcerative colitis.
In Crohn's disease, affecting above all the anorectum, and ulcerative colitis

- **Colibiogen® Kinder**
  1 tsp. 1 x/d

has proved itself over a longer period.

In metal therapy for ulcerative colitis

- **Mercurius vivus nat. D6 tab.** Weleda, **Mercurius solubilis D30 or C30 pillules** (various manufacturers)
  ½–1 tab. 5 x/d, 3–5 pillules 3–4 x/d (can be administered for a longer period also in higher potencies)

is a central medicine, particularly if the familial situation and the patient are characterized by *restlessness, the need for movement, the urge for mobility* (which e. g. after flights or longer car journeys can trigger bleeding), there is an inclination for cumulative infections (which can have a very detrimental effect here – attention must be paid accordingly to the environment of the children), and a tendency to live strongly in the environment with the soul and spiritual entity and not be able to come to rest at night. Evacuation can be slimy or purulent, there is clear inflammatory activity of the intestinal wall.

In acute cases of strongly inflammatory colitis [Girke 2010, 672]

- **Apis Belladonna cum Mercurio amp./pillules Wala**
  5 pillules/0.3–0.5 ml per os up to hrly can be administered or
- **Mercurius cyanatus D6 dil./pillules**
  in individual dosage, whereby D4 can be even more effective but is not currently available in Germany. A medicine for an aggressive course.

The gold compound of mercury has a deep-seated effect in severe forms of ulcerative colitis and Crohn's colitis

- **Mercurius auratus D15 amp.** Weleda

in combination with the homologously potentized organ preparation

- **Colon Gl D12–30 amp.** Wala
  1 ml per os 3 x/wk or in adolescents also s.c./i.v.

From a homoeopathic perspective the metals mercury and gold in potentized form correspond to the "syphilitic", destructive miasma, i.e. a chronic destructive inflammation. Homologous organ preparations from the whole of the digestive tract can be indicated in Crohn's disease; the younger the patient, the more important the treatment with these preparations.

- **Ferrum hydroxydatum 5–50 % trit.** Weleda (5 %), Apotheke an der Weleda (50 %)
  ¼–½ teaspoon at the start of the main meal

can significantly contribute to maintaining remission and balance of the anaemia, the iron deficiency in patients with ulcerative colitis, after the acute inflammatory occurrence has subsided. This medicine [Engel 2006] can stimulate the activity of the I-organization in the metabolism, the individualization of the will formation in the patient, can contribute to compensating the iron deficiency and in our experience is tolerated considerably better than other oral iron preparations. It cannot, however, replace the parenteral administration of iron which may be necessary. The patient "no longer runs out" but can incorporate the forces of his individuality better and keep them inside himself or herself. Ferrum ustum comp. Weleda has a similar effect. The iron therapy can be supplemented with

- **China D12–30 pillules** (various manufacturers)
  5–7 pillules 2–3 x/d

which can e.g. effectively supplement treatment with iron at midday and in the evening and treatment in the morning with phosphorus particularly if blood loss has weakened the patient.

The *metal therapy for Crohn's disease* is dependent on which sections of the intestine are primarily affected and whether stenosis, fistulas, abscesses or diarrhoea predominate in the symptoms. The authors consider it important in this disease to compensate for the emphasis on the head with a corresponding vitalizing treatment. In this context *sulphur* is important above all as an individual preparation or as a metal combination e. g. in Cuprum sulfuricum. Thus in the case of the patient presented in the above case study, the following was administered for a longer period of time

- **Sulphur LM6 dil.** Arcana
  5–7 gtt./d in the morning

countering the desire for sweet things and unhealthy one-sided nutritional habits which are a characteristic of Crohn patients. Sulphur has a vitalizing and ordering effect, promotes anabolism after a longer period of catabolic metabolic activity and in our experience tends to be indicated in Crohn patients rather than phosphorus.

- **Cuprum sulfuricum comp. tab.** Weleda
  ½–1 tab. 3 x/d

can promote healthy boundaries in the family, have a warming, relaxing and vitalizing (sulphur) effect whereby the onset of the effect can be judged after approx. 2–3 weeks [Hannesen 2004, 49]. The medicine contains within itself the polarity of copper sulphate in low and medium potentization and was originally developed for intestinal tuberculosis as a granulomatous inflammation which tended to affect the ileo-cecal junction (ileitis terminalis is another term for Crohn's disease). The external application of copper is important, e.g.

- **Red copper ointment** Wala
  rubbed into the skin over the stomach area, especially in the evenings

stimulating the warming and expansion of the soul entity in the abdomen and thus countering the disease dynamic of Crohn's disease.

In patients with Crohn's colitis, i.e. predominantly affecting the colon and rectum (anorectal region) the authors have used

- **Iscucin Salicis Stärke A amp.** Wala
  1 ml s.c. 1–2 x/wk

several times with success. This treatment can be considered from adolescence onwards. Willow mistletoe is also effective for other Th_1-mediated chronic destructive inflammations, e.g. polyarthritis. It is particularly indicated if the patient displays a tendency for psychological introversion, if there is or was pain or if there is clear induration. The treatment can be continued for years without a break.

Fistulas in turn react to potentized silicic acid, e.g. higher potencies of *quartz*, best injected less frequently s.c.:

- **Quarz D60 amp.** Weleda
  1 amp. s.c. weekly or less frequently

If there is a tendency for abscesses and fistulas to develop in the region of the anorectum we have used

- **Quercus ointment** Wala

with success following as gentle as possible cleaning after defecation (shower, bidet, moist flannel, drying, then application of ointment). This treatment can be supplemented with

- **Mercurialis comp. supp.** Wala
  1 supp. in the evening/d

which has also shown itself to be effective if there is a tendency to bleed in the rectum in ulcerative colitis.

Diet can be of crucial importance in the course of the disease. The exclusively liquid food with special nutrition in acute stenosing Crohn's disease, which can reach the efficacy of steroid therapy, is well known. But it can be of therapeutic benefit for all patients to undertake a change of diet. In this context we have found a patient *nutritional record* to be a useful basis which makes it possible to quickly see the individual eating and drinking habits of the patient and communicate specific possibilities to optimize nutrition.

In acute cases it is worthwhile attempting to refrain from all animal protein and gliadin-containing food and exclusively to eat *mashed food in soup and porridge form* until clear improvement of clinical symptoms (approx. 1–2 weeks) – the effect can be decidedly astounding!

Abstention *from all sugary foods and juices is important and helpful.* Spelt instead of wheat flour, fish and poultry from strictly organic sources instead of the normal meat and sausages, individual avoidance of foods which are not tolerated, above all milk and cheese.

The possibility of a trace element and vitamin deficiency in the patient must always be borne in mind. Thus *zinc deficiency* is a frequent symptom and at the same time an indicator for the presence of chronic inflammatory bowel disease. Selenium, iron, vitamin D in the event of a longer disease phase and others must be monitored in laboratory tests if necessary and substituted. Care should be taken with oral iron substitution; parenteral iron substitution is often tolerated much better.

4.7.4 Constipation in infants

It is generally known that – particularly in breast fed infants – the stool frequency physiologically strongly fluctuates at this age. Yet problems also occur at this age, predominantly in non-breast fed children, with infrequent and painful evacuation of stool when the stool is too hard; or (above all in breast fed children) there is the phenomenon that bowel movement takes place very infrequently, detracting from the wellbeing of the child and parents.

In non-breast fed children bowel movement can be regulated by

- adding **oat gruel** (e.g. Demeter Haferschleim)

to the bottle feed. For moderate constipation start with 10%, for severe constipation with 20% oat gruel supplement which can then be regulated depending on the course of the constipation. As a rule, no problems have been observed with regard to the gluten avenin contained in oats but the remarks in ▶Chap. 4.7.2 should be observed.

In *breast fed children* the first thing which should always be checked is whether the quantity of milk is sufficient. Mostly there is a *constitutional* constipation (frequently there is a positive family anamnesis for one parent).

The most important medicine is

- **Calcium carbonicum LM6 dil.** (various manufacturers)
  2 gtt./d in the morning.

Above average birth weight, rapid weight gain in the first year of life, an even-tempered friendly disposition also when bowel movement is long overdue are characteristic for this constitution. The actual stool passed is soft even after ten days or more. The parents generally suffer more with these children than the infant.

Significantly more rarely
- **Lycopodium LM6 dil.** (various manufacturers)
  2 gtt./d in the morning

is the indicated medicine.

These children embody the opposite of the calcium-carbonicum type in every respect: they often display a below-average birth weight and above all sluggish weight gain. The mother reports that although the child appears eager to drink, he or she quickly tires during breast feeding and stops drinking – and is then bad tempered. Flatulence and constipation complete the picture of an infant with *impaired liver-gall bladder activity.* If Lycopodium has a positive effect, the drinking behaviour normalizes first, followed by better weight gain and a normalization of bowel movement.

A similar effect can be seen in (▸Chap. 4.4.4)
- **Magnesium muriaticum D4-6 pillules** (various manufacturers)
  3–5 pillules 3 x/d

This medicine is indicated if the infant suffers from persistent colicky pain and *does not appear to tolerate the breast milk* (may even throw up). The stool is very hard; there is a clear functional weakness regarding the liver and gall bladder and a strong tendency for food intolerances. Here Magnesium muriaticum can produce a profound turnaround!

4.7.5 Constipation in pre-school and school-age children

If parents report constipation problems of their child at this age, *family anamnesis and a detailed consultation* are the first steps towards diagnosis and treatment, followed by an examination of the child.

The anamnesis shows not infrequently that several family members have sluggish bowel movement (constitution; imitation). Other families pay excessive attention to this subject which can have a very negative effect on the child, above all in those developmental phases in which the child itself acquires a conscious perception and control of bowel movement. Here the style of toilet training is also of importance. Problems are caused by an authoritarian or alternatively over-protective training style (in both cases the necessary trust in the child is missing!).

The consultation can reduce the psychological pressure on the child and parents and a new basis of trust can be created for all parties. Then, once the child has individually reached the necessary maturity, the parents can specify a rhythm for going to the toilet; on the other hand it must be left to the child – which sometimes requires great patience – as to the point when it starts to do a "number 2" on those occasions.

In children who are already older, the recognition of psychological stress through grief or pressure from authoritarian or unpredictable adults is also of great importance alongside constitutional causes.

There is a wealth of literature today on *nutritional anamnesis* and, as necessary, *changing diet* to whole food. But in each individual case this does not replace detailed questioning and advice by the physician or a trained specialist if we really want to achieve a change of habits in the family.

Finally, a disability of the child, above all through spastic cerebral palsy, can represent an important cause of constipation.

Medicinally the focus in the first instance is on medicines which stimulate the activity of the liver, gall bladder and pancreas. In our own experience the list is topped by

- **Lycopodium comp. pillules** Wala
  3 × 5–7 pillules/d.

In this composite medicine low potencies of Natrium sulfuricum, Mercurius dulcis and Berberis e rad. stimulate the activity of the gall bladder while generally sluggish liver function is positively influenced by Lycopodium and Carduus marianus. Lycopodium comp. is also always indicated if the liver and gall bladder function has been toxically burdened and inhibited e. g. by allopathic drugs. It applies as a general principle that medicines with a choleretic action have a positive effect on constipation.

- **Magnesium muriaticum D4 dil.** (various manufacturers)
  3 × 5 gtt.

is also a relevant medicine for older children with constipation, particularly with milk intolerance, meteorism, general fatigue and a basic mood of anxiety and depression (▸Chap. 4.4.4).

When starting treatment, the following is suitable for *spastic constipation* (stool like sheep's droppings, hard) combined with a mostly soft abdominal wall, palpable scybala, *stool retention* in the phase of learning autonomous stool control, *involuntary voiding disorders of the intestine,* neuronal disorders, locally in/following Hirschsprung disease, systemically e. g. in Rett syndrome.

- **Carpellum Mali comp. trit.** Weleda
  1 saltsp. before each meal

This medicine goes directly back to Rudolf Steiner and consists of the grated nut skins of fresh walnuts and grated apple core and according to Steiner counters a deformation in the activity of the astral body in the intestinal area: an interesting and, with the right indication, effective medicine, which can regulate the activity of the astral body in the intestinal wall (ENS, enteric nervous system) (▸Chap. 4.1.3! Cf. in detail with short case study [Kummer 2004; Soldner and Sommer 2007, 34; Vademecum 2010, 282])

In the course of the treatment, Carpellum Mali comp. can be supplemented with the following in the event of *spastic constipation*, particularly when there is severe stomach pain

- **Nux vomica/Nicotiana comp. pillules** Wala
  3–7 pillules 3–4 x/d.

This medicine is fundamentally indicated when a spastically contracted intestinal section prevents stool transport; it works spasmolytically and thus in individual cases also analgesically.

At this point we also refer to the problem of *constipation in children with infantile cerebral palsy* in which the spasticity of the lower extremities is not infrequently accompanied by spastic constipation (▸Chap. 9). In this situation, too, the use of Nux vomica/Nicotiana comp. pillules Wala in combination with oat gruel (see above) and, as appropriate, symbiotic control can result in a significant improvement.

Symbiotic control (▸Chap. 4.6.4) is worthwhile above all when there is a dysbiosis of the intestine (anamnesis, stool findings) as a result of the wrong kind of food or e.g. prior antibiotic treatment.

In these cases introducing the treatment with a potentized sulphur preparation should always be considered, e.g.

- **Sulphur D6 trit.** Weleda
  3 × 1 saltsp.

or potentized silver sulphide,

- **Sulphur D6 trit.** Weleda
  3 × 1 saltsp.

In children with Down's syndrome the authors were repeatedly able to observe a positive effect of silver in habitual (atonic, associated with connective tissue weakness) constipation:

- **Argentum met. praep. D6 trit.** Weleda
  1 saltsp./d in the morning [Vademecum 2010, 116]

If psychological grief underlies the constipation, the administration, particularly in girls, of

- **Ignatia D12 pillules** (various manufacturers)
  5 pillules 1–2 x/d.

should be considered if the triggering event does not lie far back; in a deeply rooted depressiveness, which may go back as far as the pregnancy and birth phase (▸Chap. 2.4, case study)

- **Natrium muriaticum LM6** (various manufacturers)
  5 gtt./d in the morning

is the most frequently indicated medicine.

Children (of both sexes) who easily feel insulted and humiliated by parents or siblings, but at the same time themselves display a difficult psychological disposition (bad tempered, fierce, but on the other hand timid and shy if they are put under pressure), can also come to attention in this connection through a persistent constipation.

In this case the administration of

- **Staphisagria LM12 dil.** (various manufacturers)
  5 gtt./d in the morning should be considered.

If the constipation develops after a shock or general anaesthetic in an operation,

- **Opium D30 pillules** (various manufacturers)
  2–3 × 5 pillules for 2–3 days is indicated, followed by
- **Argentum/Rohrzucker pillules** Wala
  5–7 pillules/d in the evening (▸Chap. 2.2.3, case study)

4.8 Anal fissure

During infancy, particularly in the teething phase and the phase in which the child learns conscious stool control, a painful fissure of the mucosa may develop as a result of aggressive acidic stools (teething), hypertonicity of the sphincter ani and disharmonious interaction between the rectum and sphincter. Constipation with large-volume hard stools is particularly conducive to this disorder. If as a consequence the parental attention is fixated on the pain and difficulties of the child during evacuation, a vicious circle threatens to ensue as every form of increased attention on this area (pain, parental observation) leads to further hypertonia of the sphincter and thus a painful blockage in this area.

Therapeutically it is therefore necessary to advise and support the parents in such a way that they are not fixated in a harmful way on the child's problem. It is important to remedy any constipation through the appropriate diet and quantity of drink. Sugar and sweetened drinks should be avoided until the fissure has healed as they disrupt the intestinal flora, lead to abnormal colonization (candidiasis!) and increase the child's pain. Taking the temperature rectally should be avoided for a sufficient period of time under all circumstances. Cleaning the sensitive mucosa after bowel movement should be done if possible without paper by washing and subsequent care of the sensitive mucosa with fatty ointment.

Medicinally the following have proved successful

- **Mercurialis comp. supp.** Wala
  ½–1 supp./d in the evening (unfortunately there are no children's supp.!) for ten days before going to sleep
- **Acidum nitricum D12 pillules** (various manufacturers)
  3–5 pillules 3 x/d.

and, in persistent cases,

- **Medorrhinum C200 pillules**
  2 × 3 pillules/d for 3 days

The following is recommended to strengthen the mucosa

- **Quercus ointment** Wala
  apply carefully 1–3 x/d.

The latter has also proved successful for children undergoing chemotherapy (with associated mucositis).

4.9 Oxyuriasis

An attack of worms in the child's gastrointestinal tract as such represents a normal "childhood disease" which probably also has a protective effect: it stimulates the eosinophile granulocytes to undertake their "physiological task". Children in regions in which worm infections frequently occur, tend to be less prone to allergies while children with allergies display an "a-topical" – dislocated – over-activity of the eosinophile granulocytes (e.g. in the bronchial system) with simultaneous frequent other disorders of the intestinal flora, e.g. mycoses and dysbacterioses (▸Chap. 4.6). There are other clear indications that temporary worm infections in the first years of life can protect against chronic inflammatory bowel diseases – the therapeutic administration of the eggs of the pig worm Trichuris suis was able to remedy Crohn's disease and ulcerative colitis [Koletzko and Uhlig 2010]. Such information and the thought that acute worm infections can play a role in the development of a healthy immune system help many affected parents to overcome their initial shock and adopt a rational therapeutic attitude which does not measure the treatment one-sidedly by its rapid success but primarily has the child's learning process in overcoming the worm infection in mind.

Worms tend to infest children whose catabolic forces in the upper gastrointestinal tract have not yet fully developed in comparison to adults. But also weakened adults, e. g. mothers after pregnancy and breast feeding (often with simultaneous iron deficiency), are more susceptible to worm infestation. The source is mostly organically grown salad; careful washing and maybe also a change of supplier if necessary can significantly reduce the probability of an infection. Therapeutically it is important to strengthen the action of the soul and spiritual entity in the upper digestive tract.

The basic method to achieve such a "terrain change" and thus also to counter reinfection is the administration of

- **Sulphur D6 trit.** Weleda
  3 × 1 saltsp. for 4–6 weeks.

Immediate suppressive treatment with antihelminthics is not the most advisable course of action from an allergological perspective; it is associated with a relatively high recurrence rate. More sustainably effective is a proactive treatment which puts the child in the position of being able to get rid of the unwelcome guests by himself or herself. In this sense the administration of potentized sulphur is efficacious.

Acutely the administration of *garlic* (Allium sat., which displays a strong affinity with sulphur) acts against the worm infection with such power that it often represents a real therapeutic alternative to the antihelminthics which are frequently purchased in a fit of panic when faced with the – in themselves hardly pathogenic – threadworms. It is possible to administer 1–2 garlic cloves, crushed in a garlic press, with milk or yoghurt (every third day repeatedly for 14 days). The following is suitable medicinally

- **Allium/Cuprum sulfuricum comp. dil.** Weleda
  3 × 10–15 gtt.

In persistent cases, an enema based on a garlic-carrot preparation is suitable: allow 20 garlic cloves and 500 g carrots grated into 1 l of water to boil for ten minutes as a "soup" and put through a strainer; administer lukewarm as an enema with an irrigator; quantity 200 to maximum 500 ml depending on age.

References for Chapter 4

(every reference marked with a ■ Bullet point indicates the English translation of the reference above it)

Bartick, M., Reinhold, A. : The Burden of Suboptimal Breastfeeding in the United States: A Pediatric Cost Analysis. published online : www.pediatrics.org/cgi/doi/10.1542/peds. 2009–1616 (2009).

Bovelet M., Bräuer M.: Phänomenologie des Antimons. Der Merkurstab **63,** 143–149 (2010).

Buderus, S.: Epidemiologie und klinische Besonderheiten der pädiatrischen CED. Chronisch-entzündliche Darmerkrankungen bei Kindern und Jugendlichen. MSchr Kinderheilk **158,** 745–751 (2010).

Bühlbäcker, A.: Zur Verwendbarkeit von Stutenmilch, Kumyss und Eselsmilch als Diätetika und Heilmittel unter besonderer Berücksichtigung der Bedürfnisse des Säuglings und des Frühgeborenen. Deutsche Hochschulschriften 1104. Verlag Hänsel-Hohenhausen 1996.

Buhr et al.: Temperature as a Universal Resetting Cue for Mammalian Circadian Oscillators. Science **330,** 379–385 (2010).

Busse, B.: Der Anbau metallgedüngter Pflanzen. Weleda Korr.bl. 138 (1994).

Caspi A. et al.: Moderation of breastfeeding effects on the IQ by genetic variation in fatty acid metabolism. National Academy of Sciences of the USA. published online www.pnas.org/cgi/doi/10.1073/pnas.0704292104.

Diederich, K.: Die Wegwarte. Der Merkurstab **59,** 169–177 (2006).

Dornes: Der kompetente Säugling. Die präverbale Entwicklung des Menschen. Fischer, Frankfurt/M. 1993.

Emmrich, P.: Notfälle im Kindesalter, 12. Aufl. Thieme Verlag, Stuttgart 1998.

Engel, W.: Kalium aceticum comp. – Die Vielfalt des Weines im pharmazeutischen Herstellungsprozeß. Der Merkurstab **63,** 112–122 (2010).

Engel, W.: Eisen, Wein und Essig – zur Herstellung von Kephalodoron® und Ferrum hydroxydatum. Der Merkurstab **59,** 154–162.

Engelen, R.: Komplementäre Therapie gastroösophagealer Reflux. In: Schönau, E., A. Längler, E. G. Naumann, J. Beuth: Pädiatrie integrativ, Urban & Fischer, München 2005.

Fintelmann, V.: Intuitive Medizin. 3. Aufl. Hippokrates, Stuttgart 1994.

Forlenza G. P. et al.: Ankyloglossia, exclusive breastfeeding, and failure to thrive. Pediatrics **125,** 1500–1504 (2010).

Friedrichsen, H. P.: Ganzheitliche Allergiebehandlung in der Spezialklinik. Erfahrungsheilkunde **4,** 216 (1990).

Fuchs, T.: Das Gehirn, ein Beziehungsorgan. Kohlhammer, Stuttgart 2008.

■ Girke, M.: Innere Medizin. Salumed Verlag, Berlin 2010.

English translation in progress at this time – Ed.

Goebel, W., M. Glöckler: Kindersprechstunde, 15. Aufl. Urachhaus, Stuttgart 2005, 17.Aufl. 2008.

Grandgeorge, D.: Homöopathische Arzneimittelbilder in der Kinderheilkunde, 2. Aufl. Sonntag Verlag Regensburg 2004.

Gray, B. et al.: Homöopathie mit der Hahnemann Medical Clinic. Kai Kröger Verlag, Rendsburg 1991.

Grohmann, G.: Die Pflanze, Bd. 2. Verlag Freies Geistesleben, Stuttgart. 2. Aufl. 1968, 3. Aufl. 1983, 4. Aufl. 1991.

Hahnemann, S.: Reine Arzneimittellehre. Bd. V. Haug Verlag, Heidelberg 1995.

Hannesen, R.: Anthroposophische Therapie der chronisch entzündlichen Darmerkrankungen. Abschlussbericht zum CDDV-Ausbildungsstipendium "Komplementärmedizin und Gesundheitswissenschaft" Univ. Herdecke (2004).

Hondares E. et al.: Hepatic FGF 21 Expression is induced at birth via PPARalpha in Response to Milk Intake an contributes to thermogenic activation of neonatal brown fat. Cell Metabolism **11**, 206–212 (2010).

Horwood, L. J., D. M. Fergusson: Breastfeeding and later cognitive and academic outcomes. Pediatrics **101**, E 9 (1998).

Huber, R.: Phytotherapie bei Colitis ulcerosa. zkm **1**, 8–11 (2009).

Husemann, F.: Das Belladonnagift und seine Wirkprinzipien. Beitr. z. Erw. d. Heilk. **6**, 198–206 (1979).

Husemann, F.: Anthroposophische Medizin. Verlag am Goetheanum 2009.

Husemann, F., O. Wolff: Das Bild des Menschen als Grundlage der Heilkunst, 4. Aufl. Verlag Freies Geistesleben, Stuttgart 1986.

- Huseman, F. Wolff, O.: The Anthroposophical approach to medicine: v. 1, 2. Steiner Books, Great Barrington, M. A. 1983, v.3 Mercury Press, Spring Valley, N. Y. 2003.

Imhäuser, H.: Homöopathie in der Kinderheilkunde, 12. Aufl. Haug Verlag, Heidelberg 2000.

Keller, W., A. Wiskott: Lehrbuch der Kinderheilkunde. 6. Aufl. Thieme Verlag, Stuttgart 1991.

Keller, K.-M.: Klinische Symptomatik: „Zöliakie, der Eisberg" Mschr. Kinderheilk. **151**, 706–714 (2003).

Keller, K.-M.: Transition bei Jugendlichen mit CED. Mschr Kinderheilk **158**, 738–744 (2010).

Koletzko, S.: Erkrankungen des Ösophagus. In: Therapie der Krankheiten im Kindes- und Jugendalter. Reinhardt, D. (Hrsg.). 7. Aufl. Springer, Berlin 2004.

Koletzko, B. et al.: Säuglingsernährung und Ernährung der stillenden Mutter. Mschr Kinderheilkd **158**, 679–689 (2010).

Koletzko, S., Uhlig, H. H.: Hygienehypothese: Schlüssel zur Ätiologie und Pathogenese von CED? Pathogenese von chronisch-entzündlichen Darmerkrankungen im Kontext evolutionärer Adaptation und aktueller Umwelteinflüsse. MSchr Kinderheilkd **158**, 759–765 (2010).

Koutroubakis, IE et al.: Role of appendicitis and appendectomy in the pathogenesis of ulcerative colitis: a critical review. Inflamm Bowel Dis **8**, 277–286 (2002).

Kummer, K. R.: Zur intestinalen Mykose – Versuch einer Klärung. Der Merkurstab **51**, 65–73 (1998).

Kummer, K. R.: Die Darmflora des Menschen. Der Merkurstab **58**, 448–457 (2005).

Lewin, L.: Gifte und Vergiftungen, 6. Aufl. Haug Verlag, Heidelberg 1992.

Madaus: Lehrbuch der biologischen Heilmittel, Bd. 2, Bd. 3. Olms Verlag, Hildesheim 1999.

Madeleyn, R.: Anthroposophische Kinderheilkunde. Der Merkurstab **50**, 270 (1997).

Madeleyn, R.: Die vegetabilisierten Metalle in der Kinderheilkunde. Weleda Korr.bl. **138**, 62–72 (1994).

Mezger, J.: Gesichtete homöopathische Arzneimittellehre. 12.Aufl. Haug, Stuttgart 2005.

Pahlow, M.: Das große Buch der Heilpflanzen. Gräfe und Unzer, München 1993.

Papousek, M., M. Schieche, H. Wurmser: Regulationsstörungen der frühen Kindheit. Huber Verlag, Bern 2004.

Papousek, M.: Persistierendes Schreien. MSchr Kinderheilk **157**, 558–566.

Portmann, A.: Einführung in die vergleichende Morphologie der Wirbeltiere. Schwabe, Basel 1983.

Rauber, A., F. Kopsch: Anatomie des Menschen, Bd. II Innere Organe. Leonhardt, H. (Hrsg.). Thieme Verlag, Stuttgart 1987.

Rißmann, W.: Grauspießglanz (Antimonit). Der Merkurstab **63**, 123–127 (2010).

Rist, L. et al.: Influence of organic diet on the amount of CLAs in breast milk of lactating women in the Netherlands. Br J Nutr **97**, 735–743 (2007).

Rhoads, J. M. et al.: Altered Fecal Microflora and Increased Fecal Calprotectin in Infants with Colic. Journal of Pediatrics, published online 10.1016/jpeds.2009.05.012 (2009).

Schikarski: Morbus Crohn und Colitis ulcerosa Teil I. Der Merkurstab **46**, 9–28 (1993).

Scholten, J.: Homöopathie und Minerale. Stichting Alonissos, Utrecht 1993.

Selawry, A.: Metall-Funktionstypen in Psychologie und Medizin. Haug Verlag, Heidelberg, 1. Aufl. 1985, 2. Aufl. 1991.

Simon, L.: Das Zusammenwirken von Arzneisubstanz und pharmazeutischem Prozeß in der anthroposophischen Heilmittelkomposition Kalium aceticum comp. Der Merkurstab **63,** 135–142 (2010).

Sinkiewicz, G et al.: Occurence of Lactobacillus Reuteri, Lactobacilli and Bifidobacteria in Human Breast Milk. Pediatric Research **58**, 415.

Soldner G., Sommer, M.: Allantois und Astralleib – wie können wir Rudolf Steiners Forschungsergebnisse nachvollziehen? Der Merkurstab **60**, 27–35 (2007).

Soldner, G., J. Wilkens, M. Sommer: Magnesium chloratum. Der Merkurstab **59,** 112–122 (2006).

Sommer, M.: Die Reiseapotheke. Urachhaus Stuttgart 1999.

Sommer, M., G. Soldner: Die Farne in Natur und Mensch – zum Verständnis von Digestodoron. Der Merkurstab **5**, 289–296 (1990).

Steiner, R.: Geisteswissenschaftliche Gesichtspunkte zur Therapie. Gesamtausgabe Bd. 313. Rudolf Steiner Verlag, Dornach, 3. Aufl. 1963, 4. Aufl. 1984a, 5. Aufl. 2001.

- Steiner, R.: Anthroposophical spiritual science and medical therapy: second medical course, nine lectures to physicians and medical students, Dornach, April 11–18, 1921. GA (complete works) 313. Mercury Press, Spring Valley, N. Y. 1991.

Steiner, R.: Gesamtausgabe Bd. 318. Rudolf Steiner Verlag, Dornach 1984b.

- Steiner, R.: Pastoral medicine: the collegial working of doctors and priests: eleven lectures delivered in Dornach in September of 1924. GA (complete works) 318. Anthroposophic Press, Hudson, N. Y. 1987. Also published as: Broken vessels: the spiritual structure of human frailty. Anthroposophic Press, Great Barrington, M. A. 2003.

Steiner, R.: Geisteswissenschaftliche Menschenkunde, 5. Aufl. Rudolf Steiner Verlag, Dornach 1988.

- Steiner, R.: Fundamentals of anthroposophical medicine. GA (complete works) 314. Mercury Press, Spring Valley, N. Y. 1986.

Steiner, R.: Physiologisch-Therapeutisches auf Grundlage der Geisteswissenschaften. Gesamtausgabe Bd. 314, 3. Aufl. Rudolf Steiner Verlag, Dornach 1989.

Steiner, R.: Geisteswissenschaft und Medizin. Rudolf Steiner Verlag, Dornach, 5. Aufl. 1976, 7. Aufl. 1999.

- Steiner, R.: Introduction to anthroposophical medicine. GA (complete works) 312. SteinerBooks, Great Barrington, M. A. 1999.

Steiner, R.: Das Initiatenbewusstsein, 5. Aufl. R. Steiner Verlag, Dornach 1993.

- Steiner, R.: True and false paths in spiritual investigation. GA (complete works) 243. Rudolf Steiner Press/Anthroposophic Press, London/New York 1985.

Steiner, R.: Anthroposophie – ein Fragment. Gesamtausgabe Bd. 45, 4.Aufl. Rudolf Steiner Verlag, Dornach 2002.

- Steiner, R.: Anthroposophy: A Fragment. GA (complete works) 45. Anthroposophic Press, Hudson, N. Y. 1996.

Steiner, R.: Vorträge und Kurse über christlich-religiöses Wirken V, Gesamtausgabe Bd. 346, Rudolf Steiner Verlag, Dornach 2001.

4

- Steiner, R.: The book of Revelation and the work of the priest : eighteen lectures, conversations, and question-and-answer sessions in Dornach from 5 to 22 September 1924, reconstructed from notes taken by the participants. GA (complete works) 346. Rudolf Steiner Press, London 1998.

Steiner, R., I. Wegman: Grundlegendes zu einer Erweiterung der Heilkunst nach geisteswissenschaftlichen Erkenntnissen. Rudolf Steiner Verlag, Dornach 1977, 6. Aufl. 1984, 1991.

- Steiner, R., Wegman, I.: Fundamentals of therapy: an extension of the art of healing through spiritual-scientific knowledge. GA (complete works) 27. Mercury Press, Spring Valley, N.Y. 1999. Also available as: Extending practical medicine: fundamental principles based on the science of the spirit. Rudolf Steiner Press, London 1996.

Steiner, R.: Eine okkulte Physiologie. Gesamtausgabe Bd. 128, Rudolf Steiner Verlag, Dornach 5.Aufl. 1991(b).

- Steiner, R.: An occult physiology: eight lectures given in Prague, 20th to 28th March, 1911. GA (complete works) 128. Rudolf Steiner Press, London 1983.

Stellmann, H. M.: Belladonnawirkung beim Kranken. Beitr. z. Erw. d. Heilk. **32**, 207–210 (1979).

Stockhausen, H. B. v.: Indikation zur Therapie eines Ikterus neonatorum. päd. praxis **45**, 385–392 (1993).

Stübler, M., E. Krug (Hrsg.): Leesers Lehrbuch der Homöopathie, 3. Aufl. Haug Verlag, Heidelberg 1987.

Subbotina, M. D. et al.: Effect of oral administration of termentil root extract (Potentilla tormentilla) on rotavirus diarrhea in children: a randomized, double blind, controlled trial. Pediatr Infect Dis J **8**, 706–711 (2003).

Tannock, G. W.: The acquisition of the normal microflora of the gastrointestinal tract. In: Human health – The contribution of microorganisms. Gibson, S. A. W. (ed.). Springer Verlag, 1994.

Vademecum Anthroposophische Arzneimittel. 2.Aufl. Der Merkurstab **63**, Supplement (2010).Vademecum of anthroposophic medicines, CD format. Medical Section of the School of Spiritual Science, Dornach, Switzerland 2009. Vennemann et al.:Does breastfeeding reduce the risk of sudden infant death syndrome? Pediatrics **123**, e406–410 (2009).

Vogel, H. H.: Die vier Hauptorgane. Natur Mensch Medizin, Bad Boll 1995.

von Volkmann, H.: Über den Stinkasant und seine besonderen Beziehungen zu den Erkältungskrankheiten. Beitr Erw Heilk **13**, 85–94 (1960).

Wilkens, J.: Misteltherapie. Differenzierte Anwendung der Mistel nach Wirtsbäumen. Sonntag Verlag, Stuttgart 2006.

Wotschke, C.: Die operationslose Behandlung der Appendizitis. Nachdruck in: Beiträge z. Erw. d. Heilkunst **1**, 1–14 (1963).

Zimmer, K.-P.: Pathophysiologie der Zöliakie. Mschr. Kinderheilk. **151**, 698–705 (2003).

Zwiauer, K.: Langzeiteffekte der Ernährung in den ersten 2 Lebensjahren. Mschr. Kinderheilk. **149**, 71–74 (2001).

Zwiauer, K: Nutritive Einflussfaktoren auf die Entwicklung von kindlicher Adipositas und mögliche Präventionsansätze. Mschr. Kinderheilk. **151**, 84–88 (2003).

5 Inflammatory Diseases

Perhaps the most convincing way to determine if fever is protective is to study its effects on morbidity and mortality. We believe that the evidence overwhelmingly points to the role of fever in enhancing specific and nonspecific immunity.

M. Kluger [2006]

In animal models, treatment with antipyretics for influenza infection increases the risk of mortality.

S. Eyers et al. [2010]

Reduce a fever? Preferably not!

A. Lohse, S. Schmiedel [2009]

Inflammation is an activity of the body, it is the child's own activity. It has an *essential connection to warmth*; and in a similar way in which vigorous, outwardly directed bodily activity raises the temperature – in marathon runners to over 40 °C – the temperature can reach over 40 °C when inflammatory activity is directed at the body itself. We know from physiology (the 'normal' temperature) that in fever this warmth does not arise as a 'side effect' of activity, but that the organism is aiming to reach a particular level of warmth: "Fever is an example of a *regulated* change in homoeostasis." [Kluger 2006, Preface, emphasis in the original.]

Every activity of the self must be questioned as to its *meaning* – in contrast to an effect caused from outside; fever, and inflammation in general, is "there for a purpose" and is not just an "effect" to be "normalized" and suppressed unquestioningly by the doctor.

If one concentrates initially on straightforward observation of an inflammatory process, for instance in the skin or the tonsils, one can discern the classic qualities

- calor,
- dolor,
- tumor,
- rubor.

In *warmth, the organism's own degree of activity,* which has increased in the inflamed area, becomes perceptible, even measurable. In pain, which is perceptible only in the patient's soul, not outwardly, an *enhanced perception in the soul of his/her own body* comes to expression – an enhanced presence of the soul in the inflamed area of the body. In extreme cases pain can completely overwhelm the soul andstrongly bind it to the body (for instance in toothache).

"*Tumor*" originally signified a fluid, semi-solid swelling: a manifestation of *enhanced, vital, metabolic processes* in the inflamed area and of enhanced exudation and transudation. Where such hyperthermic, painful swellings occur, there is a risk too of *dissolution processes,* the loss of structures and tissues that have already been differentiated. Inflammation initially tends to dissolve something of the corporeality that has come into being.

'Rubor' is an expression of hyperaemia, i. e. increased blood flow that is both a precondition for all enhanced activity in the body and a consequence thereof. The body reddens, particularly where there is an outer threat of being overwhelmed, as in blushing; as well as in the region of the mouth and the mucous membranes, where there is an intense encounter between inside and outside.

As an apparent deviation from our theme, let us compare the above with cancer, which is very rare in childhood and common in adults:

- *Cancer patients lack warmth*: in a study of 150 patients, Witzel [1970] found that, if they had not developed a fever above 38.5 °C in the previous five years, the relative risk of cancer increased by a factor of 11.4 compared with a control group. At the Cancer Research Centre in Heidelberg, Abel [1986, 1991] found the association of risk between a lack of feverish infections and cancer development, "although not generally known even among cancer researchers", to be "well founded; the evidence fulfils the most important epistemological criteria that have been established for evaluating associations of risk." [Cf. Hobohm 2005; Kienle and Kiene 2004, 174–193]
- The cancer itself develops – for all too long – painlessly and unnoticed by the soul. People with cancer often have a disturbed or poorly integrated inner relationship to their body, possibly because of fears and negativity about their own body and/or through being too strongly drawn out and outwardly engaged. (The understanding here is that the soul is therefore less sensitive and perceptive when it is 'drawn out'.)

By contrast, inflammation leads to an inward concentration of one's own forces and perceptions, thus strengthening the connection of soul and body, if the illness is given its space to develop in peace.

- With cancer, the swelling or tumour expresses neither the organism's own vital activity, nor the whole organism's dissolving or digestive processes; rather it constitutes primarily a hard, immovable mass, resistant to the whole organism, which grows through the body dissolving its structures instead of being dissolved by it.
- Thus rubor, which is the expression of the organism's own alert immunological activity, is also absent.

Seen against this background – here too the paediatricians must go beyond the borders of their specialist field in order to learn to measure the consequences of their action – the very real question arises today of how to understand inflammation and how to deal with it appropriately in children.

Is not inflammation a manifestation of the living, independent striving to overcome an exogenic disturbance of bodily order; to paralyse and eliminate or excrete an activity that has intruded from outside (for instance bacteria, toxins and so on)? Is there not something in the power and ability to assert itself in this way, through its own activity, that is indispensable for the human organism?

At the same time as the question of the *meaning of fever and the meaning of inflammation,* the question also arises as to the *originator* of these processes [Girke 2010, 115–128]. A glance into nature shows that, even as living organisms, plants cannot generate these processes. In experiments, lower cold-blooded organisms show that they are more likely to survive infections if they are able to find areas warmer than the temperature of their usual environment. Only warm-blooded organisms can produce a fever. The *capacity to generate fever correlates with a high degree of ensoulment and autonomy.* The human warmth organization's unique degree of freedom gives the human being broad scope, including in relation to fever.

Inflammation, and particularly feverish inflammation, always involves an *increased breaking down of bodily substance.* In the crucial phase of convalescence, this subsequently enables a *building up again* of the body which, without the fever, would doubtless have remained in its 'old' state. The frequency of feverish illnesses in childhood is significant in another way: It is not just the alien world outside that is dissolved and excreted in fever, but also something of the corporeality inherited from one's parents.

Whoever believes that health is best maintained by protecting the child as far as possible from such processes (as in the trend towards vaccination, antibiotics, antipyretics and so on) takes as a starting point a concept of health that has *no need for development* and *no connection with the individuality.* In reality, the child needs to learn to exist in relation to nature; and the individuality of the child cannot take on a body that has originated via heredity without shaping and reminting it individually. *Individual health has to be attained in the course of childhood; it cannot be acquired from the parents and then preserved for the rest of the child's life.*

Against this background, the prime concern of individual paediatrics is to regulate the child's inflammatory activity and support its processes; and to resort to measures which suppress the inflammation (or have the effect of suppressing it) only when the former do not succeed.

5.1 Respiratory tract inflammation

5.1.1 Pneumonia – a paradigm of inflammation during childhood

The knowing doctor administers each medicine at the right time.

Karl Stauffer

5

5.1.1.1 Symptomatology

The onset of pneumonia in children is often sudden and not necessarily preceded by an infection; the child does not always appear to be seriously ill. A certain sense of restriction and "tightness" is nevertheless evident: respiration is less free than usual and cannot unfold fully; the inspired breath becomes more and more limited (shortness of breath); breathing rhythm fluctuates, either becoming rapid or appearing laboured (nasal flaring as a sign of dyspnoea is sometimes noticeable). Mild anxiety often accompanies these symptoms; the child tends to avoid strenuous movement; extreme restlessness is evident in certain cases. A short cough, especially in the early inspiratory phase, is an early sign of pneumonia. Pain may be completely lacking, although severe, acute pain in the right hypochondrium is a typical early sign of pneumonia of the right inferior lobe. – One usually observes a change in general condition. Except in neonates, fever (mostly acute and rising to high temperatures) is a typical symptom of pneumonia.

A gradual illness course with slowly escalating clinical symptomatology and fever is less common, although it can be observed for example in some mycoplasma pneumonias that occur at school age. If untreated, the latter only come to full (and then often severe) expression after 5 to 7 days. Tracheobronchitis can develop into focal pneumonia, the latter mostly characterized by acute deterioration as described above.

Approaching the child with care, conscientious observation and attending to the anamnesis and physical examination are more important for achieving an accurate diagnosis than any investigative techniques. In this way, the all too frequent (mis)diagnosis of pneumonia can be avoided. Medium moist crackles heard on auscultation tend to be ambiguous in children, and when important questions regarding fever, breathing behaviour and general condition are not considered, respiratory infections are misdiagnosed as pneumonia too often (and likewise, antibiotics are unnecessarily prescribed too often!). – On the other hand, middle lobe pneumonia can be diagnosed on the basis of a typical combination of observational clues (i. e. distraught, seemingly endless coughing, absence of fever, good general condition) and clinical findings (pertaining to the middle lobe region).

With regard to focal pneumonias and acute lobar pneumonia, initially auscultation may not offer any clues. One must search very carefully and patiently for late-inspiratory, fine-to-medium moist crackles. Only later in the illness course can one hear dull or dampened sounds or the scratchy tones of an accompanying pleural friction rub.

Diagnostic radiology of the thorax carried out during the first hours of illness onset can be false-negative or inconclusive. As a rule, x-rays are not essential in order to establish a positive clinical finding for pneumonia. However, they are especially indicated when the diagnosis must be urgently clarified and the further illness course cannot be "waited out": This applies to acute onset of lobar pneumonia where appendicitis is the differential diagnosis, for example, or in patients with pleural effusion, anatomical anomalies or chronic pulmonary infections.

5.1.1.2 Causes and the question of warmth

The classic cause of childhood pneumonia is *the cold*: primarily cold weather and hypothermia. Of all the large internal organs, the lungs are most widely exposed to the outside atmosphere and usually protected from its effects by means of *intact nasal breathing*. Bypassing of nasal breathing due to intense physical exertion in cold weather or a nasal breathing disorder, for example, increases the lungs' exposure to the cold. According to the authors' observations, this factor should be given more attention in current paediatric practice (▸Chap. 5.1.2). According to the authors' observations, this factor increasingly deserves close attention in current practice. (▸Chap. 5.1.2).

The organism's own warmth organization provides the necessary compensation for these challenges originating "outside" the body. Impairments or primary weaknesses in the warmth organization are indicative of a predisposition to pneumonia. This gives rise to important questions:

- Does the child lack *exercise,* i. e. movement?
- Considering that sunlight and sun-generated warmth stimulate the muscles of the limbs and provide an essential source of nourishment for the activity of the warmth organization, is the child exposed to sufficient sunlight and warmth during the course of the year?
- Is there a lack of *warmth preservation*? (e. g. because of inappropriate or insufficient clothing?)
- Have *previous* febrile illnesses been treated in such a way that the child generated too little of its own warmth? (e. g. due to administration of *antipyretics and antibiotics*.)

- *How active is the child?* In contrast to creative play in nature, passivity of every kind has a cooling effect on the organism: for example, intellectual sedentary activity (schoolchildren!), watching television and playing video games.

During a home visit – essential in the case of pneumonia – it is essential for the doctor to gain a sense of the presence of warmth in the house. Today many homes do not have a central warmth-generating source such as a stored-heat stove (for example, an AGA or Rayburn that store heat from a continually burning source, or a masonry heater i.e. 'Kachelofen' as it is known in Germany and Austria). Under-floor heating functions in the opposite way and is a frequent cause of chronic irritation of the airways. Immaculately furnished, perfectly ordered living spaces often have a cooling effect as do certain materials such as stone, glass and metal. However, the most important factor is undoubtedly the *soul warmth amongst those living and relating in the home space* (ultimately reflected in the home environment and furnishings) – not only in the way the children are treated but also how adults, especially the parents, relate to one another.

Constitutional aspects of the child's warmth organization are equally important: A tendency to *rickets* in infancy, perhaps even only an intimation thereof, indicates that too much warmth has been absorbed by the skeleton on the one hand, and on the other that the child's ability to sustain its own warmth and immunological defence is weakened (▸Chap. 3.2). *Vitamin D deficiency* due to lack of exposure to sunlight creates a predisposition to pneumonia and promotes a severe illness course.

Case study

An eleven-month-old infant presented at the practice with a clinical picture of acute pneumonia. The case history reveals that the child already had pneumonia at five months of age and at nine months, the latter occurrence an abscess-forming staphylococcal pneumonia. The child was hospitalized on both occasions. On closer enquiry it becomes evident that the parents had not taken sufficient measures for rickets prevention; furthermore, due to illness the child had not spent very much time in the sun. These factors had been overlooked up to that point because there was no evidence of manifest rickets. Once this aspect was addressed, however, the child's clinical condition improved rapidly and the improvement could be sustained. (Pneumonia or bronchiolitis in late infancy can be the manifestation of a clinically relevant vitamin D deficiency.)

Many children exhibit basic abnormalities in the warmth organization, e.g. insufficient warmth penetration in the limbs, disturbances in warmth distribution, abnormal sweat production.

Hence, it is fundamentally important to examine the state of warmth in every child with pneumonia, as the case study below illustrates. Furthermore, a healthy digestion contributes to the vitality of the lungs, especially through the activity of making warmth in foodstuffs accessible to the organism.

If cold is understood as the central cause of pneumonia, for the purposes of diagnosis and treatment it is essential to ascertain the cause of the hypothermia. At the same time, pneumonia (a highly febrile form of inflammation), already represents an attempt of the organism to overcome the hypothermia (irrespective of whether the cause is external or to be found in the child's constitution).

Case study

A ten-year-old girl with a previously unremarkable anamnesis developed pneumonia from a 'flu-like' infection. There had been problems at school during the preceding weeks: despite good performance, she was anxious about the imminent transition to the next school level (called Gymnasium in Germany). Too much family discussion but the child did not feel understood. Treatment of the pneumonia proceeded as described below (▸ Chap. 5.1.1.4). Nevertheless, the child still had high fever on the 5th day following onset of the pneumonia, even though the inflammation was already dissipating (increasingly productive, "loosened" cough).

Examination of the child's warmth shows that despite high fever she has ice-cold feet and a localized cold zone in the back region. Following intensive warmth treatment with two hot-water bottles at her feet and light-rhythmical back massage with Argentum metallicum praeparatum 0.4 % ointment (Weleda), the fever began to decrease the next day; two days later the fever had abated completely. There were no grounds for adjusting the medicinal treatment any further. It is worth noting that the transition to the Gymnasium (next school level) was unproblematic.

5.1.1.3 From pathology to treatment

Initially the basic pathological process underlying pneumonia is capillary hyperaemia, i. e. *centralization of blood and warmth in the lung.* This brings about an *active metabolic process, i. e. effusion of a protein-rich exudate* into the alveoli which results in fibrin formation. This applies to lobar pneumonia (generally occurring after age 7) and to the so-called "focal pneumonias" [Remmele 1997, 622].

The term "hepatization" is actually an expression of how the lung *becomes similar to a gland* for a time (the lung as a liver-like organ at this point in the pneumonia is consistent with the increased metabolic activity in the lung, resembling liver activity). This condition dissipates again during the course of recovery: "Antibiotic treatment can diminish the febrile phase. But it does not affect the reabsorption of alveolar exudate which only ceases after 21 to 28 days and in the case of an uncomplicated illness course, leads to *restitutio ad integrum.*" [Remmele 1997, 624]. – The pathologist identifies a typical cyclic course of about three to four weeks in this process – a time-frame also observed in a number of classic childhood illnesses (▸ Chap. 5.3).

Embryologically, the lung is a derivative of the proenteron (foregut). At first it takes on a gland-like form (pseudo-glandular phase) [Hinrichsen 1990, 581] and only during the last trimester finally transforms into a respiratory organ (alveolar phase). The bronchi and alveoli lumens are filled with fluid until the child is born, and then in the moment of birth the lungs undergo the most extensive transformation of all the visceral organs. – From this point of view, pneumonia may be understood as a "regression of the lung" to the pseudo-glandular embryonic stage that had already been overcome at birth [Vogel 1995, 179]. Thus the reabsorption and expectoration of exudate and the consequent re-ventilation and revitalization of the diseased sections of the lung may be likened to a rebirth in this area of the organ.

Autonomous body-soul existence becomes possible through the lung's acquired capacity to breathe in outside air into the organism and to breathe it out it again. In Genesis we read how Adam's life began when God "breathed life" into him. The Greek word "Pneuma" refers both to the "breath" and to the soul's interplay with the physical-etheric body. The child's experience of pneumonia – that is, enduring the illness and overcoming it with his or her own strength and life forces – amounts to a birth experience for the soul. This experience transforms not only the affected organ (which is re-formed during the recovery process) but also the entire being of the child:

- From a psychological point of view, the process of recovering from pneumonia strengthens the child's self-confidence, especially in relation to his or her own body. Thus, the child experiences its own physical nature more intensely and integrates the experience more deeply on a soul level – to the degree that physical substance was broken down and reformed by the child during the illness.
- Facial features often mature following recovery and the child takes huge strides in motoric and mental development.
- The children often become less immunologically susceptible to infection.

This applies when treatment is carried out in such a way that the child's own capacities (for overcoming the illness and recovery) are placed in the foreground and the illness is only suppressed to the degree that it threatens to overwhelm the organism. – On the other hand, the authors have *also* experienced important developmental progress in their patients when antibiotics had to be administered due to an advanced illness course. In the vast majority of cases, however, pneumonia can be treated without antibiotics.

Within the context of the treatment approach presented here, pneumonia is not understood as a fundamentally desirable experience for the child, *but in certain cases it is often a necessary experience*. The human being can only truly individualize through experience. The currently widespread endeavour to shield children from any form of "illness experience" by means of antipyretics, analgesics, antibiotics and immunization actually weakens the child's immunological competence and soul capacities. Not least of all, the relatively frequent incidence of recurrences after premature antibiosis of inflammatory diseases raises the question as to whether the prevailing ideal of preventing illness experience is realistic.

In fact, these measures promote chronic illness. This is confirmed by recent observations of pneumonia cases treated with antibiotics[1] and above all, by the increase of chronically relapsing, inflammatory-allergic diseases associated with the "western lifestyle" (which, amongst other things, cultivates the objective of preventing illness experience – ▸Chap. 6.1). However, the kind of "illness experience" brought about by these chronic diseases is far more of a burden and discouraging to the soul than the process of overcoming acute pneumonia.

5.1.1.4 Treatment

The doctor's personal approach to diagnosing pneumonia and communicating the diagnosis to the parents or older child has a significant effect on progression of the illness. If the doctor conveys fear in any way, or the notion that the patient's own strength and internal forces cannot overcome the pneumonia, a completely different situation will arise than

1 "There are various perspectives on whether delays in decongestion of exudate and chronic pneumonia become more frequent during antiobiotic treatment (emphasis by original author). According to patho-anatomical findings, they have increased, at least in the case of lobar pneumonia." [Remmele 1997, 628]

if the doctor takes the following approach, accompanied by a clear and intelligible diagnosis (!):

- Pneumonia is an opportunity for the child to become healthier than prior to the illness.
- The child's body – initially bestowed by the parents as a "guiding principle" or a "model" – can be transformed by the inflammatory process in such a way that the body increasingly becomes a manifestation of the individuality. Consequently, the child feels more at home in his or her body, with all the positive effects on physical and soul-psychological health.
- For this to be possible, however, it is essential for the child to truly *experience*, i. e. to *"go through"* the pneumonia. Premature curtailing of the illness by means of hastily administered antibiotic treatment or high potency aconite at illness onset, for example, ultimately prolongs the recovery process and increases the risk of recurrence.
- Longstanding experience shows that complications rarely arise because of the treatment approach described here (below); or if complications do arise, they are usually easier to recognize and treat.
- Pulse oximetry enables a simple, quantitative monitoring at onset and during the course of the illness. One needs to gain experience in estimating the degree of hypoxaemia a child can tolerate without oxygen therapy. In contrast to the statemtents in recent reviews, [Schroten and Tennenbaum 2011, Schmit-Grohé 2011], when asked personally, H. Schroten shared the opinion of the authors: "I am not aware of any data to substantiate the idea that a home-based pneumonia treatment is not justified when initial oxygen saturation is below 92 %." This technique is helpful and highly relevant within the scope of a home visit: The degree of hypoxaemia and the degree of severity of the pneumonia closely correlate. One can expect saturation values below 90 % in the context of pneumonia. At school age, children can cope with an ambulatory situation without oxygen therapy for a short time with values just under 85 %. It is essential for the doctor to bear in mind the child's general condition at all times, especially with regard to the child's own internal activities in relation to the illness process. A gradual increase in saturation values is an important early sign that the child is responding to treatment. Competent monitoring and helpful commentary on the part of the doctor can also be of great support to the parents.
- Gaining the parents' cooperation and conscientious assistance is essential; thus a clinic referral is almost always avoidable. The child needs the warmth of the parents' and doctor's attention as well as their dependable management of the situation.

A first conversation with the parents as described here conveys both basic information about the illness and clarity regarding the individual situation, thus enabling trust to develop. In this way, the fear surrounding a "lung infection diagnosis" is transformed by the knowledge that the illness is a potential opportunity for the child and has a positive purpose. *Once the parents have been fully informed, however, it is essential that they be left free to decide on the path of treatment to be taken.* The doctor has to accept that the parents may not be able to consent to the treatment approach described here.

Within the context of the path of treatment described here the parents become essential partners with their child and the doctor. For many, accompanying their child in overcoming the illness in a proactive, self-determining way, with medical guidance and supervision, is often a new and decisive experience. The sense of empowerment, i. e. the possibility to be personally active engenders courage and overcomes fear. The parents' engagement in the situation, their love and attention, reinforces not only the child's trust, but also the parents' faith in the child's strength to overcome the illness.

The authors' approach to treating a typical case of pneumonia is described in three steps:

5.1.1.4.1 General nutrition measures

The way the fever is treated and managed is of significant consequence for the pneumonia patient (see above, inflammatory illnesses). From the point of view of anthroposophic medicine and homoeopathy, fever is a core expression of the child's own self-directed internal activity. Fever is the *fundamental transfomative principle that enables the illness to be overcome:* Today we can follow this principle right into the metabolism of cytokines, (Interferon and so on). Fever should only be restricted in its "breaking down" effect and will abate of its own accord during the course of the illness. *During a fever, the 'I' – i. e. the core individuality of the child – is at work in the body. This* statement contains the guiding leitmotif for treating and managing fever and "warmth" generally.

To begin with, the child needs warm, breathable clothing. Wool is actually the only fabric that best meets the requirement, ideally as underclothing or at least as a thin woollen pullover. *Bed rest* is essential, even in the inherently strenuous infancy and toddler years. While adequate bedclothes will help the child to conserve and sustain its own warmth, excessive covering and too much heat build-up should be avoided.

If the periphery of the organism remains cool at the same time as body temperature rises, an external heat supply such as a hot water bottle can sometimes be helpful. Whereas the child will probably refuse solid foods at the beginning of the illness, *warm drinks* are nevertheless important. Tilia-blossom tea (also called lime, linden or basswood) and elder-flower tea with lemon (or the like) have proven to be helpful. These teas stimulate warmth penetration as well as sweat and kidney secretion, thereby encouraging the body's elimination processes. Adequate *fluid supply* is essential! Furthermore, in the case of *infants and children around 2 years of age*, one should ensure that during the first phase of illness the children receive sufficient *nourishment* (gruel or cereal gruel with a little salt).

Parents generally need some initial guidance in how to *observe their child* during the entire illness course, especially with regard to warmth (noticing warmth penetration and warmth distribution) and circulation (noticing breathing and skin colour). Therefore, cold feet and ankles should not go unnoticed: This is an unfavourable sign if occurring after the first increase in temperature and requires immediate medical attention and treatment. This also applies to increasing dyspnoea, cyanosis etc. In all cases, elimination is especially important: Diuresis and bowel movements should normalize rapidly and sweat production should be observed.

On no account should parents administer *antipyretics* out of their own initiative because this type of intervention interrupts the natural course of illness and can have a negative influence. The following rule strictly applies: No self-medication during pneumonia!

Nowadays it is especially necessary to mention that children with pneumonia should not have any contact with media such as television, video games and so on, until they have recovered completely. The doctor must also enquire about planned visits from family and friends and strongly advise a quiet home atmosphere during the anticipated period of illness (which does not exclude the presence of a genuinely helpful third person, of course). The sick child should be sheltered from any social tensions and stress as far as possible.

5.1.1.4.2 External treatments

External applications are of *decisive significance* for the progression of pneumonia. Two interventions are applicable here: Enema and mustard chest compresses.

Enema treatment

Generally, enema treatment is most beneficial at illness onset and particularly in cases of sluggish bowel function, extreme fever peaks, and sucking-weakness in infants. Initially the purpose of the enema is to substantially ease the burden on the immune system by means of stimulating bowel voiding. From a physiological perspective, the immune system is usually at work on the surface areas of the gastrointestinal tract. In the case of pneumonia, however, the main conflict between the external world and the body is taking place in the lungs and therefore it is beneficial to relieve the gastrointestinal organs of any encumbrances as far as possible. The body absorbs the majority of enema fluid so that administering several enemas during the course of the treatment achieves the effect of a saline infusion, thereby supporting circulation and mucolysis (many children are able to expectorate better after the enema). Thus, the enema supplies a considerable part of the fluids required. Enema treatment can *regulate body temperature* and reduce extreme fever peaks, without having a purely physical "cold water effect", i.e. the enema has an effect that is not explainable solely on the basis of heat exchange with the enema fluid.

The perceivable modulation in body temperature is in an area above that expected in the purely physical area. "This supports the assumption that the enema has an effect on temperature regulation itself" [Moeller, Ulbricht 1991, 968]. This is indicative of a "dialogue" between the intestine-associated nervous system and the central nervous system (▸Chap. 4.1.3). The enema can restore balance in the warmth organization, thereby re-enabling the child's own capacities to regulate fever without exerting any physical force on the body. The enema temperature should be about 3–4 °C below body temperature.

As a rule, the authors use a physical saline solution for the enema, i.e. 9 g NaCl: 1000 ml water (9 g ss approx. equal to1 level tablespoon of salt, or can be weighed using a letter scale, for example). If the child is having difficulties eating, one may use a solution containing 1 tablespoon sugar + 1 teaspoon salt per 1000 ml water.

A rubber enema of about 130 ml is suitable for infants and toddlers. Administer about 90 ml to infants, about 130 ml to toddlers, and up to 250 ml to kindergarten age children. An irrigator is recommended for children of school age onwards so that up to 400 ml can be administered. (see also: Goebel and Glöckler 2008, 669)

The enemas should be administered repeatedly (up to max. 3–4 x/day), especially to infants and toddlers who drink poorly, run a high temperature and are restless. A chamomile tea enema is more beneficial for the latter; otherwise, water (with the addition of salt as indicated above) is adequate. As a rule, the child will feel a lot better following the enema, and many children fall asleep afterwards. In fact, the greatest difficulty is to convince the parents of the necessity for enema treatments. A comparative study carried out by Moeller und Ulbricht [1991] can be of help here: In this study, relatively large amounts of fluid were administered to the treatment group (30 ml/kg body weight, 0.9 % NaCl).

In a critical review of this study Kienle reports: "The parents of children in the treatment group reported that their children were significantly calmer following the enema, most fell asleep afterwards, and their general sense of well-being clearly improved...". After one hour body temperature differed by an average of 0.59 °C between the treatment group and non-treatment group; after six hours by 1.12 °C (treatment group with an average of *−0.88* °C and non-treatment group with +0.24 °C). "From 1990 onwards the doctor who had mainly worked on the study refused to continue to participate because *he could no longer take responsibility for withholding this treatment from any of his patients.*" [Kienle 2006, 153; emphasis by author].

The mustard chest compress is the second essential external treatment and should be applied in *all cases of child pneumonia.*

Mustard compress

The mustard compress relieves effects of the pathology in the lungs and circulation, taking effect via the skin – the skin being the third "interface organ" besides the intestines and respiratory tract. Through hyperaemization of the skin areas directly associated with the lungs – which manifests in a mildly painful sensation (burning) – inflammation and congestion in the thoracic cavity are hindered and thereby restricted, and displaced to the surface of the skin so that the strain on internal circulation is eased. (Increased resistance in the lung caused by congestion makes more demands on the circulation). Stimulation of consciousness, i.e. of the soul's awareness in the skin area (brought about by the mild, burning pain sensation) further intensifies and strengthens the "disencumbering" effect of the treatment. *Inflammation is always accompanied by increased consciousness, i.e. soul awareness of the affected organ.*

Those who shy away from the effort involved in this intervention are strongly advised to consider the broad experience base emphasizing that the beneficial effects of the mustard compress on inflammation and circulation cannot be replaced by internal medication. The first application should be carried out under the supervision and guidance of a doctor or other appropriately trained and qualified personnel because the mustard compress can cause burns if applied incorrectly, Thereafter it is normally unproblematic for the parents to prepare and apply the compress on their own, once a day. Fresh black mustard power, up to three months old and stored in airtight packaging should be on hand at the medical practice (weekends!) and the pharmacy associated with the practice. The materials required for a chest compress should also be available at the practice so that the first application can be demonstrated.

Chest compress: Preparation and application

Due to the importance of this treatment, practical aspects regarding preparation and application of the compress are described briefly here. [See Goebel and Glöckler 2008, 666–668; Vagedes and Soldner 2010, 57.] First, lay out on the bed: a woollen cloth and a swansdown cloth for insulation (both wider than the compress cloth when spread out), at the level of the child's back (○ Fig. 5.1). If administering the treatment to schoolchildren, protect nipples and armpits with Vaseline and cotton wool pads. Sprinkle black mustard power down the centre third of a thin compress cloth (e.g. a thin cotton nappy (diaper)), completely covering the surface (see drawing), fold over the two free sides of the cloth so that the mustard powder is covered and roll up from both sides.

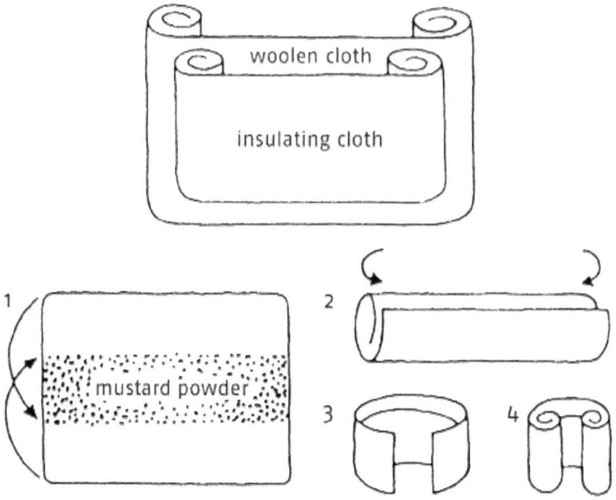

Fig. 5.1 Mustard compress. For detailed description see accompanying text.

As soon as the child is ready, immerse the mustard cloth in hot water, about 40–45 °C (note: allyl mustard oil remains effective at somewhat higher temperatures, contrary to previous assumptions), squeeze out the water carefully and when at body temperature, quickly wrap the cloth around the child's chest, from the back to the front (Fig. 5.1.). Then immediately wrap the insulating cloth and woollen cloth around the chest in the same direction so that the mustard cloth is completely covered (no exposure to the air whatsoever) and then close the compress firmly over the breastbone using sticking plaster, for example.
In the case of infants and children up to the age of two years, leave the compress on the body for only three minutes, using a kitchen timer, for example. It is not practicable to check for skin reddening during the application because children at this age tend to be disquieted. However, an adequate response is achieved after three minutes if a good, fresh mustard powder is used. In the case of children older than two years, one should check for skin reddening after three minutes and then every minute thereafter. Once the skin has reddened, much like mild sunburn, remove the compress immediately. Tolerance may increase with repeated use for several days. Once the compress has been removed, cleanse the skin of any bits of mustard powder and massage lightly with a mild oil (e.g. calendula 10 %). Then dress the child carefully. Without exception, even the babies and toddlers who cry or complain (they can be carried in one's arms during the compress) feel much better after the treatment: breathing is freer, circulation stabilizes and they often fall asleep peacefully.

The ginger compress is milder and has a warming, calming effect (▸Chap. 2.3.2.2 for preparation and application; [see also: Goebel and Glöckler 2008, 669, Vagedes and Soldner 2010, 58]). This treatment is particularly indicated for febrile bronchitis tending towards-bronchopneumonia with an obstructive component, and especially for children whose own warmth-generation capacities are weakened and previously damaged lungs (e. g. prematurely born children with bronchopulmonary dysplasia [▸Chap. 2.3.2.2], status post severe RSV infection). However, the ginger compress is not as effective as the mustard compress when treating acute pneumonia!

5.1.1.4.3 Medicinal treatment

- The more sudden and the more highly febrile and assault-like the onset of the pneumonia, the more likely the indication for blue aconite (monkshood) as the first medicine to be administered:
- **Aconitum D6 pillules/dil.** Wala (Aconitum e tubere Wala DE: Weleda UK import), Weleda (▸Chap. 2.2.3).

Aconitum napellus thrives particularly impressively in high mountainous and alpine regions where cold spells occur regularly. The aconite flower, with its intensely light-filled appearance, develops its deepest blue shade at great altitudes of up to 3000 m. The flower seems shy and reserved as it inclines its head downwards, away from the heavens. On the other hand, the root – where the highly toxic aconitine (an alkaloid) concentrates – seeks out damp, nitrogen-rich soil. Aconite belongs to the Ranunculaceae family and is easily identified by its sharply serrated leaves; plants of this family also often display radical leaf metamorphoses [Grohmann 1981, 19ff.]. The Central European representatives may flower in any season – even in winter, e. g. the Christmas rose. The "mercurial" gestures of adaptability, flexibility and balancing activity between opposite qualities, and the capacity to self-metamorphose, are evident in the aconite's characteristic strong upward growth and its capacity to produce remarkably striking, conspicuous flower forms, despite the location and damp conditions. (The marsh marigold is one example within the Ranunculaceae family that has a polar gesture to that of aconite.)

The *toxic action* of the aconite tuber on the human being causes the soul entity to abruptly "fix" into the physical-etheric – like a jolting shock – thus causing one-sided centralization of blood and warmth, i. e. congestion, with the consequence that the blood-warmth organism is in danger of suffocating and choking. The main symptoms of aconitine poisoning are severe shivering and chills, centralization of circulation, cessation of diuresis and increase in body temperature, accompanied by extreme fear.

Conversely, *low potency Aconitum (D6)* has a *"mercurially" balancing effect* on the blood-warmth organism: In counteraction to the centripetal tendency that occurs at onset of the pneumonia, low potency Aconitum activates *centrifugal processes*, i. e. diuresis, sweating, warmth penetration, and dissipation of warmth at the periphery – *to the right degree*. The mercurial "bringing-into-movement" nature of the Ranunculaceae comes to true expression here. As a result, the fever does not dissipate and nor is it suppressed (as would occur with strong doses of antipyretics, for example) but it can carry out its "task" in overcoming the sudden rush of cold coming from outside that has caused the congestion in the lung region. This is possible because the "poisoning" effect of that promotes warmth centralization is still available in the D6 potency: At this potency level, the poisoning effect is just about in balance with the counter-effect so that *during the fever* the organism receives what it needs at the time in order to restore balance between centre and periphery.

Higher potencies of Aconitum mainly have the effect of "drawing out to the periphery" whereas *substantial* doses emphasize the "centralizing" effect. (Hence, *higher potencies* are useful for treating shock because they have the capacity to release the soul's sense of being deeply imprisoned in the body.) Therefore, high potencies may initially cause warmth to dissipate too strongly. In the event of such a response, the fever will decrease rapidly but will also be lacking in the area of the body that is battling to overcome the illness, i. e. the

5

lungs, and complications may arise as a result. On the other hand, the authors also consider the very low potencies of aconite (e. g. in Pneumodoron 1 [Aconite/Bryonia drops, Weleda UK]), as having unfavourable, one-sided effects on children based on their observations in practice and also the knowledge and understanding of the medication as described above. However, after the age of 9–12 years, Pneumodoron 1 (Aconite/Bryonia drops, Weleda UK) and Pneumodoron 2 (Phosphorus/Tart. Stib. Drops, Weleda UK), i. e. medicines containing low potencies of Aconitum, Bryonia, Phosphorus und Tartarus, are remarkably effective without the mentioned "one-sided" side effect: This is possible because the soul organization and I-organization are more strongly anchored in the metabolism at this age, corresponding with the more challenging stimulation of the stronger substance in the medication [see also, Vademecum English edition 2009].

Aconite restricts the inflammatory congestion process, thereby ensuring that sufficient blood and warmth drain away from the lungs. Hence, it simultaneously *counteracts the child's anxiety and restlessness* because the latter is directly related to restriction of breathing due to hyperaemia and exudate formation, and to the congested build-up of heat.

Regarding *dosages* of Aconite D6, the following approach has proven to be effective:

At onset of illness (rising fever, chills, shivering): Every 15 minutes.

Following onset of action (diuresis, warming of the periphery): Hourly.

Later, following the first reduction in fever: 5 x/day *until the fever subsides completely* – and not only at illness onset as is often recommended in homoeopathy, for example. A clear stabilization of the disease course can thereby be observed. This can perhaps be understood as a consequence of the fundamentally "mercurial", balancing effect of Aconitum on the blood-warmth organization, which is of such importance during the entire fever phase.

Aconitum D6 can be diluted in water as follows: 50 gtt. or corresponding amount of pillules diluted with usual daily water requirement; administer by teaspoon or coffee spoon during the course of the day as directed above or administer 2–5 pillules for each individual dose.

In addition to aconite, bryony is another essential medicinal plant for administration during the early phases of pneumonia (and pleurisy, see below):

- **Bryonia dioica (e rad.) D6 dil./pillules** Wala, Weleda.

Bryonia belongs to the Curcubitaceae (gourd) family (including pumpkin, squash, cucumber, melon etc.) and just as alpine Aconitum is one of the high-altitude "border hoppers" in the Ranunculaceae family (there are several), Bryonia is the "northern border hopper" within its family [Simon 1987, 43–51]. Thus, both these medicinal plants have the *capacity to survive despite the cold* in their natural setting, pointing to the central significance of this aspect for the course of pneumonia. Usually Curcubitaceae thrive in warm, subtropical climatic zones; typical formation and ripening of the swollen, watery fruit takes place above ground in the warmth, in the part of the plant that serves reproduction and where a highly dynamic metabolic process occurs.

If one compares the physical structures of plant and human being, this part of the plant may be likened to the organ area below the diaphragm in the human being. – In contrast to this, in Bryonia (a different kind of Curcubitaceae), the location of the expansive fruit formation gesture described above is *displaced:* The pumpkin character is to be found underground (while the fruit is a tiny, almost fleshless berry!) The huge, turgescent root is fluid-rich; its signature is its pungent, sharp-bitter taste and its constituents have an inflammatory and potentially inflammation-inducing character.

Thus, Bryonia displaces a dynamic, fluid-accumulating metabolic process into the root, i. e. underground, evidently in response to cold exposure in the regions where it grows. Once again comparing this part of the plant to the human, one discovers many similarities to the head pole of the human organism [Steiner 1976, 123]. The root of the plant relates more closely to the human nervous system while fruit and flower formation can be likened to generative and active metabolic processes.

Bryonia dioica thus displays a pneumonia-like process: After the plant is exposed to the cold, a fluid containing inflammatory and metabolically-active qualities (related to intestine, gall and pancreas secretions in the human being, i. e. the area of digestive activity), is displaced to the root. In the human being, this compares to the space above the diaphragm, i. e. *in the direction of* the head pole. Like the Ranunculus, Aconitum, Bryonia also displays a "mercurial" gesture in its leaf system, but in a completely different way: The plant does not hold itself upright; instead the young leaf shoots above the ground send out long runners that then climb energetically up solid structures such as gates and fences, anchoring themselves like a leaf blanket or a "second skin" [Simon 1987, 44].

Bryonia is particularly effective when *inflammatory exudate* begins to develop in preformed body cavities such as the thorax or in the vicinity of the (larger) joints in which serous membranes (pleura, peritoneum, synovia) usually enable *high internal flexibility* and mobility (or, for example, when a rib fracture irritates the serosa, also to the extent causing inflammation [Simon 1987, 47]). The clinical effect of these processes is that every movement is painful (although this may not be present in pneumonia) and consequently the patient tends to avoid movement. Typically, this kind of pain is described as "sharp and stabbing" and can be located precisely: The very same words could be used to describe the taste of Bryonia root juice extract! Here the inflammatory fluid accumulation caused by infiltration of protein-rich blood constituents and leukocytes into areas normally carefully isolated from such events (articular space, pleural cavity, alveoli, subarachnoid space) occur side by side with extreme dryness of the mucosa.

The kind of pathology that responds to potentized Bryonia root characteristically causes *redistribution (i. e. dislocation)* of fluids within the fluid organism and *alters the qualities of the fluid.* That which is "pathological" for the alveolus and the pleural cavity is "physiological" for an organ such as the *liver.* In the liver, a form of exudate is continually being discharged from the blood into the peri-sinusoidal space of Disse: Here the free passage between intravascular and extravascular space is a normal circumstance, and there is no basal membrane to separate hepatocytes from the exudate. Reciprocal fluid exchange of this kind in the lungs, however, would amount to an acutely pathological situation. But the liver is more than the centre of metabolic activity in the organism: *it remains lifelong in the most embryonic form of all the human organs.* This attribute is even observable in the blood gas tensions that correspond to that of a foetus (arteriovenous mixed blood!) and, of course, in the unique self-regenerating capacity of the liver. As a gland that originally formed out of the midgut mesenteron, physiologically speaking the liver is the type of organ that the lung threatens to become when its regresses to the pseudoglandular state – a condition that is expressed by the term "hepatization".

With this perspective as a starting point [Vogel 1995, 179] one can attempt to understand the *mercurial balancing effect of potentized Bryonia* thus: Parallel to dissolving the inflammatory, protein-rich fluid congestion that has accumulated in the "wrong place" in the body (i. e. above the diaphragm, in the relatively cool lung region that has been exposed to the cold), Bryonia also intensifies glandular activity in liver and gall secretions in the intestinal/bowel region (i. e. the region below the diaphragm), which, in turn, stimulates digestion and elimination of stools (in the same way that Aconitum activates diuresis via the kidneys). Thus, administering Bryonia D6 during the entire inflammatory process will simultaneously limit the extent of the inflammatory exudate and activate the metabolism so that the exudate is completely digested and reabsorbed. This occurs primarily via the lymph system[1] – just as the liver is particularly active with regard to lymph formation.

Bryonia is particularly indicated when clinical signs of thirst arise (as a consequence of internal fluid loss, also a typical symptom of liver function disorders); the patient avoids movement and in some circumstances will complain about pain when coughing or even in relation to respiratory movement (Bryonia is the most important medicine when treating pleurisy; if administered early enough during a pneumonia it can even prevent pleurisy). The cough is generally dry and painful when Bryonia is indicated. On the level of soul, the patient is irritated, annoyed and unapproachable (typical when the liver-gall function is affected), withdraws socially, tends to lie very still in bed and feels intensely unwell. In Bryonia-type cases, the fever does not rise as rapidly as typically occurs in response to Aconitum and the fever is rather high and lengthy – the kind of fever that is necessary to resolve and resorb the large amounts of exudate that can occur in these patients if Bryonia D6 is not adminisetered early enough.

In practice the different "mercurial" balancing effects of Aconitum and Bryonia are an excellent complement to each other: In this way diuresis and digestion, i. e. kidney and liver-gall functions are activated and excessive centralization of warmth and consolidation of the blood and inflammatory exudate in the area of the alveoli can be avoided.

Therefore, following initial doses of Aconitum, Bryonia and Aconitum should be administered **together** e. g. 50 gtt. of each, in D6 potency, in a glass of water, administered by teaspoonful during the course of 24–48 hours. Alternatively administer

- **Bryonia/Aconitum pillules,** Wala
  2–5 pillules per dose.

Pneumonia is the result of a challenge to the *juvenile warmth organization.* In many respects, the *blood* is the centre of this warmth organization. Warmth distribution and blood flow are closely connected, but the capacity of the organism to self-generate sufficient warmth for its own purposes is also related to the *breathing function of the blood via iron-containing haemoglobin.* The release of energy – also in the immune system – is ultimately related to iron-carrying enzymes and energy-rich *phosphates.*

The onset of a pneumonia is usually preceded by *a weakness in the juvenile warmth organization.* The illness itself poses a fundamental threat to this warmth organization: As the mercurially mobile "interface organ", the lung is the centre of the body's breathing function and is responsible for activating organically-bound iron in the blood, absorbing oxygen and releasing carbon dioxide. When the lung becomes immersed in fluid, the soul and spirit lose their vehicle for activity in the organism and the body loses its capacity for autonomous physical existence. Byway of iron the lungs and red blood components enable independent bodily existence: they enable the soul-spiritual entities of the human being

1 "The bulk of the exudate is reabsorbed via the lymph system" [Remmele 1997, 624].

to incarnate, i. e. to become active in the dynamic, physical will-activity that breaks down substance and releases energy by means of the warmth that has been procured via the breathing process.

In this respect iron is *the metal that facilitates physical incarnation of the individuality.* During the course of a pneumonia, the individuality is in a conflict with the forces of outer nature and the weaknesses in the existing bodily constitution, and is fighting for the leadership role in formative and developmental activity. Here the individuality is battling for the *highest* – physiologically speaking – for the *warmth organization* (▶Chap. 2.1) and its vehicle, the blood: The iron content of the blood is the body's highest priority when regulating its iron stores. Consequently, the course of pneumonia is critically dependent upon the strength of the warmth organization and blood circulation.

Potentized iron phosphate (ferric phosphate) is an essential medicine in this sense. As a natural iron(II)-phosphate in the form of striking blue-crystals, it is the primary constituent of:

- **Vivianit D6 trit./amp.** Weleda
  e.g. 1 saltsp. (generous), 3–5 x/d.

The form of iron phosphate used in homoeopathy, Ferrum phosphoricum (i.e. iron(III)-phosphate), is laboratory produced. However, Weleda uses natural starting substances for procuring the iron and phosphoric acid, and produces the substance basis for potentized Ferrum phosphoricum by means of an intricate pharmaceutical process (in which ferrous carbonate is converted to iron phosphate via iron chloride, thus becoming a pharmaceutical "iron conductor") [Vademecum English edition 2009,; Engel 1994]

- **Ferrum phosphoricum D6 tabs./amp.**
  e.g. ½–1 tab., 3–5 x/day (the authors prefer using Pulmo/Vivianit comp. Wala for injection, see below).

Ferrum phosphoricum is the more acute, metabolically-oriented medicine (the starting substance does not have a crystalline character and is yellow in colour) while Vivianite has a stronger structural quality and forming tendency (crystal forms) and displays a finer, more harmonizing character in comparison to Ferrum Phos. (▶Chap. 6.5).

The main indications for Vivianit/Ferrum phos. are as follows:

- *Unstable circulation:* Skin colour and state of circulation vary depending on whether the child is sitting or lying down; every movement is strenuous; alternation between flushing and pallor.
- *Weakness in the warmth organization:* The pneumonia only develops a fever after 2 days; it develops from a descending 'flu-like infection that cannot be overcome (typical for focal pneumonia with less infiltration).
- *Insufficient care of the warmth organization:* Consistent with previously mentioned viewpoints, case histories do confirm that a lack of sufficient rest and warmth during an otherwise insignificant infection can lead to pneumonia as a complication.

Weakness or lability in the warmth organization and circulatory system may already be present constitutionally prior to the illness as is often the case in infants and small children, although this is also still possible during puberty.

Administration of potentized iron or iron phosphate and other iron composition medicines by *injection* is particularly effective for treating pneumonia. – The original rationale

5

for parenteral application of potentized medicines can be attributed to Rudolf Steiner who indicated that a direct effect on the rhythmic system could be achieved in this way (with effects on breathing and circulation and thereby on the warmth organization). This has proven to be the case in practice.

Administration of *potentized iron compounds by injection has* proven to be an essential component of pneumonia treatment. The authors recommend administering the injection subcutaneously, between the shoulder blades, and as a rule, paravertebral on the right side. For the purpose it is best to use a *short* (½") needle (26 or 27 G – even finer guages can be found, such as 29 guage or 30 guage), a so-called insulin needle. The effect on breathing and circulation is impressive. As a rule, the authors administer the injection at the time of diagnosis and daily thereafter if the illness course includes unstable circulation, unstable warmth conditions and/or excessive infiltration.

The following combination of medicines is most frequently administered:

- **Pulmo/Vivianit comp. amp.** Wala (composition medicine containing of potentized Vivianit D7, Bryonia e rad. D5, Tart. stib. D5, Pulmo Gl D16), 0.7–1.0 ml s.c., 1 x/day.

This preparation unites four basic medicinal substances indicated for typical problems related to pneumonia nowadays [Vogel 1994, 688–691]. Combined potentization of the components produces a completely new medicine, i.e. its efficacy is not a result of the mere addition of substances. Through the combined potentization of components (that are partly polar to each other but also complementary), the new preparation has a unique broad-spectrum effect that could not be achieved in the same way through administration of the single natural substances.[1]

Pulmo Gl D16 is a basic ingredient in the composition of this potentized organ preparation. The use of homologous potentized animal organs for parenteral administration (in this case produced from the calf lung) can be traced back to Rudolf Steiner [Sommer 1996, Roemer 1993]. In the present case, the potentized lung directs the medicinal effect organotropically to the lung. At this potency level, the organ preparation Pulmo specifically strengthens the organ's formative forces, proportionate to the escalation of the inflammatory exudative process, and promotes restoration of organ function. This may appear to be a mere claim, but since publication of the first edition of this book, many colleagues have repeatedly verified the authors' extensive positive experience in this regard.

Higher potencies of homologous organ preparations have a stronger formative effect in the above-described sense, while lower potencies (Gl D4–8) intensely stimulate vitality and vital regeneration processes in the affected organ area.

Whereas Bryonia counteracts overly excessive displacement of inflammatory-exudative processes to the lung tissue and simultaneously activates the liver-gall area, Tartarus stibiatus promotes break-down and reabsorption of exudate and supports circulation,

1 In the final step of the potentization process for Pulmo/Vivianit comp. amp. (Wala) all four components are potentized together. Even a composite medicine such as Arnica montana is not a "single substance" in the chemical or toxilogical sense: this is a natural composition with specific medicinal effects. Similarly, the pharmacist can also create a medicinal composition with specific effects that cannot be achieved by any of the individual components.

especially in the phase when the right ventricular load increases due to inflammation and oxygen saturation decreases (see below).

Pulmo/Vivianit comp. primarily strengthens activity of the rhythmic system in the circulation and in the lungs. At the same time, the organ preparation substantially reinforces the iron phosphate action. The addition of Bryonia and Tartarus stibiatus to the treatment will specifically counteract extreme or persistent inflammatory metabolic processes and the danger of circulatory insufficiency.

- If the doctor wishes to avoid composition medicines on principle, the following preparation administered by injection can achieve good results for the given indication:
- **Ferrum met. praep. D8 amp.** Weleda or Vivianite D6, Ferrum phos. D8 amp. already mentioned above.

Nevertheless, the broad-spectrum action of Pulmo/Vivianit comp. offers a very safe and reliable treatment option to both less experienced doctors as well as those more experienced with this kind of treatment.

Pulmo/Vivianit comp. may become an essential oral medicine when the main indications for Vivianite predominate during the illness course and for most pneumonias occurring in the first three years of life (at this age Aconitum only needs to be given 3–5 x/day; therefore Bryonia as a single substance medicine can be excluded). In addition to the injection, administer Pulmo/Vivianit comp., 0.5 ml, 2–4 x/day, per os[1] – beginning at the stage when Aconitum only needs to be given 3–5 x/day; administration of Bryonia as a single substance can then usually be omitted.

If it is necessary to stimulate reabsorption of exudate (or pleural effusion; ▸Chap. 5.1.1.3 below) and elimation processes via the kidneys (usually the case in the second half of the illness course) the following medicine, administered by injection, has proven to be effective:

- **Equisetum/Stannum amp.** Wala
  Administer s.c., on its own or preferably in combination with Pulmo/Vivianit comp., between the shoulder blades, on the side most severely affected.

If it is not possible to administer an injection, oral administration of these medicines will also be effective, although with reduced effect.

In the case of acute pneumonia in school age children and teenagers, with a severe course and accompanied by *severe chills and circulation insufficiency,* an i.m. (!) injection (use a large enough cannula, e.g. Nr. 2, i.e. 0.8 × 3.8 mm 21 Gauge) using

- **Oleum camphoratum comp. amp.**, Wala

1 amp. i.m., upper thigh, lateral can be of significant therapeutic benefit. This preparation is particularly helpful for children with psychomotoric retardation and cerebral palsy in whom spontaneous movement and respiratory movement are inherently restricted.

1 In the experience of the authors and countless medical colleagues, oral administration of potentized medicines licensed and approved for parenteral application can lead to good results, although per os administration cannot be equated with injection for acute treatment.

Phosphorus is fundamental to a treatment program for pneumonia:

- **Phosphor D6–8 dil.** Weleda or **LM6 dil.** Arcana®,
  2–5 gtt., single dose in the morning; possible to repeat in the afternoon.

However, the authors advise against using higher potencies during the acute phase of pneumonia. An understanding of the action of the substance can shed more light here: Phosphorous does not usually exist in nature as a free element and has only been produced chemically since the modern age [Emsley 2001]. Even when exposed to indoor air conditions and normal temperatures, so-called "white phosphorous" oxidizes spontaneously – gradually at first, in a greenish-blue glow that can be seen in the dark, and then igniting into an intensely luminous hot white flame. The Greek word *phosphor* means "light-bearer": chemically the substance has the quality of maximal propencity for spontaneous release of light and warmth imponderables. (Sulphur is related to phosphorus in some respects but when burning it releases much more warmth than light.) In this respect, phosphorus displays the same tendency intrinsic to oxidative metabolism in the animal and the human being, i. e. the use of energy-rich phosphates for energy transference.

The lower potencies of phosphorus have the effect of fostering *light-imbued integration of the soul-spiritual entities with the physical-etheric body.* In this way, Phosphor supports the incarnation process that is being challenged by the pneumonia. An aesthetic effect is not meant here: On the contrary, this effect can also be understood as – the structured! – "action of light" in the metabolic process through which oxygen radicals are released for the oxidative attack of granulocytes on e.g. bacterial pathogens (which occurs via iron containing enzymes). Administered in the dosage indicated here, phosphorus makes an essential contribution to ensuring that the pathogens can be destroyed by the inflammation – ultimately assisting the *pneumonia in fulfilling its purpose.*

During the *wintertime when there is a lack of light,* administration of Phosphor LM6 can be used a prophylaxis against *pneumonia.* This form of phosphorus is particularly indicated for delicate, sensitive children who are susceptible to infection, and always when one notices that the child appears "lacking in light": easily tired, inattentive (lacking in concentration) and sickly. Here one is reminded that the brain is especially rich in phosphates and functionally requires extremely intensive oxidative metabolism in order to enable the internal light process underlying consciousness. This explains the special relationship of the human individuality to the processes associated with phosphorus.

Phosphorus is always indicated when the individuality is unable to anchor itself sufficiently in the body so that light can be released internally. [Vademecum English edition 2009, 534, German edition 2010, 655f]. This problem expresses itself in the following way in pneumonia:

- Despite frequent high fever, the children do not appear to experience the illness process on a soul level; they get out of bed and want to move about and do not appear very ill at the practice.They can appear emotionally excitable, unrealistic and demanding, and may run around aimlessly.
- They are unable to be alone and have a strong need for affection (i. e. they are loving and ask for caresses) and become anxious when it becomes dark outside (lack of light!).

These patients are often shockingly pale when asleep and give the impression that they are burning themselves up (instead of "burning" what is infiltrating the body). Here the cough is more likely to be dry and painful; there is a tendency to nose bleeds and presence of blood admixture in the sputum; and the thirst for cold water reminds one of the attempt to put out a fire (it is barely possible to extinguish chemically-generated phosphorus fires).

In summary, the picture developed here shows that the aimless darting about of the soul and the lack of sensation (self-awareness) and activity is related to what is happening in the body. In this case *lower potencies of phosphorus administered in the morning have an incarnating effect;* on the other hand, higher potencies, particularly taken at night, can certainly have a calming effect on the "soul" aspect – but rather in the sense of initially freeing it even more from the body (as is evident at sleep onset) (▸Chap. 7.1). However, there are risks attached to this effect during an acute pneumonia!

Whenever the doctor recognizes the need to strengthen the phosphorus process in the patient as described here, phosphorus (in the suggested dosage) is indicated as an adjuvant treatment. The complete clinical picture as described above and in homoeopathic principles does not have to be present: the decision to administer phosphorus depends more on one's sense of soul-body integration in the patient rather than on isolated symptoms that one can "fix" in writing.

Once the fever has abated, meteoric iron (as indicated below) can be administered until the end of the convalescence phase, i.e. for about 4 weeks following illness onset, in order to consolidate and continue the above-described effects. This medicine has also proven to be effective as prophylaxis against a relapse:

- **Meteoreisen (meteoric iron) pillules** Wala
  5–7 pillules, 2 x/day, mornings and afternoons.

A difficult treatment situation arises when *exudate consolidates* in the alveoli to a great degree during the pneumonia. In this case the child has a mucous cough that is insufficiently productive and will not loosen easily; circulation threatens to become hypotensive; skin colour is pale and may be slightly cyanotic; the periphery of the body is cool; the child has symptoms of severe nausea (or describes such a sensation) and is unable to eat. The expression "bogged down" – the feeling of being unable to free oneself – is an apt description and a helpful catch phrase for understanding this situation. Paracelsus understood this pathological state as belonging to the "tartaric illnesses": that is, when fluids go over into a solid state and cannot be dissolved again by the organism [Lüth 1989, 64]. The concept "Tartarus" stems from the tartar sediment deposited on the bottom of a wine vat during the fermentation process in wine making.

For Paracelsus, the main medicine for treating tartaric illnesses was Tartarus stibiatus (antimony tartrate): a compound produced from a complex chemical reaction between tartar and antimony oxide. The intrinsically insoluble Tartarus becomes soluble through the reaction with antimony and extremely poisonous. Through potentization (D6–8), however, it becomes non-poisonous and an extremely effective medicine for the above-described circumstances (it is very probable that Paracelsus applied a form of homoeopathic potentization of Tartarus stibiatus, unlike his immediate successors).

The strong and rapidly noticeable effect of

- **Tartarus stibiatus D6 trit.** Weleda
  1 saltsp., 5 x/day

has been indicated elsewhere. This is the most important potentized medicine for treating postpartum asphyxia (▸Chap. 2.2.2), again underlining the parallel of pneumonia to the birth process. In teenagers and adults, D4 can have an even stronger effect (see also Pneumodoron 2, Weleda [Phosphorus/Tart. Stib. Drops, Weleda UK]).

The doctor will seldom encounter the difficult situation described above if Pulmo/Vivianit comp. and/or Equisetum/Stannum are administered by injection as indicated, and especially if *mustard compresses are applied conscientiously.* The same applies to support of the circulation during pneumonia, already been addressed to a large extent in the medications and interventions described above.

If it is still necessary to support the circulation over and above the measures described so far or to tone the circulation at the beginning of the convalescence phase, administration of Skorodit has proven to be effective:

- **Skorodit Kreislauf glob.** Wala
  5–7 pillules, 3–5 x/day.

5.1.1.5 Treatment options in case of inadequate treatment response

5.1.1.5.1 Lack of vitality

There is always the possibility that the illness course will come to a standstill and stagnate at a particular point, mostly at the start of lysis and exudate reabsorption, or when these processes should be rounding off. The doctor may have the impression that the organism is “flagging” and in need of new impetus in order to bring the illness process to completion.

In this situation one can ask oneself the following questions:

- Was the fever high enough and sufficiently prolonged?
- Is the child still affected by previously administered anti-inflammatory medications such as antibiotics and corticosteroids?
- Constitutionally speaking, does the child have a tendency to “tidy up” inadequately, i. e. are there issues with “completion”? This may be evident in disorderly behaviour that is difficult to influence. Similar to the phosphorus indication, in this case one also notices that the child does not feel as ill as one would expect given his or her physical status.

In these cases, administration of

- **Sulphur D30 pillules/trit.** DHU/Weleda
  5 pillules or 1 saltsp., 1–3 x/day max., 12-hour intervals between each dose

is often an effective intermediary medicine, both with regard to revitalization and for structuring of the life processes.

Another important intermediary medicine is

- **Lycopodium C30–200** Gudjons

Dosage as for Sulphur: 5 pillules or 1 saltsp., 1–3 x/day max., 12-hour intervals between each dose.

Lycopodium is particularly effective for those children who fundamentally do not generate much vitality and who are intellectually lively but have weak digestion and poor appetite. They also have a hardening tendency (e.g. constipation) with the result that in the event of a pneumonia they are unable to dissolve inflammatory exudate sufficiently (in this respect, this constitutional type is generally prone to "tartaric illnesses").

These children appear to be more ill than those who need sulphur; their warmth build-up is sluggish and generally inadequate. They often have a close but demanding relationship to their mother (mostly boys need this medicine).

5.1.1.5.2 Inhibited course of illness due to soul-spiritual and constitutional factors

Particularly in schoolchildren age 9 to 12 years, the illness frequently stagnates on the 3rd–5th day after onset, and possibly even worsens for no apparent reason.

- The 5th day of the pneumonia generally has special significance. The doctor should always examine the patient at this point in order to establish how treatment will continue and to ensure that mistakes or errors of judgement do not creep in at this crucial junction in the illness course.

It is essential for the doctor to be prepared for a potential crisis and to advise the parents in advance that such a situation may arise. The key question in relation to the child who has just developed pneumonia is:

- Why does this child need the pneumonia now?

The answer is usually very individual, although it usually incorporates completion of a developmental step in the soul life or processing of an experience at the level of soul that is not yet complete (the second case example 5.1.1.2. illustrates this). The child's soul-body constitution will often factor in the answer.

- In these cases, thorough and lasting success of the treatment is especially dependent on the doctor identifying *the individual reason for the illness* – which ultimately means that the doctor has perceived and understood the child. The patient wants to be "seen" and recognized.
- Of course, the right therapeutic response will vary greatly, but usually it can be identified (note use of silver ointment [Argentum 0.4 %] in the above-mentioned case study, 5.1.1.2).

Case study

A 10-year-old girl with pneumonia is seen in the outpatient clinic. It is already the 4th day of illness: After three days the fever has only reached temperatures of 39.5–39.8 °C. On auscultation end inspiratory fine-to-medium bubbling crackles can be heard over both lungs. She has a mucous cough, mild dyspnoea and right dorsal dampening of 3 finger's breadth. Considering the child's age, the illness course so far, and the relatively extensive clinical findings, a mycoplasmal pneumonia was probable (confirmed serologically later on). The girl had already seen the doctor prior to onset of the pneumonia because she had concentration problems at school coupled with inconsistent performance and results that were obviously below her potential. (Extensive investigations had been carried out by a child psychiatrist because of problems with calculation and a moderate reading and spelling learning difficulty.) The girl often needed the whole afternoon to do her homework; she increasingly displayed an attitude of passive avoidance was most happy playing with dolls on her own or doing nothing. Slightly adipose body, blonde hair, wide face – middle region of the face not greatly differentiated for her age, tending to heavier movements and not particularly fond of exercise. Psychosocially, the girl was restrained, shy and cautious with a "wait and see" attitude, but not negative or rejecting.

The course of the pneumonia seemed to correspond with the girl's intrinsic way of being: sluggish, lethargic and protracted. When the expected improvement failed to materialize after the 3rd day of treatment (initial treatment as described above) the whole case history was reconsidered. Now a more complete picture emerged: When the girl was 2 ½-years-old, a parking car ran over her brother (5-years-old at the time). He was severely injured and died within hours following the accident. This event triggered severe, long-term shock in the girl and both parents. The mother subsequently suffered from depressive disorders and the father developed asthmatic bronchitis.

The mother was pregnant at the time of the accident and so a little boy was born six months later, a new little brother for the girl. He often exhibited very lively behaviour; later on he developed migraines and asthmatic bronchitis. The child psychiatrist had already established depressive tendencies in the girl. In addition to the difficult experiences surrounding her brother's death and her parents' subsequent health problems, the girl also had to cope with her own clumsiness, consequent teasing at school and the feeling of not being understood because of her reading, spelling and math learning difficulties. The girl's lethargy and inertia was barely tolerable for the mother, herself diligent and hard working. The mother's lack of trust in her daughter's development was a strain on the girl.

Taking the history into account, a medicine was sought that would address the child's given constitutional situation and above all, a medicine that would contribute to overcoming delayed development (due to suffering and grief that lay years back); a medicine that would address the child's paralyzed capacity for aggression, thereby freeing the forces needed for overcoming the pneumonia infection. *Causticum D30* was administered as a single substance medicine. There was a tangible improvement already within 12 hours after the first dose, and thereafter the pneumonia ran its course without further difficulty or delay.

It was only years later that the mother spontaneously described how her husband had not involved himself in the question of how his daughter's lung inflammation should be treated and had left the responsibility to his wife. Initially this had been very difficult for her. However, during the course of the illness she developed renewed trust – trust in the treatment approach and trust in her daughter. Consequently, she remembers this illness as a turning point for her child and for herself. In the meantime, the girl is doing well at secondary school, the depressive components are no longer present, and the mother has a normal and relaxed relationship with her now 15-year-old daughter.

Case study

A 9-year-old girl, tall and slender with a sanguine temperament, developed broncho-pneumonia from a 'flu-like' infection. She is a very lively child and it has been difficult to keep her in bed during the infection. Typical findings on auscultation (fine, bubbly crackles), no dampening, fever up to over 40 °C, severe hardly productive coughing, worse when lying down and when speaking. The child is very communicative and cooperative, talks a lot, and most of all would like to get out of bed immediately.

Following an injection of Pulmo/Vivianit comp. and oral administration of the same, there was initially rapid improvement in the child's sense of well-being, the fever decreased and coughing became milder and looser. Two days later, however, the fever began to rise again and the previously improved auscultatory findings were again more pronounced; the child's general condition was clearly affected and she was feeling very ill. Further enquiry revealed that she had pronounced night sweats.

The mother was made aware that it is not unusual for such a situation to arise at this age and that all the circumstances surrounding the illness needed to be reviewed once again. The girl's father was ill at the time and had been hospitalized for two months owing to a depressive episode. He was due to come home soon; the most recent contact with him had been on the same weekend when the 'flu-like' infection (preceding the pneumonia) started. Family relationships were stable otherwise but strained under the current circumstances. The girl's grandfather (on the father's side) had suffered severe tuberculosis.

While it is not possible to describe all the intermediate steps in the case, one can recognize the background coherences: The father's lability strongly affected the very delicate, sensitive girl who was easily thrown off balance. His illness prevented him from fulfilling his fatherly leadership duties, which, in a certain sense, represents the above-described iron process necessary for stable anchoring of will activity. If one considers the girl's leptosome constitution (mother and father had the same constitution), her mildly excitable soul disposition combined with the lack of self-awareness of her illness (which also applies to the father's way of being, and is also typical for many tuberculosis sufferers), limited elimination during the day and severe night sweats, one gains a sense of the connections between the three generations (although this cannot be described in any further detail here).

– *Tuberculinum* C200 (Gudjons)[1] was administered, 3 pillules, 3 x/day, at 12 h intervals and led to an overall improvement with sustained decline in fever within 24 hours.

Considering these two cases in retrospect, both doctor and parents had the sense that it had been essential for the children to experience the pneumonia – and the crises. The individual constitutional medicine only became evident (and necessary!) through the crisis, and perhaps also because the child had matured sufficiently for the breakthrough to a new and individually acquired state of health that could then be consummated with the support of the appropriate constitutional medicine.

1 Unfortunately the very effective Gudjon preparation is only available as part of a therapist's set or packaged for medical practice use (likewise Med., Psor.). Swiss, Belgian and Austrian manufacturerers offer alternatives.

The most frequent **constitutional medicines** that come into consideration are:

- Sulphur
- Causticum
- Phosphor
- Silicea
- Ferrum phosphoricum
- Pulsatilla
- Tuberculinum
- Lycopodium

each administered in D20–30 potency, C200 in individual cases.

5.1.1.5.3 Pleurisy

Pleurisy usually accompanies lobar pneumonia, even if it is not clinically ascertainable, [Remmele 1997, 624] but rarely arises in the focal pneumonias and is mostly a sign of a protracted inflammatory process. The paediatrician will rarely come across pleurisy as a primary illness.

The most important measures and medicines for treating pleurisy within the context of pneumonia are:

- **Mustard compress**
- **Bryonia (e rad.) D6–12 dil./pillules** and **amp.** per os, dosage as above (▸Chap. 5.1.1.4.3).

Bryonia is especially effective at the onset of exudative pleurisy (restricts development of effusion) and for treating the drier, more severely painful pleurisy that is identified as a classical pleural friction rub on auscultation. When administered by subcutaneous injection, the effect of Bryonia is impressive, especially on the pain (this applies to most inflammatory or trauma-related pleural pain).

The main medication for treating pleural effusion is stibnite, a sulphur compound also called "antimonite":

- **Antimonit (antimonite) D6 trit.** Weleda
  1 saltsp., 5 x/day.
  In severe cases: i.v. injection using 1 ampoule [10 ml] (Weleda) is very effective.

Finally, the following medicines may also be considered:

- **Equisetum/Stannum amp.** Wala
  daily s.c. injection for pleural effusion and to support reabsorption in cases of protracted infiltration.

These three medicines can be combined with a higher potency (and therefore anti-inflammatory) organ preparation:

- **Pleura Gl D15–30 amp.** Wala.

If the patient has insufficient light and warmth forces – evident in a protracted, effusive inflammatory process, delayed lysis, purulent and foul-smelling sputum and the presence of atypical pathogens – Sulphur iodatum is an extremely beneficial medicine:

- **Sulphur iodatum D4–6 dil.** DHU
  3–7 gtt., 3 x/day.

Sulphur iodatum primarily promotes reabsorption but also intensifies the efficacy of the immune system. The latter effect is evident when the sputum clarifies and the foul smell disappears, and bacteriologically when pathogens that are difficult to control (especially those of bacterial origin) reduce or disappear [Stiegele 1981]. The iodine component is the key to this effect [Kunze 1965].

Physiologically speaking, *iodine* forms a substantive basis for thyroid activity in the development and functioning of the organism [Girke 2010, 375–377]. The same organic precondition enables the amphibian to survive on land, as is evident in the ontogenesis of the tadpole, for example. Here the development of lungs and limbs takes place ontogenetically and phylogenetically at the same time [Husemann 1993, 168ff.] and is thyroid-dependent (and therefore hormone-dependent). This process can be artifically accelerated and stimulated through administration of thyroxine; the lung primordium in the 3rd and 4th pharyngeal pouches coincides with the area of the thyroid primordium [Vogel 1995, 571ff.].

Iodine-containing thyroxine is crucial for so-called "basal metabolism", i. e. for respiratory chain activity in the mitochondria that transforms the inspiration process into a metabolic event that frees up the energy needed by the soul entity for its activity in the body. This is the same dynamic that has already been described in relation to phosphorus.

The pathway taken by phosphorus leads right into physical form – into the skeleton on the one hand, and into the nervous system on the other. That is, where phosphates are functionally and structurally crucial. Hence, phosphorus has significance in an area where the human individuality imprints its specifically human expression in the skeleton on the one hand, and shapes the nervous system into an instrument of human waking consciousness on the other. In contrast, iodine enables activity of the soul entity in the human being and the animal by mediating between breathing and metabolism. The soul is even active in the body's immunological processes that are like the release of light effects inside the organism – such as occurs in the formation of oxygen radicals, for example.

- In its substantial form iodine has an antiseptic effect, similar to that of sunlight. Whereas iodine enables the soul entity to carry out its work in the fluid life body of the organism, phosphorus is active where the spiritual individuality is present and extends right into the most physical part of the body.
- Potentized iodine is effective when excessive inflammatory secretions threaten to "drown" the lung in fluid, thus endangering its adaptation to "land conditions" (i. e. ventilation of the airways and the lung at birth) and when these secretions become the breeding ground for alien microbial life. Potentized iodine promotes reabsorption and has a sterilizing effect, especially when combined with sulphur. For this reason Sulphur iodatum D4–6 is also an important medication for treating mucoviscidosis (▸Chap. 10.4), for delayed decongestion in pneumonia, pleural effusion, existing bronchiectasis and also for facilitating a complete recovery from sinusitis (▸Chap. 5.1.2).

5

5.1.1.5.4 Recurrent pneumonia, prophylaxis

Case study

A four-year-old boy attended an outpatient clinic in March after developing four consecutive pneumonias within six weeks (all treated with antibiotics). Two days following completion of the last antibiotic treatment (carried out i.v. at the clinic) the boy's temperature rose again to over 40 °C, he has a cough and displays typical findings for pneumonia on examination. He is extremely active while the history is being taken, running around the room and clambering on the examination couch. He has a slim body build, tending to a small frame; shows signs of early dental decay of the incisors; he has large, expressive brown eyes with a very lively gaze – and in contrast to this, very pale blue skin colour. According to his mother, his temperature tends to rise very rapidly. Within the context of the previous pneumonias, many aspects had already been investigated and clarified; the clinic is considering a bronchoscopy once this pneumonia has subsided. At the request of his mother, the child was referred to our practice so that alternative treatment options couldbe explored.

The boy was principally treated with Pulmo/Vivianit comp. and mustard compresses as well as Ferrum phos. as a single substance medication. The child recovered from the pneumonia within five days, without any further problems. At the outset, phosphorus was clearly indicated as a constitutional medicine, especially following the multiple pneumonias and antibiotic treatment. In the light of the uncomplicated course, however, this basic medication was not immediately necessary and was only administered once the child had fully recovered. On the same day the boy started phosphorus treatment, he suddenly developed a 40 °C temperature, clearly in reaction to the medication (i.e. no cough or any other symptoms). The high temperature lasted for 12 hours and then subsided rapidly. The boy's health was subsequently much more stable and he never developed a pneumonia again (during the course of 17 years of follow-up), even though he has retained his extremely lively way of being. Phosphorus was administered again during the two years following the last pneumonia occurrence when his overall condition became distinctly more labile and he developed severe pallor (iron deficiency was excluded).

In the first instance, pneumonia recurrences differ with regard to whether or not a permanent physical-organic disorder is the underlying cause. If this is *not* the case – as in the case study just described – relapses mostly occur *when the pneumonia has not run its course properly in the first place or when the illness has been suppressed.* This seems to indicate that these patients intrinsically need to overcome the pneumonia themselves – and indeed, experience does show that relapses rarely occur following the treatment process as described above. *Hence, the treatment already encompasses the most effective prophylaxis against a relapse in that it steers the illness course and supports it in such a way that the purpose of the pneumonia for the organism can be fulfilled.*

In the case of a pneumonia recurrence, two potentized medicines in particular can be considered as basic constitutional remedies:

- **Phosphor LM6** Arcana® or
- **Sulphur LM6** Arcana®

One can distinguish between the two medicines according to two basic constitutional pictures:

- The child who is in need of phosphorus tends to be more strongly affected on a soul level and appears delicate and sensitive; at the same time the child lacks awareness of his or her own body, is unable to penetrate it adequately and appears vulnerable (see description of phosphorus in ▸Chap. 5.1.1.4.3).
- The child who needs sulphur tends to follow his or her own vital urges in a disorderly way and with little regard for others; the metabolic system itself is disorderly (erratic stools, flatulence). Bad posture, drooping shoulders, skin that appears unclean and a tendency to supperations are symptomatic of a disorderly, off-centre metabolism, which, in turn, strongly affects the soul disposition.

Thus sulphur and phosphorus are juxtaposed in such a way that potentized sulphur primarily has an ordering, structuring and centering effect on the metabolism – thereby liberating the breathing organization of excessive metabolic activity, both in body and soul – whereas potentized phosphorus incarnates the soul-spiritual aspect of the child more strongly in the physical-etheric body and strengthens the forces of light *within* the organism's functioning – thereby enhancing the child's immunity to the outside world. From time to time it may be necessary to administer one medicine after the other to the same child (in homoeopathic application, both medicines are closely complementary).

- **Roseneisen/Graphit glob.** Wala
  5–10 pillules, 2 x/day (▸Chap. 5.1.1.6)

strengthens the warmth organization in the lung region and is therefore an important medicine for counteracting a pneumonia recurrence.
Roseneisen/Graphit is also of benefit in the treatment of measles, both as prophylaxis and treatment. As a rule, this medicine is effective for the measles-related cough and can be administered as a preventative measure for measles-related pneumonia.

Physical-organic causes of a pneumonia recurrence include:

- Mucoviscidosis
  Longterm treatment with Sulphur iodatum is especially important here (▸Chap. 10.4).
- Anatomical anomalies (e.g. tracheal stenosis, bronchiectasis)
  In addition to the individual medicines mentioned elsewhere, treatment with *organ preparations* in combination with quarz and low potency Echinacea come into consideration, especially during the first years of life.

In the case of a child with status post operationem of oesophageal atresia Vogt IIIb and narrowing of the tracheal lumen by 60 % due to tracheal stenosis (caused by vascular anomalies), the frequency of pneumonia was significantly reduced by treatment with:

- **Trachea Gl D12 amp.** Wala in combination with
- **Quarz D12 amp.** Wala
- **Echinacea e pl. tota D3 amp.** Wala

The three medicines should be administered as a mixture (in equal parts), 0.5 ml/day, per os, for several months. In such cases, the pneumonia is due to the inflammation just below the stenosis.

The following additional measures have proven to be effective in the context of tracheal stenosis with recurrent pneumonia (Note: A ring-like tracheal stenosis due to vascular anomalies can be difficult to identify, even with a CT scan!):
A daily mustard compress every time an airways infection occurs, healthy nutrition, Vitamin D supplementation in winter and daily inhalation with

- **Pulmo/Vivianit comp. amp.** Wala
  1:1 mit NaCl 0.9 % or Emser Sole, if necessary also 5.85 % NaCl.

- Gastrooesophageal reflux
  Gastrooesophageal reflux disease is a significant cause of recurrent pneumonia in children status post operationem of oesophageal atresia, or with spastic tetraparesis and/or severe cerebral handicap (compare with 4.6.1).

In the case of premature babies who have been mechanically ventilated for a long time, children with cerebral palsy and children with psychomotoric retardation and relapsing pneumonias, the frequency of pneumonia can be substantially reduced with daily per os or inhalative administration of

- **Pulmo/Vivianit comp. amp.** Wala
  0.5 ml per os or inhalation using 1 ml 1:1 with NaCl or Emser brine, 1 x/day, afternoons.

Especially in winter, combine with

- **Phosphor LM6**
  2–5 gtt. 1 x/day, mornings.

All forms of recurrent pneumonia can benefit from complementary use of **potentizedautologous blood, administered** per os in increasing potencies [see. Imhäuser 2000]:

- C5: 3–5 gtt., 1 x/day for 4 weeks.
- C7: 3–5 gtt., 3 x/wk for 4 weeks.
- C9: 3–5 gtt., 2–3 x/wk for 4 weeks.
- C12: 3–5 gtt., 1–2 x/wk for 4 weeks.

Best to administer mornings, 10 mins. before meals.

5.1.1.5.5 Necessity for antibiotics

At the beginning of this section, the authors pointed to the fact that the majority of pneumonias in paediatric practice can be treated without antibiotics – and that this approach can be immensely beneficial for the child's further development and immunological competence.

- In individual cases, however, it can become necessary to treat with antibiotics. This especially applies to:
- New born and premature babies.
- Bronchopulmonary dysplasia.
- Mucoviscidosis and similar diseases.

- When pneumonia is diagnosed at a very advanced stage – which is not rare in mycoplasmal pneumonias in children at school age.
- When the inflammation is not restricted to the lungs but encompasses e.g. the paranasal sinuses, middle ear and lungs. (These children are usually very weak; frequently there is a difficult social situation in the background).

The doctor's experience, knowledge and engagement as well as the parents' decision are essential here. If the parents' decision would force the doctor to undertake a form of treatment with incalculable risks or one that he or she could not take responsibility for, then the treatment should be declined. But even when antibiotic treatment is undertaken, the treatment options presented in this chapter are nevertheless relevant and beneficial, as the following case study illustrates:

Case study

A five-year-old girl was severely brain damaged on the 17th day of life following a group B-streptococcal meningoencephalitis: bilateral amaurosis, microcephalia, treatment-resistent symptomatic epilepsy, diabetes insipidus neurohormonalis, lack of statomotoric development, 80 % to 90 % of nourishment via PEG, gastrooesophageal reflux.

The child normally lived at home and was lovingly and optimally cared for by parents and nursing staff; she clearly responded to her environment and her presence was a significant and deeply positive human experience for the parents and friends of the family. The child contracted peracute pneumonia about three times a year, mostly beginning on the right side and probably caused by gastro-oesophageal reflux (aspiration of acidic stomach juices). Despite prompt administration of antibiotics, immediate hospitalization had always been necessary because her general condition deteriorated rapidly and especially because hypoxaemia developed.

This time, at onset of the current episode – an acute, severe pneumonia of the right side – antibiosis with Amoxicillin + Clavulanic acid per PEG was administered simultaneously with Pulmo/Vivianit comp., s.c. injection between the shoulder blades, a daily mustard compress and oral treatment with potentized medicines as described above (including Tartarus stibiatus und Skorodit comp.). In the meantime, an oxygen concentrator was made available at home. Within 36 hours the 3 litres O_2 requirement had already reduced. The child recovered considerably more quickly from the pneumonia in comparison to all other clinic stays in the past when the pneumonia was treated exclusively with allopathic medicines and conventional physiotherapy.

5.1.1.6 Convalescence

The most important aspect of the convalescence phase following pneumonia is *awareness* that this phase is a reality and a necessity. If the doctor has a conscientious approach to convalescence, the child and parents will be favourably influenced; if neglected, secondary illnesses are likely to occur soon. The entire course of pneumonia spans three to four weeks, similar to measles for example.

- Adequate bed rest is essential; duration once the fever has subsided depends on:
- Coughing: Has the cough definitely started to loosen and relax or is an additional medication necessary e.g. Sulphur D30 or Tartarus stibiatus D6 or Tartarus stibiatus comp.?

- Circulation: Is it stable, for e. g. when the child sits up or goes to the bathroom?
- Medicines do not replace bed rest!
- Appetite: Has the child increasingly developed a good appetite? (This indicates that forces previously needed for the inflammation are again available for digestion.)

Bed rest is *imperative* and has a *decisive influence* on the course of the pneumonia: One must be aware that when antibiotics are not administered, the child overcomes the pneumonia – not the active substances in a medicine. All external treatments and internally administered medicines as described here serve only to stimulate and support. Therefore, with this approach, *everything depends on the child and the available system of forces.* Moreover, this system of potential healing forces is usually still *labile* when the fever subsides. Bed rest decisively fosters the necessary cohesion of body, soul and spiritual organizations. Today there is little awareness of this fact (in contrast to the pre-antibiotic era).

If too little attention is paid to this aspect, the novice doctor is likely to experience a setback precisely at this point, even if treatment has been effective up to then. The convalescence phase should be discussed with the parents and expectations set with regard to bed rest, how long the child will need to remain indoors, at what point he or she can go outdoors again, and when (in this sequence!) the child can return to kindergarten or school. The doctor can only fully support the latter from a medical point of view once the convalescence phase has come to a conclusion. In this context, "convalescence" actually means that *all* the body's forces – including the soul-spiritual forces – should be free to serve the recovery process. This becomes possible through adequate rest, maintaining of daily life rhythm, temporary withdrawal from social contexts and avoidance of any external intellectual challenges and demands.

If there is a need to generally build up and strengthen the child during or after the acute phase of the pneumonia, blackthorn elixir has proven to be beneficial, e. g.:

- **Schlehenelixier** Weleda
  5–15 ml, mornings, midday and possibly afternoons (disturbs sleep if given at night).

A good alternative:

- **Sanddornursaft** Weleda
  5 ml in the juice of ½ – 1 fresh orange, 1–2 x/day.

If the child has inappetence and a continued, productive cough that does not seem to progress to complete decongestion of exudate (which means that the child is ultimately unable to access and release sufficient warmth), the following medicine provides essential support during the convalescence phase following pneumonia:

- **Roseneisen/Graphit pillules,** Wala
  5–7(–10) pillules, 2–3 x/day.

In order to provide overall support for anchoring of the soul-spiritual individuality in the body and for the associated need to strengthen the warmth organization in the rhythmic system, administer:

- **Meteoreisen glob.** Wala
  5–7 pillules, mornings and aftertoons, augmented with:

- **Prunuseisen (iron prunus) pillules** Wala
  5–10 pillules, mornings and aftertoons.
  The latter is indicated for children with weak up-building capacities (excluding anaemia) and susceptibility to recurrent airway diseases (including obstructive airway disease).

For delayed decongestion of exudate and related symptoms (coughing, expectorate), the following medicines may be considered:

- **Sulphur iodatum D6 dil.** (▸Chap. 5.1.1.5.3)
  3–7 gtt., 3 x/day and
- **Tartarus stib. comp. trit.** Weleda (▸Chap. 2.3.2.2)
  1 saltsp., 2–3 x/day.

For labile circulation, the following medicines may be considered:

- **Skorodit Kreislauf glob.** Wala
  5–7 pillules, 3–5 x/day.
- **Cardiodoron® dil.** Weleda
  5–15 gtt., 3 x/day.

5.1.2 Rhinitis and sinusitis

5.1.2.1 Development and relevance of the body-soul relationship in the upper respiratory tract

"... thus one finds that just as ideation relates to nerve activity, the activity of feeling must be understood in relation to the life rhythm that is centered in breathing activity."

R. Steiner, Von Seelenrätseln
[Riddles of the Soul]

The midface of a newborn baby is hardly developed: The root of the nose does not yet project from the face and the paranasal sinuses are only beginning to pneumatize. The way in which the paranasal sinuses, teeth and jaw develop is as decisive for the individual shape of the midface as cephalization for the form of the neurocranium. The form of the newborn infant's face displays almost no interrelationship between the forehead and the eye area (nerve-sense pole of the head) on the one hand and the mouth area on the other. Physiologically, the brain and digestive/metabolic activity undergo rapid growth and development characterized by an immense dynamic. Many aspects of behaviour and pathology are the result of the infant's incapacity to form a balancing middle realm between the two poles of its organism. This is evident in the baby's irritability in relation to digestive processes (▸Chap. 4.3) and susceptibility of the sense organs (e. g. in the middle ear) and the central nervous system (e. g. bacterial meningitis) to inflammatory processes.

The rhythmic system – expressed in respiration, blood circulation, core areas of the immune system and related rhythmic processes in the body (e.g. hormone secretion) [Steiner 1921, 230–252; Rohen 2000] – is at work between the nervous and metabolic systems and is responsible for ensuring the necessary division, interplay and balance between these two systems. The rhythmic system gradually gains autonomy and stability after birth – and to the extent that the child's own rhythmic system has strengthened and can fulfill its tasks of division and mediation between metabolic/digestive processes and nerve-sense processes, so the child's susceptibility to illness decreases and mortality reaches its absolute lifetime minimum around the age of 12, i.e. before onset of puberty. [1] This process comes to expression in the shaping and refining of the midface and thorax, and inside the nose, in the forming of the nasal conchae – appearing "as if shaped by the rhythmically alternating stream of inhaled and exhaled air" [Girke 2010, 136].

During infancy, the adult – especially the breastfeeding mother – provides the child with important qualities of the rhythmic system, "lending" these qualities, so to speak. Organization of the sleeping-waking rhythm and the feeding rhythm are fundamental to this early parent-child symbiosis and breast milk itself is vitally important for development of the infant's own independently functioning rhythmic system (▸Chap. 4.1, 4.3).

The activity of the rhythmic system reveals itself most clearly in the breathing process. If one observes the infant's respiratory activity, freely and without preconceptions, one can perceive directly how *all sensations, feelings, emotions – that is, all soul states, from pain to dreaming – are reflected by changes in breathing:* Indeed, there is a direct correlation between respiration and the soul's experience of feeling. Breathing is the primordial expression of soul activity in the body.

The child does not breathe on its own while living in the maternal uterus; placental circulation is more like being ventilated. The first breath of life signifies the awakening of the soul in the body: The soul actively takes up residence in the body and begins to express itself via this bodily instrument. Breathing enables the human being's most personal form of expression: Speech.

At the moment of birth, active mediation between "outer" and "inner" through breathing becomes necessary for the first time. At the same time, breathing influences the division of the blood circulation into arterial and venous systems – which merge again with one another inside the lung as well as in the periphery. Thus breathing and blood circulation are responsible for the necessary division of and mediation between the unconscious metabolic region and the nerve sense organization that forms the basis for consciousness.

Purely from a phenomenological point of view, a major cause of infant death (in highly industrialized countries) is the cessation of rhythmical breathing activity (SIDS, ▸Chap. 2.2.2). Sudden Infant Death Syndrome (SIDS) does not occur after the age of 9 to 14 months (the phase during which the child usually begins to be able to stand up): At this developmental point, the child's own breathing rhythm has become more constant and the rhythmic system has stabilized the presence of the soul entity within the physical-etheric organism.

The infant is wholly dependent on nasal breathing for respiratory activity: Total obstruction of the nose is life threatening! Therefore pronounced rhinitis at this age can be a serious illness. During early childhood, rhinitis is often the starting point for otitis media, laryngotracheitis, sinusitis (ethmoidalis, maxillaris) or bronchitis. As the child gets older, the common cold or "sniffles" are considered to be mundane, everyday ailments and chronic rhinitis are often neglected as unimportant symptoms. Yet, these illnesses are usually a sign of a deeper lying disturbance – of possible adenoids and tonsillar hypertrophy, and increasingly today, also of allergies and occult chronic sinusitis.

1 During the past 100 years this minimum has moved forward from 14 to 12 years of age, parallel to the earlier onset of puberty [Keller und Wiskott 1991, 67; Husemann und Wolff 1991, 37].

Chronically obstructed nasal breathing and hampered pneumatization of the middle ear and paranasal sinuses compromise the child's soul-body lucency: Consciousness becomes duller, speech loses its timbre and clarity, hearing ability can be restricted and sleep is interrupted and less refreshing. Fatigue, irritability and weakening of individual will are the consequence.

Nasal and nasal sinus inflammation

Every acute nasal and paranasal sinus inflammation should receive proper attention and thorough treatment. Given environmental conditions today, acute rhinitis frequently develops into a progressive or chronically persisting disorder that tends to be exacerbated by purely suppressive "symptomatic" treatment.

The outside air becomes saturated with water vapour through physiological processes taking place via nasal breathing; it is perceived by the soul organization by means of the sense of smell and is warmed according to the individual's own warmth capacity (even at –20 °C outdoor temperature, the air temperature can rise to +34 °C within seconds). The nasal passages create a bridge – a meeting point – for the inhaled air with the life-soul imbued organism. Oral breathing, on the other hand, assimilates the outside air inadequately. Therefore chronically obstructed nasal breathing actually causes illness and is often the root cause of relapsing infections of the lower airways or of bronchial hyperreactivity.

The significance of the paranasal sinuses for the body-soul organization is not as obvious [Niewind 1992, 31–43]. *Pneumatization* of the cranium through the formation of air-filled cavities – i. e. the paranasal sinuses, middle ear and mastoid cells – *comes to completion at the same time that the soul entity awakes within the physical-etheric organism*. Typically, the paranasal sinuses are ventilated during the *exhalation phase*, i. e. the phase of breathing that also facilitates *human expression* in singing and speech. This type of air-filled cavity is the physical expression of *inner ensoulment of the living (i. e. of the life entity)*: The plant does not usually create such inner spaces but only approximates these in its flower formation, the latter bearing a relationship to the soul/animal sphere.

During the process of pneumatization (i. e. after birth), *breathing* – and thereby the child's individual soul activity – is directly involved in further formation of the body, especially transformation of the midface and development of its unique form. The form of the mouth-chin region is influenced by activity in the metabolism and limbs, while the forehead and eye region are created in tandem with formation of the central nervous system. It can be diagnostically helpful to observe the human face in this differentiated way [Glas 1935, Lievegoed 1995].

This suggests that it can be diagnostically relevant to know whether the rhinitis or sinusitis is: (▸Chap. 5.1.3, similar for otitis media)

- an expression of an *excessively vital* metabolism that has overshot its boundaries and now, in the form of a "metabolic process in the wrong place" (in the maxillae, for example), sets a process in motion that would typically form part of the physiology of the intestinal region (glandular secretion, cessation of pneumatization);
- or if the rhinitis/sinusitis *already represents a reaction* to overly strong formative and breaking down processes in the organism that cannot be countered because of insufficient vitality in the organism (compare with ▸Chap. 5.1.1.2).

If the rhinitis/sinusitis tends to be chronic (chronically compromised pneumatization with few or no acute signs of illness), consider if the problem is rooted in:

- nerve-sense activity overload
- a constitutional weakness in the warmth and metabolic organization.

The approach to treatment will be very different depending on the answers to these questions. As always, when dealing with a disease of the rhythmic system, the situation of the two interplaying polar systems that potentially influence and overtax the rhythmic system must be evaluated, and then stimulated, supported and formed therapeutically in such a way that they continue to develop in their rightful location in the body. *From this point of view, the treatment for rhinitis and sinusitis aims to free the "breathing middle" of the human being – not only of the one-sided predominance of inflammatory and metabolic processes, but also of the excessive breakdown caused by activity (and overload) of the consciousness pole.*

In addition to medicinal treatment for rhinitis and sinusitis presented below, recommendations are also made for nutrition, home environment and holiday arrangements; singing and artistic therapies for older children (eurythmy therapy, speech therapy) as well as how to address soul aspects of the child's living environment. The language of everyday life itself indicates that psychosomatic factors can also contribute to chronically compromised pneumatization (pneumatization could be freely translated from the Greek as "ensoulment"): What has the child "had enough of" (translation of the German idiom "die Nase voll haben" [to have a full nose!]) and what is it the child is "sick and tired of hearing"?

5.1.2.2 Acute rhinitis and rhinoconjunctivitis in infancy

During the first year of life, acute rhinitis can cause sleep disturbances that may include night-time respiratory distress and feeding difficulties. The basic medication to be administered at this age is:

- **Sambucus nigra D4–6** (various manufacturers)
  3–5 pillules before each breastfeeding or mealtime.

The yellow-white elderflower has a pungent, unsubtle aromatic fragrance. The plant's dynamic is less refined but all the more vital, and can be described as "sulphuric" or "sulphur-related" because of its tendency to transition from a watery gesture to a more airy gesture [Steiner 1963, 122]. Elderflower has diaphoretic and mucolytic effects on the human being. The marrow of stems and branches consist of a white, spongy pulp while the bark is peppered with lenticels (airy aggregations of cells functioning as pores). The black elder has a particularly strong relationship to the air but also loves damp, partly shady locations; it absorbs a large amount of water that is subsequently "breathed out" into the air via leaves and flowers [Pelikan 1977, 121]. The leaves and flowers contain Sambunigrin which releases hydrogen cyanide (prussic acid) and other poisonous substances. The homoeopathic medicine proving for this substance suggests a relationship to airway spasms (obstructive laryngitis, bronchial asthma), whereby the symptom "awakening suddenly, struggling for air" is especially typical for *Sambucus nigra* [Stübler and Krug 1988, 793].

Case study

(D. Scholl [Vademecum 2010, 733])

A four-month-old male infant who could not be breastfed became ill with an upper airway infection for the first time. An acute cold developed a week later, causing the baby to awake with a blocked nose at about 02h00, with dyspnoea during the remainder of the night. The mother was very concerned and distraught by the situation. The next night the boy slept intermittently and was restless throughout the night. Sambucus nigra D4 pillules, 5 x/day was prescribed. The symptoms were already considerably better the following night and the dyspnea abated completely. The boy was able to sleep through the night thereafter.

In the case of infants, the airways can stenose rapidly when metabolic activity gains the upper hand, especially at night when the conscious toning activity of the soul recedes and a slight tendency to water retention and mucosal swelling comes about naturally, i. e. physiologically. The respiratory tract threatens to regress to a fluid-filled embryonal state in the process, similar to the intestinal tract that was its developmental origins. In this case the spasm-like, fearful awakening is the *soul's reaction* to the swelling up of the airways: As the child struggles for pneumatization his panic-like overreaction aggravates the situation even more. Potentized Sambucus nigra can help to avert this danger in the region of the nose and larynx (obstructive laryngitis, so-called pseudocroup) by counteracting the mucosal swelling and the pathological overreaction of the soul. *An infusion of elderflower and lime blossom tea with a little honey and lemon* has a mucolytic and warming effect, and should mostly be administered in favour of conventional mucolytics.

Every acute rhinitis may be presenting the early symptoms of a *disturbance in the warmth organization*. With regard to infants, *adequate covering and protection of the head* is of particular concern: During the first year of life the head forms 20 % of the child's body area; if uncovered and unprotected a great deal of warmth radiates out of the head. Especially in the case of delicately built, metabolically weak infants, the wearing of appropriate protective headgear – even inside the home – will reduce susceptibility to infection.

For *local treatment* of a blocked nose in infants, it is best to apply breast milk, trickling a few drops into the nose. For more severe nasal obstruction, apply strongly concentrated chamomile tea saturated with sugar alternating with breast milk or physiological saline solution. Decongestant nasal drops can usually be avoided. Some infants and toddlers react adversely to the alpha-sympathicomimetica ingredients in these products with intense general restlessness (▸Chap. 5.1.2.2).

If there is a tendency to dry obstruction of the nasal passages following the catarrhal stage of rhinitis, for infants from 6 months of age, apply a mild nasal balm to the nasal wings and vestibule, for example:

- **Nasal balm for children** Wala.

External application of the following ointment has proven effective for *persistent rhinitis*:

- **Dr. Bach Emergency Cream** (Bach Notfallsalbe)
  Apply to entire midface region.

5

If the rhinitis is accompanied by purulent *conjunctivitis*, the following treatment is so effective that antibiotic eye drops are unnecessary in most cases:

- **Pulsatilla D12 pillules** DHU
  3 pillules, 3 x/d

alternating with:

- **Silicea comp. pillules** Wala
  3 pillules, 3 x/d.

plus administration of

- **Calendula D4 eye drops** Weleda

alternating frequently (! – each preparation 3 x/d if possible) with

- **Mercurialis eye drops** Wala

The following medicines are indicated if the catarrh is greenish-yellow and the rhinitis *is tending to worsen* to the extent of (obstructive) bronchitis:

- **Natrium sulf. D6–12 pillules** (various manufacturers)
  3–5 pillules, 5 x/day,

possibly combined with Pulsatilla. This stimulates bile secretion and encourages a more intensive connection between the sentient and warmth organizations and the metabolism (compare with ▸Chap. 5.1.2.3)

- **Sticta pulm. D6–12 pillules** (various manufacturers)

may be considered if the child has a cough that initially started with a cold or the sniffles and progressed to irritation of the windpipe.

5.1.2.3 Acute and cumulatively recurrent rhinitis in childhood

The doctor is seldom asked to treat the acute cold but is frequently confronted with its more serious sequelae: otitis media, sinusitis and bronchitis. This indicates how important it is to deal with acute rhinitis in the right way from the outset. It is well worth informing parents about rhinitis prophylaxis and treatment because many secondary illnesses and recurrences can be prevented if these measures are carried out conscientiously.

Dry nasal mucosa is a central, but often overlooked problem, occurring frequently in larger cities. Helpful lifestyle measures include: a healthy living environment, ensuring adequate humidity in living areas (measure with a hygrometer! Aim for values >45%), avoiding underfloor heating – preferably without compromise (!), providing opportunities for exercise and play in clean air regions, ensuring healthy nutrition and sufficient fluids (but avoiding sweetened drinks or processed fruit juices).

The following products are suitable for *nasal care:*

- **Rhinodoron Nasal spray** Weleda
  1 spray (= 1 dose), several x/day (contains aloe vera for moisturizing care)
- **Nasal balm for children** Wala
  Apply especially at night. This is a suitable nasal balm for allergy sufferers of all ages.

An integral part of prophylaxis and treatment that has proven effective in practice is the application of a *warm footbath at night (gradually increasing temperature)* followed by a *light leg massage* with **Malva comp. oil,** Wala (▸Chap. 2.2.1), for example. This directly activates the warmth organization and simultaneously conducts any excessive tendency to inflammation downwards, away from the head pole and out to the periphery. This treatment addresses a frequently encountered root cause of rhinitis and sinusitis: inadequate *warmth generation* in the limbs, especially the lower extremities.

Stressing the metabolism through incorrect nutrition, medication (e. g. antibiotics) and toxic substances (▸Chap. 4.6; ▸Chap. 6.3.3.2) creates a disposition to illness, i. e. susceptibility to upper airways infections. With regard to *nutrition,* a light, well-balanced diet is important; a break taken from milk and fruit juices, warm drinks such as lime blossom and elderflower tea (mentioned above) with a little lemon juice or a vegetable soup (age-appropriate seasoning) provide essential support for the child's life and warmth organizations. Especially refined sugar in all forms should be avoided.

There are many different possibilities for medication; in cases of preexistent stress on the metabolism, the following medication has proven effective:

- **Agropyron Inject. amp./glob. velati** Wala
  acute: 0.5 ml per os, 4 x/day or 5–10 pillules, 4 x/day for 5 days

This medicinal composition activates the lymphatic system, primarily through the potentized mercury sulphide compound (Cinnabar D6), liver-gall function (Taraxacum D4, Potassium carb. D9) and the boundary interface function of the mucosa (Agropyron e rad. D4). It is also effective for an accompanying sore throat ("red throat") and laryngotracheal irritation. Vitalization of metabolic processes below the diaphragm (Taraxacum, Potassium carb. and Agropyron influence the liver-gall system) is accompanied by a simultaneous reduction in inflammatory processes in the nose and throat region. This exemplifies one of the basic treatment principles of anthropsophic medicine: To regulate with sustained effect.

The following medications can be administered if one wants to curtail a heavily streaming rhinitis:

- **Allium Cepa D6 pillules** (various manufacturers)
  5 pillules per dose

alternating frequently with

- **Camphora D3 amp.** Wala
  0.2 ml per dose, (total amount: 1–2 ampoules)

The strong sulphuric qualities of the kitchen onion work here together with the potentized Camphora, which powerfully activates the warmth organization.

Local treatment with decongestant nose drops is almost always questionable because these products weaken mucosa function and do not actually promote healing of any kind.

The authors prefer application of:

- **Nasenbalsam (nose balm)** Wala
  Apply 2–3 x/day. (In cases of manifest inflammation, for children from 4 years of age this preparation is clearly more effective than **Nose balm for children (Wala);** this balm is both decongestant and soothing).

For a severely blocked nose and viscous mucous secretions, alternate with

- **Emser Nasal Spray**
  1–3 sprays, several x/day (see also Emser Nasal Douche, ▸Chap. 5.1.2.4.2)
- **Heuschnupfenspray** (hay fever spray) Weleda
  1 spray in each nostril, 3–5 x/day

Containing a 1% Gencydo-solution of lemon and quince (cf ▸Chap. 6.6), this spray has decongestant and formative effects, and is helpful when the mucosa swelling is accompanied by watery secretions or nasal obstruction, and especially so for children with allergies to inhaled allergens, e. g. house dust and house mites (today this is increasingly the case early on in childhood).

If there is a known tendency to *recurrent infections of the upper airways,* there is often still an underlying relative weakness in the formative-structural forces that are crucial for maturation and stabilization of the organism's boundary surfaces. A weakness in this formative process can be effectively treated with potentized silicic acid (▸Chap. 5.1.2.4.3).

The herbal silicic acid medicine, Equisetum Silicea cultum Weleda (▸Chap. 1.2.2), has a formative and internally light-bringing effect:

- **Equisetum Silicea cultum D2 dil.** Weleda
  3–7 gtt., 3 x/day

The effect of this medicine is clearly more intense when it is administered in combination with low potentcy sulphur (which has a vitalizing and warming effect):

- **Sulphur D6 trit.** Weleda
  1 saltsp., 1–2 x/day

Administration of these medicines in combination, over a sufficiently long period can have a sustained strengthening effect on the young constitution (▸Chap. 6.3.3.3).

Complementary treatment with a daily *warm footbath (gradually increasing temperature)* and/or a light oil massage with:

- **Malva comp. oil** Wala
  at night for 4–6 weeks, from the beginning of the cold period.

In cases of strong susceptibility to infection and tendency to allergies, treatment with potentized autologous blood can bring about a considerable stabilization of immunity:

- **potentized autologous blood** according to Imhäuser [2000, 187] from the beginning of autumn.
  3 gtt. C5 per day, per os, mane for 3 weeks. Thereafter, 3–5 gtt. of the following potencies to be taken 3 x/week: C7 for 6 weeks, C9 for 6 weeks (and possibly C12). (▸Chap. 5.4.4.2)

Within the context of a rhinitis infection or rhinitis that has already developed an allergic component, many pre-school children suffer from *nasal obstruction at night* which has an adverse effect on sleep and general well-being. (This problem should be recognized as distinct from adenoids). Following the advice of Reinhard Schwarz, the authors have meanwhile found the following medication to be consistently effective [Vademecum 2010, 573]:

- **Marum verum D4 (D1–6) pillules/dil.** DHU or Weleda dispensary **(dil.)**
  5–10 pillules/gtt., 1 × (nocte) – 3 x/day.

This medicine can be administered from early infancy onwards. In some cases *nasal polyps* in older children are also be positively influenced by this medication (D1, cf Vademecum l. c.).

Individualized constitutional treatment can provide profound support for the child's respiratory system. There are various starting points for determining the appropriate treatment, including assessment of the child's own individual warmth organization, the relationship between the nerve-sense system and the metabolic system, the child's dietary preferences and habits and unique character of soul.

(Adenoids, ▸Chap. 5.2.4; allergic rhinitis, ▸Chap. 6.6.1).

5.1.2.4 Acute sinusitis

5.1.2.4.1 Aspects of history taking and diagnosis

In many cases, the primary difference between an acute sinusitis requiring treatment and rhinitis is a *decline in general condition.* Whereas after infancy rhinitis is experienced adversely in the soul sphere (adverse effects on breathing, onset of sleep, ability to concentrate), in the case of sinusitis one can immediately see how inflammation of the paranasal sinuses fundamentally compromises the child's *vitality and warmth organism* and reactively challenges it. One may suspect sinusitis if there is a general feeling of being weak and unwell, typical changes in the facial appearance, "occult" fever with variable course (can be protracted) and if other locatable causes have been excluded. The periphery as well as kidney and abdominal regions are often relatively cool (for differential diagnosis, it is important to exclude a urinary tract infection). Landmark symptoms include rhinitis (possibly prevailing for some time – although it can also be almost non-existent), streams of purulent mucous down the back of the throat, moderately pressure-sensitive swellings in the regional lymph nodes (appearing like a string of pearls), coughing when lying down and getting up, deep shadows under the eyes, a feeling of pressure on the root of the nose and frontal lobe headaches (especially when bending down). Children of pre-school age may not have any pain, also not the percussion pain associated with acute sinusitis (even in severe cases): Pain only comes to the fore as the soul entity becomes increasingly established in the organism, as with teenagers and adults who experience sinusitis pain particularly intensely.

The younger the child, the more likely that fever will be a predominating symptom. The authors observed the case of an 18-month old girl with sinusitis ethmoidalis and maxillaris (confirmed by imaging procedures) who had fever continuously for seven weeks prior to hospital admission and subsequent diagnosis. The family doctor had been unable to establish a diagnosis due to lack of clearly identifiable local symptoms! In the case of a severe infection of the upper airways – and careful exclusion of other causes – this situation shows that it is not necessarily a mistake to include treatment for a possible case of sinusitis. As a rule, a febrile illness course – during which the child's warmth organization and immune system are more active than usual – tends to result in a more thorough recovery than sinusitis with a subfebrile or afebrile course, the latter being more typical in adults (high rate of chronic sinusitis). *Antibiotic treatment* may be unavoidable at times, as in the case of an orbital phlegmona, severely compromised vitality or within the context of

5

a severe adolescent crisis. In principle, however, antibiotics weaken the life and warmth organizations with the result that in a certain sense the patient is more ill after the treatment than before. In such cases the sinusitis is only likely to heal completely after follow-up treatment which has taken the antibiotic treatment into consideration.

The following factors are aetiologically and therapeutically relevant to sinusitis in children:

- Exposure to cold draughts e. g. cycling in winter when the body's own capacity for warmth generation is insufficient.
- Rapid and unnoticed cooling down in the evening e. g. in early autumn.
- Public swimming pools: Children absorb considerable amounts of toxic chloric gases; a reduction in body temperature due to evaporating moisture is almost unavoidable, especially during swimming lessons at school; swimming pool water gets into the upper airways when the children jump or dive. Therefore a long-term ban on swimming pools visits is often unavoidable! On the other hand, sauna visits (age-appropriate) have proven to have a prophylactic effect.
- Television and particularly computer screens devitalize the eyes and midface in numerous ways, including changes to breathing and motor functions, and withdrawal of the soul, with the result that the bodily-oriented activity of the soul entity (pneumatization!) is weakened.
- Bad teeth and defective dental fillings with local pain in the upper jaw (possibly only on palpation), purulent fistulae etc. should be treated by a dentist and not left unattended because of purely orthodontic considerations (so-called "placeholder" argument).

All the above-mentioned factors are of relevance for history taking and when advising parents regarding treatment.

Recent studies [Dykewitz 2010] consider that most acute upper airway inflammations with paranasal sinus involvement are usually viral during the early illness phase. "Bacterial sources are more probable" if the illness course exceeds 7–10 days.

5.1.2.4.2 External and local treatments

As with acute rhinitis, treatment of sinusitis begins with *warmth treatment* that aims to have a stimulating and draining ("drawing out") effect (▸Chap. 5.1.2.3):

- A warm footbath (gradually increasing temperature) with the addition of *mustard power* (3 tablespoons of fresh black mustard powder, water to about calf level); when the skin begins to redden, remove the feet from the footbath and rinse briefly with water.
- Follow by massaging the legs lightly with **Malva comp. oil (Mallow oil)** Wala.
- Dress warmly, with wool clothing if possible.

In terms of diet, the principles outlined in ▸Chap. 5.1.2.3 apply. An infusion of elderflower and lime blossom tea with a little lemon and possibly honey is as least as effective as conventional mucus dissolvers, and simultaneously has a strongly warming effect.

Local application of a nose rinse can be very helpful; for children from age 5 years use:

- **Emser® Nasal Douche**
  Mix about 250 ml water (body temperature) + 1 dosage packet of Emser® Sole. Use the nose rinse 1–2 x/day, at the washbasin [Michel 2005].

Nasal breathing can be further supported by

- use of a spray containing **Emser Sole** or sea salt solution

as well as application of

- **Nasal balm** Wala
  1–3 x/day, for children over 4 years. For children under 4 years use **Nasal balm for children**, Wala).

If the effect is insufficient, in cases of acute mucous build-up and congestion, short-term use of emulsions or peanut oil nasal inserts with menthol oil (0.2; max. 2% for nasal inserts) and eucalyptus oil, possibly combined with infrared light treatment, can be helpful.

Very helpful in cases of acute sinusitis is to lightly massage the forehead and midface region with:

- **Vespa crabro 1% ointment** Weleda
  Apply mane, especially for pain and build-up/congestion of purulent
  Apply up to 3 x/day

For a mild or abating illness course:

- **Carex arenaria 1 ointment** Weleda dispensary
  Apply 1–2 x/day, especially nocte

In acute cases, a horseradish compress is suitable for the above-mentioned body areas, especially when there is acute pain.

5.1.2.4.3 Medication

Potentized silicic acid is a centrally important substance for internal treatment of sinusitis. Pneumatization of the paranasal sinuses and the middle ear takes place in the direct vicinity of the bones (mucosa and periosteum are directly involved). This process is refined and reduced to a physically indispensable minimum in the midface region (where the skeleton is partially translucent and some areas are only divided by a membrane). A barrier to the outside air is formed inside the middle ear via the pneumatization process. The resulting structure has the capacity for "vibration", thus providing the basis for sound perception (i. e. the process of becoming conscious of rhythmical vibrations in the outside air). The middle ear and paranasal sinuses also form their *own interior air space* as a kind of "living-room" for the soul (within which the exhaled breath pneumatizes!). The nature of this space significantly influences how the soul element comes to expression in the body (▸Chap. 5.1.2.1). From the point of view of anthroposophical medicine this formative process is intimately connected to the quality of silicic acid as "physical basis of the I-organization" [Steiner und Wegman 1977, 76–80].

In nature, the silicic acid found in quartz crystal has a tendency to develop completely transparent but solid and chemically inert forms that have released all their internal warmth. On the other hand, an aqueous dispersion of silicic acid will form *colloids.* Even in their inorganic state, these colloids are already reminiscent of unique, living organizations. All living, structured liquids in the human body such as blood plasma have a colloidal character. It is remarkable that already in an inorganic state, silicic acid colloids have a relationship to *rhythm and rhythmical structure.* During the formation of agate, silicic acid oscillates rhythmically between the life-like gel condition and the strictly tetrahaedral crystallization of the quartz form.[1] Therefore each agate – each colloidal system – develops an *irreplicable individual form.* This is unusual in an inorganic substance and is fundamentally related to the aspect of rhythm [Roemer et al. 2009]. Silicic acid also has a specific tendency to *delicate, symmetric* form: this is illustrated by the comparison of the (carbonic) calcium skeleton of foraminifers with the silicic acid-containing skeletons of the radiolariae.

In 1925, when many of these scientific facts were still unknown, Rudolf Steiner emphasized the significance of silicic acid for the *individual* aspect of formation of the human body. During formation of the body, specifically in those areas where "the living becomes lifeless" [Steiner und Wegman 1977, 76–80] (for example, internally in bone formation and externally in the epidermis, hair and nails), the human individuality – via the I-organization – uses the kindred silicic acid to ensure that the formative process proceeds in favour of its own individual program. In fact recent research has confirmed, for example, that a relative accumulation of silicic acid during bone formation *before* calcium deposition can induce periosteal ossification[2] [Ciba Foundation 1986].

The human organism needs the qualities of silicic acid – (i. e. colloidal organization of fluids, receptivity to rhythmical processes, an intrinsic tendency to release warmth and, in contrast to calcium carbonate, the tendency to create a solid but transparent form) – so that it can isolate itself from the vital metabolic processes internally and the processes of nature externally in such a way that a space is created between the two poles in which *consciousness* can develop. The sense organs and the entire periphery of the human organism isolate the body from the outer environment and, via the process of perception, enable the human being to become *"consciousness of this environment"*– that is, they enable soul-spiritual transparency of the physical boundaries of the body. The human I-organization forms the human body and its boundaries inwardly (e. g. skeleton formation) so that the organism can become an instrument and expression of free human will (e. g. in being able to walk upright) thus enabling the light of human consciousness in self-determined activity to radiate outwards. Silicic acid is a kindred substance to the human individuality because it can form solid, finely shaped boundaries out of the fluid-life element while on the other hand it also enables transparency between the unconscious inner and outer worlds and human consciousness.

A pathological situation can arise in this respect when the formative process related to silicic acid does not assert itself sufficiently, and inadequate pneumatization creates a breeding ground for inflammatory processes. The middle ear and paranasal sinuses remain "too embryonic" [Vogel 1995, 178f.], catarrhal processes block out the air and thus a hothouse for autonomous inflammatory illness processes is created.

1 The body of agate is formed by means of an internal rhythm – not by global external rhythms (emphasis in original text). As emphasized by A. von Zuzaghi, already early on in 1936, agate has the same inclination as every colloidal system: the tendency to individuality. Each [...] colloidal system appears as a unique, one-off individual; all its characteristics and the changes that it undergoes are individual; its entire life is individual [Wimmerauer 1992, 158].

2 The authors are grateful to B. von Laue for this indication.

In this situation, high potency silicea may strengthen the organism's formative capacity in the fluid-life element, thus containing the inflammation and helping it to abate. The anthroposophic composition medicine

- **Silicea comp pillules/amp.** Wala

moderates reactive oversensitivity in the soul and inflammation-inducing activity by means of combined potentization with Argentum nitricum and Belladonna [see also, "Leitgedanke und Indikation von Silicea comp." (medicine principle) in: Vademecum 2010, 748].

Even though closely related, the above-described situation must be distinguished from that in which the entire organism displays an "aging" tendency, thereby cultivating too little growth, movement and warmth, and where form predominates over vitality. As a result the areas of the body occupied by the rhythmic system *cool down internally* and thus the organism becomes susceptible to outer cold and other devitalizing influences. Here the inflammation has a secondary character but will relapse and become chronic (with increasing age) if the root cause is not remedied, and if vitality and the warmth organization are not sufficiently strengthened. The mucous has a viscous nature and discharge is sluggish. In these cases, it has proven effective to initially use *sulphur-containing medicines* (Hepar sulfuris, Kalium sulfuricum, Cinnabaris) to restore the balance between vitality and form in the paranasal sinsuses followed by potentized silicic acid to stimulate the I-organization in both its formative and warmth-generating effects.

Suitable *basic treatment* for acute, febrile sinusitis with few local symptoms:

- **Silicea comp. pillules** Wala or **Argentum/Berberis comp. dil.** Weleda
  5–7 pillules, about. 5 x/day or 5–10 gtt., 5 x/day

After fever abates until full recovery:

- **Berberis/Quarz pillules** Wala
  5–10 pillules, 3 x/day for 2–3 weeks.

As a rule, a *sulphuric-dissolving* component is vital during acute treatment nowadays. A universally suitable extension of the above-described treatment is

- **Myristica sebifera comp. pillules** Wala
  Acute: 5–7 pillules, 5 x/day; during illness course: 5–7 pillules, 3 x/day for about 1 week up to 10 days.

Myristica sebifera comp. (also contains Kalium bichromicum and Argentum nitricum) dissolves congested mucous and supports drainage of viscous, purulent discharge. An evergreen tree growing in the tropical forests of South America, Myristica sebifera produces a glowing red bark sap ("Kino") in the cambium-like layers of bast and wood, thereby bringing a sulphuric quality (belonging to the flowering pole) into the saline-woody ligneous trunk. Local inhabitants drain the tree sap by scoring the bark and use it to treat inflammatory conditions occurring in the head area (aphthae, dental decay). The relationship of this plant process to sinusitis becomes clearer if one considers the nature of the inflammatory changes in the mucoperiost of the paranasal sinuses and also the image of reddened, swollen mucosa directly adjacent to boney structures [Bartke-Anders 2003, Girke 2010, 137, Seideneder 2008, 7848–50, Vademecum 2010, 604–605].

5

If pain is clearly apparent at the beginning of the illness course, arnica is effective as a supplementary treatment (compare below, injections):

- **Arnica e pl. tota D12 pillules** Wala/Weleda
  5 pillules/gtt., 3–5 x/day

Arnica and Silicea comp., or Argentum/Berberis comp. and Myristica sebifera comp. can be administered initially, until there is some improvement in the symptoms.
In cases of febrile, purulent inflammation in the paranasal sinuses and/or middle ear, beneficial supplementary treatment is offered by:

- **Echinacea/Mercurius comp. supp.** Wala
  Especially nocte, for fever: 1 suppository, 2 x/day.

By means of supplementary medication with this composition of Apis Belladonna and Mercurius solubilis combined with Echinacea and Argentum, it is often possible to control a therapeutically challenging febrile inflammatory process with severe mucous congestion and bacterial superinfection without antibiotics – also in severe cases. Treatment of rhinosinusitis with these suppositories belongs to the authors' standard treatment repertoire for children with mucoviscidosis, Down's syndrome, other limitations in midface respiration and susceptibility to infection.

Subacute, purulent sinusitis with a decline in general condition and relatively low inflammatory activity is evidence of insufficient and weakened vitality. This condition can be treated initially with:

- **Agropyron Inject amp./glob. velati** Wala
  ½ ampoule per os, 3–4 x/day or 5–10 pillules, 4 x/day (▸Chap. 5.1.2.3) and
- **Vespa crabro Gl D6–8 amp.** Wala/Weleda
  ½ ampoule per os, 2 x/day

Vespa crabro, derived from the hornet, specifically stimulates pneumatization and self-cleaning of the paranasal sinuses [Husemann 1989, Vademecum 2010, 821f.] and is suitable for combination with other medications should the illness course become too protracted.

From age 5 to 7 years onwards the inflammation increasingly *localizes* in specific sinus cavities. Manifestation of the illness becomes more and more differentiated. Nowadays *reduced vitality* – as a preexisting illness disposition – is on the increase, with the result that treatment needs to address two aspects: Strengthening of the organism's formative powers in relation to the inflammation, and stimulation of the metabolism. Specific single substance homoeopathic medicines have shown to be effective for this situation: Lower potencies should be administered initially in order to release the mucous congestion, bring it into flow and maintain the moving discharge. These medicines are an alternative to Myristica sebifera (see above).

The most important single substance medicine for sinusitis maxillaris:

- **Kalium bichromicum D6 dil.** (various manufacturers)
  5–7 gtt., 5 x/day

For sinusitis ethmoidalis and frontalis:

- **Cinnabar D6 tab.** Weleda
  ½–1 tablet, 5 x/day

For viscous, purulent mucous, combine with

- **Hydrastis D6 dil.** (various manufacturers)
  5–7 gtt., 5 x/day

to further support internal treatment.

If the patient experiences *sensitivity to cold and pain* as described above, or the anamnesis suggests toxic overload (e. g. antibiotics, amalgam) consider:

- **Hepar sulfuris D6 trit.** Weleda
  1 saltsp. 2–5 x/day

This medicine is also suitable when a cough is a major symptom from the beginning of the illness course.

Injections are an essential component of the treatment program for teenagers (and adults), especially at the start of treatment in order to rapidly alleviate pain, improve the patient's general condition and thus avoid antibiotic treatment. *Potentized organ preparations* play an important role in this form of treatment: The mucosae respond more reliably and more rapidly to specifically targeted treatment with a homologous organ preparation. Higher potencies have a decongestant-deturgescent and formative effect, whereas lower potencies stimulate vitality and mucosa functionality.

When both pain and inflammatory activity are severe, the following combination is suitable in a mixed injection:

- **Silicea comp. amp.** Wala
- **Membrana sinuum paranasalium Gl D15 amp.** Wala
  Administer mixed injection s.c., nuchal at C7 – Th2 (ipsilateral when clearly one side is affected).

For ondontogenous sinusitis:

- **Periodontium/Silicea comp. amp.** Wala
  Administer mixed injection nuchal or locally in the fold of the gingiva (only possible from a certain age; otherwise administer per os)

For a tendency to mucous congestion and weak mucosa function

- **Vespa crabro Gl D8 amp.** Wala
- **Myristica sebifera comp. amp./pillules** Wala

are suitable supplementary treatment, s.c. aa mixed injection, nuchal. 2 x/week; or Vespa crabro per os 3 x/day, Myristica sebifera comp. 7 pillules/day for 7 days.

If the illness course stagnates within the first 3–4 days, internal medication for one day, the following is suitable as an intermediary medication:

- **Mercurius sol. D/C30 pillules** (various manufacturers): dissolve 10 pillules in 30 ml water; sip the solution.
- This measure may contribute considerably to leading from the first acute-inflammatory illness phase into the second phase of dissolving and resorption.

5

If the patient appears weakened and distressed during this illness phase, among other things, this suggests a weakness in the digestive activity of the liver and pancreas, indicating that light forces are not taking sufficient effect within the life processes (immune system function is fundamentally dependent on this as illustrated previously by the link between Vitamin D-metabolism and the immune system). An important, cleansing/purifying remedy in such cases is

- **Sulphur jod. D6 dil.** DHU
  5 gtt. 3 x/day

This medicine is also very effective in cases of *sinubronchial syndrome* and *mucoviscidosis*.

- In case of (sub)-acute sinusitis with thick, greenish-yellow mucous, laryngeal irritation (compare with Hepar sulf.) with coughing, throat-clearing possibly an impending wet bronchitis and the tendency to eustachian salpingitis and mucotympanon:
- **Kalium sulfuricum D6–12 dil.** (various manufacturers)
  5–7 gtt. 2–3 x/day

is an important homoeopathic remedy.

5.1.2.5 Chronic sinusitis

Weakening of bodily vitality – especially due to acute inflammatory processes that have been suppressed, toxic influences or problems of a soul/psychological nature (in the broadest sense one may speak of a limitation in exhalation) – often creates the basis for chronic sinusitis to develop. Chronic-degenerative inflammation in the roots of the teeth is a significant cause of chronic sinusitis, especially in adults. If 5 %–10 % of all adults are affected by this condition nowadays, then the root of the problem can often be traced back to childhood. In paediatrics, it is important to be continually aware of the long-term consequences of one's actions.

In addition to an accurate diagnosis (frequently not achieved), clarification of aetiology [compare: Dykewicz 2010] and a full understanding of the patient's unique and individual constitution (as far as possible) are most important (▸Chap. 5.1.2.1). *Nasal polyps* should be diagnosed or excluded by an ear, nose and throat specialist, patho-genesis of allergies should be diagnosed and appropriately treated if necessary (▸Chap. 6.6). Full recovery from a chronic illness is rarely possible without truly individualized diagnosis and treatment. The following indications for treatment are provided only as general suggestions for a therapeutic approach.

In order to counteract "aging" in the organism and internal cooling down in the area of the upper respiratory tract which form a foundation for chronic sinusitis, all the medicinal measures and external preparations described in ▸Chap. 5.1.2.4 also constitute the treatment basis for this condition:

- Attention to nutrition, avoiding public swimming baths, cold draughts etc..
- Daily footbath followed by a light oil massage – until full recovery from the sinusitis!
- Promoting adequate outdoor activity, sauna, possibly planning a holiday in a warm sea climate.
- Daily application (light massage) with **Vespa crabro 1 %** and **Carex arenaria 1 % ointment.**

Combined potentization of Hepar sulfuris and Membrana sinuum paranasalium in a low potency has a very reliable effect on vitalizing the organs:

- **Hepar sulfuris comp. amp.** Wala
  Initially ½ – 1 ampoules per os, 1 x/day, possibly already in combination with
- **Formica D6 dil.** Weleda
  7 gtt., 2 x/day

In persistent cases with adolescent and adult patients the effect can be intensified with a mixed injection of

- **Hepar sulfuris comp. amp.** Wala
- **Formica ex animale Gl D12 amp.** Wala
  s.c. injection, level C7–Th2, each side of the spine

Following intial treatment with Hepar sulfuris comp., the most important internal medication is

- **Quartz D20 trit.** Weleda
  1 saltsp., 2 x/day (alternatively **Berberis/Quartz** Wala, 10 pillules, 2 x/day)

For weakened vitality, supplement with

- **Prunus spin. e flor. et summit. D3 pillules** Wala
  5 pillules, 2–3 x/day and
- **Formica D6–12 dil.** Weleda
  7 gtt., 2 x/day

The decayed remains of plants and animals in nature are processed, transformed and brought back into the earth's life and growth cycle with the help of red ant colonies. The red ant, Formica rufa, also cleanses surfaces where 'the living' pass over to 'the lifeless' (e. g. bark of trees) and protects these surfaces from parasitic occupation. As a colonizing insect, the ant embodies the digestive and immune systems of nature! This is evident in the excellent health of the trees in the vicinity of red ant heaps. "Therefore formic acid is an essential remedy for the exhausted, overloaded astral body that is unable to adequately fulfill its task in supporting the life organization with respect to warming, ventilation, movement and elimination […]. Internal and parenteral applications of formic acid have proved to be particularly effective for patients who, as a result of neurasthenic overload, tend to chilling, sclerosis and deposition in the respiratory system and connective tissue […][Vademecum 2010, 446, English edition 2009, 372]. This is often the case in children and teenagers. Formic acid can stimulate the organism to become active where the immune system has given up and where chronic inflammation arises due to insufficient vitality and chronically disturbed warmth conditions.

Nasal polyps are not easy to treat. Nevertheless, positive experience has been achieved with

- **Hay fever spray** Weleda
  1–2 sprays in the affected nostril, 3–5 x/day
- **Marum verum D1 dil.** Weleda dispensary10–15 gtt., 3 x/day [Vademecum 2010, 573]

5

With regard to injection treatment for school age children, an attempt can be made with a mixed injection combining

- **Tunica mucosa nasi D30 amp.** Wala
- **Citrus pericarpium D1 amp.** (special preparation, Weleda dispensary) 5 ml or 10 ml bottle (Durchstechflasche) with sterile filter, store in a cool place, not inhalative in this case, apply s.c)
  Each 1 ml in a mixed injection, 2–3 x/week, s.c. upper arm

In addition to dental treatment, the following medicines are appropriate if there are causes of dental origin

- **Magnesium fluoratum D12 pillules** Staufen pharmacy
  5 pillules, 1 x/day, alternating with
- **Periodontium/Silicea comp. amp.** Wala
  ½–1 ampoules per os, 1 x/day or every second day.

5.1.2.6 Eurythmy therapy for recurrent and chronic ventilation disorders and inflammation of the upper respiratory tract

Therapeutic *eurythmy exercises* provide effective treatment – with sustained effects – for relapsing, chronic inflammation and ventilation disorders of the upper airways, and can lead to far-reaching constitutional changes in school age children and teenagers. The patient learns specific movements that should be practiced regularly at home for a time (critical for success of the therapy). These movements directly affect breathing and ventilation of the paranasal sinuses and middle ear and have a stimulating, deturgescent effect on the life processes in these regions. The exercises also relax the often tense muscles in the neck and shoulders and improve posture and depth of breathing.

The main indications for eurythmy therapy are as follows:

- Pneumatization disorders of the middle ear, seromucotympanon, recurrent otitis media (frequently related to adenoids).
- Recurrent and chronic sinusitis.
- Chronic-recurrent or impending upper respiratory tract infections.

In addition to individual-constitutional exercises, the basic sound sequence "L – M –S" was given by Rudolf Steiner for this purpose [Steiner 1989, 191, Hachtel 2007, 436]. The vowel "U" can also be employed as a concluding movement, especially for older children and teenagers. It is important that the movements are carried out as they are learned in the eurythmy therapy session and practiced daily at home at an individually chosen time. As with physiotherapy, eurythmy therapy sessions are much more effective when daily practice at home can be integrated into the treatment program.

- "L" initially stimulates inhalation (the in-breath) and the life organization, thus providing the up-building processes in the fluid element with strengthened formative power. This reduces swelling.
- "M" regulates the balance between breathing and metabolism, directly promotes the pneumatization process (▸Chap. 5.1.2.1), intensifies the breathing process (especially

exhalation, the out-breath), and enables an overflowing metabolic process (secretion, discharge, inflammation) in the "wrong place" (in the respiration tract) to recede.

- Eurythmy therapy brings sluggish secretions into flow, helps the organism to bring chronic-inflammatory exudative processes to a conclusion and has a comprehensive eliminatory and cleansing effect. Activity of the formative soul forces that form the basis for development of the respiratory tract is intensified by the "S". These forces can be addressed as "mercurially" active forces. If acute inflammation is still present, the sound movement should only be carried out from above to below.
- "U." has an ordering and consolidating effect on the soul organization of the child and prevents nervous overactivity.

5.1.3 Otitis media

Acute otitis media is the most frequent grounds for parents taking their children to a doctor: the incidence of this condition doubled between 1975 and 1990. General trends show that acute otitis media (AOM) tends to be diagnosed too often and is also the illness that is most frequently treated with antibiotics in outpatient settings: 42 % of all antibiotic treatments for children are justified on the basis of AOM. At the same time antibiotic resistance is becoming more and more evident. Whereas almost all children are treated with antibiotics in Germany, the United Kingdom, Australia and the USA, less than 32 % is the case in the Netherlands

[Leitlinien 2010, N 6,1]

The ear displays a three-fold form: While the inner ear has already "achieved its final form and size" at birth [Rauber und Kopsch 1987, 570], the outer ear or *auricle* still continues to grow, even in old age. The outer ear varies individually with respect to size, position and form. Between the poles of birth and old age the mastoid cells craft out a space in the middle ear that is *actively pneumatized by the individual's own soul activity* during respiration: "Prior to birth the tympanic cavity is filled with a clear, yellow fluid. The mechanical apparatus that transmits sound should only become functional when the tympanic fluid is replaced by air, after several hours of breathing" [Rauber und Kopsch 1987, 593]. Primary pneumatization continues to progress in the mastoid[1], especially during the first three to four years of life, *but the process is not stable* and must continually be regained anew, especially during infancy and early childhood. "The growth processes in the middle ear are quasi opposed to each other. Epithelium "battles" connective tissue with its rich blood supply, the latter being pushed out to the edge of the bone in the process. If the connective tissue is victorious, however, a thick, vascular mucosal membrane remains in the middle ear that is prone to becoming inflamed and thus a disposition for middle ear infections in children can arise" [Rohen 2000a, 268]. In the reference quoted, Johannes Rohen impressively captures the drama of middle ear and mastoid pneumatization.

Especially during the teething phase, the middle ear is vulnerable to regression to an embryonal stage (Eustachian salpingitis/tubal catarrh, seromucotympanon). This patho-

1 Pneumatization of the mastoid proceeds individually: While in about 37 % of cases investigated the mastoid was fully developed by age 3–4 years ("pneumatic type"), in 20 % of cases the air-filled spaces had not yet been formed at all. The question remains as to what extent medical treatment of pneumatization disorders can have any influence on this process [Rauber und Kopsch 1987, 594].

5

logical tendency escalates when there is an *acute inflammation,* although simultaneously the inflammation – much in the sense of the connective tissue being limited and pushed back – has the purpose of prompting elimination of excessive secretions and any pathogens that have invaded this feeding ground, *so that the pneumatization process can be regained.* This explains more clearly how spontaneous perforation of the ear drum at the climax of the acute otitis media is a natural consequence of the organism's self-oriented activity, thus hindering development of seromucotympanon. – Hence paracentesis was frequently employed to cure otitis media during the pre-antibiotic era. Studies undertaken in recent years [Del Mar et al. 1997, van Buchem et al. 1985] have shown that when treated allopathically – also without any antibiotic treatment – acute otitis media will subside under purely antiphlogistic and analgesic treatment. This also indicates that a catarrhal change in the "terrain" (Pasteur), apparently a ventilation disorder (i. e. not infectious pathogens) is the primary problem in otitis media. Every disturbance in nasal breathing and every form of catarrh jeopardizes the presence of respiratory air in the middle ear and therefore also the pneumatization process. Thus the link between consciousness and the air space that mediates hearing of sounds and human speech is also jeopardized. Suppressive antibiotic and antiphlogistic treatment does not support the organism's efforts to eliminate and pneumatize – two functions that are primarily supported by bodily-oriented soul activity via the respiratory organization[1]. Bearing in mind the cause of otitis media, the *pneumococcal conjugate vaccination* (and Hib vaccination) are limited in their effects considering the drama of the pneumatization process in the middle ear during the early years of life. It is probable that these vaccinations primarily cause microbiological changes, i. e. replacement of the bacterial flora, but they certainly do not address the otitis media directly. Whether the illness course is more benign after such a replacement is still to be determined (see also: ▸ Chap. 3.5.1; [Coker et al. 2010]). In contrast, breast-feeding promotes pneumatization and has a prophylactic effect with respect to the risk of acute otitis media; on the other hand, use of a dummy increases the risk (and, as with so many health issues, smoking in the home is also a risk factor).

Therefore it is not surprising that "in this country during the last 20 years [...] so-called secromucotympanon" as a "form of chronic otitis exsudativa" [von Harnack und Koletzko 1997, 395f.] has become increasingly evident. More and more frequently today, suppression of the *organism's own purposeful febrile-inflammatory activity* is the cause of an illness course characterized by chronic stagnation, without fever and without the body's own excretory activity – that is to say, a condition in which the physical life processes have become independent of the breathing and warmth organizations. Thick, gelatinous mucous effusion that refuses to resolve spontaneously is usually treated with paracentesis. This intervention takes the form of an iatrogenic eardrum perforation that tends to become chronic due to the frequently employed eardrum tympanostomy tubes (grommets). The risk of permanent eardrum damage with persistent hearing impairment of 2–8 dB and tympanosclerosis appears to have increased four- to five-fold [Stenstrom 2005].

The fact that complications such as a mature, softening mastoiditis or otogenic meningitis can be conservatively treated today is unquestionably due to the current possibilities offered by antibiotics, provided that the intervention is timely. Nevertheless, if employed

1 The bodily-oriented formative activity of the human soul organization (the "astral body" in anthroposophical terms) comes to expression – during the day in healthy individuals – in all processes related to respiration, and has a formative, up-building and excretory effect [Steiner und Wegman 1991].

as routine treatment, antibiotics do not reduce the risk of complications (!); in fact, acute new problems arise in 4–10 % of children receiving treatment [Coker 2010], due to antibiotic resistance development and side effects such as vomiting, diarrhoea and allergic exanthema[1] (see introductory principle). Allergy development can be considered as a further long-term sequela of antibiotic treatment.

Antibiotics and further specialized ear-nose-throat interventions are indicated when:

- The patient has not responded to the anthroposophic-homoeopathic treatment and especially if the child presents with fever, a marked rise in CRP (according to laboratory values) and reduced general condition at the follow-up visit on the 5th day (as a rule we already monitor the illness course on the 3rd day).
- Several levels of the respiratory tract are simultaneously heavily inflamed (e. g. as in pneumonia and otitis media).
- Adequate response to anthroposophic-homoeopathic treatment cannot be expected because of a weakened immune system due to preexisting illness, immunodeficiency, cytostatic treatment etc., and reduced general condition.
- Signs of the onset of mastoiditis or osteomyelitis which required immediate hospitalization.

Acute otitis media within the context of scarlet fever should also be treated with caution (▸Chap. 5.3.4.4.1).

The authors and other colleagues [Büttner 1973, Sommer 1998] have observed in practice (also in large numbers of cases[2]) that acute otitis media can generally be treated *without antibiotics* and without an accumulation of complications. However, comprehensive exploration of the anamnesis and physical examination findings, repeated monitoring of the findings (continual in some cases) and particularly careful attention to general condition are prerequisites for the treatment approach described below. The aim of this treatment approach is to guide and support the respiratory and warmth organizations. Thus it is possible to control an excessive, painful inflammatory process without inhibiting development of pneumatization (in some cases pain can be more rapidly alleviated with the approach outlined here than with antibiotics). Hence the risk of recurrent inflammations and development of a chronic-exudative otitis media is also considerably reduced in patients receiving this treatment and antibiotics become necessary in less than 10 % of all cases. In a prospective-comparative outcomes study investigating acute airway and middle ear infections [Hamre et al. 2005], in the case of childhood illness, the individualized anthroposophic treatment approach was clearly superior: Pain and other symptoms were more rapidly alleviated (!) and the illness course proved more favourable, also due to reduced antibiotic consumption and drug side effects. *This study provides sufficient up-to-date evidence that the anthroposophic-homoeopathic treatment of acute otitis media – on the basis of its efficacy and significantly lower rate of side effects (difficulties with antibiotic resistance, allergy development, medicine side effects) – is the treatment of choice when compared to the antibiotic and antiphlogistic treatment still employed in most countries in the West.*

1 Symptoms increase two-fold with antibiotic treatment [Del Mar et al. 1997].
2 Written report by ENT specialist, K. Niewind [see also: Niewind 1992] based on more than 5000 cases of acute otitis media.

5.1.3.1 Treating acute, uncomplicated otitis media

Prognosis without antibiotic treatment: About 80 % of all otitis media cases heal spontaneously when treated symptomatically. Complications are rare. There is currently no evidence that complications can be significantly reduced with antibiotic treatment.
[Leitlinien 2010, N 6,1]

The acute middle ear inflammation is characterized clinically by acute onset within a few hours, fever (especially in infants and toddlers) and pain; symptoms vary individually in relation to physical examination findings. Onset of illness is mostly unilateral, but one must reckon with a spread of the inflammation to the other ear. An otoscopic examination can distinguish between an uncomplicated form of the illness, i. e. with reddening, retracted or bulging eardrum and serous effusion; an inflammation that has progressed to a severely painful bulging eardrum within the context of a viral infection; or a suppurative otitis media (▸Chap. 5.1.3.2). Assessment of the child's general condition and behaviour is equally important, as well as thorough examination techniques so that possible complications can be excluded.

5.1.3.1.1 Injecting potentized medicines

In the authors' daily practice, *injections administered over the mastoid* at the beginning of treatment have proven to be exceptionally effective – in all cases of otitis media, and not only those presenting with a mild, partial reddening of the eardrum. The injections are administered subcutaneously (shallow) with a short insulin needle (0.45 × 12 mm). The prick of the injection needle is hardly painful, especially if the child has earache, and the effect on pain (after a few minutes!) and further development of the inflammation is impressive. If it is probable that the other ear will also become infected – especially likely in children with pronounced catarrhal infection – this can often be prevented with the primary injection treatment *on both sides.*

The following medicinal composition is particularly suitable for this form of treatment (compare with ▸Chap. 5.1.2.4.3):

- **Silicea comp. amp.** Wala
  Approx. 0.3–0. 5 ml, s.c. (calculated on the basis of bilateral application over the mastoid, on both sides of the head)

For a severely painful illness course (and also cases of influenza-related otitis with bubble-like bulges in the eardrum) and high fever, combine Silicea comp. with

- **Apis mell./ex animale D30 amp.** Weleda/Wala
  Approx. 0.5–0.7 ml s.c.

in a mixed injection.

If one expects a poor response to treatment or the tendency to a complicated illness course – due to constitutional factors or previously frequent suppressive treatment, for example – the effect of Silicea comp. can be intensified by combining it with the following organ preparation, in high potency:

- **Cavum tympani Gl D30 amp.** Wala
  Approx. 0.5–0.7 ml s.c.

5.1.3.1.2 External treatments and nutritional measures

A well-known initial treatment measure often undertaken by parents at home is the

- **onion pack or compress** [Goebel und Glöckler 2008, 661, Vagedes, Soldner 2010, 58]

containing finely chopped fresh onion which is placed over the painful ear.

- A warm **enema** i. e. 30–35 °C (e. g. using chamomile tea)

is less common but very helpful and effective for acute-febrile otitis, especially for infants and small children. Parents can use a rubber enema for infants and small children (see also: ▸Chap. 5.1.1.4.2).

At the medical practice, following injection treatment,

- a 1 × 1 cm **cantharides plaster** (only available on prescription[1])

can be placed over the mastoid and left in place for 8 to 12 hours. There are no risks or dangers attached to a plaster of this size. The plaster draws out air bubbles and has a draining and limiting effect on the internal inflammatory process. Application of this plaster is particularly important in cases of a bulging eardrum or formation of bubbles.

With regard to nutrition measures, the same principles apply to otitis media as for acute recurrent rhinitis (▸Chap. 5.1.2.3). *Local treatment for impaired nasal breathing* (almost always a symptom) is the same as described in ▸Chap. 5.1.2.2 to 5.1.2.4, thus dispensing with the need for decongestant nose drops. The same applies to *mucolysis* which is adequately stimulated and supported by lime flower and elder tea and a little lemon (from age 1 year upwards with honey) as well as a reduction in milk consumption (complete abstention from toddler age onwards).

- **Aconite ear drops** Wala
  1–2 gtt. (body temperature), 3–6 x/day and
- **Levisticum H 10 % Oleum** Weleda.
  Soak cotton wool inserts with warmed oil

Can be helpful in cases of painful acute otitis media; after exclusion of an eardrum perforation.

5.1.3.1.3 Options for internal treatment with potentized medicines

The root of the lovage plant, *Levisticum officinale*, is generally effective for treating ventilation disorders in the middle ear as well as their acute and chronic sequelae. What strikes one about Levisticum is that the plant internalizes air to an unusual depth (tubular, hollow stems, up to 2 m in height) and loves sunny, south-facing locations in mountainous regions up to 2000 m. The roots of this hardy perennial weed grow to great depths and contain essential oils, resin, monosaccharides such as galactose and fructose and various plant acids. The lovage (known as Maggikraut in Germany) has long since found its way into the kitchen and can be added to soup, for example – with the effect of stimulating soul

1 Prescription:

Spanish fly (pulvis)	1.57 g
Yellow wax	3.07 g
Peanut oil	0.77 g
Turpentine	0.77 g

Mix and put on textile 9 × 12 cm
(Central-Apotheke, Bad Tölz, Germany are experienced with the prescription.)

activity in the digestion (compare with: ▸Chap. 4). Phytotherapeutically speaking, lovage stimulates diuresis and secretion of digestive enzymes and is therefore used to treat deposition diseases and mucous congestion of the respiratory tract [Madaus 1979, 1746–1752]. – From the point of view of anthroposophic medicine, Levisticum stimulates excretory and exhalative activity of the human soul organization, i. e. the astral body, and also activates the warmth organization. Due to its immense vitality, the lovage plant has an unusually deep connection to the air element and is also able to internalize warmth qualities, right into substance formation [Pelikan 1980, 94].

The rationale for using Levisiticum to treat otitis media stems from Rudolf Steiner [1989, 190]: "In the case of an ear inflammation one is dealing with an etheric organization that has gained the upper hand in this local canal. [...] We can best come to grips with the problem if we *activate the respiratory process* again (emphasis by authors). Internally administered Levisticum in the appropriate dosage can activate the respiratory process so that the out-breath becomes livelier." At the beginning of treatment of acute otitis media, lower potencies of Levisticum (D3, D4) should be administered frequently; only in this way can one best utilize the plant's medicinal effects: *Levisticum does not suppress the inflammatory process but rather enables the inflammation to fulfill its purpose, which in turn brings about its abatement.* The authors have found that a composition of Levisticum and Apis mell. has proven to be effective in treatment: the decongestant, anti-oedematous and excretion promoting effect of potentized honey bee postively strengthens the organism's relationship to air, light and warmth, which also correspond to the effects of Levisticum.

In practice one can prescribe

- **Apis/Levisticum II** (= D3/4f) **pillules** Wala
  3–5 pillules, initially every 15–30 mins.; after onset of action, gradually reduce number of doses
- **Levisticum, Radix Rh. D3 dil.** Weleda (alcohol free)
  5–7gtt./dose, same frequency [Vademecum 2010, 547]

If the otoscopic examination reveals a sharply defined, bright red eardrum, it is better to combine Levisticum with

- **Belladonna Rh D6 dil.** Weleda (alcohol free)
  For example, 30–50 gtt. Belladonna Rh D6 in 50 ml water, 5 ml/dose.
  Alternatively, dissolve 30 pillules (D6) in water.

For severe *catarrhal* symptoms *(nose, conjunctivae)*, serous bulging of the eardrum, and relatively moderate pain in relation to findings, one may consider the following in addition to the Apis/Levisticum treatment:

- **Pulsatilla D4–12 pillules** (various manufacturers)
  5 pillules, initially every 1–2 hours

This medicine can be administered in very low potency for treatment of acute catarrhal otitis (▸Chap. 5.3.2).

In cases of acute uncomplicated otitis media, if there are no clear indications for an individualized single substance, Apis and Levisticum can be combined with

- **Silicea comp. pillules** Wala
  5–10 pillules, 3–4 x/day

When treating acute otitis media one is always concerned with guiding and steering the bodily-oriented *soul activity of the child* and therefore the child's behaviour on a soul level during the medical consultation is always of interest. Administration of an appropriate single substance homoepathic remedy in a high potency can provide the child's astral body with a corrective impulse that will positively influence progress of the illness and the possibilities for relating to the child.

For children who are extremely sensitive to pain and appear irascible and aggressive – and especially when they are teething at the same time:

- **Chamomilla (e rad.) D30 pillules** Wala, Weleda
  5 pillules/dose, as required (short acting remedy; compare below: Fieber- und Zahnungszäpfchen [**Chamomilla comp. supp. for children,** Weleda UK]).

The child who is weepy and clings to its mother can be treated constitutionally with

- **Pulsatilla D30 pillules** (various manufacturers)
  1 × 5 pillules; subsequent treatment better with lower potencies (see above)

An immediately helpful first medication for anxious children who suddenly develop high fever at the onset of otitis media, possibly accompanied by severe pain, administer

- **Aconitum (e tub.) D30 pillules** Wala, Weleda
  5 pillules, 1–3 x/day, at brief intervals

For longstanding ventilation disorders with the tendency to recurrent otitis media, a single dose (select according to constitution) at the start of treatment (see also: ▸ Chap. 3.2.5) can improve the response to the subsequent acute medications

- **Calcium carbonicum D30 pillules** DHU
  1 × 5 pillules or
- **Silicea D30 pillules** (various manufacturers)
  1 × 5 pillules.

During the course of treating acute otitis media, in addition to the above-described animal (Apis mell.) and plant medicines (Levisticum, Belladonna, Pulsatilla), the following metal and mineral remedies can be considered in order to consolidate the treatment outcome[1].

- **Ferrum phosphoricum D12 pillules** (various manufacturers)
  5–7 pillules/gtt. 2–3 x/day

is especially indicated for left-sided otitis media, general weakness, pallor and labile circulation (with the need to lie down). The activity of the warmth organization (which mainly comes to expression in blood circulation) and soul activity appears inconstant-variable and appears to have little resilience. This medication is of central therapeutic importance when treating school age children.

- **Plumbum met. praep. D10 trit.** Weleda
  1 saltsp./day, mane

5

1 Both homoeopathy (see Hahnemann's Materia medica with regard to chronic diseases) and anthroposophic medicine have the view and experience that potentized metal and mineral medicines have the most far-reaching and long-lasting effects on the functioning of the human organism [Steiner 1982, 126f.].

is especially indicated for right-sided otitis media; treatment can begin after to a single dose of

- **Sulphur D30 pillules** (various manufacturers)
  3–5 pillules.

Sulphur and Plumbum met. administered in the above-described sequence particularly counteract *chronic inflammatory and degenerative tendencies* in the *middle ear*, when exudative processes have become increasingly autonomous and mucous secretions have taken on a dense, gelatinous consistency. Anthroposophic medicine employs potentized lead when excretory activity has weakened and self-contained depositions have formed within the organism due to insufficient engagement of the warmth organization [Steiner und Wegman 1977, 126f.]. At the present time lead is also an effective medicine for children with allergies, large-headed children who are slow to awaken intellectually and also for children with adipositas. These indications have certainly become more frequent in daily practice during the past 20 years.

Suitable supportive medication during acute otitis media with nightly pain, fever and intense restlessness can be provided by

- **Fieber- und Zahnungszäpfchen** Weleda. **Chamomilla comp. supp. for children,** Weleda UK
  Administer 1–3 x/day, especially nocte and during the night

Containing Argentum and Echinacea in the 3rd decimal potency (D3), as well as Belladonna, Chamomilla Radix and Papaver somniferum, this composition is to be preferred above antiphlogistic and antipyretic drugs.

For purulent rhinitis, fever, especially with accompanying sinusitis the authors favour

- **Echinacea/Mercurius comp. supp.** Wala
  1 supp., 1–2 x/day, especially nocte

5.1.3.2 Suppurative otitis media

Contrary to the prevailing school of thought [Harnack und Koletzko 1997, 395], it is indeed possible to treat clinically diagnosed suppurative otitis media with potentized medicines. The specific risks involved, such as scarlet fever-related otitis media, have been dealt with separately (▸Chap. 5.3.4.4). Thorough physical examination techniques, the doctor's availability to patients, *daily* follow-up examinations at the beginning of treatment, and above all, personal experience, determine what is in the realm of the possible. If these conditions can be complied with and each individual case is carefully considered, there is no need to be concerned with an increase in complications in comparison to standard antibiotic treatment. In most cases antibiotics can be avoided altogether.

If the otoscopic examination reveals a reddened, bulging eardrum with yellowish, purulent contents gleaming in the tympanic cavity, intial treatment should be carried out as described in ▸Chap. 5.1.3.1.1 (injection with Silicea comp. amp. Wala) and ▸Chap. 5.1.3.1.2 (including use of a cantharides plaster after the injection).

Internal medication with

- **Mercurius solubilis D/C30 pillules** (various manufacturers)
  5 pillules, 3–5 x/day

followed by

- **Hepar sulfuris D12–C30 pillules/dil.**
  5 pillules, 2–3 x/day.

In this situation lower potencies of Hepar sulfuris should not be used. Further treatment can be determined after about 3 days, depending on whether a spontaneous eardrum perforation has occurred or not. If the former is the case, proceed with administration of

- **Quartz D6 trit.** Weleda
  1 saltsp. 3 x/day for 1–2 weeks.

While under this treatment, the patient's condition and sense of well-being should steadily improve; within 8–10 days the otorrhoea must cease completely and the eardrum should close spontaneously. When assessing the illness course, it is critical to be aware if the eardrum has become adhesive and if the fever has resumed. In such cases antibiotics must be seriously considered (see above, ▸Chap. 5.1.3, indications for antibiotic treatment)

If the inflammation and general symptoms have subsided without perforation after about 3 days of treatment with Hepar sulfuris, treatment can continue with

- **Silicea comp. pillules** Wala
  5–7 pillules, 3 x/day

Alternating with the above-mentioned medicines, consider the following in cases of otitis media purulenta, especially as supportive treatment:

- **Capsicum annuum D6–12 dil.** (various manufacturers)
  5 gtt. 3 x/day

Administer if the illness course has stagnated, hearing has clearly diminished, mucous congestion has arisen following a perforation, or if there is pain or tenderness on pressure of the mastoid (manifest mastoiditis requires appropriate clinical treatment). Capsicum and Hepar sulfuris are the most important acute medications for suppurative otitis media in order to counteract possible complications later on.

- **Lachesis D12 dil.** Weleda
  5 gtt., 2–3 x/day

Administer Lachesis if the symptomatology is defined by *noticeably reduced general condition with ashen pallor, fever and possibly a livid tinge to the mucosa*. A mixed injection of the following two preparations is particularly effective for this indication:

- **Lachesis D30 amp.** Wala, Weleda
- **Argentum D30/Echinacea D6 amp.** Weleda
  Mixed injection, 2 ml i.v.

For suppurative otitis media, extremely effective support is offered by

- **Echinacea/Mercurius comp. supp.** Wala
  1–3 x/day, especially at night (▸Chap. 5.1.2.4.3)

5

If the acute illness phase subsides in response to the treatment described above, and especially if the eardrum has not perforated, support for further recovery and resumption of pneumatization can be provided with the following prescription developed by the authors:

- **Levisticum-Paukenmischung** Weleda dispensary, Germany (Hydrastis D6, Levisticum D10, Mercurius dulcis D12, Sylvin (=Potassium chloratum nat.) D6 aa)
  7–15 gtt., 3 x/day (see following Chap.)

5.1.3.3 Seromucotympanon

Effusion [following acute otitis media] should disappear within 3–4 weeks; in about 20 % of children effusion is still in evidence after two months [Leitlinien N 6, 9 2010]

The occurrence of seromucotympanon (glue ear) is always a sign that the fluid element in the etheric body, i. e. the life organization in the region of the upper respiratory tract, has become partially autonomous (regressive). In assessing this condition one must first clearly establish whether the child has *adenoids* or *tonsil hypertrophy* (▸Chap. 5.2.4 for treatment of these conditions). Seromucotympanon can also be a sequela to *sinusitis* (including those forms with an occult course) with accompanying swelling of the Eustachian tubes (▸Chap. 5.1.2.4).

Treatment should stimulate engagement of the warmth organization and the formative, up-building and excretory functions of the astral body, i. e. the formative activity of the soul in the body. These treatment aims can be supported artistically through singing (parents initially, child together with parents or teacher later on) and making music (e. g. mother or father playing the leier, recorder playing from pre-school age onwards). On the other hand, a hearing overload, for example, noise pollution at kindergarten (> 70 dB!) or due to electronic media have a deadening and paralyzing effect on the soul activity engaged in hearing – and thereby also on the process of pneumatization! Diagonstically it is essential to pay attention to the child's level of speech development. If there is evidence of stagnation or regression, therapeutic intervention must seriously be considered – and early on enough; if the level of development is satisfactory, this is the right time for treatment (medicinal and eurythmy) that will stimulate further development. The basic principles for nutrition and local treatments for the nose and ear are the same as outlined in ▸Chap. 5.1.3.1.2 (see also: ▸Chap. 5.2.4, Hay fever spray or topical Citrus/Cydonia treatment). Regular mustard footbaths (▸Chap. 5.1.2.4.2) are particularly worthwhile; local redlight treatment may also be considered.

Current research sounds a note of caution with regard to paracentesis, and especially the insertion of tympanostomy tubes (grommets). In the context of a study, toddlers who had bilateral middle ear effusion for longer than 90 days were randomized into two groups. Grommets were immediately given to one group; the second group had to wait 6 months, and only those children who still had effusion after six months were provided with grommets. Performance at school, attention and social competence were the same in children aged 9 to 11 years [Paradise 2007]. On the other hand, eardrum grommets can leave permanent scars with discrete hearing loss. Topical steroids (nasal sprays) do not contribute anything to recovery from seromucotympanon [Williamson 2009].

In the experience of anthroposophic paediatrician K. R. Kummer, local application of the following ear drop prescription has proven effective for treating suppurative otitis media:

- **Glycerin. anhydr.** 9.0
  Cetiol 0.5
  Ol. ricini ad 10.0
  M. D. S. Ohrentropfen [ear drops]

Thereafter, consolidate with:

- **Quarz 1 % ear drops** Weleda dispensary
  1 gtt., 1–2 x/day in the affected ear/s; additionally massage 1 gtt. over the mastoid [Vademecum 2010, 709]

With sufficient prior treatment and after the acute inflammatory processes have subsided, pressure equalization can be attempted, for example, using a special nasal balloon or a Politzer balloon.

A combined approach of internal and external treatments according to the above-described treatment aims has proven effective for many children: Stimulating engagement of the astral body and I-organization, thereby activating pneumatization in the middle ear.

- **Levisticum-Paukenmischung [Levisticum-tympanic mixture]** Weleda dispensary, Germany (In equal parts: Hydrastis D6, Levisticum D10, Mercurius dulcis D12, Sylvite (=natural potassium chloride) D6)
  7–15 gtt., 3 x/day
- **Oleum Salviae 10 %** (in olive oil special preparation obtainable from e. g. the Weleda dispensary, Germany)
  3 x/week, mane, for 3–6 months. Apply to torso and limbs (excluding head/face and nappy (diaper)/underwear area), massage lightly. (Mostly used during the cooler half year and not in the hot summer months)

The principle underlying the authors' Levisticum-eardrum mixture can be summarized as follows [Vademecum 2010,549]: "The treatment aim is to bring congested mucous secretions in the middle ear [due to the Eustachian tubes] into flow (the potentized chloride compounds of potassium [Sylvin] and mercury [Mercurius dulcis] are particularly effective here) and to provide the mucosae of the upper respiratory tract with formative, decongestant, deturgescent impulses (Levisticum, Hydrastis). Remarkably, all the medicines mentioned here take effect at the same time in the upper gastro-intestinal tract (especially in stomach and gall bladder regions), strengthening digestive and excretory activity. Thus the excessive metabolic activity in the head region causing the swelling and congestion is activated in "the right place", i. e. below the diaphragm. The medication stimulates and strengthens the formative breathing function of the sentient organization (astral body) in the middle ear and paranasal sinuses with the result that mucosal swelling subsides, secretion is regulated, and the process of pneumatization is promoted. Digestive activity is improved at the same time owing to stimulation of secretion in the "lower human being". Ensoulment of the organism – the differentiated way in which the sentient organization takes hold of the life organization – comes to expression in both qualities."

The massage with sage oil for children with adenoids and glue ear developed by a Dutch colleague, Joop van Dam [van Dam 2006, Soldner 2007, Vademecum 2010, 628] has proven exceptionally effective in the authors' practice. The treatment applies a "below-outwards" technique to achieve an "above-inner" effect, which corresponds to the basic dynamic of the constantly polarized astral body (see Girke 2010, 29 for a clear description). The formative effect of sage stimulates the process of pneumatization and relieves the swelling in the mucosae and lymphatic tissue in the area of the Eustachian tubes.

The following single substance remedies may be considered:

- **Kalium sulfuricum D6–8 dil.** (various manufacturers)
  5–10 gtt., 3 x/day

for purulent rhinitis/sinusitis with thick yellow discharge and the tendency to laryngitis and bronchitis

- **Sylvin D6 dil.** Weleda dispensary, Germany
  5–10 gtt., 3 x/day

if all airways are severely congested and mucous is visible in the throat but not purulent.

If there is no response, the diagnosis should be reassessed (adenoids? sinusitis? allergy?) and the treatment correspondingly reorientated. In the author's experience, it is generally becoming more and more difficult to treat mucotympanon. Nevertheless, it is possible (although not in every case) to avoid paracentesis or tympanostomy tubes (grommets).

Treatment can continue with individual constitutional remedies, i. e. potentized single substances:

- **Calcium carbonicum LM12 dil.** (various manufacturers)
  3–5 gtt./day, 3 x/week.

Calcium carbonicum can be administered to the classical *exudative-lymphatic constitution* in which excessive vitality from the metabolic region cannot be sufficiently formed and "breathed through". This constitutional type is characterized by (acidic) sweating on the head, chronic rhinitis, possibly delayed teething with good appetite, and above all, rapid weight gain in the first year of life, accompanied by the tendency to regress to an embryonal, uncomplicated state where the mother takes care of everything – which is relatively easy to observe. Administration of potentized oyster shell calcium stimulates teething and intensifies exhalation; both sweating and the exudative diathesis in the respiratory epithelium recede. This constitutional type – almost physiological in infancy and early childhood – is increasingly rare.

Potentized lead (in the form of a metal mirror = met. praep) can be administered when the middle ear effusion has stagnated completely and has progressively developed a firmer consistency (compare: above ▸Chap. 5.1.3.1). If the Calc-carb constitution of the infant is dominated by an overflowing metabolism that proliferates in the fluid element – in cases where Plumbum met. is indicated, decaying (i. e. moving towards the lifeless state) substances precipitating from the physical will become autonomous within the organism. This leads to a sclerotic process in the middle ear, a condition that seems to occur more and more frequently nowadays. In such cases it is especially important to vitalize the metabolism *before* the formative effect of Plumbum met. becomes active.

In the treatment of seromucotympanon, this can be achieved by administering, for example:

- **Sulphur D12 trit.** Weleda
  1 saltsp., mane, and
- **Plumbum met. praep. D10–12 trit.** Weleda
  1 saltsp., in the afternoon.

In addition, Tuberculinum as a single substance can be considered (▸Chap. 5.1.3.4) as well as Apis mell. and Pulsatilla. If one changes over to one of these medicines in the treatment plan, their effect on pneumatization of the middle ear can be guided and strengthened by appropriate supplementary application of *potentized silicic acid* (▸Chap. 5.1.2.4.3). Silicic acid has a *complementary* relationship to the effects of the above mentioned medicines. *Equisetum arvense*, i. e. horsetail actively precipitates silicic acid in an opal-like form, using it to build a skeleton of silicic acid (this becomes visible after the correct ashing process). Its rhythmically organized, clearly-cut radiating form shows how silicic acid builds the relationship of this medicinal plant to the light and rhythmically-oscillating processes, which, in the human being, are centred in breathing. The Equisetum plant has a major influence on drainage where it grows, especially counteracting stagnating, wet conditions; in the human being Equisetum stimulates the water-eliminating function of the kidneys. This can be effective when fluids have become autonomous in the organism, where air should be drawn in and "the land drained".

Pharmaceutically, Equisetum can be processed through combined toasting with sulphur in order to intensify the excretory effect and stimulate [the warmth organization's] capacity to "warm-through" the organism (▸Chap. 1.2.2):

- **Equisetum cum Sulfure tostum D4–6 trit.** Weleda
  1 saltsp., 2 x/day, mornings and afternoons

This administration is suitable, for example, when Plumbum met. has been prescribed. (▸Chap. 6.4.3.5).

In contrast, in the case of excessive, overflowing vitality and warmth generation with swelling of the mucosa and chronic catarrh, the formative effect of Equisetum can be intensified when the plant has been pretreated with silicic acid:

- **Equisetum Silicea cultum D2/Rh D3 dil.** Weleda
  5–7 gtt., 2–3 x/day.

Also in these cases, the efficacy can be increased through administration of

- **Sulphur D6 trit.** Weleda
  1 saltsp./day, mane

Onyx, a dichromatic, stratified subcategory of agate, is a mineral silicic acid preparation with a specific relationship to the *sense of hearing*. From the point of view of anthroposophical research, Rudolf Steiner was explicit about the relationship of this *rhythmically organized mineral form* of silicic acid to the hearing sense [Lit. Schwarz, see below]. In practice, potentized onyx is suitable for children with delicate vitality and a slowly emerging individuality, who are consequently overtaxed by "what they hear" in their social environs. Children with recurrent or *persistent seromucotympanon* have the impression that onyx provides them with self-protection and substitutes for their inadequate capacity to maintain boundaries. Recurrent otitis can occur in all kinds of demanding situations. "*The hearing sense needs to be strengthened* so that not only hearing, but also the boundaries in relation to what is heard are improved." This is how the Austrian anthroposophic paediatrician, Reinhold Schwarz characterizes this aspect of the indication for onyx, and for which onyx has proven to be an effective treatment in cases of seromucotympanon and recurrent otitis media [Schwarz 2005; see also: onyx and the treatment concept developed by Schwarz: Vademecum 2010, 632].

- **Onyx D20 trit.** Weleda
  1 large saltsp./day, mane

provides a suitable extension following the above-described possibilities for treatment with potentized silicic acid. Here the treatment also requires a simultaneous vitalizing component:
A suitable option is provided by bathing (R. Schwarz) with

- **Thuja essence** Wala
  2–4 tablespoons/full bath, 2 x/week.

Eurythmy therapy is a treatment possibility that has a thoroughgoing and profound (!) effect on children of kindergarten and school age (▸Chap. 5.1.2.6). The dynamic of breathing in the area of the paranasal sinuses and the middle ear can be stimulated through practice of the sound sequence "L-M-S" or "L-M-S-U" – with lasting effects.

5.1.3.4 Chronically recurrent otitis media

If taken into account, the above-described process (▸Chap. 5.1.3.1 to ▸Chap. 5.1.3.3) encompasses all the essential viewpoints and possibilities for treating chronic recurrent otitis or for providing prophylactic measures. One of the first and frequent causes of otitis media today is *suppression of acute inflammatory* processes in the respiratory tract – for example, through use of antibiotics and anti-inflammatories, and medicines that relieve swelling of the mucosae and mucous congestion: These medications can inhibit and block the active process of pneumatization. *Chronic ventilation disorders* of the middle ear as a disposition for recurrent otitis has been discussed in the previous section (▸Chap. 5.1.3.3); with regard to adenoids ▸Chap. 5.2.4.

An *individualized choice of medicine* is essential and must be determined in view of the comprehensive anamnesis (prior illnesses and treatments), the child's constitution and immediate environment.

The most important single substance constitutional remedies are:

- **Calcium carbonicum LM12/Conchae D20–30 trit.** Weleda (▸Chap. 5.1.3.3 and generally ▸Chap. 3.2.2.1)
- Potentized silicic acid preparations **Quartz D20–30 trit./pillules** Weleda/Wala,
- **Onyx D20 trit.** Weleda (▸Chap. 5.1.3.3 and generally ▸Chap. 3.2.2.2),
- **Aurum met. praep. D12 trit.** Weleda (see below)

and for this indication, of particular importance is

- **Tuberculinum (Koch alt) LM12 dil./C30–200 pillules** Gudjons

Tuberculinum in the form of a homoeopathic nosode can be considered in all cases of chronic, constitutionally related susceptibility for inflammation in the respiratory tract (possibly also the tonsils and urinary tract organs.

Furthermore, these children display a certain *restlessness* on a soul (psychological) level: they are excessively orientated towards their surroundings, inquisitive and adventurous, but also a strain on their parents and can behave provocatively. On the other hand, they display exceptional artistic gifts, for example, and respond very well to their surroundings on the level of soul. Whereas these children overexert themselves in relation to the outer world, they lack their own bodily-oriented formative strength. As a result of the deficiency in up-building processes in the body, too little vitality is generated: Consequently these children often have a delicate build while disproportionately shooting up in height at the same time; they tend to strong sweating, particularly at night and with minimal physical exertion.

With regard to vitality and responsiveness, the surface organs, especially the respiratory epithelium, have developed to an "inferior standard" and are therefore unable to create or assert boundaries around the organism's indispensable autonomous existence, which provide resistance to adverse environmental factors. Stormy, cool and damp weather or stresses and strains on body and soul rapidly flare up into inflammatory happenings that the children are often incapable of fully overcoming by means of their own strength. Whereas these children are "too young" on a soul level and inadequately incarnated (which bestows them with something very charming and attractive), their bodies are threatening to become "too old" and are incapable of developing the vitality and warmth (above all) necessary for healthy growth. People with this constitutional type were, and still are susceptible to tuberculosis in the applicable environments as described above. Furthermore, experience gained the field of homoeopathy (and the authors' own experience) indicates that if the parents or grandparents had suffered from tuberculosis, the disease will arise frequently in descendants who have this constitution.

5

In cases of chronic recurrent otitis media

- **Tuberculinum (Koch) LM/Q12 dil.**
  2–3 gtt. x/day, in about 1–2 cl spring water; after clearly observed onset of action, reduce to 2–3/week

Can be administered, ideally in combination with a silicic acid preparation (▸Chap. 5.1.3.3).

An essential diagnostic-therapeutic aspect of recurrent otitis media is the *child's relationship to his or her immediate environment*: home, kindergarten or school, parents, siblings and grandparents (! – especially when a festering conflict situation with one or other parent exists). *A determining factor is the degree to which listening is cultivated in the family: at the dinner table, for example, how much care is taken to ensure that each person has a chance to speak without being interrupted? To what extent do parents truly listen, without already thinking about a reply, contradiction or something else entirely?* One can consider whether children are able to digest everything that they hear, or whether they are overtaxed and psychologically under pressure as a result. This is not unusual these days. In the body, this results in inhibition of exhalation (▸Chap. 6.5, asthmatic bronchitis). Parents' guilt feelings and overanxious parents tax the child's capacity to breath freely. Hence conversations between parents and doctor are decisively important for diagnosis and treatment within the context of recurrent otitis media (and sinusitis): Time should be taken to breathe and listen!

The child's psychological state can be immediately strengthened and centred with

- **Aurum met. praep. D12 trit.** Weleda

This remedy can provide fundamental support, but should not diminish the focus on improving the aggravating psychosocial factors.

5.1.4 Obsttructive laryngitis (pseudocroup)

As a rule, stenosing laryngitis manifests as a *night-time, spasmodic illness accompanied by great anxiety on the part of the child and their parents.* It is experienced as a threat to the presence of the soul in the body which can evoke sudden fear of suffocation and death. The triggering swelling of the mucous membrane below the vocal chords is apparently exacerbated by falling asleep, is connected with the withdrawal of the formative forces of the soul at night in favour of the vital up-building processes, which are more at home in the fluid element and tend toward swelling. The latter are centred in the *liver,* an organ which sucks in fluid (portal circulation!) and has its maximum activity at night, swelling physiologically by up to 20 % in volume (glycogen storage). By contrast, the soul controls the fluid organism through the *kidneys,* in whose function the clearance and excretion of fluids interweave with perception (for instance in the formation of erythropoetin in proportion to the concentration of O_2 [Husemann 1989]) and the regulation of gas pressures in the blood: the kidney function thus forms an essential foundation for breathing. In contrast to the liver, kidney activity is minimal in the middle of the night – that is, in just the same period of time when stenosing laryngitis mainly manifests. It is thus understandable that waking up is actually the child's means of self defence against the illness in the larynx, because every awakening directly stimulates the kidney function and thus, in the whole organism, the processes of fluid excretion which reduce swelling.

From this point of view, stenosing laryngitis reveals a kidney activity that is either insufficient or disturbed by soul experiences, combined with too strong a manifestation of vitality in the living, upbuilding processes proceeding from the liver. Possibly connected with the foregoing may be that, on going through puberty (in which the soul's taking possession and shaping of the body mature), the timeframe in which the disorder can arise comes to an end – on the other hand, stenosing laryngitis often takes a dramatic course when it does appear in pre-puberty. The kidney is the organ which, of all the principal internal organs, is most directly affected by incidents of *shock;* this is connected to the strong activity in the kidney of the sentient organization and astral body. In the case of stenosing laryngitis, an initial attack of pseudocroup in its reaction on the kidneys can thus increase disposition to the illness through giving the child, and particularly the parents, a shock. On the other hand, a therapy that very effectively stabilizes the kidney function and harmonizes the effects of shocks on this organ prevents *recurrences and can bring healing to an existing tendency to recurrences.*

In the case of children with recurrent stenosing laryngitis, *parental anxiety* is of great significance. This anxiety may be constitutional or have arisen or been intensified through shocks during pregnancy and early childhood. The *father's anxiety* is particularly significant (including panic on his part during an attack). Parents often fear for their child's life during its first attack of croup! On the other hand, the authors were able again and again to discover serious cases of shock in the medical histories of children with recurrent pseudocroup; these had often only been revealed to their doctor, and their deleterious effect might be mitigated through a conversation or an appropriate medicine for shock (examples include a grandfather's suicide on the day planned for the parents' wedding; or a grandmother's unexpected death from a cancerous illness that had been concealed till the last moment during her daughter's pregnancy with the child in question). It is striking that Aconitum is a key medicine for shock (▸Chap. 2.2.3) and the most important medicinal plant for stenosing laryngitis.

- **Aconitum e tub. D6–30 pillules** Wala, Weleda
  for recurrent stenosing laryngitis: 5 pillules D20 daily each evening
  in acute cases of anxiety and breathlessness: 3–5 pillules D30, repeat several times according to need. Particularly effective when the attack follows a cold snap.

Aconite harmonizes kidney function, as well as acute anxiety after sudden waking at night (which can further intensify the barking cough). It is indicated in acute cases, particularly when stenosing laryngitis occurs in the *first half of the night;* it is indicated, particularly for *anxious children,* as a prophylactic or as therapy in recurrent attacks of pseudocroup. Should the triggering shock lie far in the past, C200 (three individual doses of 3 pillules at intervals of 12 hours) may be indicated.

5.1.4.1 Treating an acute attack

As there is little time to individualize the choice of medicine and one frequently has to rely on what is in the doctor's bag or the home medicine chest, in addition to Aconitum the following *medicinal compositions have proved beneficial in practice:*

5

- **Spongia comp. pillules** Apotheke an der Weleda
  (Apis mell. D2, Belladonna D4, Bryonia D4, Spongia D2)
  initially 3–5 pillules every 10–15 min, on improvement correspondingly less frequently
- **Bryonia/Spongia comp. dil.** Weleda
  (Apis mell, Belladonna, Bryonia, Spongia D3 in each case – contains alcohol)
  children under 3 years 15–25 drops in ½ glass of water/day, of which in acute conditions one sip up to 6 × per hour; when calmer less frequently.
  Children over 3 years: 3–5 drops per dose, initially every quarter hour, when calmer considerably less frequently.
  [Cf. Madeleyn 1996, Vademecum 2010, 235]

or

- **Apis D6 pillules** Weleda/DHU
  Rumex D6 pillules DHU
  Spongia D6 pillules DHU
  Sambucus D6 pillules
  5 pillules each in five-minute alternation, extend intervals as improvement sets in.

This sequence of homoeopathic medicines, available in many home medicine cupboards, has proved beneficial in a wide range of cases in the authors' experience. Sambucus is indicated particularly for children up to 2 years; Rumex for tendencies to catching cold and for croupy cough in the context of a descending viral infection of the airways; Spongia for hoarseness; and Apis as a medicine that reduces swelling.

For a bad attack of pseudocroup, the therapeutic effect is noticeably increased if the potentized organ medicine

- **Larynx Gl D30 amp.** Wala
  ½–1 ampoule is given orally at the outset of treatment, repeated if appropriate. Also applicable as *inhalation* (with **Apis mell/ex animale D30 amp.** Wala/Weleda and perhaps **Gencydo 1 % amp.** Weleda).

A key external application for stenosing laryngitis is a warm chest compress or chest poultice with

- **Ol. Lavandulae 10 %** Wala, Weleda

which not only reduces the urge to cough but also has a marked calming effect on the child's anxiety. Moisten the wrap, i. e. the inner cloth, with drops of lavender oil; gently warm in the oven, either before or after moistening, (protected, for instance, by aluminium foil) and apply.

- **Hepar sulfuris D12** (various manufacturers)

should also be mentioned to complement the medicines already named;
it is indicated particularly for stenosing laryngitis in the 2nd half of the night from 3.00 am onward, when there is severe pain in the larynx and pronounced sensitivity to cold.

- **Pyrit D2 tab. –D6 trit.** Weleda
  1 tab. or 1 saltsp. 3 x/d

is an important medicine for stenosing laryngitis in school-age children, particularly around or after the ninth year [Vademecum 2010, 696], which is also applicable in aftercare (D6).

Apart from medicinal therapy, the establishment of a mood of calm and trust on the part of the doctor, and the usual physical measures (warm, damp air produced by running the shower in the bathroom; or cool air from an open window, as long as the child is otherwise kept quite warm – depending on the child's constitution, either option may work better in a particular case. When following this course of action, corticosteroids (infectocortikrupp®) and adrenalin inhalations are unnecessary in the vast majority of cases.

Medicinal therapy should be continued after the attack – at reduced frequency – until the point is reached when the child is sleeping normally again ('normal' being relative to the individual case).

- **Larynx/Apis comp.** Wala
  5–10 pillules 3–5 x/d

has been found beneficial by the authors as a follow-up medicine in the days after an attack; less so at the onset of an attack (when 2–5 pillules can be given every quarter of an hour [Vademecum 2010, 534]).
Should descending laryngotracheitis develop from an attack of pseudocroup,

- **Bronchi/Plantago pillules** have been found particularly beneficial in the experience of the authors. Wala
  5–7 pillules 5 x/d

Diagnostically, epiglottitis – in spite of its greatly reduced frequency – must be carefully excluded in each case (beginning with high fever, sore throat and refusal of food, before the onset of inspiratory stridor; toxic, seriously impaired general condition in the case of septicemia; unable to lie prone).

If epiglottitis is suspected, the doctor should always immediately accompany the child and its parents to hospital while oxygen is administered. As an initial medicine, on the way to hospital,

- **Lachesis D30 pillules/amp.** (various manufacturers)
  1–2 × 5 pillules/0.3 ml per os and
- **Larynx Gl D30 amp.** Wala 2 × 0.3 ml per os

have proved markedly helpful in cases observed by the author, in order to bridge the interval before clinical treatment.

5

5.1.4.2 Follow-up treatment and prophylaxis

The most important medicines are

- **Aconitum LM12 dil. Arcana®/e tub. D20 pillules** Wala
  3–5 gtt./5 pillules daily for 4–6 weeks
  for anxious children, and abrupt attacks of croup peaking between 10.00 pm and 2.00am. In this indication for aconite, it can be beneficial to administer the medicine before the evening meal.
- **Hepar sulf. LM6–12 dil.** Arcana®
  1 × 5 gtt./d in the morning
  for children who exhibit more pronounced aggressive, wilful behaviour and who have a definite sensitivity to cold. Deterioration in the second half of the night is typical. This medicine has also been beneficial for laryngitis with serious, allergic inflammations of the mucous membrane.

As a consequence of what was said at the beginning, it follows that treating the kidneys is particularly important in attacks of pseudocroup. As an external application, rhythmical Einreibung of the back in the form of a lateral lemniscate in the kidney region with

- **Cuprum met.pr. 0.4 % ointment** Weleda

5.1.5 Acute bronchiolitis

Acute bronchiolitis represents the most serious form of respiratory syncytial virus infection (in itself physiological) in the first two years of life, and leads "clinically to dyspnoea and pronounced pulmonary overinflation with fine crackles at the end of the inspiration, or reduced sounds of breathing, to the point of silent obstruction". [Griese and Reinhardt 2004, 875] *Tachypnoea* with only breathing sounds on auscultation, falling oxygen saturation, high fever and poor drinking patterns reveal the seriousness of the situation. Conventional medical procedures have not so far proved satisfactory [loc. cit.]. In his excellent book "Homöotherapie", Stauffer suggests that

- serious courses of this disease "usually have a constitutional basis" and that "**constitutional remedies** should therefore always be given in high potencies as a basic medicine, in addition [!] to any remedies indicated for cough and inflammation" [Stauffer 1986, 333] – an experience which has been confirmed to the authors in valuable ways. Underlying constitutional conditions today are particularly bronchopulmonary dysplasia (▸Chap. 2.3.2.2) and, less frequently, latent or even manifest rickets (▸Chap. 3.2).
- the diet has to be "a roborative one" and it is important to continue nourishing the patient sufficiently during the illness.

The following case description illustrates a possible approach which has proved itself in clinical experience.

Case study

After three days of a non-specific infection of the airways, a nine-month-old girl suddenly developed temperatures of 40–40.5 °C, extreme tachypnoea with nasal flaring and pronounced mucous rattling, pallor, and a grey perioral area. The child quickly became weak and listless, and could no longer drink. On auscultation there was hardly any sound of breathing; percussion revealed that the lungs on both sides were moderately overinflated; there were no background noises suggesting obstruction. The girl was born in the 38th week of pregnancy at 2860 grams; she was breastfed exclusively for seven months; had a large, broad fontanelle that was easily palpable for a considerable time; her forehead was high; she was noticeably quiet up to the time of her illness; while still healthy, she had a clear, wide-awake look, and fine gestures. Delicate build; translucent skin; slow growth (her first tooth did not come till she was twelve months); a tendency to perspiration on the head and feet. Vitamin D had not been administered. The illness began at the beginning of December. No sign of manifest rickets, but a tendency to latent rickets.

Against this background (▸Chap. 3.2.5.2), Silicea D30 1 × 5 pillules was prescribed daily as a constitutional medicine. In the hour following each dose, a noticeable invigoration and calming of the situation were invariably apparent (the dose was given in the evening at the time of highest fever).

- As a *medicine for acute bronchiolitis*, **Stibium arsenicosum D8 amp.** Weleda 0.7 ml s.c. was injected between the shoulder blades and continued to be given orally (5 drops or 0.2 ml 5 x/d).

Within minutes of administration, the child became more alert, breathed more calmly, and it became possible to feed her. "Antimonium arsenicosum (Stibium arsenicosum) is a medicine which can activate the breathing, tone the circulation and thus bring the tendency to swelling in the etheric under the influence of the formative force of the breathing once more (swelling of the bronchioles, mucous congestion) ... The child's alertness and drinking pattern were promoted just as much as the breathing..." [Soldner 1991, 67]. The medicine contains the most strongly oxygen-compounded oxides of antimony (antimonpentoxide) and arsenic (arsenic trioxide) which counteract swelling and stimulate the formative forces of the organism in the airways, and are at their most effective when injected.

The following were also administered:

- enemas (chamomile tea, electrolyte solution) for intestinal relief, fever reduction (lukewarm enemas) and support for the circulation 100 ml 3–4 x/d (▸Chap. 5.1.1.4.2)
- chest poultices (in this case quark poultices, in similar cases mustard and quark poultices alternating)
- nutrition should consist of half-and-half milk and water with a gruel of finely-milled grains added: nutrition of sufficient calorific content is essential in treating bronchioloitis!
- supporting medicine with **Aconitum D6** and **Tartarus stibiatus D6** per os (▸Chap. 5.1.1.4).

The critical phase with this child, as is usual with RSV bronchiolitis, lasted around 3 ½ days. After that the child recovered rapidly and became a happy, extravert girl who is now making rapid progress with her motor activity. Apart from mama and dada, the first words that the child spoke were "my feet". It was deeply impressive to experience the incarnation of the individuality through a very dangerous, inflammatory illness.

In addition to Silicea/Quarz, Phosphor is the most important constitutional medicine (▸Chap. 2.3.2.2), particularly for children with bronchopulmonary dysplasia. The opportunity nowadays of measuring oxygen saturation by pulse oximeter in an outpatient setting is important in monitoring the course of the illness (▸Chap. 5.1.1.4). *It is vital when implementating the therapy described here to take into account the interplay of all the components* of medicinal therapy: constitutional, acute, internal as injection, external application as poultice; sufficient intake of fluids (including by means of enemas) and nutrition. If there should be a deterioration in the general condition or the oxygenation, and/or if insufficient nutrients and fluids can be taken in, prompt inpatient hospital admission must be implemented; the physician must always be available.

The RSV virus is related to the mumps virus; RSV infections appear to be on the increase. *Vitamin D deficiency* increases susceptibility to and worsens the course of bronchiolitis.

5.1.6 Tracheobronchitis – differential treatment indications for coughing

The many phenomena connected with acute and chronic inflammations of the trachea and bronchi cannot be described in more detail within the scope of the present work. The authors confined themselves, therefore, to the medicines which appeared essential to them. In this field, everyone will need to find their own therapeutic direction according to experience and their knowledge of the materia medica. Reference should be made to ▸Chap. 5.1.1 (pneumonia), ▸Chap. 5.1.4 (stenosing laryngitis), ▸Chap. 6.5 (bronchial asthma) and ▸Chap. 5.4 (feverish flu-like infections).

Different kinds and blends of teas loosen secretions and alleviate the urge to cough, for example blends of

- marshmallow root,
- narrowleaf plantain,
- mallow blossom.

The addition of mallow makes the tea much more acceptable to children. A tea of *lime blossom and elderflower*, honey and a little lemon has a warming and loosening effect. It should be given as a basic therapy for all feverish infections of the airways. A cough mixture that often helps, and that can be prepared by the parents, is made up of equal proportions of finely-chopped onion and honey; it can be given in quantities of a coffee spoon at a time. Studies have shown honey to be as effective as conventional mucolytics! *Coltsfoot* (leaves), which is very effective, is dispensed to parents with a health warning, based on the results of dubious animal studies. It has an antispasmodic effect and promotes secretion for dry coughs. Cowslip root is good as an ingredient to release secretion for wet, rattling coughs.

Dietetically, the principles described in ▸Chap. 5.1.2.3 for inflammations of the airways are also applicable. Reducing the intake of milk, or avoiding it altogether, drinking plenty, and consuming vegetable-based soups which have been seasoned appropriately to the age of the child – as well as avoiding sweet things – are all important and have positive effects.

As an external application, warm

- **Lavandula Oleum 10 %** (Wala/Weleda)

is useful in the form of an embrocation or compress for laryngotracheitis.
Good results have been had for bronchitis with

- **Plantago Bronchialbalsam** Wala (contains beeswax).

For wet bronchitis that is difficult to loosen, chest compresses of ginger (instructions, ▸Chap. 2.3.2.2) or low-fat quark are helpful; for dry, obstructive bronchitis a Retterspitz® chest wrap (▸Chap. 6.5.6.2) or lemon chest wrap [Stellmann 2009, 60].

Warm footbaths, increasing in temperature, generally have very favourable effects on inflammations of the airways – therapeutically and prophylactically.

Medicinally there exist numerous composite remedies. It is possible to go into only a few, important single-substance medicines here.[1]

Should the urge to cough and a worsening at night predominate, the following medicines should be considered:

- **Rumex D6–12 pillules/dil.** (various manufacturers)

for continual, short attacks of dry coughing, accompanied by (frequently recurrent) rhinitis, sensitivity to cold. If coughing predominates after 10.00 pm–11.00 pm and sometimes all night (ticklish cough). The back of the throat shows postnasal drip; the nasal secretion, as it flows down, triggers the urge to cough, particularly when changing position.

1 The authors would like to thank R. Schwarz for valuable indications.

- **Drosera D6–12 pillules** Weleda, various manufacturers

for barking, ticklish, excruciating coughing (similar as for Rumex), "throaty voice"/ hoarseness (moderately pronounced), worsening around/shortly after midnight, possibly vomiting of food and catarrh (▸Chap. 5.3.6). Medicine for whooping cough (Hahnemann). Possibly nosebleed.

- **Spongia D6–15 pillules/dil.** (various manufacturers)

for hoarseness, spasmodic barking. Coughing worsening in the middle of the night (11 pm–2 am). Coughing can be painful. Then

- **Hepar Sulfuris D12 pillules** (various manufacturers)

can be given by turn or alternating: sore throat and strong pains in the larynx when coughing, hoarseness, pronounced need for warmth and intolerance of cold air, worsening of the cough after 3.00am, ill-humoured.

- **Ammonium causticum D6 pillules/dil.** (various manufacturers)

for sustained nocturnal coughing fits with long pauses without bronchospasticity, plentiful loose catarrh, rattling breathing, weakness.

- **Olivenit D8 dil.** (=Cuprum arsenicosum nat.) Apotheke an der Weleda

for sustained, spasmodic coughing fits in the second half of the night, for instance with dry, obstructive bronchitis, bronchial asthma, whooping cough.

Should there be a tendency to obstructive bronchitis, possibly with dyspnoea (see 453), or to wet, rattling secretion, or to an urge to retch when coughing, then the following should first be considered:

- **Ipecacuanha D12 pillules** Weleda, various manufacturers

for pronounced worsening at night with the urge to retch when coughing and coughing to the point of vomiting, first dry, later with coarse catarrhal rattling. Irritable, dismissive mood. Clean tongue.

- **Tartarus stibiatus D6 trit.** Weleda

Bronchitis going deeper than with Ipecacuanha (which it is good to follow with Tart. stib.), finer catarhal rattling (on auscultation more audible dorsally – with Ipecacuanha more frontally, near the bronchi), pronounced dyspnoea, secretion difficult to loosen, general weakness, white-coated tongue.

Should the cough be painful, the following should be considered:

- **Bryonia D6–12 pillules** Wala, Weleda, various manufacturers
  for dry, sharply painful cough, accompanied by strong thirst for cold drinks; avoiding any movement (even the movement of breathing hurts). Ill-tempered, dismissive mood.
- **Phosphor D12/LM6 pillules/dil.** Wala, Weleda, various manufacturers
  for coughing, with substernal pain, laryngeal ticklish irritation, barking, hoarseness, but with inflammation reaching lower than with Spongia. In some cases bloody sputum (tracheitis!). General exhaustion, worsening in the evening, when cold; agile, restless character, extravert, but easily susceptible to anxiety.

- **Causticum D12 pillules/dil.** (various manufacturers)
  for painful hoarseness, dryness of the pharynx and larynx, possibly slight hoarseness. No tendency to bleeding, worsening when cold and in dry weather. Psychologically compassionate, but introverted, a readiness to withdraw from conflict situations, inhibited from aggression.
- **Kalium carb. D6 pillules/dil.** (various manufacturers)
  for dry, hard cough with sharp pain, a feeling of worsening appearing to proceed from a place in the upper region of the trachea when cold or lying down, or after 3.00am; improving over the course of the day.

Coughing with purulent and possibly malodorant phlegm requires, apart from diagnostic clarification,

- **Sulphur iod. D4–6 dil.** (various manufacturers)
  a medicine that is also very effective for mucoviscidosis and bronchiectasis.
- **Stibium sulf. aurantiacum** (Sb_2S_5) **D6–10 trit.** Weleda is helpful as a potentized medicine in cases of chronic, non-specific bronchitis with constant coughing day and night, without specific symptoms suggesting particular remedies.

5.2 Inflammation of the mouth, pharynx and tonsils

5.2.1 Aphthous stomatitis (stomatitis aphtosa)

Individual, perioral redness or blisters in the region of the skin, pathognomic gingivitis with redness and swelling, and foul breath enable early diagnosis of this illness, which is often accompanied by a high temperature. Accompanying tonsillitis and lymphadenitis should not tempt one to consider treatment with antibiotics, as they can be managed well by means of the suggested treatment. *Nutrition* with liquid and gruel-like foods (without sugar or acids likely to irritate the mucous membrane) is an important therapeutic task where the course of the illness is serious. The parents need careful support and advice from the physician. In the case of a high fever and/or weakness in drinking, *enemas* are very helpful, every six to twelve hours, with the help of a rubber enema bulb for infants and toddlers (instructions, cf. ▸Chap. 5.1.1.4.2). The fluid balance is thereby improved (the enema should be carried out slowly and sufficiently deeply, so that enough fluid is absorbed); the fever somewhat moderated; and the general condition improved (in a similar way to a corresponding, brief infusion). Hospital admission is hardly ever needed with the course of action recommended here, even when there are pronounced acute symptoms.

Meticulous care of the mouth is important. Cotton buds (with large cotton wool swabs) are good for cleaning the oral cavity; instead of the usual antiseptics,

- **Wala Mundbalsam** flüssig (Mouth balm, liquid)

can be used. It can also be helpful to rinse the mouth and gargle with

- **Symbioflor® 1**
  5–10 gtt. 2–3 x/d

Medicinally,

- **Mercurius cyanatus D6** pillules Apotheke an der Weleda/**dil.** DHU
  (3–)5 pillules./gtt. 4–6 x/d

is the most important medicine for herpetic stomatitis. Foul breath; salivation; aphthae and ulcers (with membranaceous surfaces) in the area of the gums, the oral cavity and

throat; severe pain on swallowing; inflamed swelling of the tonsils and lymph nodes; and a noticeably impaired general condition indicate this homoeopathic medicine.
For anxious, thin, restless (neurasthenic) children,

- **Borax D6 pillules** (various manufacturers)
  5 pillules 5 x/d is suitable in combination with Mercurius cyanatus;

for children whose behaviour is impulsive and characterized by their will,

- **Acidum sulfuricum D12 pillules** (various manufacturers)
  5 pillules 3 x/d

is particularly appropriate.
The latter is generally a principal medicine for aphthae in the oral cavity, even without generalized gingivitis/stomatitis.
With high, sustained fever; apathy; refusal of food; and an extremely impaired general condition, the most important medicine is

- **Baptisia D6 dil./pillules** (various manufacturers)
  5 pillules/gtt. 5 x/d

The following medicine from Holland is a significant innovation:

- **Baptisia/Lachesis comp. dil.** Apotheke an der Weleda
  (Apis mell. D4, Baptisia D3, Crotalus terrific. D10, Echinacea ang. Urtinktur, Lachesis D10, Quarz D6, Thuja Urtinktur)
  4–7 gtt. 6 x/d [Vademecum 2010, 189].

This medicine has proved beneficial for herpetic stomatitis (alternately with Mercurius cyanatus; for the indication, see Baptisia). Effective for oral and genital aphthae, both for acute conditions and as a prophylactic against this frequently recurrent and subjectively very unpleasant illness.
A *nosode* which is extremely effective in all forms of acute and particularly recurrent aphthae in the oral cavity is

- **Nosode FMD D30 pillules** Barlach Apotheke Boll
  3–5 pillules 3 × at intervals of 12 hr.
  (FMD: foot and mouth disease)

5.2.2 Herpangina; hand, foot and mouth disease

These symptoms, which are connected to Coxsackie viruses, can be treated well with

- **Apis Belladonna c. Mercurio pillules** Wala
  5–7 pillules 5 x/d for about 5 days.

5.2.3 Acute tonsillitis

(Scarlet fever ▸Chap. 5.3.4, lymphadenitis colli ▸Chap. 5.3.4.4.4).

In the case of tonsillitis, the doctor should always ask themself what the child is unable to overcome, what they are "unable to swallow" – psychologically as well as bodily. Socially, it is often the case that the easing of a burden or more security is needed; nutrition should be considered in the case history and in any consultation (bad chewing? Irregular mealtimes? Too much sugar, too much juice – too little fruit and vegetables?). *Sufficient peace and quiet* and *taking account of the basics of nutrition* (nutrition, movement, rhythms of life, balance of warmth) are the basis for treatment. This is particularly important for young people. The doctor has a big responsibility when guiding these patients, as they are frequently insufficiently aware of their own condition; while the parents' overview may have gaps. However, the risk of complications in puberty is particularly great!

The most important general measure is *bedrest* until the patient has had a whole day without fever – even in the absence of scarlet fever or definite streptococcal infection. Getting the patient up and about again afterwards must take into account a careful consideration of their general condition and the local situation, and varies very individually in the time taken. A *different* approach must be taken if it is actually scarlet fever (▸Chap. 5.3.4). As far as *diet* is concerned, avoiding sugar (in any form) and fruit juices is important.

As an *external application* for tonsillitis, a

- **lemon neck wrap** [Goebel and Glöckler 2008, 663–665; Vagedes and Soldner 2010, 56]

has proved helpful.

This may be applied from warm to hot (for about ten minutes or longer); or cool in cases of acute tonsillitis with high fever. One uses a halved, organic lemon which, after scoring its peel, one squeezes in the water so that the etheric oils of the lemon peel get into the poultice water (a small bowl, half full). The wrap cloth is immersed in the water, wrung out and then applied to the neck (covered by a woollen scarf). Also effective are neck wraps with salt water and, for very swollen and painful lymph nodes, neck wraps with low-fat quark [Goebel and Glöckler 2008, 665f.; Vagedes and Soldner 2010, 56]

It has also proved helpful to rub

- **Mercurialis 10 % ointment** Weleda or
- **Archangelica comp. ointment** Weleda

into the skin over the lymph nodes of the angle of the jaw and of the side of the neck.

Internally, the following single remedies should be considered before others: initially, and by far most frequently,

- **Belladonna D6 or Rh D6 dil.** Weleda
  30–50 gtt./½ glass water, sipped over 12–24 hrs.
  The following symptoms indicate this medicine:
  - *sudden* onset with high fever,
  - *crimson* tonsils, usually without a coating,
  - dry mucous membrane (with damp, normal skin),
  - little thirst,
  - sensitive to being touched; children *do not want any external application* (!)
  - buildup of warmth in the head area, cool extremities.

At the beginning of therapy, the following composite medicine is suitable for acute tonsillitis:

- **Apis/Belladonna c. Mercurio pillules** Wala
  initially 5–7 pillules 1–2 hrly, then 5 x/d.

This medicine is most broadly indicated for acute tonsillitis. The following may be taken into particular account as a follow-on medicine

- **Lachesis comp. pillules** Wala
  5–10 pillules 3–5 x/d.

General support for the course of therapy may be provided by gargling several times a day with sips of

- **Symbioflor® 1**
  8–20 gtt. in weak sage tea

and/or rinsing the mouth with

- **Calendula essence** Wala
  3 × 7–20 gtt. in water: rinse and spit out.

It is generally to be recommended that close relatives (parents and siblings) also carry out these measures, as this lowers the risk of infection.

The authors have found the following to be of outstanding benefit as a *single medicine for tonsillitis:*

- **Phytolacca D12/C12 pillules** DHU, Gudjons
  4–7 pillules 5 x/d.
  Guiding symptoms:
  - *dark red* throat (particularly the soft palate),
  - pains radiating into the ears,
  - follicular inflammation of the back of the throat,
  - painful, pronounced swelling of the tonsils and lymph nodes.

This is an important medicine in *mononucleosis* (▸Chap. 5.2.6). It is particularly effective for patients who feel weak and who give the impression during their illness of being withdrawn and depressed

- **Apis mell. D6 pillules/dil.** Weleda,
  dosage as for Belladonna, may be combined with it.
  Guiding symptoms:
  - *bright red, oedematous* inflamed throat,
  - uvula badly swollen,
  - lack of thirst.

For acute tonsillitis with coatings (follicularis, lacunaris) the focus is on:

- **Mercurius solubilis D6 trit.** Weleda pharmacy,
  D12–C30 pillules (various manufacturers)
  1 saltsp. 2 x/h or 5 pillules 4x/d
  Guiding symptoms:
  - *foul breath,*
  - spongy, slack, very inflamed mucous membranes,
  - painful swelling of the cervical lymph nodes,
  - flow of saliva, pronounced (unpleasant) sweating *particularly at night,*
  - alternate sweating and freezing, extreme restlessness.
- **Hepar sulfuris D6 trit.** Weleda **D12–C30 pillules** (various manufacturers) (under no circumstances should potencies lower than D6 be used)
  1 saltsp. 2 x/h or 5 pillules 3 x/d
  Guiding symptoms:
  - *sharp,* very strong pains,
  - unpleasantly foul breath (as for Mercur sol.),
  - strongly pronounced *sensitivity to cold;* the patient wishes to wear a scarf and avoid all draughts; and is generally *very sensitive.*

5

Hepar sulfuris is a medicine which is frequently very effective after mercury for purulent tonsillitis, when it can also be given as D30 or C30 5 pillules 3 x/d for about 3 days.
Hepar sulfuris is particularly important for *prevention of complications* (e.g. peritonsillar abscess inter al.).
Two further homoeopathic remedies should then be considered if there is a tonsillitis that is *definitely on only one side*:

- **Lycopodium C12–30 pillules** Gudjons
  5 pillules 2–4 x/d
  Guiding symptoms:
  - *right-sided* tonsillitis,
  - worsening in the late *afternoon* (4.00 pm–8.00 pm),
  - generally worse in the winter,
  - foul breath (also from disturbed functioning of the stomach and duodenum).
- **Lachesis D12 dil.** Weleda
  5–7 gtt. 2–4 x/d
  Guiding symptoms:
  - *left-sided* tonsillitis, livid mucous membrane,
  - very sensitive to being touched on the neck (see Belladonna),
  - restless, constantly in movement, and acute feeling of being ill
  - definite worsening in the morning, *after sleep*.

The constitutional aspects of the latter two remedies are considered in greater detail in ▸Chap. 6.4.3.6.1 (Lycopodium) and ▸Chap. 6.5.6.11 (Lachesis).
The more serious the course of the illness, the more individualized the diagnosis and choice of medicines must be; there is no substitute for finding the right medicine in this case. Where the effect is insufficient, one may increase the potency or proceed to the appropriate follow-up medicine.

In most cases of acute tonsillitis, treatment with antibiotics is not therapeutically necessary (▸Chap. 5.3.4.4).

5.2.4 Adenoids und hypertrophy of the tonsils

Children with adenoidal growths and hypertrophy of the tonsils are conspicuous by their *impaired inbreathing* [Holtzapfel 1982, 45–49]. Over time, this can have consequences for the formative development of the palate and jaw, and can lead to deformations; sleep is less restorative, when the disturbed inbreathing is particularly apparent (snoring, over-stretched neck). The *relation of the soul to its environment* becomes duller as a result of factors such as tiredness in the morning and disturbances to the air supply of the middle ear (seromucous tympanum); the musculature in the region of the jaw becomes hypotonic, the child's speech is often less articulated and, at the same time, there is a tendency to chronic catarrh and recurrent inflammations. It becomes apparent from this that the bodily formative force of the child's soul has become insufficiently active, and that the vital growth forces connected with inheritance are preponderating and hypertrophying. The aim of therapy must therefore be to promote incarnation, the entry of the soul into the body; to deepen inbreathing in the most comprehensive sense (▸Chap. 5.1.2.1).

Thus, what we are primarily concerned with here is a developmental hesitation of the soul in relation to the body, accompanied by exaggerated growth; the latter may also be a result of hereditary or constitutional factors. *Paedagogically,* consistent guidance of these children is important as, in their whole make-up, they are often dependent on their environment and live in a close symbiosis with their mother. On the other hand, it is important to consider that, for example, a tendency to seromucous tympanum can rapidly intensify with such children if they are overburdened in their independence (e. g. entering kindergarten too early). Cautious, consistent "cutting of the umbilical cord" by the parents can be supported by the doctor through appropriate consultation and also through constitutionally effective remedies.

The oral cavity is of central significance for pathogenesis and therapy. The oral cavity is a central sense organ and is the human being's most intimate interior space throughout life. Swallowing (amniotic fluid) and thumb-sucking have an effect on its development, even in utero. After birth, sucking on the nipple is greatly significant for the proper development of the oral cavity and the mandibular joint. Dummies and drinking bottles (higher risk of otitis media!), on the other hand, tend rather to work against this development. Sucking a dummy and drinking from a bottle should be stopped as early as possible. The *motor function of the tongue as the principal rhythmical centre of the oral cavity influences the child's entire motor development* [Girke 2010, 624]. Motor activity of the limbs, learning alternating (crossed) bodily movement through crawling and climbing stairs, through arm-leg co-ordination and so on, are of great importance. *Padovan therapy* is useful, among other things, for catching up on missed developmental stages and, for instance, for overcoming partially retained primitive reflexes. The number of children manifesting motor development deficits, and thus disturbed nasal breathing, one-sided oral breathing and corresponding deformities of the jaw is growing. For children with adenoids, with chronic oral breathing, myofunctional weaknesses or disturbance of the motor functionality of the tongue, the authors have had very good experiences with eurythmy therapy, where I-A-O with the feet is particularly effective and can be directly experienced in its effect on the musculature of the tongue.[1]

Dietetically, a break from milk can be beneficial for many children (sour milk products do not need to be avoided). The child should be guided into a *more thorough chewing* of their food, including through appropriate foods, in order to counteract hypotonia and stimulate the child's own formative and breaking-down forces. It is particularly helpful in this regard to chew raw vegetables (carrots!) and fruit (eating apples instead of drinking juice!). Diagnostically, one should be aware of the possibility of a *disturbance of the symbiosis of the intestinal flora, and consider therapeutic balancing of the intestinal flora* (microbiological therapy) (▸Chap. 4.6.4).

1 The authors wish to thank T. Schmidt, orthodontist in Munich, and their colleague and eurythmy therapist Dr Sabine Sebastian, of Pforzheim, for essential advice.

Tab. 5.1 Different types of Calcium

Calcium carbonicum = Conchae D12 trit./pillules	Calcium phosphoricum D8–12 pillules	Calcium iodatum D12
Good appetite; well-nourished as a child; large head; broad neck perspiration of the head	Variable appetite, poor eater; rapid growth in height; thin neck; large, soft lymph nodes	Mainly thirsty; beyond infancy, thin if anything; the appetite may be good; the lymph nodes tend to be small; adenoids are to the fore
Calm, peaceful slow but steady development	Inquisitive; likes to be on the move; often dissatisfied and demanding; not very consistent; tends to headaches and stomach aches	Happy, agile; needs fresh air, but has a tendency to catching cold

For children with adenoids or seromucous tympanum, the authors consider the following external application to be an essential element of therapy:

- **Oleum Salviae 10%** (in olive oil), e.g. as a dispensed special medicine from Apotheke an der Weleda
  massage the child 3 x/wk in the morning on the trunk and limbs (excluding the head/face and the nappy (diaper)/underpants area).

As a rule, the treatment is carried out during the winter months for 3–6 months (not during the hot summer months). The authors can confirm the experience of Joop van Dam, who introduced this measure as a therapy [van Dam 2006, Soldner 2007]: the incidence of adenotomy and drainage of the middle ear has been almost halved through this measure (Cf. ▸Chap. 5.1.3.3).

A further important external application for adenoids and seromucous tympanum has been developed by Henrik Szoeke of Budapest:

- **Hay fever spray** Weleda
  4–5 x/d horizontally (! – in the direction of the lower nasal meatus) 1–2 puffs into each nostril (▸Chap. 6.6)

or

- **Citrus/Cydonia solution for external use** (formerly: Gencydo® solution) Apotheke an der Weleda
  Put 1 drop/year of age in 5 ml slightly hypertonic NaCl solution (~2%) in both nostrils or, even better, apply horizontally with a spray top (screw-top nasal spray bottle) (the diluted solution may be kept 3–4 days in the refrigerator) [see also Vademecum 2010, 458]

Works well in combination with warm saltwater footbaths (2–3% salt content), where applicable with added ginger (bring 3–4 tablespoons Pulvis Zingiberis in 200 ml water gradually to the boil till it turns to a gruel, then add to the footbath). Freer nasal breathing should become apparent after a few weeks; treatment should continue for at least 4–6 weeks; efficacy may be checked through tympanometry among other means.

Potentized *calcium salts are the most important constitutional therapy* (Tab. 5.1). These have a fundamental effect on the formative forces of the soul, stimulating their effectiveness in the body. *Where the effectiveness of these is insufficient, or where the vital organization has become extremely independent of the soul's formative force, appropriate Barium salts, primarily Barium carb. D6–12, Barium muriaticum D12, Barium iod. D12 may bring the intended effect.*

Calcium iodatum is organotropically *specifically effective for adenoids;* for *hypertrophy of the tonsils,* on the other hand, Calcium phosphoricum is indicated. Nevertheless, it remains true that a radical effect will be most likely when the child's general symptoms correspond to the characteristics described. Fundamentally, in therapy one should decide on one medicine.

As an interpolation, one may give

- **Berberis/Quarz amp./pillules** Wala
  ½–1 drinking ampoule x/d or 7–10 pillules 2 x/d and possibly
- **Thymus/Mercurius pillules** Wala
  5 pillules 2–3 x/d

in order to strengthen the organism's form forces in the lymphatic system and the upper airways.

For lymphatic growths in the area of the nose and throat, an important support can generally be given by rubbing on

- **Berberis (Fructus) 10 % ointment** Weleda

(a pea-sized amount) in the region above the bladder in the evening. This measure stimulates a deeper connection of the soul's form forces with the bodily nature. This may be effected from the indicated region of the organism [see Soldner and Sommer 2007].

- **Thuja occidentalis Essence/Tincture 20 %** Wala/Weleda
  1–7 tablespoons according to age/weight in the bath (10 minutes) 1–2 x/wk

is effective for slim, soft children with adenoids, whether tending to be either dark-haired and mobile or light-haired and clinging. It vitalizes the metabolic region and removes from the head the burden of "excessive metabolism" (represented by the rampantly growing adenoids, mucotympanum etc.) [The authors are grateful to R. Schwarz, see Vademecum 2010, 209]

For hyperplasia and tendency to inflammation of the tonsils generally (and thereby ultimately their unsatisfactory functioning), particularly in the first seven years, responsiveness to the remedies mentioned has been markedly and repeatedly improved through *homologous potentized organ preparation medicines.*

- **Tonsilla pharyngea series pack III amp.** Wala
  ½–1 drinking ampoule 3 x/wk in the morning, descending from D30 to D5; followed perhaps by a second potency sequence in the opposite direction

or

- **Tonsillae palatinae series pack III amp.** Wala
  in the same dosage

For therapy for nasal polyps, ▸Chap. 5.1.2.3.

Through the therapeutic possibilities mentioned, ENT surgical intervention can frequently be avoided. In individual cases, however, an operation can have an exceptionally liberating effect on the development of a child. Should an adenotomy (hearing defect, *developmental speech disorder*, no response to potentized remedies or diet) be unavoidable, a recurrence can be counteracted through the constitutional remedies mentioned. It is very difficult to treat hypertrophy of the tonsils with chronically recurrent tonsillitis (▸Chap. 5.2.5) if the tonsils are no longer clearly defined, soft and elastic; but where the connective tissue has degenerated, has a hard consistency, is fissured on the surface. In such cases, surgical remediation may be unavoidable.

Therapeutically potentized Kalium salts may be considered for *large, fissured tonsils*; particularly

- **Kalium chloratum/Sylvin D4–12 dil.** DHU/Apotheke an der Weleda
  5–7 gtt. 2–3 x/d

if large, usually foul-smelling clots need to be detached from the tonsil cavities (a very reliable medicine). Potentized iodine compounds in particular have a cleansing effect, thus countering inflammation (Kalium iodatum D12, Calcium iodatum D12, Sulphur iodatum D6–12); the effect of these halogens may be understood such that more light forces are thereby available to the immunological activity of the organism.

5.2.5 Chronically recurring tonsillitis

Case study

A ten-year-old girl – already known to the doctor over a long period – came to the surgery every three to four weeks because of recurrent tonsillitis. There were no detectable haemolysing streptococci; locally, there was always a non-specific sore throat coated with small, grey spots. The girl is dark-haired, slender and has brown eyes; her behaviour is generally agile, happy and extravert for her age. Her mother works as a nurse; there are no problems in the girl's relationship with her parents. There are no difficulties at school. Treating the acute tonsillitis is straightforward; every attempt, however, to reduce the frequency of recurrence through constitutional treatment, diet, microbiological therapy (symbiosis guidance), or the like, founders.

It was often possible only to have telephone consultations when the illness was acute.

Only after about a year was the case history carefully taken again. When the doctor asked: "What was going on a year ago?", he learnt that the patient's maternal grandmother from Denmark had come to live with the family. She had lost her husband, and had become obviously depressed. On one hand, the patient's mother wanted to take care of her own mother; while on the other she was glad that there was a relation in the house when she went off to work in the afternoons. When questioned, the mother stated that the daughter's relationship to her grandmother was very close, and that the grandmother's depression was a burden to the child (who is very empathetic). Over the past year, the grandmother's condition had not improved at all.

It became clear that the patient was living in close and very ambivalent relationships with two female relations; and that out of love she was taking on some of the grandmother's suffering (which overburdened her), as expressed by B. Hellinger.

- **Lac caninum C60 pillules** Gudjons
  3 × 5 pillules at intervals of 12 h

was subsequently prescribed as medication with the result that the child had no more attacks of tonsillitis in the following three years (= the follow-up period). After the mother had became aware through the case history consultation of the connection between her mother's moving in and the illnesses of her daughter, a conversation between mother and grandmother took place. The latter then found her own flat in a nearby part of the town and moved out of the family. It is interesting to note that her depressive moods also improved. (The authors are grateful to their homoeopathic colleague from Austria, J. Gnaiger [1990, 1991], for her decisive contribution to their understanding of Lac caninum.)

Chronically recurring tonsillitis can present a therapeutic challenge which is difficult to resolve. Apart from the findings in relation to the organ itself (▸Chap. 5.2.4), careful clarification of the possible aetiology is important. The following diagnostic and therapeutic possibilities appear relevant to the authors:

- Consequences of vaccination

From our own observation, BCG vaccination of newborn infants can have particularly adverse effects in this regard.

- **Tuberculinum C30–200 pillules** Gudjons

should be mentioned here as it generally represents the most important nosode for chronically recurrent tonsillitis. It has been found particularly useful to give it to children whose condition follows BCG vaccination, and for children susceptible to infection, where the family medical history reveals a forebear with tuberculosis.

5

Case study

An eight-year-old boy comes to the surgery for consultation and treatment every three to six weeks, because of recurring, streptococcal-negative tonsillitis. He was born in Africa, where his father worked as an engineer providing development aid, and was vaccinated as a newborn infant. The family now lives in Germany; however the father works on large-scale construction projects in Germany and abroad and, apart from during holidays, is only at home when he has a free weekend. This puts quite a strain on mother and children (the boy has a sister). All therapeutic efforts initially bring only meagre results until the mother responds to a direct question about BCG vaccination. Subsequently tuberculinum is given twice, in a high potency (C200), with a six-week interval. Since then there have been no more problems with the tonsils, nor any new symptoms elsewhere. At the same time, the night sweats to which the boy had had a tendency ceased. The family problem remained unresolved (over a seven-year follow-up period).

- Symbiosis disturbance, particularly after repeated antibiotic treatment

With recurrent tonsillitis, it makes sense to carry out a thorough diagnosis (including examination of the stools and a throat swab for bacterial dysbiosis and mycosis) and, if appropriate, microbiological therapy (symbiosis guidance) with a corresponding diet (▸Chap. 4.6.4).

- **Sulphur iodatum D4-6 dil.** (various manufacturers.)
  5 gtt. 2–3 x/d

is particularly effective as medication after the acute treatment and as an accompaniment to the microbiological therapy.

If the tonsils are shown to be overgrown with a particular bacterial or mycotic species, it makes sense to give *the corresponding nosode,* e. g. as D6, 5 gtt. 1–3 x/d.

- Excessive psychological and social demands (must above all be recognized and addressed)

If there is a burdensome, psychologically ambivalent relationship to two female reference persons ("*two mothers*", as a rule mother and a grandmother),

- **Lac caninum D12-C60 pillules** (various manufacturers) – (see the above Case study) is a very effective medicine. If *aggression and jealousy* are an important motif, one should primarily consider
- **Lachesis D12-30(-200) pillules** (various manufacturers).

It is particularly difficult to treat those children for whom it is apparent that a constitutional *hypofunction and weakness of the organ* is the cause of the recurring inflammations. Usually there is a hypertrophy of the tonsils with a transition to degeneration of the connective tissue (see the possibilities for therapy listed in ▸Chap. 5.2.4; including particularly Barium carb., iod., muriaticum D6-12).

An approach to therapy may be undertaken here with

- **Kalium iodatum D12 dil.** (various manufacturers)
  5 gtt. 1–2 x/d
- **Thymus/Mercurius pillules** Wala
  5 pillules 3 x/d
- **Tonsillae palatinae potency sequence series pack III amp.** Wala
  ½–1 ampoule 2–3 x/wk in the morning (orally), from D30 to D5 descending, followed possibly by D5 to D30 ascending,
- **Equisetum Silicea cultum D2 dil.** Weleda
  interpolating 3 × 5–10 drops for 14 days.

5.2.6 Mononucleosis

5.2.6.1 Insight into the illness

Glandular fever does not affect a child by chance; as a rule, infection is not sufficient to cause the illness. The affected children and young people are conspicuous by their *weakness* – the older they are, the more it stands out – which is pronounced and sustained (and often goes unmentioned in conventional textbooks). In the background there is very often an *overburdening that has been going on for some time,* both from the environment (a stressful family situation and demands at school) as well as inner demands that the child places on themselves. Certain parallels with the so-called chronic fatigue syndrome (CFS), an illness of adults, are unmistakable.

Case study

A slender, ten-year-old girl of medium height attended the surgery. For some days she had had a temperature of 39 °C, complained vaguely of headaches and a sore neck, and had lost her appetite completely; after several visits to different doctors, no diagnosis had been reached. The child appeared exhausted and slightly depressed. Examination revealed enlarged tonsils with whitish coatings and markedly enlarged cervical lymph nodes; specifically, the examiner found there was a diffuse sensation of pain on pressure being applied to the upper abdomen, with distinct enlargement of the liver, but without perceptible enlargement of the spleen (which probably would have been detectable by ultrasound at that point). The subsequently expressed suspected diagnosis of mononucleosis was confirmed by a differential blood picture, raised levels of transaminases and later also serologically.

The girl is the eldest child of parents who are both teachers. She has three younger siblings, who are triplets; one of these is a boy with severe autism, while the other two manifest distinct disabilities connected with infantile cerebral palsy. The parents are chronically overburdened as a result of this situation. The patient herself is very conscientious, has too great a sense of responsibility for her age, and is ambitious at school.

After a thorough discussion of the situation, acute treatment was begun along the lines of the therapy described below. Following this the child was given

- **Causticum D12 dil.** DHU
  initially 2 x, then 1 × 5 gtt./d.

At the outset, a four-week break from school was agreed. At the end of this period, the child was in a very good general condition; psychologically, the depressive mood had completely disappeared and the child appeared considerably more relaxed and full of the joys of life. At the end of the school year the mother reported that, to her astonishment, her daughter had made good all that she had missed and had got a very good report.

Pathophysiologically, what is striking about the Epstein-Barr virus infection is that the virus that activates it persists in the nose and throat area and is not eliminated. In the course of the viraemia, B lymphocytes are "partly transformed and immortalized" (!) [Böcker et al. 1997, 999], and *a pathological, proliferative activity begins in the immune system.* Corresponding to this, the first phase of the illness, which is hard to recognize, can bring changes in the blood picture and swelling of the lymph glands, the liver and the spleen, *while the course of the fever is extremely variable* (sometimes only subfebrile or fluctuating temperatures). At the same time, pronounced exhaustion and *weakness are strongly apparent.*

The signature of mononucleosis becomes visible in the course of this: The patient's life organization, their ether body, is taken hold of by forces of the outer world; a pathological process of proliferation begins; while the soul and spiritual individuality – the forming forces of the astral body and the organization of the I – remain in a state of weakness akin to paralysis, and in a condition almost similar to sleep in their separation from bodily processes. The reason is that they were already very strongly drawn outward and loosened from a firm anchoring in the body; the life organization of these patients is, as a rule, also in a weakened state even before the onset of the illness. Should a high fever start, the individual warmth organization becomes active; this activity should be supported, not undermined by being suppressed. Supporting the life organization therapeutically is just as necessary as releasing the soul and spiritual individuality from outer commitments and obligations and stimulating its formative activity on the body through appropriate medicines. This is why a sufficiently long easing of the child's burden must be agreed from the outset and persevered with on the basis of an appropriate medical certificate.

Treating mononucleosis with homoeopathic and anthroposophic medicines is one of the most rewarding tasks in paediatric practice. Conventional medicine offers no alternatives. Even patients who present only after the acute phase of the illness, because they are still not properly recovered after months, can be successfully treated in the way indicated.

5.2.6.2 Treatment

In the acute phase of the illness, the following are suitable for the beginning of treatment (originally a recommendation by Markus Sommer, which has been beneficial in the authors' practice:

- **Mercurius solubilis D12 pillules** (various manufacturers)
  5 pillules 3–4 x/d together with
- **Vincetoxicum D6 pillules** (various manufacturers)
  3–4 x/d pillules and
- **Calendula D3 amp.** Wala
  ½ ampoule 2 x/d (for 10 days)

Potentized quicksilver has a comprehensive effect on the whole reticuloendothelial system; accelerates the forming intervention of the astral body there; and brings the healing process "into flow" [Selawry 1985, 179, 202ff.; Sommer and Soldner 1988b]. Vincetoxicum is a medicine for viral infections of the nasopharyngeal area; as a plant-based medicine, calendula in low potencies supports the effect of mercury.

Initially, therapy may be intensified through a single i.v. injection of

- **Vincetoxicum D6 amp.** Staufen
- **Mercurius auratus D15 amp.** Weleda,
- **Reticuloendothelial system Gl D30 amp.** Wala.

The authors are grateful to their French colleague R. Kempenich for a further *medicine for the treatment of mononucleosis:*

- **Phytolacca C12 pillules Gudjons**
  acute 5–7 pillules up to 4 x/d alternating with the remedies above.

The reader can find specific symptoms which indicate the choice of remedy under ▸Chap. 5.2.3. The essential aspects are extreme weakness; pronounced swelling of the cervical lymph nodes in particular; a tendency to withdrawal on the part of the patient (giving the impression of depression); tonsillitis; and the (spontaneously) torpid course of the illness.

Any acute case of mononucleosis can be very satisfactorily treated with the above remedies, *if at the same time* the strict *unburdening of responsibility for achieving anything* described above is carried through for a sufficiently long period.

Case study

The author received a phone call from a father: his 16-year-old daughter had fallen ill six days previously with a very painful case of acute tonsillitis. The antibiotics prescribed by the emergency service did not help. The girl was very seriously affected, unable to eat or drink, and had a very sore throat. She was admitted to the hospital, where she received infusions. The hospital report was as follows: the tonsils are acutely inflamed on both sides, with a yellowish coating; the lymph nodes are extremely swollen, also on both sides. Otherwise nothing remarkable (feeling ill in the upper abdomen). CRP 0.7 mg/dl liver enzymes (transaminases) raised, 27,600 leucozytes stimulated with lymphocytes; spleen and liver enlarged. Diagnosis: mononucleosis. Therapy: antibiotics (!), completely ineffective, infusion therapy. Her general condition remains very bad.

The patient was discharged two days later, and was brought to our practice on her way home: her speech was weak, and sounded as if she had a lump in her throat. Examination of her throat revealed that she still had a massive tonsillitis with white coatings similar to those of diphtheria. She still had a fever, was extremely weak and said she was unable to eat or drink. The therapy described above was implemented in full, including the initial i.v. injection. After 24 hours at home, the fever had gone; after 48 hours, the patient was able to eat and felt like a "different person". After 72 hours, the coatings on the tonsils had all disappeared (checked during a home visit).

The case history which was subsequently taken and could be summarized as follows: the patient's mother is in a new relationship. She left home five months previously and lives with her new partner in a flat 400 metres away at the end of the same street. The patient and her fourteen-year-old brother live at home with their father. The patient sees both parents regularly. Both parents are high achievers and the family is well-off. The father used to take part in competitive sport; now the daughter does. In four weeks' time she was due to represent her country in the world championships (this was very important for her). Her mother will accompany her. When she returns from a competition which she has not won, she feels she has let her parents down by not attaining her target, as she puts it. Her parents have long been worried about her ambition without being able to stop it. The patient always gets an A in her grades at school; now she is trying for an average of 15 points (which is better than straight As). She studies until two in the morning. In addition she has ballet lessons twice a week and regularly practises a musical instrument, which she also has lessons in. She has had a boyfriend for three months (her first); he does the same competitive sport as she does.

When she was four to five years old, she twice had a fever with vomiting; once when her parents were away for four days, once for two days. When the patient was six years old, she went to the doctor because of severe cervical tension and suspected migraine; at the age of eight because of a lump in her throat; and at nine she developed coxitis fugax. She had several attacks of bronchitis during this time. At the age of eleven, she had sever influenza, mesenteric lymphadenitis with vomiting and incipient exsiccosis.

In a conversation with the parents, the connection between this case history and the clinical picture was explained. Anthroposophic art therapy (painting) was prescribed as the principal, ongoing therapy. Two weeks after this therapy began, the patient's symptoms were gone.

5

- **Rhus toxicodendron e fol. D30 pillules** Wala
  3 × 5 pillules/d for 3–5 days or 10 pillules dissolved in 50 ml water given over the course of 3 days (preferably as a single medicine)

can be indicated in cases of long-lasting fever and extreme exhaustion.

During the phase of convalescence and with patients who have still not recovered from mononucleosis after an extended period, the following forms of medication are important:

- **Causticum Hahnemanni D12–30 dil./pillules** DHU
  5 gtt./pillules 2 x/d (D12) – with D30 to be administered in accordance with the dosage delivered for Rhus tox.

In the event of a Phosphor constitution, Phosphor compounds are appropriate for mononucleosis which are therapeutically specifically related to the weakness and depressive state of the patients:

- **Acidum phosphoricum D12 dil./D30–C200 pillules** (various manufacturers)
  5 gtt. 3 x/d (D12); 3 × 5 pillules (D30) or 3 × 3 pillules (C200) daily for 3–5 days (▸Chap. 6.7 – specifically in the case of lovesickness) as well as
- **Potassium phosphoricum D6–12 dil.** Weleda
  5–7 gtt. 3 × or 2 x/d

especially with substantial liver involvement (transaminases!, findings), depressiveness and nervousness.

Wherever swollen lymph glands, weakness and cardiovascular instability predominate, the following medicine is indicated

- **Ferrum iodatum D12 dil.** (various manufacturers)
  7 gtt. 2 x/d

and with simultaneous tendency of epistaxis

- **Ferrum phosphoricum D12 dil./pillules** (various manufacturers)
  2 x/d 7 gtt./5–7 pillules.

Constitutionally the *distinction between Phosphor and Causticum* is important (and difficult). That is because children who need this constitutional aid are the ones most prone to mononucleosis or to severe and protracted episodes. In both cases, the body structure is asthenic, with a highly developed awareness of the feelings of other people and of injustices (this being especially typical of Causticum), involving sensitive children and young people who have great difficulty in shielding themselves psychologically from the problems of their environment and who can become overtaxed as a consequence.

For Phosphor as a constitutional aid, this is associated with a fundamentally *extrovert* nature with *a typically sanguine* temperament and a highly developed artistic aptitude. The child is only shy initially and, once familiar with his or her environment, enjoys expressing himself or herself and tends to be ebullient in the process. In the event of illness, these children tend to develop high fevers, have a characteristic *tendency to bleed* (epistaxis, tendency to develop infection-associated purpura) and appear, while in a fever, to be consuming their own substance more than they are fighting to overcome their illness *(prolonged, debilitating fever phase).* If they are healthy, their movements are easy and smooth, almost too much so.

In contrast to this, children who require Causticum (and Rhus tox.) as remedies tend to have a *more serious* and more *introverted* character. Their movements and their gait are more ponderous and awkward, they barely defend themselves when attacked by others and endeavour to avoid confrontation wherever possible. A *pronounced aggression inhibition* is manifested and this appears to extend right to the immunological system. In terms of their finer feelings and anxieties, both types of constitution share great similarities.

Generally support of the immune system is beneficial, as shown in ▸Chap. 6.3.3.4.

The most important measure to adopt, right at the beginning of therapy, is to produce **potentized autologous blood** as developed by Imhäuser [2000, 187ff.]. In the event of mononucleosis, this can be administered in accordance with the following pattern:

- C5 3 gtt. daily in the afternoon as individual dose for 7 days, followed by
- C7 3 gtt. every second day in the afternoon for 14 days, followed by
- C9 3 gtt. every third day in the afternoon for 21 days.

To support a weakened life-organization, it is particularly advisable to administer

- **Blackthorn elixir**
  15 ml 3 x/d

5.3 Childhood illnesses

"There is certain irony in the fact that we must now search for new ways to reproduce the infectious diseases against which we have been fighting with great success over the past three decades (!). The challenge is an important one because of the high morbidity of allergic and autoimmune diseases."

F. Bach [2002]

5

In these words the renowned allergologist F. Bach summarized the results of his research into the pathogenesis of childhood diseases. He reaches the conclusion that we need to seek out new ways "to reproduce" infectious diseases in childhood. In point of fact, for a long time now, more children in Germany and other western industrialized countries have been dying from diabetes mellitus and asthma than from chicken pox and measles! In contrast to this, recent data point towards diseases such as chickenpox being a protective reaction to the development of diabetes mellitus, atopic dermatitis and perhaps even tumours of the CNS (▸Chap. 3.5.1 incl. references). The protective action of mumps against ovarian carcinoma in women, and of highly febrile diseases against malignant melanoma has now been verified (▸Chap. 3, Introduction).

Of course, no-one is going to think spontaneously that parents and doctors in a country like Germany are sceptical about a campaign that aims to eliminate measles or chickenpox. Instead, parents phone the paediatrician to ensure that their child is restored to health and then stays healthy. On the other hand, immunology and epidemiology now point – as does anthroposophical research into the nature of the human being – to acute inflammations and overcoming them as being absolutely essential for the development of healthy immunological self-regulation in childhood. Viewed in this light, acute inflammatory diseases during early childhood facilitate the incarnation of the human individuality and the individualization of the physical body, while also strengthening the identification with the own body. Anyone denying these insights is failing to take account of the current status of medicinal-immunological research (▸Chap. 6.1). In countries with a western lifestyle this manifests the value of acute inflammatory diseases *in early childhood* and of an individually reticent approach to antipyretics, antibiotics and vaccinations in support of sustainable prevention of chronic and above all allergic diseases during childhood.

5.3.1 Childhood illnesses according to disease type

Measles, scarlet fever[1], chicken pox, German measles, mumps and whooping cough complete the set of classic childhood diseases in central Europe. Roseola and apthous stomatitis also manifest the characteristics of childhood diseases, and in southern countries hepatitis A which manifests itself as jaundice.[2] What do these "cyclical infectious diseases" share in common? What distinguishes them from typical old-age diseases such as cataracts, cerebral sclerosis and coxarthrosis? Can we give the term "childhood diseases" – beyond the controversy about the purpose of vaccination – a *positive content?*

Childhood diseases *appear at the surface* of the organism: as exanthema and as mucous enanthema, as a swelling (mumps) or as (unmistakable) coughing attacks (pertussis), all of which manifest themselves to the eye, ear and probing hand of the doctor. Always in the course of the disease something from inside the body *is excreted or secreted.* In every childhood disease, this secretion and excretion activity from the organism is *typical, and indeed pathognomonic.* We know today that every one of these diseases has an underlying specific incursion from the environment, a pathogen that has penetrated deep into the organism (in contrast to typical old-age diseases). However, this pathogen by itself does not explain the symptomatology. These symptoms are generated actively by the organism. Viewed in this way, every childhood disease causes the organism to engage in a typical – as distinct from an individual – excretory activity.

Complications always tend to arise in situations where the disease process attacks organs that render problematic an activity of this nature (e. g. middle ear, central nervous system) and/or if the abilities of an organism to move independently and to perform excretory functions are themselves impaired (e. g. scarlet fever nephritis, apnoea with pertussis). On the other hand, secretion and excretion processes are always dependent on the vitality and age of the child: this means that, viewed from a global perspective, childhood diseases are problematic in cases where children grow up undernourished in poverty. Their organism is then, in many cases, simply not up to the task of combating disease using only its own resources. By the same token, childhood diseases can become really problematic if they occur *at the wrong point in time*, in other words too early (for example measles in babies with cumulatively frequent SSPE) or too late (e. g. mumps, a disease that now occurs most frequently after vaccination at ages of between 16 and 24). The latter is undesirably exacerbated by vaccinations, especially in cases where the disease does not

1 Defined here in a narrow sense as an exanthemic infectious disease with pyrogenic toxin formation and a resultant level of antitoxic immunity formation.

2 In many countries with less stringent hygiene standards, hepatitis A, which tends to propagate in an icteric manner, also exhibits characteristics the timing of which can be predicted and which does not develop into a chronic form (but which can, in rare cases, lead rapidly to a fatal outcome), typically in childhood – in contrast to hepatitis C, which remains virtually incurable to the present day, frequently leading to cirrhosis and/or hepatocellular carcinoma and which now, in central Europe, occurs much more frequently than hepatitis A.

permit itself to be eliminated (with measles, for example, elimination of the disease is a very difficult task indeed).

What organization, and what individual activity induces secretion and excretion in people? Anyone who impartially considers the simple excretory activities such as perspiration, secretion of urea – but also the large area of endocrinal hormonal secretion – will be able to identify the close relationship between these phenomena and the *activity of the soul entity in the body*. The anthroposophical understanding of the human being provides clear evidence [Steiner and Wegman 1991, ▸Chap. V, 37] of this inter-relationship, namely that secretion and excretion are caused by the soul organization of the human life processes. On the other hand, this is a causal factor in every active individual movement, in particular that of breathing. Human beings share this component of their being with animals, whereas plants only exhibit the phenomena of secretion and independence of movement in the areas bordering on the animal sphere, whereby these are brought about by different factors (e. g. turgor changes in the petals) (▸Chap. 1.3).

Childhood diseases therefore activate the soul entity of the child, and this is also often closely associated with a *specific mood of soul in the patient* (e. g. the tearful need for protection in response to measles). The dominance of this soul aspect is manifested by the fact that, more than other diseases, childhood diseases are not individualized and "typically" take the form of a clearly defined "cyclical" occurrence. This soul aspect is related to the animal where it constitutes the highest level of organization (whereas animals lack the spiritual individualizing aspect). The animal remains defined by what is typical of its kind; understood in this manner, the soul entity expresses itself in its most original form through the type-related own activity of the animal.

The sequence followed by childhood diseases manifests a strict *chronological order* (most evident in the case of measles and of roseola infantum); infection from an external source follows a proliferation of the pathogens within the organism and a phase of generalization associated with viremia or the excretion of toxins into the blood (scarlet fever, pertussis). Once specific independent activity of the organism starts to occur (measles exanthema, but also the paroxysmal stage of pertussis), the organism is already starting to gain the upper hand over the incursion of the pathogen into the body: *as specific disease symptoms start to occur* (not the prodromes), *the active healing process has already started to take place.* Childhood diseases, *in normal cases, tend to heal completely.* This is a further and a fundamental difference to typical age-related diseases. Continuous reference to rare complications in association with the discussion about vaccination conceals the true nature of the term "cyclical infectious diseases", which are only referred to as "cyclical" because their normal characteristics culminate in a state of *restitutio ad integrum*; the associated *acquisition of new aptitudes, i. e. ones not evident prior to the disease* (e. g. immunity) surpass the scope of the term '*ad integrum*'.

In terms of its reliable chronological order and predictable course, a *deep relationship comes to expression between childhood diseases and the growth of the physical body, the life organization of the human being:* life is essentially the bringing forth and the organizing of a physical body over a period of time *in accordance with an innate temporal law.* This means that every childhood disease can be understood as an active *creation of a physical body* arising from the soul entity of the child; immunologically, this can be identified in terms of the formation of memory that results from the impact of a disease process on the specific immune system which is not inherited from the parents. Every childhood disease experienced gives rise to a new and sustained *immunocompetence;* this ability on the part of an organism to overcome a disease is then never lost and remains in place for the whole of its life. That means that every childhood disease alters the physical body in a lasting manner. This is indisputably a *learning process for the physical body.* The distinction between "other" and "self" is a learned one, and not only in the abstract context of a vaccination, but instead in the form of *an activity of the organism concentrated solely on this "other". In a childhood disease, the soul entity is therefore able to direct and activate the entire organism in a uniform manner in line with its own purpose.* Indicatively, this gives rise to a sustained level of immunization whereas vaccination fundamentally only brings about "partial immunity": not everyone given the vaccination actually obtains immunity and the degree and duration of vaccine-induced immunization never achieves the level of naturally acquired immunity.

Childhood diseases are *inflammatory* diseases – in contrast to the sclerotic nature of age-related diseases (◘ Tab. 5.2). In the warmth organization of the human being that brings about fever, the doctor also encounters the physical will activity of the human individuality (cf. ▸ Chap. 5, Introduction). Through highly febrile inflammation – e. g. during measles – the person not only develops resistance towards the outside world and its pathogens, but at the same time subjects his or her physical self to a far-reaching *catabolic process.* This is why the ensuing phase of *convalescence* is necessary and must be added to the duration of the illness. This is because the physical entity inherited in the first instance from parents undergoes a *rebuilding and new building process* during this phase.

The human individuality is fundamentally designed to go further than the horizons of its forebears – not just spiritually but also in respect of the soul entity and the physical body. This can already be seen in that only the human being passes through the crisis of puberty which causes a dissolution of the bond with the parents and which therefore marks the beginning of an essentially self-determined life. At this same time, it is only the human being who experiences a growth spurt that alters the proportions of his or her body; becoming spiritually independent correlates with the individual metamorphosis and reshaping of the originally inherited physical body which becomes increasingly dissimilar from the parents. In contrast to this, the animal at the onset of puberty finally adopts the behavioural traits of its forebears and becomes progressively more similar to them as its youth comes to an end than it was during its growth phase.

The purpose of the unusually long childhood and teenage years of human beings [Kipp 1980] is to ensure that people remain *capable of change* including in their physical body. This precisely involves more than the brain and extends to the entire physical body, including the facial features and the development of the limbs. A particularly intensive reshaping of the body takes place in the course of childhood diseases; as a consequence, many doctors and parents observe [Kummer 1992] that the personality can appear more tangibly as the internally transforming being of the child, that it is able to take ownership of the body to a greater extent.

Our own medical experience has shown that success in the process set out above depends to a large extent on the disease *occurring at the right point in time for the individual.* Despite the fact that childhood diseases can occur in epidemiologically cumulative patterns, they never affect all of the children who could potentially be affected. On the other hand, many children, e. g. ones who fall ill with measles or with scarlet fever (see below), already exhibit a characteristic disposition prior to becoming infected. On the one hand, this makes them prone to illness while, on the other hand, *the illness itself* is the

Tab. 5.2 Comparison between the childhood disease type and sclerotic diseases typical for old age: the following characteristics emerge [G. Husemann 1998, 89]

Parameter	Childhood diseases	Sclerotic age-related diseases
Origin	Caused by external influencing factor and/or communicated	Without external influencing factor
Course of disease	Acute development, mostly febrile	Slow development, afebrile
	Temporary hyperaemia (inflammation and swelling)	Continuous increase in substance (sclerosis)
	Generalising progression of disease (e. g. viremia with measles)	In most cases local organ-related progression (e. g. cataract, coxarthrosis)
	Spontaneous healing, reacquisition of physically communicated competence	No spontaneous healing, loss of competence in the body

active process of overcoming pre-existing conditions of stress and/or developmental impediments.

Complications become numerous with childhood diseases if these diseases arise *too early* (e. g. chickenpox embryopathy or pertussis with young babies) *or occur too late* (e. g. measles in adults), and the increase e. g. of measle encephalitis correlates directly with the postponement of the age for contracting a disease from the first seven years of life to the following years of life[1].

The ideal for paediatrics as taught and practiced at the present time is to suppress and/or prevent acute inflammatory diseases in general during childhood and in particular to do so with childhood diseases. This means that paediatrics aims for the prematurely rapid solidification of the physical body in a pre-individual and immature stage, as has already been demonstrated by the example of generalized prophylaxis with vitamin D, K and fluoride (▸Chap. 3.2 to ▸Chap. 3.4). The *uniform disease prophylaxis* in respect of childhood diseases *limits the ability of the physical body to assimilate change and this in turn impairs the transparency of the physical body in respect of the soul and spiritual individuality of the child.*

This has extensive consequences, initially for the soul entity of the children affected, which are commonly disregarded. It was shown above that every childhood disease gives rise to an intensive appropriation of the physical body by the soul entity, and in particular to the formation of specific immunity [Witsenburg 1992]. If today allergies and autoimmune diseases are rapidly on the rise, they are fundamentally characterized by the irritation and impairment of the relationship between the soul entity and the person's own body either at a primary or at a secondary level (▸Chap. 6). Whereas a childhood disease

1 A lecture given by Stickl, who compared the prevalence of measle encephalitis among comparable collectives during the periods of 1960–1965 and 1970–1975 and, parallel to this, the increase in the occurrence of encephalitis rate, which Stickl found during the period 1960–1965 to represent 1:14,400, established that during the period 1960–1965, 80 % of recorded instances of measles occurred below the age of seven, while during the period 1970–1975 more than half of those affected were above the age of seven (from lecture notes taken by the authors).

as an acute conflict event between the inherited physical body and individuality generally heals and is able to bring about a soul-body harmonization – even to the extent of being able to bear and cope with suffering – allergic and autoimmune diseases do not in themselves deliver any such healing tendency; instead, they tend to create a division between the soul entity and the physical body (e. g. the excruciating itching associated with atopic dermatitis, the shortage of breath associated with asthmatic conditions, and in the fluctuations in blood sugar levels that attend diabetes mellitus).

Furthermore, it has been demonstrated clearly in the Introduction to ▸Chap. 5 that the current rapid rise in the incidence of carcinoma-related diseases among adults is frequently and strikingly associated with an absence of febrile diseases in the medical history. At the present time, it is an open question as to whether the type of the age-related disease – which in certain respects also includes carcinomas – arises ever more frequently and at an earlier stage as a result of the suppression of childhood diseases.

In the opinion of the authors, childhood diseases therefore constitute a significant source of help in cases where the dialectic between the soul and spiritual entity and the physical body is only progressing slowly; in cases where the individuality of a person does not have the strength to assert itself developmentally or if it only succeeds (e. g. prior to scarlet fever) in a one-sided manner. The therapeutic objective of the treatment described in the following section is not to prevent the disease but instead to guide it correctly, and to accompany the child sensitively through his or her process of change. Only in cases where the disease process threatens to progress in a destructive manner do the authors take recourse, where necessary, to a suppressive form of therapy. Having said that, the consent of the parents of the patient to this therapeutic objective is a crucial requirement, because their collaboration – e. g. in allowing the requisite bedrest – is indispensable under all circumstances. However, here too situations can arise that make it necessary to proceed down the path of conventional prophylaxis or treatment to avoid exposing the child to a risk, the consequences of which cannot be judged.

5.3.2 Measles

5.3.2.1 Symptomatology and insight into the illness

Measles progress in a clearly defined chronological sequence that extends over a total period of four weeks (cyclical infectious disease). Even before infection takes place, many of the children affected exhibit through their behaviour a *propensity* for catching measles: their behaviour is psychologically variable and tearful. They cling to their mothers and are unhappy. For the incubation period that lasts for between ten and eleven days, this psychological symptomatology is frequently evident in a pronounced way.

With the outbreak of the prodromal stage (11 to 13 days after becoming infected), swelling and catarrh-related inflammation, particularly of the face and upper respiratory passages, tends to occur; a particular characteristic feature being conjunctivitis (the measles virus enters the body through the conjunctiva of the eye), which gives rise to a high level of sensitivity to light. In this second stage, the living fluid element in the symptomatology of the disease dominates. On the fourteenth day after contracting the disease, high fever is common – up to and even in excess of 41 °C – and the large blotches of *measles exanthema* "raining down" from the head occur. At the start of the second rise in temperature, viremia stops: the activity of the own warmth organization is the only way for a child to overcome the disease. *For this reason antipyretics are severely contraindicated throughout the progression of the disease; studies in developing countries have demonstrated clearly that antipyretics can dramatically worsen that progression* [Witsenburg 1992; cf. also Lohse, Schmiedel 2009, Eyers et al. 2010]. In parallel to the activity of the warmth organization, skin rashes occur that generally for childhood diseases (which are also referred to as 'exanthematic infectious diseases') constitute a typical and, in each case, a pathognomonic symptom. This rash, like the fever, already fundamentally constitutes the *response* of the organism to the disease, the starting point for *overcoming and eliminating it* (cf. the suspended viremia). The rash gradually disappears within 3 to 5 days, once again parallel to the declining fever curve, and mutates into a bran-like desquamation. Experiences over the last few years, e. g. in Salzburg show that young people, above all, can develop *severe diarrhoea* from the fourteenth day after infection in parallel with the highly febrile climax (in view of the great weakness of patients, their beds should be located near a toilet, or appropriate precautions need to be taken).[1]

Convalescence is as frequently overlooked nowadays, as is the incubation period – which is psychologically quite evident. Generally speaking, the duration of this falls between day 20 and day 28 after infection.

In this manner, the disease exhibits a *lunar rhythm* of 28 days; the zenith and dynamic reversal point for the disease is reached on day 14 of the cycle. This is the same rhythm as the female menstruation cycle and that experienced by all fluids on earth, most obvious in the tidal movements of the sea [Endres and Schad 1997, 117–142]. In this it becomes clear that there is an ordering principle that originates in the cosmos – from the moon – that affects all fluids, and this points towards the activity of the "life organization", the etheric body that develops in children most noticeably during their first seven years of life (cf. ▸Chap. 1.1); in the human organization, however, the life processes taking place in the fluid element must be *ordered from within by the soul and spiritual entity.* Measles show this clearly because the peripety, the reversal point in the progression of the disease, is clearly affected by intervention of the I-organization in the fever.

In phenomenological terms, the child with a propensity for and already affected by measles virus *is unstable in its soul entity and is "built close to the water"*; the child becomes very dependent on the mother, ceases to apply any personal order to things and/or becomes unable to maintain a balanced self. The measles virus itself brings about a "spring tide", a surging and overflowing of the fluid element. This adversely affects the senses (conjunctivitis, otitis media) and the airways (rhinitis, measles croup, pneumonia). We therefore observe in measles a partial fluid dissolution of the previous form of the physical body, whereby the soul-ordering principle (in anthroposophical terms the astral body) reveals itself as being primarily incarnated in the body too weakly to be effective (and is therefore too dependent on the psychologically secure adult). Herein lies the typical starting point for measles as a disease.

Physiologically, this is the situation of the *small child* prior to school age, and indeed prior to kindergarten age. During this time, the physical body is still strongly determined by the properties inherited from the parents; it has still *not been sufficiently penetrated by the individuality of the child and reshaped, so the life organization (the etheric body) has not yet been individualized.* If children in general from the age of five to seven are a great deal *more healthy than in infancy and early childhood,* this is not only associated with the devel-

1 The authors thank B. Kenyeres, M.Hopferwieser and S.Görnitz for communicating their related observations of the course of this disease.

opment of newly acquired personal skills but also with the penetration and overcoming of the physical and etheric body inherited from their parents.

As the measles virus works its way through the physical body, the latter initially becomes even more alienated from the soul entity of the child, rendering it more helpless, something that can be directly experienced by the doctor in the prodromal stage. In measles, the life processes active within the fluid element threaten to make themselves independent, to crowd out other factors, and to do so to a point where pneumatization (middle ear, lungs), the sense organs of eye and ear as well as the central nervous system threaten to "get submerged". The differentiating activity of the soul entity, on which respiration and consciousness are founded, encounters restriction and the croup-like coughing of the child with measles renders this restriction caused by swelling of the mucous membrane audible in the airways. The *counter-stroke* is delivered by the *individuality of the child with the help of the fever, the warmth organization,* which along with the virus secretes and eliminates from its own physical entity those parts that it is not able completely to assimilate. With the help of this activity by the I-organization, the soul entity is anchored, incarnated anew and more intensively than before in the physical body [Steiner 1992, 102–104].

Viewed in this light, measles can be experienced as a "rebirth": the physical body dissolves partially to provide space for the individuality of the person. Research into epigenetics (▸Chap. 1.1) shows – entirely in contrast to the grand project for the "decryption of the human genome", the medical benefits of which are extraordinarily modest – just how decisively every human being in the course of early childhood shapes and reforms what he or she has inherited from his or her parents and the extent to which his or her subsequent health is dependent upon this process. It is in particular the ability to regulate immunity that is shaped in the course of this process, and acute inflammatory diseases play an important and beneficial role in this (cf. F. Bach at the start of this chapter). At a time when no scientific research had been conducted into these relationships, R. Steiner drew attention to the influence they can have on the individualization of the genetic predispositions in the context of feverish childhood diseases, especially measles. In contrast to the currently dominant theories, Steiner sees the driving force of this active conflict about the regulation of inherited genetic makeup, the genome, not simply in terms of "environmental conditions" but instead in the *soul and spiritual individuality of the child itself.* Environmental conditions create the opportunity (e. g. a virus infection such as measles), but the productive and individualizing dynamism is rooted in this individuality that did not arise on procreation but is instead a spiritually pre-existing individuality that is embodied and (re)incarnated in the physical body of a child in the course of childhood (anthroposophical image of the human being). "For this reason, this first period in the life of a human being involves an ongoing conflict between that which comes to us from a previous life and that which comes to us from inherited developmental traits. These factors are in conflict with one another. This conflict is expressed in the childhood diseases. ... One person is weaker, aligning himself more with inherited forces, ... but he did this himself by letting himself be guided more by the model. In contrast, we have people who, when they lose their milk teeth, become very unlike the people they were before that event in their lives. Then what comes to them from the pre-earthly soul and spiritual life is strong and they abide less by the model." [Steiner 2003, 149f.]. To the same extent that every reader should feel free as to whether or not to accept these ideas, these thoughts should also prompt caution when it comes to viewing acute diseases as something entirely negative, to view them as enemies and to treat them as such. Scientifically and in terms of medical ethics this attitude is not well founded when we are considering a sustainable and healthy developmental path for a child to follow: "disease forms part of individualization" (Novalis).

The therapeutic procedure is based very largely on the guiding principles that also apply to ways of dealing with the newborn child (▸Chap. 2). At the same time, it emerges plainly why measles *from the ninth year of life* (as shown clearly by statistics relating to the incidence of encephalitis over the last few years) and above all from the onset of puberty *have a much more serious impact* (encephalitis rate approx. 1:1000, plus abortive and inconsequentially healing courses which are statistically sometimes evaluated as encephalitis but which then fail to manifest a correspondingly negative outcome). To a growing extent at this age the dynamism of the small child in the living entity is absent; the fluid builds up more easily inside the individual and, on the other hand, the inflammatory counteracting influence of the much more deeply incarnated individuality can overburden and indeed destroy the possibilities otherwise open to the organism [cf. Kummer 1999]. If, similarly as at birth, the threat to the airways and the danger of what can under certain circumstances prove to be fatal brain damage are viewed as the main risks, it is also true to say that the human being is best able to contend with them if he or she has not yet become an "image" internally, if he or she is still to a large extent a "seed" and if his or her organism has yet to reach a final and differentiated organic form. Just as an excessively large head can make birth difficult, so physical differentiation which has advanced too far can adversely affect the course of measles without complications. As a consequence of the measles vaccination, ever more of the people now affected are of school age or are still infants (▸Chap. 3). However, the risk of measles encephalitis not only increases when people reach school age but can also be exacerbated by an insensitive and uninformed approach to tackling this disease (see cast study in ▸Chap. 5.3.2.2).

Contracted at the right point in time – between the ages of two and seven to nine – and appropriately supported by parents and doctors, measles in central Europe are a classic, cyclically recurring *childhood disease from which full recoveries are made.* The soul entity of the child emerges with a much more balanced temperament; there can be developmental leaps in numerous directions. By paying attention to the convalescence phase and by strengthening children in their immunity for the following four to six weeks (see below), a lower susceptibility to disease and allergy rate after measles is generally observable (not measles vaccination) [Rosenlund 2009]. At the same time the ability in the family increases to deal with inflammatory diseases without excessive fear of the child's fever. Child and parents gain in self-confidence through the disease, due not least to the basis of feeling "at home" in their own bodies and better able to contend with the challenges of a living development (cf. the practical study by Kummer in relation to this [1999]).

The GAÄD (*Gesellschaft Anthroposophischer Ärzte in Deutschland* = Society of Anthroposophic Physicians in Germany) has together with the author published a set of guidelines for measles [GAÄD 2008] and a fact sheet for parents (www.gaed.de). This contains and summarizes the current aspects of the disease, the vaccination process and the level of understanding of the disease (cf. ▸Chap. 3.5) At the present time, the exclusion of children who are not immune to measles from schools and nursery schools whenever a measles outbreak occurs imposes great pressure on parents to go and get their children vaccinated. Parents are often confronted by the statement that it is "irresponsible" not to have their child vaccinated. However, the competent health authorities have no response to the

5

question as to which attitude can be called "responsible" in the light of the fourfold to eightfold increase in bronchial asthma, atopic dermatitis, chronic inflammatory bowel diseases, type 1 diabetes mellitus and other chronic childhood diseases in the rich western industrialized countries. In any event, the anthroposophical lifestyle is not the responsible party in this context (▸Chap. 6.1). No grounds are evident in the field of measles prevention and treatment to call into question the principles of tolerance, freedom and the inviolable dignity of the human being. Over a long-term period, pluralistic societies have commonly proven themselves to be the ones most capable of learning.

5.3.2.2 Treatment

A decisive factor for the child during the entire course of the disease is *warmth,* for the physical body as well as the soul entity. Due to the fact that a high level of fever is needed in order to overcome the disease, the organism needs to be supported in its activity and it must not be prevented in any way. In practical terms, this means:

- bed rest up to one day after the fever has completely subsided,
- warm clothing capable of absorbing perspiration (wool underwear and/or a wool pullover),
- only hot drinks (e. g. linden (lime) flower tea).

From the parents' side, it is most important that the mother finds as much time as possible for her child to care for and be close to him or her. Many children with measles want their mother to join them in bed and to give them physical and spiritual warmth. The tranquil presence of parents strengthens the soul entity of the child.

While antipyretics should be avoided, an *enema* (▸Chap. 5.1.1.4.2 for guidance) can relax, gently regulate a fever and strengthen the cardiovascular system. This is advisable several times a day in all cases at the early stages of a rising fever, in response to high temperatures and poor drinking characteristics

For the treatment of measles with no complications, the following doses are appropriate for children between the ages of one and seven.

- **Pulsatilla D6 dil.** Weleda,
- **Belladonna D6 dil.** Weleda

  each 20 ggt. to half a glass of water (approx. 75 ml), to be taken orally in alternate sips and after defervescence
- **Pulsatilla D12 pillules** (various manufacturers)

  5 pillules 2–3 x/d up to the end of the convalescence phase.

The purpose of administering Belladonna is to prevent the counteraction from the warmth organization before the climax of the disease from being too robust, so that the activity of the warmth organization leads to the harmonious incorporation of the soul entity into the life processes taking place in the fluid body. It is of particular importance to administer Belladonna when dealing with *febrile convulsions* (incidence with measles approx. 1:250, cf. ▸Chap. 5.4.3.2). The frequency of febrile convulsions is not affected by antipyretics so this risk should also not prompt the application of "fever suppositories".

But susceptibility to measles as such entails the difficulty of the soul entity not being sufficiently well anchored in the physical body. The air organism of the child: nose, middle ear, larynx and lungs risk being overwhelmed by life processes; the soul entity holds fast to the mother (a Pulsatilla motif!) and must first learn to reorder itself in response to the fluid process that "has burst its banks".

If we consider *Pulsatilla vulgaris,* the first thing that strikes us is that the plant pushes its branches with their fine filigree leaves out of a strong, brown multi-headed root stock. During this time, the ground surrounding this plant that loves living on steep limestone slopes is often still brown and bare. It then goes on to grow a relatively large suspended flower the outer petals of which are purple, with bright yellow stamens inside. It can warm up strongly in sunlight, in contrast to the cool ambient temperature. The plant forms a protoanemonine toxin that can cause rashes while drying. Once dried, this is no longer toxic.

The relationship with the soul entity and to warmth is highly developed in the Pulsatilla flower. On the other hand the plant, even when it flowers, does not develop harmoniously nor does it grow strongly. There is a clear discrepancy between the large flowers leaning downwards and swaying in the wind on their stalks and the growth and development of the leaves and stalks below. The transition would be harmonious – e. g. as can be observed on the buttercup or in a noble form with the rose – if the flower grew out of the shoot when it had finished developing through leaf metamorphosis [Grohmann 1991].

Pulsatilla is a member of the buttercup family (Ranunculaceae). Generally, it exhibits a high level of vitality; in the leaf area, this family has many different forms of metamorphosis [Stübler and Wolff 1985]. It prefers *damp locations* and tends to bloom in springtime, although members of the Ranunculaceae can be found flowering throughout the year. Many (cf. wolfsbane, delphinium, pheasant's eye) exhibit intensive flower development and a close relationship to the animal kingdom. This enables them to organize and dynamize the aqueous element and bring it into a relationship with ensouled animal life [Soldner 2010, 510f.].

This relationship is as intensive as it is unstable in Pulsatilla. For this reason, Pulsatilla in its potentized form is indicated in paediatrics in cases where the soul organization, the astral body of the child, exhibits difficulties in penetrating through the fluid and in ordering it. This manifests itself on the one hand in a susceptibility to mild *catarrhs of the conjunctive organs, the nose and the Eustacian tubes (mucous tympanon, otitis media)*, and on the other hand in the associated *lability of mood* that always depends very strongly on the sympathy of others. When visiting the doctor, it is typical for children who need Pulsatilla initially to keep very close to their mothers, from where they look across at the doctor with friendly anticipation, only then during the examination suddenly to break down in tears and screaming. However, immediately after the examination and a friendly word the mood switches back to "sunshine" reminiscent of the weather in April, which is when Pulsatilla can be found to flower in nature. The mother of the child (this tends to be truer of girls) reports that the child is always hanging on to her apron strings and that she is almost entirely unable to leave her alone by herself. The disease of measles groups together all of the guiding symptoms of Pulsatilla because this constitutes *the most important medicine for this disease.*

In practice, measles, in the rare cases where they still occur, tend to be more common in the *second and third septennial and among infants.* In both cases, this disease tends in general to lead to complications. These result primarily from insufficient dynamization and excretion of the fluid element (mucoid otitis media, stenosing laryngitis). To stimulate this to a greater extent, *Mercurius solubilis at medium potency* (D12–15) is very effective. Structuring light forces act in iodine-based healing substances such as spongia tosta (the step that took amphibians from water to land, i. e. the formation of lungs, was rendered possible by the thyroid gland hormone that contains iodine) and in the potentized honey bee, apis mellifera [cf. Leitgedanke zu Apis mellifica, Vademecum 2010, 91f.]

On the basis of these considerations, the following therapy has proven effective for older children and young people:

- **Apis Belladonna cum Mercurio pillules** Wala
  5–7 pillules 5 x/d
- **Spongia tosta D12 pillules** (various manufacturers) – indicated in all cases of measles-associated laryngotracheitis ('measles croup') –
  5 pillules 3 x/d
- **Pulsatilla D12 pillules** (various manufacturers)
  5–7 pillules 2–3 x/d

The last of these is administered jointly with Apis Bell. c. Merc. With this treatment the measles in this age can almost always be treated completely and sufficiently, even if acute and/or croup-like coughing is present. The treatment of coughing and the prevention of pneumonia is effectively supported by

- **Roseneisen/Graphit pillules** Wala
  7–10 pillules 3 x/d

This medicine also stimulates the appetite. During convalescence, Pulsatilla D12, Roseneisen/Graphit and

- **Meteoreisen pillules** Wala
  5 pillules 2–3 x/d

can be combined with

- **Blackthorn elixir** Weleda
  15 ml 2–3 x/d

To treat *measles otitis,* we refer here to ▸Chap. 5.1.3; Pulsatilla (D6-12) is also of special significance here.

Measles pneumonia should always be taken very seriously (diagnosis and therapy ▸Chap. 5.1.1), but only occurs very infrequently with the following form of treatment. If there is the slightest doubt, an immediate house visit is essential [cf. Kummer 1999].

Diarrhoea among young people is frequently not something that therapy can do much to alleviate (▸Chap. 4.5.1). In particular, sufficient fluids must be administered, where necessary by means of infusion.

If we proceed as described above, encephalitis is probably going to be an extremely rare occurrence (the statistics fluctuate markedly here, very probably also related to treatment); nonetheless, the development of cerebrally-related symptoms must be taken into account particularly in relation to older children. Statistically speaking, infants appear to exhibit a higher *SSPE risk*; however, the authors are convinced that the treatment set out here for acute measles, which enhances the immunological capabilities of the child and does not suppress them, represents the best possible prevention in this respect alongside preventing the infection of infants.

- The most important forms of medication at the early stages of restlessness, drowsiness and deteriorating of general condition are
- **Apis mell./ex animale D30 amp.** Weleda/Wala and
- **Bryonia e rad. D30 amp.** Wala
- s.c. in the upper arm or injected nuchally. Also of relevance for every complication associated with measles is the acute production and administration of
- **potentized autologous blood** as developed by Imhäuser (see case study and ▸Chap. 3.5.7.2.2).

Every responsible doctor will carefully consider his or her diagnostic and therapeutic limits and, where necessary, will arrange for a hospital admission. The following case study clarifies the possibilities of a treatment involving the use of potentized medicines – and the risks if the elementary principles described above in respect of rest and warmth are not followed.

Case history

A 12-year old girl from harmonious domestic circumstances and without special features in her previous development exhibits the typical onset of measles: remittent fever with uncharacteristic catarrhal-inflammatory signs in the upper airways and an ill-tempered tone of voice.

On the third day of the disease, the fever starts to decline, prompting the family to decide to start their Easter vacation in their own weekend cottage by a lake. During the car journey there, in the early part of the morning, the girl starts to perspire copiously accompanied by a high temperature; the catarrhal symptoms worsen and moderate measles exanthema starts to appear. In her bed in the holiday home, which is still damp and cold from the winter period, she then has a shivering attack and her general condition worsened rapidly.

Late in the afternoon, she is examined at the house which is still cool: 40 °C fever, typical and not pronounced exanthema, great drowsiness and restlessness, slight convulsions.

Treatment: application of warmth despite the high temperature, per os immediately Belladonna D30 and Pulsatilla D30, s.c. Bryonia D30 and Apis mell. D30 as a mixed injection. Then production of autologous blood as developed by Imhäuser at sick bed in C5. 10 gtt. of this potency administered with a glass of water, one teaspoonful at a time (15 ml) every 5 minutes. After one hour, the potentization is increased to C12 and this potency is administered. Three hours after the start of treatment, the fever declined that evening by one degree Celsius, restlessness and convulsions also declining. On the following day, fever of 38.5 °C, no more restlessness, just slight drowsiness, but able to eat and drink unassisted. On the following day, no further indications of CNS involvement. Full recovery then ensued.

5.3.3 Exanthema subitum; three-day fever

This illness generally occurs during the first, second and even the third year of life. The guiding symptom is a continuous fever (approx. 40 °C) lasting for three days, and the occurrence of truncal exanthema *with or after the decline of the fever.* The strict chronology and very feverish course of this condition have many points in common with measles (▸ Chap. 5.3.2.1); primarily, the roseola infantum is an *expression of a good reactive capability* of the child's organism. Significant signs of developmental progress are also often apparent after this childhood disease, e. g. in terms of the statomotor development of the small child.

Diagnostically, the continuous fever which as such can hardly be influenced is indicative in the absence of local findings. With infants, meningeal hydrops can become palpable; children are often short-tempered especially in the first 12 to 24 hours and are easily irritated by external sensory stimuli. There is usually a fairly high *risk of febrile convulsions.*

Therapeutically, antipyretics should be avoided here; where necessary, an *enema* can relieve symptoms and can prove calming (▸ Chap. 5.3.2.2). Antipyretics verifiably do not reduce the risk of febrile convulsions (▸ Chap. 5.4.3.1).

If the disease progresses without complications, the adjunctive treatment will in practice be guided purely by the symptoms (initially Aconit D6, followed for the most part by Ferrum phos. D6–12). If there is palpable meningeal hydrops or severe irritability,

- **Apis mell. D12 pillules** Weleda, various manufacturers
  5 pillules immediately, thereafter 3 pillules 3 x/d and
- **Belladonna D6 dil./pillules** Weleda
  20–30 gtts./pillules dissolved in 50 ml of water, of which 15 ml hourly
  may be considered to prevent febrile convulsions.

It is indicative of the importance of the correct timing for childhood diseases that the HHV-6 virus, the pathogen causing roseola infantum among older children at the age of puberty, can produce a completely different clinical picture that can take the form of lassitude, fatigue and impaired concentration that can last for weeks or even months.

5.3.4 Scarlet fever

In a Cochrane analysis, the difference between treatment with antibiotics and a placebo amounted to 16 hours. ...If it were possible to disregard the reduced duration of the infection, and if the patient were to manage without the slightly shorter period of suffering, then, subject to follow-up examination, it should be possible to treat this condition without antibiotics.

DGPI Handbook 2009, 484 (Handbook of the German Society of Paediatric Infectiology)

5.3.4.1 Illness concept

When we define the phrase "childhood disease" as above in the Introduction (▸ Chap. 5.3.1), the key part of the disease concept is the own activity of the organism in the form of a pathognomonic and in each case unmistakable secretion activity. This activity can be identified at the barriers of the organism as a characteristic exanthema, enanthema or also as a typical coughing attack with whooping cough. The chronology of this “cyclical” type of disease is driven primarily by the immunological activity of the organism and not by the pathogen. All of these diseases are characterized by a specifically physical body-based immunological learning process with sustained immunity[1].

If with this disease concept we take the child’s organism to be the affected and active entity in the disease process and do not start from the microbiological laboratory findings, then we can clearly distinguish scarlet fever with its characteristic exanthema and enanthema from streptococci-associated angina[2] and a positive indication of streptococcal presence with clinically normal findings of the kind that affects between 15–30 % of the population during the winter months. Because the term “childhood disease” can *only be applied in full scope to scarlet fever*! This prompts the question as to what is specific in the disposition for, experience of and dealing with scarlet fever from the viewpoint of a child.

Current medical practice of the kind common to many doctors contrasts with this by placing *positive verification of beta-haemolyzing A-streptococcus* dominantly at the centre of diagnosis and treatment. A “positive swab” as a “diagnosis” ultimately leads to abandoning any disease concept at all: “It has been possible to demonstrate over the last few years that people with streptococci in Group A do not constitute a hazard to other people, and that they do not constitute an increased risk to themselves either.” [Peuckert 1988]. “The antibiotic treatment of carrier status is less successful” [Handbook of the German Society of Paediatric Infectiology, DGPI 2009, 481]. Today, many parents leave the doctor’s practice in the belief that their child has contracted scarlet fever, even in cases where the microbiological findings were obtained solely in the context of a family or kindergarten screening test and the child is in good health.[3]

Nonetheless, to a large extent (approx. ⅙ of all paediatrically prescribed) antibiotics are prescribed in response to a streptococci-positive mouth swab. To this day, any deviation from this line is viewed as malpractice. Specialist societies such as the *Deutsche Gesellschaft für Pädiatrische Infektiologie* or DGPI (Handbook of the German Society of Paediatric Infectiology) [2009] quoted at the beginning, the Dutch working group led by S. Zwart [2003], a Cochrane review on pharyngitis by del Mar [2002] and publications about rheumatic fever in western industrialized countries (versus developing countries [Cilliers 2006]) tend instead to come to the conclusion that the uncomplicated progression of a streptococcal infection does not require any treatment based upon the use of antibiotics and that an antibiotics-based course of treatment is only indicated in cases where children are seriously ill (e. g. unable to drink, risk of abscess) or face a high risk of contracting secondary illnesses (heart failure, s/p rheumatic fever, etc.). From the viewpoint of evidence-based medicine (see the works quoted), it is sufficient to treat purulent complications (0.7 % of all acute infections with beta-haemolyzing streptococci) and secondary diseases with antibiotics. Viewed in this light, it is possible to prevent many allergic reac-

1 Due to the great variance in toxin-forming streptococci (especially dependent on the M protein, of which more than 100 types are known), immunity against beta-haemolyzing streptococcal infections is a relative notion. Relapses are more common after treatment with antibiotics than they are after a course of treatment that does not involve the use of antibiotics.

2 Without the symptoms of an erythrogenic toxin effect (exanthema and acute enanthema).

3 This view is contrasted by Peuckert [1988] with whom we can emphasize: "Even if we bathe our patients in penicillin, the proportion of transiently populated children" (this is the appropriate term) "will not be affected to any great extent." It is worthy of note that asthma occurs with increasing frequency the less frequently scarlet fever manifests itself [Vargas 2006] and antibiotics also promote the manifestation of asthma (cf. ▶Chap. 6.1.3).

tions, fungal infections and symbiosis impairments, all of which proceed from the use of antibiotics. A critical approach to the use of antibiotics with otitis media and streptococcal infections could halve the quantity of antibiotics currently being prescribed. In the following section, the authors return to a clear disease concept as developed above. This should not in any way overlook the concomitant *risk* of certain secondary diseases associated with scarlet fever, contagious impetigo, streptococcal tonsillitis and erysipelas, nor should it omit consideration of shared aetiological factors in the associated microbiology. However, a *positive diagnosis by a doctor* must include the full gamut of specific characteristics of the symptoms and the progression of a disease; for this reason, it continues to be necessary to record scarlet fever as a disease entity in its own right, and to treat it as such. It should be emphasized that scarlet fever in the form described below is now a rare disease pattern, but it remains one to be taken very seriously. In particular while experience with this disease is on the wane, a detailed description may prove helpful. Otherwise, reference is made to ▸Chap. 5.2.3 (Tonsillitis).

5.3.4.2 Multi-faceted symptomatology and course of illness

The following section will present the progression of scarlet fever as presented during careful treatment and care of a patient without suppressive (antibiotic) therapy in its full picture.

The onset of acute fever, a *silken small-flecked and hinge joint-emphasized* (groin and armpits) *exanthema* on first to second day of disease, as well as a *fine-flecked deep red enanthema with swallowing difficulties* and regional lymph node inflammation are the guiding symptoms that clinically justify a diagnosis of scarlet fever. There is a clear and adverse effect on the general condition. The pattern adopted by the symptoms described can vary widely today. It is important with this to take due account of the *typical disease age* that lies between the ages of 5 and 15 (the high point of which is around the ages of 9 to 12). During *this time* scarlet fever manifests itself most obviously in contrast to the often very slight course of the disease in infancy. The exanthema can be very fleeting and can progress in a clinically almost imperceptible manner; this includes, at the predilection points, rough skin and, on closer examination, a slight rash. On the other hand, clear itching can occur. However, if all the other symptoms named, in particular the characteristic and, to the experienced doctor, unmistakable enanthema (signs of erythrogenic toxin effect specific to scarlet fever) are present, the disease can be identified as scarlet fever and not just as (streptococcal) tonsillitis. It then goes on to exhibit the following progression.

After the "flaring up" of the first days of illness, the appearance of the patient changes: the skin colour is strikingly *pale* (contrasting with a raspberry-coloured tongue and reddish tonsils during the throat inspection), vitality is greatly *weakened*, the face appears serious and *overcontoured*. After a recovery phase, often *approx. 14 days after* the onset of the illness, a new *downturn* affects general vitality and the sense of wellbeing of the child: the skin turns paler and the patient feels worn down and in need of rest. This correlates with the fact that "subsequent diseases" such as rheumatic fever and nephritis occur first and foremost in the third week of illness, even although this has now become a very rare occurrence (risk of rheumatic fever in western industrialized countries is "at maximum" 1:5000 (DGPI 2009, 484]. Only after about three weeks does the convalescence stabilize properly. At this time – and this is another pathognomonic factor! – *scaly skin* reaches its

Tab. 5.3 Comparison between scarlet fever and measles: A clear polarity emerges [Husemann 1989, 56ff.]

Parameter	Measles	Scarlet fever
Typical age of disease	First septennial, early childhood	Second septennial (pre-)school age
Infectious agent(s)	Virus that enters through the conjunctiva	Toxin-forming bacterium, infection in the pharynx area
Exanthema	Blotchy, primarily "running down" the face, emphasized at round contours body shape	Fine – fleeting, emphasis on torso and hinge joints; emphasized at concave depressions in body shape
Enanthema	(Koplik spots)	Bright red, pronounced
Overall impression of body form	Aqueously dissolute; very vital disease process	Pale and excessively countoured, weakening disease process
Psychological disposition	Dependent and lacking in independence, too weak in forming the physical body, active soul life	Intellectual, emphatically antipathic consciousness life which rushes ahead; under pressure, sentient soul processes overwhelmed externally and internally
Maximum fever	On day 14	At the onset of symptoms

worst point. In terms of coping with what a modern school pupil has to be able to manage, patients take about three to four weeks to recover (and for sport even longer).

- Which *disease disposition* tends to occur most frequently in scarlet fever?
- Here, the *age at which the disease is contracted* (see above) delivers an early indication. Often the spiritual *individuality* rushes ahead of the overall development before the disease breaks out. The soul life of the child *turns one-sided* in that the thinking intellectual side, which of necessity needs to place itself in opposition to the world in psychological antipathy, jumps ahead of the side comprising the actual mind, the imagination, free play and sympathetic connection with the world and pushes it into the background. This tendency is exacerbated, for example, at the time when the child starts school, by school-related requirements in the third and fourth primary school classes for instance, but also in response to the psychological stresses that the child is "unable to swallow or digest". In terms of the *spiritual individuality*, the child with a disposition for scarlet fever has *advanced too far*; but psychologically in a narrower sense he or she feels blocked and suppressed, overwhelmed by his or her own individuality and by the psychological stresses and demands coming from the environment.

If we compare scarlet fever with measles at this point, a clear *polarity* emerges (Tab. 5.3).

It should be noted that *both* diseases do not exhibit their turning point towards complete cure until the third week of the illness and that this is a time when the potential for complications is most prevalent – in the case of scarlet fever at a stage during which the conflict with the disease *is taking place inside the child and is hidden.* This also corresponds to the psychological constitution of the child suffering from scarlet fever.

In advance of the disease there is often a somewhat unpleasant know-it-all intellectualism or a depressed general mood. From the onset of the disease there is a need to withdraw and to be left in peace (without being left alone!). Once the acute symptoms start to recede, this phase is often followed by an interval of relative wellbeing, prompting the parents and the patient not to understand the doctor who continues to advise the urgent necessity of sustained rest. Then – as mentioned earlier – in the classic case there is a renewed need for peace and withdrawal, associated with a feeling of weakness. Not until this phase, *the one that decides the outcome of the course of the disease and lies in the third week,* has been overcome is the child able again to face the world, as though internally purified, in a much more harmonious manner than before.

5.3.4.3 Further insights into the illness

Scarlet fever typically occurs as a disease once the relative significance of physical growth as part of the development of a child and the dominance of the living etheric formative processes start to recede and the development of the soul entity emerges into the foreground when school age is reached. It is the nature of the soul entity to create polarities and initially to tend towards exaggeration, and this is particularly prevalent during puberty. In addition to the polarity already presented between a reason tinged with antipathy and an emotional life coloured by an emphasis on being liked, there is the psychological dichotomy and division between an emerging world of inner perception and sensation, a new *spiritual inner space* and the *external psychological incorporation into the community*: family and neighbourhood, kindergarten or primary school. In many cases the child in this way experiences new *internal contradictions that it is often not yet able, at this early age, to bring into balance with one another*; but which it is also unable to present externally in the way that becomes possible after puberty.

This creates the prerequisites for the psychological dissonances, the congestion of unresolved polarities to *break into the physical body,* take physical form in scarlet fever in order to be overcome and expelled with the help of all the constituent parts of the human being. If we look at the course of the diseases on the basis of this prerequisite – which we might call a hypothesis to begin with – the symptoms can be ordered and understood.

The disease begins with pain, reddening of the skin and fever: symptoms that result from the activity of the soul entity, the astral body and the warmth organization in which the I is physically active; in this way it is different from measles, which begins with catarrh and inflammation and is initially dominated by vital fluid processes. The dynamic properties of this disease originate in the soul entity that discharges its congestion onto the physical body of the patient. The soul entity does however have a differentiating, breaking down, shaping influence on the physical body and this grows as it develops consciousness.

With measles, skin symptoms move from within to without (Koplic spots – exanthema), and from top to bottom in terms of a healthy secretion reaction. The fine, hinge joint-preponderant exanthema associated with scarlet fever manifests its close connection with the soul entity in its form and predilection points; but the rash becomes flame-red *internally*, and specifically in the throat area. This is no random site: there is virtually no other place where undigested material content from the outside world can penetrate so close to the interior of the organism, to the lymph and blood system. Viewed in this light, the tonsils constitute a "physiological wound". Numerous *polarities encounter one another and cross over* in the neck region (alimentary and airways, nerve fibres to the left and right halves of the body etc.). The neck divides and also interconnects the reason-related nervous and sensory region of the head from the chest region, essential for actual soul sentience with the heart as the central organ. It is no coincidence that the dynamic of a disease is able to propagate through the body from the neck region.

To a significant extent, this process is communicated through the erythrogenic toxin of the streptococci; unlike measles, scarlet fever is a disease brought about by the *formation of toxin* (that in turn calls up a toxin-specific, anti-toxic immunity). Toxins always have a catabolic effect on the etheric body, the life processes; at the same time they have a very different effect on the soul entity in animals and human beings (cf. narcotics as toxins). Within ensouled organisms they imitate in a one-sided and extreme way *the action of the astral body, the soul organization, which can only produce perception, feeling and autonomous movement through breaking down living substance.* In this way, the toxin-forming streptococci, the pathogens of scarlet fever, mirror the incursion of one-sided catabolic soul impulses in the life organization as the driving force of scarlet fever pathology.

Once the organism reacts initially with fever to the disease through the medium of the I-organization and therefore is – currently – mostly able to contain and limit the extent of the destructive potential of toxin-forming pathogens, something then occurs during the second phase of the disease in which the toxin creation of the pathogens continues, further weakening the organism to such an extent that, in extreme cases, a kind of salt formation (precipitation of antigen-antibody complexes) and the paralyzing (joints) and destructive reactive inflammation (heart valves, kidney glomeruli) it provokes physically *threaten to paralyze the organism.* The *turning point in this phase of the disease does not emerge from the warmth organization of the child* but instead depends on *the life organization, the etheric body, of the child recovering to such an extent* that the downwards progression of the astral body does not penetrate through to the physical body. A real image of this is the living response of a striated muscle cell to the rapid influx of Na^+ followed by Ca^{2+} that triggers muscular movement; the cell is obliged to balance out this excitation event, to organize an opposing flow, or face being paralyzed by the non-compensated excitation (the influx of Na^+ and Ca^{2+}). The etheric body is expressed through the vitality-protecting outward transfer of Na^+ against K^+ and the retrieval of Ca^{2+} to an intracellular depot, an action which balances out an astral excitation event.

As in a plant, the etheric body develops its strongest impact while at rest, whereas the astral body is excited by movement. For that reason, with scarlet fever that is not being treated (and therefore shortened) with antibiotics bed rest is indispensable until the life forces are tangibly restored and until the toxin load and its adverse impact has been eliminated. There is no more intensive support for the etheric body and no better therapy than bed rest for keeping together the components of the human being (physical body, life organization, soul entity and I-organization). In a school-age child exhibiting the classic symptoms of this disease, anywhere between two and a half to three weeks of bed rest may be needed, but here the child must be individually perceived before a decision is taken. In every case, with any full-spectrum manifestation of scarlet fever coupled with an avoidance of antibiotics, three weeks of rest at home, with as much of that time as necessary being spent in bed, are crucially important! No sports activities should be embarked upon until 4 weeks have elapsed.

It is not until the strength of the life organization has been restored that the deep incursion of the soul entity can be contained and remedied. This has an immediately tangible effect on the soul entity itself. A frequent powerful sensation before and after the onset of the disease of a *physical sense of constriction* disappears, children feel themselves to have been freed as though of a great weight and then often behave in a much calmer and more self-contained manner in their environment, while many children bring a new depth of feeling (e. g. in their pictures) to expression. Internally, the disease deepens and strengthens the bond between the soul entity and the physical body in such a way that the sentient "heart" side of the soul entity is strengthened, promoting a sense of balance between reason and emotion. Perhaps the positive significance of the disease event lies psychosomatically in the internal penetration and linkage of the soul entity with the organs (e. g. the heart and the kidneys) that generally appear as locuses of potential complications in the awareness of the doctor.

5.3.4.4 Treatment

When a diagnosis is made, a *discussion with the parents* is required about the disease profile, the major complications that may be associated with it and the therapeutic approach upon which those involved should embark. In normal cases, therapy starts during the first days of the disease, during which the cardinal requirement is for enforced bed rest, and this is not often problematic: if no serious complications threaten (beware *scarlet fever otitis*!), the therapy described below works reliably and promotes the development of the child in the way set out. It avoids medication-related risks (the side-effects of antibiotics) and relapses are a rare occurrence.

What is substantially *more difficult to accomplish is to enforce the real need for sufficient bed rest and convalescence* in the treatment of scarlet fever. To the authors, this appears indispensable in the full manifestation of scarlet fever. If the parents cannot or do not wish to comply, then a course of antibiotics becomes advisable. The post-streptococcal glomerulonephritis is not prevented by antibiotics with certainty [Del Maar 2002].

Without antibiotic treatment, careful support and subsequent examination of the patient and sufficient availability on the part of the doctor to make house visits, particularly during the second and third weeks of the disease, are all necessary in order to identify emerging dips in the disease progression immediately and to balance and cancel these out therapeutically immediately.

5.3.4.4.1 Acute treatment during the first week of illness

In this phase,

- **Belladonna D6 dil./pillules/Rh D6 dil.** Weleda
  with high fever 50 gtt. or pillules/50–100 ml water taken in 15 ml portions over a 24-hour period, otherwise 5 gtt./5 pillules 5 x/d

is the basic medicine.

The deadly nightshade (*Atropa belladonna*), was introduced by S. Hahnemann [1995a] to the treatment of scarlet fever – at that time with great success (1796/7). This vital night shade growth is most at home at the edge of clearings in forests, on the boundary between light and shade. The powerful, angular stump shape of its green stem forks at about half-height, above which hang the flowers, externally brown-violet and internally a dirty yellow, each flower covered by the large oval or egg-shaped leaves ("shade plant"), and these are arranged in a precise architectural formation with offset heights (i. e. with the leaves in the gaps being half as big as the larger leaves, creating a "leaf mosaic" [Madaus 1999a, 676]). It is from these flowers that the strikingly shiny, toxic black fruits of the deadly nightshade grow. On its vital lower supporting structure, above the height of the fork in the stem, a highly venomous upper structure is arranged that exhibits a diversely dichotomous set of characteristics in a polar arrangement.

The toxic action on human beings leads to a state of increased excitation (tachycardia, fever, dryness of mouth, perspiration, cramps in the smooth muscles and, in extreme cases, hallucinations, convulsions etc.), bringing out every conceivable kind of "bloom" which in extreme cases can also be brought about psychosomatically by a soul life which is one-sidedly rooted too deeply in the organic. Scarlet fever is characterized as a disease with a similar set of dynamic properties. Through the potentization of Belladonna, this destructive tendency of the astral body can be reined in and directed [Husemann 1979; 1998; 2009, 15–30]. If at the outset high potencies of Belladonna are administered, this can under certain circumstances stop the fever stage very rapidly, if not indeed abruptly: it may, however, in the view of the authors, have a negative influence on the entire course of the disease, and harmonizing action. The initially necessary advance and territorial acquisition of the soul entity should be accompanied with patience and should not be combated immediately. Only in the event of an insufficient effect or acute exacerbations are higher potency levels than D6 required during the first phase of this disease.

With serious malaise, halitosis and swelling of the lymph nodes from day two, the therapy can be supplemented with

- **Mercurius solubilis D12-15 pillules** (various manufacturers) [Sommer und Soldner 1988a, b]
  5–7 pillules 3 x/d

The required cleansing process is introduced with frequent gargling with weak sage tea with

- **Symbioflor® 1**
  depending on age 20–50 gtt. distributed throughout the day;

This can be continued throughout the therapy period – beyond the end of the acute phase (after the acute phase, the best is 3 x/d after meals).
Additional mouthwashes can also be of benefit with

- **Calendula Essenz** Wala
  7–20 gtt./rinse.

On the seventh day of the disease after completion of the Belladonna/Mercury treatment, the following can be given for one day

- **Hepar Sulfuris D30 pillules** (various manufacturers)
  5 pillules dissolved in 50 ml of water, distributed throughout the day, 15 ml at a time.

to consolidate the initial treatment.
With peracute disease progression with poor general condition, severe tonsillitis, possibly noticeably livid inflamed mucous membrane in the oropharynx and phlegmonous tendency to septicaemia, the following has a crucial effect when administered right at the onset,

- **Lachesis D12 dil.** Weleda
  5 gtt. 3–5 x/d or
- **Lachesis D12/30 amp.** (various manufacturers) jointly with
- **Argentum D30/Echinacea D6 amp.** Weleda
  as a mixed i.v. injection.

5

Of course, if the therapy is not sufficiently successful, the inclusion of an antibiotic treatment should always be considered.

Externally, neck wraps with low-fat quark (select a temperature that the patient finds pleasant), and massaging in

- **Mercurialis 10 % balm** Weleda
  3 x/d

can be of help.

As a composite medicine for a very acute onset of the disease with a tendency towards purulence

- **Lachesis comp. pillules** Wala
  5–7 pillules 5 x/d and
- **Echinacea/Argentum pillules** Wala
  5–10 pillules 2–3 x/d

intensify the basic treatment (Belladonna/Mercurius sol.) – applied in frequent alternation.

- **Rhus toxicodendron e fol. D30 pillules** Wala
  acutely up to 5 pillules 5 x/d

is indicated in cases where *severely itching* exanthema occurs. The rash tends to be dark red, the disease is often preceded by exhaustion and restlessness, tip of the tongue is red, agitation, above all the need for warmth, and for hot drinks are characteristic of this indication. There is a growing impression that itching exanthema is becoming more frequent in scarlet fever.

If the patient tends to manifest a poor cardiovascular condition and an introverted, depressive mood, it is possible in the first as well as in the second phase of the disease for

- **Naja D12 pillules/dil.**(various manufacturers)
  5–7 pillules/gtt. 2–3 x/d to be administered.

This potentized toxin from the King cobra is the most important homoeopathic form of medication and is used to counteract the long-range toxic action of scarlet fever on the myocardial tract and the risk of a complication involving a heart valve.

During the early stages of otitis – usually towards the end of the first or during the second week of the disease, an immediate start can be made with this treatment:

- **Apis Belladonna cum Mercurio pillules** Wala
  initially 5 pillules every quarter to half an hour, then less frequently, and

in conjunction with immediately produced **potentized autologous blood** as developed by Imhäuser [2000, 187ff.]

- C5, daily 10 gtt. to one glass of water, taken one sip at a time,

can prove effective.

This can be supported by the aforementioned injection of **Lachesis D30** and **Argentum D30/Echinacea D6.** If the condition deteriorates or if there is an absence of therapeutic response, antibiotics need to be administered.

Generally with scarlet fever, the recurrent problem is that of a *poor cardiovascular system* to which patients are particularly prone during the second septennium of their lives. The reciprocal relationship between the physical and soul entities is expressed particularly directly in the condition of the cardiovascular system.

- **Cardiodoron dil.** Weleda
  3–7 gtt. 5 x/d.

not only has a supporting effect on a cardiovascular weakness which needs treatment, but also promotes the aforementioned objective of the disease process (and therefore of the therapy), which is to bring about a more harmonious connection between soul and physical processes, particularly in the cardiovascular system. Cardiodoron can also be indicated throughout the entire duration of treatment.

5.3.4.4.2 Treatment in the second to fourth weeks

In most cases, patients appear to be in very good condition after the aforementioned course of acute treatment, so the ongoing need for treatment and for continuing rest may appear less than apparent to child and parents alike. However, one should not be misled by this appearance; the cleaning/purification ("wound healing" – see above) of the tonsil area and the lymph channels, the support for the life organization and the overcoming of the toxin load all require time and specific medicines.

- **Calendula D3 amp.** Wala
  ½ ampoule 1–2 x/d per os

has a particularly vitalizing effect on the cleaning and closing of lesions in the skin and mucous membrane area where a weakness of the life forces, the etheric body, may be present, delaying the healing process.

As a Compositae, calendula exhibits a high level of internal organization and order; on the other hand, its orange-yellow blossoms provide shelter to a wide variety of insects, and does so without adverse effect to itself. The high level of order in its flower open to ensouled animal life, coupled with the robust vitality of this herbal plant, imparts constructive and ordering impulses to the life organization of the patient; an extraordinarily effective medicine that is used too infrequently. Always advisable in the form of a mouthwash (see above).

- **Apis mell. D12 pillules** Weleda/various manufacturers
  5 gtt./pillules 1–2 x/d

counteracts the danger of fluid status in lymph and kidney system.

In the honey bee, Apis mellifera, the soul entity of the creature is entirely ordered through its incorporation into the structure of the bee colony and its unconditional orientation towards the sunlight; this enables the honey bee to play such a constructive role in the plant world, e.g. through its contribution to pollination. Apis in potentized form can make a substantial contribution to transforming the catabolic process of the first phase of scarlet fever into an orderly regeneration process in the life organization. It is the most important medicine involved in *stabilizing the immunological conflict of the organism with the toxin that triggered the disease* thus preventing the classic post-streptococcal diseases from occurring (cf. ▸Chap. 5.5.4.1 for details of the treatment for post-streptococcal glomerulonephritis).

With children who have a high predisposition to lymphatism (incl. a predisposition to lymphadenitis) – typically with a blonde hair colour – the following treatment is an effective supplement

- **Ferrum iodatum D12 pillules** (various manufacturers)
  5–7 pillules 2 x/d

Unfortunately, Vaucheria ampoules are no longer available for therapeutic purposes (for indication cf. earlier editions of this volume).

A similar effect – vital strengthening of the child if it suffers a dip in vitality with renewed paleness and weakness in the second-third week of the disease – can be achieved through

- **Levico comp. amp.** Wala
  if possible once only 1 ampoule s.c., then 1 ampoule daily per os

The ampoules are more effective in this medicine than the pillules, also when given per os. *Blackthorn*, Prunus spinosa, is particularly effective if a phase that has excited the soul entity and exhausted the physical body has induced a weakening of the life organization, as is often the case with scarlet fever in the second phase of this disease.

Recovery is generally supported by

- **Levico comp. pillules** Wala
  5–7 pillules 3 x/d

Blackthorn has a dietetic strengthening effect in the second phase of the disease,

- **Blackthorn elixir**
  15 ml 3–5 x/d

During *convalescence* (fourth week of disease) it is possible – depending on findings – to stop the medicines set out here.

Gargling with **Symbioflor® 1** and the administration of **Calendula** should be continued until such time as the tonsil and lymph station findings have normalized satisfactorily.

5.3.4.4.3 Contagious impetigo

In cases of streptococcally-induced impetigo, this can be treated *externally* with a preparation that can be ordered at the pharmacy with the following prescription:

Calendula essence Wala/Weleda	10.0,
Sulphur praecip.	3.0(–4.0)
Lotio alba	ad 100.0

(i. e. 10 % Calendula essence, 3 % (or 4 %) Sulphur Praecip. and the rest Lotio alba).

Additionally

- **Mercurialis 10 % balm** Weleda can be used.

Internally administered options include

- **Lachesis comp. pillules** Wala
  5–7 pillules 5 x/d, max. 5 hrly and
- **Antimonit D6 trit.** Weleda
  5 × 1 saltsp. daily as well as
- **Calendula D3 amp.** Wala
  ½ ampoule 3 x/d per os

With regard to diet, we recall here the *absolute ban on sugar* which applies to all purulent skin infections; of course, nutrition for scarlet fever in general should take the form of a light diet without much protein and without any refined sugar.

If after three days the impetigo has not improved markedly, this can be a sign of severely diminished life forces. Treatment with antibiotics is then indicated.

5.3.4.4.4 Lymphadenitis colli

This complication can be prevented to a significant extent through the basic forms of treatment described above.

However, if the disease is nonetheless contracted, the following procedure has in many cases proven to be successful, subject to timely diagnosis and therapy:

- **Mercurius sol. D6 trit.** Apotheke an der Weleda/**tab.** DHU
  1 saltsp./½–1 tab. initially every 2 hrs
- **Calendula D3 amp.** Wala
  ½ ampoule 3 x/d

After the onset of improvement, switch from Mercurius sol. D6 to

- **Lachesis comp. pillules** Wala
  5–7 pillules 5 x/d

This form of treatment can in turn be applied when lymphatism is indicated

- **Ferrum iodatum D12 pillules** (various manufacturers)
  3 × 5 pillules

Externally **quark compresses** can be helpful, as can the application of balm with

- **Mercurialis 10 % balm** Weleda or
- **Archangelica comp. balm**. Weleda,

and this can generally be used in severe lymph node swelling in scarlet fever.

With children who do not permit the frequent oral administering of medicines, and in severe cases faced with the need to administer effective medication during the night, the authors have had very positive experiences with

- **Echinacea/Mercurius comp. supp. f. Kdr.** Wala
  1–2 x/d, especially evenings

5.3.4.4.5 Concluding remarks

From the scope and the required differentiation in the presentation of scarlet fever, it is apparent that an individualizing diagnostic and therapeutic approach requires great commitment from doctor and parents alike. Anyone comparing this against the general practice in dealing with “positive streptococcal verification” may well ask themselves why this elaborate and resource-intensive procedure is worthwhile.

General experience by colleagues who treat scarlet fever in this way has shown that the condition is much less likely to recur than would otherwise be the case (although it can still happen) [Husemann 1998, 20]. This is certainly due in part to the anti-toxic immunity that forms without antibiotic treatment; but underlying it is the fundamental soul and physical maturity that the child can only experience to this level if he or she overcomes scarlet fever through his or her own resources and this is not taken away from him or her through a suppressive form of treatment (making it impossible). F. Husemann [1998, 20], who also expresses a view on this question in his study already quoted on several occasions, then concludes by quoting a statement made by Rudolf Steiner back in 1909. The latter contributes a view of childhood diseases from the perspective of a researcher working with supersensory perceptual abilities that runs squarely counter to the currently dominant scientific view held by the medical establishment and which emphasizes the positive and meaningful significance of these diseases for the future. As such, this view may also deliver some impetus to develop their own perception and concepts to those whose conceptual grasp of these issues spans a narrower horizon than the one seen by the author of the following quotation:

"We see for example that childhood diseases occur typically at certain times. These are nothing other than the expression that the child, while navigating his or her childhood diseases, learns to gain control of certain part of his or her own organs from the inside, and to retain this ability for all subsequent incarnations. We should view these diseases as a process that makes people competent. That way, we come to think about diseases in a very different way" [Steiner 1988, fourteenth lecture].

5.3.5 Mumps

Mumps is generally underestimated during the early stages of the disease; a widespread fear of lasting damage to the testicles is however far in excess of the reality, and prior to puberty is without foundation in fact. Complications in the central nervous system and in the region of pancreas and testicles are most effectively countered by **one week of bed rest**. This can be justified very effectively by reference alone to the fact that the acute stomach aches and meningeal irritation levels associated with mumps are greatly alleviated, and can even be avoided, through simple bed rest.

In the experience of the authors, the children most prone to mumps are ones who *are still very closely attached to their mothers and who are dependent upon her*. It is often found that children become a great deal more autonomous and independent of their immediate family circle after having contracted mumps; this is particularly significant during the transition between the first and second septennium. The forces of the soul and spiritual individuality are more deeply incarnated in the metabolism; diagnostically and therapeutically, this disease progression closely involves the *pancreas* that is so significant in the control and regulation of the metabolism by the I-organization [Schulze 1998, Steiner and Wegman 1991, 50ff., 55f.]. In this way this disease is related to measles in many respects (starting with the inflammatory swelling of the head area, activation of the soul and spiritual individuality that now penetrates more intensively into the vital fluid processes, particularly in respect of secretion); the purpose here too lies in the individualization and appropriation of a physical body originally inherited from the parents, whereby this disease process anchors the forces of personality more deeply, and with stronger willpower (but because of that even more subconsciously) in the metabolism than measles. The duration of this disease from the start of incubation also amounts to 28 days, although the manifest disease event reaches its climax on day 21. We also gain the impression with mumps that those organs (such as the pancreas) that are more at risk of complications or are most affected by the disease are also the ones that most strongly experience the intense, individual penetration "from within" (as defined in the above quotation from R. Steiner, 253).

Treatment is based on bed rest, a light food regime with low fat and protein levels and sufficient warmth on the stomach (possibly a light hot water bottle).

The parotid swelling can be treated externally with

- **Archangelica comp. ungt.** Weleda.

With initially high fever and acute parotid discomfort, relief can take the form of

- **Belladonna Rh D6** Weleda
  5 gtt. initially hrly.

With *markedly lymphatic children* with a sluggish fever and disease course, the authors administer

- **Ferrum iodatum D12 pillules** (various manufacturers)
  3 × 5 pillules initially daily

The medication Barium citricum which is often recommended in anthroposophical literature – a medicine which as such is related to very resistant inertia of the lymphatic system – has in the practical experience of the authors generally not shown any evidence of effectiveness.

The disease process in the salivary glands of the head and stomach (detectable in the chemical laboratory in the form of an increase in amylase, something rapidly able to clarify the diagnosis) can be stabilized by means of

- **Cichorium Rh D3 dil./e planta tota D3 pillules** Weleda/Wala (▸Chap. 4.6.3.3)
  5–7 pillules/10 gtt. (alcohol-free) 3 x/d

In the event of *stomach pains – these can often be fairly severe* – the authors have found that the medication (orally administered)

- **Pancreas/Argentum amp.** Wala
  ½ ampoule 1–3 x/d per os proves very effective.

Manifestation of inflamed irritation of the meninges and the central nervous system can be treated effectively with

- **Apis mell. D30 pillules/amp.** Weleda and
- **Bryonia e rad. D30 pillules/amp.** Wala
  in severe cases, a mixed s.c. injection can be administered, e.g. in the left upper arm; as pillules, dissolved together (5–10 pillules on each occasion) in 50 ml of water, sipped throughout the day over a period of 2–3 days.

On young adult males, adnexitis can be treated externally with a jockstrap and wrap with **Retterspitz** and internally with

- **Testes D30 amp.** Wala together with
- **Argentum met. praep. D30 amp.** Weleda
  as a mixed injection in the abdomen (inguinal) or in the homolateral thigh.

In the case of adnexitis in young females,

- **Ovaria D30**

is correspondingly well suited (very rare). Mumps can have a protective effect against ovarian carcinoma (▸Chap. 3.5)!

5.3.6 Pertussis (whooping cough)

> Over the last few years, these diseases have mostly affected people from school age, and especially people who have received vaccinations, possibly because the vaccination failed to provide protection against B. pertussis. With this move in the disease towards an older demographic, an increase in the incidence of diseases and complications can be expected among unvaccinated infants. ... Adolescents and adults [are] in 20–60 % of all cases the source of infection for infants suffering from pertussis.
>
> DGPI-Handbook (Handbook of the German Society of Paediatric Infectiology) [2009]

5.3.6.1 Insight into the illness, associated disposition

The disease profile of pertussis commences *uncharacteristically in a catarrhal fashion* 1 to 2 weeks after incubation; 1 to 2 weeks later, the *pathognomonic convulsive coughing attacks* commence. The typical profile of this childhood disease takes the form of *spasms in the respiratory tract* and in *the stomach and oesophagus* (vomiting). These symptoms arise – as they do with scarlet fever – as a result of *toxin-forming bacteria* and their impact on the central nervous system (especially on the breathing centre) and on the respiratory epithelia. Whereas the child is highly contagious during the catarrhal ("streaming") stage, the likelihood of infecting others diminishes rapidly as the convulsions start [Keller and Wiskott 1991, 451]: clearly with the convulsive (windpipe and throat) excretory activity of the organism the pathogen is also overcome. For the most part, this takes place without fever.

The risk with pertussis is that of a severe *paralyzing action* on all organs associated with breathing and the central nervous system (encephalopathy). The fear is that infants under the age of 4 months may contract apnoea. Otitis media and bronchitis/pneumonia are not primary factors: instead they are secondary, building on the toxin-related damage to the epithelia in the airways; here too, infants are the ones most at risk.

From all of these symptoms (▸Chap. 5.3.4.2, ▸Chap. 5.3.4.3) it becomes directly apparent that it is the *soul organization*, which is primarily responsible in human beings and animals for active independent breathing and all independent movement of the organism, that brings about the main expressions of any disease. In the case of pertussis, it does this primarily without the leadership of the I-organization, as manifested by the absence of fever. A striking factor is the exacerbation of symptoms *at night* (also a pathognomonic indicator). Normally the dominant night-time factor for human beings is the activity associated with living regeneration and growth, i. e. the activity of the life organization, accompanied by a corresponding decline in soul and spiritual activity [Steiner and Wegman 1977, ▸Chap. IV, 30–34]. This is associated, especially in the evenings and at night, with the regurgitation of any excessively large quantities of food, particularly during or after a coughing fit.

On the one hand, the soul organization protects itself against anything that the physical body finds foreign to it: e. g. undigested food or even the causal agent of the disease in the throat. On the other hand, the child would appear, through these coughing attacks, to be defending itself against the physical body – inherited from its parents – the vital processes of which tend to predominate at night over its soul and spiritual individuality. At a time when this inherited physical body is still very strong, and while the connection between the own individuality and this body is still very labile through the breathing (first six months of life), pertussis can progress in a particularly critical way.

The *nature and way* in which the soul entity is active in the disease within the organism also tends to accentuate a certain degree of one-sidedness that is evident in many children *before* the disease as a certain predisposition to disease (see below). During the convulsive stage an *antipathic* activity predominates that acts against the "metabolic human being", the metabolic processes dominating below the diaphragm and against the nutrition entering the body from outside. The impression may arise that the soul individuality of the child is regurgitating everything alien from within its body and wishes to purify itself of those things. In extreme cases, this even applies to the inhaled air which is exhaled and "sicked up" with viscous mucous.

The *predisposition to whooping cough* is especially prevalent among children affected by a *disharmonious connection* between the upper, conscious and breathing self with the lower metabolic person. These children are characterized by general *restlessness, nervousness and high sensitivity*. They forever seek to change location, as though they feel uneasy in their skins; the associated changing and sensitively perceived impressions rapidly overwhelm them and increase their sense of restlessness. Appetite is often very slight, even prior to the onset of the disease, and *eating behaviour is finicky*. Frequently, they suffer *stomach cramps, and older children headaches*. Furthermore, there is a tendency towards *stagnation and swelling in the lymphatic system*, especially in the neck lymph nodes, tonsils and adenoids. This induces a predisposition to infection, especially when the weather is cold and damp. Here it should be noted that the blood becomes individualized much sooner as the central organ of the individual warmth organization, while the lymphatic system remains an expression of the physical body inherited from the parents for a great deal longer.

When we endeavour to understand this *predisposition for whooping cough*, we see *that the soul entity of these children behaves with great antipathy towards its own physical body which it is unable to penetrate and shape with sufficient vitality*. The body inherited from the parents is inadequately served by the soul entity and insufficiently individualized, left to its own devices, which is then in turn expressed through a tendency for the lymphatic system to vegetate and to contract infection. At the same time this gives rise to a surplus of soul activity in the nervous and sensory human being, in consciousness and sensitivity because the soul entity does not immerse itself deeply enough in the physical body and this in turn gives rise to the oversensitivity, nervousness and restlessness described above. A constitution of this kind will always tend to manifest abnormalities in the sphere of the rhythmical system, especially in the entire respiratory tract: e. g. *increased incidence of catarrh, adenoids, mucoid otitis, but also stammering (stuttering), for example, and a predisposition to bronchial asthma*. The common denominator of all of these is a weakness and therefore a tendency of the soul entity to spasm in response to a physical body which it is unable sufficiently to penetrate internally and form as required by the organs.

During the *catarrhal stage*, the streaming stage of pertussis, these problems arise again in connection with the etheric body, the life organization; in the convulsive stage the child's astral body drives its one-sided soul activity to extremes. Many doctors have now observed that after pertussis and "particularly among children who were fussy eaters beforehand" they "suddenly develop an exceptionally good appetite" [Goebel and Glöckler 2005, 168]. Many feel as if they have been cleansed and are much better able to unite with their own physical body, for example also through the intake of food. Pre-existing irregularities such as retarded language development, stammering or bronchial asthma can be sustainably normalized through whooping cough. The immunity acquired is a great deal more robust than any vaccination-induced form of immunity.

Case history

A boy aged 18 months develops serious bronchial asthma; medical history of eleven in-patient hospital stays in a year, of which two in intensive care (this case arose prior to the era of inhalative steroids). Difficult birth situation accompanied by large-scale parental anxiety; immediately before start of illness, toxic burden caused by an accident at a chemical factory close to the holiday location. Constitutionally the child matches the type described above in every respect; both parents tend to behave in an excessively anxious manner.

At the start of treatment at the age of 2½, only one hospital stay was still necessary at the beginning; three years of satisfactory treatment results, but recurrent periodic asthma attacks requiring intervention. At about the age of 5½, pertussis (treated without antibiotics, as described below). Since the start of the convulsive stage, no further bronchial asthma. (Eleven years of post-treatment observation). This is not an only case.

Evidently pertussis *can bring about constitutional change* in a child by exacerbating existing problems to an acute level, leading to a transformation in body-related soul activity. The harmonization brought about in respect of the life and soul organization is of inestimable significance, both in respect of the emotional development of the child and, at a later date, for the body-mediated will activity (salutogenesis).

The disposition for whooping cough described above is identical in many respects to the Calcium phosphoricum medicinal picture in homoeopathy (a form of medication that incorporates the extreme polarity of the substance qualities of calcium and phosphorous, substances that reflect one another in terms of the direct dissonance in their medicinal picture). Of course children with a different personality and character may also be prone to whooping cough, e. g. whose one-sided metabolic lymphatic constitution equates to the Calcium carbonicum medicinal picture of homoeopathy. The latter also change their constitution during the course of the illness, for example they lose their frequently emphasized "puppy fat" and emerge after a course of pertussis physically slimmer as well as more psychologically free in their behaviour. Consequently whooping cough, if properly attended by parents and doctor (see below), can provide children with a significant developmental opportunity to free themselves through their own efforts from traits of inherited constitutional one-sidedness, efforts brought about by the challenge from the bacterially formed toxin.

While there is no shortage of justified references that pertussis can endanger immunologically still very immature children, or children affected by certain organ diseases, the authors seek with these comments to focus primarily on a *positive disease concept* that may be of helpful guidance to parents and doctors when dealing with prophylaxis, diagnosis and therapy.

The centre of a whooping cough infection is the spasmodic attack (in the respiratory sphere) – often at night. An event of this kind initially often prompts *anxiety* on the part of the parents. Children tend to scream and cry before or after an attack, they are exhausted or then resume play immediately afterwards (or fall asleep again). The *anxiety primarily affects the adults*; it can quickly give rise to an *overprotectiveness* that does not release the child and becomes a problem in its own right in the disease process. For this causes the soul entity of the child to be drawn outwards and prevented from effecting the transition into a new and positive "conquest" and reshaping of the physical body inherited from the parents that it needs to transform in order to be able to "take up residence in it" properly. Excessive parental care and concern obstruct this step and it is therefore important for the doctor to understand the disease and to communicate to the parents a positive and trust-filled attitude. If we observe the children themselves, they resist the over-protective behaviour to begin with but this is not something of which parents are necessarily aware. On the other hand, if the necessary change in the soul organization of a child during the convulsive stage proves unsuccessful or if it is prevented from happening due to parental anxiety and over-protectiveness, this can cause coughing attacks to persevere for months during the defervescent stage.

The right approach to the disease is therefore one of the factors responsible for achieving what the disease process positively makes possible. This also applies to medicinal treatment. In the practice of the authors, based on treatment with potentized medicines that dispenses as a general rule with administering antibiotics for pertussis, diseases, especially of the respiratory system (bronchial hyperreactivity, bronchial asthma, pneumonia), are virtually never observed as a consequence of whooping cough – indeed, the opposite tends to be true, as the above case history of an asthma patient indicates. It is by all means a realistic treatment goal to strive for the child to be healthier through dealing with the disease process itself, and through the medicines used, than it was before the illness.

5.3.6.2 Treatment

5.3.6.2.1 Treatment options during the incubation stage

Treatment of infants up to four months of age during the incubation period is crucial; generally speaking, one must watch out for pre-existing cerebral damage and hereditary heart and lung diseases. In such cases the infection (visitors, siblings) is noticed before the outbreak of the disease more often than it is in kindergarten- and school-age children, and this increases the chance of initiating treatment before manifestation of the disease. In principle, antibiotic prophylaxis or mitigation should be seriously considered in such cases (and discussed with the parents). On the other hand, the authors' practice (see case study) has shown that the following treatment is effective even for very young infants.

- The most important medicine to be administered during the entire course of disease is potentized sundew, which Hahnemann [1995b, 228] introduced into whooping cough treatment
- **Drosera rotundifolia D6–30 pillules** (various manufacturers)

Round-leaved sundew grows on moors. It has weak roots and its hairy, spoon-shaped leaves grow circularly outwards near the ground, forming a rosette. At the edges of the leaves, a secretion resembling dew drops is produced by brownish-red, sensitive hairs. Insects attracted by the secretion are captured; the glandular hairs grow onto the insect which now adheres to the leaf, they cover it and digest it through the secretion. Drosera is a carnivore; the animal protein is sucked up and all that remains is the chitin skeleton. – As a habitat, *moors* are characterized by the fact that they do not allow air and warmth to penetrate into the soil; here a stagnating, acidic, watery milieu evolves which is hostile to life, with a wintery chill persisting all year round. Moors constitute an extreme form of "lympathism" in nature which shuts out sun and wind, the dynamizing qualities of air (respiration) and warmth, thus falling into a state of stagnation which preserves old and dead elements. – Whereas the roots of the sundew can hardly penetrate the peaty soil, the plant develops a relationship to animals which is abnormal for any plant; apart from the aforesaid ability to break down protein, Drosera has such a toxic effect on sheep, for example, that they develop a deep cough accompanied by progressive emaciation and die from it [Lewin 1962, 715]. Drosera extracts produce myogenic and neurogenic cramps of the musculature [Stübler and Krug 1987, 38]!

The parallel to the pathology of whooping cough might already become evident from this sketchy discussion of the plant: just as life on the moor shuts out the qualities of air, light and warmth, the depicted disposition towards whooping cough is characterized by a dissociation of physical-vital bodiliness, which stagnates lymphatically and is strongly oriented to the past (heredity – cf. the moor as something which preserves the past), from the soul organization. In this disposition, the toxin-producing pathogen finds its terrain, like the toxin-producing sundew on the moor.

For any child at risk who is known to be in the period of incubation one can administer a single dosage of

- **Drosera D30: 1 × 5 pillules** and if necessary the potentized nosode
- **Pertussinum D30 pillules** (various manufacturers): 1 × 5 pillules can be administered.

Through treatment using Drosera (see below as well), the pertussis still breaks out but it runs its course much more harmoniously and is over sooner without disturbing or suppressing the necessary individual maturation process and thus also the intensity of disease required for this.

Children at risk for apnoea (most of all infants under one year old) who are known to be in the period of incubation (▸Chap. 2.2.2) should be given

- **Tartarus stibiatus D6 trit.** Weleda
  5 × daily 1 saltsp. until the end of the stadium convulsivum (if need be with monitoring).

For infants 1–6-months old and for at-risk children with immunodeficiency it has proven effective to administer injections of

- **Echinacea D3 amp.** Wala/Weleda
  0.5 ml s.c. 3 × weekly during the first (and second) week.

5.3.6.2.2 General treatment during the paroxysmal stage

Starting with the onset of clearly evident coughing in the course of pertussis and at the latest at the onset of the pathognomonic coughing attacks which characterize this disease, the following treatment is indicated and has proven effective:

- **Drosera D6–12[1] pillules** Weleda
  3–4 × daily 5 pillules, for infants 2–3 pillules before each meal

From age 6–7 on:

- **Drosera D12–30 pillules** Weleda
  1–3 × daily 5 pillules.

A generally antispasmotic effect is achieved by administering potentized copper [Girke 2010, 745f], which can be combined with a dosage of Drosera:

- **Cuprum aceticum D4–6 dil./pillules** Weleda/DHU
  3–6 × daily 3–5 drops/pillules (drops have a stronger effect), for infants also more frequent dosages of 2–3 pillules.

A remedy compound with a wide range of application which offers an alternative to Drosera is

- **Pertudoron 1. dil./pillules** Weleda/Apotheke an der Weleda
  12–30 drops or pillules/per day dissolved in water (depending on the age of the patient) and administered one teaspoon at a time [Vademecum 2010, 650]

It contains Drosera in combination with low potencies of Coccus cacti, Mephitis putorius and Ipecacuanha, all medicinal plants which are effective for treatment of pertussis.

In the experience of the authors, Cuprum-aceticum-D3 drops Weleda, sold as Pertuoron 2, are too deeply potentized (D3) for children of pre-school age. Generally speaking, potentized copper acetate is a *spasmolytically effective* remedy in the area of the lower respiratory tract, particularly when the symptoms show *exacerbation at night* (▸Chap. 6.5, asthma bronchiale; [Vademecum 2010, 365 guiding idea and indication]. As a metallic remedy, potentized copper [Selawry 1985, 209–254] especially promotes the capacity of the soul to engage with the etheric body, the inner soul organization of life processes, whereas the convulsive coughing attacks which culminate during the night correspond to the soul aspect putting up resistance against the life organization that dominates during the night.

In children less than 6 months old, treatment using Drosera and Cuprum aceticum should be supplemented by Tartarus stibiatus D6; it is very important for this treatment to be continued until the end of the coughing attacks.

Case study

The sister of a 2-week-old newborn is diagnosed with pertussis. At this point in time the infant is given a single dosage of Pertussinum D30 and Drosera D30, and then on an ongoing basis Tartarus stib. D6 trit. 5 × 1 saltsp. After eleven days the first coughing occurs (stadium catarrhale); this is a clear indication that the child has been infected. At intervals of 2 to 3 days, s.c. injections of Echinacea D3, 0.5 ml follow. The coughing quickly becomes convulsive; treatment using Tartarus stib. is supplemented by Drosera D6 and Cuprum acet. D6, 2 pillules of each before each meal. During treatment normal, mild course of disease. On day 10 of the stadium convulsivum a severe coughing attack occurs at around 3:00 a. m. with ensuing cyanosis, which does not occur again after calium carb. D6 is prescribed. Three weeks after the emergence of symptoms the patient recovered from the pertussis completely and continued to flourish in the further course of time.

1 In the course of disease, a change to a higher potency might prove necessary should the remedy not be effective enough.

5

5.3.6.2.3 Differential treatment suggestions

Depending on the specific nature of the coughing fits, the treatment described in ▸Chap. 5.3.6.2.2 can be supplemented or modified. This has been depicted in homoeopathic terms in a highly differentiated way by H. Imhäuser [2000, 96–103]. However, in practice one can put trust in the general treatment described above. Only in cases where one of the symptoms described below calls for specific therapy is any further differentiation indicated (as became clear in the above case study).

If the *mucus expelled* during a coughing fit is *very thick and stringy* and the fits tend to get worse *in the early hours of the morning*, then

- **Coccus cacti D4–12 pillules** (various manufacturers)
  2–4 × daily 5 pillules
  are indicated. In cases of an extreme *urge to gag and vomiting*, the effectiveness of Drosera (which is simultaneously the most important remedy for vomiting up of food in the course of coughing fits) can be supplemented by
- **Ipecacuanha D6–12 pillules** Weleda
  2–4 × daily 5 pillules, especially before going to sleep.

In cases of pronounced *reddening of the face* (which also brings Arnica and Belladonna to mind) and clearly evident *exhaustion after the attack*

- **Corallium rubrum D6 trit.** Apotheke an der Weleda
  3–4 × daily 1 saltsp.

is effective; in cases of extremely *painful* coughing fits

- **Bryonia e rad. D6–12 glob.** Wala
  2–5 × daily 5 pillules.

A very important remedy for *severe and long-lasting nocturnal coughing fits* which culminate in *cyanosis* is the potentized arsenic compound of copper

- **Olivenite** (= Cuprum arsenicosum) **D8–12 dil.** Apotheke an der Weleda
  2–3 × daily 3–7 drops.

Case study

The brother of a twelve-week-old girl is diagnosed with pertussis; the infant is treated with Pertudoron 1. 5 drops alternating at intervals of 1½ hours with Cuprum aceticum D6 dil. Weleda, 3 drops (Pertudoron 2 = Cuprum acet. D3 can exacerbate coughing fits in patients of this age due to the potency, which is too low). After 2 ½ weeks the boy is almost free of complaints.

After the brother is diagnosed the still asymptomatic infant is given Drosera D30 and Pertussinum D30 pillules (DHU in each case) 3 pillules each as a single dosage. Three days later the first catarrhal symptoms appear and a few days thereafter a first, as yet atypical coughing fit occurs. Now a pertussis infection is assumed. Pertudoron 1, 3 × daily 3 drops, Cuprum aceticum D6 dil. Weleda, 3 × daily 2 drops, Tartarus stib. D6 Weleda, 3 × daily 1 saltsp. are prescribed. The latter is administerd as apnoea prophylaxis (▸Chap. 2.2.2). At the same time injections of Echinacea e pl. tota D3 every other day, later on D2 Wala, 0.5 ml s.c. each, are given. At first gradual increase in coughing; after

approx. 10 days onset of typical convulsive coughing but without spasmodic inspiration (reprise). The coughing fits rapidly increase in severity and frequency, occuring in the form of coughing paroxysms accompanied by a crimsom face and occasional vomiting. One week after onset of stadium convulsivum a single injection of Formica Gl D40 amp. Wala aa mixed with Pulmo/Tartarus II amp. Wala, 0.5 ml on each side of the spine are given s.c.. Two weeks after onset of stadium convulsivum, three short asphyxial phases with cyanosis occur at night, accompanied by convulsions of the extremities. In response to these symptoms, Cuprum aceticum is replaced by Olivenite (Cuprum ars. naturale) D12, 2 × daily 3 drops. The potentized natural copper arsenate is chosen to enhance the anti-convulsant effect of the copper by the arsenic component and thus to dissolve the too intense astral activity in the respiratory area. In the following night another coughing fit with cyanosis occurs, accompanied by relatively mild convulsions and in the following nights increasingly weak coughing fits with no more occurrence of threatening situations. The stadium convulsivum lasts 2 ½ weeks. Ten days later there are no neurological symptoms, the child sleeps well, has a healthy appetite, thrives.
The case study clearly shows how important individual consideration of the course of disease is.

In cases of pronounced *weakness* in older children, one can also consider using Tartarus stibiatus D6 as described for treatment of infants.
Children who react to the disease with – atypical – *antipathy, have extreme vomiting attacks and cry after each coughing fit* improve after administration of

- **Mephitis putorius D6–12 pillules** (various manufacturers)
  1–3 × daily 5 pillules

If the child is generally in a poor condition although the coughing fits are not particularly severe, i. e., if the disease process as depicted in ▸Chap. 5.3.6.1 stagnates, a single injection of

- **Formica ex animale D40 amp.** Wala
  0.5–1.0 ml s.c. between the shoulder blades can prove very beneficial.

The effect lies in the fact that Formica gives the child the impetus to develop the necessary excreting and cleansing activity – not only in regard to the pathogen but also in regard to its own inherited physicality. Although this injection is rarely necessary, in individual cases it can help the patient overcome the disease considerably.

- **Kalium (= potassium) carb. D6–12 pillules** (various manufacturers)
  daily 3 × 5, in some cases only in the evening 5 pillules

strengthens and opens up the child's vital anabolic processes to formation and differentiation through the soul aspect; the dominance of anabolic processes during the night is limited and this relieves the soul aspect in its body-related activity. A determining factor is *exacerbation at night around 3:00 a. m.*, i. e. at the time when the anabolic, body-formative processes, in particular those of the liver, reach their peak and the turnaround must be physiologically initiated which leads to awakening and the domination of the soul-spirit aspect in the organism during the day.

If pertussis triggers or exacerbates pre-existing asthma bronchiale, suitable remedies are

- **Pertussinum C12 pillules,**
- **Cuprum met. praep. D12 trit.** Weleda,
- **Formica D12 dil.** Weleda,
- **Astragalus D6–12 dil.** (various manufacturers)

in a suitable order or in combination.

If one treats pertussis without antibiotics using the therapeutic alternatives suggested here and avoids unusual strains and journeys during this time, one will quite regularly discover a strengthening of the respiratory system, improved incorporation of spirit-soul individuality in this area. This often manifests itself in progress in language development, which is reported by many parents and well-understood by the physician; this is frequently found in cases in which a susceptibility to asthma has been overcome.

5.3.7 Varicella (chicken pox)

Generally speaking, this disease pattern poses few problems in terms of diagnosis and therapy.

External treatment can usually be limited to

- **Wecesin Powder** Weleda
- washes (rapid, cool) using **camomile tea** [Stellmann 2009, 55f] or brief (½ min.) showers and wrapping up the area in a bath towel – especially in cases of severe vaginal itching on the fourth day of illness.

It is important for the child not to leave the house for seven days; bed rest in cases of fever and on the day after fever drops.

If a severe course of disease is to be expected due to immunodeficiency and most of all neurodermatitis, at the onset of exanthema it is beneficial to administer

- **Rhus toxicodendron e fol. D30 pillules** Wala
  3 × daily 3 pillules for 3 days,

possibly supplemented by single dosages of 3–5 pillules of

- **Nosode varicella D30 pillules** Staufen

In general, *varicella-cerebellitis* takes a benign course. In addition to treatment using Rhus tox. D30 and the varicella nosode, treatment using
potentized autologous blood according to Imhäuser [2000, 187ff.]: C5, daily 3–5 drops in the morning
and the homologous organ preparation

- **Cerebellum Gl D15 amp.** Wala
  daily 0.5–1.0 ml per os is effective.

In cases of immunosuppressed children, for example those undergoing cytostatic treatment, virostatics (for example Aciclovir) and a hyperimmunoglobulin can be given, the latter also in cases of varicella contracted by the mother immediately praepartum.

If *herpes zoster*, i.e. *shingles*, occur in children who are not receiving immunosuppressive treatment (in the experience of the authors, girls are more likely to be afflicted than boys), the aforesaid treatment (Rhus tox. D30, varicella nosode D30 and potentized autologous blood) also constitute a general basic therapy.

If the herpes zoster affects the thoracic region it is beneficial in some cases to treat the condition using

- **Ranunculus bulbosus D12 dil.** DHU (instead of Rhus tox.)
  2–3 × daily 5 drops,

supplemented by the organ preparation

- **Nervi intercostales Gl D30 amp.** Wala

daily 1 ampoule per os, especially in cass of severe itching or pain.

As a *constitutional remedy* for children with herpes zoster – especially girls with a positive family anamnesis, which is not uncommon – the most frequently indicated remedy is

- **Sepia C12–30 pillules**

Sepia is a homoeopathic polychrest for blistering skin diseases and pigment anomalies of the skin (also effective for treatment of vitiligo in children).

The described treatment also proves effective if the herpes zoster emerges after cytostatic treatment; *during* such treatment one will generally not be able to dispense with use of virostatic agents.

5.3.8 Rubella (German measles)

As a rule, no specific treatment is required for children.

5.4 Febrile, flu-like infections; febrile convulsions

The purpose of febrile diseases for the development of the child's warmth organization, the maturation of the immune system, and the assertion of formative individual impulses in the body initially inherited by the parents has been depicted extensively in the introduction to Chap. 5 und 5.1. – In the following, the focus will lie on treatment of acute, unspecific febrile diseases.

In terms of diagnostics and differential therapy it is always important to ascertain:

- Does the fever fulfil a purpose in the context of the disease or is it part of a destructive-autoaggressive event (sepsis, bacterial meningitis, epiglottitis) which requires correspondingly aggressive antibiotic and antipyretic treatment?
- Does the patient require special monitoring or therapeutic guidance due to pre-existing neurological, cardiac or severe pulmonary conditions?

Problems concerning convulsive fits associated with fever are discussed separately in ▸Chap. 5.4.3.

5.4.1 Nursing and external applications

In principle a physician should be consulted when a child with an acute febrile illness is being cared for and given external applications. – In any case, *rest and warmth* are the general conditions for enabling the child to overcome the disease by himself. Fever results from individual self-activity of the child and as such it requires guidance and support but no random suppression, which is not scientifically justifiable in any way (for exceptions see above). Febrile children require bed rest and very young sub-febrile children need to be kept in a quiet room in the presence of their parents at least. The toddler should not go outside or be taken out in a pram until after at least *one fever-free day*, even in summer. One generally underestimates how challenging the outdoors is for the self-forces of the human being in any season.

If the fever is rising but the periphery is remaining cool and a relative centralization of the circulatory system (and thus warmth) occurs accompanied by frequent shivering and chills, external applications are not indicated. During this phase the presence of a parent and warmth protection are important. – If the temperature level strived for by the organism has been reached, external applications can reduce temperature excesses and alleviate the complaints associated with the fever. This also holds in regard to poor consumption of fluids or circulatory weakness.

The most important measure to take and the one most often chosen by the authors, particularly for small children (cf. extensive discussion in ▸Chap. 5.1.1.4.2) is

- a slowly performed **enema** using a liquid at a temperature of approx. 30–35 °C. A saline solution (9 g NaCl for 1000 ml water, amounting to just under one level tablespoon of salt, which can be measured using a postage scale, for example) is suitable. Commercially available electrolyte solutions such as flavourless Oralpädon® are also suitable. Should the child have difficulty eating sufficient food, one can add 1 tablespoon of sugar and 1 teaspoon of salt per litre.

A rubber enema with a volume of 130 ml (Size 4) is suitable for use on infants and small children: for infants, approx. 90 ml are used, for toddlers 130 ml, for kindergarten-age children up to 250 ml. For school-age children it is advisable to use an irrigator; it holds up to 400 ml. (You will find instructions for use which are understandable for parents in Vagedes, Soldner 2010, 54) – The enema can be repeated after 2 hours and be performed up to 4 × daily.

The aim of an enema which, if performed properly, is reabsorbed to a considerable extent, is to achieve a rapid *intake of fluids*, which serves to *stabilize the circulation and consumption of fluids* and counteract feelings of weakness and nausea. At the same time, a mild but long-term antipyretic effect is achieved [Ulbricht 1991]; enemas have a calming effect and promote sleep. The emptying of the lower segments of the large intestine takes the strain off of the immune system. It is particularly important to execute this measure in cases of children with high fevers and poor fluid consumption. Some admissions to hospital could be dispensed with through this simple and very effective measure!

- **Leg compresses** using water and a bit of lemon juice are effective for older children if the periphery is warmed through.

5.4.2 Medicinal treatment

Treatment of unspecific febrile infections using homoeopathic single remedies is carried out extensively by physicians and laymen. However, it does not replace a correct diagnosis. Another problem arising from self-medication consists in the fact that very high potencies are often administered in a very uncritical manner. These prove to be problematic in various respects: they sometimes shorten the disease processes necessary for the child's maturation; response to constitutionally necessary single-remedy treatment using higher potencies is weakened by too frequent application; if the wrong remedy is selected, high potencies often lead to side effects which are perceived as unpleasant on the part of the affected person and they persistently disguise the individual symptoms during ongoing treatment. Thus for these cases of purely acute diseases, the general rule is that the potency selected should not be higher than necessary.

The guiding symptoms of the most important single remedies are listed in the brief overview below.

5.4.2.1 Sudden onset with high fever

- **Aconitum e tub. D6 pillules** Wala, Weleda
  beginning with 5 pillules at hourly intervals; if necessary 30 pillules in ½ glass of water, one teaspoon at a time for 12 h.

Aconite is primarily indicated

- while the fever is rising: the skin is dry and cool; the child shivers or has *chills;* the basic mood is anxious,
- there is as yet no localized organ finding,
- and effective particularly during *cold-dry weather* (east wind; winter)
- for anxiety

Aconite is a *very effective initial remedy* and it also improves the patient's response to successively administered homoeopathic medicines (similar to sulphur in cases of chronic diseases). Aconite plays a specific role in the treatment of pneumonia (▸Chap. 5.1). Usually one of the following medicines is suitable for successive treatment after initial administration of Aconite.

5

- **Belladonna planta tota D6 dil./pillules** Weleda
  15–30–50 drops/pillules dissolved in ½ glass of water, given one teaspoon at a time over a period of 12–24 h.

The true value of this most commonly indicated medicine is often underestimated (▸Chap. 5.3.4.4.1). It is particularly beneficial, especially in lower potencies, in regard to its *effect on the warmth organization.* Through frequent administration of small dosages of Belladonna one can effect a favourable *distribution of warmth; this reliably counteracts heat build-up in the body's core and/or the head area.* Thus in the given dosages, Belladonna can prove to be a valuable supplemental medication for many febrile diseases, including specific ones. The decisive guiding symptoms for Belladonna can be summarized as follows:

- *sudden, severe onset of fever*, especially between 7:00 and 11:00 p. m.,
- *reddening* of the skin, particularly in the face, a tendency to sweat on the head (most prominent shortly after falling asleep),
- dry, crimson mucosa (acute tonsillitis, ▸Chap. 5.2.3), painful swallowing,
- cool extremities, a hot head and core body,
- head congestion accompanied by *throbbing pain*, possibly also in the sinuses and the middle ear,

- abdominal *colic pain* (in cases of small children not infrequently in connection with tonsillitis, otitis media) with the child tending to overstretch himself backwards,
- aversion to touch, compresses and external applications,
- emotionally *agitated, violent behaviour* in particular in connection with pain and fatigue,
- a tendency towards *fever fantasies* (for discussion of febrile seizures cf. ▸Chap. 5.4.3),
- a generally *strong constitution* which sometimes has a phlegmatic tendency when the child is not unwell (cf. in particular the drug picture of Calcium carbonicum).

Belladonna-specific triggers of febrile infections are extreme *exposure to sun*, on *trips* in hot weather, after relatively long hikes in the summer. – The medicine must usually be taken for 2 to 3 days; a particularly determining factor is a course of disease with sudden onset and similarly sudden drop in fever and recovery thereafter.

5.4.2.2 Acute onset (not sudden) with moderately high fever

- **Ferrum phosphoricum D6 tab.** Weleda
  3–5 × daily ½–1 tablet, usually for 4–5 days

Symptoms *of the respiratory tract and the circulatory system* are determining factors for selection of this frequently indicated remedy:

- Sniffles and cough (painful, dry-scratchy, hard) with no purulent discharge, a tendency towards *epistaxis*
- Pallor and instability of the circulatory system (*fluctuating complexion*), tendency towards orthostasis; general improvement while lying down,
- Accompanying otitis with peripherally reddened eardrum,
- accompanying enteric symptoms involving nausea, mild diarrhoea, undigested stool.

- **Eupatorium perfoliatum D12 pillules** (various manufacturers)
  5 × daily 5 pillules

This remedy is primarily indicated by symptoms involving the digestive tract and the limbs:

- severe *nausea*, relief through vomiting accompanied by thirst for cold drinks,
- extreme *feeling of depletion, muscle and bone pain* (the latter primarily in the calves),
- specific exacerbation of fever and worsening of condition *between 7:00 and 9:00 a. m.*,
- sensitivity to cold, primarily indicated in *wet-cold weather.*

- **Bryonia e rad. D6** Wala
  3–6 × daily 5 pillules

- for stinging pain in the area of the head and chest
- slowly rising and then persisting fever
- painful coughing
- avoidance of movement, improvement while resting

- thirst for cold drinks
- Bryonia and Eupatorium complement each other in their effectiveness.

5.4.2.3 Gradually rising, moderately high fever

- **Gelsemium D12 glob.** (various manufacturers)
  3–5 × daily 5 pillules/drops for 5 days

This remedy is primarily indicated by symptoms *in connection with the nerve-sense system.* General guiding symptoms for its application are:

- extreme *fatigue*, somnolence at onset of fever (often conspicuously *hanging upper lids*),
- red, congested head, *headache*, mild meningism,
- usually *moderately high fever* (38.5–39.5 °C) with lack of thirst,
- tendency towards diarrhoea,
- in some cases conspicuous shaky hands, weakness of the extremities, muscle pains.

Gelsemium must be administered for at least five days if it is indicated; such patients tend to experience a *relapse on the fifth day;* since they often start feeling better after taking the remedy there is a risk of untimely mobilization and sustained complaints, particularly headaches if there is a relapse. For this reason it is very important to agree on bed rest (for school) and a doctor's certificate if Gelsemium is being prescribed.

Gelsemium used to be a specific remedy for poliomyelitis (and it continues to be used for neurological side effects of polio vaccinations even though they hardly ever occur in cases of parenteral administration). – In cases of **serous (virally triggered) meningitis** Gelsemium, when administered per os and parenterally, is a highly effective homoeopathic remedy and one of the first treatment options to be considered alongside

- **Bryonia D6–30 pillules/amp.** Wala and
- **Apis mell. D6–30 pillules/amp.** Weleda

The latter two primarily have an effect on the inflamed meninges, increased cerebrospinal pressure and thus accompanying pain, whereas Gelsemium is directed to the nervous system itself.

In such cases one can start by using

- **Apis mell. D30** together with **Bryonia D30,** 1 ampoule each, injected s.c. into the upper arm

and then dissolve

- **Apis mell. D6**, 20 drops/pillules
- **Bryonia D6**, 20 drops/pillules
- **Gelsemium D30**, 10 pillules

in 100 ml of water and administer one teaspoon at a time over the course of the day.

It is very important to consider Gelsemium in cases of *early summer meningoencephalitis (ESME)*, which resembles poliomyelitis in some respects (▸Chap. 5.6). In every case of meningoencephalitis one can consider treatment using Gelsemium D30, supplemented

5

by potentized autologous blood in accordance with Imhäuser [2000, 156 ff.] (▸Chap. 5.2), daily 3 drops of C5 or C7 (needless to say, this does not eliminate the necessity for clinical treatment).

Gelsemium is most frequently indicated in the *warm season* or when it is *unseasonably warm*.

An effective homoeopathicum of anthroposophic medicine for onset of *viral meningitis* and immediate application is

- **Agaricus muscarius, Cutis rubra D30 amp.** Weleda Switzerland [Vademecum 2010, 51; further bibliographical data there]
  1 × 1 ampoule s.c. in the upper arm

5.4.2.4 Single-substance medicines for severe, persistent fever

- **Arnica e pl. tota D30 pillules** Wala
  3–5 × daily 5 pillules or 15 pillules/day dissolved in water, taken one teaspoon at a time, at first hourly.

For the following symptoms, this remedy is indispensable and reliably effective:

- quick onset of high fever persisting for several days
- very pronounced *muscle pain* (specifically in cases of Coxsackie B), diffuse pain of depletion
- *severe headaches*, head congestion, pronounced prostration, urge to lie down
- aversion to touch, patient appears exhausted and hardly responsive.

Of great significance and effectiveness is the application of

- **Arnica Essence** Wala diluted 1:10
  externally used as a brief wash 3 × daily, as a poultice surrounding the head or sprayed onto the head area [Vademecum 2010, 139]

In the authors' own practice as well as the rich experience of the anthroposophic paediatrician K. R. Kummer, this has proven to be the most effective Arnica application for

- severe, hard to endure headaches accompanied by high fever,
- children with early signs and anamnestic indications of febrile seizures,
- severe headaches and shrieks as a reaction to vaccinations (▸Chap. 3.5.7.2.2),
- supplemental therapy for severe cases of pertussis (washes).

For severe headaches and early signs of the central nervous system being affected in cases of infections (and after vaccinations) in particular, the immediate effectiveness of external Arnica applications in almost all cases is amazing. Apply the cool remedy to the head.

- **Baptisia D6 pillules/amp.** DHU/Staufen
  5 × daily 5–7 pillules or 1 single ampoule i.v.

In individual cases, Baptisia can be highly effective for the following symptoms:

- moderately high to high, persistent fever without local symptoms over a period of several days,
- *apathic behaviour* with the patient appearing "as if drunk," with a red, congested head,
- refusal to eat, *poor consumption of fluids*,
- halitosis, foul-smelling stool,
- muscle pain, extremely *impaired general condition*.

- **Lachesis D12 dil./pillules/D12–30 amp.** (various manufacturers)
  3 × daily 5–7 drops/pillules or 1 single ampoule i.v.

plays a very important role for extreme, toxic *impairment of the patient's general condition* .

It is used for the following symptoms:

- pallor, livid enanthema,
- particularly hypotonic disorders of circulatory regulation,
- feeling of constriction: the ill person cannot bear wearing a scarf, aversion to weight of clothing and touch,
- exacerbation through external heat, urge for cool air,
- *exacerbation through sleep*, in the morning,
- trouble swallowing, paradoxically more when drinking than when swallowing solid foods,
- symptoms more pronounced on left side.

When administered parenterally, the effect of Lachesis is strengthened through combination with

- **Argentum met. praep. D30 amp.** Weleda i.v.

and if need be Baptisia D6. As a form of initial treatment and when given in the course of the disease, it is very beneficial in cases of severe flu-like infections with high fever accompanied by strikingly toxic symptoms.

- **Rhus toxicodendron D12–30 pillules** Wala
  3–5 × daily 5 pillules for 3–5 days

can have a decisive, thorough effect as a single remedy in cases of febrile diseases which are difficult to treat.

This remedy is indicated if

- the patient was already *exhausted* before outbreak of the disease and as a result of the fever he/she:
- exhibits extreme, often inexplicable *agitation* (accompanied by weakness),
- exhibits an anxious-depressive mood,
- exhibits a pronounced *need for warmth*,
- despite high fever the immune system functions insufficiently at first and the specific finding becomes worse ("adynamic fever"),
- the fever is accompanied by Herpes labialis.

5

(Regarding the indication for mononucleosis ▸Chap. 5.2.6 and for scarlet fever cf. ▸Chap. 5.3.4.4.1). Specific situations which can trigger this are *coming down with a cold after getting soaked* or after *profuse exertion and sweating*. This remedy should be considered for school children in particular and is certainly overlooked at times in this acute indication.

5.4.2.5 Composition medicines

In the practice of the authors, several *composition medicines* have proven to be especially effective; of all the preparations which exist in this area, each physician must familiarize himself with a few in order to be able to use them to good purpose. In particular, these medicines fulfil their purpose in cases where specific symptoms are missing; in their effect, some also show qualities which constitute a veritably new pharmaceutical creation which cannot be matched by any single medicine. – Moreover, Hepar sulphuris and Causticum, for example, are also pharmaceutically synthesized compounds; every living creature represents a "substance constitution" which has evolved through its vital activity. Thus the term "single-substance medicine" is not completely apt.

- **Gelsemium comp. pillules** Wala
  5 × daily 5–7 pillules

is a medicine which is indicated with particular frequency in practice today.

It primarily corresponds to

- *"brain workers,"* with schoolchildren counting as such today as well
- constitutionally neurasthenic patients in whom the head pole predominates and whose metabolic system is less developed than the nerve-sense system (or weakened)
- infections accompanied by moderately high fever lasting for several days,
- unseasonably mild weather,
- a tendency towards circulatory insufficiency and exhaustion,
- headaches with cervical tension,
- catarrhal respiratory symptoms with limited ventilation of the paranasal sinuses, unspecific sore throat and cough

A very beneficial remedy is the compound

- **Meteoric iron pillules/amp.** Wala
  2–3 × daily 5–10 pillules/single dosage 1 ampoule i.v.

There is also an indication for

- *flu-like infections* and susceptibility to infections in the fall,
- primary affliction of the upper *and lower* respiratory tract,
- susceptibility to *bronchitis and pneumonia* (preventative effect)
- general exhaustion.

When using this medicine one can experience how its application (most of all in the form of single i.v. injections) harmonizes something which could perhaps be described best as an "*inner lack of light*." In this respect the medicine has a much more intensive effect than Ferrum phosphoricum, for example, which is listed below.

Other suitable compounds are especially

- **Ferrum phos. comp. pillules** Weleda
  beginning with 5–7 pillules every 1-to-2 hours

For catarrhal-febrile infections in the cold season;

- **Aconitum/China comp. pillules/supp.** Wala
  5–7 pillules approximately every 2 hours

For fever with gastrointestinal symptoms, weakness, "ailing" children [Vademecum 2010, 40] in the cold season as well. At night 1 suppository can be given (for modulating fever)

All in all, treatment of flu-like infections is no "banal" task; the patient and the physician can gain access to and develop trust in a method of treatment which promotes the individual capacities of the child.

5.4.3 Febrile convulsions (infection-related)

> Antipyretic agents are ineffective for the prevention of recurrences of febrile seizures and for the lowering of body temperature in patients with a febrile episode that leads to a recurrent febrile seizure.
>
> T. Strengell [2009]

5.4.3.1 Clinical picture and insight into the illness

The term "febrile seizure" designates an ambiguous and inconsistent phenomenon in terms of origin and prognosis. Phenomenologally, 3–5 % of all small children between the ages of 6 months and 6 years develop one or more seizures in the course of a febrile infection, most frequently at onset of the illness. In such cases the child often has only a moderately high fever *before* the seizure occurs, whereas the temperature often rises quite a bit *after* the seizure. – One speaks of a "seizure with rising fever," but the dynamic relationship between the seizure and the rise in body temperature is unclear. The seizure itself can be a contributing factor but in the case of the most seizures there is no causal relation between the temperature and the seizure episode.

Thus in medical practice it is not difficult to ascertain that in most cases antipyretics *have no verifiably positive influence on the course of the seizure.* There is no reliable scientific justification for anxious fixation on rises in body temperature and suppression of such rises until the temperature falls below 38.5 °C.[1]

For the most part, febrile seizures are generalized and in part quite persistent. Thus it is all the more amazing that in over 90 % of the children affected, the seizure constitutes an age-dependent "overreaction" which occurs in connection with the febrile confrontation with an infection. The phenomenology as well as therapeutic experience with potentized remedies suggest that for this large group of patients the seizure must have something to do with an immaturity of the organism. This most probably lies in the

1 Anticonvulsants such as Diazepam given in relatively small dosages (for example 3.75 mg rectally every 12 h for the first two days) have a relatively good protective effect on recurring febrile seizures.

warmth organization itself; it finds itself in an utmost challenging situation while the fever is rising.

Clinically speaking it is striking that this large group of children often apparently finds it hard to respond to infections with corresponding warmth activity (i. e. activation of the metabolism). Many of these children exhibit *difficulties with warmth distribution* (centralization/peripheralization of warmth). They experience a delayed and then often sudden increase in warmth which can principally be seen as the result of *intensified intervention of the soul-spirit individuality of the child resulting in an increase of all catabolic, degrading-formative processes.* This intervention *is learned* in early childhood. Thus the febrile seizures experienced by the large patient group depicted do not reflect any cerebral or intellectual problems but rather primarily a problem connected with the development of *will activity* (and immunological activity can in fact be conceived of as such), i. e. the child's individuality asserting itself in the physicality inherited from the parents.

It is not surprising that antipyretics have little use in such cases for they impede the activity of the warmth organization instead of promoting it and on the other hand they interrupt the convulsive attempt of the individuality to penetrate its own physicality. In the meantime this statement, formulated by the authors quite some time ago, has been corroborated to such an extent that it has in fact been possible to show:

- Fever-reducing medicines (Paracetamol, Ibuprofen) *do not reduce the risk of febrile seizures* [Stuijvenberg 1998, Strengell 2009] – and
- In the case of fever episodes which lead to convulsions, fever-reducing medicines show no fever-reducing (or anticonvulsive) effect whereas they do reduce fever if no febrile seizure occurs [Strengell 2009]!
- A large British comparative study of 14,676 children, of whom 381 had experienced fever-induced seizures (287 simple, 94 complex febrile seizures) in early childhood, brought about the following result based on a follow-up examination conducted when the subjects were age 10:
- According to reports made by mothers, febrile children who had experienced seizures were more impulsive and excitable than the control group.
- The questionnaires on the children showed that in patients with febrile seizures, 2.6 % showed poor agility when doing gymnastics as compared to the 2 % found in the control group.
- Children with febrile seizures experienced slightly more anxiety than those in the control group.
- Children with febrile seizures had better reading skills than those in the control group.

With the exception of these 4 differences, the patients who experienced febrile seizures were comparable to the control group. The results of comparisons of simple and complex febrile seizures yielded no differences. Whether the first febrile seizure occurred before or after the first year of life was of no significance for later results. "… Children experiencing one or several febrile seizures showed no difference in regard to intellectual development or behaviour in relation to others in their group or to the control group, which had experienced no febrile seizures" [Verity et al. 1998, Wölfel 1999].

One must concede that febrile seizures can indisputably constitute *an initial symptom of epilepsy* (anamnesis, atypical course of disease or atypical age of onset, neurological follow-up examination including EEG, follow-up observation) and that children who are susceptible to convulsive fits sometimes experience febrile seizures more frequently.

Moreover, the fact that cerebrally damaged, febrile children have seizures more frequently calls for a separate study. – In this context it is not possible to go into such situations in detail.

For children who experience febrile seizures without any indication of an underlying neurologic disorder it is advisable from a therapeutic standpoint to fundamentally differentiate between

- children who tend to have seizures *while the temperature is rising,*
- children who tend to have seizures *when they have high fevers* (sometimes almost acting like a thermostat from a certain temperature threshold on, usually between 39 and 40 °C).

In the first-named group, seizures tend to be more severe; the children in the latter group generally show a more unstable, as yet disharmonic body-soul structure.

5.4.3.2 Treatment options: homoeopathic and anthroposophic medicines

This section will depict treatment of children who experience febrile seizures without there being any indication of underlying epilepsy or any organically fixated cause for the seizure. The *first treatment step* is to perform a thorough *anamnesis and carry out consultation* with the parents. For anyone who encounters a patient who is experiencing a seizure unprepared (and as a rule helplessly), it is a shocking experience – and for the parents most of all – which leaves behind deep and persistent anxiety. If one does not want to aggravate this, a physical examination and apparative diagnostics followed by informative discussion is necessary in which each therapeutic step is discussed at intervals and in the acute situation, the favourable long-term prognosis is mentioned, possible conditions leading to the episode are explained (in the sense of the aforementioned) and a clear treatment plan is laid out. – Not only in this respect does such a conversation liken ones conducted after a first so-called pseudocroup attack: this entails a "seizure episode" as well which is associated with a certain age group and which has something to do with the as yet immature soul-body structure (▸Chap. 5.1.4). In the one as well as the other case, it is thoroughly possible to prescribe an effective allopathic emergency medicine (for febrile seizures Diazepam in rectiole form) and depict its indication and onset of effect. This helps to calm down the situation even more – as opposed to aggravating unjustified fears regarding the child's fever activity.

The goal of *interval treatment* is to render the intervention of the child's individuality in terms of his I-aspect (warmth organization) as well as his soul organization (for susceptibility to seizures cf. ▸Chap. 5.1.4) more harmonious and fluid so as to avoid any escalation in the course of an infection. –During *acute treatment* the *maturation of the child's warmth organization should be supported* and through this the seizure should be made dispensable; in certain individual cases this does not rule out allopathic prophylaxis or therapy involving Diazepam, however.

In general the most important potentized remedy for febrile seizures is

- **Belladonna D6–20 Rh dil.** (alcohol-free)/**pillules** Weleda.

Belladonna has a comprehensive *mediating* effect. In regard to the warmth organization it mediates between the centre and periphery, and in regard to the soul organization, the astral body, it mediates between the catabolic, formative, consciousness-engendering activity and that which connects itself to the metabolic organization (for more detailed explanations of these concepts cf. ▸Chap. 5.1.4 and ▸Chap. 6.4.3.5).

Small children who require Belladonna as a remedy tend to dam up the forces of their soul-spirit individuality in the head area. Such children have a reddened face, a hot heat and are sweaty while the periphery remains cool. The susceptibility to sore throats results from this disproportion as well. In cases of *classic febrile seizures the brain is per se healthy; the discharging activity which occurs during the seizure reflects a build-up affecting the metabolic-limb area and does not primarily pose any cerebral problem.* Belladonna counteracts this build-up, effecting a more harmonious inflow of individual impulses into bodily processes which can even extend to limb movement.

The effect of Belladonna is enhanced by potentized *silver,* which promotes the *maturation of the warmth organization* in particular, and potentized *copper,* the metal which counteracts the *susceptibility to seizures* issuing from the soul aspect most intensively.

Of the herbal remedies suitable for treatment of small children

- **Chamomilla (e rad.) D12–20 pillules** Wala/Weleda
  produces an effect similar to that of copper.

This remedy is indicated if the child is not yet capable of converting impulses from the nerve-sense system into metabolic processes in a rhythmically mediated way but rather tends to experience "short circuits" – remarkable seizures – especially when under stress or in a state of fatigue. This remedy is especially effective for children who are constitutionally *irritable and oversensitive* while exhibiting, on the other hand, a *strong attachment to their mother.* Copper and camomile in potentized form have a harmonizing effect on the intervention of the soul aspect in the bodily-unconscious aspect, which manifests itself most of all in *kidney function* (▸Chap. 5.1.4 and ▸Chap. 6.4.3.5). This undergoes clear maturation between the ages of 2 and 5.

In view of the prognosis and the results of studies, one can generally advise the parents to approach situations in which the child develops a fever calmly rather than tensing themselves up and attempting to prevent a febrile seizure at all costs through complementary medicine. This attitude would contradict what has been elucidated here. It is primarily a matter of supporting the child in his maturation and providing an adequate framework, particularly where fever is involved, in which the child's warmth organization, his immunoregulation and immune system can mature by allowing the individualization of the body to occur with the least possible degree of accompanying anxiety.

Interval treatment is initially carried out within a period of 6 weeks to several months after the febrile seizure. One can approach this in a differentiated manner as follows:
a) in cases of children with a susceptibility to seizures while the temperature is rising:

- **Chamomilla e rad. D20 pillules** Wala
  5 pillules daily in the morning and
- **Cuprum met. praep. D20 trit.** Weleda
  1 saltsp. daily in the evening

b) for children with a susceptibility to seizures when they have high fevers:

- **Belladonna D12 dil.**
- **Argentum met. praep. D20 dil.**
- **Chamomilla, Radix D12 dil.** aa ad 60 ml special manufacture Apotheke an der Weleda
  daily 1 × 7–10 drops

If the febrile seizure occurs in a plausible connection with a *vaccination* it can prove beneficial to administer

- **Silicea D30 pillules** (various manufacturers)
  3 × 5 pillules at intervals of 12 h

and if need be the homologous *nosode of the vaccine* 1–3 × 5 pillules in C30 potentized (for example by Gudjons) as initial treatment.

As an acute form of treatment at onset of fever, an immediate measure to be taken for children at risk for febrile seizures is

- an **enema using camomile tea** (see above).

This relieves (see above, ▸Chap. 5.4.1.) the child's immune system, makes the temperature rise more gently and can also have an effect where there is susceptibility to seizures or a seizure is already beginning.

Medicinally, at onset of fever administration of

- **Cuprum met. praep. D20 trit.** Weleda
  3 × 1 saltsp. at intervals of 12 h is recommended as an initial measure.

Moreover, in accordance with interval treatment one can differentiate between:

a) Children with a susceptibility to seizures while the temperature is rising:

- **Belladonna D12 pillules/Rh D20 dil.** Weleda and
- **Chamomilla e rad. D20** pillules Wala
  at first 5 pillules/drops each hourly, then less often

Such children are relatively difficult to treat, and the indication for Diazepam is to be assessed more liberally here than for the group depicted below.

b) Children with a susceptibility to seizures when they have high fevers

- **Belladonna D6/Rh (alcohol-free) D6 dil.** Weleda
  50 drops diluted in approx. 100 ml water, at intervals of ¼ hour 1 tsp. or a small sip to begin with, then less often

The dosages should be oriented in such a way that the child exhibits a harmonization of warmth distribution (and a fever curve which is as constant as possible).

- **Argentum met. praep. D12–30 trit.** Weleda
  every 6–12 h 1 saltsp.

Here repeated camomile enemas every 6–12 h are to be recommended at first until the fever begins to stabilize.

5.4.4 Chronically recurrent febrile infections

5.4.4.1 General basis

For the physician devoted to individual paediatrics, children with chronically recurring, febrile infections are a particularly fulfilling patient group. This is not the place to go into organ-specific diseases such as chronic urinary tract infections or chronic sinusitis (see the respective chapters); instead the basic foundations of therapy for children with a general susceptibility to infection are to be summarized here in short, being discussed at greater depth in the corresponding contexts of this book.

Treatment of such children is founded on **two pillars:**

- Stimulation and promotion of immunological digestive and regulatory processes.
- Treatment of the patient's individual constitution.

Stimulation and promotion of the immune system requires:

- Directing one's attention to and promoting *warmth organization* (▸Chap. 5.1.2.4; ▸Chap. 5.1.1), particularly in the cold season, for example through woollen underwear, head coverings, house shoes, evening rhythmical Einreibungen of the limbs using a suitable oil (for example Mallow oil Wala), ascending footbaths in the evening, in cases of infection using a mustard flour supplement (▸Chap. 5.1.2.4), from an appropriate age on visits to the sauna, sufficient physical exertion and exercise.
- *Diagnostics of digestive processes, if need be symbiosis guidance and in any case extensive dietetic consultation* (▸Chap. 4.6): age-appropriate diet (one should dispense with milk bottles etc. in a timely fashion), temporary elimination of whole milk from the diet (but not fermented milk products), but most of all elimination of industrial sugar from the diet and clear limits on sweet foods (but no complete elimination except for in cases of mycosis treatment) are essential elements which are indispensable for rapid and sustainable success of treatment.
- *Elimination of vitamin and trace element deficiencies* (▸Chap. 6.3.3.1): special note should be taken of iron, zinc and selenium deficiencies. What is of primary importance is to improve the patient's diet and digestion; substitution (targeted or general, for example through use of Orthomol Immun junior and other preparations) sometimes accelerates the success of therapy at first but it does not constitute any satisfactory long-term solution.
- Rhythmization of daily routine, sufficient rest periods, sufficient exercise in sunlight. Regarding this and the possibility of a vitamin-D deficiency, which is often quite relevant for cases of chronically recurring infections, cf. ▸Chap. 3.2.

Organically speaking, the *activity of the spleen* and *the thymus* as superordinate organs of the immunological system deserve special attention. It is therapeutically beneficial to stimulate and support them, the result being particularly satisfactory (▸Chap. 6.3.3.4).

5.4.4.2 Medicinal treatment

Through use of concentrated *plant extracts,* children who are susceptible to infections in the cold season in particular can be supported and strengthened quite effectively. The strongest, most comprehensive effect in this respect is achieved by *seabuckthorn, Hippophae rhamnoides.* This plant belongs to the oleaster family. It is the member of this family most likely to grow in particularly barren, northern regions, resisting the hard winter frosts there and forming a unique combination of *fat- and water-soluble* vitamins, which are concentrated in the fruit and seeds (compare rosehip and black currants). In qualitative terms, the substances contained therein constitute a concentration of *forces of warmth and light.* One must really envision the achievement of the life organization of such a plant in order to understand its therapeutic effectiveness for human beings.

One can prescribe, for example.

- **Seabuckthorn Ursaft** Weleda: 1–2 tsp. daily (can be given in diluted form, for example in freshly squeezed orange juice),

but it is necessary to make note of the taste, which takes some getting used to and which is tolerated by most but not all children. The therapeutic effect is very convincing, however. For a sustainable effect, one can prescribe potentized administration, for example, of

- **Hippophae rhamnoides D3 dil.** Apotheke an der Weleda
  daily 1 × 7–10 drops [Fersch 2004].

Children who are weakened by illness, have a delicate constitution or a neurasthenic disposition and who are susceptible to colds – particularly those affecting the respiratory tract – will experience a strengthening of their life forces and immune system through preparations made from fruits of the *blackthorn*. This shrub also has a special relation to the cold season. On the one hand it blooms early in the year, in April, and on the other hand the fruits ripen late in the fall with the first frost. Elixirs made from blackthorn fruits (which are very tasty) primarily produce an effect on the *vitality* of the organs of the rhythmic system and the metabolism.

- **Blackthorn elixir** Weleda
  3 × 1 tsp. – 2 × 1 tab./2–3 × 1 tsp. (Ursaft)

The immunological functions of the child's organism are stimulated comprehensively and also individually through treatment using *potentized autologous blood* according to Imhäuser (▸Chap. 6.3.3.4).

5

It should preferrably be administered in the morning,

- C5: daily 3 drops for 2–3 weeks,
- C7: 3 × weekly 3 drops for 3–6 weeks,
- C9: 2–3 × weekly 3 drops for 3–6 weeks,
- C12 and C15: 1–2 × weekly 3 drops for 4–6 weeks.

Weakness of the immune system with frequent infections, recurring febrile illnesses and a susceptibility towards allergic and autoaggressive, chronically recurring diseases constitute an indication for this therapy.

A remedy with a similar orientation which has proven very beneficial in the practice of the authors is

- **Lien comp. pillules/amp.** Wala
  2–3 × daily 5–10 pillules

(▸Chap. 6.3.3.4, [Vademecum 2010, 551]. Among other things it contains potentized organ preparations of the spleen, kidneys and mesenchyme; thus it activates the immune system and the elimination activity of the organism in a comprehensive fashion. After *suppressive pre-treatment* (for example using antibiotics, cytostatics) and in cases of *susceptibility to infections* (for example after the child has begun attending kindergarten), this modern compound remedy created by H. H. Vogel is very valuable. In difficult cases (for example susceptibility to infections after bone marrow transplantation and GVHD) it

has proven beneficial to administer 1 drinking ampoule daily per os for seven weeks (prescribe N 2).
For cases of chronic susceptibility to infections of the upper respiratory tract one should seriously consider prescribing potentized silicic acid; this is found in herbal form in the preparation

- **Equisetum Silicea cultum D2 dil.** Weleda
  3 × 5–10 drops in combination with
- **Sulphur D6 trit.** Weleda
  1 saltsp. in the morning (cf. ▸Chap. 5.1.2.3).

If on the other hand a condition exists in which infections regularly affect the lower respiratory tract or the child is weakened as a result of pneumonia or bronchitis, one can consider

- **Roseneisen/Graphite pillules** Wala
  2 × daily 5–10 pillules

(cf. ▸Chap. 5.1.1.6) and the remedy mentioned in ▸Chap. 5.1.1.6:

- **Meteoric iron pillules** Wala
  1–2 × daily 5–10 pillules daily per os.

The latter remedy should preferably be given in the morning, and if need be a second time in the afternoon.
In cases of poor appetite and nutrition along with frequent infections of the (upper and) lower respiratory tract (recurring cases of bronchitis and pneumonia), the organ preparation

- **Organum quadruplex amp.** Wala: daily ½–1 ampoules per os can be given

to reactivate the life organization of the child and thus also create the foundation for enabling the soul aspect to connect with the etheric body, the vital processes of growth and organ formation, in an impulsating way again. A form of external application which is very beneficial in this situation in addition to ascending footbaths and oil rhythmical Einreibungen are

- Sulphur bath: for example **Spitzner Balneo Sulphur Bath**
  5–10 ml/10 l bath water (depending on size of tub), approx. 2 × weekly.

Many children who are susceptible to infections come in for treatment after having *been treated with antibiotics repeatedly*. In this situation *dietetics and symbiosis guidance* (cf. ▸Chap. 4.5) play a special therapeutic role.

In general one should initiate treatment with administration of potentized sulphur or silver sulphide (Argentite), for example

- **Sulphur LM6 dil.** Arcana
  daily 2–5 drops in the morning for 3–4 weeks,

possibly followed by LM12, 3 × weekly 3 drops for the same period of time or

- **Argentite D6 trit.** Weleda
  3 × daily 1 saltsp.

Herbal preparations which can be considered for supplementary treatment in this situation are

- **Aquilinum comp. pillules** Wala
  3 × daily 5–10 pillules

in cases of unspecific digestive disorders;

- **Veratrum comp. pillules** Wala
  3 × daily 5–7 pillules

in cases of dyspeptic stool and susceptibility to colicky stomach aches;

- **Lycopodium comp. pillules** Wala
  3 × daily 5–7 pillules

in cases of toxic impact on the metabolism; in cases of a tendency towards meteorism, stools which clearly fluctuate in colour, obstipation.

A second fundamental therapeutic step lies in *individualized treatment of the child's constitution through potentized single remedies.* These are elucidated more extensively in other parts of this book; at this point it must suffice to list the most important medicines in an overview.

Individualized constitutional treatment

- Silicea (Quartz),
- Hepar Sulphuris,
- Calcium carbonicum (Conchae),
- Phosphorus,
- Tuberculinum,
- Sulphur,
- Lycopodium,
- Thuja,
- Medorrhinum.

Potencies must be selected individually; from a constitutional perspective one can consider most of all LM-potencies (LM6–12; higher LM-potencies are not recommendable) and medium to high D- and C-potencies (usually 12 to 30, in case of insufficient effect possibly higher ones). Relatively high potencies can be administered in the form of pillules (for example 3 × 3 pillules at intervals of 12 h) or dissolved in water (for example 5 pillules of D30 in 50 ml water, daily 3 × 1 tsp. over a period of 3 days).

5.5 Urinary tract infections

5.5.1 Diagnostic aspects

When there is an infection of the urinary tract, it is important for the physician as for the parents of the child to start by assessing the extent and prognosis of the disease. One must differentiate between asymptomatic bacteriuria without clinical manifestation, i. e. a bacterial colonization of the lower urinary tract, and an invasive infection with concomitant inflammation. If one is dealing with a case of bacteriuria, the assessment made by W. Marget [1998] is apt:

"Although in regard to asymptomatic bacteriuria there have been heated discussions for years on the benefit or uselessness of permanent [i. e. antibiotic] prophylaxis, one now tends to view it as a more or less disturbed guest-host-relationship... It is assumed that 'permanent colonization' protects the host from the virulence of virulent germs. A progression of kidney damage does not occur in this case."

This means that in general, antibiotic treatment of asymptomatic bacteriuria cannot be convincingly justified – especially not if one weighs the consequences of antibiosis for the organism as a whole (for example disturbance of intestinal symbiosis) against the possibilities for treatment which stimulate the immunological self-activity of the organism. – In cases of *manifest urinary tract infections* it is important to make the following distinctions:

- Are the kidneys involved (pyelonephritis)? Symptoms can be pain in the kidney region, high fever, nausea, urine sediment and sonographic findings, for example.
- Are there any anatomical deformations which disturb urinary transport?
- Is the child younger than 3 years of age?

If all these questions can be negated, one is dealing with a simple urinary tract infection with a good prognosis [Marget 1998] which can almost always be controlled well using the medicines listed below without having to resort to antibiotics: "One should realize that immune defence against individual pathogens is quite pronounced and that this can result in pathogen-bound *immunity which lasts for months*" (emphasis in orig.) [Marget 1998].

If, on the other hand, one diagnoses pyelonephritis *urinary transport disorder* and the patient is an *infant or a toddler*, then treatment of this infection must aim for rapid and thorough success with close monitoring so as to prevent anatomical complications. The indication for antibiosis (and if need be surgical restoration) should be assessed more liberally even though there are therapeutic options involving potentized remedies (cf. ▸Chap. 5.5.2).

The same criteria hold for *chronic or chronically recurring urinary tract infections.* In cases of simple chronic infections it is true that antibiotic treatment is equally simple but not infrequently, follow-up problems arise. In particular, when relapses occur after antibiosis, one has observed that *the germ spectrum* starts to move in the direction of virulent, hard to combat pathogens such as Pseudomonas and Klebsiella. This is all the more remarkable insofar as such pathogens are actually typical for complex urinary tract infections: "complex infections" exhibit "a completely different spectrum of pathogens than simple ones do" [Marget 1998] (Klebsiella, Enterobacter, Proteus and others as opposed to 90 % E. coli in cases of simple urinary tract infections). This means that antibiotic treatment in cases where the organism would be capable of healing by itself providing it had the necessary support can generate problems which can only be controlled through aggressive or intensive therapy. – For this reason therapy should not be oriented towards influencing pathological urine findings but rather towards long-term development of the child's organism as a whole.

5.5.2 Acute urinary tract infections

Frequency, dysuria and foul-smelling urine are guiding symptoms of acute simple inflammations of the lower urinary tract. The findings elicited by strip tests are mostly leukocyturia, haematuria and possibly positive nitrite; in the urine culture a great predominance of Escherichia-coli bacteria is found with a correspondingly high bacterial count (10^6 and more per ml). Possible triggers are: *hypothermia* (most of all of the lower extremities and the pelvis), preceding infections of the respiratory tract, acute gastrointestinal infections, emotional tension. The constitutional disposition consists in an unstable warmth organization with a tendency to cold extremities, insufficient self-perception of the body and its warmth conditions (such children do not feel cold even though they are hypothermic), chronic disorders of pneumatization of the upper respiratory tract (! – sinusitis, adenoids and tonsillar hypertrophy), chronic disorders of intestinal symbiosis. Consumption of large amounts of sugar and insufficient consumption of fluids increase the susceptibility to urinary tract infections.

If one attempts to assess the nature of this phenomenology one will find that the *disposition for urinary tract infections* consists in an *insufficient penetration of the lower body by the forces of the child's spirit-soul individuality*. As the I-organization these forces are active in the warmth organization (cf. ▸Chap. 5.1.1), and as the ensouling astral body in the upper human being they are primarily active in the pneumatization (the air organization), and in the lower human being they are active in the kidney organization (which enables pneumatization of the body and an alert soul life in the first place (cf. ▸Chap. 6.4.3.5). In terms of purely vital growth, elimination of fluids, pneumatization and release of warmth are *catabolic-formative processes* which only mature gradually in the course of childhood, penetrating the bodily life processes with increasing intensity up to the point where they reach their final form and the growth process is actively brought to an end. The phenomenology of urinary tract infections – including age distribution – shows that in the cases of affected children, the I and the astral body do not or do not yet control the elimination processes in the lower body properly; anatomical anomalies and disposition-related dysfunctions of the epithelium can impede this penetration constitutionally. The inflammation already constitutes the attempt to overcome this weakness but it must be guided in such a way that it does not lead to a destruction of the organ's form and function.

Thus invasive urinary tract infections can develop when, relatively speaking, the *physicality and the life processes* in the kidney-bladder region take on too much a life of their own. This is what fosters the advance of Coliform bacteria, for example, which grow in the urinary tract "in the wrong place" (in the intestinal tract they are physiological). In normal cases, only the immunological activity in this organ region, which is a direct expression of the activity of the I and the astral body, prevents intestinal flora from invading the urinary tract! Paralysis of I-activity through hypothermia, insufficient bodily anchoring of the warmth organization, which manifests itself in insufficient generation and perception of warmth, and insufficient body-formative activity of the soul aspect (which also manifests itself in disturbances of pneumatization and digestive activity, for example) are factors which permit pathological life and growth processes to adopt an independent existence in the urinary tract.

Thus the *disposition for complex urinary tract inflammations* becomes more clearly graspable: the younger the child is, the less developed the process of urinary transport is and the more opportunities physical anomalies have to rob this organ region of its ordered function, the easier it will be for the depicted transition from physiological to pathological conditions to occur. Since these always consist in the fact that structure-giving individuality no longer dominates the processes in this sensitive organ region, having been usurped by disintegrating (bacterially conveyed) forces of nature, the connection between urinary tract inflammation and anomalies (for example versicourethral reflux) becomes understandable: wherever the Ego (the I) and the astral body of the child fail to overcome the advance of foreign etheric elements, there is a risk of increasing alienation and deformation of the physical organ structure as well – and vice versa!

Therapeutically it is possible to intervene on the following levels:

- organ-related stimulation of the warmth organization (external, thoroughly warming applications in the area of the urinary tract and the lower extremities, stimulation of the child's perception of warmth through corresponding paedagogical efforts and clothing). Medicinally speaking, potentized phosphorus in particular has an activating effect on this level of Ego-organization.
- strengthening of catabolic-formative immunological activity of the organism in regard to bacterial activity "in the wrong place," for example through use of potentized herbal (Thuja, Dulcamara, Juniperus) and metallic remedies (Mercurius vivus among others); the organism can also be activated in this direction through nosodes, i. e., through potentized preparations which are manufactured from the proliferating species of bacteria respectively.
- Abatement of excessive emotional irritability and perception of pain, for example through potentized animal remedies (Cantharis, Apis, Lachesis). – *Reduction of emotional strain put on* the child, for example through familial conflicts, and proper paedagogical response to nervousness and intellectuality can also contribute a lot to helping the soul forces become *physically effective* to the necessary degree of intensity rather than being drawn away from this task.
- stimulation of organ-forming forces, for example through potentized silver and potentized organ preparations, and of healthy eliminative activity of the kidneys and the urinary tract, for example through preparations composed of Equisetum, Solidago, birch leaves.
- protection of physical organ structures against dissolution and destruction, through antibiosis if necessary; correction of severe anomalies through paediatric surgery.

If one conceives of the therapeutic method *in this order,* then the physician's point of departure is the *possible self-activity of the child's organism,* which must be supported, guided and activated. Thus he will only employ *iatrogenic suppression of the infection or surgical restoration* as a last resort. Hence the physician is also compelled to take possible circumstances of the disease into account comprehensively. This generates trust in the physician-patient relationship as well as in the child's own forces.

5.5.2.1 Uncomplicated urinary tract infections

> Cold extremities are an indication of insufficiently warming intervention of the higher members in the lower human being and thus of a predominance of external conditions.
>
> M. Girke

Application of a warm poultice soaked in oil in the area of the urinary bladder has a warming, immunologically activating and pain-relieving effect. For this,

- **Eucalyptus Ol. aeth. 10 %** Wala,

can be used. It should be applied in the evening, covered with a bit of wool and left on overnight. – If the child's legs or even only the feet are cool or hypothermia was the cause, one can administer an

- ascending, warm, knee-high **footbath**

and then apply

- **Cuprum met. 0.4 % ointment** Weleda

to the soles of the feet and calves or apply

- **Mallow oil** Wala (cf. ▸Chap. 2.2.1)
  to the legs.

Diagnostically speaking, in assessing the child's warmth organization the *kidney region* is of great significance; should one find this to be a relatively cool area of skin (which is not seldom the case), then a kidney rhythmical Einreibung using 0.4 % copper ointment in the form of a horizontal figure eight which crosses the spinal column is indicated. This is done using a pea-size amount of ointment (only apply with warm hands!) applied to the skin with a massaging movement for several minutes until a clear warming effect becomes evident (concerning external applications for treatment of pyelonephritis cf. ▸Chap. 5.5.2.2).

Medicinally speaking, for cases of uncomplicated inflammation with no or low fever, oral treatment usually suffices.

A basic medicine which stimulates the catabolic-formative immune system and is suitable for children from age 2 to 3 on is

- **Thuja comp. N trit.** Weleda
  3–5 × daily 1 saltsp. for 3–5 days

The silver in low potencies which is contained in this medicine as well stimulates the organ-formative forces in the area of the efferent urinary tract [Selawry 1985, 36f.]. Thuja is a herbal medicine which is essential for "hidden, smouldering" infections which tend to become chronic (cf. ▸Chap. 6.4.3.6.5). Mercury, as a metallic medicine, is indicated when an inability to maintain boundaries is threatening to become chronic.
An alternative compound remedy

- **Argentum nitricum comp. pillules** Wala
  3–5 × daily 5–10 pillules

is suitable for small children and infants and as a follow-up remedy after initial administration of Thuja comp. This remedy contains silver as a nitrate in relatively high potentiation (D19) potentized mutually with low potencies of Thuja, Eucalyptus and Echinacea.

The highly potentized silver nitrate primarily supports the restoration of a closed boundary surface in the area of the epithelia and thus abatement of the invasive inflammatory process. Eucalyptus and Echinacea in the applied low potencies have a warming, defence-enhancing effect.

For treatment of severe burning pain in the area of the urinary bladder and the urethra, a combination of one of the two aforementioned preparations with

- **Cantharis bladder pillules.** Wala
  as called for 5 pillules hourly to begin with, later on 3 × daily 5–10 pillules

or Cantharis as a single remedy is suitable. A similar effect is achieved by the preparation

- **Berberis/Apis comp. pillules** Wala

In cases of severe dysuria it can be taken in alternation with Cantharis comp.; factors which determine selection of treatment are simultaneous manifestation of catarrhal symptoms of the upper respiratory tract and poor eliminative activity of the kidneys. – This can generally be stimulated, for example, by preparations derived from birch leaves and juniper such as

- **Kidney tonicum** (Nierentonikum) Wala
  2–3 × 1 tsp. daily

or preparations of Solidago virgaurea and Equisetum, for example

- **Solidagoren N drops**
  3 × 5–20 drops daily
- **Cranberry juice dry extract,** for example Urovit® capsules
  for school-age children 2 × 1–2 × 2 capsules daily, for smaller children juice in individual dosages

can counteract the adherence of the bacteria to the epithelia of the urinary tract and prove effective as a phytotherapeuticum for urinary tract infections and the prevention thereof (also suitable as part of a therapy concept as a prophylaxis for patients with anatomical anomalies and neurogenic paralytic bladder).

If it is possible to determine specific triggers, treatment can be modified accordingly (in particular initially):

triggered by getting drenched and hypothermia:

- **Dulcamara D6 dil.–D12 dil./pillules** (various manufacturers)
  at onset of infection hourly, then at greater intervals 5–7 pillules/drops

in cases of shock, traumatic events:

- **Aconitum e tub. D6–20 pillules** Wala
  on the first day 5 pillules several times to initiate treatment

in cases of emotional wounds, jealousy

- **Ignatia comp. pillules** Wala
  3 × daily 5–7 pillules, also as a preventative measure

after pneumonia or severe disease of the respiratory tract

- **Phosphorus LM6 dil.** Arcana
  daily 3–5 drops in the morning

5.5.2.2 Complicated urinary tract infections

Initially these include any febrile or extremely febrile inflammation of the urinary tract. One must always take into account involvement of the ureter and the renal pelvis for treatment. The less mature the child is, the more quickly the urinary tract infection will become generalized and the less local symptoms will manifest themselves. A poor general condition, nausea and vomiting and occasionally slight neck stiffness will initially leave the physician clinically in the dark about the origin of the disease; often all he will find is conspicuously foul-smelling urine. A diagnosis cannot be made until the laboratory results are in; one should always aim to examine the urinary tract sonographically (for diagnostics after abatement of symptoms cf. the respective guidelines).

The physician must weigh each individual case carefully and decide whether he can treat the ailment with close monitoring while refraining from use of antibiosis or not. Anatomical anomalies, age and the general state of the child's health are crucial factors. – On the other hand, in suitable cases it is possible to achieve rapid improvement and *an extraordinarily satisfactory long-term result* through the therapy depicted below while dispensing with antibiotics, for this therapy aims to help the child's own forces and his individuality assert themselves and not to weaken them through substitution. One can have the experience that a *change in constitution*, a thoroughly positive spurt of development is achieved. – The decision as to which therapeutic approach is the right one must be made individually for each case and be monitored closely at first through daily visits or consultations, and revising one's approach if necessary.

Parenteral administration of the medicines which are specifically effective for this case is crucial. Intravenous administration of a mixed injection consisting of

- **Lachesis D30 amp.** Wala/Weleda,
- **Argentum met. praep. D30 amp.** Weleda,

has proven effective for all cases of urinary tract infections accompanied by high fever.

Both medicines have an organotropic effect on the urogenital tract and also counteract the risk of urosepsis. They activate the effect of the immunological system and contribute considerably to limiting the invasive infection and preventing permanent damage of the urinary tract[1].

If there is clear pain on percussion in one or both of the renal beds

- **Renes/Argentum nitricum amp.** Wala
  will possibly prove more effective than Argentum met. praep. D30.

The authors deem potentized nosodes to be indispensable. Of these,

- **Tuberculinum Koch D30 amp.** Staufen
  is of universal significance for acute febrile urinary tract infections (see below); Tuberculinum is supplemented by a pathogen-specific nosode, most often or as a rule initially one administers
- **Nosode Bac. Coli D30 amp.** Staufen

1 Regarding the anthroposophic ratio of high potencies of silver in parenteral administration cf. Steiner and Wegman [1991, 116]. This indication for using Argentum met. D30 parenterally was implemented for the first time by I. Wegman in collaboration with R. Steiner and it has proven to be enormously effective.

At the beginning of treatment it is advisable to administer the medicine every 12 to 24 h i.v., for example Lachesis D30 + Argentum D30 + Bac. Coli D30 in alternation with Tuberculinum D30 + Argentum D30. If one finds pathogens other than E. Coli in the urine culture (for example Enterococci), nosode E. coli can be replaced by the homologous nosode (available from Staufen Pharma). For treatment of acute urinary tract inflammations, higher potencies have proven effective, usually D30, whereas for chronic infections deeper potencies work better (see below).

The nosode *Tuberculium* plays a crucial therapeutic role. Quite evidently tuberculosis, as a disease disposition, lies in a weakness in the soul-body structure [Steiner 1976, 39–43] which is similar to the disposition for urinary tract infections described above. Urinary tract infections often exhibit a concomitant disturbance of pneumatization in the upper human being and a connection with inflammation of the respiratory tract; in the view of anthroposophic medicine the astral body is not sufficiently active in body formation in the upper or the lower human being. This creates fertile soil for proliferating, body-dissolving processes of nature which cannot be overcome immunologically; there is a disposition towards chronically recurring inflammation. Bacterial pathogens persist at the body's boundary surfaces, are not dissolved completely and are eliminated.

It is always very impressive to see how high potencies of this pure culture of human tuberculosis pathogens manufactured according to Koch give the child the capacity to overcome an aggressive urinary tract infection and heal it himself. Apparently this medicine helps the spirit-soul individuality become more deeply anchored in the body aspect, thus taking the ground from under foreign processes of nature. Tuberculinum Koch is an indispensable medicine for acute and chronic inflammations of the urinary tract. If administered *per os* it can have a decisive effect if several of the following symptoms or decisive circumstances are observed:

- Tendency to sweat profusely at night,
- Extroversion and agitation,
- Mood instability, always needs diversion, does not rest, finds it hard to isolate himself,
- Need for fresh air and exercise but exhibits sensitivity to cold, weak warmth organization, unstable body temperature,
- Chronic tendency towards infections of the respiratory tract or tonsils,
- Tuberculosis or chronic infections of the respiratory and urinary tract in the family anamnesis.

For oral use of Tuberculum the authors have found that it is best to administer

- **Tuberculinum C200 pillules** Gudjons
  3 × 3 pillules daily for 3–4 days as a single remedy

in cases of acute urinary tract inflammation supplemented by i.v. injections of the aforesaid Parenteralia and unpotentized herbal remedies; for cases of chronic urinary tract inflammation followed by the remedies named in ▸Chap. 5.5.3.

In general, parenteral therapy of complicated urinary tract infections *per os* can be supplemented and continued using the medicines named in ▸Chap. 5.5.2.1.

As an external application, a **warm compress** in the kidney region using **horsetail tea** (Equisetum arvense): put 1–2 tab. Herba Equiseti arv. into 1 l cold water, bring the water to a boil and continue to boil it for 10–15 min.; then let steep for another 10–15 min. (dissolves the silicic acid). After straining, the water will be dark-brownish-green. Immerse the appropriately sized compress into the water, wring it out and lay in on, making sure it is comfortably warm. Wrap a woollen cloth around the child's body with a thin water bottle underneath if need be. See that the child's feet are warm before applying the compress. The child should rest for at least 30 min. afterwards. [Kusserow 1992]
For children of kindergarten and school age, the child's defence against infections can be supported acutely through internal administration of nasturtium preparations:

- **Angocin® tab.**
  2–3 × daily 2–4 tab. after (!) a meal.

or

- **Tropaeolum Urtinktur** Ceres
  2–3 × daily 3–7 drops (very effective!) dissolved in water.

5.5.3 Chronic urinary tract infections

Regarding diagnostic aspects ▸Chap. 5.5.1. Regarding surgical correction of pronounced anatomical anomalies of the urinary tract the authors do not advocate any standpoint in opposition to common practice. – Chronic urinary tract infections can also be attributed to

- vesicourethral reflux (VUR).

By the current state of scientific knowledge, moderate cases (VUR II-III) can heal without surgical correction through long-term antibiosis or prompt treatment of symptomatic episodes. The authors' experience has shown that in such cases therapeutic success can even be achieved without antibiotics if the treatment depicted below is used. Thus for chronic urinary tract infections which have no cause demanding surgery or are not attributable to severe anatomically or neurologically induced urine transport disorder there is indeed an alternative to long-term antibiosis.

Treatment is based on the options for therapy discussed above in ▸Chap. 5.5.2:

- Organ-related stimulation of the warmth organization.

As for any chronically recurring inflammation the activity of the I-organization plays a special role in treatment.

An important remedy in this context is

- **Phosphorus LM6 dil.** Arcana
  in the morning 2–5 drops daily (cf. ▸Chap. 5.1.1)

for vesicourethral reflux regularly combined with

- **Ureter Gl D8 amp.** Wala
  2 × weekly 1 drinking ampoule

Potentized organ preparations are effective for dysplastic tendencies and disorders of functional processes in small children in particular. Homologous preparations of the urethra, the urinary bladder and the renal pelvis (Renes, Regio pyelorenalis) are also available.

A new basic remedy developed by anthroposophic medicine for children with anomalies of the efferent urinary tract und recurring urinary tract infections is the medicine

- **Silex-Lapis Cancri solutus D4 (D6, D15) dil.** Weleda
  3 × daily 3–10 drops (cf. ▸Chap. 6.3.3.3).

In addition to the aforesaid clinical criteria, clinical guiding symptoms are:

- Local susceptibility to oedema, in particular lid oedemas,
- disorders of warmth regulation, most of all chilly feet and chilly kidney area,
- Susceptibility to pollinosis, atopic dermatitis,

microhaematuria can also be the basis for the indication of the remedy (similar to phosphorus). – The anthroposophic paediatrician H. Pechmann repeatedly observed a decrease in frequency of infection through long-term administration of this remedy (at least 6–12 weeks) [guiding idea and bibliographical source: Vademecum 2010, 745]. The remedy has less a pathogenetic effect than it does a salutogenetic one directed towards the development of the kidneys and kidney function (in any case this is the authors' current impression)). It is beneficial for treatment of urolithiasis.

Possibilities for strengthening the warmth organization through external applications are depicted in ▸Chap. 5.5.2.1. – It is very important to *prohibit going to swimming pools (most of all indoor ones)* and seeing that the patient wear suitable clothing and appropriate shoes (without warm feet and legs, no urinary tract infection can be sustainably healed – see the motto by M. Girke).

Penetration of the urine-producing and urine transporting organs through forces of the astral body which effect catabolic-formative elimination depends primarily on stimulation and guidance by the I-organization of the child. Insofar the treatment step described above constitutes the precondition for all further steps.

The astral body can be directly strengthened in it activity through

- **Argentum nitricum comp. pillules** Wala
  3 × daily 5–10 pillules

and through the administration of suitable, homologous nosodes, which can be given per os in cases of chronic urinary tract infections, for example

- **Sanukehl Coli D6 dil.**
  1–3 × 5 drops daily

For mixed infections, several nosodes can be combined.
In addition one can interpolate

- **Nosode Bac. Coli D30 amp.** Staufen
- **Tuberculinum Koch D30 amp.** Staufen aa 2 ml i.v.

every 4 weeks, for example.
In regard to kidney activity, potencies of vegetable carbon are specifically effective for recurring urinary tract infections (R. Steiner [1976, 214–221] made extensive note of this) [Vademecum 2010, 267]

- **Carbo Equiseti D15 amp.** Weleda
  2 × weekly s.c.

The child's immune system can be supported phytotherapeutically through administration of nasturtium extracts

- **Angocin tab.**
  2–3 × daily 2–3 tab. (suitable for children age 4–5 years and up)

or

- **Tropaeolum Urtinktur** Ceres
  2–3 × daily 3–7 drops diluted in water
- or **Cranberry**-Extract (cf. 5.5.2.1)

For cases of chronic urinary tract infections, stimulation of the organ-formative forces plays a crucial role. The activity of the kidney and immune system is stimulated in a comprehensive way through the anthroposophic compound

- **Lien comp. pillules/amp.** Wala
  1–2 × 7–10 pillules or 1 ampoule per os daily (most effective),

in which organ preparations with low potencies, among them spleen and kidney preparations, are mutually potentized with rhythmicized basic substances of Cichorium und Equisetum (cf. 6.3.3).

The specific immune system of the child is especially stimulated by

- **Thymus/Mercurius pillules** Wala
  3 × daily 3–5 pillules

The elimination process of the kidneys must be promoted dietetically through (primarily warm) drinks and daily servings of soup (warming effect and promotes elimination!) and medicinally through

- **Kidney tonicum** (Nierentonikum) Wala
  3 × 1 tsp. daily

or, better-tolerated for children with a sensitive stomach,

- **Solidagoren N drops**
  3 × 5–20 drops

If treatment was preceded by administration of antibiotics, sulphur in a suitable preparation should be given to help reactivate the child's life organization, for example in the form of

- **Sulphur LM6–12 dil.** Arcana
  2 × weekly to daily 2–5 drops

or, to specifically stimulate kidney elimination,

- **Equisetum cum Sulphure tostum D3–6 trit.** Weleda
  3 × 1 saltsp. daily [Vademecum 2010, 413]

Nutritionally speaking one should primarily prevent excessive consumption of sugar and sweetened drinks as well as large consumption of milk. Otherwise dietetic measures must be taken on an individual basis. – As was elucidated at the beginning of this chapter, the susceptibility to chronic urinary tract infections generally has to do with intestinal flora spreading in the urinary tract and destroying its own structure. For this reason the *intestine* plays the largest role here: stool and dietary anamnesis, clinical examination of the abdomen and microbiological stool diagnostics are indispensable in this connection. In cases of pathological findings symbiosis guidance (cf. ▸Chap. 4.6.4) is necessary. Recovery of the intestinal flora – in cases of long-term antibiosis this is only partially achievable

5

– also improves the chance that the organism will be able to fend off the advance of intestinal flora in the urinary tract.

The following case study illustrates which regulative options for therapy of complex chronic urinary tract infections exist.

Case study

A ten-month-old girl is brought in to the practice for a consultation for the first time. After early development of a urinary tract infection accompanied by a high fever and pyelonephritis, bilateral reflux which had started to spread to the renal pelvis is diagnosed. Surgical correction in the 8th month of life. Afterwards, despite long-term antibiosis, constantly pathological urinalysis.

Antibiosis is terminated; initial treatment comprises Sulphur LM12 dil. Arcana to reactivate the life organization, Colibiogen® Children to initiate symbiosis guidance and Lycopodium comp. pillules Wala to stimulate detoxification processes; in cases of chronically persisting infection Thymus/Mercurius pillules Wala to activate immunological self-activity and as an organotropic medicine for chronic urinary tract infections Argentum nitricum comp. pillules Wala.

One month later, after urinalysis in the clinic, only slight signs of inflammation: Leuko (+), Ery (+), protein neg., are found in the urine culture but still high bacterial counts of E. coli, Klebsiellas and Pseudomon aer. The parents reject the recommendation of the clinic to begin immediately with high dosages of antibiotics. The aforesaid medicines continue to be administered, supplemented by nosodes of all three bacterial species: Sanukehl Klebs D6 dil., Sanukehl Pseu D6 dil. and Sanukehl Coli D6 dil. as well as Fortakehl D5 dil. (a penicillin nosode). After four weeks another urinalysis and radiological follow-up: despite continuing, even increasing hydronephrosis – re-surgery proves necessary – completely normalized urinalysis! As the parents report, the colleague from the paediatric clinic is not able to explain this.

5.5.4 Nephritic syndrome

5.5.4.1 Generally indicated treatment measures for nephritic syndrome

The authors have limited experience with this indication, which does not comprise all subtypes of nephritic syndromes. The principles of clinical care [Ehrich 2004, 1178ff.] is valid without restriction. For the authors, the following aspects and measures have proven to be important and beneficial:

- Rest: nephritic diseases in small children are often preceded by emotional tension and dissonance, whether in the course of the child's own emotional development or as a result of unresolved tension in the surroundings. One should be aware of this and relieve the child as much as possible. Having respect for the needs of the life organization is also important, for example, when a nephritis emerges which results from failure to observe the period of rest necessary after a streptococcal infection (cf. ▸Chap. 5.3.4.4.2). *It is important to develop a sense of rest*!
- Attention to or purposeful change of sleeping place: for nephritis as well as for nephrotic syndrome, severe geopathic stress on the child's sleeping place has been ascertained in many cases. In one case the authors had the opportunity to observe how the healing

process set in after the sleeping place was exchanged for a favourable one! So-called water veins and other geopathic burdens are by no means figments of the imagination and can be reproducibly shown im blinded experiments by careful examiners! The kidney activity seems to be particularly sensitive to such environmental influences.

Medicinally the following are especially suitable:

- **Renes Gl D30 amp.** Wala
- **Apis ex animale Gl D30 amp. Wala**
  as a mixed injection s.c. in the kidney region or injected i.v.

Should this not be possible, both remedies can also be given to quite young children per os (1 ml/day).

It is particularly recommendable to alternate the aforesaid combination with

- **Mercurius vivus D30 amp.**Weleda
- **Carbo Equiseti D15 amp.** Weleda
  in the same way as a mixed injection i.v. or s.c. cf. ▶Chap. 1.2.2).
- **Equisetum cum Sulphure tostum D6 trit.** Weleda
  3 × daily ¼ drops/tsp. per os, promotes the elimination process most of all
- **Phosphorus LM6 dil. Arcana – D12–20 dil.** Weleda – **C30 pillules** Gudjons

is the most important single remedy for *nephritis* in the context of *Schönlein-Hennoch-Purpura*) [cf. Imhäuser 2000, 115]. For this form, external application of **Formica D1** as a bath is of central importance (cf. ▶Chap. 10.3)

External applications which can be recommended are

- **Equisetum-kidney compress** warm (vgl. 5.5.2.)
- **Cuprum met. 0.4 % ointment** Weleda

as ointment cloths applied over night.

For all external applications in the kidney region it is advisable to have them be supervised by an experienced, qualified nurse or the physician himself.

5

5.5.4.2 Haemolytic-uraemic syndrome (HUS)

Over the past years, the authors have been able to gain experience with providing consultation for several affected children. In doing so, they have observed the impressive effects of potentized remedies for the parents and the physician in individual cases. The necessity and justification of clinical treatment, mostly involving peritoneal dialysis and if need be transfusion of erythrocytes and thrombocytes, remains uncontested. In conventional medicine there is currently no evidence-based medicinal approach for this condition, however [Ehrich 2004, 1182].

Constitutionally speaking a non-coincidental number of children appears to be affected for whom

- **Phosphorus LM6–C30 pillules**

is suitable as a constitutional remedy.

These are slender, extroverted, playful and active, charismatic and artistically talented children. One characteristic of this type of constitution is that acute-inflammatory illnesses can quickly become vitally threatening diseases. Other characteristics are changes in and disorders of coagulation (cf. idiopathic thrombocytopenic purpura [ITP], sepsis) accompanied by an increased tendency towards bleeding.

The pathology of HUS corresponds to all characteristics of the drug picture Thuja occidentalis and thujone poisoning; Leeser explicitly determined similarities between thujone and phosphorus poisoning [Leeser 1987, 331/I]. In individual cases, the toxic picture involving enteritis with diarrhoea followed by severe toxic kidney damage accompanied by haemolytic syndrome [l. c.] has proven to be an impressively effective simile of the haemolytic-uraemic syndrome.

- **Thuja e summit. D30 pillules** Wala/**C200 pillules** Gudjons
for acute cases 3 × daily 3 pillules over a period of 3–5 days.

What is particularly characteristic of thuja is that this disease involves pathogenic bacteria "lodging themselves"' in the intestine, where they can form a toxin (verotoxin): bearing "foreign life in one's own," *not being able to eliminate an infection in due time* are guiding symptoms of thuja (cf. extensive discussion in ▸Chap. 6.4.3.6.5).

The authors are convinced that by taking the therapeutic measures described in ▸Chap. 5.5.1, phase-adequate administration of Thuja along with a suitable constitutional remedy, usually phosphorus (which is sometimes indicated before, but mostly after administration of Thuja), the course and long-time prognosis for HUS can be considerably improved in individual cases.

R. Madeleyn observed convincing results using

- **Stibium met. praep. D6 10 ml amp.** Weleda
i.v., several times a day.

R. Madeleyn notes: "We succeeded in avoiding imminent need for dialysis and stabilized the child rapidly" [report to the authors].

5.5.5 Nephrotic syndrome

5.5.5.1 Steroid-sensitive, nephrotic syndrome

Treatment of steroid-sensitive nephrotic syndrome in simple cases among children is almost exclusively the domain of conventional medicine. Therapy proves more difficult when it comes to children with frequent episodes, so-called "frequent relapsers". These confront any paediatrician with a difficult task which can only be solved on an individual basis. Conventional medicine approaches the problem exclusively with immunosuppressively effective medicines (steroids, Chlorambucil, Ciclosporin A, cyclophosphamide, mycophenolatmofetile), whose indication and concomitant problematic adverse effects (most of all dependence on Ciclosporine A treatment, which is problematic long-term). An article by Franke [Franke 2009] provides an overview and side effects are also listed in an overview by Ehrich [Ehrich 2004, 1188]. In individual cases the authors succeeded in achieving sustainable therapeutic success, always based on comprehensive and individualized therapy. On the other hand, the authors agree with R. Madeleyn concerning the experience that once a child has developed a clearly generalized phase of oedema accompanied by massively pronounced hypoalbuminaemia, anthroposophical-homoeopathic approaches do not prove successful alone and the children should not be exposed to any unnecessary risk. It should be expressly pointed out that sudden onset of stomach pain is always a sign of possible pneumococcal peritonitis.

The following therapeutic aspects can be conveyed to physicians performing treatment:

- *sleeping place:* geopathic burdens primarily due to so-called water veins are frequently found in cases of nephrosis. The authors were also struck by the fact that the houses affected often lay in damp areas near a canal, in moss, etc., in which there was *stagnating wetness*: a picture of the nephrotic child suffering from oedema! Changing the sleeping place is imperative!
- *generation of warmth:* it is important for the affected children to avoid cold wetness (for example trips to the swimming pool), that they are encouraged to develop warmth and absorb light (for example through mountain hiking), most of all that they are always dressed warmly in the region of the legs and the torso, that they wear house shoes and do not walk around on cold floors, for example in rooms with no cellar below. On the other hand experience with measles has shown that *infections accompanied by high fever* lead to healing of a nephrotic syndrome (minimal change) or can promote such healing.
- *eurythmy therapy*: it is striking that the children affected often have a tendency towards *infections of the upper respiratory tract* and as a result to relapses of the nephrotic syndrome. Therapeutically it has proven possible to vastly improve the ventilation of the nose, the paranasal sinuses and the middle ears and to reduce susceptibility to infections through regular eurythmy therapy exercises (daily exercises over several months are required!) (cf. ▸Chap. 5.1.2.6). The *tendency towards stagnation which takes hold of the organism during the course of the disease* is corrected through eurythmy therapy to great effect. Moreover, the "B"-exercises and the sound "A" [Girke 2010, 747] elicit a direct response from the kidneys. In the meantime we view eurythmy therapy as a necessary element of a complementary therapeutic approach for nephrotic syndrome!
- For the authors, a new rational approach to treatment of children with steroid-sensitive nephrotic syndrome has opened up through the study of *Helleborus niger* [Soldner 2010].

5.5.5.1.1 Helleborus niger

To begin with, the *characteristics of the Christmas rose* (Helleborus niger) which have become essential for the authors' understanding of the remedy effect should be briefly summarized:

Ranunculaceae literally means "little-frog plants." The family of the Christmas rose is called this because it likes to grow in places where frogs are also found,

- in damp locations.

A well-known example is the bright yellow kingcup. The locations usually have chalky soil, chalk being a water-soluble mineral originally formed by animals. Relatives of the Christmas rose form bufadienolides, cardiac glycosides which are similiar to toad poison, a fact which underscores the word "little frog" (from rana, the frog) contained in the name of this plant family. One characteristic of this group of animals is that it emerges from an aquatic larval stage onto land, developing limbs and air breathing. Thus the little frog is an epitome of the transformation, the step taken out of the dark water into the air and light.

5

This points to yet another characteristic of the Ranunculaceae, which can be most comprehensively described as a

- mercurial ability to metamorphose.

Members of the buttercup family grow out of the damp underground, transforming in a striking fashion the shape of their leaves as they move up from the soil to the blossoms. In the case of Helleborus niger in particular, the boundaries between the leaves and the blossoms become blurred in a special way; the white pseudanthium turns green as spring approaches, adopting a vegetative (leaf) character again in a regressive fashion. *The nature of the ensouled disappears in the course of the flowering period of Helleborus niger, going through a regressive metamorphosis* (this can be observed in children afflicted with a nephrotic syndrome quite strikingly during an episode).

Substantially speaking, the mercurial aspect of Helleborus types of Ranunculaceae corresponds to the formation of

- Saponines,

which promote the transition from air to water. The Ranunculaceae ultimately allow emotionally expressive blossoms to emerge from the leaf metamorphosis, with the spectrum extending from the open white of the Christmas rose blossom to the vibrant yellow of the buttercup and the kingcup and finally to the deep violet of the Pulsatilla and the dark bluish violet helmet of the aconite. This is also the most toxic plant in Central Europe. Thus Ranunculaceae have a strong effect on ensouled organisms: in the loveliness of their blossoms as in their substance formation, which ranges from rapidly disintegrating herbal toxins with a mild effect such as the Protoanemonin in Pulsatilla to highly toxic alkaloid aconitine. Substantially speaking this corresponds to the toxicity of all parts of the plant in Helleborus niger and in particular the formation and concentration in subterranean rhizome of:

- Beta-Ecdyson,

a steroid hormone related to male sexual hormones which unfolds its well-known effectiveness in the animal kingdom in particular. It is necessary for the metamorphosis of caterpillars into butterflies, for example, which is to say, for the metamorphosis of a dull, vegetatively oriented soul life into an airworthy animal gestalt which inhabits the air element and can perhaps be characterized as the most beautiful "blossom" in the animal kingdom. At the same time the principle of "*pneumatization*" appears here as an essential quality of the astral aspect: conquest of the air, which, in higher animals, is accompanied by the formation of inner air space. Functionally speaking, butterflies promote reproduction; thus the astralization in the transition from the caterpillar to the butterfly also indicates a relationship to sexual maturity and the sexual organs. Herein emerges the innermost

- *Principle of the astral body, the polarizing effect*, which realizes itself archetypically in the sexual (secare [lat.]: cutting asunder) polarity of the male and the female, just as the caterpillar and the butterfly embody mutually related polarities.

In the development of Ranunculacee a mercurial transition from the watery etheric element to the world of ensouled organisms extending into the airy astral element occurs, but always in an individual manner. The polarity and transition from life and soul organization is shaped by every Ranunculus in a characteristic and unique way. Thus as medicinal plants, these plants exert a strong effect on the activity of the soul organization, the astral body in the human being.

Generally speaking in cases of nephrotic syndrome in childhood with minimal change glomerulonephritis, guiding symptoms are

- Oedema, at first lid oedema, then pretibial oedema, later on also ascites – a relapse into a water-dominated world which the child gradually and increasingly leaves in the course of pneumatization, the appropriation of the body by the soul. Infections of the upper respiratory tract, catarrhs which make the upper respiratory tract swell up in a watery way and become congested with pflegm often precede an episode.
- Weight gain; the person develops a swollen – phytoid appearance.
- Foaming urine, proteinuria (like the effect of saponine in the wrong place)
- Hypoalbuminaemia
- Children with MC-GN exhibit a sensitivity to wetness and cold, often developing disorders of pneumatization in the area of the nose and the paranasal sinuses, often with exacerbation in the winter months (Helleborus is a winter-flowering plant)
- Episodes of nephrosis usually manifest themselves emotionally; the children affected develop emotional qualities such as irritability, lack of concentration, tendency to withdraw, strange oppositional traits which correspond to the aforesaid guiding symptoms. What is striking is that when such children are healthy, such traits are not necessarily present. Helleborus is an important remedy for promoting the child's attentiveness and ability to concentrate (cf. ▸Chap. 7.5.)

As a rule, the disease can be influenced by corticosteroids; in a third of all cases it disappears after one treatment (in one third of cases there are one or more relapses and in one third of cases the patient is at risk for developing steroid dependency). As adrenal cortex hormones, corticosteroids are essentially associated with awakening in the morning, with the intervention of the astral body in the physical-etheric body (which becomes plant-like in the night), thus also functioning as a "stress hormone." A considerable number of cases heals in the course of puberty, i. e. through the physiologically intensified intervention of the astral body into the urogenital tract and the onset of sexual maturation – in this context one should think of the function of Beta-Ecdysons for the metamorphosis of the caterpillar into the butterfly.

Thus a model for the healing process is already given, namely to *strengthen the astral body of the child and stimulate it to intervene in the kidney/adrenal system*. This happens to be the main basic effect of Helleborus. The Christmas rose forms "steroid saponine" substantially; its basic effect shows a certain affinity to corticosteroids. The *differentiating function of the astral body* must be strengthened therapeutically, especially in the area of the podocytes of the kidney glomeruli. One can speak here of a "conscious perception of the blood" if one considers the physiological function of the podoctyes in regard to the blood in the renal artery and primary urinary function.

Thus primary use of Helleborus niger for nephrotic syndrome in children by the authors was not based on older homoeopathic or other literature but rather on the understanding of Helleborus niger depicted in the framework of anthoposophic medicine and anthropology. The following case study describes the first case which was treated with Helleborus niger on the basis of the considerations formulated above. After 20 years of often unsuccessful encounters with this disease, the authors saw impressive proof of the effectiveness of this treatment in an individual case.

Case study[1]

A 4 ½ year-old girl with dark hair is brought in for a consultation. She clings to the mother, who had *nursed her for 18 months.* The mother speaks quickly and in an agitated manner; the child interrupts her constantly, making a striking appearance and drawing all the attention to herself. *At the level of the perception organization, mother and child appear excited* and threaten to lose control. The family's lifestyle is unsettled. Remarkable aspects of the prehistory are a large, receding haemangioma in the area of the right shoulder, a *duplex kidney* on the right but with normal morphology of the efferent urinary tract. The girl has a tendency to *"slide around" on her genitals once a day to excite herself*; the mother has the impression that the child takes a short sensually pleasurable "time out" from the impressions which assail her so strongly. A long phase of thumb-sucking.

What strikes the physician during the examination are *chilly feet and legs* (as if the child still lived halfway under water – a typical finding for children with MC-GN, including the fact that such children do not notice this. As the nephrotic syndrome heals, this should improve; such children should become more sensitive in this area). Dry skin.

Emotionally the child makes a very rational impression while at the same time appearing very emotional. The initial extreme fear of dogs has in the meantime been replaced by a love of these animals. She has a particular, conspicuous liking for fish and eggs.

At age 4, in August 2007, after a cold (contact with water), the girl develops a urinary tract infection involving E. coli. At this time already evidence of proteinuria. Antibiosis is administered using Trimethoprim but proteinuria persists. In September 2007 diagnosis of nephrotic syndrome, renal biopsy: minimal change. Standard steroid therapy using 60 mg/m^2 BSA Prednisolon daily for 6 weeks, then alternatingly 40 mg/m^2 BSA every other day for another 6 weeks. Relapse 8 weeks after completion of therapy, Prednisolon administered anew from late January 2008 on + ACE-inhibitor in small dosages (1 × 6.25 mg Captohexal). Since onset of the disease in 2008 she must urinate at night and is demanding (calls for the mother like an infant, regressive behaviour which is often observed in children with nephrotic syndrome).

The author begins by prescribing the child the following: rhythmical Einreibung of the body with Oleum aeth. Salviae 10 % (cf. Chap. 5.1.3.3) due to susceptibility to infections of the upper respiratory tract, which in turn tend to trigger relapses [Vademecum 2010, 628], Silex Lapis cancri solutus D6 and D15 dil. Weleda (cf. ▸Chap. 5.5.3) due to the kidney disease, Ignatia comp. pillules Wala 2 × 5 in view of the girl's constitution, which shows a pronounced hysteric aspect [Vademecum 2010, 508].

New relapse in April 2008, 6 weeks after beginning of treatment performed by author and discontinuation of Prednisolon due to infection of the upper respiratory tract (coughing and sniffles). Profuse proteinuria. At this point in time the decision was made – based, among other things, on finding out about the work of Dietrich Schlodders and Patrick Jesses

1 First published in [Vademecum 2010, 479]

[cf. Der Merkurstab **63**(6), 2010] – to treat this clinical syndrome with Helleborus niger in low potencies. The aim was to anchor the astral body, the perception organization of the child, more stably in the kidney.
Initially, Helleborus niger ampoules manufactured by Helixor were prescribed, beginning with D6, then D4 3 × daily 0.7 ml *orally*, in acute situations up to 1.0 ml before meals. Helleborus should preferrably be taken in the morning; when used more than once a day, in the morning and afternoon, otherwise in the morning, at midday and in the afternoon. Since the daily activity of the astral body is to be strengthened, an evening dosage does not seem purposeful. *During this period the child received a protein-free diet for three days.* In the further course of treatment 3 × 0.7 ml D4, reducing the medicine step by step to 1 morning dosage of Helleborus niger D6 0.7 ml, Silex – Lapis cancri solutus D6 in the morning and D15 in the evening, Kidney tonicum Wala 1 tsp. after breakfast, Pulsatilla D30 amp. Weleda and Apis ex animale D30 amp. aa 1 × daily 0.7 ml orally. This medication continued to be given in the course of treatment.
In August 2008, during a holiday on the North Sea in bad weather after running barefoot along the ocean, there was an outbreak of cystitis (precisely 1 year after onset of the disease) and a relapse of the nephrotic syndrome accompanied by proteinuria. By telephone, *Helleborus niger D4 2 × daily 1 ml was prescribed, only effecting a reduction of the proteinuria, then D3 in the same dosage; within 2 days protein-free.* Ongoing administration of ACE inhibitors, no more administration of Prednisolon. – Currently Helleborus niger Helixor amp. D6 in the morning 0.5 ml orally, Apis D30/Puls D30 in the afternoon 0.7 ml orally, Silex Lapis cancri. sol. D15 1 × daily 5 drops and 1 tsp. Kidney Tonicum. The girl's self-excitatory behaviour of sliding around on her genitals disappeared in the course of treatment but it occurred again in discrete form under stress conditions after starting school. Concerning the nephrotic syndrome the child has had no more relapses although she has contracted several infections, some febrile, since then.

In the meantime the author has had success using Helleborus niger for cases of MC-GN, which are usually difficult to treat. Its effect sometimes lies in being able to control a relapse of what is actually a steroid-dependent nephrotic syndrome treated with long-term administration of Ciclosporin A but without having to resort to steroids. In a particularly difficult case of an 11-year-old boy who was psycho-socially retarded for a long period of time and who had undergone several immunosuppressive treatments (among others involving steroids, Endoxan) and was taking high dosages of Ciclosporin A, it was possible to not only ward off relapses under immunosuppression but also to promote a very positive emotional development through Helleborus treatment, with the boy developing social skills and constantly improving his school performance. In this case it was not possible to discontinue administration of Ciclosporin A, however (which, as is well-known, is difficult after several years of treatment of steroid-dependent nephrotic syndrome). In this case the effectiveness of Helleborus niger for an infection-induced relapse in cold-wet weather was enhanced by administration of Erysidoron 1 Weleda and thus a relatively concentrated substantial dosage of Apis. After having treated several children including some with focal-sclerotic GN, the authors have determined that Helleborus niger has proven to be effective for treatment of kidney diseases involving nephrotic syndrome repeatedly.

Dosages of

- **Helleborus niger D6–3 amp.** Wala, Helixor

are usually given per os, 1–2 × daily 0.5–1 ml.

In cases of insufficient effectiveness the medicine can also be injected, but we do not generally administer it this way. In this indication the authors find the drink ampoules to be more effective than the pillules. In general, *onset of effect* can usually be assessed within 3 days, at the latest after 7 days, i. e., within a period of time similar to that needed for onset of effect of corticosteroids. It manifests itself in a *decline of the proteinuria*, stimulation of dieresis and possibly at first in *improvement of mood* in the form of more open, harmonious behaviour. Helleborus niger can also be effective if partial oedemas (lid oedemas, discrete calf oedemas, scrotal oedemas) are found.

Treatment must be continued for a long time with D6 (or D4) 0.5–1.0 ml taken in the morning usually being the suitable maintenance dosage. Side effects in the sense of undesired pharmaceutical effects have not be observed for this indication (as opposed to the first casuistic).

5.5.5.1.2 Further treatment options

A suitable external medicinal measure for external application is

- **Ferrum met. 0.4 % unction** Weleda als kidney rhythmical Einreibung in the morning.

The aim here is to strengthen the intervention of the I and the astral body in the kidney region in a different way than that required for cases of nephritic syndrome, which is characterized by a too extreme catabolic intervention of the astral body. In cases of nephrotic syndrome the individual risks becoming too plant-like; the structuring effect of the higher members of human fourfold nature must become more active in the organ.

The same goal is served through injection treatment using

- **Stibium met. praep. D20 amp.** Weleda,
- **Equisetum cum Sulphure tostum D15 amp.** Weleda,
- **Stannum met. praep. D8 amp.** Weleda

aa 1–1.5 ml s.c. on the left and right side of the spinal column in the kidney area.

Injection treatment used by M. Girke [Girke 2010, 752] which he depicts in an impressive case study is based on the thoughts developed by R. Steiner and I. Wegman. It entails activating the higher members (I and astral) in the metabolic area in the right way, which involves everything from the digestion of food in the digestive tract to elimination in the kidney organization. Indeed the instability of such intervention in children constitutes a substantial disposition for the development of steroid-sensitive nephrotic syndrome. Treatment is based on the rhythm, fundamental to anthroposophic medicine, of administering an iron preparation in the morning and potentized copper in the evening (cf. ▸Chap. 6.5), deepening the immersion of the I and the astral body into a breathing rhythm in this way:

- **Pancreas/Meteoric iron amp. Pancreas/Meteoreisen** Wala
- **Apis ex animale D30 amp.** Wala
  in the morning 1 ampoule each as a mixed injection s.c. (abdominal)
- **Renes/Cuprum amp.** Wala
  in the evening 1 ampoule s.c.

An enhancing effect is achieved by

- **Ginger-Equisetum-Kidney Compress**
  2–3 heaped tab. Pulvis Zingiberis mixed with boiling Equisetum tea, allowed to steep for 5 min. (warmth protection!). After prewarming the feet using a water bottle, immerse the cloth in the tea, wring it out well and lay it on the patient at body temperature. Cover with a woolen cloth and leave on for 20 mins.

A universally recommendable remedy for kidney disorders with development of oedema is

- **Equisetum cum Sulphure tostum D3–6 trit.** Weleda
  1–3 × daily 1 saltsp. to 1/4 tsp.,

which exhibits a clear eliminatory effect but also supports the reorganization of the kidney area. A similar effect is achieved by

- **Pancreas/Equisetum pillules** Wala
  1–2 × 10 pillules in the morning or in the morning and afternoon
- There is documented positive experience of treatment in isolated cases (R. Madeleyn and others) using **Aranea diadema D6 amp.** Weleda.

If one consults the homoeopathic drug picture of the cross spider [Seideneder 2008, 1061–1075], one finds no direct reference to nephrosis but one does find the trait of warmth which characterizes children with nephrotic syndrome: "Suitable for persons who are not able to live in a damp environment or on water… due to DAMP, most of all WET-COLD WEATHER [emphasis in the orig.]" as well as a *penetrating feeling of being cold* (but which, as the authors observe, only adult Aranea patients are generally aware of).

In this context we see a justification for attempting to treat recurring steroid-sensitive nephrotic syndrome with *potentized willow mistletoe*,

- **Iscucin® Salicis Strength A (–C) amp.** Wala
  1 × weekly 0.7–1 ml s.c.

to *strengthen the warmth organization* and differentiate the activity of the astral body in the kidneys (to which willow mistletoe has a close affinity). Willow mistletoe also has an affinity to melancholy, which has been found in a number of patients during an episode [regarding Salix and Iscucin Salix cf Wilkens et al. 2005]. It can be used to complement treatment with Helleborus niger, especially during relapse-free intervals. One often ascertains that patients who are treated with anthroposophic mistletoe preparations exhibit a much more stable warmth organization and that they contract fewer infections.

The authors have had favourable experience with supportive enzyme therapy, most of all for catarrh and tumescence of the respiratory tract. Suitable remedies are

- **Bromelain** POS (a pineapple enzyme which promotes digestion and has a detumescent effect on the mucosa of the upper respiratory tract)
  daily 1–3 × 1 tab. depending on the age and health condition of the patient [cf. Maurer 2002].
- **Wobenzym®**
  up to 3 × 3 tab. daily if Bromelain alone is not sufficiently effective.

In any case, careful infection prophylaxis, an appropriate diet with abstention from sweetened drinks and bought sweets (but not freshly prepared desserts or homemade cake on Sundays!) is necessary, as is abstention from cow's milk and very moderate consumption of milk products.

5.5.5.2 Steroid-resistant nephrotic syndrome

Most often, a focal-segmental sclerotic glomerulonephritis lies at the root of this clinical picture. If left untreated, this disease used to culminate in terminal kidney insufficiency after an average period of 5 years [Ehrich 2004, 1189]. Here diagnostics and therapy using Ciclosporin A have brought great changes and progress in treatment [Heeringa, Hildebrandt 2009, Ehrich et al 2009]. Initial observations made with use of Helleborus niger give rise to the assumption that potentized Christmas rose extracts could have a positive effect on these forms of treatment as well.

An impressive observation of a single case in which the condition healed completely was achieved through treatment using

- **Equisetum cum Sulphure tostum D4,** later on **D6 trit.** Weleda
  3 × daily 1 saltsp.

combined with

- **Olivenite D4,** later on **D6 trit.** Weleda
  3 × daily 1 saltsp.

(twelve-year observation period). M. Sommer reports of another case [Vademecum 2010, 638]. A noteworthy aspect of his report is that in cases of acute exacerbation of membranoproliferative glomerulonephritis after emotional injury (renewed onset of macrohaematuria) at age 9, rhythmical Einreibung of the kidney area using

- **Oxalis 30 % ointment** Weleda

had a prompt effect (cf. ▸Chap. 2.2.3; for small children use 10 % ointment).

5.6 Lyme disease (Lyme borreliosis) and TBE (tick-borne encephalitis)

About 30 % of all ticks in Europe currently carry Borrellia burgdorferi (subtype) [Hobusch et al. 1999, 37]. The probability of bacteriological infection of the human host organism, currently estimated at just over 2 %, strongly depends on the duration of the tick bite and/or the way the tick is removed [Hobusch et al. 1999]. Hence it is important to inspect children carefully in the evening after exposure in order to minimize the duration of the tick bite. The risk of contracting Lyme disease is considerably reduced if the bite duration is less than 12 hours. Serological investigations show that the infection often develops sub-clinically and leads to a specific immune response in the organism that is measurable as IgG and IgM values. Because IgM can persist in measurable antibody titers for a long time, sometimes for years, in principle there is no reliable serological method for diagnosing acute Lyme disease (in contrast to cerebrospinal fluid diagnosis for tick-borne viral encephalitis [TBE]). It is possible for measurable antibody titers to form years earlier within the context of a "silent dormancy" of the bacteria, yet specific antibodies are still not detectable in about half of the patients with erythema migrans or lymphocytoma [Hobusch et al. 1999, 37].

Clearly, the tick bite and its consequences for the organism are associated with a perception difficulty. Firstly, the tick bite occurs in such a way that it is not sensed (due to anaesthetic substances produced by the tick, among other things). Furthermore, the human organism appears to have difficulty in "perceiving" and responding to the invasion of spirochaetes in the blood stream. This is evident in the unusual time span of the humoral immune response to Lyme disease. Similar to syphilis, the Borrelia bugdorferi pathogens penetrate the human organism in stages, starting in the skin region and then travelling via the bloodstream into subarachnoid or articular space.

According to the authors' experience and understanding of the infection, prophylaxis and treatment of Lyme disease ultimately amounts to sensitizing the organism's "perception" of the Borrelia bacteria (and TBE viruses) and activating its immune response. In principle, an infection can also be overcome without antibiotics.

Following a tick bite, the authors currently proceed as follows:

- **Apis Belladonna cum Mercurio pillules,** Wala
  1st –10th day: 5–10 pillules, 3 x/day.

Potentized mercury is well-established as a specific treatment for spirochaete infections (there are numerous parallels between the stages of mercury poisoning and the illnesses caused by spirochaetes.)

- **Argentum/Quarz pillules,** Wala
  1st –10th(–14th) day: 5–10 pillules, 2 x/day.

This medicine sensitizes and activates the immune system, especially in the lymphatic system.

- **Nosode Borrelia Burgdorferi D30,** special preparation from the Barlach Apotheke, Boll (Germany)
- **Nosode FSME** or **Tick bite fever D30,** special preparation from the Barlach Apotheke Boll (Germany)
  1st, 2nd and 3rd day: 5 pillules, single dose/day.

These three medicines are also a suitable for treating acute *erythema migrans.* Dosage and duration of treatment can be intensified for this indication. The decision to attempt treatment without antibiotics should always be made individually.

The authors have developed the strong impression that systemic infection and disease can be more effectively counteracted following treatment with the Nosodes. In the authors' longstanding experience, none of the patients who conscientiously followed this prophylactic treatment developed Lyme disease.

5

Additional preparations that can be effective for prophylaxis against Lyme disease:

- **Mercurius auratus D15 amp.** Weleda
  0.3–0.5 ml, 1 x/day, per os as drinking ampoule; or 1 ampoule, 2 x/week, s.c. injection.
- **Thymus/Mercurius pillules** Wala
  5 pillules, 3 x/day, for 3–6 weeks.

These medicines should be considered for children who are susceptible to infection as well as children who currently have Lyme disease or have overcome the infection previously.

In case of manifest Lyme disease, the medical decision to administer antibiotic treatment should be taken together with the parents within the context of an informed conversation.

In general, the authors recommend two herbal mother tinctures to enrich and augment treatment of Lyme disease (stage II or III), during an acute phase and following antibiosis:

- **Dipsacus fullonum,** Ceres mother tincture
  3 gtt. mornings; up to 3 gtt., 3 x/day and/or
- **Geranium robertianum,** Ceres mother tincture
  3 gtt. 1 x/day, evenings.

Organ preparations can be effective for treating *monarthritis* (usually of the knee joint) and one-sided *facial nerve paresis* (after excluding all other diagnoses, including cholesteatoma!), see case vignette below. The authors recommend that antibiotic treatment also be accompanied by treatment with organ preparations, the excellent prognosis for childhood tick-borne viral encephalitis (TBE) notwithstanding, 11% of patients with facial nerve paresis retain weaknesses in the affected side [Skogman 2008] and monarthritis can be accompanied by recurrent arthralgias for many years. The D30 potency is suitable at the start of treatment. A series pack containing decreasing potencies can be used for treating facial nerve paresis:

- **Nervus facialis Gl D30, Series package II amp.** Wala
  1 ampoule per os, every 2nd day; teenagers also s.c., nuchal or upper arm
- **Articulatio genus Gl D30 amp.** Wala
  1 ampoule per os, daily–every 3rd day.

Treatment should continue until clinical symptoms come to a halt. Acute inflammatory conditions can subside under treatment with D30 organ preparations, especially in children, while the lower potencies (also) have a revitalizing effect.

Patients regularly report a distinct and rapid improvement in well-being and tend to recover more quickly than would otherwise be expected.

It is important to carry out conscientious follow-up treatment in children who have been treated with antibiotics:

- **Sulphur LM6 dil.** Arcana
  3–5 gtt., 1 x/day in the evening, continue for 3–4 weeks.

Additionally, give support to intestinal flora during and following antibiosis (▸Chap. 4.6).
If the child's life organization is clearly weakened and there is a consequent risk of the

infection spreading systemically, primary treatment can be effectively augmented with blackthorn elixir and especially buckthorn elixir (Weleda), as well as the preparation

- **Levico comp. pillules/amp.** Wala
  5–7 pillules, 1–3 x/day or 1 drinking ampoule 1 x/day.

This is especially recommended for children who are generally susceptible to infection and parasitosis.

In both adults and children, the clinical manifestation of Lyme disease, especially in Stage II and III, is often preceded by *psychosocial overload* (e. g. due to family conflicts, problems at school, adolescent crisis etc.), as well as a *difficulty in maintaining appropriate boundaries*, which, of course, correlates with the degree of subjectively-experienced overload. The infection can be seen as the "other side (the bodily side) of the coin": Alien life (related to ensouled animal life) invades the organism, sustains itself within the host, and then infiltrates and undermines the host organism's processes. Therefore, one often finds intestinal symbiosis disorders, oxyuriasis and accumulated infections manifesting alongside Lyme disease.

Case vignette

A 7-year-old boy presents at the practice with monarthritis of the right knee: 20° extension deficit, flexion up to 70°, distinct swelling and relatively moderate localized tenderness. He needs to use crutches. No recent gastroenteritis occurrence. The laboratory results indicate probable Lyme disease: CRP 10.7 mg/l, Borrelia IgG LIA > 240 U/ml, WesternBlot p 17,19,21,30,39,83 V1sE positive, serology for pathogenic intestinal flora (Campylobacter etc.) negative, ANA, CCP negative. The rheumatology outpatient department at the University Children's Clinic can only offer an appointment in 8 weeks time, after the Christmas holidays.

The boy attends an inter-year class at a Montessori school. After persistent questioning, it becomes clear that the knee joint symptomatology arose two days after a decision was taken to promote him from the 2nd to the 3rd class due to his intellectual gifts and capacities. A striking aspect of the earlier history was that in infancy and during the early toddler phase, the boy had a severe generalized atopic dermatitis and as a toddler he had recurrent croup attacks. Both illnesses had been completely overcome.

Within three weeks of treatment with Articulatio genus D30 amp. Wala per os (compare with 10.9.), Dipsacus fullonum (Ceres) and Bryonia/Stannum pillules, Wala, as well as initial administration of the Nosode Borrelia Burgdorferi D30 pillules (Barlach Apotheke, Germany) all symptoms had subsided/disappeared. The child nevertheless attended the appointment at the University Children's Clinic 8 weeks after starting treatment at the practice. The following excerpt is taken from the doctor's letter: "Because the knee joint swelling has reduced almost completely (without treatment [sic!]), we consider antibiotic treatment to be unnecessary. Treatment is not indicated in the case of raised titers without manifest symptoms." By mutual agreement with the clinic, arthrocentesis could be avoided (effusion no longer evident sonographically), and with conscientious follow-up at the practice over two years, antibiotic treatment never became necessary.

Remarkably, eight weeks after the start of treatment the boy came to the practice with acute arthralgia in the right knee. The previous day (this was after the Christmas holidays), he became aware that he now had a new teacher and had been placed in a new group – this came about after the proposed move to the 3rd class had been withdrawn on the physician's insistence in November. Treatment continued with Dipsacus fullonum, Bryonia D12 und Articulatio genus for several months.
With regard to the situation at school, the following excerpt is taken from the school report six months later: "Now the well-deserved holidays are beginning. Perhaps you will find the time to think about your goals for next year? I would wish that ..." [several classic teacher's wishes follow]. The boy's parents separated six months later. The joint pains never recurred.

In ancient Greek culture there was a belief that a part of the soul lives in the knee joint ... children with Lyme disease (possibly also with Osgood-Schlatter) can bring home to the physician how the soul breathes life into the entire body and how the body is both an "instrument" and a resonance chamber for the soul. This perspective is important when treating Lyme disease. When outer demands on the soul are too great, the soul organization is unable to stimulate the up-building life processes sufficiently. These children lack peace and quiet in their lives: Arthritis, facial nerve paresis and meningitis all enforce the much-needed rest. Reducing Lyme disease to a problem for medicinal treatment alone falls short of the real extent of the problem. This is especially clear in adult patients who do not completely recover from Lyme disease, even with antibiotic treatment.

Eliciting a response from the soul and the individualizing forces and sufficiently reducing external pressures on the patient are decisive for the success of the treatment. The authors have treated a number of children who ostensibly have chronic Lyme disease – some diagnosed and treated at the Deutschen Zentrum für Kinder- und Jugendrheumatologie (German centre for child and adolescent rheumatology) – primarily by exempting them from school pressures during the holidays, on Sundays and in the evenings, and carrying out the above-described medicinal treatment. In these cases Dipsacus fullonum Ceres has proven to be a beneficial revitalizing medicine.

In addition to rationalizing external pressures, drawing appropriate personal boundaries and ensuring a better rhythm in daily life, eurythmy therapy is remarkably effective (for both adults and children) in helping the patient to regain a sense of inner coherence.

The risk of manifest tick-borne viral encephalitis (TBE) in children is minimal, even in high-risk areas, and contrary to the rumours that one hears from concerned parents, fatalities are extremely rare (compare with ▸Chap. 3.5.4.14). The considerably higher risk for infected adults is often overlooked, however. On the other hand, children affected by TBE can be adversely affected for a long time – a fact not reflected by the statistics. The progression of TBE is most similar to that of poliomyelitis. ▸Chap. 5.4.2.3 for a possible treatment approach during the acute phase.

Once the TBE-related fever has subsided, motoric weakness following meningo-encephalitis can be treated with:

- **Arnica (= Radix) D30 dil.** Weleda
  5–7 gtt., 1–2 x/day.
- **Skorodit D20–30 dil.** Weleda
  5–7 gtt., 1–2 x/day.
- **Cerebellum comp. pillules** Wala
  7–10 pillules, 2–3 x/day.

Depending on disease progression and symptomatology, specific medicines can be administered individually. However, there is still a lack of experience of disease progression and availability of published case reports in this area.

References for Chapter 5

(every reference marked with a ■ Bullet point indicates the English translation of the reference above it)

Abel, V.: Infektanfälligkeit und Krebsrisiko. Dtsch. med. Wschr. 111, 1978–1981 (1986).

Abel, V.: Common infections in the history of cancer patients and controls. J. Cancer Res. Clin. Oncol. **117**, 339–344 (1991).

Bach, J.-F.: The Effect of Infections on Susceptibility to Autoimmune and Allergic Diseases. New Engl. J. Med. **347**, 911–920 (2002).

Bachmann, K.-D., H. Ewerbeck (Hrsg.): Pädiatrie in Praxis und Klinik. Thieme Verlag, Stuttgart 1989.

Bartke-Anders, I.: Myristica sebifera. Eine südamerikanische Heilpflanze. Der Merkurstab **56**, 16–21 (2003).

Böcker, W., H. Denk, P. U. Heitz: Pathologie. Urban & Schwarzenberg, München 1997.

Büttner, G.: Die Behandlung der Otitis media ohne Sulfonamide und Antibiotika in einer Allgemeinpraxis. Beitr. Erw. Heilk. **26**, 125–129 (1973).

Ciba Foundation Symposium: Silicon biochemistry. Vol. 121, London 1986.

Cilliers A. M. et al.: Anti-inflammatory treatment for carditis in acute rheumatic fever. Cochrane Database Syst Rev 2003 (2), CD003176.

Coker, T. et al.: Diagnosis, Microbial Epidemiology, and Antibiotic Treatment of Acute Otitis Media in Children. JAMA **304**, 2161–2167.

Dam, Jv: Zum Beitrag von K.-R. Kummer, Das Mukoserotympanon. Eine konservative Therapie. Der Merkurstab **59**,569 (2006).

Del Mar, C. B., P. Glasziou, M. Hayern: Are antibiotics indicated as initial treatment for children with acute otitis media? A meta-analysis. BMJ **514**, 1526–1529 (1997).

Del Mar C. B. et al.: Antibiotics for sore throat. Cochrane Review, The Cochrane Library 2002, www.update-software.com/ccweb/cochrane/revabstr/ab000023.htm.

Deutsche Gesellschaft für Kinderheilkunde und Jugendmedizin: Leitlinien Kinderheilkunde und Jugendmedizin. Lieferung 21, Urban&Fischer, München 2010.

Deutsche Gesellschaft für Pädiatrische Infektiologie DGPI: Handbuch Infektionen bei Kindern und Jugendlichen, 5.Aufl., Thieme, Stuttgart 2009.

Ehrich, J. H. H.: Glomeruläre Erkrankungen. In: Therapie der Krankheiten im Kindes- und Jugendalter. Reinhardt, D. (Hrsg.). 7. Aufl. Springer, Berlin 2004.

Ehrich, J. H. H. et al.: Therapie des steroidresistenten nephrotischen Syndroms. MSchr Kinderheilk **157,** 235–246 (2009).

Emsley, J.: Phosphor – ein Element zwischen Leben und Tod. Wiley-VCH Weinheim, 2001.

Endres, K.-P., W. Schad: Biologie des Mondes. S. Hirzel Verlag, Stuttgart 1997.

Engel, W.: Zu den Präparaten Ferrum phosphoricum und Ferrum hydoxydatum. Weleda Korr.bl. Ärzte **137**, 28–32 (1994).

Eyers, S. et al.: The effect on mortality of antipyretics in the treatment of influenza infection: systematic review and meta-analysis. J R Soc Med **103**, 403–411 (2010).

Fersch, B.: Der Sanddorn. In: Der Merkurstab **57**, 374–375 (2004).

Franke, I.: Therapie des steroidsensiblen nephrotischen Syndroms. MSchr Kinderheilk **157**, 226–234 (2009).

Gesellschaft Anthroposophischer Ärzte in Deutschland GAÄD: Leitlinie Masern. Der Merkurstab **61,** 601–605 (2008).

Girke, M.: Innere Medizin. Salumed Verlag, Berlin 2010.

- English translation in progress at this time – Ed.

Glas, N.: Die Formensprache des Gesichtes. Wien, Leipzig, Berlin 1935.

Gnaiger, J.: Lac caninum. In: Doc. Homoeop. **10**, 99–118. Maudrich Verlag, Wien 1990.

Gnaiger, J.: Angst, Sehnsucht und Unvermögen bei Lac caninum. In: Doc. Homoeop. **11**, 171–186. Maudrich Verlag, Wien 1991 (und Vortrag Köln 1991 zur Verl. des S.-Hahnemann-Preises).

Goebel, W., M. Glöckler: Kindersprechstunde. Urachhaus, Stuttgart,17. Auflage 2008.

Griese, M., D. Reinhardt: Erkrankungen von Trachea und Bronchien. In: Therapie der Krankheiten im Kindes- und Jugendalter. Reinhardt, D. (Hrsg.). 7. Aufl. Springer, Berlin 2004.

Grohmann, G.: Die Pflanze, Bd. 1. 7. Aufl. Verlag Freies Geistesleben, Stuttgart 1991.

Hachtel, B.: Bibliographie Heileurythmie. 2.Aufl. Natur-Mensch-Medizin Verlag, Bad Boll 2007.

Hahnemann, S.: Reine Arzneimittellehre. Bd. 1. Haug Verlag, Heidelberg 1995a.

Hahnemann, S.: Reine Arzneimittellehre. Bd. 6. Haug Verlag, Heidelberg 1995b.

Hamre, H. J. et al.: Anthroposophic vs. conventional therapy of acute respiratory and ear infections: a prospective outcomes study. Wiener Klin. Wschr. **117**, 256–268 (2005).

Harnack, G.-A. v., B. Koletzko (Hrsg.): Kinderheilkunde. Springer Verlag, Berlin 10. Aufl. 1997.

Haustein: In: Consilium infectorium, hrsg. von InfectoPharm, Ausg. VIII, Frage 3208.

Heeringa, S. F., Hildebrandt, F.: Monogene Ursachen des nephrotischen Syndroms. MSchr Kinderheilk **157,** 218–225 (2009).

Hinrichsen, K. V. (Hrsg.): Enbryologie. Springer Verlag, Berlin, New York 1990.

Hobohm, U.: Fever therapy revisited. Br. J. Cancer **92**, 421–425 (2005).

Hobusch et al.: Lyme-Borreliose im Kindesalter: Diagnostik und Therapie (Empfehlung der Deutschen Gesellschaft f. Päd. Infektiologie). Kinderärztliche Praxis **1**, 7 (1999).

Holtzapfel, W.: Seelenpflegebedürftige Kinder, Bd. I. Philosophisch-Anthroposophischer Verlag, Dornach 1982; Verlag am Goetheaneum, Dornach 1995.

- Holtzapfel, W.: Children's destinies : the three directions of human development. Mercury Press, Spring Valley, N. Y. c1977; 1981. This is the English publication of Seelenpflegebedürftige Kinder, vol. 1. Vol. 2 of Dr. Holtzapfel's work was published in English as: Children with a difference. Lanthorn Press, East Grinstead, England 1995.

Husemann, A. J.: Der musikalische Bau des Menschen. Verlag Freies Geistesleben, Stuttgart, 2. Aufl. 1989, 3. Aufl. 1993.

- Husemann, A. J.: The harmony of the human body: musical principles in human physiology. Floris, Edinburgh 1994.

Husemann, F.: Das Belladonnagift und seine Wirkprinzipien. Beitr. z. Erw. d. Heilk. **32**, 198–206 (1979).

Husemann, F.: Scharlach und eitrige Angina in zehn Jahren Praxis. Der Merkurstab **51**, 19 (1998).

Husemann, F.: Anthroposophische Medizin. Verlag am Goetheanum, Dornach 2009.

Husemann, F.: Sauerstoff und Niere: Das Erythropoetin. Der Merkurstab **52**, 52 (1999).

Husemann, F., O. Wolff: Das Bild des Menschen als Grundlage der Heilkunst. 4. Aufl. Verlag Freies Geistesleben, Stuttgart 1991.

- Huseman, F. Wolff, O.: The Anthroposophical approach to medicine: v. 1, 2. Steiner Books, Great Barrington, M. A. 1983, v.3 Mercury Press, Spring Valley, N. Y. 2003.

Husemann, G.: Sinnesleben, Seelenwesen und Krankheitsbild. Verlag Freies Geistesleben, Stuttgart 1998.

Imhäuser, H.: Homöopathie in der Kinderheilkunde. Haug Verlag, Heidelberg, 12. Aufl. 2000.

Keller, W., A. Wiskott: Lehrbuch der Kinderheilkunde, 6. Aufl. Thieme Verlag, Stuttgart 1991.

Kent, J. T.: Arzneimittelbilder, 5. Aufl. Haug Verlag, Heidelberg 1985.

Kienle, G., H. Kiene: Krebs und Fieber – epidemiologische Ergebnisse, empirische Therapieentwicklungen und therapeutische Erfolge. Die Mistel in der Onkologie, 174–193. Schattauer, Stuttgart 2004.

Kienle, G., H. Kiene, H. U. Albonico: Anthroposophische Medizin in der klinischen Forschung. Schattauer, Stuttgart 2006.

- Kienle G. S., Kiene H., Albonico HU. 2006a. Anthroposophic medicine: effectiveness, utility, costs, safety. Schattauer, Stuttgart, New York 2006.

Kipp, F. A.: Die Evolution des Menschen im Hinblick auf seine lange Jugendzeit. Verlag Freies Geistesleben, Stuttgart 1980.

Kluger, M.: Role of Fever in Disease. Annals of the New York academy of sciences, published online: 7 FEB 2006, DOI: 10.1111/j.1749-6 632.1998.tb08329.x (2006).

Kummer, K. R.: Masernverlauf in einer Kinderarztpraxis. Der Merkurstab **45**, 180–190 (1992).

Kummer, K. R.: 1001mal Masern – Prospektive Untersuchung von 886 und retrospektive von 115 Verläufen in der Praxis. Der Merkurstab **52**, 369–375 (1999).

Kunze, H.: Pneumonie-Lichtätherschwäche. Beitr. z. Erw. d. Heilk. **18**, 226–228 (1965).

Kusserow, M.: Äußere Anwendungen in der anthroposophisch erweiterten Medizin. Weleda Korrbl. f. Ärzte **133**, 122–153 (1992).

Lange, P.: Hausmittel für Kinder. Rowohlt Verlag, Reinbek 1988.

Leeser, O.: Pflanzliche Arzneistoffe I. 2. Aufl. Hrsg.: M. Stübler, E. Klug. Haug Verlag, Heidelberg 1987.

Lewin, L.: Gifte und Vergiftungen. Haug Verlag, Heidelberg, 5. Aufl. 1962, 6. Aufl. 1992.

Lievegoed, B. C.: Heilpädagogische Betrachtung. Hilfen zur Behandlung von Entwicklungsstörungen. Verlag Freies Geistesleben, Stuttgart 1995.

Lohse, A., Schmiedel, S.: Fieber senken? Möglichst nicht. Hamburger Ärzteblatt 12/2009, 28–29.

Lüth, P.: Das Ende der Medizin? dtv, Stuttgart 1989.

Madaus: Lehrbuch der biologischen Heilmittel, Bd. 1. Olms Verlag, Hildesheim 1999a.

Madaus: Lehrbuch der biologischen Heilmittel, Bd. 2. Olms Verlag, Hildesheim 1979, 1999b.

Marget, W.: Über die Ätiologie, Pathogenese und Therapie von Harnwegsinfektionen im Kindesalter. pädiatrie hautnah **7**, 446 (1998).

Maurer, H. R.: Bromelain: Biochemie, Pharmakologie und medizinische Anwendung. Erfahrungsheilkunde **4**, 223–235 (2002).

Mezger, J.: Gesichtete Homöopathische Arzneimittellehre, 5. Aufl. Haug Verlag, Heidelberg 1981.

Michel O. et al.: The value of Ems Mineral Salts in the treatment of rhinosinusitis in children. Prospective study on the efficacy of mineral salts versus xylometazoline in the topical nasal treatment of children. J Pediatric Otorhinolaryngology **69**, 1359–1365.

Moeller, H., Ulbricht, M.: Antipyretische Wirkung körperwarmer Einläufe. Z.Allg.Med. **67**, 964–968 (1991).

Müller-Mohnsen, H.: Kontroversen zur Toxizität von Pyrethrum und Pyrethroiden. Intern. Prax. **34**, 2231–2232 (1994).

Niewind, K.: Erkrankungen der Nasennebenhöhlen. Weleda Korr.bl. f. Ärzte **131**, 31–43 (1992).

Paradise J. L. et al.: Tympanostomy tubes and developmental outcomes at 9 to 11 years of age. N Engl J Med **356**, 248–261 (2007).

Pelikan, W.: Heilpflanzenkunde, Bd. 1. Verlag am Goetheanum Dornach, 4. Aufl. 1980.

- Pelikan, W.: Healing plants: insights through spiritual science. Mercury Press, Spring Valley, N. Y. 1997. Note: only this volume has been translated into English.

Pelikan, W.: Heilpflanzenkunde, Bd. 2. Verlag am Goetheanum Dornach, 1997.

Peuckert, W.: Scharlach – mikrobiologische Probleme. Pädiatr. Praxis **38**, 37–42 (1988).

Rauber, A., F. Kopsch: Anatomie des Menschen, Bd. III Nervensystem, Sinnesorgane. Leonhardt, H. (Hrsg.). Thieme Verlag, Stuttgart 1987.

Reinhardt, D.: Erkrankungen der Atemwegsorgane. In: Kinderheilkunde. Harnack, G.-A. v., B. Koletzko (Hrsg.). 10. Aufl. Springer Verlag, Berlin 1997.

Remmele, W. (Hrsg.): Pathologie, Bd. 3. 2. Aufl. Springer Verlag, Berlin, New York 1997.

Roemer, F.: Zur Therapie mit potenzierten Organpräparaten. Zschr. f. ganzhtl. Tiermedizin **4**, 113–116 (1993)

Roemer, F. et al.: Achatwasser – Opal – Bergkristall. Der Merkurstab **62**, 605–619 (2009).

Rohen, J. W.: Funktionelle Histologie. Schattauer, Stuttgart 2000.

Rohen, J. W.: Morphologie des menschlichen Organismus. Verlag Freies Geistesleben, Stuttgart, 2000 (a).

- Rohen, J. W.: Functional morphology : the dynamic wholeness of the human organism. Adonis Press, Hillsdale, N. Y. 2007.

Rosenlund et al.: Allergic Disease and Atopic Sensitization in Children in Relation to Measles Vaccination and Measles Infection. Pediatrics **123**, 771–778 (2009).

Schmitt-Grohé, S.: Virale Pneumonie. Mschr. Kinderheilk. **159**, 217–223 (2011)

Schroten, H., T. Tenenbaum: Bakterielle Pneumonien. Mschr. Kinderheilk. **159**, 208–216 (2011)

Schulze, U.: Das Pancreas als Organ der Mitte. Der Merkurstab **51**, 279–283 (1998).

Schwarz, R.: Onyx bei rezidivierender Otitis media. Der Merkurstab **58**, 307–309 (2005).

Seideneder, A.: Heilmittelarchiv 6 Bde., Narayana Verlag, Kandern 2008.

Selawry, A.: Metall-Funktionstypen in Psychologie und Medizin. Haug Verlag, Heidelberg 1. Aufl. 1985, 2. Aufl. 1991.

Simon, L.: Schmerztherapie mit homöopathisch potenzierten Heilpflanzen. Haug Verlag, Heidelberg 1987.

Skogman, B. H. et al., Lyme Borreliosis in Children. Pediatric Inf Dis J, **27** 1089–1094 (2008).

Soldner, G.: Erfahrungen in der Therapie von Atemwegserkrankungen im Kindesalter. Erfahrungsheilkunde **2**, 66 (1991).

Soldner, G.: Hinweis zu Oleum Salviae 10 % bei Mucoserotympanon. Der Merkurstab **60**, 477 (2007).

Soldner, G., M. Sommer: Allantois und Astralleib – wie können wir Rudolf Steiners Forschungsergebnisse nachvollziehen? Der Merkurstab **60**, 27–35 (2007).

Soldner, G.: Helleborus niger. Der Merkurstab **63**, 508–517 (2010).

Sommer, M.: Kopflausbehandlung – nur mit dem Risiko neurologischer Schäden: Der Merkurstab **47**, 484–486 (1994).

Sommer, M.: Gezielte organotrope Therapie der Karzinompatienten. Der Merkurstab **49**, 193–206 (1996).

Sommer, M.: Möglichkeiten der Kopflausbekämpfung. Der Merkurstab **55**, 470–472 (2002).

Sommer, M.: Behandlung der Otitis media ohne Antibiotika. Der Merkurstab **51**, 373–374 (1998).

Sommer, M., G. Soldner: Die Farne in Natur und Mensch – zum Verständnis von Digestodoron. Der Merkurstab **5**, 289–296 (1990).

Sommer, M., G. Soldner: Merkur in Natur und Mensch I. Der Merkurstab **41**, 279–289 (1988a).

Sommer, M., G. Soldner: Merkur in Natur und Mensch II. Der Merkurstab **41**, 337–343 (1988b).

Stauffer, K.: Homöotherapie. 3. Faksimile-Nachdruck. Sonntag Verlag, Regensburg 1986.

Steiner, R.: Von Seelenrätseln. 5. Aufl. Rudolf Steiner Verlag, Dornach 1921

- Steiner, R.: Riddles of the soul. GA (complete works) 21. Mercury Press, Spring Valley, N. Y. 1996.

Steiner, R.: Geisteswissenschaftliche Gesichtspunkte zur Therapie. Rudolf Steiner Verlag, Dornach 3. Aufl. 1963, 4. Aufl. 1984.

- Steiner, R.: Anthroposophical spiritual science and medical therapy: second medical course, nine lectures to physicians and medical students, Dornach, April 11–18, 1921. GA (complete works) 313. Mercury Press, Spring Valley, N. Y. 1991.

Steiner, R.: Geisteswissenschaftliche Menschenkunde, Gesamtausgabe Bd. 107. 5. Aufl. Rudolf Steiner Verlag, Dornach 1988.

Steiner, R.: Physiologisch-Therapeutisches auf Grundlage der Geisteswissenschaften. Gesamtausgabe Bd. 314, 3. Aufl. Rudolf Steiner Verlag, Dornach 1989.

Steiner, R.: Anthroposophische Menschenerkenntnis und Medizin. 3. Aufl. Rudolf Steiner Verlag, Dornach 1994.

- Steiner, R.: The healing process: spirit, nature and our bodies: lectures, August 28, 1923-August 29, 1924, in various cities. GA (complete works) 319. Anthroposophic Press, Hudson, N. Y. 2000.

Steiner, R.: Geisteswissenschaft und Medizin. Rudolf Steiner Verlag, Dornach 5. Aufl. 1976, 7. Aufl. 1999.

- Steiner, R.: Introduction to anthroposophical medicine. GA (complete works) 312. SteinerBooks, Great Barrington, M. A. 1999.

Steiner, R., I. Wegman: Grundlegendes zu einer Erweiterung der Heilkunst nach geisteswissenschaftlichen Erkenntnissen. Rudolf Steiner Verlag, Dornach 7.Aufl. 1991.

- Steiner, R., I. Wegman: Fundamentals of therapy : an extension of the art of healing through spiritual-scientific knowledge. GA (complete works) 027. Mercury Press, Spring Valley, N. Y. 1999. Also available as: Extending practical medicine: fundamental principles based on the science of the spirit. Rudolf Steiner Press, London 1996.

Steiner, R.: Meditative Betrachtungen und Anleitungen zur Vertiefung der Heilkunst. Rudolf Steiner Verlag, Dornach, 4. Aufl. 2003.

- Steiner, R.: Course for young doctors: meditative contemplations and instructions for deepening the art of healing: lectures for physicians and medical students. GA (complete works) 316. Mercury Press, Spring Valley, N. Y. 1994.

Steiner, R.: Die Offenbarungen des Karma. Gesamtausgabe Bd. 120. 8.Aufl., Rudolf Steiner Verlag, Dornach 1992.

- Steiner, R. Manifestations of karma: eleven lectures given in Hamburg between 16 and 28 May 1910. Rudolf Steiner Press, London 2010.

Stellmann, H. M.: Kinderkrankheiten natürlich behandeln. Gräfe & Unzer, München 1. Aufl. 1983, erweiterte Neuausgabe 2009.

Stenstrom, R., B. Pless, P. Bernhard: Hearing threshold and tympanic membrane sequelae in children managed medically or surgically for otitis media with effusion. Arch. Pediatr. Adolesc. Med **159**, 1151–1166 (2005).

Stiegele, A.: Homöopathische Arzneimittellehre. Reprint, Hippokrates, Stuttgart 1981.

Stübler, M., E. Krug (Hrsg.): Leesers Lehrbuch der Homöopathie. Haug Verlag, Heidelberg 3. Aufl. 1987.

Strengell T. et al.: Antipyretic agents for preventing recurrences of febrile seizures: randomized controlled trial. Arch Pediatr Adolesc Med **163**, 799–804 (2009).

Stübler, M., O. Wolff: Die Hahnenfußgewächse. Vorträge im Krankenhaus Lahnhöhe vom 7./8.12.1985, hrsg. vom Verein Quadrivum, Lahnstein.

Stuijvenberg van, M. et al.: Randomized, controlled trial of ibuprofen syrup administered during febrile illness to prevent febrile seizure recurrence. Pediatrics, **102**, E 51 (1998).

Vademecum Anthroposophische Arzneimittel. 2.Aufl. Der Merkurstab **63**, Supplement (2010)

- Vademecum of anthroposophic medicines, CD format. Medical Section of the School of Spiritual Science, Dornach, Switzerland 2009. Van Buchem, F. L., M. F. Peeters, M. A. van't Hof: Acute otitis media: a new treatment strategy. BMJ **290**, 1033–1037 (1985).

Vagedes, J., Soldner, G.: Das Kindergesundheitsbuch. 3.Aufl. Gräfe & Unzer, München 2010.

Vargas, M. H.: Ecological association between scarlet fever and asthma. Respiratory Medicine **100**, 363–366 (2006).

Verity, C. M. et al.: Long-term intellectual and behaviper os outcomes of children with febrile convulsions. New Engl. J. Med. **338**, 1723–1728 (1998).

Vogel, H. H.: Wege der Heilmittelfindung, Bd. 1, Bd. 2. Natur Mensch Medizin Verlag, Bad Boll 1994.

Vogel, H.-H.: Finding remedies: spiritual knowledge of man and naure; a contribution toward understanding anthroposophic remedies, based on the example of the Wala remedy compositions. V 1, 2 Natur-Mensch-Medizin, Bad Boll 1994.

Vogel, H. H.: Die vier Hauptorgane. Natur Mensch Medizin, Bad Boll 1995.

Wilkens et al.: Die Behandlung des Fibromyalgie-Syndroms mit Weidenmistelextrakten. Der Merkurstab **58**, 264–271 (2005).

Williamson, I. et al.: Topical intranasal corticosteroids in 4–11 year old children with persisten bilateral otitis media with effusion in primary care: double blind randomised placebo controlled trial. Bmj **339**, b4984 (2009).

Wimmenauer, W.: Zwischen Feuer und Wasser, Gestalten und Prozesse im Mineralreich. Urachhaus, Stuttgart 1992.

Witsenburg, B. C.: Masern-Sterblichkeit und Therapie. Der Merkurstab **3**, 177–180 (1992).

Witzel, L.: Anamnese und Zweiterkrankungen bei Patienten mit bösartigen Neubildungen. Med. Klin. **65**, 876–879 (1970).

Wölfel, D.: Rezension der Studie von Verity et al. päd. praxis **56**, 359 (1999)

Zwaart, S. et al.: Penicillin for acute sore throat in children: randomised, double blind trial. BMJ **327**, 1327–1328 (2003).

6 Allergic diseases

And the Lord said unto Satan, Behold, he is in thine hand; but save his life. So went Satan forth from the presence of the Lord, and smote Job with sore boils from the sole of his foot unto his crown. And he took him a potsherd to scrape himself withal while he sat down among the ashes.

Job 2:6–8

Job was righteous, exemplary in his actions, endowed with wealth and respect. But the word "Job" means "the enemy" in Hebrew! "The human being as his own enemy"?[1] Job is smitten by Satan, which translates as the "opposer". He loses all his wealth, his children, is struck by a generalized eczema, by "leprosy": a sign of impurity in the Jewish world of the time. Sacrifices and purification were deemed to be the way to liberate oneself from that. Job falls out of life. He sits down "among the ashes", the matter which remains when the living substance has burned away; his actions are tied to his suffering, he scrapes himself with a potsherd, the physical remains of a broken vessel. The period starts in which he is tested.

Job's three friends who analyze the causes of his suffering only magnify his pain, his isolation, his despair without being able to show a way out. Job himself insists that he is pure and without reproach – "Oh that one would hear me! behold, my desire is, that the Almighty would answer me" (Job 31:35). As far as Job is concerned, God himself becomes the one who has turned against him and considers him as the enemy, a view for which Elihu reproaches Job (33:10). Elihu, the fourth friend, introduces the change in Job's fortunes by speaking of God not as representing a superficial order but as the creative power underlying the world and human beings. The more the human being elevates himself, consciously or unconsciously, to be the centre of his world (the central position of Job was described at the beginning), believing in the end that he himself is responsible for this position without, in truth, himself being able to originate life, soul and spiritual existence, the more he threatens to become the enemy of that which he cannot create – namely of himself!

Elihu's words cause Job to fall silent; and at that point the voice of God is heard which Job has missed for so long and yet himself has never allowed to speak. After Job has heard God's words, he acknowledges: "I have heard of thee by the hearing of the ear: but now mine eye seeth thee." (42:5). He recants the position he has taken previously, which ulti-

1 We owe the idea for this introduction and important content to J. Gnaiger's presentation on a lecture by F. Weinreb in volume 9 of the Doc. Homoeopathica (ed. M. Dorsci), Haug Verlag, Heidelberg 1988, entitled "Krankheit und Heilung im alttestamentarischen Verständnis und die Psoralehre".

mately saw his own wellbeing as a recompense from God for his virtue[1], and he turns to God as the free creator of human existence. "And the Lord turned the captivity of Job, when he prayed for his friends: also the Lord gave Job twice as much as he had before. … So Job died, being old and full of days." (42:10,17).

6.1 Epidemiology and pathogenesis of allergic diseases

> Epidemiological studies show that prenatal exposure, such as nutrition, immunostimulating agents or smoking during pregnancy, can influence the asthma risk of the child. It was recently established for the first time that nutrition or exposure to exhaust gases during pregnancy are associated with childhood asthma via epigenetic changes and this asthma risk is passed down even to the second generation.
>
> S. Krauss-Etschmann et al. [2010]

The state of empirical research has continued to develop rapidly between the first and fourth editions of this volume; an abstract such as the one quoted in the motto would have been unthinkable in the German *Monatsschrift für Kinderheilkunde* ten years ago. This confirms key hypotheses of this chapter in a field which is rapidly changing – hypotheses which have remained unchanged but for which there is a much broader evidence base today.

6.1.1 Lifestyle and allergy

Epidemiology shows that allergic diseases "hardly occur in rural areas in developing countries" [von Mutius 2005, 254]. Whereas in rural Zimbabwe only one child out of more than 600 showed signs of bronchial hyperreactivity, the figure for the same period in the capital Harare was 5.9. A study published in 2001 [Riedler 2001] showed also for children from Germany, Austria and Switzerland that their risk of suffering from asthma and allergic rhinitis was strongly influenced by the lifestyle of their parents – *most significantly by the living conditions during pregnancy* (◻ Tab. 6.1).

The comparison in the above study was not between urban and rural but between children from the same village, some of whom still lived on a farm and others whose parents were already pursuing other occupations. This example clearly illustrates the formative influence of early childhood on the health of the adult: "There is convincing evidence that a childhood spent on farms confers protection from respiratory allergies *with a sustained effect into adulthood.*." [von Mutius 2008]. Life on a farm means directing, organizing and controlling nature as well as the simultaneous symbiosis with nature: a task which faces every person throughout life both in the digestion and in the external barriers of the skin and airways. Both tasks are originally related and can support one another, as these study results show. For allergies indicate that the patient is unable to organize, direct, and control his contact with his food and external nature or the symbiosis with his own intestinal and skin flora in a healthy way.

1 Cf. the close parallels between the above and the sermon of Meister Ekkehart on Matthew 21:12. Meister Ekkehart, Deutsche Predigten und Traktate, edited and translated by J. Quint, Diogenes, Zürich 1979, 153–158.

Tab. 6.1 Influence of living conditions during pregnancy on the subsequent development of asthma and allergic rhinitis in children [as per Riedler 2001].

	Woman working daily on farm during pregnancy	Woman not working daily on farm during pregnancy	Woman not working daily on farm during pregnancy and child with no contact with farm animals and raw milk (!) in the first year of life
Diagnosis: asthma	0%	2%	14%
Runny nose and burning eyes in the last twelve months	1%	12%	14%

The unborn child already has contact with fine traces of substances which are handled by the digestive and immune systems of the mother: *intestine, skin and airways of the mother are simultaneously the barriers between the unborn child and food and the environment during pregnancy*. The world experienced by the mother lastingly affects the developing life organization of the child up to and including the *epigenetic regulation of the child's genetic makeup,* e.g. through the nutrition and digestion of the mother. We can trace this in detail today: thus DNA methylation represents a central process of epigenetic "early programming" in the child's regulation of his or her genetic material. The DNA is given "bookmarks" (methyl groups) which determine the genes which will be active in life and the ones which will be "switched off". Studies show that children of mothers who drink "*farm milk*", fresh raw milk, during pregnancy display an *allergy preventive* methylation pattern – in contrast to children whose mothers have partaken in less healthy nutrition displaying a great number of methyl groups [Schaub 2010]. While many experts warn against raw milk (and its allergenicity! Koletzko [2009], 74) and recommend HA milk powder, the protective effect of raw milk with regard to, for example, bronchial asthma (OR 0.74) and allergic rhinitis (OR 0.56) has been very clearly shown [Waser 2008]. In terms of treatment, the attempt is made to mimic these processes by prescribing probiotics such as Lactobacillus GG preparations to pregnant women [Kalliomäki 2001] or probiotics and prebiotics[1] to infants [Kukkonen 2007], something which can in itself be seen as a substitute for lost natural resources (e.g. non-pasteurized milk products on the farm, bacterial flora in the byre or farmyard!). The same applies to the wealth of natural bacterial flora in the maternal environment as it typically exists on a farm – it stimulates the differentiation of the child's immune system as early as before birth in a healthy way. After birth, the air which is breathed on a farm is of a different quality to that on a main traffic artery: after plant pollen had been discovered in great quantities in cow dung, it was determined through animal experiments that inhaling dust from cow dung (particularly the arabinogalactans it contains) can protect against pollen allergy [Peters 2010] – the pollen predigested by the animal helps the child's immune system to come to terms with and develop a tolerance towards it. It is clearly of help for the immature organism if in its first encoun-

1 Galacto-oligosaccharides as growth factors for intestinal flora which are naturally contained in human breast milk

ters with foreign matter it is supported by its mother or other already mature organisms.[1] This is an impressive example of the original symbiosis between human beings and nature which can no longer be assumed to exist in western industrialized nations.

Yet the loss of this original world does not necessarily have to remain irreversible in our culture: the "anthroposophical lifestyle" has not only shown itself to be preventive of allergies but it has been possible to demonstrate that children from Waldorf schools show a greater diversity in their intestinal flora than children from farms which were examined in the same study [PARSIFAL Study Flöistrup 2006]. In this context *the consumption of biodynamically and organically grown foods clearly correlated with the diversity of intestinal flora* [Dicksved 2007, 2288]. The development of tolerance requires natural bacterial flora "in the gastrointestinal and respiratory system, particularly as it could be shown that no mucosal immune tolerance could be induced in mice living under sterile conditions without localized flora"! [Stock 2010] . Paediatric allergology brings all these results together in the "*hygiene hypothesis*": the increasing absence of natural challenges for the child's immune system leads to a growing deficit in immunological competence and regulatory ability and thus encourages chronic diseases. The strategy of avoiding or trying to escape from potential natural allergens (e. g. avoiding cow's milk permanently from the beginning) is not supported by these findings; on the contrary, the task is to guide the child in "reverence of life" (Albert Schweizer) towards nature, healthy food and the animal world. In this context support, trust, a "mantle" which accompanies this encounter are important factors. Parental stress has been shown to be a risk factor with regard to obstructive respiratory diseases [Wright 2002].

The maturation of the child's immunological organization is a sensitive, individual learning process dependent on culture (and treatment). *In utero*, the mother's and child's primary immune system behave in a pronounced immune tolerant way, something which is required to allow for the symbiosis between the mother's and the child's organism in the womb. Immunologically this is referred to today as a "physiological Th_2 stimulation" [Holländer 1999, 125] of the maternal and child's immune system during pregnancy. It is important that this displaced equilibrium of the immune system should in the first instance be seen in its positive meaning which lies in the possibility of pregnancy and its uniquely close symbiosis and openness between two people. The importance of an "intact maternal mantle" for the unborn child becomes clear (▸Chap. 6.5). And it is also easier to understand why the issue of a – partly at least – too close symbiosis between a child with an allergic disease and his or her mother and its dissolution often represents a therapeutic task. In principle, this applies as early as birth: the "acute crisis" of vaginal delivery (the risks of which continue to eclipse most acute childhood illnesses) protects children against allergies whereas children born by Caesarean section "more frequently have greater sensitivity to food allergens and episodes of wheezing and gasping breathing at the age of two", according to a prospective birth cohort study in Germany (LISA) [Brokow 2008, 253].

1 Elephants excrete largely undigested plant fibre and intestinal bacteria in their dung. As their first "supplementary food" alongside milk, baby elephants ingest something of the excretions of the mother and thus naturally support their intestinal flora in "guided symbiosis". It has been shown in human development that food antigens such as gliadin are tolerated significantly better if the child is still being breast fed at the time that he or she starts to eat various kinds of mashed up food containing gliadin (▸Chap. 4.)

6.1.2 The pathogenesis of allergies and autoimmune diseases in early childhood

From an immunological perspective, the *pathogenesis* of allergic diseases is rooted in *the failure during the first year of life to transform* the immune tolerance required before birth into a functional situation after birth in which the immune system and all dependent barriers of the organism can appropriately separate themselves off. The barriers and the immune system of the allergic child can be characterized in a first approach as too open to the environment, as qualitatively delayed in their development. At the same time this gives rise – important for the consultation with the parents! – to a fundamentally favourable prognosis with regard to early childhood allergies if it is possible to help the child's immune system to mature through individual paediatric support. According to the current state of knowledge, the learning process required in this respect is decisively dependent on external living nature being present before birth and in the first year of life – in the right way, at the right time and in its most unadulterated form – so that it can be perceived and overcome by the mother's and child's organism. Because everything that human beings take in from the outside leads physiologically to them "being able to develop activity of their own" [Steiner and Wegman 1991, 49] – and this activity itself is just as essential for maintaining human health as the substance taken in and transformed through such activity. An initial impulse to develop the immune system in early childhood and unfold the capacity for separation (in which the Th1 cells play a key role) comes from the natural substances which the child encounters in the mother. Infections overcome through inflammation and fever in the first and second year of life present a further important stimulus to achieve a balance between aggressively inflammatory separation and immune tolerance, a balance between Th1 and Th2 mediated immune processes. The key thing in this respect is *the balance, the active* immune regulation of these polar qualities of the child's immune system which can only be achieved and obtained through the individual learning process of the child, through actively overcoming external (and as far as possible natural) challenges to his or her immunological capabilities. At a cellular level, regulatory T lymphocytes (Treg) play a key role in the regulation of the immune balance.

The close connection between intact barriers and this immunological transformation from a tolerant state open to the environment (Th2 regulated) to a healthily separated, regulated (Th1/Th2 balanced) state is becoming increasingly clear, for example in an understanding of atopic dermatitis. If today epidermal barrier dysfunction is understood as a key dysfunction (▸Chap. 6.4), it has in the meantime been shown that the maturation of the nonspecific and specific immune system exercises a regulatory influence on the structure of the epidermis and thus also on epidermal barrier dysfunction. In a Th_2-dominated state (typical for people suffering from atopic dermatitis) the maturation and filaggrin formation of the keratinocytes, the antimicrobial resistance of the epidermis against staphylococci, for example, is "down regulated" [Jung 2008] by the child's immune system. Not (just) genetic circumstances but a dynamic developmental process in the child's life organization determines the extent of the barrier dysfunction of the skin. And the latter is accessible to treatment. The same applies to all barrier organs of the child's organism.

In this context it is necessary to adjust one's thinking in line with the plasticity of living things and to take into account that "the Th1 and Th2 T cells each represent extreme variants of different effector T cells and that particularly in the human immune system" (!) "*fluid transitions* (emphasis as in original) are possible and can be shown to exist ..." It can today be considered as verified that the resting naive (!) "T cell (Th0 cell) is able to differentiate both into the one and the other effector type and that there is no fixed genetic programme here in the sense of Th1 and Th2 precursor cells" [Renz 1999, 123]. In this context recent research has shown that such significant immune regulatory polarization of T helper cells extends as far as "opening the chromatin structure" [Holländer et al. 2005, 117], i. e. *a transformation of the lymphocytes extending as far as the DNA*. This contradicts any genetically-based determinism! Here existing antigens and infections exercise a switching function together with the organism's own activity; thus bacterial infections above all promote Th1 differentiation in this sensitive phase of immune development. The active management of acute infections in early childhood represents an indispensable challenge for the developing immune system of the child. At a very early stage in the comparatively tempestuous development of early childhood a "stability in the functional dichotomy" of the T helper cells is formed which is of fundamental importance for further development. The *plasticity of the (thymus-dependent) T cell system, which plays a key role in immune regulation (see Section 6.3), is strongest and has the greatest effect precisely in those phases of life in which in the last 30 years allergies (atopic dermatitis) and autoaggressive diseases (early childhood type 1 diabetes mellitus, coeliac disease) have increased the most – namely in the first two years of life*. As well as in specific immunity, which can become derailed in allergies and autoimmune diseases, the T cellular system also plays a regulatory role in inflammatory processes of the *nonspecific* immune system. This system is physiologically important for example in the resistance against bacterial infections through neutrophil granulocytes. If this part of the immune system, regulated through so-called Th17 cells, is derailed, it can for example turn into the basis of an inflammatory but non-allergic asthma in the form of a neutrophilic granulocyte infiltration and inflammation.

6.1.3 Allergy prevention and paediatrics

In parallel to the acquisition of upright gait and independent walking, an initial and always individual balance of the child's immune system – the immunological individuality of the child – grows to maturity in the course of a healthy development. That is also the reason why anthroposophical paediatrics and many other colleagues working with homoeopathy are sceptical about the massive "education" of the child's immune system through immunological manipulation in the first year of life (▸Chap. 3.5). For with regard to the development of the immune regulation there is a fundamental difference between the effect of vaccination and the effect of naturally occurring infections to which the child responds with an acute inflammation; this could be shown, for example, with regard to the mumps vaccination (protection against ovarial cancer only as the result of mumps, not vaccination [Cramer et al. 2010), or the measles vaccination (protection against allergies stronger after measles than after vaccination [Rosenlund 2008]). Furthermore, vaccines present numerous problematical aspects with regard to the sensitive digestive and immune systems of the young child, for example through the preservatives and allergy-promoting additives such as aluminium hydroxide which they contain (▸Chap. 3.5). Thus Canadian epidemiologists were able to show that vaccination with pertussis antigen and aluminium hydroxide (DPT) in the first year of life can produce a clear statistical rise in the risk of asthma *depending on how early the (same!) vaccine was used in infancy* [McDonald 2008]: "The risk of asthma was reduced to ½ in children whose first dose of DPT was delayed by more than 2 months." In the light of epigenetics, such results, published in Pediatrics, are more plausible than the current German S 3 guideline for allergy prevention [Muche-

Borowski 2009] which claims: "There is no evidence that vaccination increases the allergy risk, but there are indications that vaccination could reduce the allergy risk." If that were the case, then, in view of the explosive rise in vaccinations recommended by the German Standing Vaccination Commission (STIKO), the allergy risk should have fallen dramatically since the 1980 s. Unfortunately the opposite is the case. If groups of children are compared *who in the first and second year of life are deliberately vaccinated less frequently/ later and are treated differently in the event of acute diseases* [Alm and Swartz 1999: children with an anthroposophical lifestyle were given 80 percent fewer antibiotics in the first year of life, very many fewer antipyretics and they were vaccinated against measles a lot less frequently], the result is a *very clear allergy-preventing effect* (see below). In contrast, the wording of the allergy prevention guideline contradicts the epidemiological facts and many of the studies quoted in ▸Chap. 3.5.

Vaccination, the use of antipyretics and of antibiotics is part of the standard repertoire of mainstream paediatrics in the first year of life. In the view of conventional experts, too, most prescribed antibiotics are medically without benefit during this period, for example in otitis media and tonsillitis (▸Chap. 5.1.3). There is no proven benefit of antipyretics (apart from their analgesic effect) with regard to the progression of infectious diseases, including the prevention of febrile seizures (▸Chap. 5.4), but there are considerable side effects. It is striking, then, that a study of 205,487 children from 31 countries [Beasley 2008] and a meta-analysis of this subject [Etminan 2009] produces the result that the use of *paracetamol (acetaminophen) increases the risk of asthma in childhood* (considerably if used intensively). Paracetamol can, among other things, deplete glutathione in the organism and promote a Th2-dominated immune response [Farquhar 2010]. The use of paracetamol as early as during pregnancy also appears to increase the risk of asthma; there is an observable correlation worldwide between the level of paracetamol use and the prevalence of asthma. It is remarkable how an Australian study has sought to refute this hypothesis prospectively [Lowe 2010]: the study used a cohort of children whose parents were atopic, in which 30 percent (!) of the children had "current asthma" at the age of six to seven, and in which 51 percent of the children had been given paracetamol up to the twelfth week of life (!) and 97 percent up to the second year of life! By means of this cohort, the study claims to have shown that the use of paracetamol does not have any noticeable influence on childhood asthma. There is no mention of a comparison group treated differently or, indeed, without paracetamol while the prevalence of asthma in this high-risk group lies far above the population average. This result, which in reality is not based on a comparative study and cannot be transferred to the normal population, is now popularly quoted to reject any kind of connection between paracetamol and allergy.

The quoted S 3 guideline on allergy prevention 2009 does not mention the subject of antipyresis; neither does it see any connection between the administration of antibiotics in early childhood and allergies [Muche-Borowski 2009], like many of the studies published up to 2005 [Lauener, Hansen and Wahn 2005, 316]. That claim can still be found in the review by E. von Mutius [2010], published under the editorship of D. Reinhardt, evidenced by a publication of her own from 2001, while the article does not take account of any publications after 2005 (!). Curiously the PARSIFAL study and the study by Beasley on paracetamol quoted above are missing although E. v. Mutius was involved in both of them as a co-author! V. Wahn is in the meantime taking greater care in what he says: "Although the majority of studies refer to a positive correlation between the administration of antibiotics in the first year of life and subsequent allergies/asthma ..." He also quotes a meta-analysis from 2006 [Marra et al. 2006]: "On the basis of four retrospective and four prospective studies the authors found a significant connection between the use of antibiotics and subsequent asthma" [Wahn 2006; our emphasis]. Thus the PARSIFAL study from five European countries, published in 2006, showed that the use of antibiotics in the first year of life increases the risk of developing childhood bronchial asthma by 2.79 times! Fever-suppressing antipyretics in the first year of life increased the risk of asthma by 1.54 times, the risk of atopic dermatitis by 1.32 times [Flöistrup et al. 2006]. This correlation is confirmed in other publications [Kozyrski 2007]. It is becoming increasingly clear that the way in which the treatment and prevention of acute inflammation – above all in early childhood! – is normally handled in paediatrics in countries with a western lifestyle promotes allergies and thus chronic inflammation in childhood and conflicts with current basic immunological research! The problem is not, however, restricted to early childhood.[1]

If a one-sided Th2 dominance persists, the child remains too strongly tied symbiotically to the external world and develops allergic inflammations which break down his or her barriers through chronic inflammation and put a physical and mental strain on the developing autonomy of the child (also from the perspective of too close a primary and secondary mother-child symbiosis in children suffering from neurodermatitis and bronchial asthma). Conversely, those chronic, immunologically related diseases of early childhood which are based on the opposite immune situation, above all diabetes mellitus (similarly coeliac disease), have also increased in the last thirty years. Its increase in western industrialized countries by a factor of approx. 2.5 between 1966 and 2000 has been shown not to be based on genetic causes but on environmental changes [Gillespie 2004]. The cause of the disease is thought to be a disorder of the immunological balance leaning towards a one-sided Th1-mediated immune status leading to an excessive, autoaggressively decompensated, Th1 cell-mediated degradation process (in diabetes, degradation of the pancreatic islet cells). It becomes clear that in the course of the child's immune development the identification with his or her own bodily nature must be acquired just as much as the separation from external nature. Both of these capacities support each other, both represent the reciprocal condition for the development of a stable, resilient immunological balance. There are studies which show that the clinical manifestation of either bronchial asthma or type 1 diabetes reduces the risk of falling ill with the other disease. But there are equally indications that both diseases in their rising prevalence are increasing in association with one another [Raile and Kiess 2005, 188]. If we understand the way in which individual equilibrium typically develops in the human organism, the way it underlies immune regulation (but also, for example, human upright posture!), it is no longer surprising that bronchial asthma/atopic dermatitis and type 1 diabetes mellitus/coeliac disease have increased dramatically and in parallel above all between 1965 and 2000 in western industrialized nations [2] despite their apparent polar immunological genesis: because equilibrium always mediates between polarities and when equilibrium is not achieved this finds corresponding expression in the increase of both possible extremes. It

1 In this connection we warmly recommend to all our medical colleagues the result of the study by Velicer [2004] which documented an increased risk of breast cancer of up to more than double depending on the previous use of antibiotics.

2 Thus Rosenbauer [2002] reports that type 1 diabetes mellitus among girls in the Düsseldorf area increased by 4.3 percent per year between 1987 and 2000.

has been shown that the genetic base point of the population during this period did not materially change: "Hence it is above all environmental factors – and not 'diabetes genes' – which are responsible for the rapid increase in the prevalence of type 1 diabetes in the last 10 to 20 years" [Raile and Kiess 2005, 185]. But only an understanding of the epigenetics creates the opportunity at a scientific level to approach this contemporary phenomenon on a new level, namely the way in which the child's organism regulates its genetic material. From the perspectives of anthroposophic medicine, *this process is not decided at the level of the physical body but at the level of the life organization, the etheric body*. A key point here is the understanding that these environmental factors are *not causal reasons* but necessary, if not always present, *conditions for the achievement of maturity* in the development of the immune system and thus in the all-encompassing physical individualization of the child.

Such an understanding provides a wider perspective with regard to the question: why are children in today's western industrial societies increasingly unable to achieve and maintain an immunological balance? Thus W. Kiess [2001] quotes a Swedish study [Hagloof 1994] which shows the influence of the *experience of serious loss* in childhood on the incidence of diabetes, for example moving house, divorce of parents, death of a parent or near relative. The authors have been left with the strong impression from daily practice that *mobility of lifestyle and unstable ties (*between the parents, ambivalence towards the child, ambivalence towards the place they live and the people who live there) do little to help the soul-spiritual individuality of the child anchor itself in the body (embodiment, incarnation) and thus also form an obstacle to harmonious immune regulation.[1] For the ability to create and maintain equilibrium is strongly connected in the human organism with the activity of the I-organization.[2]

The "*western lifestyle*" has been significantly influenced by the Anglo-American world which, on the other hand, also has the highest rate of children with allergies. In an American cohort study, the incidence of new cases of asthma in the first 13 years of life was determined in six cross-sectional studies: *in boys the cumulative risk of falling ill with asthma during this period was 43.6 percent, in girls 23.5 percent.* Within western countries there is a clear *gradient of incidence in Europe from west to east,* the highest prevalence of allergic diseases is in Great Britain and Australia/New Zealand; from 1964 to 1994, with identical study criteria, asthma in Scotland increased by 2.5 times, pollinosis by four times and eczema by three times in the eight to 13 age range. This increase in the frequency of allergic diseases has not slowed down in any way through the successful treatment of, for example, bronchial asthma [von Mutius 2005, 254–256]. In contrast, acute, non-obstructive inflammation of the airways in the first years of life is associated with significantly reduced serum IgE levels and skin prick test rates in later years. In children in rural Papua New Guinea, the rate of acute inflammation of the upper airways was four times as high as in comparable children in Great Britain; bronchial asthma hardly occurs in children in Papua New Guinea. *The fall in acute inflammation* in (above all early) childhood *correlates directly with a rise in chronic allergic inflammation.* Jean-Francois Bach summarizes these findings in remarkable words in a review in the *New England Journal of*

1 The same applies with regard to the need for achievement in the family which has taken on a life of its own (borne by the super-I).

2 For patients with type 1 diabetes mellitus, M.Girke [2010, 287–310] has comprehensively developed and published perspectives of anthroposophic medicine which provide a deeper understanding of this disease and the associated typical constitution.

Medicine: "There is certain irony in the fact that we must now search for new ways to reproduce the infectious diseases against which we have been fighting with great success over the past three decades (!). The challenge is an important one because of the high morbidity of allergic and autoimmune diseases" [Bach 2002]. Sociologically it has, furthermore, "long been observed that allergic diseases *are a disease of the affluent classes*" [von Mutius 1999a, 163]. Single children tend to be more affected – partly, but perhaps not only, because they suffer from fewer acute inflammations in the early years of life than children who have older siblings or grow up in close proximity with other children. But a western lifestyle is characteristic not only of the people and lifestyles in places where allergies are prevalent and manifest at an early stage, but today it is also decisively a characteristic of *the system of medicine used to treat children on the basis of natural science.* Job himself is the rich, superficially happy centre of his world, subjectively wholly god-fearing, but filled, above all, with the feeling that he is just in his actions and working in the spirit of God – so that he is due a rich reward. Is the "western lifestyle", "mainstream medicine" not characterized precisely by this basic attitude of fundamentally being on the indubitably correct path? Do people not increasingly believe in this respect in the dream of autopoiesis, in being able to give rise by themselves to wealth and happiness up to and including a carefree virtual mental world and the cloning of genetically perfect bodies? [Fuchs 1999] People of the "first world" have long left Job far behind. Job encounters the "opposer" at a time when he no longer has any outer obstacles to overcome. In the western lifestyle, human beings encounter inflammation in a new, chronic and allergic form at a time when their power and endeavour to suppress or prevent acute inflammatory diseases is at an historical high. Epidemiology shows: *preventing acute inflammatory diseases in early childhood and the rise of chronic allergic inflammation in childhood are directly related. And this suppression is "passed on" to the next generation in that individuals who suffer from allergies have many more children suffering from allergies than people without allergies.* That this has *nothing to do with the genome itself* is proven precisely by the case of the divided Germany where, with a genetically completely comparable population, 40 years of different lifestyle (at a "high level" in relation to the world as a whole) was sufficient to create a difference in the prevalence of allergic diseases between East and West of up to 300 percent – and in which after reunification 20 years were enough to make that difference disappear [Schlaud 2007]. No one to date has been able to demonstrate a physically and morphologically recordable change in the genetic material of people with allergies; the fact, however, that the *parental allergic process, which functionally takes place in the life sphere, affects the children virtually in a "dose-effect relationship"* is of the greatest importance. Clearly the aspect of the life sphere, the human life organization, must be distinguished from the physically describable genome. The suppression of acute inflammatory diseases *weakens living immunological capacities, not the genome.* Hahnemann already referred to this in his "psora doctrine", in which he explains that the suppression of acute inflammatory diseases – illustrated using the example of parasitic skin diseases – leads to a *weakening of the organism's living capacity to react,* which is transferred as such to the next generation: which is why in the treatment of chronic diseases according to Hahnemann it is fundamentally a matter of countering the incorrect handling of acute inflammatory diseases in the medical history of the patient and in the life of the preceding generation [Hahnemann 1985, 131.]. *"Inherited characteristics"* thus contain a *physical aspect which can be crystallized out* and a *living functional aspect.* That is also supported by the idea of so-called "maternal imprinting": both manifestation rate and degree of seriousness of childhood atopic eczema are more strongly influenced by whether the mother also suffers or suffered from a similar illness than by a corresponding allergic disease of the father [Höger 2005, 144]. The reason lies in the sustained influence exercised by the maternal organism on the epigenetic development of the unborn child which has already been shown to exist as early as conception (as part of IVF research). In the meantime, the so-called "agouti model" regarding epigenetically influenced risks of disease passed on over generations says:

"Passing on epigenetic marks from one generation to the next is fundamentally possible." [Krauss-Etschmann 2010, 147]

That corresponds precisely to Hahnemann's psora doctrine (if it is related to "suppression" *in early childhood* and the epidemiological observations on the incidence of allergic diseases. At the same time, however, the following applies:

In principle, atopic syndromes are *reversible* when looked at over several generations; there is *no underlying chromosomally and genetically* set deviation of the body but a historically induced *weakness, an epigenetically acquired regulatory disorder of bodily functions*. Such a disorder of the child's life organization can be rebalanced through diet and treatment and is not inevitably passed on from one generation to the next. To achieve this, foods and medicines are required which do not have a suppressive but a stimulating and harmonizing effect on the child's life processes.

This aspect is also important in parental counselling, particularly if the parents themselves display atopic syndromes. The study by Alm and Swartz [1999] shows that a change of lifestyle, allowing the classic childhood diseases and reducing antipyretic and antibiotic chemotherapeutic drugs can lower the occurrence of atopic syndromes by forty to fifty percent as quickly as within one generation. The PARSIFAL study, which i. a. looked at the allergy prevalence in Waldorf pupils whose parents suffered a high level of allergies (and displayed the highest educational standard among all the comparison groups, i. e. a further risk factor) [Alfven, Brown-Fahrländer et al. 2005], was able to show that through an "anthroposophical lifestyle" these children at risk displayed fewer allergies than the control group: *The increase of allergies does not have to be an irreversible process!* The details of the study already referred to above show that i. a. the paediatric treatment of acute febrile inflammation with the minimum amount of suppression possesses a decisive prophylactic quality with regard to allergies. Epidemiology thus provides evidence that a suppression-focused medical approach to treatment can have an effect which *exacerbates the problem* and leaves the opportunity unused of developing *a treatment which in the long term can provide a way out of the increasing prevalence of allergies – both as regards the individual patient and subsequent generations. The findings of the "hygiene hypothesis" must finally be included in the treatment of children and not just remain something with which epidemiologists are familiar*!

The natural science-fixated paediatric medicine of the western world continues to see its mandate as the *a priori* minimization of inflammatory pathological processes in childhood through vaccination and hygiene – and stokes scientifically unfounded fears of fever and acute inflammatory diseases. The losses which are caused through hygiene to normal skin flora,[1] through antibiosis to intestinal flora and through the absence of inflammatory diseases to immunological competence are known – yet nevertheless continue to be accepted. At the same time allergology, in the context of the hygiene hypothesis, has shown the negative impact of such measures on the long-term health of children. If, then, allergic diseases occur as a result of this situation, which is no more than a part of wider social allergy-promoting developments, *the therapeutic approach of paediatric allergology is in turn once again fixated on suppression and elimination.* No one will want to claim that the "immune deviation" of people with allergies would as such be positively corrected by topical steroids, antihistamines etc.; the uncritically propagated success of steroids in the treatment of bronchial asthma and allergic rhinitis is already being countered in the treatment of atopic eczema, where steroids have been used for a long time, through the gradual withdrawal of corticoids from widespread use – not least because of negative long-term experiences of patients.

Western-oriented societies *and purely natural science-oriented* medicine must wake up to the realization that *they themselves are significantly responsible* for the problem of the rapid growth of allergic diseases. Since the training and skills of every doctor today are significantly the result of such an orientation and the services associated with it, this represents a painful moment of self-awareness for everyone. *Just because we can acutely suppress a problem does not by any means imply that we are not involved in the creation and perpetuation of the problem.*

Clear consequences can be derived from what has been set out above with regard to a reduction in the incidence of allergic diseases, i. e. with regard to disease prevention, even at this still little differentiated level of understanding of the diseases. In the view and experience of the authors, the perspectives developed in ▸Chap. 2 to ▸Chap. 5 with regard to our understanding of diseases, their prevention and treatment – perspectives which have as their objective to strengthen the child's individuality down into his or her physical capacities actively to overcome illness and identify with his or her own physical body – entail a relevant approach to the prevention of allergic diseases.

This is empirically shown most clearly in a comparative study from Sweden by Alm and Swartz which was published in May 1999 [Alm and Swartz 1999]. The authors from the Swedish Karolinska Institute compare a total of 675 pupils with the result that the Waldorf pupils, particularly those with an "anthroposophical lifestyle", suffer from allergies to a significantly lesser extent than pupils at a conventional school (13 percent versus 25 percent). The study describes an "anthroposophical lifestyle" as a form of living which resulted in the pupils in the study being given "decisively fewer antibiotics and vaccinations", having caught "infectious diseases such as measles, rubella and chickenpox to a greater extent" and having eaten "more organic food, above all preserved by fermentation with lactobacilli". With regard to so-called genetic risks, passive smoking and owning furred animals there were no significant differences. In detail, only 18 percent of the Waldorf pupils had been vaccinated against measles/mumps/rubella (93 percent in the comparison group); 61 percent of the Waldorf pupils had had measles (compared to four percent in the control group). So far only 39 percent of Waldorf pupils had been given antipyretics in contrast to 89 percent in the control group, for antibiotics this was 52 percent versus 90 percent. With regard to their medical history, 5.1 percent of Waldorf pupils had

1 The physiological skin flora comprises approx. eight million micro-organisms/cm^2 of skin [Jachens 1999a, 52]; with regard to intestinal flora ibid. 61ff.

suffered from atopic dermatitis (compared to 8.2 percent of the control group); *to date only 2.7 percent displayed atopical dermatitis compared to 8.9 percent in the control group. This shows that the lifestyle and style of treatment of the families had a very clear effect on the risk of falling ill from an allergy.* With regard to bronchial asthma, 5.8 percent of Waldorf pupils and 17 percent of the comparison group were affected. *The effective prevention of allergic diseases requires a change in the way that parents, teachers and doctors think and act* and thus *a transformation of paediatric medicine as a whole* – not just paediatric allergology.

Allergic diseases represent a testing time for patients, parents and doctors. In its concrete form, an allergic disease is always individual. It challenges the soul through suffering and reveals a deviation in the life processes. People with allergies are restricted, unfree, thrown back on their own resources in their sensory experience of the world, in overcoming and separating themselves from the world as well as in uniting with the world. Historically, allergies are found as potential illnesses where the individuality has become detached from its integration into nature, into the cosmically determined rhythms, into ongoing traditional ways of life. Allergies accompany human beings who seek the way to freedom and as a result are at risk of losing the connection to their own body and to nature – and thus the connection to the foundation of their own creation.

A general phased treatment plan which responds to the allergic inflammatory activity of the child's *own* organism in a uniform and suppressive way cannot meet the requirements of this situation. Not the inflammation but the failure in the *management of the immunological event* (which, being allergic, is typically afebrile!) is the basic problem of people with allergies. Only an individual approach to paediatrics can strengthen children in their developing individuality in such a way that in the long term an *increase in health* replaces the current shocking rise in allergic diseases.

6.2 Atopic syndromes and nutrition

> We will not come to an understanding of the healthy and sick human organism if we imagine that any kind of substance from external nature taken in with nutrition simply continues to work in the same way inside the organism. It is not a question of continuing the action observed in the substance outside the human organism but of overcoming it.
>
> R. Steiner, I. Wegman [1991, 25]

Klemens von Pirquet in 1906 coined the term "allergy" for the phenomenon that people do not always respond in the same way to substances which they imbibe or with which they come into contact from the outside but that they can develop both a – substance-specific – *over-sensitivity* and excessive activity or, indeed, the opposite (cf. for example desensitization). Oversensitivity can develop above all with regard to *substances containing protein:* "Proteins, particularly those which are clearly distinguished from the body's own proteins" [Holländer 1999, 58], are the most important so-called "antigens". *In their specific configuration, these proteins are the result of foreign life activity.* "The absorbed protein is initially a foreign body in the human organism if it is taken as food. It contains the after-effects of the etheric processes of the living being from which it has been taken. They must be completely removed from the protein. It must be absorbed into the etheric activity of the human organism" [Steiner and Wegman 1977, 55]. A classic example of the development of an allergy is the infant cow's milk allergy. The human newborn is completely oriented towards the mother and her breast milk, which is directly related to the inner environment of the infant. If, for example, the newborn is fed in the middle of the night by a well-meaning nurse on the maternity ward with a bottle of milk which still contains intact cow's milk protein, then, in the first instance, *the child is tricked:* it does not receive what it is expecting; it is *irritated* in its perception. The child's digestive system is still immature, it is still developing; foreign protein cannot yet be sufficiently broken down and can all too easily permeate the intestinal wall. Thus it can often happen in cases such as the one described above that the cow's milk protein penetrates the inside of the organism *untransformed, i. e. in the specific protein structure formed by the cow,* and must then be *broken down, digested and excreted at the wrong location.* This fact is reflected in the meaning of the term *"atopic syndrome"* (topos: a place).

Today "atopic syndrome" describes a substance-specific IgE synthesis of the organism. But the latter is a consequence of the atopic syndrome presented in the example which arises from the presence of something foreign, a substance specific to foreign life, inside one's own organism. *The atopic syndrome initiates the formation of a pathological memory in the organism* which is expressed in the synthesis of antigen-specific IgE. In the event of renewed contact, this immunoglobulin catalyzes *"excess digestive activity"* which is intended to prevent, *at the barriers of the organism already,* the repeated penetration of the substance which triggered the atopic syndrome in the first place. Thus the same infant who drank a bottle of milk after birth can develop diarrhoea, eczema or indeed obstructive bronchitis during weaning after renewed contact with cow's milk – although at that point he or she might well be in a position to digest the offered cow's milk. But he or she is prevented from doing so by the pathological memory which has been created as the result of the *premature contact, the premature overpowering of his or her integrity.*

This formation of a pathological memory represents a decisive deviation from healthy forgetting. It is noteworthy purely from a language point of view that the word "for-get" contains the word "get"; the syllable "for" as a prefix means away, opposite (e. g. forbid, forbear, forswear). The organism can forget what it "got" in the right way, for example through nutrition, and was able to break down fully in the digestion process. (Similarly, the German word "ver-gessen" contains the reciprocally intensifying preposition "ver" – found in "vergeben", "vergleichen", vertragen, etc. – in front of the word "essen", to eat). Here the focus is on the digestive and *nonspecific immune system.* The later, for example, is activated by every febrile infection so that it is not surprising that these acute inflammatory diseases fundamentally promote immunological normergy. A healthy digestion arises from the *correspondence between perceptual and digestive activity, between learning and forgetting.* Learning assumes a corresponding perceptive ability and an active interest; and those people learn best who can develop their own activity from what they have learnt. We can forget what we have mastered; abilities are developed in a rhythm of learning and forgetting in "digesting what we have learnt".

Nutrition – and, more comprehensively, every sensory impression – gives cause for our organism to develop activity of its own (ergy). This starts at the barriers (skin, intestinal and respiratory epithelium) and is primarily *perceptual.* There are sense organs in all barriers of the organism. Every sense organ is organized in such a way that it allows the external world to penetrate it in a controlled way, only allowing in a specific "impression" fixed and selected by the organ. The latter then generates a corresponding internal activity, a perception, while the entering stimulus or substance is broken down. *It is not allowed to penetrate the barriers, the sense organs untransformed; on the contrary, in the process of perception it must become a complete part of the organism's own activity.* Sensory perception on the one hand links the soul and spiritual element intensively with the external world – up to and including conscious perception which only forms a part of the perceptions of the organism – while on the other hand separating the inner life of the body from the environment. The human organism is dependent on absorbing from the environment *in a suitable form* ponderables (e. g. from nutrition) and imponderables (e. g. light effects). To this end it must transform and break down what comes from the outside in such a way that it no longer has any quality imprinted by a foreign organism adhering to it (e. g. protein structures of cow's milk or chicken protein) and that what is absorbed from the outside fully integrates into the organism's own activity. This breakdown, this transformation starts with the activity of the organism at its barriers and the associated organs (glands, teeth, etc.). The organism can be relieved of breaking down foreign substance to a certain extent through the preparation of food (e. g. cooking, baking) but it can also be made more difficult (e. g. through gluten in modern types of grain that is difficult to digest, through food additives). Each foreign substance must be broken down in a specific manner, which can only happen in the right way where previously and simultaneously the foreign substance has been properly "grasped" in a timely way in the process of perceiving it. For children, food must be "comprehensible" and transparent – in a way that is appropriate for their age and the maturity of their digestive tract. This quality is often questionable in the foods commercially available today. Thus there has to date been almost no research on whether carrots from hybrid seeds developed using advanced technology purely with yield in mind are less easily digestible than traditional single-origin carrots – yield-focused agricultural seed research does not currently consider how well human beings can tolerate the resulting produce but follows purely commercial criteria. Indeed, most carrots, including organic ones, today come from hybrids! The increase which has been observable in practice of intolerance reactions to carrots may to a considerable extent also be due to this change in the seed stock.

The same applies to the homogenization of cow's milk which changes the protein distribution in the milk, shortens the time which the milk spends in the digestive tract and makes the necessary break down of the cow's milk protein in the digestive tract more difficult [Beck and Forster 2002] – while studies show that raw "farm milk" which has not been processed in a dairy has a protective effect against allergies in the children of farmers (▸Chap. 6.1.1). Here the influence of such milk on the intestinal flora of the mother during pregnancy is already of significance, a finding which has inspired allergy prevention through prebiotics and probiotics, such as giving Lactobacillus GG to pregnant women and children in the first year of life [Kalliomäki 2001]. It is also assumed that the vegetables preserved by fermentation with lactobacilli given to 70 percent of children with an anthroposophical lifestyle in the study by Alm and Swartz [1999] quoted above played a role in the outstandingly positive study results, while conversely the clear increase in allergic asthma after the administration of antibiotics in the first year of life is linked to the sustained disorder of intestinal flora in childhood, the physiological development of which requires the first three years of life (!)[cf. Kummer 2005b]. These studies sugggest that the trend towards the devitalization of food, and towards disorders of the mother's and child's intestinal flora through industrially modified foods and medicines, prepares the ground for allergies (90 percent of all German infants aged nine months are or were already given preserved foods – the usual baby jars – that are often older than the child itself. The only conclusion to be drawn from this is that *foods which are as natural, fresh or appropriately preserved as possible* (e.g. dried cereals, stored fruit) should be used in the nutrition of mothers and children, thus giving the child the necessary impulses and possibilities for building up his or her digestive system. If, for example, a pregnant woman eats raw sauerkraut in quantities she can tolerate, probiotics become largely superfluous and the tendency for fungal diseases during pregnancy is also reduced. The tragedy of the allergic child is that in advanced stages of the disease extensive restrictions to, for example, hydrolized foods may become necessary. But even then we should ask: through which natural sensory experiences in the digestion can the zest for life and the child's own activity in the digestive tract be stimulated again and supported?

In small children, the ability to digest in the right way substance taken in from the outside and adapt it to the inner environment is only just developing. Here *sensory perception is working directly to form the body in a specific way* [Goebel and Glöckler 2005, 309] as the organs only develop fully through perceptual stimulation and the child's own activity – irrespective of whether we are looking at the brain or the intestine. From this perspective, *breastfeeding* provides an ideal mental and physical education: the human mother breastfeeds her child face to face and she should do it with the same concentration on the drinking child as the suckling child normally concentrates with all its power on taking in the nutrition. Initially, the breast milk itself takes on the digestive activity of the intestinal tract to a large extent; it supports both the perceptive and digestive ability of the infant (▸Chap. 4.1). It is breast milk which enables full development of the *barrier function* of the intestinal mucous membrane. The protein of the breast milk can be assimilated by the child almost completely because it is configured in such a way that it integrates into the child's organic activity almost seamlessly; among other things, it places very little burden on the *kidneys* (low burden of nitrogen substances that must be excreted). We know today that breastfeeding – which as an interpersonal act represents more than just the passing on of breast milk – is of key importance in developing the immune system. Inextricably linked with breastfeeding is its importance with regard to the soul and spiritual development of children and their ability to relate to the world around them. Breastfeeding has an allergy preventing effect [allergy prevention guideline, Muche-Borowski 2009] and in particular prevents autoimmune diseases such as Crohn's disease, diabetes mellitus and celiac disease (▸Chap. 4.7). Lifestyle and nutrition of the mother are also reflected in the composition of breast milk and influence the child's immunological development: "Epigenetic marks can in principle be influenced by nutrition" [Krauss-Etschmann 2010, 147]. In practice this means that already from a gynaecological perspective detailed nutritional advice for pregnant women is important – including, as appropriate, the optimization of intestinal symbiosis as well as the avoidance as far as possible of antibiotics and toxicologically damaging dental procedures (amalgam removal!) or similar things. Nutritional advice for pregnant and breastfeeding women should not lead to a fearful attitude of avoidance but open up positive possibilities of healthy enjoyment.

6.3 General treatment of allergic diseases

Throw away the stone of today. Forget and sleep. If it is light you will find it again tomorrow, before dawn, transformed into sun.

J. R. Jiménez

In their impaired immunological development, in the changed interaction between the soul elements and the body, children with atopic dermatitis, bronchial asthma and pollinosis display common fundamental aspects, even if the manifestations of the disease are different and the over-sensitivity to certain antigens is not the only triggering cause. From a therapeutic point of view these common elements must first be grasped before gradually individualizing the treatment.

In the treatment of children suffering from allergies, adhering to a *sequence of basic therapeutic steps* and clearly discussing this with the parents before the start of the treatment has been effective. The intensive collaboration which will be required makes it necessary to give the parents an idea of the *time* that the treatment will take and, as far as possible, the prognosis of the disease. When there are pronounced symptoms, successful treatment will generally comprise a period of two to four years; even where there is rapid therapeutic success, the child's development must be carefully observed for the whole of the period indicated above and situations which could trigger an allergic response avoided as far as possible. In most cases the allergic inflammation can be largely or fully cured; that must be the clear aim of the treatment. On the other hand the doctor must try to be as realistic as possible with his or her prognosis in each individual case. In key aspects the amount of time required and the possibilities of the treatment depend on the child's development: in infant atopic dermatitis the aim should be to complete the treatment by the third year of life, in bronchial asthma in a child of school age every effort must be made to achieve a cure by the onset of puberty. By setting the timeframe of the treatment broadly enough for the parents at the beginning, the – otherwise almost unavoidable – pressure created by the expectation of rapid success, which would otherwise prevent the realignment of the child's constitution and his or her environment, is avoided.

6.3.1 Basic therapeutic steps

In the *first stage of treatment*, it is necessary to *remove* the child from the *causes which trigger allergies*. The aim of this measure is to relieve the organism of what it cannot manage, what it cannot actively "forget" (▸Chap. 6.2). Abstention in the case of allergies entails two things: exclusion from the uninhibited involvement in life and fasting – and thus simultaneously a restriction to what is essential and elementary. This is only possible if the parents actively support this measure, which must be guided and directed by the doctor in a very sensitive way. Then the discovery of new essential, life-supporting qualities can be set against painful abstinence already in this first step. This therapeutic step is intended to enable the child to "forget", initially in a passive way through external restrictions; if the period for this is sufficiently long and if the general immunological competence of the child is strengthened, the reaction caused by the atopic syndrome (e. g. to cow's milk) will disappear in many cases.

As the *second stage of treatment*, it is necessary to restore *the equilibrium* in the child's organism at every level:

- through restoring missing trace elements with regard to matter and substance, for example through appropriate nutrition;
- through supporting and regulating the digestion and vital regenerative processes which are generally impaired in children with allergic diseases and are insufficiently grasped by their soul organization;
- through the stimulation of the immunological digestive and regulatory organs;
- through creating a fundamental constitutional balance in the interaction between perception and consciousness on the one hand, digestion and regeneration on the other (nervous and sensory pole and metabolic pole) which typically become one-sided in children with allergic diseases;
- through *strengthening the physical presence of the child's individuality* and thus the ability of the child to regulate and regain the required equilibrium at the level of the warmth organization, feeling and movement, the regulatory rhythmical processes, the immune system.

In the third stage it is necessary to integrate the child harmoniously back into life. The first two therapeutic stages already make it possible for the soul aspect to find a new relationship to the body, to learn to intervene in the right way. Now it is important for this soul aspect also to connect properly with the environment. Finding the right integration into the family, into a social context, into nature and the world of matter is the objective with which the child and his or her parents are supported in this phase.

The extent of therapeutic intervention and its duration will be different in each case; but using the general sequence of stages as a guide for treatment is necessary and helpful in maintaining the required alert attentiveness and orientation towards the patient, his or her parents and oneself in what can often be very changeable range of symptoms.

Even Hahnemann as he grew older came round – after decades of strictly individualized simile treatment – to treating chronic diseases initially with "typical remedies" (above all sulphur in a low LM potency), following this with a more individualized therapy [Seiler 1988]. As his reason for doing so he cited the *curtailment of the organism's ability to react which always precedes chronic diseases.* This means that it can no longer overcome harmful influences from the environment, for example, with an acute inflammatory response but enters a chronic state of weakness which it can no longer manage without help. In this situation a general lifting and support of the organism's vitality, combined with stimulating elimination is a prerequisite in Hahnemann's view for the organism to be able to react properly to an individualized homoeopathic remedy.

In their introduction to the chapter "Typical cases of illness", R. Steiner and I. Wegman make a similar point [1991, 98f.]: "The remedies must therefore be so constituted as not only to roll back the process of the disease but also support the decreasing vitality again. The latter action will have to be undertaken in part by diet during the illness. In more serious cases of illness, however, the organism is not in a fit state to develop sufficient vitality as it processes the food. It will therefore be necessary to organize the treatment itself in such a way that the organism is given support in this respect."

It is recommended for all children with allergic diseases to start with a general basic therapy which fundamentally activates and supports the digestive, elimination and regenerative processes of the organism and thus the physical foundation of the immune system.

Any subsequent individualized treatment will be all the more effective and thorough – and this next step may not even always be necessary.

6.3.2 Unburdening the organism – ordering and eliminating allergenic causes

In principle, people are generally familiar with this method of treatment today; it presumes that a careful medical history has been taken. In detail, the following is involved:

- *Foods* which have been identified through exposure and/or testing as being allergenic must be eliminated or, where possible, reduced to a manageable level. Food with a strongly allergenic effect must be given up for a sufficiently long period of time; but it should be checked regularly in any case whether the initially allergenic food can in fact be tolerated again. Food additives and preservatives should be avoided as a matter of principle; organic and, in particular, biodynamic foods are recommended. Genetically modified foods represent a further burden for the organism; the best tolerance is produced by grains and vegetables which have not been cultivated as hybrid seeds to produce greater yields but which are of a single variety.
- *Inhalation allergens:* when looking at mattresses, floors and curtains, etc. (house dust/mites) we should also always check whether there is *underfloor heating* which can produce particularly unfavourable air conditions and exposure and it should be switched off wherever possible. In these cases there is generally a considerable lack of moisture in the air when the heating is on; taking a measurement using an (inexpensive) hygrometer is to be preferred over guesswork (ideal is 50–60 % humidity and sufficient ventilation). On the other hand, modern insulation measures can promote mould formation and too much humidity in the air so attention should be paid to that as well because mould in the house can have a detrimental effect. The way in which ventilation and heating are used is of material importance, also with regard to pollen and ozone levels in living areas.
- When ensuring that the bed is "*decontaminated*", care should be taken to ensure that the child is kept suitably *warmly covered* at night – there is almost always a natural alternative to a synthetic bed cover. A study by Woodcook et al. [2005] showed that synthetic pillows, for example, had more fungal colonies than down pillows! That does not mean recommending down pillows; but natural and washable materials should be given preference. This all the more so as in many studies and one meta-analysis [Götzsche 2008] *no benefit from the recommended "decontamination" (encasings, etc.) could be shown to exist for patients, e.g. the FEV_1 each morning in children with asthma, despite its action on the house mites contamination*! [arznei-telegrammt 5/2008] If the attempt is nevertheless made to reduce the number of mites, the neem product milbiol® has shown a positive effect in reducing house dust mites e.g. on mattresses and soft furnishings [Rembold 2004]. In its traditional use in India, neem has for centuries shown that it can be well tolerated by humans as opposed e.g. to the benzyl benzoate-containing acaricides (e.g. Acarosan®)…
- *Animal hair, feathers:* keeping animals *inside* the house tends to be unusual on farms! It has generally been shown in recent years to be the case that contact of the mother with animals during pregnancy does not have a negative effect and that working in the byre on farms can be protective. On the other hand, a proven allergy of the child to a pet, above all when it lives in the house, represents a strong argument for removing the

animal from the family. Allergies to cat [Muche-Borowski 2009.337] and horse hair pose a particular problem.

- *Pollen*: here holidays or a cure, for example in the birch pollen season, can provide temporary relief until the treatment begins to take effect. On the other hand, travel during the pollen season can particularly promote allergies!
- *Environmental medical site appraisal:* the collaboration with a reputable, experienced assessor is becoming increasingly important in practice. Exposure to formaldehyde and similar things corrupts the barrier function of the organism and weakens many different organ functions. If the sources of the exposure remain unknown, there is a risk of long-term, cumulative chronic poisoning which is difficult to reverse. We refer to energy-saving light bulbs, introduced as a result of the EU, which contain mercury vapour: if such a lamp breaks, toxic mercury with high vapour pressure is released and quickly spreads throughout the whole room. That is precisely why mercury thermometers were originally abolished. The authors expressly warn against the use of such bulbs in rooms in which children are also present.

If, backed up by blood and urine tests as necessary, a toxic load has been determined in the patent, the elimination of the poison can be stimulated through

- **Okoubaca D(2–)4**
- **Berberis D3 aa dil.** (various manufacturers)
  3–7 gtt. 3 x/d and
- **Coriander** ∅ Ceres
  1–5 gtt. 1 x/d (gradually increase dose)

combined, as necessary, with a single daily administration of the relevant poison in homoeopathic form potentized to D6–30 (made up by Staufen or other pharmacies equipped to do so), 5–7 pillules.

Particularly with regard to atopic dermatitis in infancy, *an amalgam burden of the mother* should be considered (for example if the mother has amalgam fillings and gold crowns at the same time) (▶ Chap. 6.4.3.1.3).

A toxic burden in the mother or the child should fundamentally be considered when well-chosen, usually successful treatments fail to show any effect. Experience shows that in such cases it is often necessary first to carry out suitable "draining off" procedures so that the organism becomes sufficiently capable of reacting.

- *Electromagnetic pollution where the child sleeps*, for example, can also be determined and corrected. There can be high toxic burdens in modern, non-organic agriculture. The exacerbation of allergic symptoms can also be observed in people who live next to fields and meadows which have been sprayed with pesticides and insecticides.
- *Avoiding situations which promote allergies:* we should particularly mention chlorinated *indoor swimming pools* here which are often visited as part of primary school activities. Here sufficient time out is indispensable for the allergy treatment to work. But chlorinated swimming pools and indoor swimming pools also pose a problem from a preventive perspective: "Swimming pool attendance during infancy is associated with a higher risk of bronchiolitis, with ensuing increased risk of asthma and allergy sensitization" [Voisin 2010]. Learning to swim has reduced deaths through drowning among children by 75 % since 1970. On the other hand, studies show that

e.g. in 10-year-old children the effect of swimming as a baby can still be shown to produce increased inflammatory markers, a rise in bronchitic and asthmatic symptoms in comparison to non-baby swimmers [Nickmilder 2006, overview in Argiroffo 2006]. Conclusion: children should if at all possible learn to swim outdoors – but they should learn to swim!

If we look in summary at the points mentioned, it becomes apparent that the allergic child poses a challenge to his or her fellow human beings to adjust their thinking, to become sensitive and perceptive to what a "western lifestyle" means for the life and development of a person. Only when this dimension enters the awareness of doctors, parents and children will the initial therapeutic step indicated here really become a step towards healing, will the associated need to give things up be something we are willing to do of our own accord – thereby mediating a new, permanent understanding.

Nutritional advice (▸Chap. 4.6)*is particularly important with regard to therapeutic success and future collaboration.* That is why it should at first be given by the doctor, even if working with a nutritional advisor, the formation of patient groups, information from a relevant cookery course, etc. can be very helpful and important in putting it into practice further down the line. In order to determine the tolerance to food of the individual patient, a thorough nutritional anamnesis (nutritional record, ▸Chap. 4.6) can lead the way. In the ongoing process the mother herself should above all creatively learn to discover what new nutritional opportunities exist for her child and the whole family which have not so far been explored. The regular repeated check of nutritional records allows the doctor to check and enhance the sustainability of his or her advice.

Milk substitute for infants with cow's milk intolerance following weaning or if there is insufficient breast milk remains a particular problem. *The first requirement is that there should be clear signs of a cow's milk intolerance as this often exists only in the imagination.* The authors recommend starting with breast feeding and (only![1]) after the age of six months to begin the attempt to build up nutrition with non-homogenized fresh demeter milk in a suitable dilution, starting with 2/3 milk [Goebel, Glöckler 2008, 340]. This is because the protein in non-homogenized cow's milk is easier to digest than after homogenization (e.g. powdered milk) as the fat treatment of the milk is of key importance with regard to the presentation and digestion of the milk protein and the speed at which the milk passes through the intestine [Beck and Forster 2002].

Unfortunately, *mare's milk* – under other circumstances an ideal replacement for breast milk [Bühlbäcker 1996] – may not be tolerated either by infants suffering from allergic diseases (there have been individual instances where there has been an excellent treatment course with tolerance of mare's milk). The advantage of mare's milk (with sufficient (3–4 %) substitution of oil and carbohydrates (e.g. corn starch) is that it causes the susceptibility to infection in children to fall strongly and supports the maturation of the immune

6

1 If breast feeding is impossible, mares milk (with added fat and starch) is not tolerated or too expensive and breast milk is not accepted or available from a donor, the authors advise the use of a supplemented adapted milk in the first six months of life. The benefit of hypoallergenic nutrition in allergy prevention is negligible, its negative effects e.g. on the sense of smell and taste in children (and thus their long-term eating and instinctive behaviour with regard to foods) has not been investigated.

system, something which can be clinically observed. This is especially the case if it has not been pasteurized, which is possible with mare's milk due to the low bacterial count. If mare's milk is tolerated, many observations of our own show that it promotes the development of the child's immune system. Mare's milk can be given without a problem to premature babies weighing as little as 1800 g (information from R. Madeleyn). Following many positive experiences, the authors explicitly adopt a position which varies from the recommendations currently in force [Koletzko 2009, 73]. *Goat's milk* is a possible replacement in some cases with the corresponding substitution (particularly folic acid); Holle is one of several companies offering goat's milk products from the second year of life. *Soy milk* is not recommended by the authors, in agreement with current recommendations, and has become suspect in view of its worldwide genetically modified cultivation. In serious (often multiple) protein allergies, particularly to cow's milk, amino acid mixtures (Neocate®, Pregomin AS® are safer than highly hydrolyzed protein (Alfare® etc.). A clear decision should as far as possible be taken because tolerance can only be induced through the regular administration of (optimally suitable and presented) protein while on the other hand an allergy which can no longer be counter-regulated by the organism requires a sufficiently long and consistent (!) abstention period. (A comparison might help: when you use plaster you cannot just put it aside for five minutes half-way through). Premature intermittent re-exposure carries high risks and prevents a "forgetting" which in the case of cow's milk allergy is mostly a realistic treatment aim.

One should always try to stay as close as possible to the model of breast milk; on the other hand relief must be provided if there is a serious intolerance. In these cases one should at least try to offer a "dessert" (e. g. based on white almond butter) and an easily digestible green vegetables along with and after the industrially produced hydrolyzed food in order to provide positive "nutrition" above all for the *sense of taste and smell* while on the other hand stimulating the intestinal flora through natural food. Otherwise there is a great danger that food which has had the allergens – but also any positive taste – removed promotes subsequent eating disorders, a dislike of natural foodstuffs with vitality.

Mostly well tolerated are green *vegetables* (above all courgettes, broccoli), whereas tomatoes and peppers should be avoided; with regard to carrots, tolerance can vary a great deal and is dependent on the variety. Tropical and kiwi fruit (list individually, mandarins are the least-well tolerated!) should be avoided in favour of mild local *varieties of fruit* (apples, pears), whereby – as for *potatoes* – tolerance can vary considerably from one variety to another. Thus one eczema patient reacted very strongly to a particular variety of potato, scored RAST class 6 in in the RAST test for potatoes at the age of one but was able to digest another variety of potato without difficulty! – *Sausage* in general and pork in particular is not to be recommended while particularly *lamb and veal* are easily tolerated almost without exception.

Alongside the intolerance of cow's milk and hen's eggs, the most frequent over-sensitivity is to *breadstuffs,* above all wheat and rye (cf. also Chap. 4.7.2, Coeliac disease). If this is very pronounced, the corresponding flours must be used very sparingly in the household (the dust from the flour already has a detrimental effect). Quinoa and buckwheat (Tau® from Erdmann-Hauser is a suitable product) are well tolerated above all; spelt, oats and amaranth are frequently tolerated, whereas tolerance can vary with maize, rice and barley. Millet is of great benefit for people with allergies if it is tolerated. It is a gluten-free cereal rich in iron and minerals which is an excellent base cereal in all Th_1-mediated diseases, not just celiac disease. In eczema, too, a clear improvement is often evident in response to a millet diet; on the other hand millet can also be too "irritating" and provoke a deterioration, which is why careful monitoring is required following exposure. Often the mother might learn to bake suitable *bread* if there is a pronounced intolerance to cereals; bakers also increasingly offer suitable products for people with allergies. Gliadin-free products for patients with coeliac disease have proved their worth also for many atopic patients (in many chronic-inflammatory diseases it is worth trying to reduce gliadin in the food or leave it out altogether temporarily under careful clinical observation).

Fats are mostly less problematical. Cream and butter made from sour cream may still be tolerated even with a cow's milk allergy. There is generally no problem with olive and thistle oil which can even be used for spreading on bread. Rape seed oil has many benefits from a biochemical perspective but there are nevertheless fundamental concerns with regard to rape seed as a food crop due to the erucic acid content in native rape plants [Wolff 1998, 137ff.]. *Linseed oil* and *walnut oil* are ideal due to the ratio of omega-3 and omega-6 fatty acids they contain, but also due to the characteristics of the plant (cf. in comparison to Juglans regia, the walnut tree [Rispens 2010]). These oils can counter chronic inflammatory processes. Fatty fish is in the meantime recommended even for infants as well as for pregnant and breast feeding women as a source of high quality fatty acids. The authors also recommend high quality cold water fish, from sustainable fisheries (!), for children after teething at the earliest. The fat quality of meat from conventional agriculture is so unsuitable because today's "concentrated feed" results in an excess of omega-6 fatty acids in the meat. Beef from naturally reared cows with much green fodder is tolerated much better.

Cocoa and ordinary chocolate should fundamentally be avoided; juices, if used at all, should only be freshly squeezed as they otherwise disrupt both eating behaviour and the intestinal flora: because it activates the nervous and sensory pole, chewing an apple has quite a different effect on the gastro-intestinal tract from dirking apple juice which, for example, clearly promotes intestinal mycosis. *Refined beet sugar* frequently has a negative effect even if the child is not allergic to it (intestinal flora, blood sugar activity etc.) and can therefore indirectly worsen both the susceptibility to infections and allergic inflammations. But the child should not have to be deprived of an *experience of sweet things* altogether! Because this experience is of fundamental importance with regard to the needs of the small child, and for the way that human beings experience themselves. Fruit sweeteners, honey in small quantities (from age two onwards), maple syrup or small quantities of cane sugar can be used in the preparation of an evening dessert which also takes account of the need of the mother to give "material" expression to her love for the child.

◻ Tab. 6.2 provides an overview of the degree to which various foods are tolerated. Otherwise we refer to the wealth of specialist literature on the nutrition of the allergic child; but we warn against dogmatically prescribed or implemented diets and medical support of parent and child. There should be no diet without a good reason and if possible no diet which is not re-examined after an appropriate interval.

Tab. 6.2 Tabular overview of selected foods and their toleration.

Very well tolerated	Valuable, less frequently tolerated	Frequently not tolerated
Broccoli	Kohlrabi (German turnip)	Tomatoes
Courgettes	Carrots – better tolerated if from open-pollinated varieties[1]	Pepper,
Chard	Beetroot	Ketchup and similar things
Potatoes	Oats	Wheat (spelt, einkorn better tolerated)
Quinoa	Rice	Rye
Buckwheat	Maize	Cow's milk
Millet	Barley	Eggs
Amaranth	Quark	Hard cheese
Veal*	Soft cheese	Pork, particularly from conventional agriculture
Lamb*	Fish	Conventional sausage varieties,
Pears	Beef sausage* without problematic additives,	Nuts (hazelnuts, peanuts, walnuts),
Mild apples	Almonds, almond butter	Kiwi fruit, strawberries
Cultured butter	Cream	Citrus fruits
Olive oil	Cane sugar in small quantities	Many spices
Thistle oil		Ready-spiced foods
Light-protected linseed and walnut oil (watch out for rapid oxidation) in small quantities		Cocoa-containing foods
		Refined beet sugar

6.3.3 Strengthening the organism's equilibrium

6.3.3.1 Redressing trace element and vitamin deficiencies

The first requirement for creating an inner balance in the organism of the allergic child is of a purely physical kind. When treatment is started, many of these children display *typical deficiencies in trace elements and vitamins*. There are many reasons for this:

- Deficiency through insufficient supply during pregnancy and lactation.
- Deficiency through disorders of the intestinal flora (e. g. selenium deficiency in intestinal mycosis) and intestinal function (e. g. iron, folic acid and vitamin B_{12} deficiency).
- Deficiency through losses at allergically inflamed barriers (e. g. selenium and zinc deficiency in eczemas).
- Deficiency through one-sided nutrition, also through diets (e. g. calcium and magnesium deficiency).

Serious cases of atopic dermatitis in the first year of life can lead to protein deficiency and oedemas; thyroid function, for example, can also be temporarily impaired. All of this indicates that in allergic children with pronounced inflammatory symptoms (above all of the skin) who are underweight and failing to thrive, with a noticeable susceptibility to infection or with a typical aspect (e. g. of iron deficiency), a corresponding *laboratory diagnosis*

1 cf. S. Schäfer [2009]; most carrots found in supermarkets are from hybrid seeds and may be less well tolerated and qualitatively less valuable.

and, particularly when treatment starts, a *substitution* of those substances is helpful which are not available to the organism for its own activity.

In practice the most important substances are:

- *Selenium* [Schrauzer 1998]: the most frequently missing trace element, particularly in atopic dermatitis (e.g. Seltrans peroral drink ampoule; dos. 3–5, max. 10 µg/kg kg/d; substitution for a limited period, check the serum level as necessary). Stimulation of selenium absorption can be achieved through **Sulphur selenosum D6 trit.** Weleda, 1 saltsp. 1 x/d.
- *Zinc:* improves the course of the treatment above all in eczema; serious deficiency is rarer than with selenium, but there is frequently a slight deficiency (e.g. zinc orotate 20 tab., unizinc amp. oral, approx. 10–20 mg zinc/d). Has shown its efficacy in children with malnutrition incl. in the prevention of pneumonia [Götz 2004, 921]. Zinc deficiency accompanies (and indicates) chronic inflammatory bowel diseases. A valuable biological substitute for zinc and vitamins is *wheat germ powder* if it is tolerated (resorption can be better than with common zinc preparations and can be improved through the administration of **Zincum met. D6 trit.**, Weleda, or **Zincum met. D3 trit.**, Apotheke an der Weleda).
- *Vitamin B12* and *folic acid*: children of vegetarians are at risk (insufficient maternal nourishment) as infants (consequences for the differentiation of the nervous system!), as are children who drink goat's milk and children with a one-sided diet (e.g. Folgamma tab., amp. oral and separate substitution of vitamin B_{12}/folic acid). There is often plenty of folic acid in fresh (!) green vegetables. If there is a lack of tolerance to the substitute (diarrhoea) or a recurring B_{12} deficiency, supplementary (!) administration of **Cobaltum D6 trit.**, Apotheke an der Weleda, 1 saltsp. 1 x/d [Soldner 2004].
- *Calcium* and *magnesium*: particularly a problem with poor assimilation in the bowel, tendency for rickets, absence of milk *and* meat in the diet (calcium). Magnesium substitution shows a positive effect in children with asthma (300 mg/day during school age).
- *Iron*: iron deficiency in the mother, lack of balanced diet, poor assimilation through impaired bowel function – the substitution of substances causes particular problems in people with allergies in this instance. the best is an appropriate diet (meat) and above all treatment of stomach and bowel function. A well-tolerated and strengthening iron preparation in anthroposophic medicine is **Ferrum hydroxydatum trit. 5–50 %** (5 % Weleda, 50 % Apotheke an der Weleda) [Vademecum 2009, 357]

Conventional vitamin-mineral mixtures almost always contain vitamin C which can have a detrimental effect on allergies. On vitamin D cf. ▸Chap. 3.2. In short: active movement in sunlight, particularly of the mother during pregnancy and breast feeding, as well as sufficient maternal vitamin D levels have a preventive effect, whereas vitamin D substitution in the first year of life can also have an allergy-promoting effect (also accords with our own observations).

In practice, the substitution of selenium, zinc, magnesium and, as necessary, calcium have a noticeably calming effect on allergic inflammation and the mental state of the child in the corresponding deficiency.

6.3.3.2 Regulation of organ functions disorders in the digestive tract

This task is of *central importance* in the treatment of children with allergies. As already set out above (▸Chap. 6.2), atopic syndromes develop on the basis of inadequate catabolic and digestive processes *of the substance which has not yet been absorbed inside the organism. Protein digestion* is particularly important in this context. Rudolf Steiner and Ita Wegman [1991, 56] pointed out as long ago as 1925 that if the breakdown of the protein in the duodenum is incomplete, human beings run the risk of taking in protein "which still contains external etheric effects". Human beings then have in their own life organization "a range of effects which do not belong there. They have to be eliminated in an irregular way. This gives rise to pathological excretion."

Therapeutically the action of the exocrine pancreas can be strengthened, something that plays the most important role in the complete breakdown of food and the elimination of its potentially allergenic character. *In order for such strengthening to take place, the forces of the individuality must be strengthened in this organ:* "Now it is necessary, if human beings are to digest the food protein (formed and determined by foreign organisms) in a healthy way, for them to have an I-organization which is strong enough so that all the protein required by the human organism can be transferred to the sphere of the human etheric body ... The strength of the I-organization in the pancreatic gland, which is too weak, must be increased" [Steiner and Wegman 1977, 57]. Elsewhere in the same volume (116), reference is made for the first time to the therapeutic possibility of stimulating the activity of the pancreas in the patient through the oral administration of (low potencies of) *organ preparations* [1] [Jütte 2009; Vademecum 2010, 916ff.] produced from animal pancreas.

The activity of the *pancreas* can be observed i. a. by

- the tendency to meteorism of the children (percussion of the abdomen),
- the extent to which the stool contains *insufficiently* digested elements (fats, food elements – floating stools resulting from impaired fat digestion),
- the tendency to diarrhoea, massive, badly smelling stools,
- the impaired feeling of wellbeing of the child, above all in the corresponding digestive stages,
- the findings on palpation in the region of the duodenum.

Although all the symptoms specified can also be associated with other organs, particularly the gall bladder, it is nevertheless necessary with each child suffering from allergies to assess the function of the pancreas as precisely as possible. The possible laboratory examination of the stool (utilization, pancreas elastase-1, etc.) only play a supplementary role. The experience of the authors and many colleagues shows that therapeutic support of pancreatic activity and the general catabolic digestive activity connected with the duodenum has an effect not just on the digestion but beyond that positively affects the allergic and inflammatory events and the general wellbeing of the child.

1 On the rationale of potentized organ preparations in anthroposophic medicine cf. in detail the special issue on organ preparations of the journal *Der Merkurstab* published in 1999. In the experience of the authors, these preparations represent a valuable extension of the therapeutic repertoire in paediatrics.

The authors primarily use

- **Pancreas Gl D4 amp.** Wala
  0.5(−1.0) ml/d per os in the afternoon

or, acting more strongly on the periphery

- **Cichorium/Pancreas comp. pillules/amp.** Wala
  5–7 pillules 3 x/d or ½–1 ampoule per os 1 x/d

Low potencies (D3-5 and Gl. D7) of Cichorium intybus, chicory (▸Chap. 4.6.3), Stibium met. (antimony) and of the Pancreas organ preparation have been jointly potentized in them. Potentized antimony is a basic medicine for inflammatory disorders of the intestinal mucosa: above all, it strengthens the barrier function of the intestinal mucosa while Cichorium and the potentized Pancreas organ preparation reinforce the catabolic activity of the gall bladder and pancreas. Cichorium also addresses the activity of the spleen (▸Chap. 6.3.3.4).

In contrast to substitution therapy e. g. with pancreatic enzymes, the latter as well as the medicines mentioned below do not work directly as "active agents" but have a *stimulating* effect on the organ's own function. They engage the soul and spiritual activity in the organ through *the perception of the potentized medicine;* it starts to unfold its action as early as contact with the oral mucosa. That, however, strengthens the organism, the interaction between soul and body in the digestion, while pure substitution therapy tends to weaken the organ's own activity. From this perspective, potentized antimony stimulates the intervention of the I-organization in the digestive tract.

Cichorium/Pancreas comp. is particularly indicated if

- "chronic inflammatory processes at the periphery of the organism (e. g. atopic eczema, chronic rhinitis) and
- digestive weaknesses, diarrhoea tendency and stools containing insufficiently digested foodstuffs" occur as parallel symptoms. [Vademecum 2009, 267]

The effectiveness of Cichorium/Pancreas comp. can be recognized in that the digestion becomes less obtrusive overall, meteorism and, as relevant, an existing tendency to diarrhoea is reduced, digestion is improved, there is a reduction in the general restlessness of the child and a rise in wellbeing during the digestive phases. The duodenum is less distended and painful on palpation. Peripheral occurrences of inflammation improve.

- **Pancreas/Equisetum pillules/amp.** Wala
  5–10 pillules/½ ampoule per os 1–2 x/d

If the pancreas function and protein tolerance is too weak, Pancreas/Equisetum works particularly if there is

- *weeping eczema* or, indeed, a tendency towards oedema with an albumin deficiency.

A further indicative symptom can be a

- *tendency to constipation* (with simultaneous weak digestion) which can often be remedied with this medicine.

The effect can be recognized through increased diuresis, a reduction in the tendency for fluid retention and "displaced" excretion (e.g. weeping of the eczema) and, after initial diarrhoea, in the improvement of stool quality; the dosage should be adjusted accordingly.

The treatment with Cichorium/Pancreas comp. is usefully supported through the administration of

- **Taraxacum e planta tota D3 pillules** Wala
  3–7 pillules 2–3 x/d

Taraxacum, the dandelion, is also a composite (compositae) like Cichorium intybus, chicory. If we compare the shinning yellow of the dandelion which blossoms in May with the blue of chicory, we are reminded of the relationship between the sun and the blue of the heavens. The dandelion has been used phytotherapeutically for a long time to "stimulate the metabolism and cleanse the blood". The liver is stimulated therapeutically in all its metabolic functions: the carbohydrate metabolism (helpful concurrent medication for diabetes mellitus), bile production (also proven for intrahepatic jaundice, e.g. hepatitis A) and loss of appetite which may be connected with the liver metabolism are favourably influenced. Taraxacum produces the mild, harmonious stimulation of the metabolism with the same effect which is also aimed for with the administration of low potencies of sulphur (see below). In the practical experience of the authors, the interaction of this medicine with Cichorium/Pancreas comp. has shown itself to be very effective in children with allergies for producing a balanced digestive and metabolic situation.

Disorders of the liver and gall bladder are frequently diagnosed in children suffering from allergies. The following symptoms indicate disorders in this area, whereby the top of the list primarily relates to disorders of *liver activity*[1], the bottom three symptoms above all to disorders of *bile secretion*:

- Constipation
- Stool colour changes, alternation with too light stools
- Preference for cold drinks, food rich in carbohydrates, strong desire for sweet things
- Fatigue, depressiveness
- Worse in the afternoon (between 15.00 and 16.00) and at night between 02.00 and 04.00
- Insufficiently digested stools, constantly changing stool quality
- Irritability, bad mood, tantrums in children
- Worsens after fatty foods

Coloured and lactiferous roots (roots which augment sulphuric secondary plant matter related to the blossom) such as berberis, celandine, curcuma often have a stimulating effect on *bile secretion*. Plants with impressive upper parts resulting from the great vitality of their *anabolism* (and which therefore also play an important role in human nutrition and enjoyment) are important for stimulating the liver metabolism: in the *leaves*, vines are prototypical with their strong sugar formation, thistles in the development of oil-rich *seeds*, e.g. the milk thistle or artichoke.

1 On the liver, gall bladder and pancreas in anthroposophic medicine from the perspective of the anthroposophical knowledge of the human being cf. Girke [2010, 683–732]

Typical basic anthroposophic medicines for young people and adults in this respect are:

- **Hepatodoron tab.** Weleda
  chew (!) 1–3 tab. before sleep above all in the evening

The tablets contain dried vine and strawberry leaves. Their use for children with allergies is restricted on the one hand through their lactose and wheat starch content, on the other through their taste of vine leaves. Taking them before sleep supports going to sleep and sleeping through the night.

Preparations from the milk thistle, e.g.

- **Carduus marianus caps.** Weleda
  1 capsule after meals 1–2 x/d,

represent valuable stimulation of the liver, above all with regard to *toxic burdens* and disorders of the fat metabolism which are evident for example in a polar way in atopic dermatitis and acne (▸Chap. 6.4, ▸Chap. 10.7). In dry eczema and generally in hepatopathies following strongly toxic therapies (e.g. chemotherapy in oncological diseases) concentrated Carduus marianus preparations represent a valuable and effective treatment. For small children who cannot swallow capsules very well the mother tincture from Ceres is suitable.

- **Choleodoron dil.** Weleda
  from age 9, 10–15 gtt. 3 x/d before or after meals diluted in water (contains 64% alcohol)

is made from celandine root and curcuma root (main spice in Indian curry) *and is a strongly gall-stimulating and* effectively detoxifying medicine. Alongside the improvement in the stool quality (colour, consistency), a reduction in peripheral local inflammations and a positive stimulation of the will is evident. These medicines play an important role in puberty and adolescence today. Other celandine preparations (e.g. Chelidonium Ferro cultum) are suitable for younger children (▸Chap. 2.3.2.3, ▸Chap. 3.3).

In the general basic treatment of weakened organ functions in children suffering from atopic dermatitis with regard to the liver/gall bladder, intestine and kidneys, anthroposophic medicine uses *preparations from the three oldest land plants club moss (Lycopodium clavatum), ferns (bracken, buckler fern and hart's tongue fern) and horsetail (Equisetum arvense) as a very effective basic medicine.* Aqueous plant extracts proved particularly effective for the authors, treated rhythmically with light and warmth (heated to 37 °C and cooled to 4 °C) whereby they undergo a bacterially mediated acidification process. With the exclusion of all environmental factors apart from the controlled action of light and warmth, the harvested plants undergo a breaking down and simultaneous vitalization process leading to a stable aqueous basic substance (without conservation agents). Ludger Simon has shown how this process on the one hand corresponds to the digestive and metabolic process in human beings and on the other hand specifically supports the development of an independent life organization in the infant during the first septennium. Anthroposophic pharmacy and medicine here in practice follow the principle that the effect of a medicine on the human metabolism is dependent not only on the substance but also on the "structure of the substance-transforming processes to which the substance is subjected during its pharmaceutical preparation into a medicine" (i. e. on the pharmaceutically applied metabolic process) [Simon 2007]. In view of the metabolic weakness and disorder in children with allergies, this aspect occupies a very important position in prac-

Tab. 6.3 Organotropic area of action of the three oldest land plants.

Lycopodium clavatum	Pteridium aquilinum, Dryopteris filix-mas, Phyllitis scolopendrium	Equisetum arvense
Liver metabolism	Intestinal activity	Kidney function

tice. The medicines characterized below are significantly more effective as a result of the quality of their pharmaceutical processing than would be expected on the basis of the plants used alone. The concept of potentizing applies here in a comprehensive manner to the whole pharmaceutical process which aims to uncover the effect of the medicinal plant on the human organization. The objective is the organ-specific activation and regulation of the organism's own activity. It is worth noting that the three oldest land plants correspond in their action to the three basic digestive and metabolic organs in ensouled organisms and even today still act on them in a deeply vitalizing and regulating way (Tab. 6.3).

Stag's-horn club moss, Lycopodium clavatum, displayed extraordinary vitality in the early periods of the earth. Lycopodium very strongly enriches *aluminium* in its spores. Aluminium is a basic component of clay and enables the soil to store moisture and salts – corresponding to the problem of children suffering from atopic dermatitis who often cannot keep enough moisture in their skin. The germling of the plant, consisting of spores, lives in a symbiotic relationship with fungi and the prothallium is also dependent on saprophytic nutrition. The development of the plant requires a period of ten to 15 years [Stübler und Krug 1987, Pflanzl. Arzneistoffe I, 265]. Thus club moss today represents *increasingly slowed down and inhibited metabolic activity* in the course of evolution, although it embodies the purest form of plant growth in the shape of the green and non-blossoming club moss winding its way along the ground (▸ Chap. 4.3.1).

Constitutionally, Lycopodium is indicated in children where a primary weakness of the liver function, delayed weight gain, inhibited digestive function ("had enough after a few mouthfuls") are observed. There is often constipation which can turn into diarrhoea at each dietetic challenge, the stomach is strongly distended, particularly towards the evening, there is a tendency for mycosis also due to the preferred easily digested carbohydrates and sweets. The *bond with the mother remains close,* to which the inhibition of the anabolism and the corresponding weakness of will contribute; quite often *competitive and egotistical behaviour* can also be observed at the same time. Prolonged jaundice in the corresponding constitution can provide an early pointer towards this medicine. Typical allergy symptoms are above all the early appearance of dry, strongly itching *eczema* with a tendency towards generalization as well as persistent, not just seasonal rhinitis with a *nightly blocked nose.*

With the appropriate constitution, ascending homoeopathically potentized potencies of

- **Lycopodium C6–30 pillules,** Gudjons
  in chronic, persistent cases up to **C200.**

In this expensive but very effective preparation, the strongly mineral (aluminium rich) club moss spores are produced in the first potency levels through trituration like mineral homoeopathic agents.

Lycopodium is broadly indicated for children with allergies if there is a toxic burden on the liver and the liver-gall function is globally weakened (e. g. as the result of antibiotics, toxic environmental substances or also Candida albicans and its fusel alcohol formation which is reabsorbed in the intestine).

In general, the following has proved itself in practice as the corresponding basic treatment

- **Lycopodium comp. pillules/amp.** Wala
  3–7 pillules 3 x/d or 1 × ½–1 ampoule per os/d

It contains deep, liver metabolism-stimulating potencies of extracts of club moss (whole plant) and milk thistle seeds, Carduus marianus, with gall-stimulating deep potencies of Mercurius dulcis, Natrium sulfuricum and berberis root, potentized together and processed into a composite medicine.

Lead symptoms for the indication of this medicine are

- tendency towards constipation and meteorism, lack of appetite,
- colour changes of the stools, alternating stools which are too light, intercurrently occurring diarrhoea,
- discomfort, bad mood, irritability of the patient.

Lycopodium comp. obtains its indication significantly from reduced function of the liver and gall bladder.

Its effect can be significantly supported by the *external application of heat in this region*: e.g. by a

- **warm liver compress with yarrow tea** [Goebel and Glöckler 2008, 675]
  for 20–30 min. during the afternoon "siesta" with additional rest 2–3 x/wk.
  The way in which this compress supports an anabolic effect is always astonishing.

Alternatively suitable, but less effective is

- **Malvenöl** Wala (▶Chap. 2.2.1).

Apart from an improvement in the indicative symptoms above, the effectiveness of Lycopodium comp. can be seen in that the patients appear brighter, more awake, as if cleansed.

Ferns probably represent the oldest land plants. In their origins they display a close therapeutic relationship with the first step of human and animal bodily development, the digestion of food in a rhythmical and peristaltic process and the absorption of vital substances into the own metabolism [Sommer and Soldner 1990]. Medicines which contain extracts and potencies of ferns are suitable for stimulating and stabilizing the central functions of the digestive tract – a cardinal task in the treatment of children with allergies (and autoimmune diseases).

The following is suitable as a universal composite medicine to support bowel function

- **Aquilinum comp. pillules/amp.** Wala
  5–10 pillules 2–3 x/d or ½–1 drinking ampoule 1 x/d (▶Chap. 4.6.3.3).

It is a suitable basic medicine particularly for infants and at pre-school age to treat intestinal disorders in children with allergies.

Stool irregularities decline, intestinal flora is positively influenced particularly e. g. in bacterial dysbiosis. This medicine can also be administered for disaccharidase deficiency, e. g. post-infectiously occurring lactose intolerance. The fern species listed in the overview above, which particularly vitalize the bowel function, are jointly potentized in this composition with the low potentized rhythmized basic plant substances of Chelidonium (▸Chap. 4.6.3.3) and Taraxacum to stimulate liver and gall bladder activity as well as Solidago virgaurea which supports the excretory function of the kidneys. Hence Aquilinum comp. works primarily on the intestine but also includes the large parenchymatous organs in the background whose function significantly influences intestinal activity. The reason for this composition is to stimulate and harmonize the activity of the astral body, the unconsciously working soul organization in the area of the gastro-intestinal tract [Vogel 1994, 123–127], on which the activity of digestion is dependent to a high degree – knowledge which can also be beneficially applied in practicing table manners when eating because that also promotes concentration on the digestion. The fact that the enteric (ENS) and vegetative nervous systems in the abdomen have almost the same scope and dimension as the CNS, and that thus the intestine is the most strongly innervated organ outside the brain, underlines this perspective. The rhythm of the intestinal movement, the secretions of gall bladder and pancreas, but also the differentiation in the functions of the small intestine and the development of the so-called mucosal block are dependent on the unconscious presence and activity of the astral body, the soul component which humans and animals have in common (▸Chap. 4).[1] That can also be seen in that the development of the digestive tract as an internal hollow organ and the absorption and digestion of food in the digestive tract is an expression of original activity in all ensouled animal and human organisms which is absent in this form in the typical plant. Interestingly, in German (Adlerfarn, Wurmfarn, Hirschzungenfarn) all the names of the ferns which stimulate such activity (such as hart's tongue fern in English) relate to animals. Even if there may be different reasons for that, it can remind us that the human organism can experience the stimulation of its own "animal" activity in the digestive tract when these medicinally prepared plants are digested.

Archetypally, fern and willow leaves are together processed into a "typical medicine" of anthroposophic medicine, based on a recipe from Rudolf Steiner for the *vitalization and rhythmization of intestinal function*, in

- **Digestodoron® tab./dil.** Weleda
- **D/Aspidium/Salix tab./dil.** Weleda Switzerland
  from school age: chew 1–2 tabs. 2–3 x/d;
  infants 5 gtt. 3–4 x/d dissolved in a little water
  (Aspidium/Salix can have a lower dose)

The function of willows in nature is to stabilize river banks in hitherto unformed regularly flooded landscapes (primary colonizer); at the same time they dynamize moisture exchange between water and air in that they absorb enormous quantities of fluid which then evaporate. As an early blossoming tree with a lot of pollen, the willow for example

1 The impression can arise clinically that many food intolerances, for example, are influenced by disorders in the activity of the soul organization such as depression for instance (and improved by anti-depressive therapy). This perspective should also be considered in many a case of disaccharidase deficiency (fructose and lactose intolerance).

provides food for bees in early spring, thus revealing an intensive relationship with the soul element (in poetry it also stands for grief and depression if one is "prone to tears". Digestodoron represents a proven medicine in

- *disorders of the intestinal rhythm*: tendency towards constipation but also recurring diarrhoea as part of enterocolitis or chronic-inflammatory bowel disease. A tendency for gastroesophageal reflux is also positively influenced. Peristalsis (auscultation) becomes more regular, less strained.
- *disorders of the mucosal functions* and differentiation (e.g. postenteritis syndrome, damage to the mucosa as part of celiac disease). It is worth noting that some patients have a feeling of warmth in the abdomen through this medication [Kohlhase and Fintelmann 2009]. In the experience of the authors children with celiac disease, for example, often lack sufficient warmth in this area.
- *damage of the intestinal mucosa* e.g. following chemotherapy, but also as part of treatment for candida mycosis (▸Chap. 4.6). Restorative medicine during and after symbiotic control. A tendency towards flatulence and lack of appetite is positively influenced, the soul element can noticeably immerse itself in the digestion.
- If the medicine is chewed in tablet form, it is even more effective in older children and young people. The Swiss preparation contains bracken which is missing in the German preparation. This is also a primary colonizer with a strong connection to light (therapeutically that means a strong connection to the kidneys) and can in some cases play a key therapeutic role. Digestodoron® [Vademecum 2010, 390f.] or Aquilinum comp. should be taken for several months to properly develop its effect.

The extent to which healthy gastro-intestinal activity is dependent on the harmoniously unconscious activity of the astral body in this region can become particularly clear when such activity is disrupted. Thus it can be observed not infrequently in allergic children that the unconscious body-related activity of the astral body is irritated – e.g. through shock experiences in early childhood, nervosity and lack of experience in the adult reference person, or recurring disruption of the daily rhythm – and becomes too consciousness-like in character. These children are inclined to develop insufficient activity in breaking down, digesting and resorbing food and literally to take hold of the gastro-intestinal activity only externally: hypertonic disorders of the intestinal wall occur with a colic tendency and dysrhythmic disorders of the passage (diarrhoea tendency, irregular stool behaviour) with simultaneous maldigestion.

If against this background infants and small children display above all

- increased irritability and a tendency to develop spasms in the upper abdomen,
- weaknesses of the catabolic digestive functions in the duodenum,
- possible underweight/dystrophia,

the following medicines can provide support (▸Chap. 4.4.4)

- **Belladonna Rh D4(–6) dil.** Weleda
- **Oxalis Rh D4 dil.** Weleda
  3–5 gtt. 3 x/d each
- **Siderit D6 trit.** Weleda
  1 saltsp. 3 x/d.

6

Apart specifically from the digestion in the area of the duodenum, *balancing impaired intestinal flora* and normalizing intestinal function as a whole is of considerable importance in children with allergies. We refer in principle to ▸Chap. 4.6 in this context. Special attention must be paid to mycosis and bacterial dysbiosis as part of a manifest allergic disease; the appropriate *symbiotic control* (▸Chap. 4.6.4) can contribute significantly to a balanced intestinal function.

If no clearly visible harmonization of the catabolic and digestive process occurs in the patient, although there was a change of diet, intestinal activity was stimulated using the possibilities mentioned and serious deficits in the substances were compensated, the administration of sulphur

- **Sulphur D6 trit.** Weleda
  1 small saltsp. 3 x/d

over a period of 14 days, for example, can reactivate the metabolic organization as an interim measure. In (often reddish-blond-haired, "high-sulphur") children with a tendency for strongly hyperergic inflammatory exacerbations of atopic dermatitis, for example, a careful dosage (LM6, 1 gtt. in 100 ml, of which 1 tsp. every 1–2 days) can be effective and is tolerated better while "low-sulphur" children (dark-haired, tending to look more Mediterranean) tend to benefit from a stronger dose of sulphur (on the "high-sulphur, low-sulphur" aspect which measurably corresponds with the sulphur content of the skin cf. F. Husemann, "Die Haarfarbe als Spiegel des Stoffwechsels" [2009, 99–116 with case studies]).

Sulphur as a natural mineral displays an intensive *relationship with warmth:* it is formed as a mineral in the environment of volcanoes which release a lot of sulphur out of the earth. The yellow sulphur crystals contain so much energy that they are completely combustible. On heating, sulphur constantly changes its colour and viscosity in an impressive way, depending on temperature, and is qualitatively very dependent on heat in its behaviour. The sulphur flame is simultaneously very hot with very poor light output (in contrast to phosphorus for example). In living things, sulphur is an indispensible and dynamizing element in the *protein metabolism*, in building the living functional spatial structures of the proteins (through sulphur-hydrogen bridges), and on the other hand in detoxification processes. Upon death of a living creature the sulphur becomes volatile and is released from the decaying organism in the form of the most energy-rich sulphur compound of hydrogen sulphide. In the therapeutic stimulation of vitality, protein anabolism and detoxification, it is a matter of integrating sulphur more intensively into the metabolic sphere. This is done by particularly low potencies of the substance, initially in its mineral form. They have a *warming effect* in the "metabolic human being"; this can also be supported through appropriate external applications (see above). As we have already mentioned, Hahnemann towards the end of his life began the treatment of patients with weakened reactive power (in his terminology "psoric diseases") using sulphur in LM potencies, some starting with LM1. In their basic work on anthroposophically extended medicine already quoted, Rudolf Steiner and Ita Wegman [1991, 85f.] refer to sulphur as the basic medicine for the protein metabolism: "That enables it to play an important role also within the protein substances ... harnessed into the etheric actions" (of the organism) "... if the body cannot itself utilize protein substances introduced from the outside such that they are incorporated into its own activity because of a diseased state." [Steiner and Wegman 1977, 85f.] The latter statement refers to the antimony compound of sulphur:

- **Antimonit D6 trit.** Weleda
  1 saltsp. 3 x/d

which is indicated therapeutically above all when *inflammatory disintegrating processes* in the digestive tract, recurring diarrhoea, insufficient formation in the sphere of the intestinal content, the intestinal flora and the intestinal mucosa are determined.

The simultaneous or vicarious appearance of "pronounced metabolic" skin rashes, e.g. purulent super infections, impetigo, but also allergic contact eczema e.g. on contact with metals or disinfectants indicate Antimonit (cf. the indications in [Vademecum 2010, 76f]. The children tend to have a "hysterical" constitution; the lack of integration of the soul entity in the digestive and metabolic sphere comes to expression, as described by homoeopathy, particularly in the easily grumpy and bad-tempered mood (actually these forces should come to expression in the digestion of food and not be directed at the doctor). A coated white tongue can be an indication for this medicine.

Pronounced metabolism-related skin rashes up to and including acne (▸Chap. 10.7) and maldigestion also indicate the iodine compound of sulphur,

- **Sulphur iodatum D4-6 dil.** (various manufacturers)
  3 × 3–5 gtt./d.

This medicine is indicated if

- the catabolic pancreas activity is insufficient and there are signs of maldigestion (very unpleasantly smelling, massive stools; failure to thrive),
- at the same time there is a chronic inflammatory tendency in the sphere of the upper and lower airways with abnormal bacterial colonization and sometimes *unpleasantly smelling* nasal discharge and expectorant.

Sulphur iodatum has a very strongly cleansing effect, stimulates *nonspecific immunity* and supports the digestion – something which illustrates the direct link between these functions.

6.3.3.3 Regulation of kidney activity – Equisetum arvense

Examine me, O Lord, and prove me; purify my reins and my heart.

Psalm 26

The indication of the third group of original land plants, the horsetail (Equisetum) is focused in the sphere of kidney activity which occupies a central place in the treatment of children with atopic dermatitis, bronchial asthma and pollinosis. The activity of the soul entity with regard to the welling up vitality of the etheric is expressed directly in the *excretory activity of the organism*: if the vitality of an organism is generally reflected in turgor, then the intervention of the animalistic soul entity, the astral body is expressed in all exocrine and endocrine glands and excretory organs which thereby simultaneously limit and regulate the welling up vitality of the living element. In general we can differentiate between various qualities here; in patients with atopic dermatitis, for example, *excessive secretory processes which take on a life of their own, "dislocated" secretion* (weeping eczema, tendency to perspire, catarrhal infections, tendency for diarrhoea) *or retained secretion insufficiently connected with the metabolism* (dry eczema, little perspiration and only cool, sticky, unpleasantly smelling, stress-related perspiration at the corresponding predilection sites). In the latter case we generally find *elevated nerval activity around the sweat glands* whose excretory activity is thereby changed (generally inhibited); the *itching* is particularly intense at the moment when perspiration (nevertheless) starts and the sweat issues through the skin; it "mostly tends to ease once the sweat flows" [Jachens 1999b].

The underlying factor in these phenomena is that *the soul entity can combine in various ways with the body.* It can be immersed unconsciously wholly in the "metabolic human being", the sphere of the metabolism and movement, stimulate vital processes like the digestion and limb activity and thus be taken hold of too strongly by the inherent dynamic of the metabolic human being; it can thus lose its ordering and differentiating power and be overwhelmed by the influences of external nature, e. g. food which has not been fully digested, foreign protein and suchlike. There is then a trend for the *metabolism to make itself independent, a lack of guidance of the etheric body which becomes too independent and subject at the same time to foreign influences.* The breaking down of foreign matter, of external nature at the barriers of the organism becomes inadequate, the barriers themselves tend to lose form, to swell, to increase permeability and secretion; psychologically, too, a tendency to "flow out" and a mood which is strongly dependent on the metabolic situation is noticeable. Catarrhal infections and diarrhoea, *"exsudative lymphatic diathesis"* and *weeping eczema* tend to belong to the picture of this type. This constitution is described anthroposophically with the term *"hysterical constitution"*. But it is also accompanied by an *abnormal sensitivity at the barriers because they are too open to the environment and thus take on the characteristics of a wound* [cf. Steiner 1985, 66]. The image of the wound and wound healing can be particularly helpful in the treatment of allergic diseases of the skin and mucosa in children with this constitution.

The organ which shapes the fluid balance of the organism in that it excretes water and salts in a differentiated way and regulates the gas tension ratio in the blood over the medium and long-term is the *kidney.* Located retroperitoneally behind the central metabolic organs, *the pair of kidneys limit the sphere of up-welling vitality.* The metamorphosis of the kidney from an organ supplied with veno-venous blood in primitive sea creatures into the organ containing an arterial rete mirabile [Portmann 1983, 225–233] is crucially connected with the *move to land* of the higher animals in the course of evolution and occurred in parallel to increasing alertness and perceptual and movement activity of the higher animals: awakening is centrally connected with physiological kidney and adrenal function. The development and incarnation of the astral body in the organism can be directly seen in the evolution of the kidneys and the closely associated adrenal glands. Internally, the kidneys make it possible *for parts of the organism to dry out* and thus *for the respiratory organ of the lung to develop* – only from this perspective is it possible to understand why the kidneys play a key role in CO_2-bicarbonate regulation and through erythropoietin formation in the regulation of oxygen respiration. Externally, kidney activity makes *life on dry land* possible, among other things through the accumulation of high *internal salt concentrations* in the renal medula. The desert mouse, which has a salt concentration of 7,000 mOsmol/kg in its renal medula, can thereby maintain its internal milieu in an extremely dry environment while at the same time minimizing external secretion, i.e. holding back the secretory processes to the maximum. This animal illustrates simultaneously a high basal metabolism and a *catabolically* determined metabolism (the kidneys themselves have an enormous oxygen requirement primarily for differentiated excretory activity) with behaviour characterized by *alert nervousness.*

Pulmonary respiration, high oxygen turnover, control of the acid-base and sodium-potassium balance, which plays a key role in the course of all excitation processes in the organism, limitation of the liquid-based anabolic metabolism – all these kidney-dependent functions show that this is *where the possibility of higher, wakeful soul life* begins. Accordingly the kidneys display a clear day-night rhythm in their activity (which is greatly dependent on the hormonal activity of the adrenal glands) and kidney activity is particularly affected by any psychological shock extending as far as shock kidney. None of the other large parenchymatous organs of the human metabolism are so directly connected with the *bodily* activity of the soul entity, the astral body, as are the symmetrically paired kidneys and the spatially and functionally closely associated adrenal glands.

If patients now display a correspondingly one-sided kidney activity, this comes to expression physically in the *tendency for dryness, induration and overformation.* On the skin, it corresponds to subacute chronic eczema, xerosis of the skin (which is also connected with a lack of urea in the epidermis); the Dennie-Morgan fold, increased lip folds and hyperlinear palms point in this direction. In psychological terms, elevated nervous tension, difficult (or only explosive) expression of inner emotions, an often above-average intelligence which is analytically accentuated, and a tendency for introversion are characteristic of this constitution which is described in anthroposophic medicine as *"neurasthenic"*. The opposite pole is represented by the hysterical constitution which is characterized by an inadequately controlled "leakage" of the organism: one example of this is the nocturnal enuresis of a child which sleeps too deeply with exsudative lymphatic diathesis (and nasal breathing often disrupted through adenoids); another is the weeping "wheezy bronchitis" of well-fed infants and small children whose airways tend to swell and produce excess mucous secretions with every infection because there is still too little activity in the draining background kidney activity.

Disorders of the secretory activity can be found in all allergic diseases:

- with pollinosis it is typically the increased nasal secretion but also the chronically blocked nose in allergic rhinitis,
- with bronchial asthma the interconnection between elevated bronchial secretion and abnormally tenacious, solidifying secretion.
- with atopic dermatitis in the polarity set out above between weeping eczema and often predominantly dry skin with its tendency of overformation.

This leads to the conclusion – confirmed in therapy – that a constitutional imbalance of kidney activity as reflected in the extended meaning developed here can be found in almost all childhood allergic diseases; its treatment can lead to the effective harmonization of the formative and excretory activity of the soul entity, the astral body, in the child's life organization. This can help us to understand how a medicine which in homoeopathy and phytotherapy is mostly only used in connection with a pathology of the urinary passages plays an important role in the anthroposophical treatment of allergic children – above all with atopic dermatitis – as a basic medicine, namely

- Equisetum arvense, the common horsetail [Husemann 2009, 79–98]

In contrast to the ferns with their emphasis on the leaves, the horsetail embodies *a purely axial stalk principle* (extension originally always indicates the influence of light in nature). It has in common with Lycopodium and the ferns that these plants as primary land colonizers were forced to protect themselves against drying out – just like the newborn who has left the amniotic sheath – and were the first to develop a vascular tissue system which acts in a very special way in Equisetum: 9/10 of the plant lies under the earth as a draining, cross-linked underground conduit system which drains the surrounding soil to a high degree. As one of the three original land plants, Equisetum here develops a kidney-like activity with regard to the earth.

In terms of its substance Equisetum arvense displays a high proportion of ash substance (16–20 %), of which approx. 60–70 % is silicic acid *in opal form,* whereby *"every species of horsetail displays its very specific pattern of silicea* which occurs with such diversity in no other plant family" [Strüh 1989, 174]. On the other hand, the ash contains *sulphur* (approx. 4.2 % in the ash) whereby the sulphur content of E. arvense exceeds that of any other species of horsetail by about tenfold [Strüh 1989, 175, 177]. The importance of sulphur for activating the metabolism was already discussed above; silicic acid is closely related in turn to all the form-giving processes in the human organism. Rudolf Steiner emphasized repeatedly the silicic acid and sulphur content of the common horsetail, whereby he spoke of the dynamism which the plant metabolism lends to the substance: "Silicic acid is, however, turned into a process in a certain sense in Equisetum arvense ..." [Steiner 1994, 49]. The *phytochemical inner polarity of E. arvense has its correspondence in a morphologically specific polarization* of the spatial and chronological form as a whole: The fleshy and chlorophyll-containing sulphur-rich *spring shoot* which serves reproduction highlights the archetypal vitality in the growth and reproduction of this archaic plant genus – "the sulphate content appears all the higher the more the fertile ... and vegetative shoots grow spatially and chronologically apart from one another" [Strüh 1989, 178]. In contrast the silicea-rich vegetative *summer shoot* – the actual "horsetail" – almost "compulsively" emphasizes the form, the light beam-related stalk principle (the relationship between silicic acid and light is directly evident). The dual relationship of the kidneys to the conscious soul life on the one hand and the metabolism and procreation on the other is qualitatively reflected in the summer and spring shoot of E. arvense. Pharmacologically a rise in diuresis has been shown for E. arvense as a drug [Stübler and Krug 1987, Pflanzl. Arzneistoffe I, 284].

Steiner describes the action of Equisetum arvense such that it displays a great affinity with the kidneys – something which can be understood from the ecological drainage function of the plant alone – and intervenes in the kidney organization similarly to the way that the soul and spiritual organization does in the human being. Whenever the activity of the kidneys takes an abnormal course – cf. the constitutional observations above – the administration of Equisetum can introduce a harmonization in that it takes over control of kidney activity for a time so that the soul and spiritual organization of the child can be relieved, thus enabling it to reorient itself and aim for a new equilibrium [Steiner 1987, 21]. The importance of silicic acid with regard to barrier development in allergic children is particularly highlighted in the account by Ita Wegman and Rudolf Steiner in the book

Grundlegendes für eine Erweiterung der Heilkunst. The function of the silicic acid metabolism in humans is described as follows: "It shuts out the external effects of nature from the inner organism so that the latter does not have to perpetuate the effects of nature within its sphere but can develop its own" [Steiner and Wegman 1991, 76–80]. That expresses the healthy antithesis to allergy also in line with current scientific findings. But it is also important to understand that such an exclusion of the outside, the regulation of separation and excretion in humans, is not purely a physical issue but is dependent on the actual intervention of the soul and spiritual entity in the metabolic processes of the organism.

Equisetum in rhythmized form can assist the kidneys in finding a better balance in the relationship between the metabolism-oriented "sulphuric" element and the form-giving, light-related activity of the soul and spiritual entity. Here the sulphur content of Equisetum supports the assimilation and distribution of silicic acid. In therapeutic terms, rhythmized aqueous plant extracts of Equisetum are suitable for allergic children with a hysterical and neurasthenic constitution, e.g.

- **Equisetum ex herba pillules** Wala//**Equisetum arvense Rh D3 dil.** Weleda
  5–7 pillules/5–10 gtt. 3 x/d

Equisetum D3 and Aquilinum comp. represent the perhaps most frequently indicated basic medicine in the first phase of atopic dermatitis therapy.

The medicine has a slow and mild action which generally makes itself felt after two to four weeks and the treatment must be carried out over several months. Weeping processes regress, the inflammation of the skin and mucosa as well as the quality of nails and hair can improve, as can mental restlessness and the hypersensitivity of the skin and mucosa (e.g. itching and coughing), and excretion and detoxification through the kidneys is stimulated.

Especially if the skin is too cool in the kidney region and the child finds it difficult to let go with his or her soul in the evening and becomes restless, *an rhythmical Einreibung in the kidney region* is indicated in addition to the administration of Equisetum, e.g. with

- **Cuprum met. praep. 0.1%–0.4% ointment** Weleda

The detachment of the soul entity from the kidney region in the evening and the associated deeper sleep can, as necessary, be supported by *a foot rub* with copper ointment (most effectively by a trained nurse as a rhythmical Einreibung).

The action of Equisetum can be significantly modified by the *pharmaceutical process*. If the Equisetum plant is treated over several years with silicic acid or the correspondingly prepared plant ash, a preparation can be obtained which emphasizes the formative, silica-related side of Equisetum.

The greatest effect is produced by

- **Equisetum Silicea cultum D2 dil.** Weleda
  5–10 gtt. 3 x/d [worth reading from a paediatric perspective: Vademecum 2010, 411f.]

This medicine is indicated in allergic diseases

- if there are accompanying chronic-inflammatory processes of the upper or also the lower airways[1]
- there is a tendency for weeping and inflammatory eczema, for "soreness" also in the accompanying sensitivity at the barriers

The effectiveness of Equisetum Silicea can be enhanced through the administration of

- **Sulphur D6 trit.** Weleda
  1 saltsp. 1x/d

If, on the other hand, the Equisetum herb is *roasted* with 1% sulphur additive and the preparation is then potentized through trituration, a medicine is created which has a stronger excretion-stimulating and sulphur-related effect:

- **Equisetum cum Sulfure tostum D3-6 trit.** Weleda
  1 saltsp. 1–3 x/d [cf. the instructive Equisetum case history in Husemann 2009, 95f.]

Equisetum Silicea cultum tends to stimulate the formation, the immunological management of the barriers of the skin and airways, Equisetum cum Sulfure tostum the management of the protein metabolism and excretory activity of the kidneys (cf. also ▸Chap. 5.5.5, Vademecum 2010, 413f.]

There is a certain similarity between Equisetum cum Sulfure tostum and the medicine mentioned above **Pancreas/Equisetum** Wala (▸Chap. 6.3.3.2).

If there is insufficient warmth development and a clear deterioration in the winter, but also a toxic burden and deterioration after vaccination (reference from K. R. Kummer), if there is a tendency to develop infections and *severe itching or coughing*, Formica, the potentized forest ant, can positively reinforce the action of Equisetum and stimulate excretion through the kidneys, e.g. in the form of

- **Equisetum/Formica pillules., amp.** Wala
  5 pillules 1–3 x/d, s.c. injection 1–2 x/wk,

or also as a single medicine

- **Formica D6-12 dil.** Weleda
  5–7 gtt. 1 x/d

In this context the following preparation, introduced in 2004 as a new proprietary medicinal product, is particularly valuable and effective as a basic medicine to stimulate and stabilize kidney activity

- **Silex-Lapis Cancri solutus D4, D6, D15 dil.** Weleda
  D4 and D6: 5–10 gtt. 2–3 x/d, D15: 3–7 gtt. 1–2 x/d.

1 Indicated as an injection in D2 for bronchiectasis and bronchiolitis obliterans!

This medicine goes back to a suggestion from Rudolf Steiner [notebook entry R. ST. No. 1300]. The preparation entered paediatrics primarily through the anthroposophical specialist Heidi Pechmann [Pechmann 2002] who was involved both in its new development and who carried out an application study. Its production from flintstone (a silicate which can be found in chalk cliffs, for example) and gastroliths (calcium carbonate stored in a stomach fold of crayfish during molting) is undertaken with careful control of the acid-base ratio so that the silicic acid is not precipitated: the pharmacist himself or herself carries out the "kidney process" in which substances with a strong mineralization tendency are kept in liquid and "completely combined" (as required by Rudolf Steiner in the quoted notebook). This creates a profoundly effective mineral composite medicine made of calcium carbonate (from crayfish) and potassium silicate (from flintstone). The primary indication for this medicine is to counteract and prevent mineral precipitation in the wrong place, i. e. *stone formation* (e. g. kidney stones; but there are also positive experiences including, for example, recurring stone formation in the excretory duct of the parotid gland). In the context of allergic diseases, the following lead symptoms indicate this medicine in accordance with clinical experience:

- proneness to oedemas, specifically *proneness to lid oedemas*, above all also affecting the upper lids, but also swollen hands,
- disorders of the warmth regulation, above all of the feet and kidney region,
- proneness to urinary tract infections, anomalies in the excretory urinary passages, but also e. g. asymptomatic micro-erythrocyturia,
- pollinosis, particularly also clearly affecting the eyes,
- atopic dermatitis,
- proneness to stone formation above all of the urinary passages (for which this medicine is the specific in anthroposophical treatment).

It should in any case be used over a longer period of time, 6–12 weeks as a rule. Its effectiveness can be well evaluated by a positive change in the quoted lead symptoms.

6.3.3.4 Stimulating immunological digestive and regulatory organs – spleen and thymus

6.3.3.4.1 Spleen

The spleen is "a lymphatic organ which is directly integrated into the blood circulation *and filters antigens out of the blood*" (emphasis in original) [Holländer 1999, 79]. About half of the total blood volume is filtered by this organ in a 24-hour period. More familiar is its cleansing function, for example of pathogens which have penetrated into the bloodstream (splenic macrophages) and the function of the specific antibodies formed in the spleen which, among other things, considerably increase the effectiveness of hepatic phagocytosis (through so-called opsonization). Even the effectiveness of the alveolar macrophages of the lungs is clearly dependent on the function of the spleen [Schulte-Wissermann 1999, 510]. This contrasts with the organism's susceptibility to and defencelessness against serious infections through haematogenous dissemination following the loss of the spleen, familiar above all in connection with pneumococcal infections.

The experience of the authors in practice shows – confirmed, not least, by successful treatment of the spleen – that an *abnormal rise in the susceptibility to infection* is a significant symptom of *impaired or insufficient splenic function*. The catabolic, digestive activity of the spleen with regard to all pathogens *and antigens* which have penetrated the blood clearly illustrates its central connection with the problem of atopic syndrome.

The organism has created an organ in the spleen whose function it is to break down everything which has broken through the barriers of the organism in an untransformed state and develops an irritating or destructive activity in respect of the body's own life processes within the organism.

This activity is not yet "atopic"; because here the organism has created the right place (Greek: topos) for a problem which clearly always exists in demarcating the inner milieu from the environment: that traces of this environment can always penetrate the interior of the body, that living barriers can never be completely impenetrable from the outside. *An atopic syndrome really only occurs when this function of the spleen fails* because then a function which the spleen would normally do has to be performed in the wrong place.

Rudolf Steiner [1999, 298] noted as long ago as 1920 that the spleen performed a crucial "background function" for the digestion. He localized its activity at the transition from the metabolic sphere to the activity of the rhythmical system, i. e. to the cardiopulmonary system. The spleen regulates and limits what the digestion and metabolism do with regard to the blood circulation. Nothing must penetrate into the latter which has not been transformed by the digestion. A crucial cleansing function accrues to the spleen *after* the ingestion of food. Steiner points out how this function can, for example, be supported by *resting after a meal*, how some animals do this instinctively "who keep healthy by lying down and not letting the digestion be interrupted by external activity; in reality they are protecting the activity of the spleen. People do not protect the activity of their spleen if they are engaged in external, nervous, catabolic activity. People who eat constantly induce quite a different spleen activity in themselves than people who also leave periods in between. That can be particularly observed in the fidgety splenic activity in children if they are constantly snacking …" [Steiner 1976, 294].

These words, spoken in 1920 in true clairvoyance, precisely correspond to the knowledge and observable reality today. We know that atopic syndrome is a problem of people who cannot digest properly, who are distracted mentally from the task of digestion, whose mind is elsewhere when they are eating; we know the extent to which "constant snacking" promotes a susceptibility to infection and at the same time undermines the right instinct for beneficial food. Rudolf Steiner emphasized that supporting the spleen has an unconscious effect on appetite behaviour, on a "more healthy relationship with what serves people in the organism and what does not" [Steiner 1976, 296].

We will briefly summarize once more diagnostically the symptoms which point to impaired spleen function:

- cumulative susceptibility to infection,
- improvement of the allergic symptoms in fever (in fever the activity of the spleen is intensified by the I-organization),
- strong tendency to develop an atopic syndrome, imbalances in the humoral (B cell-dependent) resistance (e. g. IgG subclass deficiency, high overall IgE, etc.),
- conspicuous states of restlessness following eating, lack of rhythm in eating behaviours,
- general "fidgety" restlessness, tendency for food intolerances,
- addiction-like craving for foods which are not tolerated.

In terms of treatment, specific advice on lifestyle (breaks between meals, rest after meals, elimination of foods which are not tolerated, etc.) is the prerequisite for treatment of the spleen. The primary medicine in the practice of the authors is

- **Lien comp. pillules** Wala
  5–10 pillules 1–2 x/d, e. g. between meals.

This composite medicine, developed by H.H. Vogel [1994, 516–518], contains a low potentized spleen organ preparation as well as the mesenchyme organ preparation, among other things, to stimulate the metabolic activity of the spleen. The kidney organ preparation and Equisetum in medium-high potency regulate renal excretion, Cichorium intybus in medium-high potency regulates the activity of all the digestive and excretory processes associated with the duodenum. Its *efficacy* can be primarily recognized in the reversal of the tendency to develop an infection; the preparation can be given for a very long time if necessary and can easily also be combined with more individualized therapies.

Rudolf Steiner suggested as long ago as 1920 that the spleen should be treated with *external organotropic rhythmical Einreibungen* which should, however, be applied by an expert (rhythmical Einreibungen) and can then show a very sustained effect.

Ointments which are suitable for these organ rhythmical Einreibungen on the skin above the region of the organ include

- **Cuprum met. praep. 0.4 % ointment** Weleda and
- **Oxalis 10 % ointment** Weleda

Oxalis directly links the soul entity more intensively with the organ activity, above all in cases where the anabolic forces are weak or have been weakened and there have been psychologically stressful experiences in early childhood (we might think of the delicate, green common wood sorrel which folds up when touched in the shade of the forest), while the copper ointment with its warming action stimulates the I-organization to control the activity of the astral body and the latter can thus more strongly immerse itself in its unconscious organotropic activity.

The active forgetting of the organism reaches its peak in the immune activity of the spleen: what was initially imbibed, eaten is completely broken down in its own particular nature and can thus be forgotten and integrated into building up our own living substance or excreted. In general, this activity of the spleen can be supported with potentized lead, e. g.

- **Plumbum met. praep. D10–12 trit.** Weleda
  1 saltsp. in the morning

Potentized lead is a profoundly effective medicine for allergies (lead as a metal is used, among other things, to create a barrier against the external world in the form of red lead to protect against rust, a lead apron to stop radioactive radiation). *It is constitutionally* effective in macrocephalic, clumsy children with slow movements who have difficulty in concentrating [Vademecum 2010, 673]. At the same time there is a weaknesse in the digestion and they are easily distracted and cannot separate themselves from external stimuli. The I-organization is too little present and can be significantly strengthened through potentized lead particularly in its metabolic function.

6

If the activity of the metabolic pole, the digestive organization has too little vitality and if this is associated with inflammatory allergic "outflowing" phenomena in the nervous and sensory pole (e.g. pollinosis) or the skin, the sulphur compound of lead can be administered:

- **Galenit D10 amp.** Weleda
  ½–1 ampoule per os in the morning

If there are also food allergies and allergies against inhalation allergens (pollinosis, house dust mites), the following is suitable

- **Plumbum D14 2 parts/Stannum D14 1 part trit.** Weleda

The authors with increasing frequency use lead in vegetabilized form as

- **Cichorium Plumbo cultum Rh D3 dil.** Weleda
  5–10 gtt. 3 x/d (alcohol-free) [Vademecum 2010, 318]

This produces a refined lead action aimed at supporting the boundaries of the body and soul entity. The medicine is indicated above all for children

- who are hypersensitive (look out for hypersensitivity to smell)
- with weak resistance and a tendency to develop allergies
- with weak digestion, tendency to have undigested stools
- tendency for addictive consumption of (not tolerated) foods

The direction in which the treatment with *potentized autologous blood* as developed by Imhäuser [2000, 187ff.] acts can be directly understood on the basis of what has been explained here: for the activity of the spleen is related specifically to the patient's own blood which (e.g. with regard to the ageing of the erythrocytes) is literally "scanned" and critically purified. *This process is stimulated through the administration of the patient's own potentized autologous blood;* and the effect of this therapy is also initially evident in the reduction of the tendency to develop infections and in the further regression of allergic inflammations, particularly in pollinosis.

Autologous blood can be potentized in centesimal stages (1:100), the respectively administered potency made non-perishable with an 18–30 % alcohol-water mixture. Sweet tasting glycerine (40 %) can also be used as an additive to preserve the medicine.
According to Imhäuser, the potencies C5–18 can be used (▸Chap. 5.1.1.5.4, ▸Chap. 5.1.2.3), initially 3–5 gtt. 3 x/wk (C5), in higher potencies from C9 upwards correspondingly less frequently. In acute situations autologous blood can be used more frequently (cf. the diagram in ▸Chap. 5.2.6.2)

For the following description of the thymus, the authors owe key suggestions to the collaboration with M. Sommer.

6.3.3.4.2 Thymus

The *thymus* is embryologically the *first lymphatic organ* to develop at all and the "primary lymphatic organ of the T cell system. The thymic primordium is built up … from epithelial material of entodermal and ectodermal origin as well as from mesodermal elements. Only the interaction of these various components leads to the differentiation of the functioning organ" [Gaudecker 1990, 340ff.]. In a probably unique way the *organic development of the thymus includes all three germ layers of human embryogenesis.* In terms of its origin, the thymic primordium belongs to the nervous and sensory pole and moves from the neck region into the chest cavity in order there to assume a central position between the heart and lungs. Observation of the organ formation and localization itself can already lead us to perceive a close, indeed direct relationship of the living formative process with the whole human individuality.

This impression is strengthened when we look at the function of the thymus in the human immune system. After the differentiation of the thymus structure into the cortex and medulla, through which the blood-thymus barrier is also developed, the necessary space is created in the thymic cortex for a unique occurrence in the organism: prethymic precursor cells mature there – independently of antigens! – into T lymphocytes. In doing so, *the inherited genome is acted on* using a specific enzyme [Holländer 1999, 34–39; Gaudecker 1990, 347–350] and partly regrouped through "rearrangement", thus producing a wealth of different surface structures which are crucial for later functioning (the number of possible antigen receptors is estimated at approx. 10^{16} [Holländer 1999, 37]). In this way the organism achieves a creative potential within the thymus which can intervene in the hereditary stream in a unique way, partially dissolve it and create own structures on that basis.[1] This process *is the prerequisite for the development of a specific immune system which is capable of learning for the whole of life and is individual to each single person. There is an "opening of the chromatin structure" and thus a transformation extending into the DNA of the lymphocytes* [Holländer et al. 2005, 117] also in the *Th_1-Th_2 differentiation. The same applies with regard to the regulatory (Treg) T cells and Th_{17} cells whose function is dealt with in greater detail in* ▸Chap. 6.1.2. Allergies are an expression of an abnormal equilibrium within this differentiated structure.

At the same time the thymus has the ability to compare all *cell surfaces in the organism* which come into contact with the bloodstream with the newly formed, specific surface receptors of the T lymphocytes. In a healthy person this comparison, which occurs immediately after genetic rearrangement and the development of these specific T cell receptors in the thymic cortex, leads to all T cell lymphocytes dying which react to the body's own surfaces. Immunologically we refer to the "intrathymic preservation of self-tolerance" [Holländer 1999, 39]. Here approx. 95 % of all newly formed T cells die off – namely those which would potentially introduce an autoaggressive inflammation in the body – and this happens by apoptosis: after the cells have received a corresponding signal from their environment in the thymic cortex, they actively dissolve their genome and then die off.

If we follow these events, it becomes clear what a key role the thymus plays in ensuring that the body, all living surfaces, *is perceived* in an organ of the nervous and sensory pole and, on the other hand, that the central regulatory organs of the immune system are formed on the basis of this perception in such a way that an *autoaggressive inflammation is normally avoided.* The thymus is the key to the individuality positively ("in self-tolerance") combining with the body. *At the same time* the prerequisites for maintaining the integrity of the body against all influences from outside which might endanger it arise from the thymus. The T cells populate all lymphatic organs from out of the thymus *where they mature to their full functional capability.*

The activity of the thymus thus forms the basis for the virtually unlimited learning ability of the human specific immune system with regard to the outside and immunological self-tolerance with regard to the inside. Breast feeding supports the development of the

1 The anthroposophical view that the child must partially dissolve and individualize the body inherited from the parents through his or her own individuality down as far as the form of the physical body has its empirical evidence here. It is of particular importance that this takes place specifically in connection with the specific immune system which is also connected in its importance and development with subjects such as, for example, protective vaccination and childhood diseases.

thymus in a measurable way: the volume of the thymus is higher in breast fed children than in children who have not been breast fed [Koletzko 2009, 71].

The thymus assumes a central position in the regulation of the immunological balance. This is where we find the organic centre of the perceptual, memory and control functions of the human immune system. The development of "competence", the active immunological digestion of foreign matter, is based on the activity of the spleen, the lymph nodes and tonsils, i.e. all "peripheral" lymphatic organs, and reaches its peak in the spleen. Only what has been competently digested can be forgotten.

It is characteristic of children with allergies that the breakdown of foreign, antigenic or infectious agents takes place to the wrong extent in the wrong place. The allergy is characterized by impaired immune regulation, insufficient perception and differentiation of "self" and "foreign", partially insufficient and partially excessive immune responses. Both individual learning and being able to forget are impaired.

That is why in the practice of the authors it has proved worthwhile to treat the spleen *and thymus* in order to stimulate the immune digestive and regulatory processes so that the child's individuality is better anchored in the immune system. That can create a *new equilibrium of learning and forgetting* in the child.

Fundamentally, medium to higher potencies have proved their value in the treatment of allergic (Th_2-dominated[1]) as well as autoaggressive (Th_1-dominated) inflammatory diseases with the organ preparations of anthroposophic medicine. They can be given in childhood per os with good effect, in young people and adults they are more effective s.c. or i.v.. In autoimmune diseases (▶Chap. 10.9, rheumatoid arthritis), D30 has proved successful for the authors as a general potency, for allergies and cumulative susceptibility to infection lower potencies can also be indicated (in the sense of an activating effect).
If allergy and a cumulative susceptibility to infection predominate,

- **Thymus/Mercurius pillules** Wala
  3–5 pillules 2–3 x/d

can be combined with the medicine already mentioned

- **Lien comp. pillules** Wala
  5–10 pillules 1–2 x/d.

In an *acute episode* of atopic dermatitis,

- **Thymus Gl D12 amp.** Wala together with
- **Amnion Gl D30 amp.** Wala
  as a mixed injection of 1 ampoule each i.v. or s.c.

can provide rapidly effective help (Vademecum 2010, 802]. In acute episodes of autoimmune diseases, injections of thymus D12–30 ampoule s.c. can also be indicated, e.g. with the homologous organ preparation (▶Chap. 10.9) or a medicinal plant with steroid-like action such as Helleborus niger D12 (▶Chap. 5.5.5.1.1, [Vademecum 2010, 802])

1 The Th1 and Th2 dominance is a guiding perspective. It can also be found in chronic-inflammatory bowel diseases (▶Chap. 4.7.3). The clinical phenomenology and treatment of ulcerative colitis as a Th2-dominated chronic inflammation reveals a connection with eosinophilic colitis but cannot itself be classified as an allergic inflammation.

The development of thymus activity reaches its climax *in the first year of life* and already starts to recede in infancy. That is in accord with the findings of epidemiological research which shows the paramount importance of pregnancy and the first year of life with regard to the pathogenesis of allergies. The development of the thymus thus takes place chronologically directly in parallel with the development of the higher sense organs (eyes and ears) and the central nervous system. Accordingly this period is also particularly important for the treatment of insufficient thymus activity.

Any treatment with corticosteroids in a sufficient concentration leads to the immediate restriction of thymus activity and a reduction in size of the organ. Hardly any data are available regarding the consequences for the thymus of long-term inhalation treatment with topical steroids or external steroid applications in acute eczema undertaken with the correspondingly detailed diagnosis. The inhibition particularly of T cell mediated immune processes through corticosteroids and topical immunomodulators (e.g. Tacrolimus) is generally known. Perhaps this account will also contribute to *the development of a greater sensitivity in dealing with the child's individuality, which can be affected just as much by medicines as the way in which we deal with the child on a human level. Against this background, the current trend of immunosuppression in allergic children in line with a graduated scheme should be questioned with regard to its long-term consequences.*

6.4 Atopic dermatitis

> As we look more closely at such a miracle of construction and gain a greater insight into the way it arises, we encounter another principle of organization: that no life can work on the surface and express its generating force there, but all of its life activity requires an envelope which protects it against the rough external element, be it water or air or light, preserving its delicate being so that it can complete what lies in its specific inner nature.
>
> J.W. von Goethe, "Die Absicht eingeleitet"

6

6.4.1 Typical inflammatory skin diseases during childhood

If we look at typical inflammatory skin diseases in childhood today, we can highlight three typical clinical pictures which in view of their frequency and in their mild form can still be considered as typical attendants of the respective phase of life, but in their more severe and chronic form lead to pronounced distress:

- *Atopic dermatitis*
  Atopic dermatitis manifests in the majority of cases between the third and twelfth month (◘ Tab. 6.4) – the phase in which there is a profound transformation of the immune system in parallel to the eruption of the teeth and the achievement of upright posture; a new balance is formed between symbiosis and separation from the environment. The child with atopic eczema remains one-sided in the sense of being too open to the environment, with too great an emphasis on symbiosis (▸ Chap. 6.1; "Th2 dominance"). Atopic dermatitis itself is an *epidermal inflammation*. In two thirds of all cases there is an improvement *in the second year of life*, particularly *after eruption of the canines*. As the child begins to separate himself or herself, digest food and explore the world with increasing independence, the inflammation often starts to recede. Febrile

Tab. 6.4 Time of manifestation and characterization of typical inflammatory skin diseases in childhood.

Atopic dermatitis	Urticaria	Acne vulgaris
Most prevalent age 1–2	Most prevalent mid-childhood	Most prevalent age 16–18
Epidermal inflammation	Vascular reaction of the dermis	Inflammation of the oil glands in the subcutis

inflammations, with appropriate treatment, reinforce the healing tendency and exanthematous childhood diseases often reduce the atopic eczema and also have a preventive effect (e. g. varicella, measles). Perhaps exanthematous childhood diseases represent the physiological skin rash of the first septennium, the disappearance of which has been replaced by the increase in atopic eczema. (In old age – with the loss of the own teeth, reducing vitality, less ability to run a fever – the tendency to develop dry skin, itching and itchy eczema reappears). On the other hand, atopic dermatitis has a tendency to become chronic: according to Ring [2005, 391], only a third of cases of atopic dermatitis really heal properly. The experience of the authors with homoeopathic and anthroposophic medicine presents a more favourable impression but the treatment of atopic dermatitis nevertheless remains a demanding task.

- *Acute urticaria*
  Acute urticaria as an inflammatory skin phenomenon occurs relatively more frequently at kindergarten and school age up to puberty (Tab. 6.4). If the triggers of the acute form are primarily acute infections and food intolerance, psychological stresses and vegetative lability are present in the background in most children, as can be observed more frequently particularly at this age, and are connected organically with the development of the rhythmical system. The urticaria itself represents a vascular, inflammatory allergic reaction in the region of the upper dermis (urticae) or the lower dermis (angioedema, Quincke's oedema), i. e. an event in the sphere of the vascular supply of the skin in the dermis, the middle zone in the structure of the skin. Physiologically this is the region in which blushing and growing pale occur, psychologically-related changes of cutaneous perfusion, which can also occur in a particularly pronounced way at this age. *As the rhythmical system matures, the soul entity is increasingly anchored in the physical body and the circulation stabilizes in puberty and adolescence, the tendency to develop urticaria reduces.*
- *Acne vulgaris*
  Acne affects up to 90 % of all young people to a greatly varying degree and reaches its climax between the ages of 16 and 18 (Tab. 6.4). It occurs as a secondary *inflammation in the region of blocked oil glands in the subcutis.* Its appearance is related to sexual maturity; the blockage in the emission of fatty secretions through the skin plays an important pathogenic role. *As the metabolic and limb system matures,* the I increasingly controls the will, own warmth (and thus conversion of the fats) is created in meaningful work, but also through fulfilled interhuman relationships, *the general tendency for acne wanes.*

The skin itself is characterized in atopic dermatitis by a fat deficiency, *sebostasis* ("dry skin"), as the basis of inflammatory skin changes (impaired barrier function of the epidermis), while acne is characterized by *seborrhoea*, a fat blockage as the basis of inflammatory phenomena.

6.4.2 Atopic dermatitis and the warmth organization

The naked skin makes us human.

N. Jablonski

An observation of the polarity of acne vulgaris and atopic dermatitis opens a groundbreaking perspective on our understanding of atopic eczema as an illness: both clinical pictures concern not just polar layers of the skin but there is also a common factor in the polarity, namely *the pathogenically crucial importance of the fats. The latter are uniquely important for human beings among all land creatures.* It is only through the wealth of (primarily subcutaneous) fat on the one hand and the (dermal-epidermal) regulatory ability of the naked skin on the other that human beings can do without fur, feathers or scales, turn their epidermis into naked skin and stabilize their temperature homoiothermically at 37 °C.

The importance of the naked skin in connection with the soul and spiritual individuality is only gradually coming to the attention of science. Anthropological research has meanwhile recognized that it was only the transition from the fur of the primate to the naked skin which enabled the comparatively huge *enhancement of the human brain*: the loss of fur and the doubling (to the present day tripling) of brain volume occurred in parallel. *The reason for that lies in the warmth organization*, for the brain as the most heat-sensitive organ of the human organism (!) will only tolerate an expansion in volume typical for humans in the context of a warmth organization which permits temperature regulation through the naked skin (adult humans can evaporate up to 12 litres of sweat per day through the skin and the perfusion of the fingers and toes can vary by a factor of 600). At the same time erect humans developed longer limbs and thereby another efficient opportunity to dissipate more heat through the surface.

The human epidermis thus represents tissue which is unique in nature and arose in evolutionary terms at the same time as the development of the human brain.

At the same time there is a key change in the communicative character of the organism's surface. Descartes, as the founder of a purely scientific way of thinking, already had to come to terms with the fact that the *Passions de l´ame* (thus the title of his posthumously published last work) are reflected in humans by the skin and particularly the face. Mitschenko [2008] calls his article in *Der Hautarzt* on the neurogenic origins of atopic dermatitis "Wie kommen die Gefühle in die Haut?" (How do feelings get into the skin?). The psychological encounter between human beings is communicated and enabled physically through the naked skin as the "mirror of the soul": touch, warmth, correspondence through gestures assure us of the presence and affection of the other and enable us to understand him or her. "The naked skin makes us human" the anthropologist Nina Jablonski concludes [Spektrum der Wissenschaft 10/2010, 60–67] her review article "Warum Menschen nackt sind" (Why humans are naked) to which this account is significantly indebted.

But against this background we can understand and empathize with the suffering of the patient and his or her nearest and dearest when the mirror of the skin becomes dulled through eczema, the warmth flows away unchecked, the sensitive response to touch is transformed into itching and hypersensitivity and the security of the human envelope flips over into the shirt of Nessus of exacerbated atopic dermatitis.

Fur, feathers and scales are protein structures: the human skin owes its barrier abilities largely to the fats both in the importance of the fats for the epidermal barrier and in the warmth protection which is enabled by subcutaneous fat. While mammals living in the wild (e.g. a three ton hippopotamus) have 2–3 % body fat, an infant physiologically doubles his or her body fat to a maximum of 28 % in the first year. This is then reduced up to the age of nine in order then to rise again after puberty to 18–28 % depending on gender (the problem of obesity has to be excluded here). Using fat in this way (something which only the large marine mammals come close to doing) emancipates humans from the comparatively rigid warmth organization of the furry or feathered animals. If we consider the perspective already set out in ▸Chap. 5 that the warmth organization represents the highest physiological regulatory level of the human organism which is crucial for the expression of free will, then Rudolf Steiner's and Ita Wegman's account of the importance of the fats for the human organism becomes understandable and takes us forward. They explain to begin with that the fat which human beings ingest with food contributes nothing to the human being "other than its ability to develop warmth". And "of every substance contained in the human body only so much is relevant for the I-organization as heat is developed through its action" [Steiner and Wegman 1991, 59].

If we look at the energy (=warmth) reserves of a healthy 75 kg person from this perspective, then we find the following distribution of available heat:

- ATP: 4 kJ,
- Creatine phosphate: 15 kJ,
- Carbohydrates: 4,600 kJ,
- Fats: 300,000 kJ = 98.5 % of all available heat reserves! [von Laue 2005].

It is striking how, in contrast, protein – the substance which is particularly critical for people with allergies – does not represent any available heat reserve at all!

With birth, the skin together with the blood becomes one of the main organs of the human warmth organization. Before birth, the foetus lives in the warmth envelope of the amniotic fluid which according to more recent research also plays a central role in uniformly warming through the foetal organism (whereas the embryonic warmth regulation is located in the placenta). Only when the amnion is lost at birth does the skin start to function as a barrier organ; at the same time the newborn must double his or her own warmth generation on the first day of life in comparison to during pregnancy. The subcutaneous fatty tissue which does not develop until late in pregnancy assumes its central task as warmth envelope of the human organism on birth, initially still in the special form of the brown adipose tissue. The fats allow human beings largely to emancipate themselves not just from the immediate symbiosis with the maternal organism but also from any type-related epidermis which would otherwise determine the warmth organization (fur, feathers, scales).

If we look briefly at the importance of the fats in nature – the authors owe this aspect to Markus Sommer – they appear in the plant realm particularly in seed development, for example in thistles, sunflowers, flax and rape. They no longer serve the life of the plant itself but its descendants. Human beings have obtained oil from oil-forming plants since time immemorial which provided (and provides) food as well as skin care. Here the consistency, the melting point of vegetable fats displays a remarkable relationship with the warmth organization of the earth: linseed oil as a very northerly vegetable oil remains fluid to very low temperatures whereas palm oil generally solidifies outside the tropics. In the animal realm, bees wax represents a particularly striking fatty substance sweated out by the bees when they build their hives in a hexagonal form, which can only be understood from a cosmic perspective. A noticeable feature here is that bees are the only colony forming insects which can realize homoiothermy all the year round in a way which approximates to humans. Here, too, we can see the close relationship of fat creation with the warmth organization which is not represented by the individual animal but the swarm as a whole. Finally, in cold water fish the fats enable active mobility under extreme temperatures; the fats in whales and dolphins approximate almost to human conditions, something which can throw a remarkable light on these companions of human beings in evolution.

Our observations so far support the hypothesis of Rudolf Steiner and Ita Wegman that the fats are of qualitatively unique importance for human beings and must be seen in close connection with the action of the I-organization. We note only in passing that fats represent up to 40 % of the dry weight in the central nervous system and cholesterol – as the fat which is so important for the development of consciousness in humans (e. g. as starting substance of the steroid hormones) – is found in its highest concentrations in the adrenal cortex and the central nervous system. The fats are thus as important in human physiology with regard to awakening and the development of consciousness as they are for the development of warmth and the will. In this context Rudolf Steiner's and Ita Wegman's hypothesis is interesting, that the secretion of fats by the breast feeding mother is of special importance because she transfers forces from her own I-organization to the child through these fats which are not consumed by her: "The shaping force of breast milk is based on that. The mother thereby transfers her own shaping forces of the I-organization to the child and in that way adds something to the formative forces which have already been transferred through heredity." [Steiner and Wegman 1991, l. c.] (cf. ▸Chap. 4.1.1) We can gain an initial understanding of this puzzling statement if we bring to mind that in contrast to plants and animals the fat of the human being's own organism represents the most important substance for the I-organization, for body temperature. The mother thus sacrifices in the fat of breast milk the most important substance of her own organism, something which becomes immediately evident where people are forced to live in conditions of malnourishment. The above quote is also interesting from the point of view that it has been empirically shown today that if the mother and father are similarly prone to atopic syndromes, the maternal influences act more strongly on the child than the paternal ones ("maternal imprinting"). This consideration is deepened through the observation [reference from Markus Sommer] that when the newborn is put to the breast for the first time, the breast warms up strongly at the same time and the child is warmed as far down as into his or her feet. There is a strong rise in the maternal prolactin and oxytocin and the bond between mother and child is positively reinforced throughout the whole of childhood. In the presence of the father, similar endocrine inner reactions are also apparent (!) and his bond with the child is also positively influenced accordingly.

A fundamental characteristic of atopic dermatitis is an anabolic disorder of the fats in the epidermis: The lamellar bodies, which synthesize the barrier lipids in the skin and "exfiltrate" them into the Stratum corneum, are reduced in the Stratum granulosum, the reduced ceramide content is simultaneously additionally supplemented by enhanced degradation of barrier lipids and the development of atypical ceramides [Höger 2005, 145]. *As a result the skin loses excess moisture and body temperature and becomes susceptible to super infections.* A light is thrown on these circumstances by Steiner's and Wegman' characterization, who describe *a situation of "heat starvation"* as a possible extreme manifestation of the fat metabolism: "If the animal forces" – which make the fats available to the organism through digestive activity – "transport too little fat for the I-organization, the I-organization suffers heat starvation. The latter has to withdraw the heat it requires from the activity of the organs. That makes them brittle, rigid, in a sense. … We will then see disease processes arising here and there in which it will be necessary to discover whether their cause lies in a general fat deficiency" [Steiner and Wegman 1991, 60]. That is precisely what happens in early childhood atopic dermatitis! The key thing here is the imbalance between the warmth requirement of the I-organization and its ability to make this warmth available to itself, above all from the fat in food.

Many phenomena support this hypotheses:

- The majority of all atopic eczemas worsen in the cold seasons of the year.
- At the same time external heat can mostly not be tolerated – because the I-organization has the need to generate sufficient warmth itself.
- In exacerbating atopic dermatitis in the form of a generalized erythroderma, there is the risk of life-threatening heat and fluid loss.
- Supporting the gall bladder and pancreas, in particular, has shown itself empirically to be helpful for children suffering from atopic dermatitis – and these are of crucial importance for making the fats available through the organism.
- Contact with foreign protein which cannot be completely broken down, as well as the increased consumption of rapidly digestible carbohydrates – we can speak about food which is "too cool" in this respect – can promote allergies (while in the beginnings of food allergy research fatty meat turned out to be the food which by a long way triggered the least intolerance reactions – a strongly heat-bearing food also in the sense of ancient Chinese dietetics for example. Cf. also today's recommendation regarding fatty fish).
- After all, the appropriate substitution of missing epidermal fats through creams is a generally practiced measure for eczema which in itself indicates the underlying deficiency but does not fundamentally cure it but only substitutes it temporarily.
- It becomes apparent that the deficiency in fats and antimicrobial peptides (epidermal barrier) is crucially caused (in western societies) by a **breaking down** *of the fats* (ceramides), a *process actively stimulated by the sentient organization (astral body)*: "The synthesis of ceramides is reduced in patients with atopic eczema and their enzymatic splitting is increased." [Höger 2005, 10] "The skin barrier is destroyed under stressful conditions through an elevation of the cortisol level…", and there are several case reports which show that in flaccid pareses a systemic atopic dermatitis no longer occurs on the paralyzed extremity! [Mitschenko 2008]. The term neuro-dermatitis (as an alternative term for atopic dermatitis) is therefore more fitting than allergologists have sometimes thought. With asthma and chronic inflammatory bowel diseases, too, it is certain that a neurogenic inflammation plays or can play a role in them, leading to an inflammatory disorder of the barrier organs through, for example, the secretion of proinflammatory neuropeptides (substance P) or mast cell-nerve interaction. Thus the skin of atopic children contains more intraepidermal A and C nerve fibres which in turn secrete stress-dependent neuropeptides to a greater degree. In summary, this is an expression of the excessive catabolic activity of the astral body which dominates in respect of the integrating I-organization; the latter comes to expression in a healthy and specifically human fat anabolism and catabolism connected with the human warmth organization.
- In adults, the degree of seriousness of the atopic dermatitis is reflected in the intensity of the inner feeling of penetrating cold.

In childhood atopic dermatitis, the *degree of sleep disturbance as a measure of the seriousness of the eczema* corresponds to the above symptom. Here, too, the *circadian daily rhythm of the human warmth* organization forms a significant background for the comprehension of the pathology. *Waking up* is physiologically associated with *centralization* and an increase in warmth with reduced perfusion of the periphery; physical movement (and fever!) produce a general warming through during the day. *Fatigue* and *falling asleep* are associated with *peripheralization* (with simultaneous central reduction) of warmth. If we trace this movement of warmth throughout the course of the day, it makes the relationship between the human I and the body directly apparent: the immersion in the body in the morning, its complete penetration with physical will activity has as its counterpart the gradual separation as we grow tired and go to sleep. *This rhythm threatens to be lost in parallel with the extent of the atopic dermatitis because the outflow of heat and the fluid loss make themselves independent in the skin area on the one hand, while on the other hand an increased temperature deficiency impairs the warming through of the body core and makes the uniform warming through from the inside out towards evening as a prerequisite for going to sleep more difficult (cool acra in serious atopic dermatitis!).* The rhythm of waking and sleeping reveals itself to be dependent on being inwardly filled with warmth during the day and self-controlled discharge of heat during the night. Inner hypothermia and the loss of heat which has taken on a life of its own prevent falling asleep and lead to pathological awakening.

A "counter test" also confirms the thesis that early childhood atopic dermatitis is primarily a disorder of the warmth organization in the sense of a warmth deficiency: acne vulgaris. Let us start by following the description of what Steiner and Wegman characterize as an excess of fat in the organism: "An unhealthy path is when the fat is not used up in warmth processes by the I-organization but is transferred to the organism unused. Such fat forms an excessive possibility of generating warmth here and there in the organism. … Parasitic heat sources arise, we might say. These contain the tendency for inflammatory states within them.. The origin of such sources must be sought in that the body develops the tendency to create more fat than the I-organization needs for its life in the internal warmth" [l. c.]. This very well characterizes the situation of the young person with acne vulgaris. He or she forms excess fat in the oil glands, the subcutis, which has the tendency to cut itself off and is then secreted in a secondary inflammation. At the same time there is often a life of the will which has not yet fully unfolded; the young person "hangs about", his or her I only fully incarnates around the age of 21 (the threshold when we reach the age of majority under criminal law in Germany – in many countries it is earlier, but in no country later), and at this age, in which the inner warmth potentials are increasingly transformed through action guided by the I, the acne disappears.

If we focus on the immaturity and impairment of the warmth organization in the child with atopic dermatitis, we can link that with further basic insights into the pathogenesis:

Immunologically, atopic dermatitis is based on a persistent immune position which is symbiotically open to the environment ("Th_2 dominance"). Ring characterizes this in brief as follows for atopic dermatitis: "The elevated Th2 reaction goes along with weakened Th1 resistance" [Ring 2005, 382], i. e. weak resistance above all in the skin with regard to bacteria, viruses and fungi.

- This corresponds to the fact that the main manifestation period for childhood atopic dermatitis lies between the third and twelfth month of life – the time in which this one-sided immune tolerance is normally overcome in favour of a balanced Th_1-Th_2 equilibrium. Here the formation of this equilibrium can be seen as a central function of the human I-organization (which evidently comes to expression in the individualization of human immune development). The subsequent maturation of such impaired immunity is of curative importance for the child with atopic dermatitis and is crucially dependent on the positive support of the child's warmth organization – also by the doctor! At the same time this aspect makes clear how unjustified it is to talk of atopic dermatitis as being incurable in childhood.

Febrile, non-suppressively treated (!) infections frequently improve an eczema; during fever, the I works more actively in the body and the consequence is often a consolidation of the human warmth organization and, in association with that, of the immune system. Therein lies the preventative and curative importance of acute inflammatory diseases particularly in early childhood (▸Chap. 5). The Swedish study by Alm and Swartz [1999] as well as the PARSIFAL study [Alven, Braun-Fahrländer et al. 2005] were able to show that that suppressive antipyresis increases the tendency for atopic eczema. The key to understanding this situation is offered by the *development the individual warmth organization of the child.*

The importance of warmth also becomes clear through a central *sensory function of the skin*, namely the

- *sense of warmth*, the profound importance of which can be experienced particularly in the closeness and touch of a trusted person: the presence of the I, of the person, is felt in warmth (whereas a corpse is experienced as devoid of warmth), in the quality of a human attachment and relationship, in the quality of human affection.
  Just as crucial is the perception of physical warmth which in excess, just as with extreme cold, damages the skin and can call forth an inflammatory reaction (to which acute eczema is remarkably similar).
- A second sensory area registers *changes in the vital context of the skin itself* in the form of *pain* (e.g. in an injury) or also an *itch* (above all if the epidermis dries out). The itching in atopic dermatitis reflects the consequences of the impaired build up of fat (desiccation) and the impaired warmth organization of the skin (local hyperthermia). This sensory area can be included under what anthroposophic medicine calls the "sense of life" which in the healthy person communicates an almost subconscious feeling of well-being but which also includes, for example, the healthy feeling of tiredness at night and freshness in the morning [Goebel, Glöckler 312; Steiner 2002, 23]
- Finally, the *sense of touch* enables a fundamental experience that something has a material, physical existence. The experience of support is significantly connected with the sense of touch.

Perhaps the above considerations will enable a better understanding of the *localization of the eczema reaction.* To begin with, it is generally known that eczema in infancy affects "the convex face and body areas" [Henz and Grabbe 1999, 324] above all. Convex means curving outwards. Eczema at this age particularly often takes an acute course, ranging from weeping to extensive crusting and purulent super infections. The epidermis, particularly the epidermal lipid barrier, remains immature, "too young", too embryonic and cannot sufficiently take on its immunological barrier function or the protection of the inner warmth and fluid space. At the same time there is a nonspecific inflammatory immune response from the underlying dermis, the blood and warmth pole of the skin, *which faces outwards and can thus lead to a further loosening and dissolution of the epidermis and severe warmth, fluid and protein losses.* The physiology of the human warmth organization illuminates why this tendency often breaks out most strongly in the sphere of the face and head: nowhere can human beings restrain their heat dissipation less than in the area of the upper face, above all the forehead and scalp.

"In *childhood* the distribution of eczema moves to the concave body regions with particular emphasis on the body folds and hinge joints of the extremities; the back of the hands are often affected as well. In terms of its morphology, eczema tends to be subacute or chronic and infiltrated with scratch marks" [Henz and Grabbe 1999, 324]. Concave means curving inwards; that is fundamentally the direction of the sensory processes. In the hinged joints the skin always touches itself and there is a kind of self-perception. With regard to the skin, eczema in the hinge joints affects *locations of elevated sensitivity. The orientation of the sensory processes from the outside to the inside correlates histologically with a pathology which with regard to the epidermis displays greater scaling, cornification and drying up of the upper layers of skin and, looked at from this perspective, also represents an orientation from the outside in.* In this second, subacute state we thus have a sclerosing tendency in the epidermis; the skin in terms of its aspect appears slightly aged and dull with dry flaking. But at the same time the epidermal lipid barrier continues to remain immature. Whereas the acute weeping eczema on the head is not rarely associated with little itching, the sensation of itching is prominent in the subacute chronic eczema of the hinge joints.

The interpenetration of the disease tendencies as described is particularly characteristic of atopic dermatitis. The human sensory organization reaches its apex in the region of the eyes and forehead. On the other hand, the human warmth organization comes to particularly intensive expression on the skin in facial blushing and going pale, in the continuous heat dissipation particularly connected with the region of the forehead. It is no accident that regions are often particularly affected by eczema which have a particularly intensive relationship with both the warmth and the sensory organization, such as for example the periorbital area in which many stigmata of atopic dermatitis are familiar to us. The perioral region of the face is further particularly affected; but large, warmth-bearing blood vessels run close to the sensitive surface of the skin in the frequently affected hinge joints, too. *Overall, the skin of the nervous and sensory pole* predominates, corresponding to the concentration of sense organs in this sphere. The "nervous and sensory pole" is dominant in the first septennium; the brain, eyes, ears and also the epidermis already mature to a large extent during this septennium whereas the "metabolic pole" (and also the further development of the subcutis, cf. acne or the development of the female breast) do not mature until the second half of childhood and the second septennium is the crucial maturation period for the rhythmical cardiopulmonary system (of relevance for bronchial asthma).

From clinical experience we can add that eczema with a perioral emphasis indicates the consumption of foods which are not tolerated, particularly also a milk intolerance. Eczema with a periorbital focus is primarily often connected with stress, nervous tension and overload; but it can also be an indication of an intolerance of breadstuffs, particularly wheat and rye.

6.4.3 Treatment

6.4.3.1 Age considerations

It can often be experienced in practice that parents also describe very localized eczema as "terrible" and "very bad". Such remarks are not helpful for the affected children in whose presence such comments are often repeatedly made, particularly if we consider the (catabolic) hyperactivity of the soul entity in the skin of the person suffering from atopic dermatitis.[1] Therapeutically it is necessary to give the parents and the child appreciable support, to calm the emotional perception of the situation, the reaction of the parents to it, *and thus to create an atmosphere in which the skin of the child can heal and a stable physical and psychological boundary can develop between the mother and the child.*

As a first necessary stabilization measure, it is helpful to create a common awareness in the parents and doctor – and with older children and adolescents also in the patient himself or herself – which can be used as a criterion to judge the seriousness of the eczema. The best orientation is the extent of all disorders associated with the warmth organization, particularly

- the extent of sleep disturbance,
- the inner cooling down of the child as revealed in cold hands and feet, for example,
- the susceptibility to infection and frequency of super infections (which can both simultaneously bring about an improvement trend).

These qualities, some of which are only indirectly captured in the "SCORAD" score commonly in use today for atopic dermatitis [Höger 2005, 154], take priority from a curative point of view and initial sustained therapeutic success can best be identified from them whereas the purely visual findings can fluctuate a great deal for a long time. Thus initial *therapeutic goals* can be formulated together with the parents which can lead to a new and comprehensive perception of the child including warmth. Highest priority should be given in this respect to *reestablishing a stable day-night rhythm*; the frequent failure to thrive of the child also mostly stabilizes once sufficiently long and undisturbed night-time sleep returns. Similarly the itching is related to overtiredness to a large degree, and that includes both the fatigue of the child and his or her parental carer.[2]

A realistic prognosis (▸Chap. 6.3.1) is important, which can fundamentally be favourably determined for atopic childhood eczema under anthroposophic and homoeopathic treatment because the underlying cause is an immunological learning disorder and not an irreversible genetic defect. This knowledge can lead to an initial stabilization as the diagnosis of atopic dermatitis is associated for many parents with catastrophic impressions.

1 When talking to the parents without the child, they can be told what it means to have one's skin constantly inspected and negative comments about it. Such "paradoxical intervention" in the sense of Frankl can help the parents to develop a greater awareness of their child again and to be more mindful that the soul is present in the skin and feels very precisely how it is perceived.

2 Chronic parental fatigue facilitates the development of depressive disorders above all in the mother, with all the consequential problems for mother-child interaction, the couple relationship and the care of siblings. The symptom of insomnia is just as much a symptom of profound depressive disorders as of pronounced atopic dermatitis and should be given a higher value in treatment considerations than the look of the skin.

6.4.3.1.1 Physician-parent-child relationship

In the treatment of childhood atopic dermatitis, it is particularly necessary consciously to distinguish between

- support,
- attentiveness,
- own activity

as qualities in the parent-child relationship and the doctor-patient relationship and to learn to handle them in a practical way [cf. Largo 2000]. *Here the quality of the support which is experienced in consolidating the child's life organization and thus also in the subsequent maturation of the skin acquires the greatest importance.* Frequently the (exhausted!) parents fail to understand support as an independent quality while they are plagued by worry and fear in constant attentiveness to their child. In this situation an image can help to clarify what is meant: when a sailing ship encounters a storm on the high seas, it does not calm the passengers if the captain hurries over to them, enquires in detail about how they are feeling and finally asks them what course he should steer or whether he should turn around. A much more calming effect comes from the captain who steadily takes the wheel, issues orders to the crew and has a comforting word and understanding look for the passengers while instructing them not to wander about the unprotected deck. The eczema of a small child can quite easily create a "high seas" situation for the whole family and the most important thing to advance the cure of the child is that during the illness the familial framework, the rhythm of family life is kept stable and does not fall victim to surging emotions, attacks of scratching and immediate countermeasures, and increasing exhaustion!

In practice this means that to begin with the doctor creates security and stability by establishing a clear awareness of the nature of the disorder, its prognosis and the necessary therapeutic steps and periods (!), including also the necessary restrictions (diet). The parents can support their child by clearly differentiating between day and night, a structured daily rhythm, through planning and adhering to a menu and other measures set out in 6.3. That also includes *not responding immediately and instinctively to each behaviour of the child*, e. g. not interrupting through physical intervention or commenting on every bout of scratching. For the underlying pathology is an *excessive activity of the soul entity in the child's skin* (with catabolic effect) which is charged and reinforced with additional soul energy (from the parents) through their mesmerized and reflexive (animal-like, typical for the astral body) actions (e. g. preventing scratching). *What needs to be strengthened, however, is the presence of the I* which comes to expression in the ability to inhibit one's own reflexive actions and the striving for balance.

Parental attentiveness should, as far as possible, not (just) be in response to demands of the child but also happen spontaneously and regularly. It also includes the external applications for the child, particularly when treatment starts, which can give the child a "second skin" for instance through fatty moist wraps under which the child's own skin can recover. *The important thing is the right degree of attentiveness which can best be found if it is practiced in rhythm.* Thus the child should experience intensive physical and psychological attentiveness and care in the evening before going to sleep; but the parents should also work intensively to ensure boundaries during the night and sufficiently long periods of sleep and rest for the child and mother except in the case of acute diseases and exacerbation (▸Chap. 7.1). *What is absolutely vital is that the child does not sleep in his or her par-*

ents' bed and that thus the persistent embryonic symbiosis (which is reflected immunologically in a Th2-dominance) comes to an end. Only if the parental attentiveness possesses a rhythm, and thus also has breaks, will there be success in achieving the most important treatment goal, activating the child's own activity:

- learning to calm himself or herself, going to sleep and sleeping through the night,
- learning to approach the world actively and thus learning to forget to scratch,
- regular digestion and utilizing the fats in food, learning to break down the protein completely (dependent on observing breaks between meals),
- learning to transform the close symbiosis with the mother or the main caregiver in an age-appropriate way.
- own activity matures where no substitute is provided and the child encounters a boundary. Separation (from the parents) can be painful at first, a gesture of antipathy, but without a balance between attentiveness and separation the child's immune system cannot find and regulate a balance between too great an openness to the environment and aggressive/autoaggressive separation (which is in turn reflected at a cellular level in the Th2-Th1 balance).

Such rhythmicity is also supported by regular appointments with the doctor which are not "catastrophically" determined but give the parents support in a four-weekly or, in difficult phases, a weekly rhythm, as well as by the ability to reach the doctor on the telephone.

6.4.3.1.2 Stress during pregnancy – early childhood attachment disorders

This subject acquires great importance with regard to *atopic dermatitis manifesting soon after birth*. Loss of support for mother and child during pregnancy is a serious factor in this respect. There can be very different reasons for this:

- *Relationship conflicts and separation of the parents:*
  Here mother and child lose a supporting existential base, very often associated with grief and anger of the mother, which affects the developing physical organization of the child as a reality reflected in the soul entity. The soul quality which the mother – and father – experience during separation acquires key (and in individual cases also pathogenic) importance, not just the fact of the separation itself. Relevant medicinal treatment possibilities for the affected child are set out in ▸Chap. 2.4. Something which is important for the physician to look out for is that the child is not tied into a symbiotic relationship as a substitute partner (cf. above, mother-child symbiosis).
- *Shock experiences of the mother during pregnancy*
  Together with road accidents, unexpected deaths in the family or other events which must be asked about when the medical history is taken, the experience of so-called prenatal care can be particularly significant. Many mothers today report about shock experiences when they are told by the examining doctor that the head of the child is too small, the nuchal fold conspicuous, growth too slow and much else. The subsequent checks can reinforce that experience still further – mothers reporting about it burst into tears even ten years later! If in this connection the question of amniocentesis or chorionic villus biopsy arises, and possibly of a termination of the pregnancy, then it is very clear that here the symbiosis of mother and child has been deprived of its foundation – very often leading to the impairment of that symbiosis after birth if the child survives the prenatal care. While in India and China millions of mothers and fathers

face terrible conflicts when they are told that the foetus is female, parents in western industrialized nations are affected when they are told that their child might have Down's syndrome, a diaphragmatic hernia or another anomaly. In parallel to the ever more sophisticated fight to keep extremely premature babies alive, and in vitro fertilization with its demonstrable rise in foetal deformity rates, the uterus has become a platform on which the scrutinizing spotlight of medical, social and, more or less voluntary, parental selection is thrown at an ever earlier stage. It has never been systematically investigated whether and to what extent this type of medicine contributes to the increase of postnatal allergies and autoaggressive diseases.

In this connection potentized embryonic organ preparations as original treatment possibilities of anthroposophic medicine are particularly effective.

Essentially three *embryonic organ preparations* are available today which relate to organs which humans and every mammal lose at birth and which therefore cannot be related directly in their use to homologous organs of the child. The question as to the reasoning behind their use therefore needs to be asked all the more clearly.

The *placenta* is created extraembryonically out of the decidua basalis of the *chorion*. This only occurs in the most highly developed group of vertebrates, the mammals, and in humans. In rodents, beasts of prey and ungulates there is a specific developmental tendency (much more clearly evident than revealed by the embryo at the beginning) and the human placenta comprises features of all these three different placental types in its formation [cf. Schad 1971].

The *umbilical cord* develops in a very complex way, enveloped by the amnion, and contains the body stalk with the allantois as well as the yolk stalk and the umbilical coelom. We can *indeed see all the germ layers of the embryo as well as the chorion being involved in the creation of the umbilical cord.* (It links the "amniotic umbilicus with the chorionic umbilicus" [cf. Hinrichsen 1990, 140].) But the development of the umbilical cord clearly starts with the body stalk and the *allantois* (an organ which is little developed in humans but strongly in bird embryos, for example, and still has clear functions in the latter, in gaseous exchange for instance).

The *amnion* most clearly represents a purely embryonic structure, although not an inner embryonic one but also a sheathing organ (which is lost at birth), which is clearly related to the *ectoderm – and thus the epidermis.* The internalized liquid of the cerebrospinal fluid preserves the composition of the amniotic fluid; the aqueous humour of the eye also represents a section of "isolated amniotic fluid", an inland sea we might say, which retains a similarity with amniotic fluid throughout life. All vertebrates whose offspring develop primarily on land require such an amnion at the start of their development with which they organize a fluid, sea-like buoyant space which allows for the primary development of the body with a negligible effect of earthly gravity. The amnion thus limits the fluid and warmth space of the unborn child and is, at the same time, a buoyant space liberated from gravity.

These three organs have in common that they are shed at birth and die. At the same time the higher forces of the human being which formed them (etheric body, astral body and I) unite with the born body in a new way [cf. Steiner 1998, 75–93]. Rudolf Steiner explained the embryonic situation in these words on 23 April 1924: "The situation is this, we have to know that the amnion is the physical correlate of the etheric body, allantois is the physical correlate of the astral body, chorion is the physical correlate of the I-organization of the adult person" [Rudolf Steiner 1989, 308].

In the experience of the authors and other experienced anthroposophical paediatricians, the following is specifically suitable for embryonic shock experiences of the mother, s/p amniocentesis and a difficult birth associated with massive maternal anxiety

- **Amnion Gl D30 amp.** Wala
  0.5 ml to be administered per os in the evening, daily to every two days.

At the same time this preparation has an anabolic action on the "epidermal insufficiency" of the child suffering from atopic dermatitis due to the relationship between amnion and epidermis.

If the mother is under profound psychological stress during pregnancy leading to *psychological ambivalence* towards the child going as far a latent alienation,

- **Funiculus umbilicalis Gl D15–30 amp.** Wala

is suitable in the same dosage as specified above for Amnion. This medicine is more strongly related to disorders of the lungs (bronchial asthma), the urogenital tract and motor functions (cf. also the fourth case of sickness in [Steiner and Wegman 1991, 107–114])

With such a background, premature labour, failure to thrive of the child in utero and pre-eclampsia are often revealed in the medical history and indicate the choice of this medicine [cf. Soldner and Sommer 2007].

In the experience the authors, Amnion is by far the most important embryonic organ preparation for allergic diseases of the child and represents the most important organ preparation of any for atopic dermatitis – alongside Pancreas (!) (its introduction as a treatment is due to M. Sommer). The authors lack sufficient experiences of their own for the use of Placenta; one possible indication is s/p placental insufficiency (Gl D12-30, dosage as above) [cf. Kummer 2005a, 19–6–19–26].

- *Early childhood attachment disorders*
  Attachment disorders in early childhood often have their initial cause in the disorders during pregnancy described above. Alongside relationship conflicts, an ambivalence towards the mother role and other stress factors, *the postpartum depression of the mother* represents an important and often insufficiently diagnosed cause of early childhood attachment disorders; such a depression can lead to the sustained impairment of the correspondence between mother and child and strongly facilitate the manifestation of childhood eczema – which in turn places a burden on the relationship between mother and child. Feelings of guilt and the depression itself contribute to the mother not speaking about these stresses herself; Fathers[1] often find it difficult to understand the situation as they themselves primarily feel rejected, and after the occurrence of the child's eczema at the latest the paediatrician will see the depression of the mother as a reaction to the skin rash. Understanding the sequence in which the disorders appear is important here, asking the right questions of the mother or the father. The triggers of such disorders can be very different and are not easy to determine in postpartum

1 Fathers, too, show double the rate of depression after the birth of their child than would otherwise be expected by age.

depressions. But from a therapeutic perspective everything depends on the paediatrician not overlooking the situation of the mother and the impairment of the mother-child attachment. It is not infrequently up to the paediatrician to initiate competent care for the mother – and thus to introduce the most effective therapeutic measure for the child.

6.4.3.1.3 Further causes for the early onset of eczema

Other important causal reference points for the early onset of eczema can be:

- the *constitution of the child* (▸Chap. 6.4.3.6) as well as
- *organic functional disorders* and *weaknesses:*
  The more pronounced the eczema is rooted in these physical predispositions and conditions, the earlier it mostly manifests, which is why this aspect is of primary importance in infancy and early childhood. Important lead symptoms and their basic treatment were already set out in ▸Chap. 6.3.3.
- *Toxic burdens through the maternal organism* (amalgam! – prior antibiotic treatment, etc.):
  Toxic burdens from the mother also make their presence felt through the early appearance of eczema. The eczemas resist treatment with apparently indicated potentized medicines and have a tendency to increase with continued breast feeding. The paediatrician should not be afraid to take a precise medical history of the mother in this respect and even to examine the status of her teeth himself or herself: not infrequently gold crowns will be discovered next to amalgam fillings in the mouth of the mother – with all the familiar consequences resulting from the increased disintegration of the amalgam caused by the gold.

If there is a suspected amalgam burden, the child can be treated with

- **Silberamalgam D30 pillules** Staufen Pharma
  regularly repeated, e.g. 3 pillules 2 x/wk
- **Hepar Sulfuris D6 trit.** Weleda
  1 saltsp. daily in the morning
- **Berberis e rad. D3 pillules** Wala
  3–7 pillules 1–3 x/d

The root and bark of the barberry are processed in the preparation, which has "cholagogic and cholekinetic as well as uricosuric" characteristics [Bäumler 2007, 81], i.e. promotes drainage through the gall bladder and kidneys. Berberis e rad. is a good "opening medicine" in treatment for atopic dermatitis if there is a pre-existing toxic burden. H. H. Vogel has pointed out that promoting bile secretion has a positive effect on itching of the skin (just as conversely a lead symptom of biliary cirrhosis is itching). Berberis e rad. is also contained in Lycopodium comp. Wala (see below).

Success of this treatment is another indication if a toxically-caused eczema reaction of the child is suspected.

- *Toxic and allergen burden on the child's organism after birth:*
  Avoiding the corresponding burdens is of particular importance in atopic eczema – we refer here to the perspectives set out in ▸Chap. 6.3.2. Thus the introduction of solid food and weaning are known to frequently represent a time when eczema first manifests itself and careful individual nutritional advice and support is required through the treating doctor. Mould, wood preserver in interior spaces, air which is too dry and many other things can place a particular burden on the still immature skin of the infant.

  Antibiotics can also promote the manifestation of eczema and require a corresponding detoxifying treatment and above all attention to and, as necessary, restoration of the childhood intestinal flora, something which is of overriding importance for the development of a healthy immune regulation (▸Chap. 4.6). In infants we can consider to begin with:
  Bacterial lysates, e. g.
  - **Pro-Symbioflor®**
    5–10 gtt. 3 x/d, or
  - **Colibiogen® Kinder**
    ½–1 tsp. daily

  followed by the administration of *Lactobacillus*, e. g.
  - Lactobacillus Reutteri **BiGaia® Tr.**
    3–5 gtt daily or
  - **Symbiolact comp.®**
    ½–1 bag daily

  and *E. coli preparations*, e. g.
  - **Mutaflor® Suspension**
    0.5–1 ml daily

  (For the reasoning cf. Kummer [2005b] in detail)
  But antipyretics and other allopathic medicines (e. g. used for anaesthetic purposes) can also lead to allergies and require corresponding compensation. We specifically refer in this context once more to
  - **Lycopodium comp. pillules** Wala (▸Chap. 6.3.3.2)
    3–5 pillules 1–3 x/d

  which is also indicated if a toxic and allergenic burden from vaccines is suspected.

- *Protective vaccinations* (▸Chap. 3.5)
  The repeated multiple vaccinations recommended today place a burden on the child's immune system in first year of life through the unphysiological and premature stimulation of the development of specific immunity, while nonspecific immunity has not yet matured, thus promoting the impaired development of the child's immune regulation with all the consequences. Attention should also be paid to the allergenic adjuvants and preservatives contained in vaccines. It is the experience of many paediatricians that early childhood eczema manifests more frequently after (above all repeated) protective vaccinations in infancy.

Starting treatment with potencies of the vaccine used or its particularly problematical components should be considered here, e.g.

- **Hepatitis B vaccine C30 pillules** Gudjons
  3 pillules at an interval of 12–24 h each

The schematic administration of Thuja following vaccination often does not work (cf. ▸Chap. 3.5.7.2). Particularly helpful in general is the potentized administration of silicic acid – e.g. as Equisetum Silicea cultum (▸Chap. 6.3.3.3) or Opal. In terms of differential treatment Conchae, Mezereum and Thuja may be considered (▸Chap. 6.4.3.6.2, ▸Chap. 6.4.3.6.5).

Specifically indicated after a vaccination-related worsening of allergic diseases is the composite medicine

- **Lien comp. pillules** Wala
  3–7 pillules 1–3 x/d (depending on age) – (▸Chap. 6.3.3.4)

Parents suffering from allergic diseases, the manifestation of childhood allergies or the worry about them often motivate parents to take an *individual vaccination decision* in respect of *what and above all when* to vaccinate. Detailed advice for the parents on this subject and the recommendation of suitable literature is important in the context of allergy prevention and treatment. More detailed information in this respect and references can be found in ▸Chap. 3.5

- *Clothing and body care*
  Protecting the body temperature of the infant is protectively and therapeutically of central importance with regard to the development of atopic dermatitis. Thus the recommendation not to leave the home in the first four weeks of life in itself already represents warmth protection, but also protection against sensitization if the child is born in the pollen season and against fine particles and other pollution (assuming the appropriate equipment for ventilating the home). Woollen bodysuits and clothing particularly in the winter months protect the body temperature of the child, but can often not be the right thing with manifest eczema or individual skin intolerance which can trigger itching – it is therefore all the more important that the clothing as a whole supports the balanced warmth distribution in the infant. This point is very often insufficiently taken into account. Oil rhythmical Einreibungen have been part of the culture of human skincare since time immemorial and are very important for infants particularly in the winter months. Questions should be asked about the use of soaps and shampoos (mostly unsuitable) and washing powder (fragrances and brighteners etc. should be avoided for example) as much as about unwashed new clothing. For special textiles for atopic dermatitis (e.g. overalls with silver fibres) see www.allergate.de.
- *Teething*
  Almost every early childhood eczema grows worse during dentition and parents should be made aware of that beforehand if possible. Dentition itself occurs physiologically as an acute inflammation, acute infections occur simultaneously in this vulnerable phase. It is important to avoid as far as possible any new challenge to the child's organism, such as the introduction of new foods (or, indeed, protective vaccinations)

during acute dentition, and to treat acute infections themselves carefully without the use of allopathic medication as much as possible. On the other hand, the eruption of the canines announces a radical stabilization of the child's organism, his or her digestive ability and ability to set boundaries. Breast feeding should end at this time at the latest to give way to the child's own activity in the digestion of foreign foods. The symbiosis of the infant with his or her mother can now be overcome in favour of a growing mutual autonomy. If this is done successfully, what might be the crucial foundation for the atopic dermatitis to heal will have been laid.

6.4.3.1.4 Appearance of eczema after infancy

Second and third year of life

In eczema which occurs for the first time after dentition, a *specific trigger* can often be discovered. Here all the factors referred to so far individually come into question. If they can be easily eliminated (newly introduced foods which are not tolerated, medicines, body care and detergent products, clothing and so on), the prognosis is very favourable. The medical history, taken with thorough detective work, and consistent avoidance are of crucial therapeutic importance here. Diagnostically, *allergy testing* should build on a careful medical history and be carried out specifically. More difficult to treat are iatrogenic and/or disease-related weaknesses of the child's immune system, e.g. as the result of repeated antibiosis and serious infections during dentition which have led to the "dam breaking" on the child's barriers of skin, intestine and/or airways. Here careful organ diagnosis and restorative, salutogenically oriented treatment (in the sense of ▸Chap. 6.3) are necessary, leading to the restoration of the immunological balance. Most difficult to treat, and not rare at this age, are serious family conflicts and stresses through the separation of the parents.

Kindergarten and school children

Particular attention should be paid to the quality of the mother-child attachment if the atopic dermatitis occurs for the first time at this age. Anxiety disorders *play a particular role in (often generalized) atopic dermatitis in the early school years.* These display two components: at the primary level, a considerable maternal anxiety disorder can mostly be determined which can originally have arisen independently of pregnancy and the maternal role. When asked (!), the mother can frequently specify very precisely which situations give rise to her anxiety which then acts on her like a compulsion (e.g. if she has to take a longer trip alone in the car). In a second step, this anxiety can attach itself to the child – particularly in a close mother-child attachment – for example when he or she starts to go to school on his or her own. In such cases the mother might continue to drive the child to school each day and collect him or her again even when in terms of age the child has long been in a position to go to school himself or herself or use a bicycle. The maternal anxiety can remain hidden as the child develops anxieties (which he or she cannot explain) and not infrequently atopic symptoms, e.g. a dry and itchy eczema. In a new manifestation or pronounced exacerbation of eczema between the ages of six and nine this can be a main cause which very frequently is not recognized and treated.

- **Aconitum D30–C200 pillules**
  dissolved in water (5–10 pillules) administered over three days (1 tsp. 3 x/d)

is an effective initial treatment for both sides in these cases.

Providing clarification and an explanation of the connection in a meeting with the parents in itself already has a therapeutic effect. In many cases qualified psychotherapy proposed by the paediatrician and initiated by the mother can represent significant relief and help. Behavioural therapy must work on a gradual resolution of the anxiety-related "overprotection" of the child. The increased involvement of the father (who often sees himself marginalized in such constellations by the close mother-child attachment – in several cases the affected child was sleeping with the mother while the father slept in another room) is mostly helpful and improves the balance within the family. It is just as necessary to explain to the child that his or her anxieties will gradually disappear if he or she masters his or her life independently (and that he or she should not wait for the reverse to happen). In doing so, the mother must not be exposed in front of the child; it is sufficient to enable the child to take a hold of the independence of which he or she is capable through, for example, a reward system and with the permission of the mother (doing homework independently, going to friends, going to school, going on an excursion with the father, etc.). Lastly, carefully carried out *constitutional treatment of the child* can be of crucial importance (▸Chap. 6.4.3.6). In general, every mother-child attachment which is too close at this age has the effect of promoting anxieties, social withdrawal, lack of attachments to children of his or her own age and professional educators (kindergarten teachers, teachers) and the disposition for allergies. The cause of the too close attachment can lie in the child's constitution or the familial system and should not be attributed one-sidedly to the mother.

Other age-specific issues are sibling rivalry, experiences of isolation and bullying[1] in his or her own age group, stress through parental, school and political performance expectations. In addition, all the aspects listed for infancy and early childhood can still be of relevance later on.

Puberty and adolescence

The new onset of serious cases of atopic dermatitis at his age tends to be rare, a renewed exacerbation or the recurrence of early childhood eczema very much more frequent. On the one hand, this is connected with what anthroposophy calls the "birth of the astral body", or in simple terms the development of independence of the young person's soul organization at around the age of 14. This event corresponds in a global cultural and religious context to the performance of an initiation rite (e.g. confirmation in the Christian church), a ritual which in societies with a western lifestyle is increasingly just a consumer event which no longer gives backing to the soul of the young person.

The loosening of the strong parental attachment and the growing importance of relationships with his or her own age-group faces the young person with great psychological

1 In the observation of the authors, children with a close or close and ambivalent maternal attachment at this age tell with above average frequency of experiences which are reported to the doctor as "bullying". The doctor should not directly adopt this judgement but carefully determine the interaction of the child with children of his or her own age.

challenges. When they are experienced as becoming too much, this can be reflected in a resurgence of eczema. Thus own anxieties have to be overcome in the detachment from the parents which is now due – it happens not infrequently that there will be an exacerbation of eczema before or when the young person moves out of the parental home. The same applies to exam situations especially if there are ambitious parental or internalized expectations. Far-reaching decisions have to be taken while the lack of life experience and fragile social relationships provide shaky ground for the adolescent's new independent responsibility. The western lifestyle does not necessarily reinforce the young person in this respect: the immunocompetence of female adolescents is lastingly weakened through contraceptives (Th_2 stimulation), facilitating serious infections and allergies, without the prescribing gynaecologist as a rule raising this issue.[1] At the same time the psychological and cognitive pressure on young people to appear perfect has increased in the last decades. The skin, not least, should look perfect! Contact eczema from cheap jewellery (ear studs as a young child promote the onset of contact eczema in later years), allergic reactions to questionable cosmetics and skincare agents must be taken into account as much as the psychological hyperactivity of the adolescent in his or her skin which is constantly inspected in the mirror. Then there are the demands of school and the labour market, the lack of support in broken homes, the stress of partnerships entered into at an ever earlier age with sexual contact, and the frequently lacking meaningful work for others. Nutrition lacks rhythm and often high quality fresh food. Nicotine and recreational drugs are a further issue; smoking has a detrimental effect on atopic dermatitis because, among other things, it causes the skin periphery to age prematurely.

Alongside providing the necessary support for the young person in acute exam situations for example, the avoidance of recreational and lifestyle drugs, as well as the necessary basic therapy and constitutional treatment, therapeutic counselling is now unavoidable. The required backing for the newly to be acquired autonomy grows if the adolescent learns to find occupational orientation through practice placements and doing meaningful things for others, to overcome own anxieties through visits abroad, and to detach himself or herself from the parental home and acquire new skills, whereby the resilience of the patient always has to be taken into account and assessed. The aspect of *own activity* becomes most important therapeutically at this age.

6.4.3.2 Climate change and reconvalescence treatment

The question of *holidays* is of general importance and finding a *suitable spa* where relevant. Here it is to be recommended in the first year of life that *quiet*, the creation of a lovely home environment, avoiding technical media (radio, TV, CD and similar things) – which flood the child with sense impressions for which there is no physically present correlate – and avoiding longer trips are most helpful for the development of the child's barriers and sense organs. Mobility promotes allergies.

Sun and a *maritime climate* have a healing effect on many eczema patients from toddler age. This can only be understood in its wider significance if, alongside the physical aspect, we begin to perceive the importance of sun and sea *for life*. All the action of *warmth and light* which is crucial for life comes from the sun; in the sea, on the other hand, we have the

1 The Society of Anthropsophical Physicians in Germany GAÄD www.gaed.de has published an information sheet "Pille" (The Pill) which is suitable as a source of initial information.

original *fluid and salt environment* for the evolution of living things [cf. a comprehensive account of this aspect at the level of the life organization in Steiner 1963, 32].

On this basis we can say the following about holiday destinations – at least as a hypothesis to be tested in practice:

- *Maritime climate* generally stimulates the *anabolism, the vitality* of the child: above all it promotes appetite and sleep. A coastline with sandy beaches (North Sea, Atlantic, parts of the Mediterranean) is preferable, not a karst coast e. g. in Croatia.
- In the *high mountains* – primitive rock is suitable, mountains with geologically younger limestone (e. g. German Alps) should be avoided – sunlight is dominant but, in contrast to the maritime climate, not in a calming but a stimulating way. This mainly strengthens the *formative forces* which come from the nervous and sensory pole; in this way the *digestive activity* for example and the *barrier function of the boundaries* can be strengthened towards the environment.
- *Southern locations* (Mediterranean, Canary Islands) directly support the child's *warmth organism*. All those atopic dermatitis patients whose eczema grows worse during the winter, who develop insufficient body temperature, who psychologically tend to be introverted (up to and including depressive tendencies), show an improvement in the south (as a rule) which can last for very different periods.
- In contrast, *the north or also the high mountains fundamentally challenge the child's warmth organism.* A visit to the North Sea in particular should therefore be for a sufficiently long time (four to six weeks) so that the child has time to respond with his or her warmth organization to the natural environment. Then such convalescence treatment can have a particularly sustained effect because it strengthens the own activity of the child's organism.

In general, the length of the holiday of people with allergies in a climate which is fundamentally different from home should correspond to the rhythms of the organism. Just as the human I (cf. the section on the circadian temperature regulation above, ▸Chap. 6.4.2) lives in the daily rhythm, a four-weekly rhythm applies to the human life organization, the etheric body [Steiner 1988, 187; Hildebrandt 1986, 170–221]. That is also what in the past underlay the period of four weeks for a cure. Anyone who wants to achieve anything in the living organism must know about these periods and adjust to them. Otherwise it can happen, as it not infrequently does, that a worsening of the clinical picture after a one or two-week holiday together with an elevated susceptibility to infection can be observed – after four weeks it might have been possible to observe the opposite effect with the same holiday destination.

After all, convalescent stays are particularly suited for dealing with chronic disorders in the relationship between child and mother or child and parents in the continuous presence of nurses and doctors with the relevant training. That applies particularly with regard to the so frequently *impaired sleep behaviour.* With atopic dermatitis it is generally necessary to give the parents *periods of respite* which allow them to step back and retrieve their inner equilibrium. In practice it happens, however, that mother and child are so symbiotically closely connected (above all if both of them are completely tired out through sleep disturbance) that good outpatient suggestions no longer helps either. Convalescent facilities[1] which offer thorough advice on food and surroundings, age-appropriate sleep training (for child, mother *and* father), a suitable diet, with symbiotic control as necessary, under favourable climatic conditions (proximity to the sea) can make a valuable long-term therapeutic contribution.

6.4.3.3 External treatments

External treatments for atopic dermatitis have an *alleviating, supporting, balancing effect but not a healing one.* That applies to every treatment, including conventional dermatological ones. But since a *curative aim* is pursued in the therapeutic concept set out here – and not just the symptomatic suppression of the disease – the position of the external therapy changes fundamentally: it assumes an auxiliary function (in relation to the internal treatment) and in general does not need to be individualized as much as the latter. It is important to tell the patient and/or the parents in advance about this approach in order to avoid a fixation on the external therapy. External treatments should be used with restraint as a matter of principle – the too frequent application of fatty external agents only leads to the further irritation of the already hypersensitive organism, further impairment of its warmth organization and beyond that not infrequently to a maldevelopment in the relationship between parents and child. The constant application of creams "on demand" only makes the situation worse. In contrast, when applying the cream or a bandage on the weeping section of skin each evening, the mother should focus on the child with calmness and concentration – in order then to release him or her into sleep.

This therapeutic goal is derived from the holistic understanding developed above: namely to activate the competence of the child's organism in digestion, in building up the fats, developing his or her warmth organization and immune system, thereby guiding the soul forces "inwards and downwards" which are otherwise active in a one-sidedly catabolic way "outwardly on top" on the skin. This goal is explicitly different from "control" through anti-inflammatory substances in which externals (and allergen avoidance) play the dominant role. As important as skin care is, the parental attention and care should nevertheless gradually move away from a one-sided fixation on the skin. That was already discussed in detail above (▸Chap. 6.3). On the other hand it applies that a sufficient measure of skin care is necessary so that the skin can be "forgotten" and the child is not trapped psychologically by its own physical boundaries.

6.4.3.3.1 Acute exudative eczema (weeping or wet eczema)

In general, external treatment follows the dermatological principle that weeping eczema should be treated moistly and dry eczema drily. Each doctor has to make his or her own restricted choice from the great range of possibilities and thereby build up and expand his or her personal experience.

1 Convalescent stays in convalescence clinics should be avoided in the months when infections are most prevalent as there is otherwise a high risk of having to deal mainly with the consequences of infection.

With weeping inflammatory acute eczema, moist wraps are suitable to begin with as well as fatty-moist bandages: a non-heat retaining cream should be applied directly to the skin whereby in recent years the authors have found the newly developed

- **Imlan® Creme Pur**

to be successful. It was developed for skin diseases by A. Scheffler [Scheffler 2004] on the basis of medicinal suggestions by Rudolf Steiner [Steiner 1994, lecture of 4 April 1920]. In *intertriginous skin rashes* this completely non-toxic cream is a masterful external application.[1]

The cream is based purely on the extract of white birch bark, which contains betulinic acid and other triterpenes with wound-healing, antiseptic, anti-inflammatory and antiproliferative characteristics and at the same time functions as an emulgator of oil and water. It has the benefit that

- it does not contain any allergenic substances (e.g. emulgators) but only water, jojoba oil and betulin,[2]
- super infections are becoming rarer and can also be treated with it if used early enough,
- with regard to its function in the plant, birch bark precisely fulfils the task (protection against cold and water loss) which is a central role of the lipid barrier in the epidermis and thus in terms of its process represents a "model" for the skin which it is used to treat,
- there is no occlusive effect.

This newly developed external application shares a basic problem with a number of other external plant applications mentioned below: it is not, or not yet, licensed as a medicine (the same applies to Bedan® and Intensiv Creme/Lotion Mittagsblume). The extreme costs of licensing medicines, including nontoxic herbal medicines, (currently approx. 15 million euros) will ensure that this unsatisfactory situation continues to exist in the next few years.

6

Tubular bandages (e.g. Tubifast®, washable, available in five size) are often suitable for moist bandages on skin which has had cream applied, moistened by placing them in lukewarm tea,

for *weeping inflamed* eczema:

- **Pansy tea** (Viola tricolor),

for *weeping itching* eczema:

- **Horsetail tea** (Equisetum arvense)

add to cold water 6 h, then boil for 10–15 mins. and allow to draw for a similar period to allow the silicic acid to be released from the horsetail. The exudation and itching is countered by the addition of oak bark essence, e.g.

1 The authors owe this reference to intertriginous eczema originally to Prof. C. Schempp, University Dermatological Clinic Freiburg i.Br. The Imlan cream has in the meantime proved itself many times for this indication.

2 It does, however, have to be said that the original Birkencreme® with almond and sunflower oil appeared to have a somewhat stronger effect.

- **Quercus Essenz** Wala (astringent)
  15 ml/250 ml water 1 x/d

while an essence of Calendula is suitable for eczema with threatening or acute super infections, but also to stimulate skin regeneration:

- **Calendula Essenz** Wala/Weleda
  15 ml/250 ml water 2 x/d

or also use some oak bark tea. For older children green tea is also suitable.

- **Silicea coll. comp. Gel** Wala
  apply e.g. after fatty-moist bandages for acute, weeping, itching eczema as *cooling* gel to calm itching

is suitable for *cooling* and calming itching ([Vademecum 2010, 747]; confirming reference by F. Roemer).

Horsetail forms silica in opal form and enriches it. *Silicic acid in opal form* hardens out of an *aqueous colloidal* state; opal always contains up to 10 % water and changes its water content through contact with the air (precious opal which is created out of aqueous solutions containing silicic acid over long, undisturbed periods loses its former vivid colour play when removed from water and regains it if it is placed back in it). Living organisms such as horsetail or bamboo can concentrate silicic acid in opal form in a concentrated mineral way which they produce in a comparatively very short period of time themselves. The basic relationship between silicic acid and the epidermis, to develop the barriers, was already discussed in ▸Chap. 5.1.2.4. Equisetum in aqueous form limits, if externally applied, the inflammatory dissolution of the skin by means of the action of the silicic acid.

Oak bark, on the other hand, acts above all through its *tannin content*: "Tannin has ... the ability to form more of less stable complexes with proteins. That is what their anti-inflammatory, astringent, slightly locally anaesthetizing and drying out action on the skin and mucous membranes is based on. They stabilize the always labile "barriers" of a person which with weeping eczema for example becomes too porous and too closely related to metabolic activity in the development of secretions" [Meyer 1997].

A second, dry layer is pulled over the moist bandage layer and the bandage is kept on for 6–8 hours or overnight. Too much cooling down through bandages which are kept on for too long must be avoided; a precise control of the acra is required to prevent the moist bandage being applied too tightly. Such a "second skin" can have an effective calming effect, particularly for the night, which allows the soul to separate from the body and thus enables going to sleep. Wearing the corresponding coveralls, if necessary with silver fibres woven into them, which enclose the hands can be a further help for self-calming and the avoidance of excessive scratching during the night.

- **Imlan® Creme pur**

can, as the acutely moist eczema heals and if there are dry spots of eczema, be *mixed* with

- **Quercus Salbe** Wala
  (contains extracts of Hamamelis and Borago alongside oak bark extract).

This mixture, suggested by K. R. Kummer, has proved very useful for the authors and others experienced in treating atopic dermatitis. For small children, moister skin, during the warm periods of the year, a mixture of 2 parts Imlan Creme pur and 1 part Quercus Salbe; for older children, dry skin, during the cold periods of the year, a ratio of 1:1 is recommended. In dry eczema and children from the age of 3–4 the following is suitable

- **Imlan® Creme plus**
  (contains 3 % urea and beeswax).

Urea-containing external applications do not benefit children under the age of three.

6.4.3.3.2 Dry eczema

With the latter external applications mentioned above, we are already getting close to dry eczema. A new external application, available since 2009, has shown itself to be excellent when used by the authors and others for dry to very dry acute eczema:

- **Intensiv Lotion/Creme Mittagsblume** Dr. Hauschka
  apply several x/d to begin with, later on clearly less frequently

The lotion can be applied very easily and quickly improves the dryness of the skin and itching; if the skin is constitutionally dry with acute eczematous exacerbation, this cream represents a very effective herbal external application.

Mesembryanthemum crystallinum, the common ice plant, is native to the South African cape flora and the Canary Isles. The anthroposophical nurse Waltraut Marschke discovered it there as a medicinal plant and introduced it to atopic dermatitis treatment (as a prescription preparation) as long ago as the 1980 s. In this respect there have been positive therapeutic experiences for a long time. The plant itself grows on a saline substrate (near beaches) and in "disturbed places" and displays a pronounced resistance against drying out. "Stalk and leaves are covered with numerous transparent blisters which are needed to store water and give the plant a shiny appearance." [Maddaus 1979, 1901] The common ice plant thus represents a natural model for the barrier function of the skin. The preparation has also proved its value for patients who suffer from episodes of eczema through long baths, chlorine baths and dry heating air in winter and for children with constitutionally ichthyosiform dry skin. (Information from Prof. C. Schempp).

- **Bedan® Creme**[1] (contains hyperforin-rich St. John's Wort extract)
  apply as required

1 The suggestion to use this cream comes from Prof. C. Schempp who was the first doctor in decades to write his habilitation on herbal medicine (the ingredients of Hypericum and their effectiveness in dermatology).

The lipophilic main active agent of St. John's Wort, the phloroglucinol derivative hyperforin, possesses pronounced antibacterial, antiinflammatory and differentiation-promoting characteristics [Schempp 1999, Müller 2008]. Bedan cream has worked well in many cases of dry, sub-acute eczema and prevents super infections through its herbal ingredients. It cannot be predicted with certainty whether common ice plant or Bedan or the mixture of Imlan cream/Quercus ointment is tolerated better – but almost every patient with dry eczema will experience a clear to very clear improvement with one of these alternatives.

Very suitable with dry eczema particularly in the winter six months is

- **Rosatum Heilsalbe** Wala
  several x/d or at night as an ointment bandage

This ointment, which is licensed as a medicine, is strongly lipid replenishing, calms itching and boosts regeneration and is experienced as very pleasant by many patients.

- **Dermatodoron® Salbe** Weleda
  apply once or several x/d

has proved successful for dry eczema in the winter six months, above all for areas exposed to the cold (face, hands) with dry, itching, eczematously changed skin [Vademecum 2010, 388].[1] Its indication is the polar opposite to the internal application of Dermatodoron® drops which have shown their value for pronounced metabolic, exudatively disintegrating skin phenomena [Vademecum 2010, 386).

The following is very oily and enriched with the valuable fat-soluble substances of sandthorn berry oil (costly to produce)

- **Salbengrundlage SK** Apotheke an der Weleda

It contains almond oil, sandthorn berry oil, yellow wax and lanolin and was developed by the anthroposophical dermatologist Lüder Jachens [Vademecum 2010, 730].

The authors have not so far been able to come to an empirical judgement on the hydrophilic vitamin B_{12}-containing cream Regividerm® [Hung 2010].

In principle, the action of the cream or ointment used to alleviate itching can be enhanced through the addition of potentized additives which thus represent an alternative to the otherwise commonly used Polidocanol (5 % additive).

The following for example can be used especially with dry, strongly itching eczema (the authors owe this reference to Markus Sommer)

- **Berberis D3 dil.** 1.0
- **Hydrocotyle D3 dil.** 1.0
- **Argentum met. praep. D6 trit.** Weleda 1.0–2.0
- **Arsenicum album D12 dil.** 1.0
- **Equisetum arv. D4 dil.** Weleda 1.0–3.0
- e. g. in **Imlan® Creme Plus** or **Rosatum Heilsalbe** Wala.

If there is a wish not to use potentized substances for external treatment, a decoction of Equisetum is suitable for severe itching [cf. Jachens 1999b, 171]:

- **Equisetum arvense, decoction aquosum 10 %** (make freshly) 100.0
  DAC-Basis-Creme ad 200.0 M. f. Salbe [Goebel, Glöckler 2008, 699]

1 R. Madeleyn confirms its effectiveness also in the context of in-patient treatment.

Equisetum can also be used as an additive on its own; if the ointment base is not tolerated, 10 % of Equisetum 10 % Oleum (Weleda) can be added to a tolerated base. Other possibilities are: the addition of the waxy jojoba oil (2–4 %); the addition of 1 gtt rose oil to 100 g gives the ointment a pleasant scent (M. Sommer).

For moisture 85 % glycerol can be added (up to 10 %), while urea is not well tolerated under the age of five.

A valuable emulsifier-free external oil treatment which, if carried out properly, can lead to a *sustained stimulation of the child's warmth organization*, and can thus stimulate healing processes, is

- **Oil dispersion bath as developed by Junge** (www.jungebad.com),

whereby the temperature of the bath should be pleasant for the child, not cool.
In atopic dermatitis the following bath oil is universally suitable

- **Rosa e flor. 10 % Ol.** Wala

and alternatively or complementarily

- **Equisetum ex herba 5 % Ol.** Wala
  (calculated at 3–5 ml per full bath).

It is important that the baths are *given in the proper way*, if possible after competent instruction, to optimize the stimulating effect on the child's warmth organization. The bath should not be given hot, on the other hand the child must not be cold in it – the warmth stimulating effect on the organism comes from the finely distributed oils, which also pleasantly oil the skin (does not produce heat accumulation if properly applied). The subsequent rest in bed, optimally without drying, wrapped in a bath towel after the bath, is important. In this way the warmth organization of the child is strengthened and stimulated in a positive way. The oil dispersion bath is not therefore an external treatment but a medicine with a profound action.

If the paediatrician has a bath dispersion device which can be lent out, it is advisable for the parents to gather their own experience with this treatment before they purchase this comparatively expensive device which is, however, incredibly economical with regular use.

6

Chapped, hyperkeratotic-rhagadiform eczema in older children and adolescents, e. g. on the hands and fingers, responds to

- **Antimonit 0.4 % Creme** Weleda
  used occlusively overnight with the corresponding gloves [Jachens 1999b, Vademecum 2010, 81];

as does periorbital and perioral eczema in so far as an ointment is not contraindicated.

Corticosteroids can be avoided in most cases. However, this does also depend on the age and attitude of the patient. The social demand that we should all look perfect creates the necessity, particularly when treating adolescents, to balance the patient's involvement, his or her tolerance limits, on the one hand, and the requirements of a healing treatment on the other. As a short-term interim aid, the authors have used *hydrocortisone-containing creams* (e. g. Pandel, Alfason) for example in generalized, weeping infant eczema with hypoproteinaemia for long enough to allow the internal treatment with potentized medicines to start working and the protein to start rising (a few days). We should bear in mind that the resorption rate in the nappy (diaper) area is 42 times, and on the face and under occlusion 10 times the resorption rate on normal healthy skin! [Höger 2005, 162]

6.4.3.4 Superinfected eczema

The treatment of superinfections associated with atopic dermatitis can also succeed without antibiotics or antimycotics. Such treatment requires experience and everyone will draw their own boundary as to the point where they start to lose control of the disease process and its prognosis. The important thing to realize is that the weakness of the lipid barrier of the skin is of prime importance, not only the weakness of immune regulation. This is why a non-occlusive skin-nourishing treatment with a lotion or a cream is important, especially with stubborn, recurrent, or therapy-resistant superinfections.

The authors have found that for prophylactic purposes as well as during the initial stages of a superinfection the previously discussed

- **Imlan® Creme Pur**

has proven to be a valuable basic therapeutic aid.

The most frequent superinfections are with *staphylococci*, identifiable from their characteristic pustules. This should be distinguished from the much more aggressive characteristics of *impetigo,* caused by a superinfection with *streptococci.*

Pustules and abscesses can be treated during the day with

- **Clay poultices**

A suitable clay is

- **Haferkleie mit Calendula-Essenz** Wala/Weleda
  1:10 diluted and stirred until spreadable by adding ½–1 teaspoon of honey.

At night, the following ointment is appropriate:

Sulphur praecip	3.0
Camomile salve	10.0
Ol. jecoris	30.0
Zinc. oxyd.	30.0
Adeps lanae	ad 100.0 (cf. Goebel, Glöckler 2008, 699].

Alternatively, as an *aqueous cover,* a shaken mixture of zinc and appropriate additives can be used:

Sulphur praecip.	3.0–4.0
Calendula essence	5.0
Echinacea essence 10 % Wala/Weleda	5.0
Lotio alba	ad 100.0

Regarding superinfections of the skin, we are greateful to Prof. C. Schempp, Univ. Dermatology Clinic Freiburg (Germany) for showing the benefits of 1 % coriander oil. This treatment almost completely replaces allopathic antiseptics (also in the Freiburg University Hospital). We have also found it very useful. An extensive description of the antimicrobial effects of this oil can be found in C. Schempp (2011).

Superinfected skin regions can be treated with

- Oleum Coriandri 0.5
  Imlan Creme Pur ad 50.0

or

- Oleum Coriandri 1.0
  Unguentum leniens ad 100.0

Coriander oil 1% can also be added to a neutral oil lotion such as for example Imlan Lotion pur. We can confirm the statement of C. Schempp that this treatment has an excellent antibacterial effect without any side effects.
In exceptional cases, generalized superinfections must be treated systemically with antibiotics (a cephalosporine that is effective against Staphylocc.), escpecially in babies and small children.

In terms of diet, an *absolute avoidance of sweet foods* in any form is essential alongside the general principles. Equally *rest*, the avoidance of unnecessary or demanding travel are nowadays all too often forgotten essentials for curing acute and purulent inflammations.

Internally, proven medicines for *Staphlococcal infections* are

- **Hepar Sulfuris D12 pillules** (various manufacturers)
  5 pillules in the morning
- **Argentum/Quarz pillules/amp.** Wala
  5–7 pillules 2–3 x/d

Argentum/Quarz has proven its capabilities to the authors as a way of counteracting a spread of cutaneous infections through the lymphatic system (also effective with lymphangitis). This therapy can be supplemented especially in the event of acute *itching* and *severe internal lack of warmth* by the administration of

- **Psorinum C12–30 pillules** Gudjons
  acutely 5 pillules 1 x/d

In some cases, *Streptococcal impetigo* may initially require a parenteral dose of

- **Argentum/Quarz amp.** Wala, where necessary with
- **Pyrogenium D30 amp.** (various manufacturers)

mixed 2 ml or only Argentum/Quarz i.v.; with Staphlococcal infections this is usually not necessary.
With impetigo (▸Chap. 5.3.4.4.3) an appropriate internal medicine comprises

- **Lachesis comp. pillules** Wala
  5–10 pillules 5 x/d

alternating with

- **Antimonite D6 trit.** Weleda
  1 saltsp. 5 x/d

If the purulent superinfection is associated with fever, it is in isolated cases possible to greatly strengthen individual resistance by administering

- **Argentum D30/Echinacea D6 amp.** Weleda
  1 amp./d orally in 1–2 individal doses or i.v. or
- **Echinacea/Argentum pillules** Wala
  5–10 pillules 3 x/d

6

In principle, *acutely purulent* inflammation of the skin represents not just a danger for eczema patients, *but also an opportunity.* By overcoming the acute inflammation through the body's own immunological defences, the immune system and warmth organization are often permanently strengthened. In practice, this often gives rise to deep-rooted improvement of the eczema, once infections have been overcome. In isolated cases, antibiotics are required, but the frequency of their application reduces as the doctor's therapeutic experience rises.

Fungal infections of the skin with atopic dermatitis can be treated externally with

- **Wecesin Puder** Weleda
  use mornings/during the day

and

- **Melaleuca (tea tree) oil, 10 %** in olive oil
  apply in the evenings

Internally, horsetail in low potentized form has therapeutic benefits:

- **Equisetum arvense D3 dil.** Weleda
  5–7 gtt. 3 x/d and
- **Argentite D6 trit.** Weleda
  1 saltsp. 3 x/d

The sulphide form of silver supports vitality and the warmth organization in the skin, whereas Equisetum brings the formatively organizing impact of silicic acid to bear on the barrier organs of the body (cf. also above, the external application of equisetum, and ▸Chap. 5.1.2.4), fungal infections tend to proliferate where the warmth organization of the organism is weakened and the living fluid organization is no longer structured by forming or shaping forces to a sufficient extent.

6.4.3.5 Steps towards individualized treatment

6.4.3.5.1 Acute exacerbation

In daily practice, it may repeatedly be necessary when faced with *acute exacerbations of eczema*, especially in early childhood, to commence a general and *internally applied* acute therapy of the skin. There is already in practice the possibility of acute intervention involving the preparation of an *ampoule mixture* and, in response to a positive impact, continuing to administer it for a (varying length of) time. This mixture can be varied to suit the individual; a frequently tried and tested option being the basic matrix listed and explained below:

- **Calcium-Quercus amp.** 1–2 ml Wala
  Amnion Gl D30 amp. 1 ml Wala
  Argentum met. praep. D30 amp. 1 ml Weleda
  Apis ex animale D30 amp. 1 ml Wala
  Pancreas/Equisetum amp. 1 ml Wala
  drawn into a 10 ml injection, stored in a cool place, then administered orally from it, with *acute weeping eczemas* 0.5–1.0 ml 3–4 x/d.

With older children and young people, it is possible in acute situations to administer a

- **Calcium-Quercus 10 ml amp.** Wala
  10 ml i.v.

injection, supplemented as necessary by 1 ampoule **Apis D30** Wala and **Argentum met. praep. D30** Weleda.

- **Calcium-Quercus amp./pillules**

have a sealing effect on the epidermal barrier [Vademecum 2010, 247 Leitgedanke]; the more acutely this barrier dissolves in the child, the higher the dosage of this medication which can be chosen. Depending on age, a favourable alternative consists of dissolving 10–30 pillules in water and having the child take it in sips (cf. below ▸Chap. 6.4.3.6.2)

- **Amnion** (Chap. 6.4.3.1.2; ▸Chap. 6.4.3.6)

constitutes an "archetypal" embryonic organ preparation that is very effective in acute cases in that it has a stimulating impact on the anabolism of the epidermal barrier formation while relaxing the overactivity of the soul entity in the skin. Alternatively, it can be administered individually for the night in acute situations.

- **Apis D30**

acts in a structuring manner especially on seriously inflammatory and barrier-dissolving processes [Vademecum 2010, 92] and in acute allergic reactions as an important potentized medicine.

- **Pancreas/Equisetum**

has proven its capabilities to the authors in the acute therapy of weeping eczemas (▸Chap. 6.3.3.2). It stimulates digestion and renal secretion, which in turn promotes the concentration of astral soul activity "at the right location – below inside", which relieves the skin and causes the eczema to dry up. It is striking that *medicines of animal origin* (Amnion, Apis, Pancreas) can act particularly fast and be highly effective in acute cases. Rudolf Steiner attributes to them an immediate impact on the life organization (the etheric body) [Steiner 1994, 228].

- **Argentum met. praep. D30**, potentized silver,

in acute dissolving situations has a concentrating, contracting effect on the higher components of the human being, especially the soul organization and life organization. The acute dissolving tendency in acute eczema tends to move towards the periphery while central life processes (digestion, excretion, anabolism) are disregarded. The acute inflammation gives way to an excessively unhealthy catabolism and must be rebalanced so anabolic processes are once again possible [cf. Girke 2010, 115–119]. Only then will restorative sleep occur. Silver therapy is therefore of the highest value in the treatment of acute cases of atopic dermatitis alongside antimony.

- **Antimony**

is very important in atopic dermatitis when administered internally and externally. When given internally, it especially stimulates the formative forces. (Antimonit/Antimonium crudum ▸Chap. 6.4.3.6.2).

In cases of acutely protracted eczema episodes affecting older children, it can in some cases be administered as an injection

- **Stibium met. praep. D6 amp.** Weleda
  10 ml i.v.

Where necessary, this can be administered in combination with one or more of the above medicines.

6.4.3.5.2 Vegetabilized silver: acute and primary treatment for atopic dermatitis

Vegetabilized forms of silver as a medicine have an important role to play in anthroposophic medicine in the acute and primary treatment of atopic dermatitis.

The following are suitable for children suffering from atopic dermatitis with hysterical constitution and acute weeping eczema, nocturnal itching and sleep disorders

- **Bryophyllum Argento cultum Rh D3 dil.** Weleda
  10–15 gtt. up to 4 x/d
- **Bryophyllum D5/Conchae D7 amp.** Weleda
  10 ml i.v.

can be of great benefit to older children and young people in cases of acute exacerbated eczema and severe insomnia; this ampoule can also, where necessary, be administrated orally in smaller, more frequent doses, or can be combined with one of the above options.

Bryophyllum is a medicinal plant which is particularly active at night (▸Chap. 2.2.3). The purpose is so to prevent this succulent plant from drying out during the day in hot locations. The plant is therefore able to fend off the aggressive impact of the day, a therapeutic motif in the treatment of atopic dermatitis. This plant's respiratory processes occur in the cooler, moister hours of darkness (so-called crassulacean acid metabolism (CAM)) which means that by day it keeps the gap apertures required for plant respiration closed. This explains why Bryophyllum is effective for balancing the outflowing tendency of the hysterical constitution.

Vegetabilized preparations of silver should also be considered for initial treatment of atopic dermatitis.

The relationship between the qualities of silver and the moon [Sommer 1999] have been evident since time immemorial. In terms of the human epidermis, it is remarkable that it normally regenerates in a lunar rhythm of 28 days. The conscious daytime activity of people tends to cause the skin to age slightly, imbuing it with various hues of soul and especially warmth; at night, skin regenerates and regains its full turgor and vitality. It was a creative step to vegetabilize silver (i. e. through specific fertilization of a plant with silver to "potentize" the metal in the plant metabolism) through a plant that exhibits a markedly nocturnal pattern to its metabolic activity while manifesting an unusually active lipometabolism.

Since November 2005 silver has been available in a vegetabilized form with *evening primrose, Oenothera biennis* for atopic dermatitis patients. Flowering throughout early spring to summer, evening primrose does not open its yellow flowers until twilight. It flowers in moonlight instead of in sunlight. Plant processes of this kind that are nocturnally active offer a strong indication of their effectiveness in the field of the regenerative metabolism, the processes related to the moon and silver. Thus the preparation of evening primrose described here was developed by the Dutch colleague Joop van Dam primarily from a gynaecological perspective. Both the epidermis and the endometrium of the female genital tract share this 28-day rhythm. The yellow colour of the flowers of the evening primrose indicates sulphuric effects which stimulate the warmth processes and vitality. *Oenathera biennis*, the evening primrose, concentrates an oil in its seeds that is rich in unsaturated fatty acids, whose benefits on the epidermis of atopic children has long been known. By fertilization with silver during cultivation, which is absorbed by the plant and "potentized" through its metabolism, the pharmacist obtains a preparation through which the moon and epidermis-related dynamic of the silver and evening primrose can have a stimulating effect on the patient. This substantially enhances the dietetically administered effectiveness of evening primrose seed oil. It is particularly suitable for the interval treatment and aftercare of children with atopically dry skin; but it can also be administered successfully from the initiation of treatment, if *constitutionally dry skin* forms the basis for a more subacute and insidious progression. Here initial signs of eczema can be arrested from a very early age, thereby working salutogenetically with our current understanding of atopic dermatitis, to normalize epidermal lipometabolism, in which the activity of the I-organization of the human being comes to expression.

- **Oenothera Argento culta D3 dil.** Weleda and Apotheke an der Weleda
  5–10 gtt. 3 x/d combined with ½–1 tsp. evening primrose seed oil (Rp. 100 ml)

The anthroposophical dermatologist Lüder Jachens sees in this a primary medicine "for the epidermal situation of the atopic individual. ... Dryness and itching diminish significantly within four weeks. ... This effect can be seen particularly clearly (unclouded by inflammation) i*n atopic persons with a healthy skin who merely complain about dry skin with mildl variants of eczema in wintertime*" [Jachens 2006; emphasis by the authors].

With *recurrent* mycosis and superinfections in the nappy (diaper) area, *molluscum contagiosum* with atopic skin (▸ Chap. 10.8.1.3), a tendency for diarrhoea and poor immunity, Thuja provides a vegetabilized form of silver:

- **Thuja Argento culta Rh D3 dil.** Weleda
  5–7 gtt. 3 x/d.

In this preparation, Thuja has a vitalizing effect and in particular strengthens the immunological ability of the skin (and mucous membranes) to defend itself. A distinction must be made between this indication and higher homoeopathic potencies of Thuja (▸ Chap. 6.4.3.6.5).

With the latter medicines, specific to anthroposophical therapy, very beneficial forms of dynamization of silver are available for children affected by eczema.

In this context, the embryonic organ preparation

- **Cutis feti Gl D5–8 amp.** Wala
  initially 0.5–1.0 ml 1–2 x/d, thereafter 1 x/d in the evening, also alternating with Amnion D30 [Vademecum 2010, 384]

has grown in importance for the authors in primary treatment.

The reference from Karl-Reinhard Kummer to use Cutis feti – instead of amnion in a *low potency* (after high potencies had proven unsatisfactory) was crucial. Due to the fact that atopic dermatitis ultimately always constitutes a weakness of the life organization in the skin (this equates precisely to the Psora Concept of Hahnemann, that starts with itchy forms of dermatosis), it is evident that the corresponding organ preparation should be administered here in a lower and therefore more effectively vitalizing potency. In contrast to this, the universal ectodermal preparation of Amnion (the nervous system, like the epidermis, is ectodermal in origin) is able simultaneously to moderate and reduce to a healthy level the excessive nerve-related perceptual activity in the skin that causes catabolic processes there. This is probably the reason why Amnion in D30 has a better therapeutic effect than lower potencies, even when used over extended periods.

Cutis feti can provide effective support for the therapeutic intention in the application of potentized and vegetabilized silver, which is to relocate the excessively catabolic ("typical daytime") inflammation to a "nocturnal" anabolic process of the epidermis.

6.5.3.5.3 Introductory primary therapy

Based on the experience of the authors, the treatment of atopic dermatitis in children is most effective when a stepwise approach is adopted, the principles of which are described in ▸Chap. 6.3. A leading role is played here by the recognition of key individual triggers, taking account of the mother-child relationship and life circumstances, recognizing existing organ weaknesses and functional imbalances in the organism (▸Chap. 6.3). This yields viewpoints such as

- delineation of allergy-triggering causes, such as diet,
- building a new functional and psychological balance,
- solving an inhibiting, enmeshed, or ambivalent relationship of mother and child and the promotion of a child's own powers in an organic and social respect,

to be achieved in a successive and progressive sequence of steps.

Initially this requires that the doctor *takes time* to understand the child and the family situation, to explain diagnosis and therapy clearly to the parents and to identify the essential points of each individual case from the plethora of possibilities: which organ function is in a weakened state, which nutrition is not tolerated, where are psychological burdens in the prior history, etc. A great *effort of will* is demanded from the child and parents to think differently, to alter habits, to develop new aptitudes.

On the other hand, these comparatively general treatment measures will enable the child almost universally to experience a *great sense of relief*, and especially in milder illness it is often possible to achieve cure. *For this reason, treatment should be typically given for at least four to six weeks (where necessary also for much longer) under normal circumstances, prior to prescription of individual, potentized homoeopathic and anthroposophic medication.*

Firstly, this approach enables doctor and parents to establish what each step (e. g. a diet, symbiotic control) means in terms of this treatment (what for example is important in sustaining a change in nutrition, but also what impact does this have on the accurate evaluation of treatment). Secondly, the true need in terms of individual medicines can be better and more reliably discerned after such a first phase of therapy. Finally, this sequence in most cases significantly improves the patient's receptivity to potentized single-substance medicines (e. g. after elimination of incompatible foods, balancing trace element deficits and correcting impaired organ functions). S. Hahnemann [1983, 7, 129ff., 158ff.] as well as Rudolf Steiner and Ita Wegman [1977, 98f.] all make specific reference to this point in the treatment of chronic diseases; the authors have found it increasingly important to follow this approach.

6.4.3.5.4 Viewpoints on categorization of substance choice: neurasthenic and hysterical constitutional types

Leading aspects that can contribute to the selection of a single-substance medicine are derived from the preceding consideration of atopic dermatitis.

A weakness the *warmth organization* is generally found. This can be differentiated: if the child is chilly and constitutionally has *insufficient warmth,* does health deteriorate in the *cold season* (suggests Silicea/Quartz or Arsenicum album). Or is the child *sweaty, hot and worsens in the summer* or habitually declines warm clothing and bedding *while remaining warm* (Sulphur or Antimonit/Antimonium crudum is suggested). Or perhaps the warmth changes constantly, with the child alternately too hot and too cold at night, etc. (as in Mercurius sol.), which would indicate significant instability in the *warmth organization and therefore also in the I-organization* (this in turn leads us to anticipate that several different single-substance medicines may be required consecutively). In terms of the medical history, close attention should be paid to any *change in warmth response over time*, which may be constitutional or a reaction, for instance to antibiotics used to treat an acute inflammation.

From this viewpoint, a fundamental constitutional distinction can be made which can be supported and focused by the inclusion of the secretory activity of the organism, the active regulation of fluid balance (▸Chap. 6.3.3.3). At the same time, the pathogenetic aspects of atopic dermatitis form the basis for applying constitutional differential diagnosis and therapy, which promotes both understanding the child and selecting the correct medicine.

In this context, *neurasthenia* usually goes hand in hand with *a lack of warmth*, impaired digestion and assimilation of food, since catabolism and anabolism in the metabolic sphere are too weak. *Appetite* is generally less intense or is markedly *picky* ("neurotic eating habits"), something that is sometimes exacerbated by diets. In all neurasthenics, *interest in food and in digestion*, indeed in all of life, must be awakened and strengthened. Children tend towards being *underweight*; in many cases, they may manifest *nervous thirst* (day and night). Boys are more prone to this than girls. Behaviour tends to be aggressive, confrontational, even "pig-headed". *Sensory hypersensitivity* is common with dry skin and miserable itching. Intellectual precocity and the neurastenic child's basic psychological traits have already been described.

Children with a *hysterical constitution* tend to develop *excessive warmth*. But there are notable exceptions (cf. "poikilothermic" traits of Pulsatilla and the wintertime exacerbations of Conchae/Calcium carb). In particular, they have *oversensitivity to proteins*, which can involve poor catabolism and leaky barrier surfaces and, on the other hand, a *hearty appetite* and vital growth processes. *Diets usually have a favourable impact on these children*. They invariably tend to enjoy their food, and their thirst is normal or reduced. These children tend to have watery *sweat*, (even being "steamy" in heat or with physical activity) and are prone to being "runny" (with *catarrh*, loose mucous in the airways, nocturnal enuresis, etc.). In early childhood they often have obstructive bronchitis Psychologically they are happier and better behaved than neurasthenic children. Physically, they tend to be overweight, particularly as infants. Development is sometimes slowed down and their relationship to their parents may be characterized by gentle but also by demanding dependence. Their skin is prone to *weeping eczemas* with less itching, in contrast to neurastenic children.

The more decisive the tendency toward neurasthenia or hysteria, the more anxious and unsettled the child will be, frequently also suffering significant sleep disorders.

Tab. 6.5 Individualized treatment with single-substance medicines – an overview.

Neurasthenic constitution	Psychological ambivalence	Hysterical constitution
Preparations containing silicic acid: Amnion Opal Quartz Silicea	*At a soul entity level:* Sepia Natrium muriaticum	*Preparations containing sulphur:* Sulphur, Antimonit
Medicines containing arsenic: Arsenicum album Kalium arsenicosum	*At the level of the warmth organization:* Mercurius solubilis	*Medicines containing calcium:* Conchae/Calcium carb. Calcium/Quercus
Medicines containing aluminium: Lycopodium clavatum		*Medicines containing carbon:* Graphites Roseneisen/Graphit
Medicines containing silver: Argentit Oenothera Argento culta		*Medicines containing silver:* Bryophyllum Argento cultum Thuja Argento culta
Constitutionally effective nosodes: Psorinum	*Constitutionally effective nosodes:* Tuberculinum	*Constitutionally effective nosodes:* Medorrhinum
Universally appropriate medicines: Aurum met. praep., Argentum met. praep., Stibium met. praep., Oenathera Argento culta		

6.4.3.6 Individualized treatment with single-substance medicines

This section will begin by outlining the most important single-substance medicines for the neurastenic and hysterical constitutional directions, followed by medicines that should be considered in strong psychological ambivalence and tension; then additional metallic medicines, concluding with a small selection of important single-substance medicines. In view of the wealth of necessary medicines and the need to differentiate between their indications, a detailed rationale cannot be presented in each case. For a more in-depth study, we refer to the homoeopathic and phytotherapeutic literature [Eichler & Eichler 1996, Vermeulen 1999, Imhäuser 2000, Pfeiffer 2007, Kent 1985, Weiss & Fintelmann 1999, Bäumler 2007] and to anthroposophic medicine [Selawry 1991, Basold et al. 1995, Vogel 1996, *Vademecum Anthroposophische Arzneimittel 2010*, Jachens 2006, 2011]. A summary overview, making no claims to completeness, can serve as a guide to the next section (Tab. 6.5).

6.4.3.6.1 Medicines for the neurasthenic constitution

Potentized silicic acid is of universal importance in the treatment of atopic dermatitis (▸Chap. 5.1.2.4). In addition to its administration in the form of therapeutic plants containing silicic acid, such as Equisetum, it can be used in various ways. One application arises from the *significance of silicic acid for the formation of ectodermal barriers* in the sense organs, in which the silicic acid is enriched by the organism. There it facilitates the exclusion of all "ponderables" from the outside world and simultaneously, by the innate property of silicic acid not to retain heat and light, it is able to achieve transparency for imponderable effects. In the view of Rudolf Steiner and Ita Wegman [1991, 77], the healthy organism uses silicic acid to enhance "organs of conscious life, ... primarily the sense organs". Here it is remarkable that the ectodermal human amnion contains the highest proportion of silicic acid – up to 22 % in the ash.

The *amnion* (▸Chap. 6.4.3.1.2) is what enables the embryo to develop in a microenvironment created by itself in which it floats almost weightlessly – just as lower forms of animal life during their early developmental stages floated weightlessly and transparently in the sea. "The amniotes never lay their eggs in the primary medium of vertebrate development, in water" [Portmann 1983, 271]. Through the amnion the embryo is able to create for itself a *living-fluid developmental space* that at a higher level assumes the function which the sea has for the embryonic development of lower forms of animal. In this way, the amnion facilitates morphogenesis and primary growth of land-living animals that are only able to accomplish these processes if they are almost completely free of gravity in a precisely regulated, living-fluid environment. This indicates that *the amniotic envelope itself exercises a primary organizing function in the process of* embryogenesis: in the view of anthroposophic medicine, the child's soul and spiritual individuality is closely associated with the amnion right up to birth [Schad 1982, 69–77]. (In so-called primitive cultures the placenta is often buried carefully after the birth of a child.) So it is that at birth the human being sheds an enclosing organ indispensable for early development. Inside the amnion the skin is protected and its surface is usually intact. When the first breath of life awakens the soul and spiritual individuality *in the* body, the skin becomes the barrier between the fluid living interior of the body and the physical external world. It becomes the primary barrier between "I" and "not I". The Amnion organ preparation derives its therapeutic rationale and indication where this boundary is damaged or there is a constitutional delay in maturation or a functional weakness in the skin as a barrier organ. It also has a regulatory action on nerve activity in the epidermis since epidermis and nervous system and key parts of the sense organs all originate from the ectoderm, which forms as its first organ the amnion.

- **Amnion Gl D30 amp.** Wala
  ½ ampoule = 0.5 ml per os daily–every other day in the evening

can be a deeply effective medicine for atopic dermatitis [Vademecum 2010, 65], especially

- in early childhood, for former premature babies,
- if adverse factors arose during pregnancy (amniocentesis, premature labour, psychological stress for the mother, relationship conflicts especially in regard to letting a pregnancy go to its full term, etc., ▸Chap. 2.4),
- after a traumatic birth, including a Caesarian section,
- or constitutionally if the skin resembles that of a premature baby and is translucent, hypersensitive and prone to dryness, inflammation and infection.

Case study

Second child, normal birth. Father has pollinosis and pollen-induced asthma, mother and brother are free of atopy. From his earliest days of life, the child strikes the parents as hard and rejecting, and the mother notes "the gaze of a prosecutor". Both parents are conscientious and careful; the father works 50 km away, spending twelve to fourteen hours away from home. The baby is exclusively breastfed. At three months, generalized atopic dermatitis develops. A month later the child has a febrile bronchitis, followed by a life-threatening, highly febrile E.-coli superinfection with sepsis requiring treatment with parenteral antibiotics in hospital. Subsequently, despite a diet of breast milk and hydrolysate nutrition, the child developed chronic generalized atopic dermatitis. The parents decline corticosteroid treatment, due to concerns about the high risk of side effects given his age and severity.

At age twelve months the baby first presented to our medical practice with a generalized flare, rated as 3–4 on a severity scale of 0 to 4. Sleep was disurbed by unbearable itching. Skin had poor turgor, marked xerosis, and scarring due to past superinfection. The child had finely sculpted facial features, an alert and anxious gaze, poor appetite and digestion, a low level of vitality as well as a gentle, hypersensitive neurastenic constitution.

First medication: Cuprum met. praep. D30 amp. Weleda and Amnion Gl D30 amp. Wala aa (aa = equal parts) mixed in 2-ml injection, 0.5 ml orally twice daily for 2 days. When seen just two days later, mother reports that her child is "as though transformed" with immediate improvements in both skin and sleep. Then therapy with Amnion Gl D30 amp. Wala (0.5 ml every evening initially, then alternate evenings, later 0.3 ml; all given orally) resulted in 3 months in a 50 % eczema reduction dropping severity scale to 1–2. Nine months later, the skin remained dry, but the eczema has disappeared. Therapy was continued for 2 ½ years. At eleven year followup, he is completely eczema-free. A year into Amnion therapy, he had onset of infection-induced asthma, which occurred less frequently, and in a milder form, once the child reached school age when eurythmy therapy marked a turning point in his treatment.

A striking feature in the development of this child was that immediately after the sepsis in infancy, the parents could tell that the child had become psychologically gentler and more open. This increased further with Cuprum and Amnion treatments. The child's dependence on the mother remained excessive throughout the development of asthma, but was transformed rapidly with eurythmy therapy. The child quickly learned to practice eurythmy movements alone with the therapist, increasing both the child's self confidence and that of the mother. The child grew more independent and adjusted well to kindergarten, which had earlier seemed impossibile.

A second aspect of silicic acid is its universal importance within the organism for the *mesenchymal basic substance* [Vogel 1996, 24]. The *interrelationship between mesenchyme, basement membrane and actual barrier* (epidermis, but also respiratory epithelium of the lungs etc.) is *fundamentally loosened in people with an allergic disposition*. This causes the barriers to lose their formation and to start to disintegrate from the blood pole through inflammation, which allows foreign matter to penetrate the surface from the outside in (cf. also below, bronchial asthma).[1] Over the last few years, it has become apparent that *neurogenic factors* – the direct "footprints" of one-sided, "typical daytime" astral destructive activity – trigger most of this pathogenetic process. This disintegration has been shown to occur in many processes including chronic inflammatory bowel diseases as well as asthma and atopic dermatitis.

A therapeutically appropriate form of silicic acid for dry atopic dermatitis is potentized

- **Opal D12 amp.** Wala
  0.2–0.5 ml 1–2 x/d per os.

In Opal, silicic acid is not present in crystalline form as it is in Quartz, but is a colloidal gel (▸Chap. 6.4.3.3). The basic substance of the human organism also oscillates between a state of solution and gel and requires silicic acid to organize fluid in a living way. Geologically, opals are the youngest of the silicic acid minerals. They have a special relationship with the soul-entity of the human being through the lively interplay of colours in precious opals, which disappears through water loss.

To date, in the experience of the authors, opal has proven its capabilities in *very young children* in early-stage occurrences of *constitutionally related eczemas in neurasthenic children* in whom

- the skin has only slight vitality, a low level of turgor and appears dry, dirty, itchy and inelastic,
- there is a stressful overdependence, especially on mother, characterized by anxieties and expectations,
- the mother gave birth at a relatively late age or was burdened by the stresses of her own atopic history.

The application of *quartz* has a slightly different orientation in a simple form potentized through trituration

- **Quarz D20 trit./pillules** Weleda/Wala
  1 saltsp./5 pillules 1 x/d in the morning

In *acutely inflamed* processes based on chronically dry atopic dermatitis, school-age children and adults may find

- **Quarz D60 amp.** Weleda
  as a single dose of 1 amp. s.c.

to be remarkably effective.

In quartz, silicic acid is in its hardest, most formed state. This lifeleless form achieves both complete transparency to light (even more than does window glass, another solidified gel) and emission of all of its warmth. In its whole crystalline form quartz perfectly expresses

1 A. Fromme writes: "To begin with, purely ectodermal cells were cultivated in amphibian embryos at early stages of development. An irregular complex of atypical epidermal cells developed. But if mesenchyme cells were cultivated at the same time, a blister developed whose surface is formed by epidermal cells arranged in an epithelium-like way while the connective tissue fills the interior as a loose network." [Quoted from H. H. Vogel 1996, 109]

the relationship between the *nervous and sensory pole,* the sense organs, and human consciousness.

Quartz obtains effective medicinal properties wherever a pronounced *weakness in warmth formation* is present in neurasthenic constitutions. Quartz is primarily indicated for treatment of school-age children and young people (Opal, Amnion and Equisetum in the first septennium are often more appropriate). On patients we observe

- a lack of warmth and chronic recurrent airway infections in winter (▶Chap. 5.1.2.4), especially cold and stinky sweaty feet, sometimes also a sweaty head,
- poor nutritional absorption, stunted growth, underweight to the extent of failure to thrive, low birth weight for gestational age,
- dry and infection-prone skin as described for opal above,
- poor wound healing, slow metabolism,
- protracted upper respiratory infection (cf. Equisetum silicea cultum),
- wakefulness, psychologically on the one hand curiously objective and *inflexible, socially easily challenged*, stubborn, while on the other hand fearful, slow but with steady biographical development. Typical for neurasthenics is a certain sense of order that may already be evident in the way the child plays with dolls.

The silicic acid preparation in homoeopathic medicine, known as *Silicea,* is manufactured from quartz, which is first crushed into a powder, then turned into a liquid gel, and then precipitated again. In this remarkable recipe from Hahnemann lies a pharmaceutical process that converts silicic acid from its crystalline final condition back into a colloidal state close to life before it is potentized.

- **Silicea LM6 dil., D12–C30–C200 pillules** (various manufacturers)
  3–5 gtt. 1 x/d in the morning, 5 pillules/d (D12) or single doses

therefore takes a universal central position between Opal and Quarz.

A significant therapeutic effect is observed in the form of *thorough warming of the organism right out to its periphery*, a decline in or the healing of chronic recurrent infections, and better digestion; psychologically, children become more flexible, although affected children may long remain inflexible in their rhythmical system, seemingly trapped – tasks for artistic therapy and education.

- **Arsenicum album LM12 dil.** Arcana, **D12–C30 pillules** (various manufacturers)

is indicated for pronounced neurasthenic constitutions where problems associated with the astral body predominate. This largely affects boys.

Psychologically we can observe

- *a nervous tension throughout combined with high intelligence,* restlessness (e. g. at table), *fearfulness in the face of solitude* and at night, especially after midnight (then join parents in bed, where they immediately fall asleep again).
- *ambition*, worsening with performance stress and examinations, assiduous learning, wishing to be the best. Here parental expectations and concerns are frequently present in the background and perceived and adopted by children very strongly. In their fears

and in their ambition, children are very dependent upon their environment, and primarily upon their parents.

- a compulsive need for orderliness (e. g. schoolbag, pen case), fears of burglars, robbers in the room, betraying a basic sense of the child feeling unsafe in its own body, and latently feeling alien and divorced from it: this translates into a disproportionate sense of the previously discussed (▸Chap. 6.4.2.5) distancing process of the soul entity from the child's own physical body, all associated with kidney activity and the awakening of awareness, all a characteristic expression of the neurasthenic constitution and dominant in these children.

On the skin we can observe

- dry-red, scaly, *burning*-itchy eczema; the burning and itching sensations can be much more pronounced compared to the visible manifestation of the eczema; scratching further exacerbates this,
- dry, split lips that may be unusually red in colour,
- hypertrophy of the mucous layer, thickening of the epidermis (in contrast to the translucent skin with Silicea).

Important general symptoms that support the indication of Arsenicum album are

- *a lack of personal warmth*, a strong need for external warmth, worsening in winter,
- stomach aches, strong *nervous thirst*, pronounced *picky eating habits* among young children (only eating specific foods),
- tendency towards diarrhoea when excited, and in response to cold drinks or meals,
- often dark-haired; thin, Mediterranean skin type,
- tendency towards bronchial asthma and pollinosis.

We must understand arsenic as a substance that has an intense relationship to air, to disintegration or decay, and to all that opposes the fluid vital element which it destroys with its toxin. But arsenic's presence in trace amounts – as its accumulation in the thyroid gland and importance for the heart muscle shows (▸Chap. 10.1) – is essential for the organism to wrest a higher level of ensouled life from the living organism. Once we grasp this view, the indications for this form of medicine become much more readily apparent. Rudolf Steiner [1984, 82] has compared the active effect of arsenic to that of the astral body compared to the etheric body of the human being.

If the dominant symptoms are restricted to severely itching, scaly eczema with exacerbation of itching during the second half of the night, especially at about 02.00–03.00, the following medicines are often more effective than Arsenicum album

- **Potassium arsenicosum D6–12–30 dil./pillules** (various manufacturers)

This medicine is very significant if *an allergy to household mites* plays a trigger role, typically associated with an exacerbation at the beginning of the heating period.

Even with childhood *psoriasis*, it may be appropriate to consider **Potassium arsenicosum**; as a skincare agent, these children may benefit from **Imlan® Creme pur,** external preparation with **Colchysat® Bürger** 1:1–1:2 as well as, where necessary, a **topical vitamin D preparation** (e. g. **Silkis®**). Diagnostically, a family medical history is key!

6

A preferred option for boys with a neurasthenic constitution in the context of treatment for atopic dermatitis is

- **Lycopodium clavatum C30–200 pillules** Gudjons
  single doses (e. g. 3 pillules 3 x/d over 1–3 days),

a profoundly effective medicine. It is indicated whenever a primary vital weakness in the metabolic organization is a dominant feature of the associated symptoms (▸ Chap. 5.1.1.5).

In these cases there is a *constitutional* disorder which means that *problems of nutrition and digestion* can be recognized at a very early stage:

- weak or ravenous appetite that stops after a few swallows or bites,
- poor digestion with *meteorism* and a tendency towards *constipation,*
- in contrast to a swollen abdomen and lean body, often a comparatively large and well-shaped head,
- *failure to thrive* to the point of paedatrophy, but in contrast to Silicea,
- deterioration with a buildup of warmth (Carbo vegetabilis as a complementary medicine accentuates the effect of lycopodium, with a similar set of symptoms in respect of warmth and digestion).

In this respect, external warmth is unbearable (the patient feels better in the open air and worse in a poorly ventilated room) despite the fact that their own warmth development may vary, with some patients being clearly deficient. The *difficulty* here always lies in *absorbing* external necessities such as warmth or nutrition *into the child's own life organization.* In respect to problems associated with the *liver* and digestion, other issues can involve

- worsening of symptoms in the afternoons (*16.00 to 20.00*),
- a tendency to emphasize the symptoms *on the right side.*

Allergic symptom can often occur at a very young age, leading to

- the skin being very dry, the eczema often being extensive and pruritic.

Inflammations persist; the lack of immunological resistance corresponds to the weakness of vitality.

Intellectually the children are very wakeful, characteristic of a neurasthenic constitution, tending later to engage in purely intellectual pursuits, e. g. with the computer (which generally occurs more frequently with neurasthenic patients with atopic dermatitis) [Jachens, 1999a, 76f.]. Psychologically, they often are fearful towards the outside world together with a close attachment to their parents where, within their trusted immediate circle, their extraordinary compulsion to set the agenda for everything can be a real torment, even dictatorial. In all of this, a *deep-rooted insecurity is being expressed towards all that is living.* Later on they put tremendous efforts into presenting themselves as self-assured to the outside world, while internally remaining stressed, which has ramifications on the digestion in particular.

One gains the impression that the metabolic organization of these children exhibits a vitality that is not in keeping with their physical age. Often there are similar problems in the parents' and grandparents' generations. These children have difficulty appropriating and transforming the physical bodies they have inherited from their parents. Acute inflammations and childhood diseases tend to be severe, but can also be very beneficial in terms of their personal development.

Alpine clubmoos, or Lycopodium clavatum (cf. ▸Chap. 6.3.3.2), is a remnant of one of the oldest land plants that once formed giant, thriving woodland areas. Today, Lycopodium is a ground-crawling ('snake moss'), green, non-flowering plant whose spores can be used for medicinal purposes. "The seedling that emerges from the spores lives in symbiosis with fungi and also the prothallium is dependent upon saprophytic nutrition. The entire development of this plant takes a period of ten to fifteen years" [Stübler and Krug 1987, *Pflanzl. Arzneistoffe* I, 265]. Once again the central signature is the healing effect: the *greatly slowed vitality, dependent upon help*, evident in nature itself. In substance-related terms, the ash of these spores contains up to *15% aluminium*: the use of Lycopodium clavatum therefore constitutes a botanically organized and enriched mineral (such as Equisetum in respect of silicic acid). On the other hand, this may explain the unusually long-lasting and far-reaching impact of Lycopodium that is otherwise more typically associated with mineral-based medicines.

In view of this picture, the old homoeopathic experience comes as no surprise that for Lycopodium to be effective the help of other, vitalizing medicines is often necessary. Lycopodium should not be prescribed as a medicine of first instance. But the possibilities described in ▸Chap. 6.3 for the treatment of digestion and metabolism provide good prerequisites for the action of Lycopodium; however, the important thing is to use *medicines related to sulphur* first (Taraxacum, Argentit, Sulphur in very fine dosages).

In summary, the individual medicines specified act

- with silicic acid primarily on the *warmth organization and therefore on the I-organization* and its effectiveness on the formation of barriers within the organism,
- with Arsenicum album and Potassium arsenicosum primarily on the one-sided physically catabolic, catabolism-increasing and nerve system-related activity of the *astral body, the soul entity* within the physical body,
- with Lycopodium clavatum primarily on a constitutional weakness of the *life organization, the etheric body* in the area of liver and digestion that threaten to remain too lifeless, too physical, while internally failing fully to assimilate the impulses of the child's individuality, and externally to assimilate and break down nutrition, the life in nature.

6.4.3.6.2 Medicines for the hysterical constitution

The most frequently indicated medicines for atopic dermatitis in this type of constitution are Sulphur and Conchae/Calcium carbonicum (Hahnemanni), and these differ fundamentally in terms of their impact on the warmth characteristics of the patient.

- **Sulphur LM6–12 dil.** Arcana, **D6–30 trit.** Weleda, **C30–200** pillules (various manufacturers)

is no longer indicated as frequently as it was just 30 to 40 years ago in the older homoeopathic literature. The dosages call for great experience and caution, as does phosphorus, an element that is also entirely combustible. In cases of very acute eczema it may for example be necessary to administer 1 gtt. of LM6 to 100 ml of water and of that 1 tsp. in the mornings, and then possibly to repeat this tiny and precise dose just once every 3 days. In all cases, the Sulphur potencies should be administered in rising order (1 saltsp. D6 up to 3 x/d, D12–15 1 x/d, D30 1–2 x/wk); initial deterioration can be expected after the initial dose (advisable to inform parents of this expectation), so due care and attention to appropriate dosage is essential.
Individual doses of higher potencies (C200) should only be administered occasionally, allowing several weeks to pass between them for observation purposes.

The fundamental relationship of sulphur to warmth on the one hand, and to assimilation and the (especially protein) metabolism on the other, has already been discussed elsewhere (▸Chap. 6.3.3.2). Here sulphur can provide a balancing effect, regardless of constitution, to the *consequences of suppression, weakening of the warmth organization, and the digestion and metabolic organs* (D6, LM6). This weakening is nearly always present in some form in atopic dermatitis; this was something that Hahnemann was aware of when he identified potentized sulphur as a *general* medicine for the initial stages of therapy for chronic diseases, as well as its relationship to iatrogenic suppression of acute diseases (in particular of the skin itself!), as formulated by [Hahnemann 1983, 126ff.].

Constitutionally sulphur is indicated whenever the metabolic sphere subordinates itself insufficiently to the shaping guidance of the I and the soul entity is "flooded" and governed by impulses from the subconscious, the vital drives and pure will. Typical symptoms of affected patients indicating this choice are the following:

- *Intolerance of external warmth*, worsening of the main symptoms in bed and in summer, an aversion to hot baths and corresponding deterioration in condition,
- *Evident hunger*, especially in the mornings, also between meals, in particular for sweet things. This involves a clinically *high level of fluctuation in the blood sugar level* (this rampant hunger and the fluctuations in blood sugar with a tendency for transient dips in blood sugar level often improve markedly after just a few doses),
- multiple *nutritional protein intolerances*, especially in respect of cold milk and eggs (many of these children do not like eggs and milk),
- insufficient breakdown of foods with *malodorous flatulence* (rottenlike hydrogen sulphide!) and diaorrhoea-like loose stools,
- corresponding to the hysterical constitution, prone to catarrhic airway infections and pneumonia – the most important agent to counter recurrent pneumonia.

In terms of their *behaviour* these children are *impulsive, willful* and enjoy occupying centre stage. They encounter the doctor in an inquisitive manner (including any objects that may be lying on the desk at the time), are open, but without much sensitivity. Their intelligence may be very alert and quick to assimilat many practical and material contexts, but one glance in the child's schoolbooks, for example, shows poor organizational and design skills, with sloppy writing, smudges and even grease spots. Not just the metabolism, but also the *movement organism* becomes independent with resultant impulsivity. Boys especially often have uncontrolled and violent behaviour with *poor posture* and slumped shoulders (which should always direct scrutiny towards the digestive and metabolic organization).

All forms of atopic dermatitis can be found on the *skin*, but especially

- acute, weeping and *very itchy* eczemas,
- *tendency to superinfection*,
- deterioration in response to warming (see above), for example through contact with wool, which may be a constitutional sensitivity from infancy,
- often very early stages of eczema (cf. Lycopodium, Calcium carbonicum).

Generally boys are more frequently affected in accordance also with their greater emphasis on the limbs and will. In contast, girls are more likely to benefit from Calcium carbonicum.

An important modification affects the action of sulphur in its compound with antimony:

- **Antimonium crudum D6–12 pillules/Antimonit D6 trit.** Weleda
  5 pillules/1 saltsp. 1–3 x/d

strengthens the formative forces against a metabolism which has a latent tendency to make itself independent (▸Chap. 6.3.3.2)

This is expressed by:

- a tendency towards *purulent superinfections* of the skin, especially impetigo (▸Chap. 6.4.3.4),
- eczema of the ususally spared upper thigh, buttocks, and perioral area,
- misshapen nails, hardened *warts* on hands and feet, *verrucas*,
- *Deterioration in summer* or by bed warmth,
- Burning, itchy eczema with similar forms of exacerbation of eczema, as with Sulphur.

This medicine is more frequently indicated for boys, especially those who are unruly, willful and resistant to any form of medical examination. Antimony has great significance when applied either internally or externally to atopic dermatitis. When applied internally, it promotes the formative forces.

In contrast, when externally applied in its natural sulphur compound as antimonite it is indicated as a nightime ointment dressing for *hyperkeratotic, cracked, and rhagadiform-hand eczemas, hard warts, and lichenified dry eczema* [Jachens 1999b] (▸Chap. 6.4.3.3).

Potentized oyster shell calcium,

- **Conchae D6–30 trit.** Weleda/**Calcium carbonicum LM6–12 dil.** Arcana
  1 dose 1–3 x/d, D30/LM12 can be administered less frequently,

is indicated for constitutional eczemas in which an inadequate breakdown, especially of protein, is associated with excessive anabolic metabolism.

Physically the children exhibit

- *"great mass without firmness"*, as infants tending to be overweight, especially for as long as they are breast-fed,
- hypersensitivity especially to milk and chicken protein (typically exacerbated during breast-feeding) – but these children love milk and eggs and will cry when they learn of the diet restriction, which is actually helpful for them,
- as infants constipation without feeling unwell,
- *weepy and generally less itchy rashes*, often starting at the head and severely affecting the crevices behind the ears, at the groin, and armpits (Intertrigo, cf. Graphit),
- milk crust (cradle cap),
- *prolific sweating* particularly on the head, in response to exertion.

Oysters themselves exhibit a purely exoskeletal formation similar to the head – a human exoskeletal formation. In infants with a tendency to craniotabes Calcium carbonicum D20 is very effective. The formative hardening forces of the oyster remain external, while the interior is filled with a very vital, mucilaginous protein with high reproductive powers. The oyster's sensory organs regress to a large extent at an early age while it settles permanently on the seabed, dedicated to its metabolism and shell formation. In this way the oyster embodies an astral activity in the life entity which has remained at an early stage of development and whose waking sensory life actually manifests regressive traits,[1] dedicating itself entirely to its metabolic and reproductive activity. The catabolic and secretory activity of the astral body exhausts itself in the task of forming a shell. In terms of human I development [Steiner and Wegman 1991, 88, 93], the soul entity has, in contrast, to develop a thorough waking consciousness and autonomy of movement which is enabled by respiration and catabolism in the physical body, releasing a correspondingly high level of heat. After birth, there should not be an "oyster-like" impact, but instead it should obey the needs of the I-organization.

Constitutionally, potentized oyster shell calcium promotes development in children who have difficulties in eliminating fat and releasing *heat*, who are sensitive to cold, who have frequent infections and wintertime skin exacerbations. But most importantly, their astral body's *ability to secrete* is reorientated in response to this medicine causing the prolific sweating and weeping eczema to diminish, while simulataneously stimulating intestinal and kidney activity.

Psychologically the children manifest the previously mentioned characteristics of a hysterical constitution; in overall terms, they appear to be happier and less troubled by their eczema. Striking aspects include

- the close attachment to the mother,
- the tendency for *anxieties* – especially the fear of "losing ones shell", of embarassment in front of other children, fear of loss of home or family,
- slow but often steady development,
- the need for a great deal of sleep.

1 Here the authors wish to thank their colleague L. Simon (unpublished lecture at the conference of the German Anthroposophical Medical Association in Kassel in 1999) and F. Husemann (2000) for their valuable input.

- **Calcium-Quercus pillules** Wala
  5–10 pillules 3–5 x/d

are beneficial in less profound *springtime and food dependent* eczemas of children with a Calcium carbonicum constitution.

These children may tend, for several years in succession starting in early springtime, to develop moderately itchy eczema – and they love Easter eggs! During eczema episodes, the avoidance of milk and eggs is beneficial (usually this abstention is sufficient during the period leading up to Easter).

Calcium-Quercus combines the effectiveness of oak bark tannin with the calcium organized in the oak bark [Selawry 1966] both in low levels of potentization. A detailed current characterization of this interesting vegetable-mineral medicine is provided by Ulrich Meyer [2005]. Based on the experience of the authors, it is primarily indicated in cases of

- acutely exacerbating weeping eczemas,
- acute urticaria,
- acute allergic reactions to an *insect sting*,
- forms of eczema that worsen in springtime and in response to nutritional factors (especially milk and eggs).

Finally, this series includes

- **Graphites D12–30 pillules** (various manufacturers)
  5–7 pillules 2 x/d–2 x/wk

In terms of its characteristics, graphite represents a certain polarity to quartz with its slightly greasy-metallic sheen, dark grey colour (pure carbon is the purest black that exists in nature), lack of hardness, and suitability as a lubricant. In contrast to the extremely hard diamond, which is also made of carbon, the carbon in graphite is only interlaced in a laminar fashion, so the different layers of the mineral only bond slightly. Particularly noteworthy in this context is graphite's *response to warmth or heat.* Graphite consists of more than 98 % pure carbon (an entirely combustible substance) and so from that perspective has not released its heat in contrast to fully oxidized silicic acid. And yet there is no substance which is more thermostable (up to almost 4000 °C). Graphite is therefore the ultimate mineral expression of the *ability to retain heat internally*. Noteworthy features in the patient are:

- worsening of condition in response to warmth from an external source, but little independent release of heat (internally chilly, with heat locked into the substance),
- yellow weepy, viscous skin rashes, particularly on the *head, behind the ears, in intertriginous area, also with eye inflammations* extending all the way up to *herpes cornealis* [Grandgeorge 2004, 94],
- no tendency to sweat, the skin tends to be *dry and cracking*, the *nails are often misshapen* (atrophic peripheral area alongside central hypertrophy),
- slow-healing skin prone to suppuration,
- sticky, yellowish, crusty secretions; in some cases fetid-smelling secretions under a plaque or kerrion,

6

- pronounced itching, exacerbated by bed warmth,
- most important single-substance medicine in pronounced, also generalized infant *seborrhoeic eczema* [cf. for diagnosis Höger 2011, 180]

Psychologically, these children *have a tendency to enjoy breaching all boundaries,* to refuse to follow rules and to withdraw from the moral influence of the people bringing them up. This expresses a basic characteristic of the medicine – the insufficient presence of the I (and the correspondingly poor response to the I of the caregiver). This trait of "laughing when being told off" (Hirte in [Pfeiffer et al, 876]) is more characteristic than many of the more frequently reported features of the medicine.[1] Grandgeorge reports on a characteristic case study and defines the essence of the medicine as follows: "He could have become a diamond" [l. c., 94f.]. But the philosopher's stone, the diamond for human beings is the presence of the I which enters into a relationship with the other.

A very universal application of graphite is the anthroposophic medicine

- **Roseneisen/Graphit pillules** Wala
  3–5 pillules 2–3 x/d

in which graphite is jointly potentized in D15 with an extract of rose petal, produced through the addition of haematite (iron oxide) [Vogel 1994, 728–731].

The authors have found this medicine to be effective with

- *intertriginous* infant eczema (cf. Conchae),
- seborrhoeic dermatitis,
- appetite problems,
- slower than usual convalescence after severe airway infections.

A significant feature is the way that the iron-tinged rose petal extract strengthens the rhythmic system and the warmth organization of the child – an outcome that cannot be achieved using only graphite.

In summary, the individual medicines specified relate

- in the case of *sulphur* primarily to the *assimilation* of food and to the *metabolism* up to and including *warmth formation;* potentized sulphur – depending on the dosage and situation of the patient – both counteracts excess independence of these processes and reactivates and balances this sphere, for example after intoxication or suppressive medication,
- with *Calcium carbonicum* (and *Pulsatilla,* ▸Chap. 6.5.6.11) primarily to the insufficient action and formative activity in the life organization of the *astral body, the soul entity in the physical body,*
- with *graphite* primarily to the *warmth organization* and therefore on the *I-organization,* that develops an insufficient level of activity in catabolism.

6.4.3.6.3 Medicines for the child with a predominantly ambivalent soul disposition

The next two medicines are especially indicated for *girls,* as are also Pulsatilla and by tendency Calcium carbonicum. This becomes more comprehensible if we consider the

1 The authors thank their gynaecological colleague H. v. Löwensprung for a valuable insight

underlying condition of psychological ambivalence, with its equally intense experience of contradictory feelings, experiences and drives. The male constitution typically works more "in series" in that one psychological condition *follows on* from another (and what happened before is then often forgotten!), whereas the female constitution is characterized to a greater extent by a *simultaneous experience* of different psychological conditions which may be contradictory.

- **Sepia D12–C30 pillules** (various manufacturers)
is one of the single-substance medicines now commonly indicated for atopic dermatitis; when given to an appropriate constitution, it may be the decisive medicine, one that (like Natrium muriaticum discussed below) proves reliable even years later with a relapse or recurrence. Here, medium potencies can be of lasting benefit.

In isolated cases Sepia may be indicated primarily by the physical constitution rather than by the psychological ambivalence; however, in these cases a situation mostly exists with the parents that led to a psychological burden in the way described below, and in which either Sepia or Natrium muriaticum would already have been indicated.

Sepia is indicated for children who

- *are lively, enjoy dancing* and movement (and feel clearly better as a result),
- as a rule stare at the doctor with large eyes, open wide, emitting an intense and steady gaze,
- who at the same time emit "*noli me tangere*" and who do not enjoy having their skin examined – resisting more aggressively and persistently than is the case for children typical of Pulsatilla.

In these characteristic traits we are reminded of the cuttlefish (Sepia officinalis). It is one of the most highly developed of all the invertebrates and has the largest eyes of any member of the animal kingdom, but is not yet capable of any inversion of the retina. Its states of excitation are strikingly reflected in various skin patterns. If approached too closely, it reverses at high speed, concealing itself in a cloud of ink, hence the German name *Tintenfisch* (or "ink fish"). The ink is used for medicinal purposes and, like the shell of the oyster, constitutes a broadly mineral complex organized by the creature itself – it is therefore also a mineral-based medicine with correspondingly deep action.

With children who respond therapeutically to Sepia, a form of psychological ambivalence is frequently present in the family, with *affection/sympathy often accompanied by underlying initially concealed aggression.* The ambivalence of the mother between a work orientation (calling for a "cool head" and ambition) and the maternal-feminine role; the frequent ambivalence today in the psychological relationship with the husband (by whom the mother – as mother – feels left alone, and who claims for himself the outgoing work oriented role and also occupies that terrain); as well as the rising level of ambivalence in respect of the increasingly masculine leading role of the wife in a family where the male role model is weak (i. e. with the father, the man, frequently being away from home, and often working only in purely intellectual professions); in short, the *ambivalence in which many women today find themselves for social reasons* clearly has a problematic impact on the children. In this respect the conflict in the family increases to the extent that exhaustion rises ("I feel nothing for my husband", "I would prefer never to see any of them ever again"), although these admissions are only forthcoming in response to sensitive ques-

6

tioning. In this respect, advice and support is indispensable for the mother, and not infrequently Sepia can be a supportive medicine for her in cases where *exhaustion*[1] resulting from pregnancy, breast-feeding and possibly also eczema in the child are dominant issues.

Sympathy and antipathy, will impulses and (premature) intellectual development (constitutionally: hysterical and neurasthenic traits) are related in a contradictory and psychologically unmediated relationship. We can refer once more to the cuttlefish and the cephalopod family which, among the invertebrates, display a *rushing ahead development* especially in respect of their sensory organs, giving these animals a tense behaviour which is simultaneously *dependent on the environment* in its impulses.

This culminates in a situation where children are overwhelmed by the ambivalences and conflicts that the mother herself, and parents jointly, have to overcome. If this is not recognized and dealt with, they can later display a remote, self-contained, and introverted behaviour (cf. also Natrium muriaticum that can supplement Sepia in these cases). *The skin* manifests

- dry eczema, primarily around the hinged joints; the hands are also severely affected (split skin, super infections on the hands and wrists),
- severe itching,
- thickening epidermis,
- tendency to staphylococcal skin infections,
- generally a tendency for increased pigmentation or vitiligo.

In *vitiligo* in childhood, the administration of Sepia, where necessary after treatment for shock, has been confirmed as by far the most dependable homoeopathic medicine, even reversing vitiligo if treatment is started early enough, as could be observed on several occasions. The cause of vitiligo in childhood can almost always be deduced through a medical history and is psychological in nature. Experiences or conditions of tension express themselves on the skin of the child in a polar pigment quality to the cuttlefish, which squirts out a cloud of black ink when it is about to flee the scene.

A very important and indicative aspect of the picture of Sepia is the tendency for

- *blistering skin diseases*, e. g. herpes zoster (especially in children with a positive family medical history, less in the context of an immunosuppressive therapy), but also dermatitis herpetiformis and others,

for which Sepia (as well as Rhus tox. and Natrium mur.) represents one of the major single substance medicines (cf. also homoeopathic specialist literature).

- **Natrium muriaticum LM6 dil.** Arcana/**D12–C200 pillules**
  5 gtt./d/high potencies as individual doses

is perhaps the most deeply active and healing potentized medicine for psychological ambivalence, grief, consequence of psychological injury as the cause of atopic dermatitis

Cooking salt, Natrium muriaticum, as a substance manifests the remarkable property in nature of crystallizing into perfect cubes (with a high degree of transparency) while on the

1 Exhaustion is an important symptom among adults for this prescription, but not in childhood.

other hand dissolving in water comparatively easily and completely (a unique quality in this form). In human culture, cooking salt has long been important as a unique *preserving agent* alongside drying. Physiologically, impulses of *excitation* in the organism are driven primarily by the extracellular concentration of sodium. *Psychological excitability and sensitivity, psychological isolation* and the *long-term retention of an unforgotten grief* in the child, or in the mother closely attached to that child, characterize at first approximation the constitution of a child who needs Natrium muriaticum.

A very striking and telling symptom displayed by these children is that they *avoid exposure to direct sunlight* (which may causes headaches or a general deterioration in condition). This expresses a deep-rooted impairment in the absorption and assimilation of incoming warmth and light – the child rejects what he or she innately most strongly craves. In a similar manner, *direct consolation exacerbates his or her* condition although the child is *very easily offended.* In some cases they may have hysterical and tearful episodes, but try to cry alone and unseen. The child avoids any discussion of anything that weighs heavily upon its soul, even though it can be of great relief to these patients if the doctor is aware of their grief and very cautiously raises it to the surface. *Painting* is of great therapeutic benefit as a way of learning to express what is innermost and which will otherwise injure the soul like a sharp-edged crystal.

The triggers for such grief can be many and varied (▸Chap. 2.4) and often extend back as far as pregnancy (cf. also the case study in [Pfeiffer et al. 2007, 319]). The threat of abortion, or of termination as a result of parental conflict or of the mother being left alone, isolation as a newborn, parental divorce, troubling deaths in the family, assaults on the child, as well as failure in communication, in expressing oneself fully and freely, can all impact on these children. They feel deceived and abandoned while others would get over a loss or a perceived slight. A characteristic feature is the tendency of these children to have only "a few good female friends" to whom they like to cling (and whom they consequently often lose again). The most important source of solace for these female patients is often *music* for which they have a deep sensitivity.

Psychological precocity and grief, but on the other hand a high level of sensitivity are what characterize these children, whose problem of the ambivalence between excessive distance and excessive closeness is frequently reflected at the barrier of the skin. In general they physically have

- the tendency for a metabolic event abruptly to break through the boundary to the nervous and sensory system such as an acutely exacerbating *eczema*, *pollinosis* or also a *migraine*; a more local incident is *herpes labialis* after exposure to direct sunlight,
- significant *sensitivity in the head area* (headache after grief, sunlight, after school – in girls); thin secreting mucous membranes in eyes and nose; oral aphthous ulcers herpes,
- *the neck*[1] is frequently affected (halogens such as chlorine have a striking relationship to the neck, the "septime region" of the human being [Husemann 2010, 42–64]) and in adolescence this is a central medicine for *autoimmune diseases of the thyroid gland*
- skinfolds, especially in the periorbital region and a *markedlyy large forehead,*
- a striking appetite for salt,
- an aversion to fat, also somewhat to bread.

1 A patient whose atopic dermatitis healed completely at school age in response to treatment with Natrium mur. was operated on at the age of two for a median neck cyst.

6

Generally speaking, the patients exhibit a catabolic metabolism; the fatty tissue is not well developed. In terms of nutrition, breads are often a source of problems.

On the skin we perceive

- eczema, particularly at the nape of the neck, the hairline, the wrist and the elbow with severe itching,
- a generally dry form of eczema, which can, however, acutely display severe and weeping, burn-like exacerbations.

6.4.3.6.4 Medicines of metal origin

An affinity with the medicines described in ▸Chap. 6.4.3.6.3 for predominant psychological ambivalence is manifested by

- **Mercurius solubilis LM6 dil.** Arcana/**Mercurius vivus naturalis D12–30 trit./amp.** Weleda
  1 × 5 gtt./1 saltsp. in the morning; acutely where necessary 1 ampoule D30 i.v./s.c.

The guiding symptoms for this important remedy in atopic dermatitis are a deep-rooted lability and ambivalence in the warmth organization associated with often *foul-smelling secretion activity* of the astral body which takes on a life of its own and is insufficiently managed by the I.

Mercury itself has characteristics [Sommer and Soldner 1988a] that shows a striking ambivalence, having on the one hand a high specific weight (13.6 g/cm^3) and the ability to form almost perfectly shaped droplets; and on the other hand great volatility, high vapour pressure and an ability to atomize under external influence into a spray of countless tiny droplets. It reflects heat in its expansion characteristics (thermometer), it responds to every external impulse but does not achieve any internal consistency and strength.

With Mercurius solubilis H. this *ambivalence without a centrepoint* is even greater when linked simultaneously to a reducing and an oxidizing nitrogen group: $NH_2Hg_2NO_3$. In the medicinal picture these characteristics manifest a high level of contradiction and lability in behaviour from which the stabilizing centre is absent [Sommer and Soldner 1988b]; primarily this applies to the warmth organization:

- General *deterioration caused by heat and cold,*
- Alternately *too cold or too hot,* deterioration in eczema in response to bed warmth, at *night,*
- Severe *night-time sweating* and foul-smelling secretions worsening at night,
- Tendency to purulent, superinfected *foul-smelling* eczemas, with itching exacerbated severely by sweat,
- Very prone to infection (e. g. tonsillitis – ▸Chap. 6.3.3.4).
- Prone to diarrhoea.

The children – boys are clearly more affected than girls – display:

- Intellectual precocity, with alertness and speed, but superficiality,
- Acute need to constantly move, episodes of uncontrollable impulsivity, irritability,
- Can be overwhelmed by group situations with worsening of infections, eczemas or behaviour.

A pronounced level of *immaturity in the rhythmic system* is apparent in all of this and a weakness in the I-directed warmth organization can be detected. A different metal delivers an exemplary stabilizing effect. That metal is gold:

- **Aurum met. praep. D12 trit.** Weleda
  1 saltsp. In the evening or 1 saltsp. 2 x/d

Gold in a middle potentization is particularly effective during the *second septennium* during which the rhythmical system undergoes its decisive development. This medicine "carries" the children through a time in which the forces of rhythmical balance are not yet sufficiently available to them as a result of their immaturity and it promotes the development of their psychological maturity. It has particular significance in the case of a *depressive tendency to withdraw* at this age, and these factors may also be present or be lurking in the history in cases of atopic dermatitis.

▸Chap. 6.4.5 dealt with the effectiveness of silver as a medicine for atopic dermatitis. The vitalizing effect of silver can be enhanced by its natural sulphide compound

- **Argentite D6 trit.** Weleda
  1 saltsp. 1–3 x/d

that has proven its capabilities for example with dry eczemas on children after cytostatic therapy for xerosis. A further indication is dyshydrotic hand eczema. It is principally indicated for dark-haired, "low-sulphur" constitutions [Vademecum 2010, 108].

An important indication of Argentit in its interaction with the antimony compound of silver (dyscrasite) and formica is manifested by *allergic contact eczema of the hands*, especially after frequent contact with washing agents, detergents etc.:

- **Formica ex animale Gl D12 amp.** Wala
- **Argentite D6 amp.** Weleda
- **Dyscrasite D20 amp.** Weleda
  s.c. 1–2 x/wk in the forearm for a few weeks
- **Calcium/Quercus amp.** Wala
  1 ml, 10 ml acute i.v. (with this indication possibly together with **Argentum met. praep. D8–30** Weleda and **Apis ex animale Gl D30** amp. Weleda/Wala)

6.4.3.6.5 Other single-substance medicines for treating atopic dermatitis

Due to constraints on space, this chapter must restrict itself to a selection of medicines that omits any mention of the great many minor but in individual cases important medicines (cf. in particular the homoeopathic specialist literature). Nevertheless, a few of the latter will be set out here. The most important and most far-reaching plant-based homoeopathic medicine in this group is

- **Thuja e summit. D12–15 pillules** Wala
  5 pillules 1–2 x/d

In his lecture to doctors given on 9 April 1920, Rudolf Steiner [199, 373] characterizes a situation in which food in the stomach and duodenum is not broken down sufficiently and, to a certain extent, takes "the wrong way out". Here he cites *Thuja occ.* – and Argentum – as appropriate medicines. Hahnemann accorded this *arbovitae* ("tree of life") in its potentized form the status of a deeply effective medicine in respect of chronic and chronically progredient infections [Hahnemann 1983, 122ff.], specifying the urogenital tract and specific venereal infections as an indication for Thuja. With these indications, too, a minor tendency for self-healing and an "infiltration" – often occult for an extended period – of the organism by destructive, invasive foreign life is characteristic. Both authors thus refer primarily to a weakness in the boundary of the metabolic pole, in the area of digestion and of the urogenital system, even if it is expressed "on top and outside". The appearance and presentation of the patient is therefore far removed from the locus of the central problem, which is rooted in a very vital and subconscious region.

Thuja occidentalis belongs to the family of cypress plants. This evergreen tree is now planted frequently in hedges for visual screening purposes; the scaled or overlapping leaves have the thick outer skin typical of the cupressaceae family, inside which calcium oxalate crystals are stored. The interior of the tree is very dark, and the thuja hedge does not allow any light to penetrate. The interior of the leaves is filled with a slimy substance characterized by a high level of turgor; externally the leaves secrete an etheric oil as the result of a vegetable catabolic process that can have a highly toxic effect on all abdominal organs [Stübler & Krug 1987, 331]. In extreme cases, thuja can cause a haemolytic-uremic syndrome, similar to the verotoxin of certain pathogenic E.-coli strains (EHEC); it can trigger miscarriage (▸Chap. 5.5.4.2). The "tree of life", thuja, thus generates a level of toxicity that affects human beings primarily in the intestines and kidneys. An observation of plants that also incorporates the evolution of plant life shows, as does a morphological consideration, that thuja is a plant (as is the closely related sabina, for example) that has remained at a relatively primitive stage of evolution and that, compared to its original developmental potential, tends to exhibit *regressive traits*. The form of this plant appears petrified and monotonous. Against this background it may be possible to understand why the elements of thuja are able to develop such a high level of toxicity for human beings.

In the *homoeopathic medicinal picture* some symptoms are striking that relate to the disease pattern being presented here:

- consequence of chronic infections,
- chronic irritation of mucous membranes in intestinal and urogenital area,
- sensitive to cold and damp, freezing all the time (not enough personal warmth formation),
- dyspepsia, bloating, indigestion,
- "feels ill and does not know why",
- has the feeling of carrying "an (alien) living entity" in the body,
- tendency to exhibit chronic sinusitis, asthma, and atopic dermatitis.

Modern homoeopathy has discovered that patients who respond well to thuja suffer inside a carefully constructed façade, behind which they harbour intense dislike and rejection of themselves – a deep divide which favours a split in the subconscious soul life associated with the "metabolic pole". The patient finds this condition a puzzle and the connection between the soul entity and the physical body is burdened with such splits.

This corresponds to a poor ability of the I to integrate which is expressed in the warmth organization. Patients tend to develop insufficient warmth and exhibit an immunologic inability to distinguish reliably between "self" and "foreign". Allergies and cellular immunodeficiences, and the resultant clinical pictures at all barrier organs are observable consequences. This facilitates the penetration and persistence of chronic infections that can lead to internal intoxication.

Thuja occ. is indicated as follows:

- *sensitive to cold and damp, feels cold;* worsening in late autumn and winter,
- atopic dermatitis *and* bronchial asthma,
- initially weeping, thickened and hardened, later dry, severely itchy and generalized eczemas that are prone to bleeding,
- frequent *molluscum contagiosum* and atopic dermatitis (cf. also fluorite, ▸Chap. 10.8.1.3),
- generally a tendency for chronically persistent infections.

This substance is not an easy one to incorporate into a systematic constitutional observation, but is primarily associated with the hysterical type in its emphasis on and insufficient shaping of the metabolism, on the tendency for chronic inflammatory conditions and restlessness; then, secondly, also exhibits neurasthenic traits with poor warmth formation and frequently a slim shape (in contrast to the literature).

In practice, this relates to slim patients who enjoy sports pursuits which relieve their psychological pressures, although they do not easily access their own feelings. The restlessness, the slightly addictive need to engage in sport, the link between atopic dermatitis and bronchial asthma, the latter often triggered by infections and wet-cold weather, are all indications – in combination with the other symptoms specified. In cases where D12 has a significant effect, it is advisable to remain at this potency and to administer it over an extended period. This can result in a sustained and healing action that requires no further medicines.

In adolescence the affected patients benefit greatly from *art therapy* if the aim is to open the door to their own soul and self expression.

- **Formica D6–12 dil.** Weleda
  1–3 × 5 gtt.

counteracts *itching with dry eczemas* and assists with the regeneration of the skin, especially in the case of a neurasthenic constitution (▸Chap. 6.3.3.3; [Vademecum 2010, 446]). Indicated among other things after an impairment of the life organization caused by the interventiopn of allopathic forms of medication (e.g. cytostatics) or worsening through contact with washing agents, detergents, etc.[1]

The patients do not generate *enough body temperature* and tend to be thin and chilly (worsening in winter).

- **Mezereum D12–20 pillules** (various manufacturers)
  3–5 pillules 1–2 x/d

1 Cf. also Equisetum/Formica

Mezereum is indicated for

- extremely itchy, weeping, purulent, crust-forming eczema caused by severe scratching and blood-smeared eczemas of the face and scalp in infancy and early childhood, particularly if
- vaccinations are the trigger behind acute exacerbation (cf. Quarz, Conchae, Thuja). This substance can also be indicated with
- *herpes zoster* in the area of the first trigeminal branch, especially around the eyes.

D. Grandgeorge [2004, 128f.] points to the relationship of Mezereum to febrile, purulent bilateral sinusitis. It contains the motif of the concealed, latent infection that does not want to heal, an alien quality inside the organism that can also indicate the consequences of vaccination. It is therefore also possible to attempt to formulate the indication in such a way that the organism (initially unsuccessfully) tries to expel an alien quality in the head area. The massive inflammatory symptoms that frequently accompany this, and that can be observed in the indication for Mezereum, then present themselves in a different light.

- **Petroleum D8–12 dil/pillules** (various manufacturers)
  5 gtt./pillules 1–5 x/d

Petroleum is indicated for eczemas that

- very clearly get worse in *winter*,
- especially relate to the *acral periphery – nose, ear lobes, fingers* – that have a tendency for hypothermia,
- exhibit *acutely painful cracks* in the skin.

In many individuals with severe or treatment-resistant atopic dermatitis, a breakthrough can occur using *homoeopathic nosodes.* The preparations of Gudjons have proven to be particularly reliable.

- **Psorinum C12–200 pillules**
  with primary *weakness of the life organization and warmth formation* (extremely frosty people, worsening in cold weather); neurasthenic constitution [Pfeiffer et al. 2007, 314].
- **Medorrhinum C12–200 pillules**
  for hysterical constitution with impulsivity, chronic-allergic rhinitis, *stubborn, recurrent dermatitis in the nappy (diaper) area, recurrent anal fissures* (cf. Hirte, in [Pfeiffer et al. 2007, 912–915].
- **Tuberculinum C200 pillules** (▸Chap. 6.5.6.11)
  in the combination or *vicariation of atopic dermatitis and bronchial asthma* or *obstructive bronchitis;* constitutionally there is a hybrid form of hysterical and neurasthenic traits here [Steiner 1976, 43ff.].

Administer high potencies (C30-200) in single doses (1–3 × 3 pillules every 12 hrs,) then wait, where possible at least 1 week, and in some cases much longer, for the response.

The individualized approach to treatment with potentized single-substance medicines allows for the most thorough and sustained treatment successes with atopic dermatitis. It must, however, remain part of a holistic course of treatment that embraces all aspects of this disease, from nutrition to psychological and social family relationships.

6.5 Bronchial asthma

We can have a low opinion of homesickness. It can, of course, be explained on the basis of so-called psychological habits and suchlike. But I do ask that you take into account that there can be physiological consequences as a result of so-called homesickness. ... It can come to expression in asthmatic manifestations. ... Please take that together with other things which do not normally prompt scientific consideration – unfortunately not.
Rudolf Steiner [1921]

"The story told by the biography is retold in shorthand by the attack, just like in the story book the picture captures the critical moment and gives it permanence in our mind. ... If we now take the concealed psychological anxiety and asthma together and imagine a kind of dependency, we can say: fear creates something that in turn creates fear."
Victor von Weizsäcker [1947]

6.5.1 Towards a clinical picture

In 1946, Victor von Weizsäcker in a lecture to his medical students in Heidelberg presented a fifty-year-old female cigar maker suffering from asthma:

"We now see this disease remarkably often in the clinic. At first she only suffered from severe bronchitis which would not heal properly. It may be that at the time the severe unemployment which affected whole industries at the end of the War threw its first shadow on the thoughts of this patient as well. Then her company did, indeed, also close down – she became unemployed and lost her livelihood. Shortly after this event, which deeply affected her, the asthma attacks started in full strength. After twenty-six years of steady work a disaster struck her for the first time ... Her pride was gone, but also her feeling of security. Pathological physiology teaches us that bronchial asthma is a form of vagus neurosis, is accompanied by secretion of the bronchial mucous membrane and contraction of the bronchial muscles which are both often triggered by an allergy, a hypersensitivity to plant and animal proteins (! – 1946) ... But that tells us nothing about why the effect occurs in this organ precisely here or precisely now ... 'Precisely now' – in that respect we hear that her soul suffered a serious loss of security in the critical period. ... ...

If we ask, what is asthma, then we ask: what is respiration, what does respiration mean in psychological regard? And how does it happen that this complex of functions becomes the sphere in which the loss of security is expressed?

To examine these matters, let me give you a guiding thought. As an experiment, always look at organic diseases *as if the ill person were creating their illness themselves* (emphasis as in original). This is a complete reversal of our normal way of experience and thinking because it says that the ill person does not get his or her illness but creates it. To begin with, we resist such a thought – the patient, those around him or her and medical thinking do not want to accept it. And yet there are individual occurrences which point in this direction and which are not easy to forget. I remember a serious melancholic who one day developed a cystitis with urinary retention ... during catheterization the treacherous words escaped her: 'Isn't it dreadful that I have to do this!'

I said she was behaving like a child. How do children behave? Let us take a specific, although common scene. A child is to go for a walk but does not want to do so. He or she prefers the comfort of staying at home. He or she resists having their coat put on; the child struggles, screams, cries. Finally he or she says: 'Serve you right if I get a cold.' Or sometimes he or she might even say: 'Serve you right if I die.' The child's imagination already imagines an illness, uses the threat of an illness in defiance or as retaliation; but ultimately it arises from anxiety, the anxiety of the loss of security. This anxiety must be very powerful if it gives rise to such terrible threats."

At this point Victor von Weizsäcker briefly summarizes Gogol's famous novella *The Overcoat* which tells of an impoverished government clerk who saves for months for a new overcoat – his old one is threadbare. His colleagues celebrate with him when he gets his new coat from the tailor. On the way home after the celebration he is mugged and his coat is stolen. He awakens with a fever, develops a serious inflammatory disease – perhaps pneumonia – and dies.

"Hence Dostoyevsky later wrote to a friend: we all come from Gogol's 'Overcoat'. The overcoat is a symbol of the protection which even the poorest need – vitally need. You will now understand how this relates to the child …

Let us apply this to the disease of asthma and respiration. Respiration is a vital function. … It consists of two parts: inhalation and exhalation. It is also a taking in and giving out. The muscles have to effect first the one, then the other; if both were to happen at the same time, a stoppage, a retention would occur.

So what does every child do? He or she cries and screams. His or her tear glands secrete and the laryngeal muscles block the airway. … And what happens in an asthma attack? Something equivalent only one level lower. The bronchial mucous membrane secretes, and the involuntary bronchial muscles block respiration. *We can say that there is crying and screaming in the depths of the lungs. The attack is a kind of tantrum in the lungs* (author's emphasis) as an expression of that anxiety, that defiance, that retribution with illness and perhaps death. The whole thing has merely been relocated. What happens in the child in the upper sphere takes place here in the involuntary depths. The attack does not last forever, just as the tantrum is just an episode … But in both cases the scene is simply a discharge of tension which has been building up for a long time, circumstances which have been a long time in the making. An episode to which there is a background." [Weizsäcker 1947, 94ff.]

In 2010, the *S2-Leitlinie Asthma bronchiale im Kindes- und Jugendalter* (Guideline on bronchial asthma in childhood and adolescence) defined asthma as an "illness with an elevated sensitivity of the airways with regard to various irritants (hyperresponsiveness), based on a chronic inflammation of the bronchial mucous membrane, particularly in the region of the small airways. There is a complex interaction between endogenous (genetically determined (!)) factors and exogenous irritants of a physical, chemical pharmacological and/or immunological type (triggering mechanism or inducer) resulting in hyper/dyskrinia, bronchospasm, mucosal oedema and, under certain circumstances, remodelling. Beyond that there is a close connection between bronchial asthma and an atopic disposition. Bronchial asthma is **clinically** (emphasis in orig.) characterized by a largely paroxysmal, in rare cases also constant, expiratory inhibition of the respiration which is either spontaneous or variable as the result of treatment." [Berdel 2010, 1f.]. After reading von Weizsäcker, the reader may well ask himself or herself: *Who* is there? If we look for the subject of the pathopsychological definition in a strictly grammatical sense, genetic factors are the most like ones in the sense of an "endogenous" dimension which is part of the affected person. If we look at the 38-page guideline, we come across the term "psychosocial factors" on p. 33: "Although psychogenic comorbidities or psychosocial constellations of problems do not cause asthma, they can make treatment and self-management more difficult as well as preventing the achievement of good controls. In such cases psychological/psychotherapeutic help can be indicated. Patients with insufficient asthma control in particular should therefore be specifically investigated for psychosocial problem constellations/psychological comorbidities." [Berdel 2010, 33]. So what causes bronchial asthma? Who suffers from bronchial asthma – and who disrupts successful treatment?

"There are also psychological and spiritual dimensions underlying these phenomena such as insufficient boundaries, autonomy conflicts, traumas (including worries and grief), slights or obstacles in the development the individuality of the person. Their relationship with the bodily physical manifestation can be described with the cognitive tools of anthroposophic medicine, the functional tripartite structure and the fourfold structure of the human being." This is how the *"Leitlinie zur Therapie des Asthma bronchiale in der Anthroposophischen Medizin" (Guideline for the treatment of bronchial asthma in anthroposophic medicine)* of the Arbeitsgemeinschaft Anthroposophical Pneumologie (Working Group for Anthroposophical Pneumatology) supplemented its guideline published in 2010 [AAP 2010].

Against this background, differentiated paths of access to this clinical picture open up which in the period from 1946 to the present day has become the most frequent chronic clinical picture in childhood and is also the most costly to treat.

6.5.2 Observations in practice

> The good news first: many affected children are very sensitive with above-average intelligence. They are often also artistically gifted and as adults know better than others what they want. It is important that parents should keep this reassuring message in mind despite all the worries about a child suffering from asthma.
>
> J. Vagedes, G. Soldner [2010]

The experience in the encounter with children suffering from asthma can vary a great deal and cannot be reduced to a single statement. But it is the material starting point for *learning to understand* these children and their families and thus to get away ourselves from *just our knowledge*. An individual approach to paediatrics which aims to heal this disease cannot do without this starting point.

Children suffering from asthma noticeably also touch the soul of their counterpart outside states of acute breathing difficulty. They have an intense presence of soul which outside the states of acute dyspnoea can be awake, charming and bright. At the same time we frequently gain the impression that there is an increased *basic tension* between the body and the soul entity, movements and reactions are often somewhat jerky and lack freedom, the action of the muscles and joints in some regions (particularly the neck and shoulder girdle) is tense – this inner tension and movement blockages are also noticeable in temperamentally pasty and rather sluggish asthmatics [Vögler 1987]. Most of the affected children are very sensitive and have above-average intelligence in common. Many show themselves to be artistically gifted. A considerable number are inhibited in aggression, in the ability to fight back, particularly against children of the same age. That, incidentally, clearly changes if the treatment of the asthma is successful (it is a good thing to point this out in advance).

The doctor will often notice a pale face; rings under the eyes indicate an obstruction of nasal breathing or a disorder of the digestive tract (dysbiosis, food intolerances). Pulling up the shoulders during ascultation, even when there is no obstruction of the airways, is a characteristic feature during the examination. Constitutionally boys outweigh girls before puberty, as does a *neurasthenic constitution* (▸Chap. 6.4.3.5.4). With increasing frequency we also encounter chubby, slightly overweight boys with often close bonds to their mother who during physical exercise quickly start to sweat and develop breathing difficulties. These children also frequently display impaired concentration and attention; their restlessness and weak feeling of self-esteem is also apparent during the consultation (▸Chap. 7.5.3.6.2).

In the *relapsing obstructive bronchitis* of infancy (which is known to have a better prognosis and responds better to therapeutic measures than bronchial asthma), a *hysterical constitution* (as set out in ▸Chap. 6.4.3.5.4) and excessive metabolic processes in the lung are prominent: the swelling of the mucous membrane in the region of the bronchioles and the secretion of mucus primarily contribute to the symptoms. As triggers, the focus is on infections which the child cannot, or not yet, overcome in the form of an acute inflammation and food intolerances (particularly to milk protein). The ability to generate a fever and break down and overcome foreign matter immunologically, to control digestion and the metabolism, is not (yet) sufficiently developed; but the metabolism as such is very active in these children. It is a characteristic feature that as a rule they *suffer little anxiety and shortage of breath.* The disease generally takes a less dramatic course with fewer attacks and rather takes a course of subfebrile, subacute bronchitis with whistling and rattling respiration.

In contrast, bronchial asthma is conspicuous through the *linkage* of inflammatory, often tough, rapidly solidifying mucous secretion and muscular bronchospasms in the form of a *paroxysmal* disease. *Psychologically,* there is mostly a *clearly different kind of behaviour and feeling during an attack* than at other times which is characterized by anxiety, agitation and motor unrest. A *conflict* of polar, contradictory tendencies can thus be clearly experienced at various levels. In individual cases this already develops in the first two years of life; then it is diagnostically and prognostically more correct to refer to "bronchial asthma" from the beginning and not "obstructive bronchitis".

Although food intolerances (and therapeutic diet plans) do not play such an important role in bronchial asthma as in atopic dermatitis, the *relationship* of asthmatic children *with food often stands out.* There are, above all, extreme preferences and aversions; unrest and lack of concentration when the family is eating together; the circadian rhythm of the appetite is displaced; food *means little to many children.* They eat outside meal times, one-sidedly, "as if in passing". The increasing lack of appetite and nausea as the bronchial obstruction increases is familiar. In children with an *hysterical, markedly metabolic constitution* there is also abnormal eating behaviour in the sense that certain foods are one-sidedly preferred and the children eat frequently between meals; except that here there is the tendency to be overweight behind which there is not infrequently also a depressive, psychologically inhibited development (on digestive disorders, assimilation and warmth generation cf. ▸Chap. 6.3 and 6.4). In contrast, pleasure in eating and intensive digestion are indicative of an intensive connection between the soul entity and the living element of the food as well as with the life-bearing sphere of the own organism, which cannot digest without the impulses of the soul and I (▸Chap. 4). Eating together and living in the rhythm of the community strengthens this *connection with life* which in children suffering from asthma is often insecure at the beginning and underdeveloped.

Asthmatic children *fall out of rhythm* not just in their own respiration: they tend to be restless in the evening, often find it difficult to let go of their own inner tension to go to sleep and wake up during the night, frequently with anxieties (even when there are no breathing difficulties). The rhythm of their bodily movements is often jerky and speeded up or blocked, inhibited; their breathing does *not flow freely* even outside asthmatic attacks. They stand out through their *hypersensitivity,* in the first instance to *meteorological influences* – almost every asthmatic disease in this respect displays typical modalities under which it worsens, and this *fact as such* reveals an abnormal sensitivity to the environment and dependence on the climate. That in itself is an expression of the labile connection with the body. The all-too-free appearance of the soul entity of these children corresponds to weakness at the point where this soul entity has to become active in the body: above all in breaking down and overcoming food and in building up the barrier organs which create the boundary of the body with external nature. Hypersensitivity as pollinosis, to dust mites and other things is an expression of the problem of retaining a relationship with nature while at the same time emancipating oneself from it. It is intimately connected with the way the soul entity is linked with one's own living physical body.

In summary, the soul entity of asthmatic children is revealed – in different ways – in our encounter with them: often it appears to the other person as too intense – while at the same time being unable to immerse itself in its own physical body, giving a vulnerable and hypersensitive impression. Equally it can appear restrained and inhibited at first; but then, too – perhaps at the second look – the child's homelessness and tenseness can be felt. The mother of twins, a colleague, whose twin daughter has asthma while the twin son shows no trace of it, was asked by the author how she would draw her two (9-year-old) children with the soul entity in mind: with the son the legs and body were strongly represented; they became diffuse in the picture of the daughter while the upper half of her body was depicted in impressive size. The mother: Well, here her soul is too large – and at the same time it became clear how closely this soul, which was not quite at home in the body, was connected with the mother. The mother experienced the relationship with her twin son in quite a different way, felt psychologically more free in this relationship.

The interaction between the soul entity and the physical body in the human being is crucially dependent on the activity of the I-organization and thus the *individuality of the child itself.* The latter lives in the warmth organization (▸Chap. 6.4.2). Asthmatic children often display a noticeable discrepancy between their own feeling of warmth in relationship to their body temperature and to the warmth in the environment. They also have difficulty in distributing their body temperature harmoniously. Here their own lower organism is particularly affected (e. g. cold feet and lower legs). Therapeutically a warm footbath or mustard footbath [Girke 2010, 157] and the corresponding treatment of the feet very oft have a antispasmodic and beneficial long-term effect (▸Chap. 6.5.6.2). *Suppressive pretreatments* of the child's warmth organization (e. g. antibiotic, antipyretic treatment of infections of the airways, etc.) and corresponding weaknesses or weakening of the parent generation ("atopically loaded family medical history") – cf. the previous ▸Chap. 6.1 to 6.4 – play an even greater role in bronchial asthma than in atopic dermatitis. Many children with bronchial asthma have atopic dermatitis in their own case history. As well as growing older, anti-inflammatory measures, not least against the eczema itself, can promote the transition to bronchial asthma.

The relationship with the family, above all the mother, is of great importance in asthmatic children. Putting it into words like this alone expresses the problematic position of the father in the family.

It should be said here that the following remarks no more apply to all children and their parents than any of the previous ones; neither can it be the intention to apportion blame, particularly as we are dealing with *correspondence relationships* which are developed by both sides from birth. The brief description of the colleague and mother of twins can perhaps already make that clear. The child, too, brings its independent individuality (and destiny) with him or her and at conception and birth is more than an empty sheet waiting to be written on.

An important reason for problems between father and mother as well as father and child exists if the father rejects the pregnancy or even wanted the child to be aborted; and if he left the mother during the pregnancy or she felt psychologically abandoned. That is something which can frequently be experienced when taking the medical history of children with chronic-obstructive respiratory diseases. It can equally be the case that only the mother wanted the pregnancy, did not connect inwardly with the father of the child and soon detached herself from him, keeping him at a distance (▸Chap. 2.4). Separation or the threat of separation of the parents – this is often the background against which mother and child create close bonds and the father moves to the periphery, particularly in the first years of child's life. Other reasons for a such a development can lie in the immaturity of the father, occupational and financial worries, a weak position of the father e. g. with regard to his mother-in-law, etc. *In any event, a weakened position of the father* is much more prevalent in families with asthmatic children today than a paternal position which is too dominant. On the maternal side, the reason for an *imbalance between the parents with maternal dominance* or *too close a mother-child attachment* can lie both in a dominant, possessive personality or a basic anxiously depressive outlook.

Here it can be observed that since the Second World War and the disappearance of pre-industrial agriculture, the *absence of the father throughout the day has become the norm in societies with a "western lifestyle"*. It also gives pause for thought that boys are more frequently affected with childhood bronchial asthma.

Childhood bronchial asthma more frequently occurs in families with labile and tense relationships (whereby the grandparents and the importance of the siblings must also be considered – the systemic family therapy approach [Weber 1995, ▸Chap. III, IV] can be of crucial help here in clarifying the medical history and diagnosis, even if we wish to go a different therapeutic path). But the greatest importance accrues to a *psychological ambivalence of the mother towards the child.* Here the aggressively rejecting element is frequently concealed behind a very concerned and formally protective (but not warm) style of upbringing. The little story above can illustrate that the quality with which the child bonds with the mother can trigger or reinforce such ambivalence. In such a situation the maternal love does not provide any warmth: without the latter the child's soul remains unenveloped, is lacking the covering which allows it gradually to venture into the open and survive there. But this warmth flows from a deeper source than the always ambivalent emotions of the pure soul entity (the astral body): *warmth flows from the identification of the human individuality with itself, with the circumstances of its own life, its fellow human beings.* If the parents cannot generate this warmth for their child because such identification is impossible for them – as a result of the characteristic mid-life conflict with the partner, with that which the person himself or herself has not been able to realize in life, with what acts in the present because it has not been resolved in the past – *then the parents themselves are in trouble.*

Be it at a primary or secondary level, the parents of asthmatic children require psychological support from the doctor. That is not always possible: because it cannot be admitted, because e.g. the father cannot be reached, because the doctor's life experience and training are still insufficient. But that does not change anything in the true significance of these processes.

Case histories

A boy, the first of two children, has been a patient of the practice from birth. From as early as the first year of life relapsing obstructive bronchitis which turns into asthma with sometimes frequent attacks of breathing difficulty. No cure despite intensive treatment with homoeopathic and anthroposophical medicines.

Problematic family relationships: the father is an amiable, soft musician, the mother a teacher at an anti-authoritarian private school (1968). There is a lot of tension in the marriage.

From the father devoted antiauthoritarian upbringing, going so far as the boy screaming at his father at age 7: "When are you finally going to punish me?" Bad pupil despite intelligence, leaves Waldorf school early. Apprenticeship.

Only when the patient was able to liberate himself from home and successfully pursue a career (ship builder) was the asthma cured.

When the pat. was 15 years old, the doctor was informed by a third party that the family father was not the biological father, which the mother despite much effort from others – as far as known – has been able to tell neither her husband nor her son nor her doctor (in a cautious conversation held in this regard).

A boy, second of two children, obstructive bronchitis for the first time at age two without a detectable trigger. Development of bronchial asthma with serious attacks of breathing difficulty which repeatedly had to be treated in hospital.

When the boy was four years old, the family started going to Greece twice a year for their holiday. There he was always immediately free of complaints. Whatever the length of the holiday – be it two or six weeks – the breathing difficulties returned mostly as soon as the return flight.

At the age of 7 (pat. was in class 1 of primary school), the parents (both teachers) decide to build a house in Greece. The father takes leave and under primitive conditions (father and son live in a VW camper van) he starts to realize the project with the patient. The boy goes to school there, learns modern Greek and together with his father builds the house with great enthusiasm, whatever the weather and difficulties, which is finished two years later.

No more asthmatic complaints, either during the building period or after the return to Germany.

A girl, a third child, is presented at the surgery aged 7 months with the full picture of bronchial asthma. Obstructive bronchitis for the first time at the age of a few weeks, antibiotically treated infections of the airways, increasingly severe attacks of breathing difficulty, ongoing treatment for months with beta2-sympathomimetic drugs and inhaled steroids, but severe episodes of dyspnoea continue.

The girl comes to the surgery with pronounced dyspnoea and correspondingly pronounced auscultation findings. She has a noticeably friendly look, is alert and physically thin and delicate.

The mother is a colleague, working; a tall, serious, psychologically introverted woman. The father is a doctor, currently not in permanent employment, pursuing various scientific and professional interests. He displays a sanguine temperament with a neurasthenic constitution; his position with regard to his wife and child appears labile. A phlegmatic, sympathetic, somewhat overweight nanny takes over the care of the child when the parents are not at home and brings the pat. to the practice when the mother is prevented from doing so through work. A medical history reveals that the first child has been suffering for years from bronchial asthma; after the child had been conceived, the father felt a strong ambivalence towards the pregnancy. The second child is healthy; here the pregnancy period was "OK" between the parents. During the pregnancy with the pat., a conflict in the relationship began between the father and mother which remains totally unresolved; the mother wants a separation, the father cannot decide.

The mother is successfully transferred to a colleague who helps her to clarify her attitude in the family conflict; today, four years later, the parents live harmoniously together. The significance of the parental conflict was discussed with both parents. Under the corresponding medication (▸Chap. 6.5.5, ▸Chap. 6.5.6) the permanent allopathic medication with steroids could be brought to an end within weeks and totally (stoppage also of DNCG and beta-sympathomimetics) finished after some months. No more asthma attacks in the last two years. No other allergic diseases, for the last two years only normal infection frequency (at the beginning strongly cumulative infections of the airways; acute pneumonia in the course of that).

6.5.3 Pathogenesis

Embryologically, *an anterior section of the gut is transformed gradually into a respiratory organ* in lung development [Hinrichsen 1990, 579f.]. During the process, the formative impulses on the epithelium – this applies in general to morphogenesis, the form-giving processes of the organs in human embryology [Hinrichsen 1990, 19f.] – are conveyed by the *extracellular matrix*. The *contact and cohesion of the epithelial cells with the basement membrane*, in which "integrins" play a mediating role, allows for maturation into a *respiratory* epithelium. The cohesion of the epithelial cells between one another – and thus the unity of the epithelial surface – is also produced with the help of these integrins: the contact with the extracellular matrix through the basement membrane, the unity of the epithelial surface and the differentiation into (internally polarized) respiratory epithelial cells are thus directly connected.

This connection becomes labile and inflammatory in bronchial asthma (reversible obstruction) and can give way in "remodelling" to a profound, irreversible process of sclerosis with goblet cell metaplasia, thickening of the subepithelial basement membrane, hyperplasia and hypertrophy of the smooth muscles and an increase in connective tissue in the subepithelial space. The obstruction of the airways is partially irreversible. The established asthma treatment consisting mainly of beta-agonists and inhaled or, as necessary, systemic corticosteroids does not prevent remodelling (cf. below, ▸Chap. 6.5.5.3). The living coherence of bronchial organ development can only be depicted today in its pathogenic aspects, its disintegration but not at the level which creates and maintains its coherence. This connection has its origin in the life organization, in the etheric body of the organism (▸Chap. 1.1). A salutogenetic understanding of bronchial asthma with the aim of healing must be guided by the maintenance of this activity and the coherence it constantly generates between epithelium, matrix, vascular and nervous supply of the bronchial system. That does not reduce the value of being able to implement the effective control of potentially life-threatening asthma attacks but directs our attention to the underlying reality of the living organism which is not reached by conventional fine-tuning treatment (several clinical studies are in agreement on this) and upon which the long-term prognosis is crucially dependent.

While the lungs in the first third of pregnancy still appear "pseudoglandular" as a glandular appendage to the gut, bronchia and bronchioles develop by the twenty-fourth week of pregnancy. From this point the alveoli appear, first as air sacs until birth, and then begin to develop in the alveolar period, up to the end of the first septennium [Hinrichsen 1990, 595; Girke 1997, 282]. Here bronchia and bronchioles take a middle position between the alveoli, which are closest to the metabolic organization and function, having acquired an elastic, physically not fixed shape through surfactant and other substances (closely connected with the sphere of the metabolic organs), and on the other hand the large bronchia and the trachea, which morphologically comes close to the head with its fixed exoskeleton. *In the spasm, in the thickening of the smooth muscles during asthma, the small bronchia and bronchioles tend towards the head organization* (in parallel, the thorax as a whole becomes bell-shaped and stiff); the *hyperresponsiveness* resulting from the irritation of free-ending fibres of the vagus nerve in asthma (as a result of the loss of covering epithelium) also points in this direction. Here a nerve originating in the head is irritated which is important in the pathogenesis of asthma [Reinhardt 1996, 70f.]. In the meantime, proinflammatory, neurogenic influences can maintain and reinforce the bronchial inflammation. In the spasm, the lungs threaten to become too similar to the head, to stiffen in inspiration.

In *eosinophilic inflammation*, the secretion of protein-containing mucus starts to have a breaking down effect like a digestive enzyme, and the bronchia come close to a gut-like digestive organ (in parallel, mucus becomes audible in the respiration and sputum occurs). It is noteworthy that the original role for eosinophilic inflammation lies in the resistance against intestinal parasites (e.g. in worm infections) – and that in countries in which this is frequently necessary, allergic inflammations occur significantly more rarely (▸Chap. 4). The radical elimination of intestinal helminths has been shown to increase the rate of allergic sensitization to house mites [Biggelaar 2004]! Eosinophile inflammations of the bronchia thus represent a physiological process – at the wrong place, for the "wrong" reason: the lung "becomes a quasi 'intestine'" [Schnürer 2006, 58]. The head-like tendency comes to the fore in the neurasthenic, the intestine-like tendency in the hysterical constitution, but there is always an *interpenetration of both tendencies* with individually different weighting. This can take on a constitutional accentuation which for adult COPD has been set in the familiar images of the "pink puffer", the neurasthenically tense, over-alert emphysematic person and the "blue bloaters", the prominently metabolic adipose chronic bronchitic person. The head-related, awake "day side" associated with spasm, lack of appetite and tension contrasts with the inflammatory "night side" of asthma associated with mucous secretion and swelling [Girke 2010, 153].

From a current allergy perspective, key factors for the development of bronchial asthma are an initial increase in the permeability of the respiratory epithelium on the one hand and the vascular endothelium on the other [Schuster and Reinhardt 1999, 291], to which the neurogenic inflammation must be added as a third component. This process is only possible in that the cohesion, the functional integrity of epithelium and vascular endothelium with the extracellular matrix loosens [Renz 1999, 121–132; Vogel 1996, 63–94]. This cohesion is, on the one hand, simply an expression of healthy function, an intact etheric body in the respective organ. On the other hand, it cannot be separated from the human I-organization and thus the warmth organization. Immunologically, the matrix is a decisive place for the preservation of the "self" in physical form; inflammation as an expression of the increased struggle for a person's own integrity is significantly determined in its course by the matrix – including in bronchial asthma.

All the consequences for the bronchia arising from *the loss of cohesion between the matrix, epithelium and vascular endothelium* are familiar and will only be set out briefly here:

- From the lumen, *foreign matter* (pollen, viruses, animal epitheliums, toxins in the air, etc.) *penetrates into the sphere of the matrix* where it triggers "dislocated digestive processes"; through the inflammatory response with the release of the corresponding mediators in the matrix there is a
- Change in the vascular endothelium with consecutive leukocyte infiltration,
- Irritation of the free endings of the vagus nerve fibres (whose irritation up to and including triggering a muscular spasm of the bronchioles and coughing is reminiscent of the itching in atopic dermatitis which correspondingly triggers scratching),
- Further oedematous loosening of the barrier to the airways through which an increased number of antigens can permeate,
- And finally, the development of inflammatory mucus, desquamating degenerating epithelial cells, disintegrating eosinophilic granulocytes etc. leading to abnormal viscosity, a tendency to solidification and once again barrier-damaging action of the mucus through its content of e. g. eosinophilic cationic protein (ECP), major basic protein (MBP), etc.

Surface loss and hypersensitivity interpenetrate and reinforce one another with the inflow of inflammatory dissolving elements from the blood pole; in epithelium destruction, basement membrane thickening, muscular hypertrophy, mucus hypersecretion and nerve "imbalance" with elevated vagal tone the various qualities and components of the lungs become independent of one another – like the pieces of a whole breaking apart – in pathological interpenetration. That, however, is an expression of the loss of the integrating and formative I-activity in the body which is at work in warmth.

Another issue with regard to bronchial asthma has arisen under the keyword "united airways disease". Thus the current S 2 guideline concludes on asthma:

"The *upper airways* play an important role in bronchial asthma. The pathology of the nose should always be included in diagnosis and treatment. Thus the frequent co-reaction of the upper airways can lead to a worsening of the course of the asthma and vice versa. In accordance with the close interaction of the upper and lower airways, the consistent treatment of the nose clearly improves the course of asthma." [Berdel 2010, 38]

"In each case of bronchial asthma and chronic bronchitis the simultaneous presence of chronic sinusitis should be clarified as the latter can strengthen the bronchial symptoms and must be treated without fail." [Girke 2010, 139]

How can this clinically unquestionable phenomenon be explained? One clue for an understanding is revealed by research into NO, nitrogen monoxide. Lundberg [1994, 2008] and others were able to show that a considerable measure of NO is released in the (healthy) paranasal sinuses and reaches the nasal meatus through the paranasal sinus ostia. There it is nasally inhaled and physiologically exercises an "aerocrine" vasodilatory influence on the lungs (and thus on measurably elevated oxygen intake). In contrast, mouth breathing has the opposite effect, particularly with exercise-induced asthma in relatively cold air, namely an inflammatory irritation of the bronchia through the alien quality of the non-assimilated respiratory air[1]. From this perspective, nasally inhaled air often has a polar effect on the lung from mouth breathing; inflammatory changes to the mucous membrane in the upper respiratory tract change the quality of the inhaled air, as does violent inspiration. From this perspective, hectic (costal) mouth breathing represents the pathogenic opposite of quiet, nasal inspiration which results from the activity of the diaphragm.[2] "It must additionally be taken into account that children and adolescents not infrequently have pulmonary overinflation as the only characteristic of asthma."[Bredel 2010]. How often do asthma patients stand out, also in the intervals without an attack, through a one-sidedly changed, costally accented, jerky inspiration! Lastly, *anxiety* fundamentally changes the act of inhalation as well as the relationship, the rhythm between inhalation and exhalation which is fundamentally impaired in bronchial asthma. The authors draw the following consequences from the current state of research:

- The respiratory process of the asthma patient should diagnostically and therapeutically be considered as a unity.
- From a therapeutic perspective, free nasal respiration and, on the other hand, the calm deepening of the breathing with mobilization of the thorax and activation of the diaphragm level is of material importance.
- Only the calmly and adequately inhaled air through the nose has the warmth and humid quality as it enters the lungs which is suitable for the integrated activity of the bronchial and alveolar mucous membrane, the nerve and vascular activity in the bronchoalveolar sphere, and does not burden it with alien qualities.

1 It is noteworthy that the eosinophilic inflammation of the lower airways can go along with elevated NO exhalation (while often at the same time the NO exhalation in the paranasal sinuses is reduced or impaired).

2 There are whole schools building on such an understanding and approach and regard bronchial asthma as inflammatory-obstructive "resistance" against excessive qualitatively insufficiently assimilated inhalation (cf. on the Internet for example the theory and practice developed by Buteyko). The author does not mean such a one-sided understanding (see the following section).

Not just corticosteroids but also anthroposophical medicines which counter an inflammation of the airways (on the basis of lemon and quince) are just as effective, and sometimes more so, when applied nasally rather than as an inhaler.

Thus the *therapeutic goal* of asthma treatment can be comprehensively described such that the patient's *whole respiratory process*, in which his or her soul entity is active, must be taken hold of therapeutically and re-integrated. The corresponding level in this respect is the level of the *I-organization* which is involved in evenly warming through and integrating all of the organs involved in the respiratory process. The aim must be to strengthen its leading role with regard to respiration and thus to promote the coherence of the life processes in the upper and lower airways. A balanced rhythm of the qualities of inhalation and exhalation, consciousness and trust [cf. Arbeitsgemeinschaft Anthroposophische Pneumologie 2010, 57], daytime waking activity and nightime rest and security is the expression of this treatment goal. Since the human rhythmical system takes shape at school age between the ages of seven and 14, this age is of crucial importance for receiving a salutogenetic medicine with the aim of curing bronchial asthma.

6.5.4 From pathology to treatment

> Clinical pathology in general still attempts today to differentiate diseases by *physio*-pathological and *psycho*pathological perspectives and assign them to the corresponding specialist areas. Such a dualistic way of looking at the disease is bound to fail with bronchial asthma because here we can see with all intensity that physiology is in truth psychology. Organic activity and soul activity turn out to be a functional unity.
>
> H. H. Vogel [1984]

Speaking to doctors, Rudolf Steiner [1989, 203ff.] in 1924 responded in detail to a question about the pathology and treatment of bronchial asthma. He began by pointing out that *psychologically-based resistance opposes the exhalatory stream,* "hooks into" the airflow as it were. How is this a pathological counter-image and distortion? It distorts the formation of the air we exhale when we speak, which is carried out by movement of the muscles with the help of the soul entity. The "dislocation" which Victor v. Weizsäcker refers to from the level of the deliberately shapeable muscles in the mouth and throat down into the involuntary spasm of the smooth bronchial muscles is also dealt with by Rudolf Steiner. The soul entity "injects itself" into the airflow; "that is the diagnosis" (Steiner).

Asthma is located hard at the boundary of purely psychiatric diseases; "but under psychiatric diseases I understand those where ... there are real underlying psychological effects such as shock effects, anxiety and suchlike. ... And with asthma it is indeed the case that we often have to go very far back in the psychological causes ... even as far as the embryo. And the external causes often really do lie in the embryonic life. They lie in the mother (!) having had shocks or tribulations which have been repeated at irregular intervals (!) during pregnancy. Such things have an exceptionally strong action on the whole of the mucous membrane system in the respiratory tract ..." [Steiner 1989, 203f.]

The paediatrician will find this declaration by Rudolf Steiner frequently confirmed in a thorough medical history:

- Accidents, deaths in the family,
- Conflict at the time of conception,
- Relationship conflicts during pregnancy,
- Stress at work particularly during the first pregnancy,
- House moves which are difficult to cope with as a result of the pregnancy,
- Rejection of the pregnancy by parents/parents-in-law,

and many other things are frequent stresses in the medical history. And is it not remarkable that an iatrogenically, e. g. through Fenoterol, triggered beta-sympathomimetic stress suppresses premature labour in the same way as an acute bronchospasm?

Furthermore

- premature labour, tocolysis,
- amniocentesis (incl. the associated psychological ambivalence of the mother),
- pathological ultrasound findings during pregnancy (irrespective of their accuracy),
- preeclampsia of the mother,
- premature birth,
- disorders during delivery, anxiety and shock situation during birth

are often an expression and sign of stress in the mother in the sense stated by Rudolf Steiner (▸Chap. 2.4). Above all, all these things express the "loss of the envelope" of security for the child to which Victor v. Weizsäcker refers.

The soul of the child is not connected with the body during pregnancy in the same way as after birth, once breathing starts, after the first sound, the first cry. And it only gradually and increasingly deeply combines with the body during childhood, culminating in puberty: only then does the adolescent become psychologically independent, is "born" in his or her soul [Treichler 1981, 23–35]. Until that time, and particularly during pregnancy, the child's soul entity surrounds his or her body and from the beginning is involved in forming it, initially imprinting itself on the morphogenesis of the body.

Here we encounter the soul entity in a way in which it is present – as can definitely be perceived by many mothers – but not yet immersed, already forming but not yet actively present: a situation of the soul organization, of the astral body, which can be experienced has having certain similarities with the asthmatic child. And in this situation the soul entity is always particularly closely connected with the mother, is particularly dependent on her and forms the physical body in dependence on the envelope with which the mother surrounds it.

A separation process starts at birth in which the soul entity of the child immerses itself in the body. In a healthy situation the impulse for that comes from the child itself. During that process the child undergoes a physiological process which is close to asphyxia; the lung is squeezed out, permanently loses its gland-like, fluid-filled shape and is transformed into a respiratory organ.

A very experienced pulmonologist once spoke at a conference about her experience with many asthma patients. The calls during the night, the anxiety and breathing difficulty of the patients and their calls for support, increasing into the early hours of the morning, and finally the almost always successful resolution of the attack reminded her of her early work in the delivery room. Every night the soul entity separates to a certain extent from the body, the breathing changes – and each morning on waking human beings combine themselves again more deeply with their physical body until they are fully awake. This dream situation of the night and this process of ensouling the body and waking up by oneself [Steiner 1975, 23–35] touches on the fundamental problem of the asthmatic child. He or she has a tense and labile relationship with the body which often originates in the phase of pregnancy described above, in processes at birth: "Because the story told by the biography is retold in shorthand by the attack, just like in the story book the picture captures the critical moment of the story and gives it permanence in our mind" [Weizsäcker 1947].

Rudolf Steiner further explains in the quoted passage that as a result of the processes described, *the "inner appetite" is impaired in many asthmatics* – whereby Rudolf Steiner characterizes the affinity of the astral body with the etheric body. "And a lack of appetite of the whole organism occurs with the asthmatic ... The organism first has to be given back its appetite again" [Steiner 1989, 205]. He refers to a *cure of rhythmized tea*: in the morning oak bark tea – for the tannin content which "expands" the activity of the soul entity to the life organization and particularly stimulates the breaking down and control of foreign protein [Meyer 1997]; in the evening tea from speedwell leaves (Veronica off.) which has to taste bitter and thus gives the life organization a positively stimulating impulse above all in the hepatobiliary sphere so that it can be more easily penetrated by the soul entity.[1] It is noteworthy that current research has discovered bitter taste receptors in the (human) bronchial smooth muscles which have a bronchodilatory action independently of the beta receptors (and experimentally to a greater extent) [Deshpande 2010]. It is currently an open question whether this could also offer a way of treating bronchial asthma through inhalation; in any event it confirms the emphasis on the importance of bitters in asthma treatment in anthroposophic medicine. It also recalls that the lung itself originates in the anterior gut and is thus a transformed (ento-mesodermal) part of the human digestive system in which bitters have a strong effect.

Rudolf Steiner points to the fundamental therapeutic need of asthmatic patients by means of the example of rhythmized treatment with tannin and bitters: guiding the soul entity into life through rhythmizing treatment, initially into its activity in its own body, its own life organization; and leading the latter – primarily weakened, hurt, not properly provided for by the soul and spirit – in turn towards the soul entity by elevating and strengthening vitality. This principle has proved successful therapeutically in anthroposophic medicine: the rhythmical application of polar substances (centrally: iron and copper), catering in alternation for "day and night qualities" has shown itself to be effective with a particularly sustained effect in asthma treatment. Thus the harmonious interaction of body and soul can develop in the child's rhythmical system. As the soul entity combines with the physical body to an ever greater extent in stages up to puberty, the *treatment can support a maturation process which* each person goes through.

This explains why bronchial asthma which starts with and after puberty, or continues beyond it, has a fundamentally worse prognosis (also in treatment extended by homoeopathic and anthroposophic medicine). Paediatrics thus has a unique therapeutic opportu-

1 The practical application of this reference by Rudolf Steiner was particularly worked on at the Gemeinschaftskrankenhaus Herdecke and successfully used on many patients [Knol 1998, 8] (▶Chap. 6.5.6.8.2).

nity with bronchial asthma. Its therapeutic goal must be to shape this period in the maturation of the child with curative intent.

6.5.5 Treatment basics

If we compare bronchial asthma with atopic dermatitis, important differences become apparent alongside the similarities which are important for understanding the treatment and how to apply it.

6.5.5.1 Obstructive bronchitis and asthmatic bronchitis

Looked at in terms of *age*, the typical time when patients with bronchial asthma fall ill is at kindergarten age; in atopic dermatitis persisting beyond the end of dentition, the subacute dry, itching, eczema particularly in the joints comes to prominence at this age (in 70 % of affected children bronchial asthma today manifests by the fifth year of life). With this type of eczema the direction *from outside in* takes the lead, the hypersensitivity of the soul entity and neurasthenic constitution come into focus. With bronchial asthma, *the atopic, inflammatory event is dislocated to a barrier organ of the nervous and sensory human pole further inside;* it therefore represents a pathological metamorphosis, an "internalization" of the atopic (a-topos: in the wrong place) event.

It is true that the same can be said about the so-called "obstructive bronchitis" of infants; but a comparison quickly makes clear that in the latter *exudative processes combined with mucous congestion and swelling of the mucous membrane* typically take place, i. e. the focus is on excessive inflammatory metabolic processes *from the inside to the outside* – similar to the frequently exudative weeping infant eczema (▸Chap. 6.4.2). The lungs in these children are "too embryonic", the barrier function still immature – and accordingly there is a favourable prognosis which is characterized by the subsequent maturation of these still immature barrier organs.

Therapeutically, the approach, sequence and emphasis in the *general basic treatment of (recurring) obstructive bronchitis* correspond to the procedure for atopic dermatitis at this age – cf. the explanation in ▸Chap. 6.4.3.1. In accordance with the immaturity of these children, great importance accrues to the *care and subsequent maturation of all the barrier organs* of these children. Thus *diet* is significantly more important and effective here than at a later time; a *milk intolerance* in particular can play an important role here (but not necessarily) (▸Chap. 6.3). *Constitutionally* the *hysterical* constitution as explained in ▸Chap. 6.4.3.5 is still dominant here; a tendency *to get worse in winter, when it is cold* and *an elevated susceptibility to infection* is noticeable.

Care of the warmth organization thus is very important at this age in the typical, relapsing (infection-triggered) obstructive (wheezy) bronchitis: particularly rhythmical Einreibung of the whole body (only the head is excluded) in the evening, e. g. with

- **Malvenöl** Wala (▸Chap. 2.2.1) or
- **Ol. Lavandulae 10 %** Weleda/Wala,

whereby the mallow oil (Malvenöl) has a stronger warming effect, the lavender oil (Ol. Lavandulae) a stronger calming one – thus also on coughing fits.

In contrast, the approach for atopic dermatitis patients at this age applies with regard to *children with bronchial asthma* who have already reached early childhood or kindergarten age or are older: here *the first step is* to obtain the *trust of the child and parents.* This also means that a pre-existing treatment e.g. with beta-sympathomimetics and inhaled steroids must not be abruptly reduced or interrupted. To begin with, trust can also be created in that the doctor without much ado supports an acute asthma attack allowing the parents to see the effect of externally applied and potentized medicines. In this way the doctor gradually gets to know the child and family better and this also enables access to the psychological ambivalences and conflicts which to begin with often lie concealed in the background or in the past.

Therapeutically the focus is on the *restoration of equilibria* (▸Chap. 6.3.1). That assumes a comprehensive medical history, examination and diagnosis. Here the doctor will often experience that the *impairment of the equilibrium in bronchial asthma is more complicated, contradictory and deeper* than with atopic dermatitis. We are dealing with a "second order" chronic disease tendency.

Thus constitutionally there can to begin with be a tendency for a hysterical constitution which in the course of the disease – be it through suppressive treatment, accelerated intellectual development, the experience of shock and grief or other things – can change into a prominently neurasthenic picture. In such cases the doctor will have to take both tendencies into account in the treatment, which can penetrate one another or come to appearance one after the other or in alternation. Rudolf Steiner [1976, 43ff.] explained this in a lecture on chronic inflammatory lung disease, the pulmonary tuberculosis which was still common in 1920; in classic homoeopathy, too, the phenomenon of various layers ("miasmata") in chronic disease trends which surface consecutively during treatment is familiar and has been described in detail [Köhler 1983, 169–220].

Thus tasks arise in the treatment of bronchial asthma *which in themselves are polar opposites.* The simple therapeutic example which Rudolf Steiner gave with a tannin-containing morning and bitter-containing evening tea already indicates that a *therapeutic rhythm* is needed to achieve a new equilibrium, the reintegration of polar tendencies. The tasks required in this respect are listed below:

6.5.5.2 Acute, interval and constitutional treatment

In *acute treatment* the focus is on the direct pathological penetration of the spasm and solidification on the one hand and inflammatory mucous congestion and swelling of the mucous membrane on the other. It is a matter of mediating directly between *astral and etheric body, soul and body* and in doing so to support the parents. In the *interval* after an attack, lasting as a rule several weeks or months, a modified symptom-related treatment continues to be necessary to avoid a renewed paroxysmal escalation. But a start can be made in parallel to balance the *impaired equilibrium* in digestion and metabolism and immune system on the one hand and the psychological familial sphere on the other. Here the general treatment of allergic diseases set out in ▸Chap. 6.3 *is of vital importance.* Anyone who fails to observe this step will experience many more setbacks or dislocation of the disease in the medium term. But the question as to the *cause which triggered the disease* also becomes very important here. *Constitutionally* the focus is on the *individuality* of the child and the structure of the components of its being. Here the main task in asthma is above all to integrate the soul entity in such a way that the *I-organization* itself can restore the equilibrium with the life processes. Constitutional treatment should follow *after* acute and interval treatment. It can then take place on the basis of a more comprehensive knowledge, with less haste and after the interval treatment it has a deeper and more sustained effect.

6.5.5.3 Conventional and anthroposophic-homoeopathic treatment

Many children are already treated in accordance with the current step-by-step plan of mainstream medicine when they come to surgery for the first time. Allopathic treatment in many *acute situations* of bronchial asthma is necessary and helpful. But we can meanwhile consider it to be proven that the inhalation steroid treatment does not have any preventive effect in early childhood regarding the development of chronic asthma and does not have a healing effect at any age which is certain to stop the "remodelling" of the airways [Guibert et al. 2006, Martinez 2006, Murray et al. 2006, Bisgaard 2006]. There is no dispute about the suppressive effectiveness of steroids, particularly in allergic asthma, and their preventive value with respect to asthma exacerbations. As a result *mortality due to bronchial asthma in childhood has been decisively reduced.* The central argument with regard to fine-tuning treatment in bronchial asthma is thus not the healing effect but

- enabling normal daily activity and a better quality of life,
- the reduction of stressful bronchial hyperresponsiveness, the normalization of pulmonary function and, above all, the far-reaching reduction of mortality from asthma [Berdel 2010, 9]

It is true that the quoted guidelines also strive "to avoid of the progredience of the disease", but this goal in particular has not so far been underpinned by clinical evidence.

If we analyse the allopathic, fine-tuning asthma treatment, the substances used reveal a *one-sided* quality which directly correlates with the human awakening process: adrenaline and cortisol form central hormones in the human awakening process. Here the former has an immediate effect whereas the latter by comparison has a "delayed reaction" which puts a sustained end to the anabolic night metabolism and transforms it into the catabolic day metabolism which is necessary for the conscious activity of human beings. When experienced pulmonologists say: "Never stimulate a receptor permanently without good cause," they are indicating that health particularly in the cardiopulmonary system is defined by rhythm: "Rhythm bears life" (R. Steiner).

In current allopathic pharmacological procedures, there is an absence of an adequate "night quality" which could stimulate the healthy, i.e. organ-building life and anabolic processes (which probably in reality counter any remodelling) in the same way that they can suppress pathogenic moments (e.g. allergic reactions). One of the strengths of homoeopathic and anthroposophic medicines and anthroposophic therapies such as eurythmy and art therapy is that they can actively strengthen precisely these healing "night processes", the vital coherence, the growth and regeneration processes. In contrast to conventional pharmacotherapies, anthroposophic medicine in particular adopts *rhythmical* procedures in that polar medicinal and non-medicinal treatment principles are applied primarily in a "*morning-evening rhythm*" (whereby the mid-afternoon has a morning quality, the siesta after lunch an evening quality). The authors are very much in agreement with the guideline of the Arbeitsgemeinschaft Anthroposophische Pulmunologie that inhalation correlates with the quality of consciousness, of awakening, and exhalation with the quality of trust [AAP 2010, 57]. In this sense homoeopathy and anthroposophic medicine can today effectively supplement the treatment of bronchial asthma and thereby strengthen the envelope of trust, of security for the affected children.

During the *interval treatment*, the attempt should be made to reduce the anti-inflammatory and bronchodilatory treatment, particularly steroids and potentially long acting beta-agonists, followed, as necessary, by treatment with Montelukast (Singulair®). But that does not always succeed until the constitutional treatment phase has been reached. Disodium cromoglycate [Ecker 2009] and, as required, beta-agonists will frequently be necessary for a longer period of time. The goal of the *constitutional* treatment is to reduce the need for allopathic medicines initially to occasional use ("crisis intervention") and finally to make them unnecessary. But the child will require a readily available, allopathic "intervention backup" for many years, which the parents and, above all, the young person should be precisely instructed how to use. In the fatalities from asthma in childhood today ("currently 1–3 per 10,000 asthma patients and year (!)" [Hansen, Schuster and Reinhardt 2005, 377]), the non-availability but also the wrong use of such emergency medication (particularly beta-sympathomimetics) plays an important role – alongside the general tendency to underestimate this disease. The basic way that *homoeopathic and anthroposophic* medicines work is not intended to replace or suppress (patho) physiological processes but to *stimulate, control and develop own, in this case rhythmical abilities* in the child's organism. The child's own activity is addressed even more strongly by eurythmy therapy (see below) and art therapies (the long-term result above all improves). But also a change in lifestyle (e. g. through dietetics in a wide sense) can stimulate and harmonize the own activity of the child if carried out in the right way.

6.5.5.4 Fears and expectations – asthma "training"

> These treatment goals can only be achieved through the combination of medicinal and non-medicinal measures.
>
> Leitlinie Asthma bronchiale im Kindes- und Jugendalter [2010]

The paediatric focus will always be on the examination and treatment of the child. But the side of the parents, family (possibly including the grandparents) requires its own perception and guidance. The parents need to be supported during the acute phase, especially in relation to the anxiety which is associated with this disease. Precise instructions regarding treatment, personal availability and security are key factors in this respect. During the interval treatment, the time is ripe for a consultation with the parents without the child. This serves initially for a direct acknowledgement of the parents and enables them to express themselves emotionally. Crucial things regarding the course taken by the treatment can happen here without it being possible to say in advance what that might be. Ultimately it is about the parents regaining their *trust*: in the treatment, in their child, in the child's future and in themselves. A detailed medical history, revealing and discussing conflicts, reorientation in the way the child is brought up and conflicts in the family form the content of such conversations.

Alongside the *anxieties, the expectations* of the parents are particularly important. To begin with, they relate to the disease itself: the treatment of bronchial asthma takes *years;* two to four years of joint work are mostly a realistic period. This should be clearly stated at an early stage. It will be noted in general that there is a great *weight of expectations* in families with children suffering from asthma: the parents with regard to themselves – possibly linked with guilt – the parents with regard to the child (all the greater the fewer children there are in the family), finally with regard to the doctor ("getting to grips" with the illness). Anxieties and the weight of expectations can block the child in its development like Scylla and Charybdis – a development which can sometimes seem like an Odyssey.

Significant help in treatment is offered by the possibility of *asthma training* in small groups as is generally offered today and is part of established treatment. The perspectives set out in this book can be integrated into it, something which B. Ulrich (Saarbrücken) has long practiced successfully. It has been shown that trained patients ultimately use fewer allopathic medicines to achieve asthma control (from a given starting point) but do so earlier and more adequately while requiring ambulances and emergency doctors significantly less. Although the pole of consciousness, daytime activity and control determines the conventional treatment approach in a one-sided way, it is nevertheless vital as one moment of asthma treatment. As ultimately paediatric asthma patients cannot be medically guided without at least themselves or through their parents having been told about the possibilities of asthma control by conventional treatment possibilities, and having learnt to use them as necessary, such training through the doctor or professional in an asthma training is of fundamental importance.

The work in the group enables many of the participants to take a first step out of the constriction of their own experiences, anxieties and expectations and to come to a learning stance which enables a return to health. But in carrying out the training, it is also important to see that *the quality of the doctor-parent-patient relationship plays a crucial role in asthma treatment* (and not just control-oriented "management"). If control always means consciousness, but also distrust (and bronchial asthma as a disease evokes this), parents and patients can experience what support means in a trusting relationship with the doctor and how this quality is different from mere emotional attention – which in asthma is often characterized by anxiety and expectations. *Support means reliable availability and competence in managing crisis situations, but setting clear boundaries also enables anxieties to be overcome and trust to be gained.* The child requires support which takes him or her as he or she is and not as he or she should be. That can be communicated in the training. If we consider how often in the medical history of children with bronchial asthma the trust of all family members to one another has been shaken, then the significance of reliable support from the attending doctor for the whole family becomes clear. Asthma training can significantly strengthen such support in that it communicates clear information, strengthens own competence and thereby makes anxieties recede. On the other hand it also becomes possible in some cases that hidden and stressful experiences from the medical history, psychological feelings of ambivalence and conflicts are expressed for the first time and can become accessible to treatment. Seizing these moments in a wakeful, individual and sensitive way can be crucial for the long-term success of the treatment. Words which can heal, conversational work which enables the parents to fulfil their role properly and create an atmosphere of warmth and trust in the family are perhaps the most profoundly effective medicines in the treatment of bronchial asthma.

6.5.6 Treatment

> Three trials reached identical conclusions: clinical and functional outcomes after 2–4 years of therapy did not differ in children treated with inhaled corticosteroids or placebo.
> F. D. Martinez [2006]

6.5.6.1 Overview

The intensive international collaboration of the authors with experienced paediatric colleagues and paediatric pulmonologists as well as their own practice has produced a further deepening in understanding and handling of complementary medical as well as anthroposophic-homoeopathic medicines and therapeutic possibilities for bronchial asthma. The sequence of the following presentation is derived from that.

The management of acute asthma crises is in crisis today in the face of the allopathic treatment possibilities, and the fine-tuning of the patient is more rarely the starting point for his or her treatment. This allows a greater overview at the start of the treatment but on the other hand presents the doctor with greater challenges from the outset. The phenomenological impression of the crisis is often missing, truly indicative symptoms come to appearance less frequently and are concealed by a running step-by-step plan for the asthma. On the other hand a constitutional orientation of the treatment has become very much more important because it is not so much the acute moment but sustained therapeutic and curative success which today justifies the cost of extended asthma treatment.

Prognostically and therapeutically we distinguish the infection asthma of the small child from the asthma of a child with proven allergies, particularly frequently inhaled allergens, and the child with exercise-induced asthma: if a five-year-old child displays

- no exercise-induced and allergic asthma, then according to a current British study the probability is almost 90 % that he or she will not display any asthma 6–11 years later,
- but if at the age of five he or she suffers both from exercise-induced and allergic asthma, the probability in contrast rises to more than 50 %,
- if he or she display only exercise-induced or allergic asthma, the probability lies at just under 20 %. [Frank 2008]

That shows clearly that the treatment of the mostly well-fed "happy wheezers" in early childhood suffering from infection-related bronchitis can be undertaken in a therapeutically relaxed way and that steroids are not really necessary in this group as a rule and bring no real benefit if we ignore the sometimes annoying irritation of the throat. *It is very practice-relevant to be medically clear that this large patient group can largely be sufficiently and sustainably treated with anthroposophic-homoeopathic medicines.*

The authors see very good medium and long-term results in children with *exercise-induced asthma.* The following treatment concept works reliably in the majority of cases over the period of one to two years. In acute cases, trained handling of exertion (warming up phase, use of short-term beta-sympathomimetics, etc.) is required at the start of treatment particularly when it is cold and wet outside.

Allergic asthma incl. pollinosis asthma and mixed forms present greater therapeutic difficulties above all at school age, during puberty and in adolescence. The use of inhaling steroids must constantly be rechecked and managed here, and therefore asthma training is particularly important for these patients. The goal of the step-by-step plan to prevent escalating crises through the corresponding fine-tuned treatment is evident. In this connection, but with reference to all forms of asthma in middle to higher school age, we refer to the subject of "under reporting" by the patient: only the correct *diagnosis of pulmonary function* with regular checkups will reveal the extent of the asthma; a considerable percentage of girls in puberty, in particular, display restrictions in pulmonary function which are not reported to anyone and can remain hidden for a long time through a quiet restriction of their own activity. Limbs and lungs develop in parallel in evolution and restrictions of everyday physical activity should not be accepted (however, sport which takes place under the training of performance-fixated adults does not have a healing effect). Also important in this respect is the question of the *nutritional state*, as the lungs as an organ are particularly dependent on it (malnutrition and chronic pulmonary diseases occur globally in parallel; illnesses such as cystic fibrosis and others also show the therapeutic relevance of sufficient food). Being overweight in turn elevates the incidence of asthma, is associated with less exercise and increased television consumption which both have been shown to worsen the asthma prognosis. A tested setting is therapeutically necessary here in childhood [cf. e. g. Streber 2010]

External applications (asthma massage, footbath, chest wrap, rhythmical Einreibung, oil dispersion bath) are vital in the acute treatment of bronchial asthma and sometimes also work where even schemes based on a step-by-step plan do not produce a sufficient response. But they also work constitutionally above all through their action on the warmth organization.

Medicinally *potentized metals* occupy a central position in asthma treatment in anthroposophic medicine. Their effectiveness covers all levels of the patient and all stages of the disease:

- Metals are effective in the acute situation, have a wide indication and can, given over the long term, produce a particularly deep-seated constitutional effect.
- They can be used orally, by inhalation, parenterally and externally.

Antimony, iron, copper and lead represent the most important potentized metals in asthma treatment. Levico water occupies a special position.

Potentized organ preparations and animal medicines are of great therapeutic importance in asthma in particular, also as part of composite medicines. Their strength is that they are often *rapidly* effective, that they support the *life organization* and thus also affect and support the medium and long-term after-maturation of organ functions.

Herbal potentized medicines have a direct effect on the activity of the astral body, the soul organization, which is of crucial importance in bronchial asthma. They can have a formative strengthening effect in their body-related activity with regard to the vital anabolic processes (e. g. Citrus), and they can have a relaxing effect on a spasmodic tendency, anxiety, the need to cough and nausea (e.g. Nicotiana tabacum). Lastly, they can effectively support regeneration and stability in the face of infections (e. g. Prunus).

Mineral medicines have a particularly profound effect constitutionally on the activity of the *I-organization* but as a rule require a longer period for their effectiveness.

Eurythmy therapy and (anthroposophical) speech therapy are of central importance for the sustained healing of asthma in childhood; but in both forms of therapy techniques for acute treatment can also be learned.

6.5.6.2 External treatments

Asthma massage

When there is acute shortage of breath, to deepen calm inhalation and release spasms which prevent exhalation, asthma massage is universally applicable which should be mastered by the doctor and the carer of the patient. It should be carried out by and can be learned from a correspondingly trained nursing specialist:

"Both hand start with the massage in parallel next to one another on the erector spinae muscles (M.erector spinae)...[place the hands on the back at the height of the seventh cervical vertebra] going down as far as the lower third of the thoracic spine. Thereafter they divide and follow, rising and falling once more, the course of the [lower] ribs as far as into the flanks [where they are deliberately and gently lifted, communicating space].

At the start of an asthma attack, the first strokes should be adapted to the respiratory rhythm of the patient in order to "collect" him or her at the point where they are. After a few strokes the attempt can be made to gradually reduce the speed together with the patient." [Fingado 2002, 121]

This simple initial measure can guide the clenched astral body (rigid, overinflated thorax, hunched shoulders, anxiety) back deep into the body and in the second part of the movement enable it to experience exhalation, release from behind, laterally and below: a deep experience which removes anxiety! The massage occurs essentially over the kidney region and affects the harmonization of the soul entity's activity in this organ area, with which spasms and agitation, waking consciousness and anxiety are closely connected. An experience of support can be felt.

It is just as important to activate the *warmth organization* of the child, on which the inner guidance of the activity of the astral body is dependent.

- An effective method both in an acute attack and as long-term therapy and preventively is the
- **Footbath** (also hip bath for the small child), at a temperature of 37–38 °C, if possible in suitably high 10 l bucket or similar,
  - either rising to 40 °C over approx. 15 min.
  - more effective with the addition of a handful/3 × 15 ml *("black"[1]) mustard powder* (with a constant temperature), until the skin starts to burn slightly and a line becomes clearly visible between the reddish skin in the bath and the other skin (then briefly shower off the mustard and massage in a warming and calming oil, e.g. lavender oil 10 %. The child must be kept warm during the application (e.g. when sitting on the edge of the bath), particularly kidneys/bottom/thighs must be well covered).
- In this way the higher components of the human being – the soul entity and the I active in the warmth – are addressed elementally by the metabolic pole. That allows the I to take control of the activity in the metabolic pole, thus having a relaxing effect, as well as allowing the inflammatory and hyperergic processes in the nervous and sensory pole to dissipate. The effect can be particularly sustained if the following ointment is thinly massaged into the feet and calves:
- **Cuprum met.praep. 0.4 % Salbe** Weleda or **Kupfersalbe rot** Wala

1 Mustard powder is yellowish, but milled from black mustard.

A relaxing effect both in acute situations and long-term treatment is achieved with *massaging copper ointment into the kidneys*. A profoundly healing effect can be achieved in children with bronchial asthma, particularly with a neurasthenic constitution, by a regular rhythmical Einreibung of the kidney area through a trained specialist once or twice a week.

Chest wraps (for precise instructions cf. Lange [2005], Goebel/Glöckler [2008]]) assume a bit more instruction, material and, in the dyspnoeic child, also experience, but are very effective – the external measures are mostly underestimated by doctors! Here acids have a particularly direct effect on the activity of the astral entity, while warming applications directly address the I-organization. Chest wraps are a direct part of treatment particularly in infants as well as small and kindergarten children with obstructive bronchitis and infection asthma; they replace considerable parts of normal standard treatments, give parents and children security, promote sleep and reduce bronchial swelling and coughing. Most parents are happy to apply this wrap after brief familiarization and a direct experience of the effect on their children.

The following have a specific effect on asthma

- **Retterspitz wrap** diluted 1:10 at body temperature (with water or camomile tea)

It has a relaxing effect on *dry asthma*, hard coughing, reduces coughing.

- **Quark wraps** (body temperature, warm low-fat quark on wrap in oven (100 °C) for 3–4 min., check temperature with back of hand, for wrap technique cf. Goebel and Glöckler [2005, 671], must be wrapped in such a way that no air penetrates under the wrap and the outer cloth of the wrap, e. g. a scarf, must be able to absorb much humidity)

are effective in *wet, inflammatory asthma and slimy-obstructive bronchitis*, help to reduce the swelling of the oedema of the mucous membrane and have a calming effect on mucous secretion; afterwards the children often find it possible to get to sleep, whereby the wrap (for a period of at least 1 hour) can also be left on for longer (possibly the whole night).

- **Lemon chest wraps**

have a milder, nonspecific effect both on coughing and mucous congestion and are also indicated where quark is not tolerated.

- **Warm lavender oil wraps** (and rhythmical Einreibungen)

with 10 % lavender oil (infants 2–5 %) primarily have a relaxing and calming effect as well as promoting sleep (mainly with *dry asthma, dry-obstructive bronchitis, bronchial hyperreactivity syndrome*).

An important aspect in obstructive bronchitis and bronchial asthma (up to and including serious asthma attacks! is the *intake of fluids* [cf. Berdel 2010, 27]. If the infant, small child or pre-school child is not drinking well, there is circulatory hypotonia and shortage of breath, an *enema at body temperature* (▸Chap. 5.1.1.4) is a great help: mucolysis, circulatory support, relief through emptying the bowels, reduction of nausea are only a few of the key effects of this measure. At school age a drip can offer crucial help and security during an asthma attack through which anthroposophic medicines (cf. below Cuprum aceticum comp., ▸Chap. 6.5.6.3.3) can also be administered as necessary. The author will never forget the nine-year-old boy with a serious asthma attack who after the failure of all conventional and complementary medicines and with critical oxygen saturation of 84 % pointed to the hanging infusion bag and forced out the words: “That helps!” while the saturation rose by the minute.

A relaxing measure which loosens the muscles (particularly of the back and the intercostal muscles) and has a warming effect is *rhythmical massage therapy* [Kummer 1990, Börner 1989], developed by Dr I. Wegman and Dr M. Hauschka, and rhythmical Einreibungen [Fingado 2002], warming, organ-specific treatments which have been developed in anthroposophical nursing. These therapies make it possible to give the child an "envelope" in the sense of Victor v. Weizsäcker and thereby to strengthen the trust pole, the "nightly" anabolic and growth processes. These therapies are suitable in early stages of the course of treatment as a treatment of the rhythmical system.

6.5.6.3 Treatment with metals

6.5.6.3.1 Antimony

If the obstruction of the airways

- is caused by (e. g. infection-related) *swelling of the mucous membrane* and mucous congestion of the airways, if the lungs threaten to be become "gut-like",
- with simultaneous weaknesses of the circulation, problems coughing up mucus and low tone,
- the formative differentiating toning activity of the astral body is low (physiologically in infancy, later acute or constitutionally),
- the bronchial obstruction worsens when it is cold and/or there is an infection,
- there is weak digestion,

potentized antimony compounds acquire a central position in any treatment.

On the basis of the above characteristics, a very rapidly acting medicine in *acute* obstructive bronchitis in infancy and early childhood, in RSV bronchiolitis and infection asthma at pre-school age is

- **Stibium arsenicosum[1] D6 trit., D8 dil., D8/15 amp.** Weleda
  - D8 acute 0.5–0.7 ml s.c. between the shoulder blades;
  - continuously 1 saltsp. 5 x/d D6 (above all, if at the same time there is a tendency for diarrhoea) or 5 × 3–5 gtt daily or 0.2–0.3 ml of the amp. per os D8

The medicine contains the most strongly oxidized stages of antimony (antimony pentoxide, Sb_2O_5)[2] and arsenic (arsenic trioxide, As_2O_3). The starting substances can be described as "metal ash" of antimony and arsenic (W. Engel) and as such have a particular relationship with the lungs. The medicine stimulates the formative swelling-reducing forces of the organism in the sphere of the airways and at the same time tones the circulation, acutely most effective as an injection between the shoulder blades (▶Chap. 5.1.5, case history; [Vademecum 2010, 770 incl. Leitgedanke]. In low potencies (D6–8) it is effective for debilitating diarrhoea and is particularly indicated if obstructive bronchitis and a tendency for diarrhoea exist simultaneously.

---

1 = Antimonium arsenicosum (various manufacturers)

2 *We encounter antimony* in nature as a sulphurous compound in the form of the radiating "stibnite" (antimonite, Sb_2S_3), from which through melting and renewed solidification – "liquation" – the even more finely radiating "Antimonium crudum" is produced. This shows its relationship with the formative-shaping forces to which Rudolf Steiner and Ita Wegman [1991, 130–132] referred many times. The sulphur compound of antimony is active above all in the metabolic sphere and at the "primary" barriers of intestine and skin, cf. the indications for antimonite). The pharmacist converts antimonite into the oxide form through combustion whereby it precipitates as smoke on cool surfaces in finely formed "flowers of antimony" (Sb_2O_3). In homoeopathic prepara-

Two different antimony oxides are used for treatment:

- In the **maximum oxidized** form (as pentoxide) in *Stibium arsenicosum* loosely mixed with *Arsenicum album* (As_2O_3), also an oxide. In the lower potency Arsenicum album has the effect of engaging the astral entity more strongly in the body; a similar effect is also achieved by Levico water described below in which arsenic is also contained in concentrations corresponding to low potencies together with other trace metals (particularly copper and iron).
- In **weakly oxidized** form as part of *Tartarus stibiatus* (▸Chap. 2.2.2). This medicine *works against the living element becoming too physical* ("Tartarus" corresponds to a concrement formation), particularly in
  - tough solidifying mucous which is only coughed up with difficulty,
  - circulatory adynamia and nausea;
  - respiratory regulation disorders, apneas.

The focus of the indication of Tartarus stibiatus also lies with children with infection asthma and obstructive bronchitis (cf. ▸Chap. 5.1.1.4, Pneumonia).

- **Tartarus stibiatus D6 trit.** Weleda
  1 saltsp. 3–5 x/d. (for e. g. young people with serious disabilities and adults with pulmonary mucous congestion D4 can be even more effective)
- **Pulmo/Tartarus stibiatus II amp.** Wala
  (Tartarus stib. D7/Pulmo D16)
  - acutely 0.5–1.0 ml s.c. or also mixed with Stibium arsenicosum D8 s.c. between the shoulder blades or in thigh;
  - inhalation (e. g. PariBoy®) very well proven with tough mucous congestion and obstruction 1–3 x/d 1:1 mixture with NaCl 0.9 %–3 % [Vademecum 2010, 689]
  - and/or administered per os 0.5 ml 2–3 x/d.

6.5.6.3.2 Iron

Potentized iron represents a central medicine above all in infection and exercise-induced asthma. The *warmth organization and the integrating activity of the I-organization* can be stimulated with particular intensity through its activity. From a salutogenetic aspect, iron is perhaps the most strongly curatively acting metal for bronchial asthma because it supports the maturation of the organism and the connection of the soul entity with the metabolic pole, the digestive tract, and it strengthens the power of the life organization. Iron acts against anxiety. It is particularly effective in exercise-induced asthma. This action of iron reveals the therapeutic quality of potentized iron compounds: exercise-induced asthma is triggered by the cold stimulus (through the mouth) of inhaled air on the bronchia – iron strengthens the warmth organization and tolerance of cold. Exercise-induced asthma paralyzes the child in his or her will impulses, in his or her limb activity – iron strengthens the anchorage of the soul and spiritual individuality in the activity of the limbs (which in turn is strongly warmth generating).

---

tion the *oxygen compounds* of the metal have a *stronger effect on circulating and respiration*. The finely radiating antimonite and the flowers of antimony in their appearance directly reveal their relationship with the formative forces.

Iron strengthens the child and young person in a "typical daytime" way in his or her physical roots and activity: warming through, movement, toning ability are strengthened. It has been shown to be very valuable to apply iron preparations in asthma therapy, particularly in long-term treatment, in the morning and, as necessary, afternoon (15.00–16.00).
A relaxing and releasing therapy particularly with copper preparations (▸Chap. 6.5.6.3.3) should, in contrast, preferably be given at midday and in the evening. A treatment rhythmized in this way potentizes the effectiveness of iron.

Iron in obstructive bronchitis and infection asthma

In children mainly *in the first septennium* with (possibly relapsing) *mucous inflammatory obstructive bronchitis, infection asthma and asthma crises* with (inspiratory and) expiratory rattling and correspondingly wet adventitious sounds during auscultation, the lung threatens to become too gut-like (whereas in the dry-obstructive form it becomes too far removed from its origins, becomes too head-like). It is therefore a *regressive* disorder (the lungs remember that they originate from the (anterior) gut). Here coldness, infections, changes in the weather stand in the foreground *as triggers*; in the *background:* there is an immaturity or weakness or suppression of the warmth organization.

Potentized siliceous iron has a favourable effect with this indication:

- **Nontronit D15 amp.** Weleda
  - acutely s.c. 0.5–0.7 ml injected between the shoulder blades or in the thigh,
  - inhaled 1:1 with NaCl 0.9 % 1–2 x/d or
  - per os 0.5 ml in the morning and afternoon

This medicine is also suitable for former premature babies. It strengthens the immunological power to separate oneself from the environment and makes the susceptibility to infection particularly of the lower airways recede. [cf. Vademecum 2010, 621]

Iron as basic medicine in exercise-induced asthma

Potentized iron is a reliable medicine for *exercise-induced asthma* at kindergarten and school age.

Depending on the constitution, the natural, bluish-green iron (II) phosphate has proved successful as a basic treatment particularly for

- *sensitive*, open, easily irritable children (aged 5–12) with a
- tendency to develop *inflammatory infections of the lower airways*, possibly with fever and sputum,
- tendency for *epistaxis*,
- tendency for school headaches, exhaustion after intellectual exertion,
- *labile circulation*.

- **Vivianit D6(–10) trit.** Weleda
  1 large saltsp. in the morning, (and afternoon) [Vademecum 2010, 833]

If used for a sufficiently long period of time (several months), Vivianit can have a very sustained effect. In this indication Vivianit should be given in alternation with a potentized copper compound (▸Chap. 6.5.6.3.3). Natural copper arsenate is frequently suitable for the constitution described above,

- **Olivenit D(8–)12 dil.** Apotheke an der Weleda
  5–7 gtt 2 x/d in the afternoon and evening,

for the indication of which a clear natural nervousness and strong mother or parent attachment, a tendency to tense up, long coughing fits especially in the second half of the night, anxieties in the evening when going to sleep are typical [Vademecum 2010, 630f.].

For

- restless children of school age (aged 7–14)
- possibly with an allergic tendency (and not so good asthma prognosis)
- hyperactivity, impetuousness or more female varieties of a hysterical emotionality characterized "by the metabolic pole"
- conspicuous use of language (e. g. unclear, hectic, slightly hoarse, stuttering)
- possibly a tendency for inflammation in the pharyngo-laryngo-tracheal sphere

the natural, energy-rich iron sulphate has proved successful in the form of

- **Pyrit D6 trit.** Weleda
  1 large saltsp. 1(–2) x/d in the morning (and afternoon)

Here, too, the alternation with a copper compound or potentized metallic copper is to be recommended, e. g. blue vitriol

- **Cuprum sulfuricum D12 dil.** Apotheke an der Weleda
  5–7 gtt/pillules 1–2 x/d in the afternoon and evening

a copper compound which is suitable for restless, "high-sulphur" (slightly reddish/blond) children with a tendency for asthma and laryngo-tracheal-bronchitic incessant coughing, possibly with stomach and gastroesophageal reflux problems [cf. Seideneder 2008, 4504–4508] and tensions in the family. [Cf. also Vademecum 2010, 382]

A composite medicines that combines iron, sulphur and quartz:

- **Ferrum/Sulphur comp. pillules** Wala
  10 pillules 1–2 x/d in the morning and afternoon

is effective preferably for exercise-induced asthma in children with a

- strong compulsion to move, hyperactivity,
- uncontrolled excessive metabolic processes, e. g. in the form of migraine, or
- blood sugar fluctuations with headaches and a strong desire for sweet things (cf. Sulphur).

Potentized iron mirrored at high temperature and then potentized

- **Ferrum met. praep. D6-8 trit.** Weleda
  1 large saltsp. 1–2 x/d in the morning and afternoon

strengthens the I forces particularly

- at puberty between the ages of nine and 15
- in exercise-induced asthma above all with feminine boys who may have a tendency for corpulence and are closely attached to their mother/have a feminine father
- with a general lability of the rhythmical system, *circulatory lability,*
- weak posture and
- defensive, insecure social behaviour.

Stimulating the gall function is often additionally relevant (▸Chap. 6.3.3.2).

Potentized oyster shell calcium, as a medicine which also has copper characteristics, can be suitable here (at midday and) in the evening, particularly for anxieties and strong sweating on exertion:

- **Calcium carbonicum LM6 dil.** Arcana
  5 gtt 1–2 x/d.

Levico: universal iron preparation for bronchial asthma

A further very suitable medicine for inhalation therapy is made from *Levico strong water. We can see this water as a model for an anthroposophical composite medicine* [Steiner 1999, 228]. Only human intervention (through mining) made it possible for the therapeutically valuable composition, stable in water, of primarily bivalent *iron and sulphuric acid* as well as traces of numerous metals and minerals, including *copper, zinc and arsenic* to be created which comes to the surface in the spring of Vitriolo. Its action as a bath (at the Levico Thermal Bath, Roncegno, Vitriolo/South Tyrol) is strongly toning and very effective for *states of exhaustion.*[1]

Medically and pharmaceutically, Levico water represents a vitalizing iron sulphate solution which through traces of arsenic (we can speak of a natural low potentization through the spring) shows a toning and with copper traces, shows a relaxing, vitalizing aspect. *The connection of the astral body with the metabolism and the limbs, the "inner appetite" of the soul entity is strengthened* through Levico water. The activity of the soul entity in the metabolism, but equally the action of the I-organization in warmth generation and movement, is stimulated through Levico water. "The preparation stimulates the interaction and rhythmical meshing of the soul and spiritual entity with the vital anabolic processes of the organism." [Vademecum 2010, 541 incl. detailed References].

1 Its balancing effect on states of hyperfunction and hypofunction of the thyroid gland is famous. This shows that Levico water exercises a balancing and overall incarnating effect on the astral body, the component of the human being which is of central importance in respiration and thus in connection with thyroid function. The thyroid gland enables embryonic lung development and crucially functionally regulates cellular respiration. The thyroid gland forms a central organ for the respiration to take effect in the metabolism and it is worth noting that the thyroid gland (and the heart) is an organ particularly rich in arsenic (▸Chap. 10.1).

The Levico application as an inhalation in anthroposophic medicine goes back as far as Rudolf Steiner [Werner 1983] and, because of the better technical possibilities, is today an important therapeutic option in acute and above all invigorating interval treatment.

- **Levico D3 amp.** Weleda[1]
  1:1 with NaCl 0.9% inhaled 1–2 x/d (more frequently at the beginning, as necessary) for 4–6 wks

is effective particularly for children
  - with loss of appetite, "weak stomach", possibly gastroesophageal reflux
  - weak warmth generation
  - infection asthma
  - bronchial hyperresponsiveness
  - too weak intervention of the soul and spiritual entity in the digestion, metabolism and movement
- **Levico D1 dil.** Weleda/**"strong" water** (from Roncegno/Trentino)
  5–12 gtt daily in the morning in 2 cl. water over 4–6 wks

has a pronounced strengthening and appetite stimulating effect on children with a profound weakness in the digestive sphere and the anabolic metabolism against the background of a chronic cardiopulmonary disease (bronchial asthma, chronic myocarditis). There are also positive experiences in individual cases of children with chronic *gastroesophageal reflux* and relapsing bronchopulmonary infection/bronchial asthma in s/p oesophageal atresia.
- **Levico comp. pillules/amp.** Wala (contains Prunuseisen D2 and Hypericum D2)
  1 ampoule 1 x/d per os in the morning/7 pillules 2 x/d
  - has a strengthening action through the blackthorn flower and shoot tip extract with ferric oxide (haematite) in
  - an *etheric weaknesses of the respiratory system* (e.g. s/p premature birth, after pneumonia, as part of a growth spurt, for exhaustion at school) particularly between the ages of seven and 12.
  - school children tending towards exhaustion in winter with weak circulation and
  - recurring pulmonary problems
  - frequent low iron levels and light deficiency.

(Most effective as ampoule per os in the morning, also suitable for inhalation.)

6

1 The Apotheke an der Weleda provides a 10 ml ampoule with a sterile filter for multiple dispensing for inhalation purposes

The following is suitable as an *external application*

- **Ferrum met. 0.4 % ointment** Weleda
  massage in a pea-sized quantity between the shoulder blades or into the calves in the morning, alternating with
- **Cuprum/Nicotiana ointment** Wala
  in the evening

This stimulates the incarnation and leading role of the I-organization in the morning and strengthens it in the rhythmical system, and in the evening the separation of the astral body, thus aiming to achieve a relaxing effect. Ferrum has a toning action, strengthens inhalation, copper releases and enables a good transition into sleep. This balance overall positively addresses the *circadian rhythm of the human warmth organization* connected with the I.

6.5.6.3.3 Copper

Potentized copper, copper salts and vegetabilized copper are part of basic anthroposophic-homoeopathic asthma treatment. If iron treatment corresponds to the *weakness* of the "day side" of the I-organization, the development of body temperature and management of the metabolism which can rise up into the lungs and turn them "gut-like", and finally to the weakness in active movement, an opposite quality characterizes the copper indication: the lungs, rib cage and ultimately whole physical body become "head-like", bronchial spasms dam up the air in the rib cage, the cough is dry and racking. The soul entity does not separate from the physical body on going to sleep to make room for the etheric anabolic processes; but during the day it is not sufficiently immersed in the physical body. It therefore cannot now separate from it while the child physically has been unable to assimilate enough soul and spiritual impulses in his or her etheric body during the day. The soul and spiritual individuality remains "on the outside" and does not penetrate the physical body but is placed in a state of tension with it. This is not released during sleep but only exacerbated during the night. The "Queen of the Night" in Mozart's *Magic Flute* represents the soul aspect of this occurrence, a close maternal attachment which at the same time takes on a backward-looking, psychologically one-sided and destructive character and draws the child into emotional abysses which place too many demands on him or her and fill him or her with fear. Potentized copper has a profoundly releasing effect if the deceased are "too close to the child", nightmares are reported by the child or experienced as happening by the parents, and if experiences occur during the night which create a psychological burden [cf. Steiner 2004, 75f., Sommer 2001]. It represents an important medicine for the exhalation process which simultaneously enables the transition into the night. It "brings the cough to light", dissolves anxieties, blockages and spasms. It has increasingly proved successful for the authors in the evening in *low* potentization (D6). It can be indicated for all ages.

Universally effective, also as the "partner" of an iron medication for exercise-induced asthma (▸Chap. 6.5.6.3.2) is the potentized metal

- **Cuprum met. praep. D6–20 trit./D10–30 amp.** Weleda
  1 saltsp 1 × in the evening (–3 x/d), acutely 1 ml D30 i.v.

The most important potentized copper salt is *copper acetate, Cuprum aceticum.* The "Vademecum of Anthroposophic Medicines" describes its indications: Conspicuous is

- the tendency for spasms, the difficulty to relax and let go when breathing out, to relax the tension in the muscles,
- particularly on going to sleep and during the night.
- Spasmodic coughing is a classic symptom which can escalate into a seizure (in whooping cough and bronchial asthma). (…)
- In children there is often a noticeable clinging relationship with the mother and a general tendency for dammed up, aggressive psychological impulses which are somatized." [Vademecum 2010, 365].
- In auscultation a *dry asthma* with hyperdistension, whistling on expiration and dominating *bronchospasm* is highlighted.
- The main period of nocturnal deterioration lies in the second half of the night.
- Psychological causes and stresses play an important role as *triggers* while in the *background* there are early disorders during pregnancy and birth, loss of security and shocks.

- **Cuprum aceticum D4–6 dil.** Weleda
  5 gtt. 3 x/d up to hrly

is a basic medicine per os in the acute situation for dry asthma which worsens during the night/with nightly attacks. If the above criteria also apply to a large extent in the soul entity, higher potencies can also be administered, as can a constitutional treatment of LM6 (5 gtt. 1 x/d in the evening) in the interval. *Prolonged* nightly coughing fits are more effectively treated with Olivenit (see below)

- **Cuprum aceticum comp. amp.** Wala. (contains Cuprum acet. D5, Nicotiana tabacum D9 and Renes D5)
  - acutely 1 ampoule s.c. between the shoulder blades paravertebrally or in the thigh, can as necessary also be repeated 1–2 x/wk (adolescents). Also i.v. and in an acute nocturnal asthma attack by infusion in 250–500 ml NaCl 0.9 % (very effective also for severe attacks).
  - 0.5 ml per os 3–4 x/d and/or
  - 0.5–1.0 ml 1:1 with NaCl 0.9 % inhaled 1–3 x/d

Cuprum aceticum in combination with potentized tobacco, *Nicotiana tabacum*, has a more profound action on the bronchial spasm but also on the neurogenic asthma component with *nausea and vagotonia* and has a strong effect on *deformation of the lungs.* The component organ preparation *Renes* can – like the asthma massage – stimulate and deepen the connection between the astral body and the life organization, thereby also enabling an easier separation. The medicine represents a central anthroposophic medicine for "hypertonicity of the astral body in the rhythmical system". The injection, also in the thigh, can be very effective in acute situations.

In children where there is psychologically prominent

- anxiety, particularly at night, alone,
- suppressed aggression, severe agitation and anxiety
- great pressure of expectations
- prolonged sustained coughing fits
- particularly in the second half of the night
- the natural arsenic compound of copper is even more effective[1]:

- **Olivenit D8–12 dil.** Apotheke an der Weleda/**D6 amp.** Weleda
  acute 1 ampoule s.c./i.v.; 7 gtt. 2–3 x/d, above all administered at midday and in the evening

Olivenit and Cuprum sulfuricum are particularly suitable when given in alternation with iron preparations for exercise-induced asthma (▸Chap. 6.5.6.3.2).

6.5.6.3.4 Lead

Allergically triggered asthma, with predominantly *sensory hypersensitivity* (cf. G. Husemann [1983, 156–164], Geruchssinn und Allergie, incl. an impressive case history) and a simultaneously weak barrier function of nose and lungs (these patients often display *inflammatory allergic symptoms* of the nose in advance of an attack) characterize the indication of this metal.

Here potentized lead is a very effective medicine to distance the soul entity from its direct experience of and being dragged along by the environment and to focus it more strongly on its formative function in the physical body (▸Chap. 6.6). Here the natural sulphur compound of lead, galenite, has shown its therapeutic value. The latter is remarkable in that two such different starting components (amorphous and crystalline respectively) as lead and sulphur together form a strictly cubically shaped mineral: the reinforcement of the formative power in the mineral is shown here in an exemplary manner.

Lead treatment is of the greatest importance in school children and young people. In allergic asthma the lead treatment s.c. or by inhalation is, as a rule, combined by the authors with preparations of lemon and quince, the basic medicines in anthroposophic medicine for allergic rhinitis and asthma (cf. ▸Chap. 6.5.6.4.1 as well as ▸Chap. 6.6)

- **Galenit D10 amp.** Weleda
  - acutely 1 ampoule s.c. between the shoulder blades or in the upper arm.
  - 1 ampoule per os 1 x/d in the morning
  - 1 ampoule 1 x/d as inhalation with NaCl 0.9 % or **Gencydo** 1–3 % Weleda or **Citrus pericarpium** D1 (1 ml each) (▸Chap. 6.5.6.4.1)

The guiding symptom for the application of galenite is the "switch" from allergic rhinitis to allergic asthma (typical in pollinosis) or the simultaneous occurrence of allergic rhinitis and allergic bronchial asthma.

1 Cf. also the case history on whooping cough ▸Chap. 5.3.6.2.3

A lead composite medicine for allergic bronchial asthma is

- **Lobelia comp. Weleda amp./dil.** (contains Plumbum met. D8, Lobelia infl. D6, Quercus D4 and Veronica D4)
  - acutely 1 ampoule 1 x/d inhaled 1:1 with Gencydo® (see below),
  - 10–15 gtt. 3 x/d [Vademecum 2010, 554]

This medicine has an internally vitalizing effect through the plant extracts as well as a "sealing" effect, strengthening the barriers to the outside in the sense of the action of lead.

- **Plumbum D14** 2 parts/**Stannum D14** 1 part **trit.** Weleda
  1 saltsp. 1–2 x over 4–8 weeks

can be particularly recommended as a basic medicine in the combination of pollinosis and food allergies and intolerances.

In vegetabilized form, lead can be used as **Cichorium Plumbo cultum Rh D3 dil.** Weleda (▸Chap. 6.3.3.4.1). It represents a basic medicine for the treatment of allergies above all if the digestion is weak and in sensory hypersensitivity. A guiding symptom for this medicine is, indicatively, a "nasal symptom": *hypersensitivity to smells.*

6.5.6.4 Basic plant-based medicines for treating asthmatic bronchitis

The basic medicinal plants in anthroposophic medicine for allergic asthma and pollinosis are quince and lemon. [Steiner, Wegman 1991, 133f.].

6.5.6.4.1 Citrus and Cydonia: primary medicines for allergic asthma and pollinosis

A specific medicinal plant for allergies is the *quince.* It shows an extreme of fruit development within the Rosaceae: a strongly inferior ovary which is enclosed by swelling stalk tissue as happens in accessory fruit development. The fruit contains so-called stone cells and calcium and is not edible for humans without cooking. The calcium binds the plentiful pectin in the quince fruit. Humans can prepare the quince for consumption by cooking it; it has an astringent and refreshing taste. The substances which are organized by the quince fruit – particularly calcium – have a similar effect on the astral body as for example the administration of oak bark preparations but in a form related to pollinosis and allergic inflammation (fruit process). The loosening of the epithelium and the tendency to mucous membrane swelling is countered, the soul entity concentrated inwards. It can be a valuable experience in this respect to allow the sight of a flower and fruit bearing quince tree to work on us.

There are profound common features and differences between the quince and lemon. Both are at home in a southern sunny climate and require a lot of warmth to ripen. The fruits display a strongly inwardly directed and closed organization. In terms of substance the *quince* has a strong relationship with *calcium* and forms mucilage whereas the *lemon contains traces of silicic acid* and mainly forms acids and essential oils.

This fruit, the lemon, which ripens over the year in four cycles, displays a very remarkable shape *oriented from the outside to the inside.* The leathery yellow shell containing therapeutically important essential oils, forms a *stable barrier* in relation to warm, southern, sunny nature (filled with active metabolic life). The acid of the fruit has an astringent effect on human beings.

The underlying pathological situation of pollinosis – and this can be extended to all allergic inflammations of the airways – is characterized by Rudolf Steiner and Ita Wegman [1977, 134] such that "the etheric body dominates with its forces". This observation, which might appear surprising at first, is however meant relatively: the soul entity, the astral body, is hypersensitive and drawn away to the outside, to the environment and surrounding nature in its allergic reaction because it is not (yet) associated formatively with the vital metabolic processes in its own body in an orderly way. That is why it can be distracted in its activity by metabolic processes in nature (e. g. excretions of the house mite). "The healing process must therefore accommodate the astral body and help it to intervene in the etheric body correctly" [Steiner and Wegman 1977, 134]. It is also significant that all the formative processes in the lemon are associated with *warmth*; extending as far as its substantial content of silicic acid it thereby acts not just on the soul entity but "at the same time effects the support of the I-organization" [Steiner and Wegman 1977, 134] (cf. in this context ▸Chap. 6.6.2).

This describes the intention of a medicine made from quince and lemon (Gencydo®, Citrus/Cydonia) which is suitable as a primary medicine for the treatment of all principally allergic/inflammation-related forms of asthma which are associated with inflammatory swelling and mucous congestion (relative hyperactivity of the etheric body) of the nasal mucosa and the respiratory epithelium in the lower airways. We can always consider this preparation when we think of the action of steroids.
With the prevalence of obesity in childhood, our experience that Gencydo® (lemon and quince) is particularly effective in prominently metabolic adipose patients is relevant.
It has been shown in recent years that the *nasal application* of this medicine (Heuschnupfenspray, Weleda) is particularly effective for all forms of asthma with an inflammatory component: exacerbations become less frequent or stop altogether; the bronchial inflammation slowly recedes. That confirms empirically the importance of nasal breathing and activity in connection with bronchial asthma (cf. ▸Chap. 6.5.3).
A further innovation for cases of pollinosis and allergic asthma which are difficult to influence is a preparation made from lemon peel (Citrus pericarpium). It can have a very positive effect also in strongly neurasthenic patients and barely hurts when applied subcutaneously. As an extract of lemon peel it has a slightly bitter character (cf. bitters and asthma, ▸Chap. 6.5.4).
The name "Gen-cydo" includes gentian, the yellow gentian, a plant with the strongest bitters of all indigenous plants. It was one of the original intentions of anthroposophical allergy treatment to use *bitters* therapeutically (▸Chap. 6.6.2). This intention has received a boost through the discovery of bronchospasmolytically effective bitter receptors in the bronchia; the oral and inhaled application of bitters (e.g. in Gentiana 5 %, Gentiana Magen Inject ampoules) will most likely grow in importance in the coming years.

We summarize the therapeutic indications of these medicines below [cf. Vademecum 2010, 454–457 incl. References, 330–332]:

- **Heuschnupfenspray** Weleda (corresponds to Gencydo 1 %)
  1–2 sprays/nostril 1–5 x/d

represents primary medication for all inflammatory allergic forms of asthma. The action is not acute, including for hay fever (for pollinosis the treatment must be started 6–12 wks before the season with application 1 x/d to achieve a clear effect), but the medicine produces a clearly noticeable continuous stabilization. It does not replace careful nasal care (▸Chap. 5.1.2). Here the following have above all shown themselves to be effective in people with allergies and pollinosis patients

- **Nasenbalsam für Kinder** (nasal balm for children) Wala
  several x/d, particularly with dry nasal mucous membranes
- **Rhinodoron®** Weleda
  to keep the nasal mucous membranes moist and clean, with Aloe vera
- **Emser® Nasendusche (Nasal shower)**
  1 x/d with 1 dosage envelope Emser® Sole and water at body temperature to clean and reduce the swelling of the nasal mucous membranes

The primary medicine for inhaled and subcutaneous (thus always parenteral, directly aimed at the rhythmical system) application of lemon and quince is Gencydo® or Citrus/Cydonia:

- In *allergic bronchial asthma associated with swelling of the mucous membrane* (for *pollinosis* cf. ▸Chap. 6.6) inhalation has been therapeutically proven for more than 30 years) [Belart 1978].
- In *stenosing laryngitis,* too, the so-called pseudocroup, the medicine is suitable because of its swelling-reducing effect.
- An allergy-related *bronchial hyperreactivity syndrome also reacts positively* (cf. also the case study below).

It is an effective treatment for acute allergic asthma and pollinosis and – if used early enough – also has a preventive effect. One or two inhalations per week before the start of the season is sufficient. When pollinosis starts, inhalation should be once or twice a day, supplemented by the use of the nasal spray and, as necessary, the eye drops. The result can be very satisfactory in many cases, not only alleviating the symptoms or getting rid of them altogether, but also including a gradual abatement from year to year. The preventive injection treatment can be even more effective for overweight or plump school-age children and can also give a psychologically important boost. On the other hand, the authors tend to refrain from the injection with neurasthenic and anxious patients suffering from pollinosis and allergic asthma or only infrequently give injections of Citrus pericarpium – with positive success – which cause little pain in the upper arm.

- **Gencydo® 0.1–3 % amp.** Weleda/**Citrus-Cydonia amp.** Wala, (corresponds approx. to a 1 % solution)
  - As inhalation for allergic asthma in children up to age 5 (0.1–)1 % 1:1 with NaCl 0.9 %. From school age 3 % each 1:1 with NaCl 0.9 % or (max. 1 x/d.) **Galenit D10** Weleda (see above) acutely 1–3 x/d, preventively 1–3 x/wk. Supplementally **Heuschnupfenspray** (see above) acutely 2–3 x/d, preventively 1 x/d.
  - As inhalation for *infection asthma* in younger children with inflammatory obstruction and mucous congestion combined with **Stibium arsenicosum D8 amp.** Weleda in metabolically pronounced slightly formless children or **Realgar D30 amp.** Weleda in neurasthenically slim and nervous children. Supplementally and on a continuing basis **Heuschnupfenspray** Weleda 1–2 x/d.
  - Subcutaneously (can burn) especially for pollinosis and pollinosis-triggered asthma in advance of the season in ascending dosage 0.1–3 % from age nine [Vademecum 454] 1–2 x/wk with **Galenit D10 amp.** Weleda. Acutely in the season **Citrus pericarpium D1** is often tolerated better and more effective especially in slim patients.

Lemon without quince extract can be very effectively used as an *extract from the lemon peel* as

- **Citrus pericarpium D1 amp.** Apotheke an der Weleda
  - s.c. (do not inject too flatly) 0.5–1,0 ml, with **Galenit D10 amp.** as necessary. Weleda (see above) 1:1 mixed, in the upper arm (best tolerated) in single doses, max. 3 x/wk.
  - As inhalation 1.0 ml with NaCl 0.9 % or **Galenit D10 amp.** Weleda

The Citrus pericarpium preparation can be obtained individually on prescription from Apotheke an der Weleda in 5 and 10 ml pierceable ampoules with a sterile filter. If properly used, the sterile filter allows the ampoule to be used several times without a problem (store in fridge). It was mainly developed by the pharmacist P. Pedersen [Pedersen 1991]. The preparation is an extract of lemon peel, 10 %, which still has a strong scent but which is well tolerated both as an inhalation and subcutaneously and causes little pain on injection despite the high concentration. "The ampoules are intended for inhalation. Medical experience shows that their use as an s.c. injection often has a quicker and stronger effect." [Vademecum 2010, 332]. There is a rapid onset of effect, it can be judged after 3–4 hrs at the latest.

Case history

by K. R. Kummer: Bronchial hyperreactivity syndrome

The eight-year-old boy has been treated for severe atopic dermatitis, followed by recurring asthmatic episodes, since birth. Significant stabilization was achieved through the long-term oral administration of Amnion GL D30 amp. Wala. Most recently the boy suffered a massive dry cough for a four week period. On presentation, a twice-daily inhalation with 1 ml Citrus pericarpium D1 (Apotheke an der Weleda) was prescribed. Presumably there was an acute exacerbation of a previously diagnosed mould allergy. Two days later the boy was free of the complaint on a sustained basis. No further medicines were administered.

The interval between needed injections is very individual; frequently the occasional injection is sufficient (every 1–2 weeks) or injection treatment is only necessary at the start of the allergy season; in this way otherwise treatment-resistant pollinosis can be treated by the means set out here.

6.5.6.4.2 Nicotiana tabacum

It is well known today that smoking during pregnancy can exercise a profound influence on the pulmonary development of the child in utero [Mutius 1999a, 170], up to and including a measurable restriction of the vital capacity of the lungs in the newborn. The tobacco plant itself lives in the warmth and on the one hand possesses exceptional vitality with great assimilative power [Stübler and Krug 1987, Pflanzl. Arzneistoffe II, 743]; on the other hand it forms nicotine in the roots in parallel to the plant's own protein synthesis from where it transports the nicotine for storage in the leaves. Toxicologically nicotine acts directly on the *warmth organization* (centralizing) and the circulation, on the respiratory centre, the vagus nerve, the adrenal gland and the kidneys. Nicotine very quickly penetrates the skin and mucous membrane of the airways and *is concentrated in the lungs, brain, adrenal gland, kidneys and stomach*. It thus displays a direct relationship with the astral body which "intervenes from above" and is directly linked with waking consciousness; the toxic effect highlights a neurasthenic, spasmodic, warmth centralizing (rousing) state.

What the plant can assimilate (warmth, light), what it can separate within itself and thus also combine: toxin production and accelerated growth are interlaced in humans pathologically in a *deformation of the rhythmical system*. That is the origin of the profoundly destructive action of tobacco as the cardiopulmonary system ultimately makes possible the inner vitalization and ensoulment of the human being. Potentized Nicotiana tabacum is effective in cases in which the soul entity acts in a deforming way on the life organization. "Nicotiana tabacum is used for patients whose etheric forces are weakly configured in relation to the astral intervention" [AAP 2010, 59]. The effectiveness of potentized tobacco for bronchial asthma is easily explained by the familiar toxicology of the plant, including its tonicizing and spasmogenic effect on the vessels and bronchia. The application of Nicotiana is thus close to copper (▸Chap. 6.5.6.3.3). The most important medicine in asthma treatment is **Cuprum aceticum comp.** Wala, as an external application **Cuprum/Nicotiana ungt.** Wala, both of them described there. Nicotiana tabacum has taken a leading place in anthroposophical asthma treatment since the 1930 s. Specific guiding symptoms are:

- slim, stressed, nervous patients with a cool periphery, pale
- spasmodic, dry asthma with a lack of appetite, nausea
- possibly sneezing attacks, rhinorrhoea
- racking cough
- general tendency for spasms, e. g. epigastric colics, dysmenorrhoea

For older children and adolescents and, as applicable, for asthma patients who smoke, the vegetabilized application of copper in tobacco has proved successful:

- **Tabacum Cupro cultum Rh D3 amp./dil.** Weleda
  acutely 1 ampoule s.c., as relevant repeat 1 x/d–1 x/wk, 5–10 gtt. 3 x/d

This medicine is also of considerable importance if there is a concern that a "remodelling" of the bronchia could develop in the sense of a chronic obstructive pulmonary disease [Vademecum 2010, 791]. Its therapeutic use is intended to enable healthy regeneration during the night. "Although this is a low potentization, D3 also has a constitutional effect" [AAP 2010, 60]

A widely indicated, spasmolytic medicine for dry spasmodic coughing, especially from the age of nine, with the above guiding symptoms is

- **Nicotiana comp. pillules/amp.** Wala
  acutely to hrly. 5–7 pillules, 1 ampoule s.c. 1 x/d

As well as Nicotiana, it contains Carbo betulae in higher (D19) and Chamomilla e rad. in lower (D2) potency.

6.5.6.4.3 Prunus spinosa

"On the one hand, blackthorn is subject to strongly catabolic forces, something which is evident in the shoots rapidly dying off to become thorny, the relatively small leaves and the creation of cyanogenic glycosides in the leaves. On the other hand it reveals considerable vitality in the intensive tiller formation, [the expansion full of vitality at the boundaries in nature to form impenetrable thickets], the resistant wood as well as ample nectar secretion which is so important for the insect world in early spring. Blackthorn can thus stimulate the life forces of the etherically weak patient, particularly in the form of the shoot tips and flowers harvested in early spring." That is how it is formulated in the asthma guideline of the Arbeitsgemeinschaft Anthroposophischer Pulmunologen [AAP 2010, 60]. It is indeed the case that blackthorn simultaneously acts

- to vitalize the cardiopulmonary sphere,
- to strengthen the immunological competence and resistance of the organism,
- at a soul level it effects a better, deeper integration of the astral body in the life organization, thus promoting appetite and elevating mood,
- thus it also promotes convalescence after debilitating infections,
- it strengthens the vitality of the rhythmical system if familial circumstances place a stress on the soul entity and weaken the child.

The authors have found the joint product of blackthorn flowers and shoot tips with iron oxide, haematite, (cf. above **Levico comp.** Wala, ▸Chap. 6.5.6.3.2) particularly effective for children with bronchial asthma in the form of

- **Prunuseisen amp.** (= D6)**/pillules**(= D3) Wala
  1 amp./d by inhalation or ½–1 ampoule 1 x/d in the morning per os;
  5–10 pillules 2–3 x/d

This form of etheric support is of particular importance at the age of nine to 12. Rudolf Steiner spoke about the importance of "iron with plant acid" to support lung development at this age [Steiner 2001, 77]. But this metal is also very valuable for very much smaller children for example with bronchopulmonary dysplasia following premature birth, for psychologically burdened children with weak vitality and for many children of school age who are prone to infection and weakened through overintellectualization.

Thus blackthorn is therapeutically related to iron, Nicotiana tabacum to copper and lemon and quince mediate qualities which can also be supported with potentized lead. Gencydo® injections between the shoulder blades, Tabacum injections in the kidney region and injections of Prunus spinosa, Summit., in the neck area, each one once a week, represent the original treatment schedule for bronchial asthma in anthroposophic medicine, also in childhood [Suchantke – well worth reading – 2000]. The authors rarely use them in this way but the medicinal plants contained in them continue to represent the central primary plant medicines for the treatment of asthma.

6.5.6.5 Animal or insect-based medicines for treating asthma

The current debate within homoeopathy has also developed an awareness of the qualitative differences between medicines from the animal, plant and mineral realms (▸Chap. 1.2, e. g. Sankaran's Materia medica). In the potentized organ preparations from healthy mammals which are relatively close to humans (cattle, pigs) and colony-forming (related to the I) insects (bees, ants), anthroposophic medicine has created its own group of animal preparations in which the focus is not necessarily on "survival" (Sankaran) as in Lachesis, but on an action which strongly supports anabolic activity in the etheric body and moderates the intervention of the astral body. They all have the perspective in common that these medicines often act quickly and are therefore important and reliable medicines in acute situations. The spectrum of their action is relatively broad, corresponding to the nature of the etheric body, whose sculpting formative power is of a different kind from the strongly differentiating power of the astral body and individualizing action of the I-organization. That makes the use of potentized organ preparations and preparations from colony-building insects both clear and comparatively simple. Hence the authors devote the following section to them.

6.5.6.5.1 Organ preparations for treating asthmatic bronchitis

We can differentiate between

- Primary *spasmolytically active* organ preparations which anchor the astral body more strongly in the system of the kidneys/adrenal glands (Renes, contained in Cuprum aceticum comp. Wala, Glandulae suprarenales),
- Organ preparations which act on bronchial and parenchymatous (remodelling) *inflammation* (Pulmo; surface-related bronchia),
- Organ preparations which act on the *neurogenic component of inflammation*, often with a particularly *racking cough* (Plexus pulmonalis)
- Embryonic organ preparations which are indicated for early childhood disorders/traumas particularly in the case of atopic patients (Amnion, Funiculus umbilicalis as required).

The specified organ preparations are available either as mono preparations or in the form of composites with metal salts (Tartarus stibiatus as antimony oxide, Vivianit as iron phosphate and Cuprum aceticum as copper acetate) or metals. The therapeutically most important are briefly characterized below in an overview:

6

- **Pulmo/Tartarus II amp.** Wala
  is described above under ▸Chap. 6.5.6.3.1in respect of indication and handling.

It is a particularly broadly effective basic medicine in bronchial asthma with *tough mucous congestion* when the lung threatens to regress into a "gut-like" state. Effective at all ages, as necessary also acutely s.c. between the shoulder blades or in the thigh, acute and subacute as inhalation and per os.

- **Pulmo/Vivianit comp. amp.** Wala
  1 amp./d 1:1 with NaCl 0.9 % or with 1 ampoule **Prunuseisen** Wala

is a very effective medicine *for the prevention of infection asthma*, also for previously damaged lungs (s/p artificial respiration, bronchopulmonary dysplasia, s/p relapsing pneumonia, etc. ▸Chap. 5.1.1). Used together with Prunuseisen, it is particularly effective for underweight, etherically weakened children (▸Chap. 6.5.6.4.3).

- **Cuprum aceticum comp. amp.** Wala
  indication and application described above under ▸Chap. 6.5.6.3.3
- **Glandulae suprarenales Gl D4(–5) amp.** Wala
  0.5–1 ml per os in the evening or together with Cuprum aceticum comp. as inhalation, as necessary also s.c./i.v. (D5)

are the most important organ preparations for *dry spasmodic bronchial asthma*. The addition of Glandulae suprarenales is particularly valuable for

- nightly exacerbating asthma (in the physiological depths of the body's own cortisol formation)
- children with inhaled steroid treatment (ICS), to stimulate the activity of the adrenal gland and be able to excrete steroids as necessary
- children with bronchial asthma in the early hours of the morning

An important organ preparation introduced by M. Sommer to the treatment of asthma [Sommer 1994, Vademecum 2010, 671] is

- **Plexus pulmonalis Gl D15 amp.** Wala
  acutely 0.5–1.0 ml s.c. or per os, also suitable s.c. or per os (administered more frequently at 0.4 ml spread over the day) as mixed injection with **Cuprum aceticum comp. amp.** Wala and **Bronchi Gl D30 amp** Wala. Can be administered 0.5 ml per os 1–2 x/d over a longer period of time.[1]

The most important indications of this medicine are

- a racking, dry cough which "becomes worse through coughing".
- *bronchial hyperreactivity syndrome*
- primarily nightly exacerbating asthma with nausea and agitation (cf. Tabacum, Cuprum aceticum; vagus activity).

Plexus pulmonalis may often be considered as a "second line" medicine if a lot has already been done against coughing and can also be effective where both allopathic and homoeopathic standard preparations have failed.

1 Cf. also the antitussive pharmacological characteristics [Gilani 2008] and the homoeopathic medicinal picture of Hyoscyamus [Vademecum 2010, 496].

- **Bronchi D30 amp.** Wala
  0.5–1.0 ml per os 1–2 x/d or acutely 1 ampoule s.c. between the shoulder blades

may be considered supplementally or alternatively especially if a shallow, dry and unproductive irritating cough during or after an infection does not allow the child to settle down.

It can also be indicated and valuable for *acute swelling* of the mucous membrane (allergy, RSV bronchiolitis).

- **Amnion Gl D12–30 amp.** Wala (▸Chap. 2.3.2.1; ▸Chap. 6.4.3.6.1)

may be considered for the treatment of bronchial asthma if disorders during pregnancy and delivery play a role, particularly if in atopic diathesis *atopic dermatitis and asthma* exacerbate at the same time. It can be helpful after obstructive bronchitis in premature babies (cf. case history in ▸Chap. 2.3.2.1). It can also be of value after oligohydramnios.

6.5.6.5.2 Apis mellifica

The effectiveness of the potentized worker bee, Apis mellifica, is valued in homoeopathy and anthroposophic medicine. H. H. Vogel has repeatedly pointed out that the use of this medicine can be considered in all those situations where the use of *steroids* is also being considered. Apis can help to save on steroids, particularly for:

- inflammatory swelling and dissolution of barriers, inflammatory bronchial asthma,
- lack of separation of the inner warmth organization from the environment,
- physical and psychological tendency for metabolic overreaction, e.g. in the form of *urticaria* at school age, rapid blushing and changing skin colour, *hysterical constitution*,
- possibly with *pasty* bearing (typically: venepuncture is difficult), tendency for obesity.

A detailed guiding principle is contained in the Vademecum of Anthroposophic Medicines, second edition, 2010 [91f.]. It is easy to see that the bee colony as a whole, as the hive, masters and overcomes all of these qualities – not the single bee but the "Bien", the colony, thus represents a model for the relatively too great independence of the etheric body in these patients and an astral body which is still too little incarnated, too strongly dependent on environmental stimuli. The use of social insects thus has an integrating action at several levels of the components which make up the human being and strongly addresses the I, the I-organization: just as the bee colony at a comparatively primitive stage of development of the individual insect can as a whole create a homoiothermic organism, the I-organization also transforms the "cellular state" of the body into a higher whole which is integrated and stimulated by the warmth organization. From this perspective Apis mellifica can be used for a very long period of time and supports the maturation of the child's organism.

- **Apis ex animale Gl D20 amp.** Wala/**Apis mellifica D30 pillules** Weleda
  initially 1 ampoule 1:1 with NaCl 0.9 % 2 x/d and as necessary Salbutamol, then inhale 1 ampoule 1:1 with NaCl 0.9 % in the evening 1 x/d [Vademecum 2010, 93] and/or subsequently 5 pillules in the evening (for girls often together with Pulsatilla D30, 5 pillules over months – proven).

for s/p asthma attack, allergic moderate asthma, in the tapering period of corticosteroids (together with Glandulae suprarenales as necessary).

6

6.5.6.6 Acute treatment

The anthroposophic-homoeopathic treatment possibilities for acute obstructive bronchitis and acute bronchial asthma arise largely from the medicinal possibilities and external applications described. The authors also use them when the patient is being treated allopathically. The possibility of monitoring treatment using *pulsoxymetry*, which in contrast to the pneumonia guideline can also be found in the current asthma guideline for acute attacks [Berdel 2010, 26] and which provides valuable guidance about the degree of seriousness of the attack, should not be forgotten. A valuable contribution can be made with the complementary medical treatment set out here to

- reducing the degree of seriousness of the attack (thus also saving indicated allopathic medicines of the step-by-step plan as the current degree of seriousness under treatment is the crucial factor),
- being able to avoid, as relevant, allopathic dosages or medicines which are not tolerated,
- providing a saltugenetically oriented treatment approach alongside suppressive treatment which is of crucial long-term importance, thus introducing a sustainable interval treatment between acute exacerbations
- directly improving the state of the child and reducing anxieties,
- integrating the parents further in the treatment, particularly through external applications,
- supporting the vitality of the organism and thus also minimizing the risks of allopathic treatment,
- reducing hospitalizations

6.5.6.6.1 Use of medicine compositions for acute treatment

In acute cases it is often necessary to pursue various treatment goals at the same time (mucolysis, spasmolysis, anxiolysis…). *Ampoule mixtures* put together by the doctor at the time (per os, inhaled, i.v. or s.c. if necessary) can be used for this purpose which can be mixed from the medicines listed under ▸Chap. 6.5.6.3 to ▸Chap. 6.5.6.5 and others. But for frequently recurring (typical) treatment situations readers can themselves have a *mixture of homoeopathic dilutions* compounded by the pharmacy for such initial treatment. The authors will set out one suggestion here as an example:

- **Cuprum aceticum D6, Ipecacuanha D6, Stibium arsenicosum D8, Thenardit D6** (= Natrium sulf. naturale) aa ad 50 ml dil. Apotheke an der Weleda, prescription number 5125
  hourly to begin with, 5–10 gtt. 5 x/d on improvement.

It contains the antispasmodic Cuprum aceticum, Stibium arsenicosum for swelling of the mucous membrane and circulatory insufficiency (for both medicines cf. Chap.6.5.6.3) and a medicine which acts strongly on the vagus:

- **Ipecacuanha D6(–12) dil./pillules** DHU/Weleda

made from a strongly bitter tasting alkaloid-containing root extract, the medicine is effective for *nausea, coughing with an urge to gag*; its action is directed more at the metabolism (as is the case with many bitter tasting root extracts). Specifically in low potency it is therefore particularly effective for *wet bronchial asthma* and *mucous congestion* which is difficult to cough up; *deterioration during the night* is very characteristic.

- **Thenardit D6–12 dil.** Weleda (= Natrium sulfuricum)/**Natrium sulfuricum D12** (various manufacturers)

is a medicine which works primarily in the *hepatobiliary sphere* and stimulates excretion there. It is an important medicine especially for childhood bronchial asthma [Blackie 1990, 216f.]. These children do not sufficiently break down the food in the digestion, and have difficulty extracting warmth from fat digestion [Steiner and Wegman 1977, Chap. X, 58ff.]. They are correspondingly susceptible to catarrhal infections, particularly in cold and damp weather, infection asthma, asthma during/after rhinitis/sinusitis.
This mixture is particularly suitable for acute infection asthma in the first seven years. It can be well supplemented by

- **Petasites comp. pillules** Wala
  dissolve 20–30 pillules/d in water, administer in sips, alternatively 7–10 pillules 3 x/d. (err on the side of higher dosage)

The medicine contains butterbur among other things which is distinguished by antispasmodic and mucolytic characteristics, buckhorn which has a positive effect on coughing, among other things, and Abies nigra (black spruce) which produces deep-seated warmth in the lung and stomach region (copper region). It is a universal medicine for infection-related obstructive respiratory diseases in childhood, acting simultaneously to roborate and relax.
In *allergic asthma*, **Lobelia comp.** Weleda dil, and in strongly *stress-related and convulsive dry asthma* **Nicotiana comp.** Wala pillules each represent an available model as finished medicines for a suitable mixture in acute treatment (▸Chap. 6.5.6.3, ▸Chap. 6.5.6.4).

6.5.6.6.2 Other medicines for acute treatment

We can only refer briefly here to a number of important single-substance medicines for acute treatment. Their indication is given especially by the circumstances which have triggered the acute attack. Like all medicines for acute treatment, they can also be important in interval treatment.

If as part of an *asthma attack* in adolescent patients acute *anxiety and panic* are prominent, particularly with a *hysterical markedly metabolic constitution* the administration of

- **Bryophyllum 5 % 10 ml amp./50 % trit.** Weleda
  10 ml i.v., supplementally/alternatively 1 dosage spoon/saltsp. 50 %

can have a rapid calming effect as "anthroposophical valium" without the side effects of (risky) benzodiazepines. "Bryophyllum holds on to the etheric in the metabolic pole" (Rudolf Steiner), it reliably prevents anxiety and feelings of panic from "rising" and at the same time has an antispasmodic effect [Vademecum 2010, 238 incl. Lit.]. Also suitable, particularly for attacks in the evening of at night, is

- **Bryophyllum D5/Conchae D7 10 ml amp.** Weleda
  10 ml i.v. (if not possible, per os)

which has proved effective for states of agitation in the evening/at night with sleep disturbance, also for acute hyperventilation disorders – see also sleep disturbance in atopic dermatitis in acute episodes ▸Chap. 6.4.3.5.2.

If there is a complex of symptoms of *allergic rhinitis, eczema and asthma attacks*, the treatment is deepened, especially with *house mite allergy* by the administration of

- **Kalium arsenicosum D6 dil.** (various manufacturers) (▸Chap. 6.4.3.6.1)
  up to 5 gtt. 5 x/d in combination with
- **Heuschnupfenspray** Weleda
  1–3 x/d 1–2 squirts (▸Chap. 6.5.6.4.1)

as well as inhaling **Apis ex animale D20 amp.** Wala in the evening.

If the asthma *occurs suddenly with heat accumulation in the head and neck region, possibly a fever*, sensitivity to touch (often rejects a wrap), deterioration in the evening and during the first half of the night, if the whole character of the (possibly recurring) asthma attacks is *choleric* (with pent up warmth), if there is a sudden onset, equally a sudden end to the attack, and if the child has a *strong constitution*, is direct in his or her behaviour, possibly fierce (but not resentful), then

- **Belladonna D12 pillules/dil.** Weleda
  up to 5 gtt./5–7 pillules 4 x/d

is indicated as a medicine. Godhart Husemann [1984] has published impressive case histories in this regard.

With regard to external circumstances, travel and *intensive exposure to the sun* could have been "too much" for these children; today Belladonna is indicated and effective especially if the child feels psychologically overwhelmed in a social setting (typically these children here have a tendency to develop a sore throat, possibly tonsillitis).

In comparison to the "sthenic" Belladonna (cf. the powerful way in which the shape of the plant unfolds), another Solanaceae,

- **Dulcamara D6–12 dil./pillules** (various manufacturers)
  dosage as Belladonna,

is indicated in the event of a labile warmth organization which was overwhelmed by rapid *alternation of warmth and sudden cooling*. In bronchial asthma such circumstances occur especially at the end of the summer (September).

In lively soul activity as such, but *weaknesses of the life organization*, particularly weakening through preceding diarrhoea, weak digestion in the region of the small intestine with meteorism, and *start of the asthma attack with the onset of autumn* (October),

- **China D or C12–30 pillules** (various manufacturers)
  7 pillules 2–3 x/d (D12) or 10 pillules (D or C30) dissolved in 50 ml of water, administered in sips distributed over 2–3 days

is a very effective single-substance medicine [Voegeli 1996].

Acute *slights* and *jealousy* can also lead to asthma attacks in children who are so disposed (mostly girls) who display a close dependence (particularly on the mother) on the one hand and a strong tendency to tense up on the other. After the initial administration of Cuprum D30, the following is particularly indicated

- **Ignatia D30 pillules** (various manufacturers)
  10 pillules dissolved in 50 ml water administered in sips over two days.

We further refer to two important single-substance medicines in connection with climate-related deterioration of asthma:

- **Carbo Betulae D12 trit.** Weleda, **Carbo vegetabilis LM12 dil.** (various manufacturers)
  1 saltsp. or 5 gtt. 1–2 x/d

when the weather is *warm and humid and muggy*; often simultaneous meteorism in the child is typical.

When the weather is wet and cold:

- **Thenardit D6–12 dil.** Apotheke an der Weleda or **Natrium sulfuricum D6–12 pillules/ LM6 dil.** (various manufacturers.)
  5–7 gtt. 3–5 x/d (D6–12), 5 gtt. 1–2 x/d (LM6)

Potentized Natrium sulfuricum stimulates excretory activity, the intervention of the astral body primarily in the hepatobiliary region: the "inner appetite", the intervention of the astral body in this metabolic sphere which is central to the life of the will strengthens the children, makes them less susceptibility to infection, but also less bad tempered. (Cf. ▸Chap. 6.5.6.6.1)

6.5.6.7 Inhalation therapy

Through inhalation the medicine acts *directly on the rhythmical system* (the same applies in a different way to injections). In the acute treatment, allopathic medication (beta2-sympathomimetics, steroids, ipatropium bromide) predominates today. The possibilities of managing the treatment even of severe asthma attacks without an admission to hospital have been significantly extended through these medicines. It is of course necessary to be familiar with their use (including age-appropriate help with the inhaler) and the most recent step-by-step plan for their application; these medicines have their place also in the practice of the authors. On the other hand, the person who extends his or her asthma treatment in accordance with the perspective advocated here, will have the experience that the child's own capacities are unlocked, giving the allopathic medication a different, fundamentally more temporary value. Thus also in the acute treatment of bronchial asthma and obstructive bronchitis the inhalation of natural and potentized medicines can achieve sustaining therapeutic importance (but here in combination with the treatment paths set out above).

Inhalation therapy remains an important branch of treatment for a long time in the course of the disease. In this way allopathic bronchodilatory medicines and steroids can as appropriate be reduced or replaced more quickly. The inhalations with cromoglicic acid preparations can well be inhaled in alternation with the medicines specified here [cf. Ecker 1999]. In a pilot study, Ecker [2009] was able to publish the first clinical evidence of the effectiveness of such a treatment approach.

To that extent the so-called "wet inhalation" occupies a much more prominent place in this treatment approach than in conventional step-by-step plan treatment, in which "dry" inhalation systems predominate. Many of the medicines mentioned below have already been presented in this or other chapters so that their presentation here will briefly summarize once more the important medicines for inhalation.

Medicines for inhalation therapy

The following medicines especially have a profound constitutional effect (▸Chap. 6.4.3.6):

- **Quarz D20 amp.** Weleda/Wala

strengthens the barrier function of the bronchial mucous membrane and counters the chronic inflammation of the airways in that the warming activity of the I-organization is stimulated. It is valuable above all for a *neurasthenic* constitution, for slim, delicately limbed, over-wakeful, intellectually attentive and ambitious children with weak warmth generation.

- **Conchae D30 amp.** Weleda

especially as an inhalation every evening; stimulates exhalation and is particularly suitable for children of a more *rounded, anxiously* restless type who have a tendency to be overweight, quickly start *sweating* on exertion and have a *hysterical constitution.*

The following is suitable for *dry spasmodic asthma* (▸Chap. 6.5.5.1.3), for children under stress, who are slim and have little appetite

- **Cuprum aceticum comp. amp.** Wala (▸Chap. 6.5.6.3.3)

For children with a *weak digestion, weak warmth generation, infection asthma exacerbations* and a tendency for bronchial hyperresponsiveness (▸Chap. 6.5.6.3.2):

- **Levico D3 amp.** Weleda

For children with *recurring infection asthma and (wet) obstructive bronchitis* (▸Chap. 6.5.6.3.2):

- **Nontronit D15 amp.** Weleda and
- **Pulmo/Vivianit comp. amp.** Wala

For children with *thick congested bronchia*, both in spastic and inflammatory bronchial asthma:

- **Pulmo/Tartarus stib. II amp.** Wala

For children with *allergic bronchial asthma, pollinosis* in general (▸Chap. 6.5.6.4.1) as well as all asthma types when the focus is on the reduction in swelling of the mucous membrane and bronchial inflammation:

- **Heuschnupfenspray** Weleda

and for a primarily *hysterical constitutional type*, pasty overweight bearing as relevant:

- **Gencydo® 1–3 % amp.** Weleda

For a primarily *neurasthenic constitution* and for resistance to treatment with Gencydo®:

- **Citrus pericarpium D1 amp.** Apotheke an der Weleda

Gencydo® and Citrus pericarpium can be combined for *pollinosis* with

- **Galenit D10 amp.** Weleda (▸Chap. 6.5.6.3.4)

Also worth considering are:

- **Calcium-Quercus amp.** Wala

supports epithelial regulation and "sealing", complementary to Gencydo®.

- **Apis ex animale Gl D20 amp.** Wala

has a calming effect on eosinophilic inflammation of the bronchia. Very valuable in perennial allergic asthma (e. g. with the aforementioned **Heuschnupfenspray** Weleda).

- **Bronchi Gl D30 amp.** Wala

should be considered especially for *persistent bronchial hyperresponsiveness.*

In pollinosis it is recommended to start inhalation therapy 4–6 weeks before the start of the season.

All these inhalations are undertaken with the usual inhalation device in asthma treatment (e. g. Pari-Boy). Alongside the inhalation of specific medicines, the inhalation of an Emser® Sole or table salt solution has an important, especially relaxing and calming effect.

6.5.6.8 Interval treatment

It is generally known today that after an acute asthma attack there is an elevated susceptibility for another attack with bronchial hyperreactivity and corresponding inflammatory changes for at least four to eight weeks. This accords with the therapeutic experience that in the first instance a *modified continuation of the acute treatment* is necessary in the subsequent interval – and that includes anthroposophically and homoeopathically extended treatment. The return to a purely acutely oriented, correspondingly intensified treatment can become necessary at any time.

Fundamentally the account in ▸Chap. 6.5.6.3 to ▸Chap. 6.5.6.5 makes it possible to embark on a therapeutic path which comprises acute and interval treatment and in many cases can also become constitutionally effective. That applies particularly to metal therapy. To that extent acute, interval and constitutional treatment become one in so far as it is possible to perceive and treat the patient individually under an anthroposophical and homoeopathic approach.

Some aspects however only appear in the interval, in follow-up medical histories which are less determined by the acute situation (original trigger, for example) or cannot be implemented until the calm of the interval treatment (constitutional "retuning" treatment with Quercus and Veronica for example). Such aspects will be dealt with subsequently in this chapter.

6.5.6.8.1 External treatments

Regular evening *footbaths* (preferably with the addition of mustard powder) several times per week (if done daily 3 x/wk with a mustard additive) should be given for six to eight weeks or longer especially if there is

- a deficiency in the development of body temperature,
- infection asthma with a deterioration in the winter six months,
- a general deterioration in the asthma in wet and cold weather and fog.

Carrying out this measure *consistently over the long-term* followed by massaging oil into the legs (Malvenöl Wala) or copper ointment into the soles of the feet and calves (▸Chap. 6.5.6.2) contributes significantly to healing childhood asthma, particularly if the child lives in an unfavourable location (near a river or fenland).

- While chest wraps are no longer necessary after the acute phase, the evening *rhythmcal Einreibung of the back* is particularly to be recommended for neurasthenic asthmatic children using
- **Ol. Lavandulae 10 %** Weleda/Wala

6.5.6.8.2 Continuing medication during treatment pauses

This is determined by the medication during the attack. It has shown itself to be effective to retain those medicines which proved effective when administered internally during the acute phase of the asthma, for the interval (three to six weeks, or longer) with the correspondingly reduced dose (e. g. 1–2 x/d).

A rhythm-giving basic treatment in the relationship between the soul entity and the metabolic sphere (and vice versa) is the treatment suggested by Rudolf Steiner with

- **oak bark** in the morning, best as concentrated tea
  put 1 tablespoon of bark in a large cup of cold water, bring to the boil for 10 min., administer 15 ml.
- **Veronica** in the evening, best as concentrated tea
  pour a large cup of boiling water on 1 tablespoon of leaves, allow to stand for 10 min., then administer 15 ml.

The taste experience is very tart (oak bark) or bitter (Veronica), but the effect is largely dependent on that (cf. the work of M. Knol [1989]). This application can be used especially during the interval treatment to achieve the "retuning" effect; the dose must be set such that it is adequate for the child and his or her age. While initially not so simple use, it is on the other hand an advantage that here the medicine is made by the parents themselves. The treatment makes sense above all if it is evident that the "inner appetite", the interest and joy in eating and the ability to digest are weakened or impaired.
Suitable as an alternative are

- **Quercus D1 dil.** Weleda
  10 gtt. in the morning [Vademecum 2010, 710]
- **Veronica D1 dil.** Weleda
  5 gtt. in the evening [Vademecum 2010, 820]

This therapy can be judged by an improvement of appetite and digestion. U. Meyer [2007] has published a basic article on this treatment and suggested sage tea as an alternative to the tart oak bark tea for "asthmatics who have a weak metabolism, are over-formed and tend to be too cool" [Meyer, l. c.131]. Walnut leaves (and willow bark) offer a middle way between these two polarities.

6.5.6.8.3 Triggers

The search for and treatment of triggers *even if they lie chronologically far in the past,* is very important in the interval. The general principle which applies in this case is that the further the trigger lies in the past, the higher the potency which has to be chosen; LM potencies enable medium-high and mild potentization with a mild but sustained effect.

Shock, fright, panicky anxiety states in the medical history – particularly important here are situations which have triggered such feelings in the child and mother – are important triggers in connection with bronchial asthma, even if the crucial event lies far in the past. We refer to the medicines presented in detail in ▸Chap. 2. We pick (▸Chap. 2.2.3 incl. case history)

- **Aconit D10–30 pillules** Wala

as the most important and effective medicine.

Godhart Husemann [1984] has published an impressive case history on it (bronchial asthma in a 17-year-old girl). The anxiety-triggering situation which caused the shock for mother and child occurred when the girl was 2½ years old.

Case history

The mother was involved at the time as a "singer in a church concert. Her daughter ... was also going to listen. Shortly before the music started, the child began to cry. She called for her mother and ran forwards in that direction. The wife of the clergyman came, picked up the child and carried her into the sacristy under her arm like a parcel. There the child continued to scream. The mother faltered whether she should go to help her daughter or continue to sing. She decided to complete the performance.

Afterwards she found her child in an almost inconsolable state. She was pale, cried and screamed. The mother, too, cried the whole night. ... Her whole body shakes even now when she recalls that event. As she was telling me about it, the tears ran down her face. This is a mentally and physically healthy woman ..." "Grief and worry gnawed at the mother like a chronic poison for about fourteen years. They became an 'organic counter-picture' in her daughter. In both patients the nervous and sensory pole poisoned the metabolic pole. The life forces of the metabolic pole were weakened in the child by a shock at the age of two-and-a-half" [Husemann 1984].

The asthma healed completely after only one acute attack treated by G. Husemann (four-year follow-up after a prior two-year course of the disease – the asthma had started clinically at the age of 15 with unexpectedly sudden attacks, towards the end every three to four weeks). She was treated acutely with Aconit D6, 5 gtt. 4 x/d, and in the interval with Quercus D1, 5 gtt. in the morning, and Veronica D1, 5 gtt. in the evening. The lowness of the potency of Aconit is remarkable here. In the practice of the authors it has shown itself to be the case that if in triggering events which lie far in the past there is an insufficient effect from the lower potencies, the repeated use of higher potencies of the same medicine then did after all produce the desired result (D30-C200).

This case history illustrates a basic characteristic of the pathogenesis of bronchial asthma: the triggering situation is traumatic not just for the child; *it plunged the mother into an acutely insoluble psychological ambivalence* between being a mother and giving the child the necessary envelope and covering on the one hand, and the demands of society on the other. This ambivalence developed into a pathological attachment between mother and child which G. Husemann illustrated in his case history. It is not until later, when there is an additional stress or, as in this case, when the step to maturity and independence should take place in the soul entity, that this pathological attachment turns virulent; the child himself or herself becomes subject to a pathological psychological and physical ambivalence which he or she cannot resolve acutely and which blocks the breathing. It is a moving moment as a doctor when we have the therapeutic experience that there are medicines in such a situation which in a successful individualized choice can resolve the cause of the disease and not just manage the symptoms. But what was the significance of the doctor listening, of the mother for once being able to express what she had carried with her unresolved for fifteen years, and being able to experience that the doctor was seeking a solution to this individually unique biographical event? The catharsis in the dialogue with the doctor is a dimension of medicine which should not be underestimated: for many patients and their parents the doctor is today one of the very few people where such catharsis is possible.

If the doctor notices that concealed, silent grief – grief which the patient mostly cannot come to terms with – and an inability to accept help and consolation are significant factors in the background of the asthma,

- **Natrium muriaticum LM6 dil.** Arcana
  5 gtt. in the morning

should be considered, even if not all the constitutional indicators (▸Chap. 6.4.3.6) can be detected in the child which the homoeopathic medicinal picture describes. Crucial here is the original triggering situation – in contrast to Aconit less an individual shock than sustained psychological isolation or repeated, deep-seated psychological slights (▸Chap. 2.4, incl. Case history).

If the asthma occurs after *suppressive medication* (e.g. antibiotics), potentized sulphur should be considered first:

- **Sulphur D30 pillules** (various manufacturers)
  at the start of therapy 1 × 3–5 pillules

intensified as necessary by follow-up treatment with rising potencies

- **Sulphur). D6, D12 trit.** Weleda, **LM6 dil.** Arcana
  1 × (D12) in the evening or 1 saltsp. 3 x/d (D6); 2–5 gtt. 1 x/d in the morning (LM6)

The same applies to asthma which occurs in atopic dermatitis treated with steroids.

Asthma *following protective vaccination* can be treated with

- potentized autologous blood as developed by Imhäuser (▸Chap. 6.3.3.4)
- the homologous vaccination nosode as an initial single dose (D or C30, 5 pillules),
- the constitutionally most suitable single-substance medicine from the list below (D12–30): **Silicea, Thuja, Calcium carbonicum, Sulphur,**
- supplementary treatment of the spleen (▸Chap. 6.3.3.4).

For consequences of general anaesthetic and toxic medicines the following may be considered:

- **Nux vomica D12–30 pillules** (various manufacturers)
  initially (D30) 1 × 5/d in the evening 1 × 5 pillules.

Preceding longer treatment with corticosteroids can be treated on the one hand with potentized sulphur (revitalization of the life organization active in the chemical metabolic processes) and on the other hand – particularly – with

- **Phosphor LM6 dil.** Arcana
  2–5 gtt./d in the morning

Phosphorus helps the soul and spiritual individuality to intervene itself as far down as into the metabolism (which is imitated by corticosteroids but at the same time weakened in its authenticity); it thus promotes the inflow of *light* and warmth forces from the top downwards into the child's life organization.

We refer for further details to ▸Chap. 6.5.6.5.

There is still too little practical experience with regard to the question as to the degenerative consequential damage that corticosteroid inhalations over many years can cause in the lungs. That applies particularly to fluorinated steroids. We just refer to the following medicines:

- **Formica Gl D12-15 amp.** Wala/Weleda,
- **Quarz D12-30 amp.** Wala/Weleda,
- **Pulmo Gl D8-12 amp.** Wala,
- **Prunuseisen amp.** Wala.

These medicines are indicated for all forms of *pathological premature ageing of the lung parenchyma*, be it as the result of treatment or the consequences of chronic inflammatory pulmonary processes (steroid damage, chronic bronchial asthma, later stages of broncho-pulmonary dysplasia, fibrosing remodelling processes in the lungs).

6.5.6.9 Redressing imbalances – strengthening the centre

Much of the content of importance here has been explained in ▸Chap. 6.3. and ▸Chap. 6.4. But the *emphasis* in asthma lies primarily in the sphere of the *rhythmical organization.* The emphasis shifts accordingly in relation to the treatment for atopic dermatitis.

The first thing is an ordered, regular *daily rhythm.* For school children the *weekly rhythm* is also of importance in which the possibility both of concentration and real relaxation must be created by the school (don't carry learning over into Sunday; real exhalation! – on the other hand sufficient activity at the appropriate time). Here we can recall Rudolf Steiner's [1924] far-sighted remarks about the "methodology of teaching" to which F. Husemann has drawn attention: a teacher who exaggerates the intellectual element which fails to pass over into the pictorial, suppresses the respiratory process of the child, causes the "exhalation to solidify", an "unconscious incubus" which later turns into an "asthmatic state". How is this pictorial element created?

It is created by making abstract intellectual content *vividly accessible* in the soul. The creation of such vividness requires leisure, assumes a limit on the amount of "material" that must be assimilated so that the latter can *come to life in the mind.* In relation to the organs this means becoming active not just with the brain but "understanding" something with the hands; it must not just be seen but grasped with all the senses (particularly also the hearing – cf. the remarks on language). The *rhythmical alternation* of intellectual, *artistic* and physical activity in the course of the day is a fundamental medicine for children with bronchial asthma. An atmosphere infused with genuine warmth – e.g. at meal times, in play together, work in the house and garden, reading and singing in the evening and joint festivals – creates the basis for *strengthening the rhythmical centre in the child.* It is important to start here (and also to structure taking the medical history in this field accordingly). The soul entity must be grasped, guided and reunited with the living element by the I working out of the warmth. If the focus in atopic dermatitis is on the immunological aspect of the warmth organization – organically centred in the functions associated with the spleen – in bronchial asthma it is on the *heart* as the central organ of the human warmth organization in which the living sentience of the soul, the soul entity becomes living process and rhythm. There is no bronchial asthma which is not associated with changes in the activity of the heart.

Advisory activity is the medical focus here. Medicinally, the following have proved successful for asthmatic children to strengthen the centre both in the cardiac and pulmonary sphere:

- **Prunuseisen amp. Wala, (= D6)/pillules (= D3)**
  0.5–1 ml/d per os in the afternoon/5 pillules 1–3 x/d.

For great stress in acute familial or other social conflicts and for depressive tendencies

- **Aurum met. praep. D12 trit.** Weleda
  1 saltsp. 1–2 x/d

and the inhalation of

- **Aqua Maris D3/Prunus spinosa D5 amp.** Weleda
  inhale 1 ampoule 1:1 with NaCl 0.9 % 1 x/d–every second day

are very effective medicines to support the child also in connection with bronchial asthma.

Starting from the centre, all the steps previously set out to relieve the child of asthma triggering causes (▸Chap. 6.2) and to build up a new inner equilibrium (▸Chap. 6.3) should be examined with regard to their importance for the individual patient.

The goal for the doctor is to obtain his or her own *overall picture of the child's life organization* . By this means we can ask ourselves the question which was already raised under the aspect of change of climate and convalescence (▸Chap. 6.4.3.2): how do the qualities of light and warmth in the organism combine with the forces which are connected with the chemistry of the metabolic sphere, with the anabolism and living metabolism of substances? How do the nervous and sensory pole and the metabolic pole coexist in the living, the etheric entity? For all the constitutional differences, a healthy person displays a diurnal rhythm guided by the I: at night the stream flowing from below upwards consisting of the chemical metabolic processes predominates, building up living substance, whereas during the day light and warmth are more strongly internalized (which takes place in a stream flowing from above outside inwardly downwards). The key thing is that these forces combine, that the human life organization receives sufficient impulses from both sides and rhythmically oscillates. This interaction can be seen in the formed shape of the body (form and vital fullness), in going to sleep and waking up, in colour and body warmth. Therapeutically, disorders of this interaction can be treated in many different ways: dietetically, through external applications, through a change in daily rhythm and more. Medicinally there are also treatment possibilities.

The administration of phosphorus in low potentization, possibly supplemented by a corresponding flower extract, can stimulate and strengthen the *action of the light in the* **life organization**, e. g.

- **Phosphor D5/Malva dil.** Weleda; **LM6 dil.** Arcana
  5 gtt. in the morning

This has its correspondence in the management of the treatment by ensuring that there is sufficient physical activity in sunlight (not just a floodlit pitch at night during football training in November).

The administration of sulphur, silver or sulphur-related flowers (e.g. Taraxacum) in the evening can stimulate the substance building regenerative and growth forces, e.g.

- **Argentit D6 trit.** Weleda
  1 saltsp. in the evening [Vademecum 2010, 107]

In general weaknesses of the anabolic and growth forces possibly supplemented by

- **Organum quadruplex amp.** Wala
  1 drinking ampoule 2–3 x/wkly in the evening [Vademecum 2010, 633]

For "light poisoned" children who cannot find rest and into sleep at night, the following is suitable

- **Phosphorus D24/Malva dil.** Weleda
  5 gtt. in the evening.

The health of the lungs is physically greatly dependent on the qualities considered here. In ▸Chap. 5, the connection between the susceptibility to infection of the lungs and a deficiency in light and warmth qualities in the child's life organization was considered (cf. also the corresponding dependence on the climate of this organ). But the lungs react just as sensitively to malnourishment from the metabolic sphere (as can be seen in an exemplary fashion in children with cystic fibrosis). An equilibrium which is important for the treatment of asthma thus concerns the nourishment of the pulmonary organ by the organism as a whole ("inner appetite", cf. ▸Chap. 6.5.6.8.2)

The question about *change of climate and convalescence* can be answered in the wake of these diagnostic and therapeutic considerations. The leading perspectives in the view of the authors were set out above in ▸Chap. 6.4.3.2. The corresponding holiday planning or convalescent stays can be therapeutically very valuable in many forms of asthma if they are of the right duration; particularly in the first septennium, in which the child's own physical organization is completely engaged in building itself up (cf. also the growth of the lungs themselves), they can have a sustained positive effect on the child's organism.

6

6.5.6.10 Eurythmy therapy and art therapy for asthmatic bronchitis sufferers

In the context of strengthening the centre and the rhythmical system, the authors refer to *eurythmy therapy and artistic therapies* as a result of their own impressive and sustained experiences. These are some of the *most curatively effective forms of therapy* in childhood bronchial asthma and are indispensible for many children to avoid or bring to an end suppressive allopathic treatments [cf. Ecker 1999; with case studies]. In the meantime there has been a first, elaborate study, financed by health insurance companies, on the long-term effectiveness of these forms of therapy [Hamre 2004].

In *eurythmy therapy* the exercise is based on a certain sequence of sounds. Certain speech sounds are not spoken by the child but carried out in a way that corresponds to the sound *as a physical movement* [cf. von Laue 2007, 59–64, 79–86]. In the consonants, the sequence of the movements corresponding to the sounds "L" and "M" release tension and blockages in exhalation, and inhalation and exhalation are brought into a more balanced relationship; through the movements corresponding to the vowels "A", "O", "U", the centre of the soul entity is more strongly internalized and stabilized (L-A-O-U-M). The movement corresponding to the consonant "B" can be carried out in such a way that it supports and harmonizes the immersion of the soul entity in the metabolic processes connected with the kidneys which has a beneficial effect on children's hypersensitivity. The children themselves acquire new skills as part of the eurythmy therapy treatment; they learn to exercise a positive effect on their body and the link with the soul entity through their own, consciously guided movements. That promotes their self-confidence and their joy in life. *It has been possible to observe repeatedly that children gain greater independence in general through eurythmy therapy and the previously observed excessive dependence on the mother is therapeutically corrected.*

Therapeutic success can often be judged simply through the number of visits to the doctor – in the reduced dependence on medical intervention, the *effectiveness of eurythmy therapy* (as explained above) on the child's independence is evident. The children's inner ability to maintain or restore an organic equilibrium in their rhythmical system is supported and formed by this therapy in a sustained way.

Of the *artistic therapies*, *painting therapy* releases tension in the soul in bronchial asthma. This applies in particular to forms of asthma in which a psychological trigger, a psychological ambivalence or a neurasthenic constitution are of pathogenic relevance. To that extent painting therapy corresponds to medicinal copper applications – corresponding to the world of Venus, of copper as the most richly coloured of the metals.

The starting point for the therapeutic process lies, as with eurythmy therapy, in the *discussion between doctor and therapist,* in which the diagnostic and therapeutic motifs leading to a prescription are presented in a generally comprehensible language. In the course of the artistic therapy which builds on that, the child experiences a free space of his or her own for the soul entity in which he or she learns to move. In that space her or she can bring his or her inner life to expression in colour, form and arrangement; he or she learns to embark on new experiences of the soul, to create new equilibria and harmonies. The child takes his or her own steps towards healing through artistic activity.

The salutogenetically most effective artistic therapy alongside eurythmy therapy is probably (anthroposophically oriented, holistic) *speech therapy.* Its action can be compared to a greater extent with medicinal iron therapy. Anyone who has learnt to express themselves through language can best assert themselves socially by that means. To the extent that bronchial asthma is connected with inhibited aggression and intelligence, this particularly corresponds to speech therapy. It enables the children to assert themselves socially (aggressive capability) without coarsening their abilities and sensibilities. At the same time "emergency techniques" can be learnt in speech therapy from pursed lips breathing to certain exercises which are also suitable in an attack.

6.5.6.11 Constitutional treatment

The goal of the therapeutic path set out here is to achieve the healing of bronchial asthma; to reintegrate the child into his or her life context. This can only be achieved with patience; to begin with, a period is required in the acute phase of the treatment which has some similarity with periods of fasting, cleansing and reflection which are of importance in the religiously marked course of the year. It is not just a phase of relinquishment in which, for instance, harmful allergens are avoided and a new inner equilibrium is gradually constructed, but it is also a time in which a new attention to and perception of the child and its true needs can arise.

The aim of the constitutional treatment is to enable the child's organism itself to maintain its equilibrium – also in stressful situations – and to restore it after external disorders. It is necessary to be patient in preparing the time when this therapy becomes possible. It

Tab. 6.6 Constitutional treatment with single-substance medicines – an overview.

Neurasthenic constitution	Psychological ambivalence	Hysterical constitution
▪ Arsenicum album ▪ Causticum ▪ Nux vomica ▪ Lycopodium	▪ Natrium muriaticum	▪ Calcium carbonicum ▪ Lachesis ▪ Pulsatilla ▪ Sulphur
Penetration of hysterical and neurasthenic constitutional characteristics		
▪ Tuberculinum ▪ Thuja		

may be possible at the start of treatment, but it may also be necessary first to gain control of the asthma largely within the framework of the conventional step-by-step plan and gradually to dismantle obstacles through acute and interval treatment until the organism is capable again of responding to the impulse of a constitutional treatment. On the other hand it also requires that the doctor is familiar with the individual problems of the child. This also requires time and patience in order to recognize the crucial constitutional lever in the often complex pathogenesis.

▸Chap. 6.4.3.6 sets out the key constitutional medicines for the treatment of atopic dermatitis in a specific order. In bronchial asthma the treatment possibilities set out in ▸Chap. 6.5.6.3, ▸Chap. 6.5.6.4, ▸Chap. 6.5.6.5 (selected metallic and plant medicines and medicines from the animal realm) *at the same time represent key possibilities for a constitutional treatment.* The authors and other paediatric colleagues were able to achieve particularly reliable results in a *rhythmical therapy*, particularly a *rhythm of copper and iron medicines.* Non-medicinal therapeutic methods can also be included in that: thus speech therapy works analogously to an iron medication; in eurythmy therapy very different qualities can take effect. The medication can take account of that. It particularly correlates with bronchial asthma as a disorder of the rhythmical system, that a therapy which is in itself polar, gradually training the ability to achieve a rhythmical balance, should turn out to be particularly sustained. To this extent we refer the reader once more back to the account of the central asthma medicines in ▸Chap. 6.5.6.3, ▸Chap. 6.5.6.4 and ▸Chap. 6.5.6.5.

Below we will now set out additional basic constitutional medicines. Here mineral medicines predominate (cf. e.g. Sankaran "Struktur" 2010]) which have a slower but deeper effect on the activity of the I-organization in relation to the other components of the human being. ▫Tab. 6.6 summarizes the most important single-substance medicines which come into question in the view of the authors.

For childhood asthma

- **Natrium sulfuricum LM6 dil.** Arcana, D12–C200 pillules (various manufacturers)

also represents a sustainably effective medicine (for acute therapy cf. ▸Chap. 6.5.6.6).

Constitutionally *the emphasis in* the indication of Natrium sulfuricum is on *the physical,* what happens in the metabolism, particularly in the hepatobiliary system. The children

6

can display a certain inertia, indolence, a phlegmatic trait; temperamental eruptions come completely out of the sphere of the will. *The soul entity is less differentiated and sensitive*, and rather more dependent on the child's own life processes and climate and season (deterioration also in mood in the autumn and winter). *The activity of the warmth organization is weak* – and it can be seen not infrequently that very strong will activity emanates from parents or siblings in that regard.

As small children, the patients appear uncomplicated; the child "is who he is". In adolescence, in contrast, serious *depressive* situations can arise. The patients appear withdrawn and difficult to approach psychologically; they withdraw socially with single intensive emotional attachments; eating disorders, depression and also suicidal tendencies which should be taken seriously can be discovered on questioning and if a careful medical history is taken; but they are rarely expressed spontaneously.

It is very important for these children that the soul and spiritual individuality should be enabled to engage better with the metabolic sphere, which constitutionally leads a life which is too independent, at the earliest possible time. Alongside an improvement in the clinical symptoms, the observable expression of a positive medicinal effect is that the child opens up psychologically, becomes more perceptive and capable of relationships; he or she develops greater warmth and the susceptibility to infection is significantly reduced.

■ **Lachesis D12–30 dil./pillules** (various manufacturers)
is indicated as a constitutional medicine if the unconscious soul entity of the child associated with the metabolism impulsively drags everything along with it, if a *hysterical aggressive constitutional type* predominates.

Passion, jealousy, particularly of siblings, with openly aggressive characteristics, possessive, expansive behaviour which rejects any control by an authority, dominate the presentation. The child appears to possess "a *precocious attentiveness* with regard to the people around him or her. He or she is able to find the sorest point and strike verbally – like a snake" [Morrison 1995, 390]. Warmth development is excessive and cannot be sufficiently controlled by the child himself or herself. The asthma appears in connection with the overwhelming hysterical dynamic, e. g. after jealousy, intensive emotions (cf. also Hyoscyamus, Stramonium).

It accords with the situation described that these children cannot tolerate *external warmth* (e. g. scarf or shawl, heat of the sun) and generally feel warm. The asthma improves in the open air and cold; it *gets worse when lying down and above all during sleep* (both conditions strengthen the dominance of the metabolic pole, of the metabolic events through the rhythmical system – cf. also dislocation of parts of the blood volume into the thorax when lying down, during sleep, and the reduction in kidney activity during the night). It *improves with the onset of physical excretions* – which are connected with the formative intervention of the soul entity in the dynamic of the metabolism (▸Chap. 6.3.3.3).

A remarkable trait in this connection is the frequent fear of snakes which we encounter in these children; this motif can also appear in nightly nightmares (similar: Lac caninum).

This medicine is made from the potentized venom of the bushmaster, the most venomous viper living in the South American tropical jungle. The venom gland is formed as a metamorphosis of the salivary gland and in Lachesis can swell enormously and significantly determine the outline of the head. The action of the venom of Lachesis is especially *liquidating* in character (while Naja naja, the King cobra, secretes a primarily *paralyzing* venom); when it bites its prey, the snake sets a liquifying digestive process outside its body in motion and can thus unfold its digestive and metabolic potential beyond the limits of its body. On the other hand Lachesis, like all snakes, is *cold blooded* and therefore fundamentally not independent in its own activity but dependent on the warmth conditions of its environment. But it has developed an extremely sensitive organ in this respect, the *pit organ* (between nose and eyes) which can perceive temperature differences of 0.003 °C: "For example, a pit viper" – to which Lachesis belongs – "can detect the heat radiating from the human hand at a distance still of ½ m. The most highly developed venomous snakes have here developed a sense organ for heat for which zoologists have not found any equivalent elsewhere in the animal kingdom" [Husemann 1999; 2009, 53–62]. In the work quoted here, F. Husemann has published a comprehensive account of this venomous snake and the therapeutic use of its potentized venom. The sense to perceive the human I lives in the sense which perceives warmth. The mythological relationship of the snake and the Fall is connected with its delicate warmth sense behind which, however, there lives a dynamic of psychological drives which arises from the metabolism. The sentience and activity of the snake are not guided by an internalized warmth organization; thus the body temperature of another creature becomes a trigger for the snake to launch a destructively possessive activity.

The effect of the potentized medicine can accordingly be recognized in the child's warmth organization, an internalization and calming of his or her soul life and a reduction in his or her excessive metabolic dynamism – which can now be transformed into positive strength of will and engagement.[1]

- **Causticum D12-30-200 pillules** (various manufacturers)
  is indicated in a constitutional *neurasthenic* situation of quite a different type. The child encountered by the doctor seems quiet, restrained, modest and serious. His or her warmth development is reduced; his or her health generally worsens in the winter six months.

Questioning reveals that the child is sensitive and *displays great empathy*: for his or her fellow human beings and often also for nature. He or she suffers greatly from injustice, even if he or she is not affected but for example a sibling or fellow pupil. He or she is a careful and fearful person. Particularly noticeable is his or her *inability to defend himself or herself; his or her* inhibited *aggression.* All of these things are also the symptoms of a close maternal attachment, perhaps to a mother who feels great psychological ambivalences in herself.

Bronchial asthma is very much connected with aggression turned against the child's own body; as part of the healing process, this aggression must be removed from its pathological context and transferred into a meaningful relationship with the environment as a necessary separation.

This inhibited aggression often causes a noticeable *susceptibility to infection* in the affected children (e. g. relapsing otitis media, which can also take a purulent, perforating course; increased susceptibility for serious bacterial infections, e. g. pneumonia and a *neurasthenic* tendency. Physically these children tend to be slim and tall; in the sphere of

1 On the possible metamorphosis of constitutional disharmonies into positive character strengths and characteristics cf. Coulter [1989, 375–431].

the rhythmical system they tend to laryngitis with *hoarseness,* a dry racking persistent cough and also to *stammer*. The excretory activity is also inhibited or delayed: *spastic constipation* on the one hand, *nocturnal enuresis* on the other are part of the constitutionally important symptoms.

At school age a *quiet ambition* and perfectionist behaviour is often revealed in the fields in which the child is interested while in contrast the sense of orientation and order in other partial areas is noticeably lacking.

The impressive feature of these children is their quiet sensitivity, their idealism, their moral *ideal of purity* for which they strive. On the other hand it cannot be overlooked that they partially suppress the side of the soul entity connected with the unconscious, the vital drives; the nervous and sensory pole threatens to get into a state in which it exhausts itself in resisting the vitality rising from below and becomes cornered. Thus externally a somewhat awkwardly insecure gait (and in terms of the medical history a slow gross motor development) is often evident, according with the often uncertain orientation in space. Psychologically these children are characterized especially through *fear of the night, of darkness, of dogs, of something terrible happening. Nightmares* can turn the night into an ordeal.

Case history

An eleven-year-old girl is presented at the surgery because of nocturnal enuresis. She has a gentle, quiet, modest appearance with warm, brown eyes. In response to being asked, the mother reports that the child has woken up screaming in the second half of the night in the last three to four weeks; that is when the bedwetting was noticed.

Only in response to further questions does the girl herself describe the – always recurring – content of her dreams, of which the mother was also unaware until then: she dreams that she is standing in line with other people at the edge of a pit. On being struck from behind, she falls – with the other people standing next to her – into the pit without feeling any pain on landing. Lying in the bottom of the pit, she perceives people at the top who step to the edge of the pit and start to fill it with earth ... – and wakes up.

The child had never until then told her mother about the dream. After the administration of Causticum in D200 the dreams and enuresis disappeared in direct chronological proximity with taking the medicine (several years of follow-up observation). This dream of a child at the end of the twentieth century can give us an inkling how far the prior history of the ailment can extend into the past which children with this constitution suffer.

The bronchial asthma occurs in them above all when they feel overwhelmed by emotional overload and distress from outside or through (suppressed) own feelings. Physical exertion can also trigger asthma.

If Causticum brings about a clear improvement or healing of the asthma, the behaviour of the children as a rule also changes such that they resist encroachments more clearly and also separate themselves off better – also from the parents. It is important in asthmatic children with inhibited aggression to make the parents aware in advance that the children will become more healthy through the treatment but not necessarily "simpler" to bring up. Here the child requires the support of the doctor to begin with so that the people around him or her understand the changes and learn to respond to them properly.

Only individual aspects will be supplemented or repeated with regard to the following constitutional medicines which have already been described.

- **Thuja. e summit. D12–15(–30) pillules** Wala
  (cf. in detail ▶Chap. 6.4.3.6.5)

is indicated in children who are *restless* inwardly and in their compulsion to move, suffer from *lack of self-esteem*, fight for *recognition* e. g. among their siblings or fellow pupils. The *warmth organization is weakly* developed with a tendency for chronic infections particularly in the region of the airways and a pronounced *deterioration in fog, when it is cold and wet.* All barrier functions are affected by this weakness: tendency for rhinitis, *nasal polyps and sinusitis*; bronchial asthma, atopic dermatitis, molluscum contagiosum, warts and finally digestive disorders, morning diarrhoea, disorders of the intestinal symbiosis. These disorders can manifest in different order and several of them at the same time.

Case history

A five-year-old boy is presented for the first time at the surgery. He is thin, lanky and displays clear motor restlessness, has difficulty keeping still. It is not possible to establish more intensive eye contact; the child gives a very insecure psychological impression. The atopic dermatitis is localized particularly in the hinged joints, typical for this age; the skin is dry and scratched. After relapsing bronchitides, the asthma developed under purely allopathic treatment and has existed for some months, the atopic dermatitis for approx. two years; it worsens during infections, when it is cold and wet.

During his early years of life, the parents had great money worries as self-employed people in a newly established small business (which went bankrupt); the mother is a strong woman but also with a choleric and temperamental inclination. The patient's older sister suffered from a stammer in kindergarten and primary school which she later lost.

Therapeutically Thuja was the constitutional medicine which completely healed the atopic dermatitis and bronchial asthma (D12, initially 5 pillules 2 x, then 1 x/d; 18 years of follow-up observation).

- **Tuberculinum Koch C200 pillules** Gudjons
  is a widely effective, constitutional medicine for bronchial asthma.[1]

The children initially display an impaired warmth organization with night sweats, recurring infection of the middle ear, the tonsils and/or the bronchia up to and including pneumonia and urinary tract infections. Their behaviour is restless, provocative – including in the surgery – but it can equally appear attractive and charming; that clearly reveals the lack of integration of the soul entity. They give the impression of being psychologically

1 Bronchial asthma has replaced tuberculosis as chronic inflammatory lung disease in western industrialized states. Tuberculosis continues to be rampant in countries where there is starvation, malnutrition, overcrowding and also, where e. g. women have to veil themselves too much against the sunlight. Both extremes, the materialism and excess of the West as well as the poverty in other parts of the world, create a disposition for chronic disorders of the middle. It is remarkable that the most money in paediatrics is meanwhile spent on children with asthma in the western industrialized countries while most children on earth continue to die in poverty and starvation. Illness is also a social question.

without roots and always require new impressions, need other people, which makes their behaviour appear somewhat obtrusive and hyperactive. The family medical history very often reveals chronic or recurring inflammatory diseases of the lungs, particularly bronchial asthma or tuberculosis. Among foods, milk is particularly badly tolerated; there can also more frequently be an allergy to animal hair (particularly cats).

In these children bronchial asthma is the most frequent and typical chronic inflammatory disease of the barrier organs, but frequently atopic dermatitis and bronchial asthma can also appear in alternation (▸Chap. 6.4.3.6).

Almost all possibilities can be considered as asthma *triggers* ("mixed asthma"); in most cases no single trigger can be determined. Constitutionally hysterical and neurasthenic traits interpenetrate. These children fundamentally have difficulty in *combining light and warmth with the metabolism.* Nervous and sensory pole and metabolic pole do not sufficiently work together in the etheric entity. That accords on the one hand with their susceptibility in the region of the airways and on the other hand with weakness in digestion and anabolic metabolism of these children, but also with their compulsion. A suitable climate is particularly a warm and sunny one (e. g. southern Alps, Canary Isles).

- **Calcium carbonicum LM12 dil./Conchae D12–20 trit.** Weleda
is the most important mineral medicine for the *hysterical constitutional type* in bronchial asthma. (▸Chap. 6.4.3.6.2)

That applies particularly with regard to *recurring obstructive bronchitis* in infants and small children; in kindergarten and school children the *tendency to sweat and catch a cold is apparent; worsening of asthma during physical exertion; tendency for catarrhal infection, particularly when cold and wet.* The further north the children live, the more frequently Calcium carbonicum is required: inhabitants of the Mediterranean region almost never require Calcium carbonicum. Nasal breathing is impaired or completely blocked through excessive metabolic activity in the region of the head (catarrh, swelling of the mucous membrane, adenoidal growths).

Psychologically, the children develop slowly, tend to have many *anxieties,* especially *about showing weakness in front of others* or *being exposed.*

- A further important single-substance medicines for allergies which can also harmonize the relationship between the soul entity and the physical body arising from a *hysterical one-sidedness* is
- **Pulsatilla vulg. D6–30 dil./pillules C200 pillules** (various manufacturers)

The plant itself, Pulsatilla vulgaris, loves limestone; it flowers in the spring, before unfolding its finely formed leaves, with a large violet, nodding, flower which speaks to the soul. The latter has shining yellow stamens inside; in direct sunlight the somewhat bell-shaped interior of the flower also generates passive temperatures which can lie very clearly (by more than 10 °C) above the surroundings. This bloom of the wind flower, as Pulsatilla is also known, sways in the breeze given up to the wind; the plant seeds are distributed through the air and themselves display an abnormal mobility (through turgor changes) (reference by Markus Sommer).

This *emphasis on emotional attraction* with a simultaneous strong dependence on the movement of the wind and tendency to be weighed down (nodding, noticeably large flower), and preference for a sunny, spring climate with fresh air can help one to understand the indication for this medicine:

- gets worse in heat, unventilated rooms, improves in fresh air (these children *are keen to go outside*),
- but *worsening of the overall state in winter*, clear improvement in sunny, airy climate (mood dependent on sunlight),
- *tendency for venous stasis*, the blood sinks: e. g. slightly bluish extremities. These children need physical movement, their own *warmth and circulatory organization is fundamentally labile,*
- general worsening *in the evening* and at night, in enclosed spaces (eczema, asthma),
- digestive difficulties especially with hard to digest fats, while butter is preferred,
- remarkably little thirst.

Psychologically these children are *labile, up one minute, down the next.* In the consultation they sit (like the children who require Conchae) on their mother's lap, can cry violently during the physical examination, trying a timid smile straight afterwards again and looking for sympathy. The soul entity is fundamentally excessively dependent on external factors and on the metabolic organization (for women subsequently the menstrual cycle) whereas the control of the I-organization is weakly anchored. Accordingly all barriers have a tendency to be too open to the environment (here silicic acid can be an important complementary medicine). Pollinosis, bronchial asthma and eczema as well as catarrhal infections particularly of the conjunctiva and upper airways are part of the appearance of these children. The medicine strengthens the control of the I over the soul entity; the blood circulation and warmth organization, utilization of fats and consolidation of the barriers of the organism become accordingly more stable. Pulsatilla is an important constitutional medicine especially if – with the corresponding constitution – the child is burdened with *grief* (mostly family-related).

Sulphur has already been presented multiple times and in detail (▸Chap. 6.4.3.6.2). Apart from its constitutional importance, a single dose (e. g. D30) or intermediate treatment (e. g. LM6) enables other medicines to achieve a much better effect (e. g. Calcium carbonicum Lycopodium, Phosphor, Plumbum).

With regard to the medicines for a *neurasthenic constitution* (▸Chap. 6.4.3.6.1) we can additionally note:

- **Arsenicum album**

is the most important constitutional medicine of them all.

We refer particularly to a *dependence on support* (especially from the mother), the *fear of being alone, the worsening around and after midnight, the frosty* and neurotically ambitious behaviour of the children (often also of the mothers).

As *a herbal medicine* for a *neurasthenic constitution*,

- **Nux vomica LM6–12 dil. Arcana, D6–30 pillules** (various manufacturers)
  3–5 gtt./d in the evening/individual dosage,

like Arsenicum album, displays a primary relationship with the astral body, the activity of the soul entity in the physical body. The indication for this medicine is given especially in situations where the soul entity acts in a one-sidedly catabolic way on the physical body; when the rhythm between activity and rest, eating and breaks between meals, day and night is strongly impaired by an impulsive rush, nervosity and tension. Many things in the world we live in today reinforce this tendency. Nux vomica is also a central medicine for allergic rhinitis and pollinosis (▸Chap. 6.6)

Poisons, food additives which are difficult to break down or only in the "wrong location" and allopathic medicines can have a similarly one-sided catabolic effect on the life organization. Nux vomica is therefore generally an important medicine for allergic diseases; but specific symptoms of the skin do not indicate the choice of this medicine.

The seeds of Strychnos nux-vomica contain strychnine, a poison which acts particularly on the vegetative nervous system, which is very difficult to break down and which can accumulate long-term in body. It produces a disinhibition at the level of the spinal cord with a general convulsive tendency which in severe poisoning can lead to tetanoid convulsions with a clear mind [Lewin 1992, 794ff.].

Important indications for this medicine are:

- pregnancy burdened by *allopathic medicines*,
- the outbreak or worsening of allergic symptoms after anaesthesia (e.g. hernia op in infants).

This medicine supports toxic elimination (▸Chap. 6.3.2) and reduces the irritating effect of involuntary premedication on the child. In terms of the general symptoms of the children the following should be observed:

- early, severe, long-lasting *stomach cramps* in infancy (▸Chap. 4.3.4),
- tendency for spastic constipation,
- impairment of nasal respiration, tendency for catarrh
- hyperalert ambitious children,
- nervous, tendency for choleric short-tempered outbursts, aggressive,
- yet themselves very *sensitive to criticism*, do not forgive, tendency for hypochondria,
- very tense in themselves, performance oriented, in this respect pedantic, precise.

A certain relationship with the picture described under Arsenicum album cannot be overlooked. It is also worth noting that these two medicines are frequently indicated for *pollinosis* (particularly Nux vomica) which is clearly promoted in its manifestation through nervous stress and a sedentary intellectual lifestyle (▸Chap. 6.6). But the constitution of Nux vomica is more vital, aggressive and less distinctive than the one of Arsenicum album. From an organic and functional perspective, hepatobiliary activity tends to be at the centre for Nux vomica, whereas it is the activity of the kidneys and adrenal gland for Arsenicum album.

With regard to cold *sensitivity*, the tendency to develop stomach complaints and a digestive weakness, among other things, it is the medicinal picture of Nux vomica which corresponds to the neurasthenic basic type.

The toxic character of the mother compound is characteristic for Arsenicum album and Nux vomica; in both cases, the hypersensitivity of the airways and obstruction of exhalation in the patient comes from the predominant and *catabolic dynamism of the nervous system.*

Both medicines are also very important with regard to *pollinosis* which occurs in the region in which the respiratory as well as the nervous and sensory system directly meet. On Lycopodium clavatum cf. ▸Chap. 6.4.3.6.1

- **Natrium muriaticum** (▸Chap. 6.4.3.6.3)

is one of the, also constitutionally, most important single-substance medicines for childhood bronchial asthma when there is a dominant *psychological ambivalence, long-acting grief,* dependence on the presence of others with a simultaneous inability to accept help and comfort from them; this particularly in girls (cf. Pulsatilla, see above).

it is noteworthy that these children love the warm season of the year but *avoid direct sunlight* – internally, too, in the life organization the light has difficulty in combining with the vital metabolic processes. Thus *the physical and social maturation of these children is delayed,* they are thin, tense inside, thirsty, often learn to walk relatively late (more rarely also late to speak). On the other hand they are *mostly very musical,* find in music a form of expression for their soul which can also be used therapeutically towards balance.

6.6 Pollinosis

"You see, human beings are initially of a sensory nature. They perceive things around them and then they reflect on them. They need both. They must perceive things so that they can make contact with the world. They must also think, must suppress their perceptions and in doing so develop their autonomy. If we only had perceptions we would be completely caught up in an external outlook."

Rudolf Steiner

In paediatric practice, the budding of pussy willows and the blossoming of hazel bushes and alders is accompanied by the appearance of a group of patients which *historically speaking did not come about until the onset of industrialization: children with pollinosis.* One generation ago such children were usually of school age; today hay fever, as a seasonal allergic disease, emerges with increasing frequency among kindergarten-age children and even younger ones. Of pre-school children, "7 % are currently affected, and in older children prevalence is as high as 19 %"; the incidence of new cases is highest between the ages of 6 and 15 [Bachert und Wahn 1999, 279]. Many of these patients did not suffer from any manifest allergy before and they have no history of atopy (and parents who are afflicted with pollinosis are often the first to manifest atopic diathesis in the family history).

On the part of the doctor as well as the patient, the confrontation with pollinosis is accompanied by peculiar specific feelings. Paediatricians who have experienced the dramatic course of pneumonia in late winter will be inclined to take patients who sneeze and rub their reddened eyes less seriously. They also know that such symptoms will vanish of their own accord at some point, that they need not fear any serious complications – except, perhaps, in cases of allergic bronchial asthma, which 40 % of all patients with pollinosis develop after a 10-year course of disease. Whereas children with high fever evoke the entire earnestness, focus and dedication of the medical profession, in cases of pollinosis one might catch oneself perceiving this disease initially as pesky, bothersome and inconvenient: as something disagreeable!

On the side of patients and their parents, we discover something quite similar: the children who are often healthy and active before the symptoms break out suddenly react to them with "irritation"; many are exhausted and tired, which is a cause of concern for the parents (being also worried about a decline in performance at school). For the patient and his or her environment, the sneezing and eye-rubbing develops a significance similar to that of the scratching which we observe in someone afflicted with atopic dermatitis. In the acute situation the doctor only too often develops a defensive attitude – with the result that empathy is lost, compassion for what it means to have burning and itching eyes, nose and gums, a swollen nose and a head befogged by emotional numbness – while nature is burgeoning and blossoming outside.

Are pollinosis patients really only seasonally ill? Or does a more deeply rooted disease *manifest itself* in hay fever? Should pollen really be regarded as the cause even though pollinosis was practically unknown in Europe 300 years ago and is still rare in pre-industrial societies today? The experience of the authors, like that of many anthroposophic and homoeopathic doctors, reveals that *pollinosis in childhood is an allergic disease which can be healed long-term in many cases.* Such therapeutic success can only be achieved, however, if the aversion towards the disease, often found in patients *and* doctors to begin with, can be overcome and attention can be directed to the underlying *year-round problem of the patient.*

6.6.1 Insight into the illness and relevant organs

The significance of the upper respiratory tract for the body and soul entity was depicted earlier at length (▸Chap. 5.1.2.1). The nose and the sinuses determine the form of the mid-face, lying between the forehead, the neurocranium, on the one hand, and the mouth, as the organ of ingestion, on the other; they belong primarily to the *human rhythmical system* [Lievegoed 1995]. Through this connection the insight arose in recent years that *a rhythmical process orders the physiological functions of the nose and facilitates its entire healthy interplay, the "nose cycle."* It has "a duration of 2 to 8 hours and is often disrupted long-term by diseases of the nasal mucosa. The nose cycle plays a substantial part in functions of the nose, the moistening, warming up, purifying of the breathing air and formation of airways resistance" [Bachert and Wahn 1999, 278]. Within this nose cycle there is an alteration between swelling and reduction in swelling of the mucosa inside the right and left nasal meatus that is mediated by the interplay of nerve regulation, matrix and vascular structures. In this area *health* is thus ascertainable as an *intact rhythmical organization* that integrates and orders the moistening and warming up of the air we breathe, its purification (mucociliary clearance) and its olfactory perception to create a single functional organization.

Every allergic rhinitis leads to a disturbance of the "nose cycle, mucociliary clearance and olfaction" [Bachert and Wahn 1999, 279]. As a rhythmic organization, the nose cycle mediates between the digestive and the immune function of the mucosa (clearance) and the sensory function of the olfactory epithelium. The *perception of things* and the *suppression of what is perceived,* its dissolution and digestion express themselves meaningfully here, and in cases of allergies *both processes are impaired and disturbed.*

Why do children who live in societies with a "western lifestyle" develop hay fever as an oversensitivity reaction to sensory impressions of the nose? Today, hay fever emerges most often at the age when the human sense of smell is at the height of its development (around the ninth year of life). Children who live in industrial societies are exposed to completely different worlds of smells than are those who live in pre-industrial conditions. Natural, intensive, and repetitive olfactory impressions recede. Notions of hygiene, which are strongly oriented towards odourlessness and thus also towards maintaining a distance to nature and the bodily nature of the other person, culturally suppress the natural world of smells (and emotions). Just as centrally heated or air-conditioned rooms and a lack of proper motion weaken the human warmth organization in its development, many children lack the necessary emotional experience of encounters with the world of scents during the first septennium. An insufficient connection with the world via the senses is established: *those who never had the experiences of helping to bring in the hay and playing in the fragrant piles of it as a child are the ones who most often become afflicted with hay fever.* The allergy is rooted in an overly developed *distance to life.*

As an epidemic disease process, pollinosis shows quite clearly that this development has overshot its goal one-sidedly: for olfactory sense impressions, fine concentrations of substances which are contained in the air we breathe, are what evoke a process in the nose which makes it impossible for the patient to perceive odours in an emotional sense, while at the same time being dominated by an excess of digestive and immune processes and a negatively-irritable mood. These are clear consequences of a culturally determined suppression of soul and physical needs, the development and control of which children living in western societies are increasingly unable to learn on their own.

This alienation towards nature that is felt by such children is intensified by smells which do not express the real quality of things (artificial aromas etc.), that are designed to trigger a sense of well-being but which have no experiential value. The mobility provided by bicycles and cars leads to fleeting contact with smells without any intense emotional connection, and without any real perception of what the scent or odour emanates from. Especially in city areas, technically generated fumes perpetually cover up the natural world of scents until human beings gain consciousness of it again in the pathology of pollinosis.

A *lack of adequate sensory impressions* in the first septennium subsequently correlates with a *lack of involvement with nature* in the second septennium. In pre-industrial societies the burgeoning of nature is accompanied by intensive human activity in and vis-a-vis nature. The farmer who cleaned out his stable with a pitchfork, combated weeds on the field with his rake and mowed the flourishing grass with his scythe was hardly ever afflicted with pollinosis. "Interestingly, several European studies have shown quite consistently that children who grow up on a farm are very well protected against becoming afflicted with hay fever, bronchial asthma and allergic sensitization. The risk of developing hay fever, for example, is about half as high for such children as it is for schoolchildren who have grown up in the same village but not on a farm" [Mutius 1999b].

This shows that it is not natural sensory impressions that evoke or explain hypersensitivity, but rather that the latter results from the lack of an inner relationship to nature and most of all from a lack of human activity which engages with nature.

Kindergartens and schools of the type that predominate today aggravate this problem, whereas it would appear that reforms such as Waldorf schools (cf. the previously cited study by Alm and Swartz [1999]) and kindergartens in which the children move around freely outdoors and interact with nature in all weathers contribute to a decrease in the frequency of new cases of allergies. Allergologically speaking, the latter probably constitute an optimum (albeit a somewhat one-sided one in educational terms).

In practice there is a clear historical indication that excessive one-sided strain on the intellectual life, especially through stress at school, parental expectations and the child's own ambitiousness, foster pollinosis in particular. Of all the atopies, pollinosis evidences the clearest connection with excessive or premature development of intellectuality that pushes itself to the fore at the cost of emotional maturation, free play and purposeful physical activity.

Whereas *atopic dermatitis* initially involves *weakness in the area of the digestive, metabolic and immune systems* as well as the immaturity of the barrier organs, in the case of *bronchial asthma, emotional ambivalence* in regard to the patient's relationship to his or her parents and premature loss of emotional security constitute important etiological factors. And in the case of *pollinosis a one-sided emphasis and strain on the intellect* require the attention of the doctor to a particular degree.

6.6.2 From pathology to treatment

In publications and lectures on the anthroposophical extension of medicine, Rudolf Steiner [1994, 42–45] made repeated observations on pollinosis, most extensively on 2 September 1923 in London. He begins his account by drawing attention to the pronounced importance of the nervous and sensory system in early childhood, which reveals itself clearly even in regard to anatomical proportions. Thus "the entire organization of the child" is physiologically subject to "the influence of the outside world – in the widest sense ... – much more so than is the case in later periods of life." A consequence of this, he observes, is the tendency towards exsudative diathesis found in small children; this catarrhal metabolic activity, which in small children takes place physiologically in all mucosa to a certain extent (and in the lymphatic system), is not primarily an expression of inner impulses but rather of natural influences acting on the inside from the outside that evoke a counter-reaction of the digestive and immune system, this being directed from the inside towards the outside.

Physiologically speaking, Rudolf Steiner posits that exsudative diathesis, i. e., a tendency towards catarrhal inflammations, can essentially be overcome if the child develops increasingly intense limb activity in the course of maturation. This occurs in the form of movement in the external world, but it receives its impulse and formation from the inner human being. Thus the underlying organization "also strives towards the inside of the human being, just as the nervous and sensory organization strives outwards" [Steiner 1994, 43]. If a balance between the sensory process on the one hand and the heat-forming metabolic and limb activity on the other is found, the human being is healthy. Using the nose cycle as an example, this is depicted in terms of the balance between the olfactory function and mucociliary clearance.

But if the sensory process in its one-sided effect on the overall organism is not offset "sufficiently by the metabolic process"[1] [Steiner 1994, 44], exsudative diathesis can reappear and persist in transformed form, manifesting itself in a way which "specializes" in certain organ areas. For in cases of pollinosis, which is to say, in all forms of allergic rhinitis, influences of nature evoke an inflammatory secreting counter-reaction at the barriers of the eyes and the upper respiratory tract even though it has other effects than those that evoke catarrh in small children.

Thus an area in the human being exists in pathological form in which the soul and spiritual individuality is not "master in its own house," i. e. does not control processes in the life organization. "[...] the astral body withdraws and tends to refrain from intervening in the etheric and physical body. And the catarrhal symptoms are the consequence of this ... the astral body and the I-organization become hypersensitive ... Thus the healing process must facilitate the astral body and help it to intervene in the etheric body properly" [Steiner and Wegman 1991, 134].

From the perspective of Rudolf Steiner it is a matter of orienting the soul aspect of the child to penetrating its own bodily nature, to direct it initially to this task. Naturally this happens through physical activity, most of all if it occurs by virtue of the person's own emotional impetus and experience.

For medicinal treatment, Rudolf Steiner [1994, 44] recommends "fruits ... which are surrounded by leathery peel." The aspect underlying this recommendation is that in the main "pathogens" of pollinosis (grasses and grains but also birches, hazels, willows) the "fructification process ... looks out into the atmosphere in complete nakedness ... being oriented outwards towards the periphery." In these plants there is an orientation towards the periphery in the sphere of the flower (wind pollination). To put it bluntly, pollinosis can be conceived of as a tendency of the hay fever patient to "flower under the same atmospheric influences under which the Gramineae" [Steiner 1982, 43] blossom – because they are excessively determined by the periphery rather than by his own internally concentrated forces.

If we view the lemon from this perspective, for example, we can observe a process in the sphere of the blossom, fruit and seed which is the opposite of the Gramineae; lemon blossoms form fruit simultaneously; they form mature fruit in all four seasons, allowing for four harvests per year. The fruit is protected by a yellow "leathery peel" (flavedo) rich in essential oils that protects it from the environment. These essential oils have a refreshing effect on human beings. Underneath lies a white layer (albedo) containing *bitter substances* (▸Chap. 6.5.4) from which the juice sacs of the pulp grow *from the outside inwards.* The riper the lemon, the more sour its pulp will be – despite the intense southern sun which ripens it, it does not sweeten. In human beings bitters have the effect of intensifying digestive activity in the hepatobiliary sphere (an important therapeutic effect for allergy patients); the sour element has a concentrating, awakening and astringing effect on the soul entity.

1 Cf. Rauber und Kopsch [1987, 526] concerning the function of the olfactory glands (with their affinity to the metabolism): "The gland secretion simultaneously acts as a solution for the odorants and a cleanser. Failure of such glandular activity also leads to an impairment of the sense of smell as does flooding of the olfactory glands with secretion." There is a finely regulated balance between the sensory and the metabolic function to be found everywhere, and in cases of pollinosis this is persistently impaired.

According to Rudolf Steiner and Ita Wegman, "mere observation [of the organization of the lemon fruit] already shows the strong activity of formative forces working from the outside inwards" [Steiner und Wegman 1984, 134]. Through suitable pharmaceutical preparation and application it was possible to obtain a particularly effective pollinosis medicine. Injections were especially suitable [Steiner 1982, 44]. This treatment is enhanced by stimulation of the gall bladder function (bitter substances) (▸Chap. 6.3.3.2): it is especially important "for the health of the nervous and sensory system," Rudolf Steiner notes [1982, 46], "that gall bladder functions properly." What this means is that there must be a balance between the ability to overcome foreign substances and the affection of the sense organs through these substances. (Cf. the extensive discussion on Gencydo® and Citrus pericarpium, medicines that are derived from this, in ▸Chap. 6.5.6.4.1).

6.6.3 Treatment

6.6.3.1 General treatment options

In the order of basic treatment stages, the third step, that of integrating the child harmoniously back into life, has special significance (▸Chap. 6.3) An extensive (family) history and the medical finding (including nasal mucosa) should be followed by extensive consultation. This should make clear which of the child's forces need to be strengthened, where stress caused by school, kindergarten and parental expectations can be relieved, and how one should deal with the child's ambitiousness, agitation and nervous tension educationally.

6.6.3.1.1 Bitter substances

An essential step in building up inner equilibrium consists of bringing about a balanced *digestive process* through dietetic and medicinal means (▸Chap. 6.3.3.2). Promoting the catabolic and digestive activity in the stomach and the duodenum, the gall bladder and the pancreas is necessary for treatment of pollinosis and has often proven to be very effective in acute cases. *On the basis of very recent experiences* the authors use medicines which contain the bitter substance absinthium (wormwood) as first-line general treatment of acute pollinosis. Here the bitter, parts of the plant above the ground are used (flowering herbage). The flowering period of wormwood is the summer; the concentration of bitter substances in the plant is directly related to flower formation: "its pungent aroma immediately reveals some of the forces which bring together *the bitter and the aromatic aspect*, rendering a unique interaction," – "a strange synthesis of etheric oils with bitter substances" [Pelikan 1980, 264f.]. *Therapeutically speaking, absinthium*

- *has a toning effect:* "having the same effect on the stomach which it has on the bile ducts, namely that of influencing the *atonic conditions* of these two organs" in a very pronounced way [Weiß 1999, 147]; this means it guides the soul activity (tonus) more intensely into the digestive activity of the upper abdominal organs.
- *has a warming effect and increases immunological resistance* [cf. Pelikan, l. c., and Weiß, l. c.]: The *ability of the organism to isolate itself from external nature* is stimulated by absinthium (against flu-like infections and worm infections as well).

Through administration of absinthium, the upper components of the human being are strongly directed to and focused on their inner tasks in the organism: digestion of external nature, inner warming and immunological stabilization of the individual's own physical boundaries. In this way external, blossoming nature can no longer irritate the organism to the same degree and make its own sensory organs (eyes, nose) "blossom" in fits of hay fever. A strong effect can be achieved by using absinthium in the acute stage of pollinosis; the warming and toning effect of the medicine can also promote the healing process if it is used in a timely fashion before the season begins.

According to an observation by Reinhard Kindt (Hanover), a proven medicine for pollinosis, particularly if the eyes are affected to a strong degree, is:

- **Absinthium D1/Resina Laricis D3 dil.** Weleda
  5–10 gtt. 3 x/d [Vademecum 2010, 32]; it can be taken in diluted form if necessary but it should taste bitter!

The very clear effectiveness of this preparation in more than half of all treatments confirms the specific effectiveness of wormwood, which is probably one of the most effective bitter substance drugs for treatment of hay fever. Wormwood in combination with larch resin guides the activity of the astral body very strongly towards the area of the digestion and the kidneys. In this way, control of the water organism, "water excretion in the right place", is stimulated and allergic swellings are counteracted. Kidney activity directed inwards is strengthened, which is a foundation of human development of consciousness and which can be viewed as "inner light formation". Thus the therapeutic principle is to strengthen inner organ activity in such a way that the organism is not overpowered by external nature and cannot be deformed in its organ activity from the outside. The eyes, as sense organs for external light and the foundation of our objective waking consciousness, stand in a close inner relationship to kidney activity. Thus one can understand that allergic eye symptoms are a special indication for this medicine.

If pollinosis is accompanied by *a sensitive stomach, ructus* and meteorism of the upper abdomen, an alternative preparation which can be considered is

- **Absinthium/Caryophylli comp. dil.** Weleda
  3–10 gtt. 3 x/d

A further quite universally applicable medicinal plant is bitterwort, Gentiana lutea, whose root has the strongest bitter values of all indigenous plants.

Rhythmicized, non-homoeopathically potentized extracts of bitterwort, wormwood and dandelion are mutually processed with Nux vomica D4 in

- **Gentian Magen globuli velati (stomach remedy)** Wala
  5-7-10 pillules 2–3 x/d.

This medicine can be considered for any form of allergic rhinitis, not only seasonal forms. In practice it is very impressive to observe time and again how inflammatory processes in the nose region subside after careful stimulation and regulation of the digestive activity has been performed, even if it has proven therapy-resistant for a long time previously. Its effect is often supplemented by administration of Cichorium, for example Cichorium/ Pancreas comp. (▸Chap. 6.3.3.2) or Cichorium 5 % pillules Wala [Vademecum 2010, 313]

As a single medicine Gentiana can also be administered to quite small children in the form of:

- **Gentiana 5 % Rh dil.** Weleda/**Gentiana lutea e rad. 5 % pillules** Wala
  3 × 3–7 gtt., 3 × 3–5 pillules

All of the aforementioned bitter substance medicines can also be taken after meals.

6.6.3.1.2 Citrus and Cydonia for acute and maintenance treatment of pollinosis

The anthroposophic medicines derived from lemon and quince, whose rationale was developed in ▸Chap. 6.6.2, are listed in terms of their indications and discussed at length in ▸Chap. 6.5.6.4.1. Although they were primarily developed for treatment of pollinosis, they have come to play a crucial role in treatment of allergic bronchial asthma. In a considerable percentage of cases (approx. 40 %), pollinosis itself evolves into allergic asthma in the course of "allergic march". Now that the unity of the respiratory tract, the significance of nasal breathing for bronchopulmonary function, has becoming increasingly clear ("united airways"), the pollinosis treatment discussed below turns out to have a preventive role in regard to allergic asthma, which has the least favourable long-term prognosis of all forms of childhood asthma.

- **Gencydo® amp. 1–3 %/eye drops 0.1 %/Heuschnupfennasenspray** (=1 %) (hay fever spray) Weleda

is effective for acute cases of pollinosis and – provided that it is administered early on also – for prophylactic use. Repeated use for several years during childhood and accompanying therapy can constitute a central component of a curatively effective therapy concept.

Regular inhalation treatment using **Gencydo® 1–3 % amp.** Weleda in combination with 1 ml NaCl 0.9 % (or **Galenit D10 amp.** Weleda in cases of already diagnosed pollinosis-induced asthma – see below) starting approx. *6–12 weeks prior to the beginning of the pollen season* is recommended 2–3 x/wk. In cases of pronounced eye symptoms it can be supplemented with 1 gtt. **Gencydo® 0.1 % eye drops** 2–3 x/wk. If there is no vaporizer available, a suitable alternative or supplement in any case is **Heuschnupfennasenspray (hay fever spray)** Weleda, 1 puff in each nostril 3 x/wk.

At the beginning of the season one or more daily inhalations and use of nasal spray and eye drops (up to 3–5 x/d) are recommended.

Injection of Gencydo® can be considered in particular for pasty-adipose children, children and adolescents with a metabolic constitution from the age of nine onwards. For age-differentiated dosage schemes see [Vademecum 2010, 454]. If possible, this therapy should also be used prophylactically two months before the season begins.

In this way, very satisfactory therapeutic success can be achieved in many cases that goes beyond alleviating or eliminating symptoms, with a gradual decline in the pollinosis occurring from year to year. In cases where this does not succeed, anthroposophic medicine has other treatment options at its disposal that are not as well-known.

For
- lack of response to Gencydo®,
- patients whose constitution has a neurasthenic accentuation,
- quickly developing, acute symptoms

the authors have found
- **Citrus pericarpium D1 amp. 10 ml amp.** Apotheke an der Weleda (cf. for administration ►Chap. 6.5.6.4.1)

to be therapeutically beneficial in many cases. The acute effectiveness surpasses that of Gencydo® in cases of medium severe and very severe pollinosis.

This preparation seems to be most effective when administered in the form of an *injection*. As years of experience on the part of the authors have shown, this can be used in undiluted form for all age groups if the patient has been properly informed of the slight burning sensation it creates and it is injected s.c. not too superficially in the upper arm.

Citrus pericarpium and Gencydo® amp. can be used for inhalation, as well as for s.c. administration (1 ml), for acute symptoms in combination with a *potentized organ* preparation in a higher potency (1 amp.):
- **Tunica mucosa nasi Gl D30 amp.** Wala
- **Bronchi Gl D30 amp.** Wala
- **Conjunctiva Gl D30 amp.** Wala

This especially enhances the acute effectiveness of the medicines in the organ area under treatment (swelling, secretion, itching/burning/urge to cough).

The intervals between the necessary injections must be individually determined; for administration of Citrus pericarpium, injections every 1 to 2 weeks suffice in most cases; in some cases, one injection treatment at the beginning of the season is enough. Pollinosis can be treated in this way which otherwise proves treatment-resistant. The effectiveness of this medicament is not increased through very frequent injections (more than 2 to 3 x/wk); inhalations can be used more frequently, however. All in all, it should be administered as rarely and as briefly as possible in order to be optimally effective.

Gencydo® and Citrus pericarpium used for pollinosis treatment can be enhanced and increased in its effectiveness through administration of *lead* (►Chap. 6.5.6.3.4) in medium potentization (D10–12). The effectiveness of lead is closely associated with the *sense of smell* (cf. also ►Chap. 6.5.6.3.4 and Vademecum 2010, 318, 598]. In practice, when treating pollinosis alone the authors prefer
- **Plumbum met. praep. D10 amp.** Weleda

and for pollinosis accompanied by allergic bronchial asthma
- **Galenit D10 amp.** Weleda

each 1:1 with **Gencydo® 3 %** or **Citrus pericarpium D1** mixed as an inhalation or s.c.
- **Plumbum D14** 2 parts/**Stannum D14** 1 part **trit.** Weleda
  1 saltsp. 1–2 x/d for 4–8 weeks.

is a basic medicine which is particularly to be recommended for *pollinosis accompanied by food allergies* or intolerances.

6

A much more sustained effect on the course of the disease is achieved with this potentized metal or metal ore than can be effected through use of purely herbal preparations. *Grass and cereal allergies*, which are often difficult to treat, respond specifically to *supplementary* treatment using

- **Flores Tritici comp. dil./amp.** Weleda
  as inhalation 1 ampoule 2–3 x/wk, 6–8 weeks before onset of season,
  10 gtt. 1–2 x/d per os. For adolescents also 1 amp. 2 x/wk s.c. 6 weeks before onset of season. Contains extracts from Formica parva, wheat and common wasp.
- **Citrus/Quarz amp.** Weleda
  can be administered inhalatively or s.c. during the same time period for cases of *late bloomer pollinosis* (May-July). The preparation contains potentized extracts of elder, wheat and linden, quartz in D20 (intensified in isolation) and Gencydo® 1 %. This is most suitable for patients with a hysterical, metabolically accentuated constitution, especially for s.c. application.

In regard to pollinosis-induced *conjunctivitis*, very well tested medicines are

- **Euphrasia Einzeldosis Augentr.** Wala
  1–2 gtt. 3–5 x/d

or, for a more intense effect, but initially accompanied by a slight burning sensation

- **Gencydo® Augentr.** Weleda
  1 gtt. 3–5 x/d

in alternation with

- **Quarz D6 Augentr.** Weleda

For pronounced photophobia a preparation with a complicated notation which is however extraordinarily effective is

- **Aesculus, Cortex D30/Lavandula sicc. D6 aa Augentr. Weleda**
  1–2 gtt. 1–3 x/d

6.6.3.2 Interval treatment

In the discussion on "hay fever treatment" by Rudolf Steiner and Ita Wegman [1991, 117] something is striking that has maintained its validity today: it is only possible to *heal* pollinosis by having the patient undergo *repeated treatment cycles* several years in a row. If such treatment is carried out, a decline in symptoms should be observed from year to year. In fact the general treatment described above can develop a sustainable effect if this principle is followed. Rudolf Steiner and Ita Wegman describe a four-year course of treatment and the authors' practice has shown that a similar period of time is necessary to obtain thoroughly effective treatment.

What is of decisive importance in this context are *the therapeutic measures taken during the time in which no symptoms of pollinosis are observed.* During this period steps can be taken which are essential for the healing process. Fundamentally speaking, *stimulation of the child's warmth organization* constitutes the basis for treatment. Physical exercise and child-appropriate activities in nature (until the child begins sweating) strengthens the connection of the spirit and soul entity with the physical body, in particular the limbs, effecting better separation from nature in the barrier organs.

Warmth protection through appropriate clothing, age-appropriate trips to the sauna (for example 2 × monthly) and most of all

- **Oil dispersion bath** as developed by Junge [1990]
  1–2 x/wk (for more detailed information go to www.jungebad.com)

strengthen the I-organization in its physical action, which manifests itself partly in immunological digestive and regulatory processes. Some suitable bath oils, depending on the patient's constitution, are:

- **Citrus, Ol. aeth. 10 %** Wala,
- **Lavandula, Ol. aeth. 10 %** Wala,
- **Rosmarinus, Ol. aeth. 10 %** Wala.

In many cases the most important medicinal measure to be taken during interval treatment of pollinosis is *autohaemotherapy using potentized autologous blood as developed by Imhäuser* [2000, 187], which is described and explained with regard to allergic diseases in ▸Chap. 6.3.3.4.1. Treatment is initiated between November and January, approx. three months before onset of the pollinosis season. Concerning *dosages* one can proceed as follows:

- C5 3 gtt./d in the morning (2 to 4 weeks).

The remainder of C5 is used to prepare a C7 through potentization, of which

- 3 gtt. are administered 3 x/wk in the morning for approx. 4 weeks; afterwards
- C9 3 gtt. 2 x/wk for 4–6 weeks,
- C12 and C15 3 gtt. 1 x/wk each for 4 weeks.

In persistent cases it is advisable to begin with C3.

This treatment must be repeated annually for approx. three to four years. It does not constitute a measure for acute treatment; the irreplaceable value of this treatment consists in its long-term effect on the immunological digestive and regulatory organs. The organism's response can be evaluated in the second year of treatment. If there is no response to treatment within two years, it should not be continued. The authors do not administer injections of autologous blood to patients of childhood age.

6.6.3.3 Individualized treatment with single-substance medicines

The connections discussed in ▸Chap. 6.6.1 and ▸Chap. 6.6.2 already make quite clear why, among the potentized single-substance medicines for treating pollinosis,

- **Nux vomica LM12 dil.** Arcana
  5 gtt./d (often more effective if taken in the evening)

plays such a central role (extensive discussion in ▸Chap. 6.5.6.11). Not only does this medicine correspond to constitutional conditions frequently found in children with hay fever; in its effect it also harmonizes the circumstances and strains suffered by many of the children living in western industrial nations today.

We summarize once more below the major symptoms and characteristics of pollinosis which suggest that this medicine is indicated:

- *neurasthenic* and at the same time *impulsive* constitution; *Mediterranean* ("low sulphur", cf. Husemann [2009, 103]) constitution: slender, usually dark-haired, sensitive to cold, higher prevalence among boys.
- in the winter *tendency to develop catarrhal symptoms* of the upper respiratory tract,
- in cases of pollinosis *watery-irritative rhinitis during the day; at night clogged nose,*
- in a state of *constant tension*, patients have high expectations of themselves and are under great pressure due to expectations of others,
- *ambitious*, meticulous when it comes to schoolwork,
- if patients' own projects do not succeed or are impeded – in part, for example, by the pollinosis itself – patients tend to experience extreme anger,
- anger exacerbates all symptoms or can trigger them.[1]

This choleric tendency expresses psychosomatically the relationship between the medicinal effect and the *biliary secretion of the liver*. Nux vomica is a proven medicine for stimulating detoxification processes of the liver, nausea and vomiting in connection with disorders of the stomach and the duodenum and for dyskinesia of the bile ducts. A tendency for cramps of the hollow organs pervades the medicinal picture (▸Chap. 4.3.4). The one-sided, catabolic effect of the soul entity on the life organization manifests itself in all of these symptoms; constant stress in the form of vegetative tension dominates such patients. The aggressive potential of the organism accumulates within the digestive tract in the activity of the gall bladder and the pancreas. As a potentized medicine, Nux vomica helps the patient integrate the bottled-up aggressive energies into the life activity and to reduce the incidence of outbursts of rage.

Case study

An eight-year-old boy with pollinosis comes to the surgery for an initial consultation. He has a delicate physique and gives a shy impression in his meeting with the doctor. The mother reports that pollinosis started to develop when he was five years old, mostly triggered by grass and grain pollen. Since then, she says, the patient has suffered from extreme sneezing attacks, itching of the gums and conjunctivitis; at night his nose has been clogged. His mood has been irritable and there have been frequent outbursts of anger (single child). In connection with the pollinosis there have recently been attacks of shortness of breath. The mother is a housewife and is very worried about her child's health. She reports that her husband holds a job in the automobile industry which carries a lot of responsibility accompanied by a high degree of stress and that he does not come home until late in the evening. The boy performed well at school; he was very

1 The model of modern management, the first European who wore a fresh shirt every day, Napoleon I, was a typical Nux-vomica patient in every fibre. "Vitesse, vitesse" was Bonaparte's maxim. He won his battles for the most part through precise time management, which he bequeathed to France in the form of the code civile, but he was also ruthlessly capable of ordering his artillery to fire on Russian soldiers fleeing across a frozen lake to drown them. He lost the Battle of Waterloo as the result of an acute haemorrhoidal crisis [Coulter 1991, 79–82, gives an impressive account of this grand medicinal picture].

meticulous about doing his homework. He tended to be a homeboy and gets cold easily in the winter.
After this initial consultation the father was asked to come to the practice for an individual consultation. He appeared in a pin-striped suit, exhibited a very composed posture and had a striking face with a slightly grim expression. When asked about his biography, he reported that he came from a family of refugees and had worked his way up through work and adult education after having received only a formal elementary education. He said his family was very important to him, quickly adding that his son should "have it better than he did" some day. For this reason, good school performance was the most important thing, he said, reporting that his son made great efforts at school. In the course of the conversation it was possible to modify the father's expectations to a certain extent.
Treatment began with prescribing Arsenicum album LM12 but with only moderate success, followed by administration of Nux vomica C12 with very clear success. During the first two winters, autohaemotherapy as developed by Imhäuser was carried out, and during the past three years treatment only consisted of daily dosages of five pillules of Nux vomica C12, beginning four weeks after the onset of the season until the end of it. In the meantime the patient is free of symptoms during the season.

Generally speaking, it is evident that in patients who respond well to Nux vomica the *rational matter-of-fact persona* directly determines the will while circumventing healthy rhythmical mediation/emotional sensibility. The great will energy is fixated on achieving goals determined as the means to an end; with the same large measure of energy, everything is suppressed which does not comply emotionally and physically with this goal orientation. The centre, the rhythmical system, is gripped in a vice (outwardly as well as inwardly). In view of the fact that the midface belongs to the rhythmical respiratory system ("united airways"), being directly associated with the emotional life, the chronic nose problems experienced by Nux vomica patients are a sign that this centre is oppressed and weakened. J.T. Kent once remarked that all human beings could really use Lachesis at some point, and in today's achievement-oriented western society one can (almost) say that of Nux vomica as well. It is telling that a medicine with such a universally positive effect as Gentiana stomach pillules Wala, which were discussed in connection with bitter substances, contains a deep potency of Nux vomica.

For cases of pollinosis, Nux vomica is often a very effective acute polychrest as well as a *constitutional medicine* with a long-term healing effect that is frequently indicated.

Under the last-mentioned aspect, the following other single medicines can be considered for treatment of pollinosis:

- **Arsenicum album,**
- **Natrium muriaticum,**
- **Lachesis,**
- **Pulsatilla,**
- **(Lycopodium).**

(▶Chap. 6.4.3.6 and ▶Chap. 6.5.6.11)

If pollinosis has a tendency to change into *allergic bronchial asthma*, another indicated treatment option in addition to the aforementioned ones (inhalations of Gencydo® 1–3 % and Galenit D10 amp. Weleda) is the internal administration of potentized *iodine* [Scholten 1993, 213f.] or iodine compounds:

- **Iodum LM6/12 dil.** Arcana
  3–5 gtt. 1–2 x/d or
- **Arsenicum iodatum D6–12 dil.** (various manufacturers)
  5 gtt. 1–2 x/d or
- **Ferrum iod. D12 dil.** (various manufacturers)
  5 gtt. 1–2 x/d

Restlessness, a slender physique, exacerbation in heat and a tendency towards a hyperthyroid metabolism [Girke 2010, 375–377] are characteristic of patients who respond positively to potentized iodine. In patients for whom *Arsenicum iodatum* is indicated the *rhinitis is more aggressive and more likely to make the nose sore;* such patients tend to have a more neurasthenic constitution than those for whom Iodum is indicated. In both cases a tendency towards chronic inflammation of the lungs can be observed. In contrast, *Ferrum iodatum* is more likely to be indicated for *blond patients with an originally very lymphatic* constitution.

It is also possible to administer one of the three aforesaid medicines in the morning and combine a dosage of a potentized lead compound at midday (*Galenit D10* as trit. internally or *Plumbum D14 2 parts/Stannum D14 1 part trit. Weleda*, 1 saltsp. each) with the most similar constitutional medicine in the evening (for example Lachesis).

If the pollinosis worsens considerably *in the summer heat*, then potentized charcoal is often a very effective medicine (for bronchial asthma as well):

- **Carbo vegetabilis D12/LM12 dil.** (various manufacturers)
  7 gtt. 2 x/d or 5 gtt. 1 x/d

The potentized coal of horsetail:

- **Carbo Equiseti trit. D6** Weleda
  1 saltsp. 3–4 x/d

is a quite universally effective medicine for treating pollinosis.

Carbo Equiseti has a regulatory effect on very runny noses. The affinity between Equisetum and the kidneys (▸Chap. 1.2.2, ▸Chap. 6.3.3.3) shows itself here insofar as pollinosis is accompanied by an irregular secretion process which can be viewed as “kidney activity in the wrong place.” Insofar as the kidneys and the adrenal glands constitute central organs for the connection between soul and body activity, it makes sense to take these organs into consideration in connection with pollinosis.

For general hypersensitivity *and a neurasthenic constitution* accompanied by *sensitivity to heat*, relatively high potencies of horsetail coal can be used as a constitutional medicine:

- **Carbo Equiseti D15 amp.** Weleda
  1–2 x/wk s.c. or as inhalation

For acute treatment of pollinosis, some other potentized single medicines play a role which are briefly listed here:

- **Sabadilla D12 dil.** (various manufacturers)
  5–7 gtt. 1–3 x/d

in cases of patients who are *sensitive to cold, high-strung-anxious* (usually girls); allergic conjunctivitis and rhinitis with *large amounts of watery secretion*, in some cases frontal headaches due to shifts in openings of the paranasal sinuses, *itching gums*.

- **Luffa D12 dil.** (various manufacturers)
  5–7 gtt. 1–3 x/d

in cases of dry, swollen, irritated nasal mucosa.

- **Arundo D12 dil.** (various manufacturers)
  5–7 gtt. 1–3 x/d

if the pollinosis is accompanied by severe *itching of the nose and gums.*

- **Acid. succinicum Injeel** Heel
  0.5 ml orally 1–2 x/d or 1–2 x/wk s.c.

if severe *itching of eyelids and nose* occur and the pollinosis is conspicuously exacerbated *whenever the air cools down.*

It is not always possible to dispense with symptomatic allopathic treatment during the acute phase of the disease.

In closing, some acutely and constitutionally effective options for use of *eurythmy therapy* for treatment of pollinosis should be mentioned. Certain individual exercises which exhibit a noticeable effect in the pollinosis season are, for example, the so-called large "E" exercise and specific series of exercises for pollinosis patients, such as the series T-S-R-M-A [Hachtel 2007, 439], which have the potential to increase and stabilize the success of medicinal therapy considerably in intervals as well if done on a regular basis. Eurythmy therapy gives the child the capacity to strengthen the stability of his or her health through self-activity, in particular through soul-guided movement of his or her own limbs. Thus this form of therapy responds to the underlying problem of pollinosis in a deeper, causative sense.

6.7 Perennial allergic rhinitis

More and more children who suffer from allergic rhinitis all year round are coming to paediatric practices for consultation. *Diagnostically speaking*, in cases with one-sided symptoms the presence of a foreign body should be ruled out; it is also advisable to perform a routine ENT examination (check for adenoids and nasal polyps, anterior and posterior rhinoscopy, ultrasound scan of the paranasal sinuses, precise diagnostics in regard to the possibility of a disorder of tube function or of accompanying seromucous tympanum) and basic allergological diagnostics. *Dryness of the nasal mucosa* is a basic finding with a prevalence of about 60 % in children examined who live in large cities. Nose care is a basic issue of modern paediatric treatment, especially since the connection between impaired nasal respiration and bronchial asthma is becoming increasingly clear. We refer to the therapeutic recommendations made in other parts of this book (▸Chap. 5.1.2.3).

Therapeutically speaking, the steps depicted in ▸Chap. 6.3 constitute the basis for treatment. Treatment using *potentized autologous blood* as developed by Imhäuser

(▸Chap. 6.6.3.2) is specifically effective here. If other medicines are being taken as well, the autologous blood should be administered at separate times. The onset of autumn is particularly suitable for blood taking, potentization and initiation of therapy.

Further basic treatment can be given using

- **Heuschnupfenspray** Weleda (▸Chap. 6.6.3.1.2)
  as long-term treatment 1–2 x/d
- **Nasenbalsam für Kinder** (nasal balm for children) Wala [Vademecum 2010, 612]
  1–2 x/d for care and protection of mucosa, showing a long-term strengthening effect and thus indirectly reducing the swelling (with no side effects, but slow to develop effectiveness)
- **Rhinodoron® Nasenspray (nose spray)** Weleda
  for care and cleansing (contains Aloe vera)
- **Marum verum D4(–1) dil./pillules** DHU
  5–10 gtt./pillules in the evening, very effective for relief of clogged nose at night [Vademecum 2010, 573]

The most suitable constitutionally indicated medicines are the following homoeopathic medicines for the *neurasthenic type of constitution*:

- Acidum phosphoricum,
- Quarz,
- Arsenum iodatum,
- Formica,
- Lycopodium.

Of the specific medicines for perennial allergic rhinitis, we highlight as the primary one

- **Acidum phosphoricum D12–30** (in individual cases up to C200) **dil./pillules** (various manufacturers)
  5 gtt. 2 x/d, in rare cases higher potencies

In chemical terms, phosphoric acid is a weak acid; it can even be found in crystalline form at room temperature and it does not exhibit the hardly tameable activity of pure phosphorus. In physiological terms the energy metabolism of animals and human beings is closely associated with the phosphate metabolism. In general, acids have an affinity to ensouled organisms; in animals and human beings, secretion of acids – for example in the stomach – is closely connected with the activity of the soul entity in the physical body. As a substance, large amounts of phosphoric acid are contained in Coca Cola, for example; it is an (unconsciously) appealing component of luxury foods and drinks. The special affinity which phosphoric acid has to the soul organization, the astral body, becomes apparent in all of this; it is also of decisive importance for its use as a potentized medicine.

In the *homoeopathic medicinal picture* of Acidum phosphoricum, the focus lies on the following characteristics and symptoms:

- *rapid exhaustibility,* especially after intellectual exertion (exhaustion caused by school): “First intellectual, then physical weakness” [Boericke 1994, 594],
- headaches after school,

- rings under the eyes, pale face, emaciation,
- *chronically clogged, itching nose*, dry or watery, secreting mucosa; patient subjectively suffers to a high degree from impeded nose respiration,
- general tendency for shivering and feeling cold
- tendency for dizziness,
- tendency for meteorism, poorly digested stool, diarrhoea.

The depicted symptoms most often appear before and during puberty, in the second septennium. Growth spurts (skeletal growth strips the organism of considerable amounts of phosphates) can trigger this condition or aggravate it considerably. At this age the human soul organization is in the process of becoming gradually autonomous; in anthroposophic medicine we speak of the "birth of the astral body," which takes place by the age of 14. In patients who require Acidum phosphoricum as a medicine, we often gain the impression that this "birth" tends to be drawn-out, delayed, and does not receive enough impulses from the power of individuality. An important aspect for selection of this medicine is *emotional anguish*, which is not always easy to detect. Anguish in connection with the first love relationship is often responsive to Acidum phosphoricum.

The *intellectual strain* put on children often plays a major role. During the growth spurts in the second septennium, demands of school in particular rob them of more strength and energy than the organism can actually provide: the development of the body is weakened by its premature and one-sided instrumentalization. Poor posture, slight forms of depression, a decline in the ability to concentrate, especially in the afternoon, is often observed. It is important for the doctor to prevent the parents and teachers reacting with even greater expectations and admonitions, thus aggravating the situation. Instead, we should ensure that the situation is sufficiently balanced out through physical activity and stimulation of the warmth organization (for example through visits to the sauna and appropriate physical exercise), and that time limits be put on homework, for example. By involving children in age-appropriate practical tasks, their overall condition will often improve considerably.

A further important single-substance medicine for chronic allergic rhinitis is

- **Arsenum iodatum D6–12 dil.** (various manufacturers)
  5–7 gtt. 2–3 x/d

Such children initially exhibit pronounced *restlessness* and *(anxious) nervousness* as well as a tendency towards *emaciation*, with their condition tending to be subjectively exacerbated through heat (▸Chap. 6.6.3). Arsenum iodatum is a very valuable medicine if part of the respiratory tract seems to become inflamed easily of its own accord and to resist regulatory immunological processes; it can help the formative forces of the child's individuality to break through, thus simultaneously putting limits on excessive general catabolism in the organism as a whole.

- **Lycopodium C30–200 pillules** Gudjons
  3 pillules 3 x/d for 3 days on each occasion

has proven to be highly effective for chronic swelling of nasal mucosa. In predisposed constitutions (particularly among boys, ▸Chap. 6.4.3.6) it can have a curative effect. The preparation by Gudjons is the only one to be initially potentized by trituration of the seeds with their high concentration of aluminium and it proves to be most effective for this indication. In cases of perennial allergic rhinitis only high Lycopodium potencies are effective.

- **Berberis/Quarz amp.** Wala
- **Tunica mucosa nasi D15 amp.** Wala
  in combination (mixed injection) 1 ml 1 x/d per os in the morning or 1–2 x/wk s.c. during adolescence

are indicated most of all in cases where there is an inclination towards sinusitis, excrescences of the mucosa (polyposis) and of the organs of the lymphatic tonsillar ring (for example adenoids).

In otherwise therapy-resistant cases, very effective treatment can be achieved through injections using

- **Citrus pericarpium D1 amp.**, special manufacture by Weleda,
- **Tunica mucosa nasi Gl D15 amp.** Wala
  2 ml 1 x/d

Possibly alternating 1 x/wk with

- **Nux vomica D30 amp.** Wala and
- **Sympathicus Gl D30 amp.** Wala
  administered as a mixed injection.

6.8 Urticaria

Doctors almost exclusively encounter acute cases of urticaria in children. It is often impossible to determine the trigger (for example sunscreen, cosmetics, etc.) but one should always look for the cause and prescribe abstention accordingly. The child should avoid protein-rich foods and all food additives for several days.

The most important potentized medicine is

- **Apis mell. D12–30 pillules/D30 amp.** Weleda[1]

In less severe cases 5 pillules up to 4 x/d should be administered; more effective results are obtained by (mostly one) *i.v. injection*.

Depending on the trigger this can be combined with

- **Nux vomica D30 amp.** Wala,

especially if reactions to toxins or exogenous substances play a role.

- **Sulphur D30 amp.** Wala,

if suppressive medication, for example antibiotics, anti-histamines etc., was taken before the outbreak of urticaria.

The effect can be intensified if Apis and, in some cases, Nux vomica or Sulphur are added to 10 ml of

- **Calcium-Quercus amp.** Wala

and slowly administered i.v.

1 Or Apis ex animale Gl D30 amp. Wala

References for Chapter 6

(every reference marked with a ■ Bullet point indicates the English translation of the reference above it)

Alm, J. S., J. Swartz: Atopy in children of families with an anthroposophic lifestyle. Lancet 353, 1485–1488 (1999).

Alven, T., C. Braun-Fahrländer et al.: Allergic diseases and atopic sensitization in children related to farming and anthroposophic lifestyle – the PARSIFAL study. Allergy (2005). E pub September 15; doi: 10.1111/j.1398-9995.2005.00939.X.

Arbeitsgemeinschaft Anthroposophische Pneumologie: Leitlinie zur Therapie des Asthma bronchiale in der Anthroposophischen Medizin. Der Merkurstab **63,** 56–63 (2010).

Argiroffo, C.: Irreversible Schäden durch Babyschwimmen? Paediatrica **17,** 8–9 (2006.

Aristoteles: De anima. Dt. von A. Lasson, F. Diederichs, Jena 1924; zit. nach Husemann 1998.

Bach, J.-F.: The Effect of Infections on Susceptibility to Autoimmune and Allergic Diseases. New Engl. J. Med. **347,** 911–920 (2002).

Bachert, C., V. Wahn: Allergische Rhinitis. In: Pädiatrische Allergologie und Immunologie. Wahn, U., R. Seger, V. Wahn (Hrsg.). 3. Aufl. Urban & Fischer, München 1999.

Basold, A. et al.: Heilmittel für typische Krankheiten nach Angaben R. Steiners. Verlag am Goetheanum, Dornach 1995.

Bäumler, S.: Heilpflanzen Praxis heute. Elsevier, München 2007.

Beasley et al.: Association between paracetamol use in infancy and childhood, and risk of asthma, rhinoconjunctivitis and eczema in children aged 6–7 years: analysis from Phase Three of the ISAAC programme. The Lancet **372,** 1039–1048 (2008).

Belart, W.: Weleda Korr.bl. f. Ärzte **94,** 37–39 (1978).

Berdel, D.: Asthma bronchiale im Kindes- und Jugendalter (S2-Leitlinie). Deutsche Gesellschaft für Kinderheilkunde und Jugendmedizin: Leitlinien Kinderheilkunde und Jugendmedizin. Urban & Fischer, München 2010.

Bisgaard H. et al.: Intermittend inhaled Corticosteroids in Infants with Episodic Wheezing. New Engl. J. Med. **354,** 1998–2005 (2006).

Blackie, M.: Lebendige Homöopathie. Sonntag Verlag, Regensburg 1990.

Beck, A., Forster, P.: Die Homogenisierung von Milch und ihre Bedeutung für Allergien gegen Kuhmilch. Der Merkurstab **55,** 50–54 (2002).

Biggelaar, van den et al.: Long-term treatment of intestinal helminths increases mite skin-test reactivity in Gabonese schoolchildren. J. Infect. Dis. **189,** 892–900 (2004).

Boericke, W.: Handbuch der homöopathischen Materia Medica. Haug Verlag, Heidelberg 1. Aufl. 1994, 2. Aufl. 1996.

■ Boericke, W.: Pocket manual of homœpathic materia medica: comprising the characteristic and guiding symptoms of all remedies (clinical and pathogenetic). Indian Books & Periodicals Publishers, New Delhi 2004.

Börner, E. M.: Zur Behandlung spastisch gelähmter Kleinkinder mit der rhythmischen Massage. Der Merkurstab **42,** 156–161 (1989).

Brokow, I. et al: Einfluss von Lebensbedingungen und Verhaltensweisen auf die Entwicklung von Immunsystem und Allergien im Ost-West-Vergleich: MSchr Kinderheilk **156,** 249–255 (2008).

Bühlbäcker, A.: Zur Verwendbarkeit von Stutenmilch, Kumyss und Eselsmilch als Diätetika und Heilmittel unter besonderer Berücksichtigung der Bedürfnisse des Säuglings und des Frühgeborenen. Deutsche Hochschulschriften 1104, Verlag Hänsel-Hohenhausen 1996.

Coulter, C.: Porträts homöopathischer Arzneimittel, Bd. 1, 2. Aufl. Haug Verlag, Heidelberg 1989 und Bd. 2, 1. Auflage 1991.

Deshpande, D. A. et al.: Bitter taste receptors on airway smooth muscle bronchodilate by localized calcium signaling and reverse obstruction. Nature Medicine, published online: doi: 10.1038/nm.2237 (2010).

Deutsche Gesellschaft für Kinderheilkunde und Jugendmedizin: Leitlinien Kinderheilkunde und Jugendmedizin. Urban & Fischer, München 2010.

Dicksved J. et al.: Molecular Fingerprinting of the Fecal Microbiota of Children Raised According to Different Lifestyles. Applied and Environmental Microbiology, 73, 2284–2289 (2007).

Ecker, D., Bräuner-Gülow, G.: Anthroposophische Asthmatherapie und -schulung bei Kindern. Der Merkurstab **52**, 88–95 (1999).

Ecker, D. et al.: Anthroposophische Asthmatherapie im Vergleich. Ersetzt sie das inhalative Corticoid? Der Merkurstab **62,** 30–34 (2009).

Eichler, K., R. Eichler: Neurodermitis. Erfolgreich behandelt durch klassische Homöopathie. Barthel & Barthel, Starnberg 1996.

Etminan, M. et al.: Acetaminophen use and the risk of asthma in children and adults: a systematic review and metaanalysis. Chest 2009, **136** 1316–1323 (2009).

Fingado, M.: Rhythmische Einreibungen. Natura Verlag, Dornach 2002.

Flöistrup, H., J. Swartz et al.: Allergic disease and sensitization in Steiner school children. J. Allergy Clin. Immunol. **117,** 59–66 (2006).

Frank, I.: Long term prognosis in preschool children with wheeze: longitudinal postal questionnaire study 1993–2004..

Fuchs, T.: Leibliche und virtuelle Realität. Scheidewege. Jahresschrift für skeptisches Denken **27,** 182–203 (1999).

Gaudecker, B. v.: Lymphatische Organe. In: Humanembryologie. Hinrichsen, K. V. (Hrsg.). Springer Verlag, Berlin 1990.

Gilani A. et al.: Gastrointestinal, selective airways and urinary bladder relaxant effects of Hyoscyamus niger are mediated through dual blockade of muscarine receptors and Ca2+-channels. Fundamental&Clinical Pharmacology **22,** 87–99 (2008).

Gillespie, K. M. et al.: The rising incidence of childhood type-1-diabetes and reduced contribution of high-risk-HLA haplotypes. The Lancet **364,** 1699–1700 (2004).

Girke, M.: Erkrankungen der Atmungsorganisation. Asthma Bronchiale. Der Merkurstab **50,** 285 (1997).

Goebel, W., M. Glöckler: Kindersprechstunde, 15. Aufl. Urachhaus, Stuttgart 2005.

■ Gloeckler, M., Goebel, W.: A guide to child health. Floris Books, Edinburgh 2003.

Götz, M.: Pneumonien. In: Therapie der Krankheiten im Kindes- und Jugendalter. Reinhardt, D. (Hrsg.). 7. Aufl. Springer, Berlin 2004.

Götzsche, P. C., Johansen, H. K.: House dust mite control measures for asthma. The Cochrane Database of Systematic Rev. 2008 (2).

Guilbert, T. W. et al.: Long-Term inhaled Corticosteroids in Preschool Children at High Risk of Asthma. New Engl. J. Med. **354,** 1985–1997 (2006).

Hachtel, B., Gäch, A.: Bibliographie Heileurythmie. Natur-Mensch-Medizin Verlag Bad Boll, 2007.

Hagloof B. et al: The Swedish diabetes study: indications of sever psychological stress as a risk factor for type 1 diabetes mellitus in childhood. Diabetologica **34,** 579–583 (1994).

Hahnemann, S.: Chronische Krankheiten. Bd. 1, Theoretische Grundlagen. Organon Verlag, Starnberg 1983; Haug Verlag, Heidelberg 1999.

Hahnemann, S.: Chronische Krankheiten, Materia Medica Teil, 4 Bde., Organon Verlag, Starnberg 1983; Haug Verlag, Heidelberg 1999.

Hahnemann, S.: Organon der Heilkunst. Organon Verlag, Starnberg 1985; 6. Aufl. (Nachdruck) Hippokrates, Stuttgart 1999.

Hamre, J. H. et al.: Anthroposophic Therapies in Chronic Disease: The Anthroposophic Medicine Outcomes Study (AMOS). Eur. J. Med. Res. **9**, 351–360 (2004).

Hanifin, J. M., G. Raijka: Diagnostic features of atopic dermatitis. Acta Derm. Venerol. (Stockh.), Suppl. **72**, 44–47 (1980).

Hansen, G., A. Schuster, D. Reinhardt: Astma bronchiale. In: Pädiatrische Allergologie und Immunologie. Wahn, U., R. Seger, V. Wahn (Hrsg.). 4. Aufl. Urban & Fischer, München 2005.

Henz, B. M., J. Grabbe: Das atopische Ekzem. In: Pädiatrische Allergologie und Immunologie. Wahn, U., R. Seger, V. Wahn (Hrsg.). 3. Aufl. Urban & Fischer, München 1999.

Hildebrandt, G.: Chronobiologische Grundlagen der Ordnungstherapie. In: Kneipptherapie. Brüggemann, W. (Hrsg.). 2. Aufl. Springer Verlag, Berlin, New York 1986.

Hinrichsen, K. V. (Hrsg.): Humanembryologie. Springer Verlag, Berlin 1990.

Hirte, M: Impfen – Pro und Contra. 2. Aufl. Knaur 2005.

Höger, P.: Kinderdermatologie. Schattauer, Stuttgart 2005.

Holländer, G.: Aufbau, Entwicklung und Funktion des Immunsystems. In: Pädiatrische Allergologie und Immunologie. Wahn, U., R. Seger, V. Wahn (Hrsg.). 3. Aufl. Urban & Fischer, München 1999.

Holländer, G. A. et al.: T-Zell-System. In: Pädiatrische Allergologie und Immunologie. Wahn, U., R. Seger, V. Wahn (Hrsg.). 4. Aufl. Urban & Fischer, München 2005.

Hung C.: Vitamin B 12 – Wundermittel bei atopischer Dermatitis? MSchr Kinderheilk **158**, 111.

Husemann, A.: Der hörende Mensch und die Wirklichkeit der Musik. Verlag Freies Geistesleben, Stuttgart 2010.

Husemann, F.: Anthroposophische Medizin. Verlag am Goetheanum, Dornach 2009.

Husemann, F.: Lachesis. In: Vademecum der anthroposophischen Medizin. Persephone Verlag am Goetheanum, Dornach 1999.

- Tellingen, C. Ed.:Vademecum: A handbook of anthroposophic medicine. Mercury Press, Spring Valley, N. Y. 2007.

Husemann, F.: Die Austernschale oder Calcium carbonicum. Der Merkurstab **53**, 413–420 (2000).

Husemann, G.: Geruchssinn und Allergie. Beitr. z. Erw. d. Heilkunst **36**, 156–164 (1983).

Husemann, G.: Asthma bronchiale. Drei Krankengeschichten. Beitr. z. Erw. d. Heilk. **37**, 181–184 (1984).

Husemann, G.: Sinnesleben, Seelenwesen und Krankheitsbild. Verlag Freies Geistesleben, Stuttgart 1998.

Imhäuser, H.: Homöopathie in der Kinderheilkunde. Haug Verlag, Heidelberg 12. Aufl. 2000.

Jachens, L.: Hautkrankheiten ganzheitlich heilen. Verlag Freies Geistesleben, Stuttgart 1999a, 2. Auflage 2006.

Jachens, L: Die Neurodermitis. Der Merkurstab **52**, 163 (1999b).

Jachens, L.: Oenathera Argento culta. Der Merkurstab **59**, 66 (2006).

Jachens, L. (Hrsg.): Dermatologie und anthroposophische Menschenkunde. Salumed Verlag, Berlin 2011.

Jung T. et al.: Atopic dermatitis: Therapeutic concepts evolving from new pathophysiologic insights. J Allergy Clin Immunol, published online doi:10.1016/j.jaci.2008.09.042.

Junge, W.: Wie kann das Immunsystem durch Wasser und Öl aktiviert werden? Der Merkurstab **5**, 313–319 (1990).

6

Jütte, R.: Organpräparate in der Geschichte der Schulmedizin, Homöopathie und Anthroposophischen Medizin. Der Merkurstab **62**, 49–60 (2009).

Kalliomäki, M. et al.: Probiotics in primary prevention of atopic disease: a randomised placebo-controlled trial. Lancet **357,** 1076–1079 (2001).

Kent, J. T.: Arzneimittelbilder. 5. Aufl. Haug Verlag, Heidelberg 1985.

Kiess, W. et al.: Ätiopathogenese des Diabetes mell Typ 1. MSchr Kinderheilk **149,** 641–649 (2001).

Knol, M.: Die Behandlung von Kindern mit Asthma und/oder Ekzem. Ms.-Druck, Gemeinschaftskrankenhaus Herdecke 1989, 8.

Köhler, G.: Lehrbuch der Homöopathie. Hippokrates Stuttgart, 2. Aufl. 1983, 7. Aufl. 1999.

Koletzko, S.: Erkrankungen des Dünn- und Dickdarms. In: Therapie der Krankheiten im Kindes- und Jugendalter. Reinhardt, D. (Hrsg.). 7. Aufl. Springer, Berlin 2004.

Koletzko, S.: Grundlagen der Ernährung im Kindes- und Jugendalter. In: Speer, Gahr (Hrsg.): Pädiatrie, 3.Aufl., Springer, Berlin 2009.

Kohlhase, M., Fintelmann, V.: Digestodoron. Der Merkurstab **62,** 623–630 (2009).

Kozyrski, A. et al.: Increased Risk of Childhood Asthma from Antibiotic Use in Early Life. Chest **131**, 1753–1759).

Krauss-Etschmann, S. et al.: Umweltinduzierte frühe Prägung von Asthma und Epigenetik. MSchr f Kinderheilk **158**, 142–148 (2010).

Kukkonen, K. et al: Probiotics and prebiotic galacto-oligosaccharides in the prevention of allergic diseases: a randomized, double-blind, placebo-controlled trial. J Allergy Clin Immunol **119,** 192–198 (2007).

Kummer, K. R.: Zur Bewegungsentwicklung des Kindes II. Der Merkurstab **43**, 26–39 (1990).

Kummer, K. R.: Neurodermitis. In: Anthroposophische Arzneitherapie. M. Glöckler (Hrsg.). Wiss. Verlagsgesellschaft, Stuttgart 2005a.

Kummer, K. R.: Die Darmflora des Menschen. Der Merkurstab **58,** 448–457 (2005b).

Lauener, R., Hansen, G., Wahn, U.: Prävention von Allergie und Asthma. In.: Pädiatrische Allergologie und Immunologie. Wahn, U., R. Seger, V. Wahn (Hrsg.). 4. Aufl. Urban & Fischer, München 2005.

Lange, P.: Hausmittel für Kinder. Rowohlt Verlag, Reinbek, 18.Auflage 2005.

Largo, R.: Kinderjahre. 5. Aufl. Piper Verlag, München 2000.

Laue, H. B. v.: Phosphor als Substanz und Prozess im Menschen. Der Merkurstab **58,** 438 (2005).

Laue, H. B. v., E. v. Laue: Physiologie der Heileurythmie. Verlag am Goetheanum, Dornach, Schweiz 2007.

- Laue, H. B. v., E. Von Laue: The physiology of eurythmy therapy. Floris Books, Forest Row, England 2010.

Lewin, L.: Gifte und Vergiftungen. 6. Aufl. Haug Verlag, Heidelberg 1992.

Lievegoed, B. C.: Heilpädagogische Betrachtung. 2. Aufl. Edition Bingenheim, Wuppertal 1986; 3. Aufl. Verlag Freies Geistesleben, Stuttgart 1995.

Lowe A. et al: Paracetamol use in early life and asthma: prespective birth cohort study. BMJ **341**, published online doi: 10.1136/bmj.c4616.

Lundberg, J. O. et al.: Nasally exhaled nitric oxide in humans originates mainly in paranasal sinuses. Act Physiol Scand **152,** 431–432 (1994).

Lundberg, J. O.: Nitric oxide and the Paranasal Sinuses. The anatomical record **291,** 1479–1484 (2008).

Lutzker, P.: Der Sprachsinn. Verlag Freies Geistesleben, Stuttgart 1996.

Maddaus, G.: Lehrbuch der Biologischen Heilmittel. 3 Bde. Olms Verlag Hildesheim 1979.

Marra, F., Lynd, L., Coombes, M., Richardson, K., Legal, M., Fitzgerald, J. M., Marra, C. A: Does antibiotic exposure during infancy lead to development of asthma? Chest **129**, 610–618 (2006).

Martinez, F.: Inhaled corticosteroids and asthma prevention. The Lancet **368**, 708–710 (2006).

McDonald K. et al.: Delay in diphtheria, pertussis, tetanus vaccination is associated with a reduced risk of childhood asthma. J Allergy Clin Immunol **121,** 626–631 (2008).

Melnik, B. C.: Biochemie und Pathobiochemie des epidermalen Lipidstoffwechsels. Stuttgart 1990, zit. bei Jachens 1999b.

Merkurstab, Sonderheft Organpräparate **52** (1999).

Meyer, U.: Eiche und Birke – Heilmittel für allergische und dermatologische Erkrankungen. Der Merkurstab **50,** 171 (1997).

Meyer, U.: Die Eiche – Heilmittel für allergische und dermatologische Erkrankungen. Der Merkurstab **58,** 358–364 (2005).

Meyer, U.: Die Gerbstoff-Therapie des Asthma bronchiale. Pharmazeutische Gesichtspunkte zu Quercus, Salix, Juglans und Salvia.

Mitschenko, A. V.: Neurodermitis und Stress. Wie kommen Gefühle in die Haut? Der Hautarzt **59,** 314–318 (2008).

Morrison, R.: Handbuch der homöopathischen Leitsymptome. Kai Kröger Verlag, Groß Wittensee 1995.

Muche-Borowski, C. et al.: S3-Leitlinie Allergieprävention – Update 2009. Allergo J **18,** 332–341.

Müller M. et al: Specific TRPC6 channel activation a novel approach to stimulate keratinocyte differentiation. J Biol Chem **283** 33942–54.

Murray, C. S. et al: Secondary prevention of asthma by the use of Inhaled Fluticason propionate in Wheezy INfants (IFWIN): double-blind, randomized, controlled Study. The Lancet **368,** 754–762 (2006).

Mutius, E. v.: Epidemiologie allergischer Erkrankungen. In: Pädiatrische Allergologie und Immunologie. Wahn, U., R. Seger, V. Wahn (Hrsg.). Urban & Fischer, München, 3. Aufl. 1999a, 4. Aufl. 2005.

Mutius, E. v.: Epidemiologie atopischer Erkrankungen, Vortragsabstract. M. Schr. Kinderheilk. Suppl. **2,** 55 (1999b).

Mutius, E. v.: Living on a Farm: Impact on Asthma Induction and Clinical Course. Immunol Allergy Clin N Am **28,** 631–647 (2008).

Mutius, E. v.: Prävalenz und Determinanten des Asthma bronchiale. MSchr Kinderheilk **158,** 121–128 (2010).

Nash, E. B.: Leitsymptome in der homöopathischen Therapie. Haug Verlag, Heidelberg 1996.

National Institutes of Health (National Heart, Lung and Blood Institute). Guidelines for the diagnostics and management of asthma (1977); zit. nach Schuster u. Reinhardt.

Nickmilder, M. et al: Respiratory Health and Pulmonary Epithelium Integrity of Swimming babies. Proceeding of the American Thoracic Society **3,** A 23 (2006).

Ornish, D.: Revolution in der Herztherapie. Kreuz Verlag, Stuttgart 1998.

Patzlaff, R.: Kindheit verstummt – Verlust und Pflege der Sprache im Medienzeitalter. Erziehungskunst **7/8,** 779–802 (1999).

Pechmann, H.: Ein neu durchdachtes Renodoron: Silex-Lapis Cancri solutus. Der Merkurstab **55,** 56 (2002).

Pedersen, PA. Pharmazeutische Betrachtungen zu Gencydo. Weleda. Korrespondenzblätter für Ärzte **129,** 5–19 (1991).

Pelikan, W.: Heilmittel aus dem Tierreich. Der Merkurstab **51,** 54 (1999).

Pelikan, W.: Heilpflanzenkunde I. Phil.-Anthrop. Verlag, Dornach 1980.

Pelikan, W.: Healing plants: insights through spiritual science. Mercury Press, Spring Valley, N.Y. 1997. Note: only this volume has been translated into English.

Pfeiffer, H., Drescher, M., Hirte, M.: Homöopathie in der Kinder- und Jugendmedizin. Urban & Fischer, München, 2.Aufl. 2007.

Portmann, A.: Einführung in die vergleichende Morphologie der Wirbeltiere. 6. Aufl. Schwabe Verlag, Basel 1983.

Raile, K., Kiess, W. et al.: Äthiopathogenese des Typ-1-Diabetes mellitus. Kinder- und Jugendmedizin **5**, 184–191 (2005).

Rauber, A., F. Kopsch: Anatomie des Menschen, Bd. III Nervensystem, Sinnesorgane. Leonhardt, H., G. Töndury, K. Zilles (Hrsg.). Thieme Verlag, Stuttgart 1987.

Reinhardt, D.: Asthma bronchiale im Kindesalter. 2. Aufl. Springer Verlag, Berlin, New York 1996.

Rembold, H., H. Oetzel: Kontrolle der Hausstaubmilbe D. farinae durch Wirkstoffe aus dem Samen des Neembaums, Azadirachta indica A. Juss. Allergo J. **13**, 269–273 (2004).

Renz, H.: Immunologische Grundlagen allergischer Erkrankungen. In: Pädiatrische Allergologie und Immunologie. Wahn, U., R. Seger, V. Wahn (Hrsg.). 3. Aufl. Urban & Fischer, München, Jena 1999.

Riedler, J., C. Braun-Fahrländer et al.: Exposure to farming in early life and development of asthma and allergy: a cross-sectional survey. Lancet **358**, 1129–1133 (2001).

Ring, J.: Atopische Dermatitis, in: Braun-Falco et al (Hrsg.): Dermatologie und Venerologie, 5. Auflage Springer, Berlin 2005.

Rispens, J. A.: Zwischen Esche und Eiche – die Walnuss Juglans regia. Der Merkurstab **63**, 224–234 (2010).

Rosenbauer, J et al: Incidence of childhood Type I diabetes mellitus is increasing at all ages in Germany. Diabetologica **45**, 457–458 (2002).

Rosenlund, H.: Allergic Disease and Atopic Sensitization in Children in Relation to Measles Vaccination and Measles Infection. Pediatrics **123**, 771–778 (2009).

Sankaran,R.: Struktur. Erfahrungen mit dem Mineralreich. 2 Bde. Homoepathic Medical Publishers, Mumbai 2010.

Schad, W.: Säugetier und Mensch. Verlag Freies Geistesleben, Stuttgart 1971.

Schäfer, S.: Gesunde Kinder mit Freude am Essen. Der Merkurstab **62**, 476–484 (2009).

Schaub, B: Asthma bronchiale. Pränatale Einflüsse auf die Immunentwicklung im Kindesalter. MSchr Kinderheilk **158,** 137–141 (2008).

Scheffler, A. et al.: Zur Heilprozessidee von Birkenrinde und Hautkrankheiten. Der Merkurstab **57**, 453–466 (2004).

Schempp et al.: Antibacterial activity of hyperforin from St.Johns wort, against multiresistant Staphylococcus aureus and grampositive bacteria. Lancet **353,** 2129 (1999).

Schempp, C. M. et al., Koriander (Coriandrium sat.) – ein heilkräftiger und antimikrobiell wirksamer mediterraner Doldenblütler. In: Der Merkurstab **64**(4) 2011, 339–345.

Schlaud M. et al.: Allergische Erkrankungen. Ergebnisse aus dem Kinder-und Jugendgesundheitssurvey (KiGGS).

Schnopp, C.: Neurodermitis – neue Aspekte in Prävention und Behandlung. Bay. Ärztebl. **10**, 654–658 (2005).

Schnürer, C.: Mehr Luft. Atemwegserkrankungen verstehen und überwinden. Verlag Freies Geistesleben, Stuttgart 2006.

Scholten,J.: Homöopathie und Minerale. Stichting Alonissos, Utrecht 1993.

Schrauzer, G.: Selen. J. A. Barth Verlag, Leipzig 1998.

Schulte-Wissermann, H.: Milzverlust und Immundefekt. In: Pädiatrische Allergologie und Immunologie. Wahn, U., R. Seger, V. Wahn (Hrsg.). 3. Aufl. Urban & Fischer, München, Jena 1999.

Schuster, A., D. Reinhardt: Asthma bronchiale. In: Pädiatrische Allergologie und Immunologie. Wahn, U., R. Seger, V. Wahn (Hrsg.). 3. Aufl. Urban & Fischer, München, Jena 1999.

Seiler, H.: Die Entwicklung von Samuel Hahnemanns ärztlicher Praxis. Haug Verlag, Heidelberg 1988.

Selawry, A.: Silber und Silber-Therapie. Haug Verlag, Ulm 1966.

Selawry, A.: Metall-Funktionstypen in Psychologie und Medizin. Haug Verlag, Heidelberg 1991.

Simon, L.: Indikationen anthroposophischer Arzneimittel aus gesichteter ärztlicher Erfahrung. Kap. Pharmazeutische Prozesse. Hrsg. von der Gesellschaft Anthroposophischer Ärzte in Deutschland. Der Merkurstab **61**, 1, Supplement (2008) – in Druck –.

Soldner, G.: Cobaltum met. bei Vitamin-B_{12}-Unverträglichkeit. Der Merkurstab **57**, 302–303 (2004).

Soldner, G.: Erfahrungen in der Therapie von Atemwegserkrankungen im Kindesalter. Erfahrungsheilkunde **40**, 66 (1991).

Soldner, G., M. Sommer: Allantois und Astralleib – wie können wir Rudolf Steiners Forschungsergebnisse nachvollziehen? Der Merkurstab **60**, 27–35 (2007).

Sommer, M., G. Soldner: Die Farne in Natur und Mensch – zum Verständnis von Digestodoron. Der Merkurstab **5**, 289–296 (1990).

Sommer, M.: Plexus pulmonales – eine Kasuistik. Der Merkurstab **47**, 358–359 (1994).

Sommer, M.: Sonnenfinsternis als Zeichen. Der Merkurstab **52**, 222–224 (1999).

Sommer, M., G. Soldner: Merkur in Natur und Mensch I. Der Merkurstab **41**, 279–289 (1988a).

Sommer, M., G. Soldner: Merkur in Natur und Mensch II. Der Merkurstab **41**, 337–343 (1988b).

Sommer, M., Paulig, M.: Potenziertes Kupfer bei Alpträumen von Verstorbenen. Wirksamkeitsbelegan Einzelfällen. Der Merkurstab **54**,146–152.

Steiner, R.: Anthroposophie – ein Fragment. Gesamtausgabe Bd. 45. Rudolf Steiner Verlag, Dornach, 4.Aufl. 2002.

- Steiner, R.: Anthroposophy: A Fragment. GA (complete works) 45. Anthroposophic Press, Hudson, N. Y. 1996.

Steiner, R.: Die Methodik des Lernens und die Lebensbedingungen des Erziehens. GA 308, Vortrag vom 9.4.1924, in: R. Steiner Tb Bd. 658 (1924).

Steiner, R.: Das Verhältnis verschiedener naturwissenschaftlicher Gebiete zur Astronomie. Dritter naturwissenschaftlicher Kurs [1921]. Gesamtausgabe Bd. 323. Rudolf Steiner Verlag, Dornach, 3. Aufl. 1997.

Steiner, R.: Geisteswissenschaftliche Gesichtspunkte zur Therapie. Gesamtausgabe Bd. 313. Rudolf Steiner Verlag, Dornach 4. Aufl. 1984.

- Steiner, R.: Anthroposophical spiritual science and medical therapy: second medical course, nine lectures to physicians and medical students, Dornach, April 11–18, 1921. GA (complete works) 313. Mercury Press, Spring Valley, N. Y. 1991.

Steiner, R.: Meditative Betrachtungen und Anleitungen zur Vertiefung der Heilkunst. Gesamtausgabe Bd. 316. Rudolf Steiner Verlag, Dornach, 3. Aufl. 1987.

- Steiner, R.: Course for young doctors: meditative contemplations and instructions for deepening the art of healing: lectures for physicians and medical students. GA (complete works) 316. Mercury Press, Spring Valley, N. Y. 1994.

Steiner, R.: Erdenwissen und Himmelserkenntnis. 3. Aufl. Rudolf Steiner Verlag, Dornach 1998.

Steiner, R.: Heilpädagogischer Kurs. Gesamtausgabe Bd. 317. 7. Aufl. Rudolf Steiner Verlag, Dornach 1985.

- Steiner, R.: Education for special needs: the curative education course; twelve lectures for doctors and teachers given at Dornach between 25 June and 7 July 1924. GA (complete works) 317. Rudolf Steiner Press, London 1998.

Steiner, R.: Geisteswissenschaftliche Menschenkunde. 5. Aufl. Rudolf Steiner Verlag, Dornach 1988.

- Steiner, R.: Fundamentals of anthroposophical medicine. GA (complete works) 314. Mercury Press, Spring Valley, N. Y. 1986.

Steiner, R.: Physiologisch-Therapeutisches auf Grundlage der Geisteswissenschaften. Gesamtausgabe Bd. 314, 3. Aufl. Rudolf Steiner Verlag, Dornach 1989.

Steiner, R.: Allgemeine Menschenkunde als Grundlage der Pädagogik. Rudolf Steiner Verlag, Dornach 1975.

- Steiner, R.: Study of man: general education course : fourteen lectures given in Stuttgart between 21 August and 5 September 1919. GA (complete works) 293. Rudolf Steiner Press, London 2004. See also: Steiner, R.: Foundations of human experience. GA (complete works) 293. Anthroposophic Press, Hudson, N. Y. 1996.

Steiner, R.: Das Zusammenwirken von Ärzten und Seelsorgern. Pastoralmedizinischer Kurs. Gesamtausgabe Bd. 318.Rudolf Steiner Verlag, Dornach 3. Aufl. 1994.

- Steiner, R.: Pastoral medicine: the collegial working of doctors and priests: eleven lectures delivered in Dornach in September of 1924. GA (complete works) 318. Anthroposophic Press, Hudson, N. Y. 1987. Also published as: Broken vessels: the spiritual structure of human frailty. Anthroposophic Press, Great Barrington, M. A. 2003.

Steiner, R.: Anthroposophische Menschenerkenntnis und Medizin. Gesamtausgabe Bd. 319. Rudolf Steiner Verlag, Dornach 3. Aufl. 1994.

- Steiner, R.: The healing process: spirit, nature and our bodies: lectures, August 28, 1923-August 29, 1924, in various cities. GA (complete works) 319. Anthroposophic Press, Hudson, N. Y. 2000.

Steiner R.: Das Initiatenbewusstsein. Gesamtausgabe Bd. 243. Rudolf Steiner Verlag, Dornach 6. Aufl. 2004.

- Steiner, R.: True and false paths in spiritual investigation. GA (complete works) 243. Rudolf Steiner Press/Anthroposophic Press, London/New York 1985.

Steiner, R.: Geisteswissenschaft und Medizin. Gesamtausgabe Bd. 312. Rudolf Steiner Verlag, Dornach 7. Aufl. 1999.

- Steiner, R.: Introduction to anthroposophical medicine. GA (complete works) 312. SteinerBooks, Great Barrington, M. A. 1999.

Steiner, R., I. Wegman: Grundlegendes zu einer Erweiterung der Heilkunst nach geisteswissenschaftlichen Erkenntnissen. Gesamtausgabe Bd. 27. Rudolf Steiner Verlag, Dornach 7. Aufl. 1991.

Steiner, R., I. Wegman: Fundamentals of therapy : an extension of the art of healing through spiritual-scientific knowledge. GA (complete works) 027. Mercury Press, Spring Valley, N. Y. 1999. Also available as: Extending practical medicine: fundamental principles based on the science of the spirit. Rudolf Steiner Press, London 1996.

Streber, A., Egger, A.: KinderLeicht. Wie übergewichtige Kinder abnehmen und Lebensfreude gewinnen. ebook, Kösel, München 2010. www.kinderleichtmuenchen.de.

Strüh, H. J.: Equisetum und Kiesel. In: T. de Brahe-Jahrbuch für Goetheanismus. Tycho de Brahe-Verlag, Niefern 1989.

Stübler, M., E. Krug (Hrsg.): Leesers Lehrbuch der Homöopathie. 3. Aufl. Haug Verlag, Heidelberg 1987.

Suchantke, G.: Ergebnisse und Erfahrungen in der Behandlung vonAsthma bronchiale. In: Beiblätter der Zeitschrift Natura, Dornach, Natura Verlag 2000.

Traencker, I. et al.: Die Behandlung des atopischen Ekzems in interdisziplinärer Zusammenarbeit zwischen Dermatologie und Psychosomatik. Hausarzt **47**, 628–633 (1996).

Treichler, R.: Die Entwicklung der Seele im Lebenslauf. Verlag Freies Geistesleben, Stuttgart, 3. Aufl. 1981, 5. Aufl. 1995.

Vademecum Anthroposophische Arzneimittel. 2.Aufl. Der Merkurstab **63**, Supplement (2010).

Vademecum of anthroposophic medicines, CD format. Medical Section of the School of Spiritual Science, Dornach, Switzerland 2009. Velicer, C. M. et al.: Antibiotic Use in Relation to the Risk of Breast Cancer. J. Am. Med. Ass. **291**, 827–835 (2004).

Vermeulen, F.: Kindertypen in der Homöopathie. 5. Aufl. Sonntag, Regensburg 1999.

Voegeli, A.: Das Asthma und seine homöopathische Behandlung. 5. Aufl. Haug Verlag, Heidelberg 1996.

Vogel, H. H.: Ein Beitrag zur Ekzem-Therapie. Beitr. z. Erw. d. Heilkunst **9/10**, 191 (1954).

Vogel, H. H.: Beiträge zu einer medizinischen Menschenkunde, Bd. 1, Teil II. Haug Verlag, Heidelberg 1984.

Vogel, H. H.: Beiträge zu einer medizinischen Menschenkunde, Bd. 1, Teil I. Haug Verlag, Heidelberg 1987.

Vogel, H. H.: Wege der Heilmittelfindung, Bd. 2. Natur Mensch Medizin Verlag, Bad Boll 1994.

Vogel, H.-H.: Finding remedies: spiritual knowledge of man and naure; a contribution toward understanding anthroposophic remedies, based on the example of the Wala remedy compositions. V 1, 2 Natur-Mensch-Medizin, Bad Boll 1994.

Vogel, H. H.: Die vier Hauptorgane. Natur Mensch Medizin, Bad Boll 1995.

Vogel, H. H.: Organe der Ich-Organisation. Natur Mensch Medizin, Bad Boll 1996.

Vögler, H.: Asthma bronchiale – klinisch-therapeutisches Kolloquium. Beitr. z. Erw. d. Heilk. **40**, 308 (1987).

Voisin, C.. Infant swimming in chlorinated pools and the risks of bronchiolitis, asthma and allergy. Eur Respiratory J **36,** 1–8 (2008).

Wahn, V.: Fragenbeantwortung Frage 5012. Consilium infectiorum **57,** 4–5 (2006).

Wolff, O.: Biochemie. Verlag Freies Geistesleben, Stuttgart 1998.

Waser, M.: Inverse association of farm milk consumption with asthma and allergy in rural and suburban populations across Europe. Clin Exp Allergy **37,** 661–670 (2006)

Weber, G.: Zweierlei Glück. Die systemische Psychotherapie Bert Hellingers. Auer-Systeme, Heidelberg, 7. Aufl. 1995, 13. Aufl. 2000

Weiß, R. F., V. Fintelmann: Lehrbuch der Phytotherapie. 9. Aufl. Hippokrates, Stuttgart 1999

Weizsäcker, V. v.: Fälle und Probleme. Anthropologische Vorlesungen in der medizinischen Klinik. F. Enke Verlag, Stuttgart 1947

Werner, H.: Inhalationstherapie bei Asthma. Beitr. z. Erw. d. Heilk. **36**, 102–105 (1983)

Wright, R. et al.: Parental Stress as a Predictor of Wheezing in Infancy. Am J Respir Crit Care Med **165,** 358–365 (2002)

Woodcook, A. et al.: Allergy 2005; dol:10.1111/j.1298–9995.2005.00941.x

7 Psychosomatic disorders

"To attain any assured knowledge about the soul is one of the most difficult things in the world. [...] it might seem that there is some single method of inquiry applicable to all objects whose essential nature we wish to gain knowledge of. But if there is no such single and general method [...], our task becomes still more difficult; in the case of each different subject we shall have to determine the appropriate process of investigation."

Aristotle, On the Soul

The disorders described below are generally associated with the soul entity of the child and in part they are viewed as determined by it. This insight is reflected in the heading of this chapter. To the reader of the preceding chapter it will have become entirely clear, however, that *for every disorder* it is necessary to distinguish between the *purely physical aspect* and the *living self-activity* of the organism. The latter, as a complex of processes, is directed at the preservation and regeneration of organs, thus constituting the real foundation of all (self) healing processes. The *soul aspect* reveals itself directly in *sensation* (for example pain), *consciousness* and *active locomotion* (▸Chap. 1.3) and is involved in the incidence of disease in various ways. It must be distinguished from the life organization, the etheric body of the human being. Every cough, as it were, constitutes a psychosomatic disorder – and the incidence of disease rarely exists without participation of the soul entity. This participation is practically never of a purely passive nature; even the type of pain involved and its intensity depend not only on bodily factors, but also to a considerable degree on the regulating activity of the soul organization [Egle et al. 1999, 19]. Soul perception reflects itself bodily; heart and respiratory rates are examples of this.

Spiritual individuality, *the human I,* is to be distinguished from the soul aspect in the narrower sense of the word (▸Chap. 1.3). It elevates the human being out of the circle of ensouled organisms and invests the person with a capacity for development and learning, potentially empowering every human being to attain free thought and self-reliant action. The human I is the incarnation of a creatively active, spiritual individuality in an earthly being. All processes in the human organism are at its service and are influenced by it. The presence of the I can be perceived in every newborn child and even in the most severely disabled children. The intentionally will-oriented nature of the I is the foundation for child development. The capacity of the I for living and acting in mutual perception and participation of I and Thou forms the foundation of human maturation. As a practical science, as an art of beneficial action [Wieland 2006], medicine has its roots in dialogue, in mutual respect and support of I and Thou.

In the previous chapters it was repeatedly shown how the activity of the I determines the emergence and course of disease to a substantial degree, even influencing what would appear to be purely somatic diseases (such as pneumonia, ▸Chap. 5.1.1). From this perspective, every human disease is a psycho-somatic event. However, inferring the causative aspect of the disease from the level of its primary manifestation can prove deceptive. Cuts on the extremities can be caused by auto-aggressive behaviour, somnolence can be induced by brain pressure from a brain tumour. The symptoms of coeliac disease can appear qualitatively as irritability and fatigue whereas the severity of anorexia nervosa can practically be measured in terms of weight curves, amenorrhea and possibly electrolyte imbalances. These are somatic parameters which have nothing to do with the cause of the disease. Such reflections show that the concept "psychosomatic" is tentative in nature and of little use per se for diagnostic and therapeutic comprehension of human diseases. In reality it is always the task of the doctor to *include all aspects of human existence in his or her perceptions and judgments as equally real, participatory factors in disease.* Their relation to one another, their etiological significance for the incidence of disease is never completely predictable and generalizable, as little as the appropriate therapeutic response is!

In the present medical climate, when great emphasis is placed on catalogued diagnosis and therapeutic guidelines, it is necessary to point out the following: conceptually speaking, rigorous *generalizations* can only be made *within the particular aspects of medical observations and measurements,* such as reference values for sodium concentration, growth rate, child development "milestones", or benchmarks for cognitive performance. *Individual* diagnosis and therapy are only possible if intrinsically differing aspects – the soul, life, spiritual and physical aspects *have been brought into correspondence with one another by the doctor* and determined in their relation to one another. *This act is only possible if it is performed in reference to the individual, the patient in question; it constitutes the decisive quality of individual paediatrics.*

7.1 Sleep disorders

> It turned out that the greatest determining factor of sleep disturbance was the child's perception of parental conflict.
>
> Palmstierna, Sepa, Ludvigsson [2008]

> A sleep-deprived parent often experiences helplessness, frustration, anxiety, anger, self-blame, negative self-evaluation, and depression.
>
> Jan et al. [2008]

7

Many parents feel the sleep behaviour of their child is abnormal, and feel burdened by this. On the other hand, some parents only report their child's sleep pattern when relevant questions have been asked by the doctor; these parents may accept a child's sleep behaviour that from a medical point of view is clearly disturbed. Psychological ambivalence is frequently encountered: parents, especially the mothers, suffer a lack of sleep and are often "stressed", which is accompanied by a more or less conscious aggression towards the child and/or partner. The British artist Henry Moore has produced a remarkable display of the archetypical feelings of a mother who is literally being eaten up by her child (in the sculpture, the child at the mother's breast threatens to devour her like a wolf). On the other hand, a mother can in these situations induce excess binding of the child to her through lack of boundaries (e.g. lack of rhythm), insecurity, guilt and partner conflicts – this can cause or reinforce sleep problems (cf. the two works quoted in the quote above).

Within the framework of individual paediatrics, the diagnosis, parental guidance and therapy of sleep disturbances are of increasing significance. A medical practice whose spectrum is broadened by anthroposophic medicine and homoeopathy generally leads to very satisfying results.

7.1.1 Function of sleep

> Notably high prevalence of problems with falling asleep or not sleeping through the night among first-graders (15 %) as well as instances of recurring nightmares (14 %) are reported by parents. ... As regards co-morbidity ... the risk of hyperactivity or emotional problems is two to three times higher.
>
> Kraenz et al. [2004]

> The results indicate a close connection between sleeping disorders and emotional disturbances.
>
> Lehmkuhl, Wiater et al. [2008]

Falling asleep and waking up are profound psychosomatic changes of state in human beings, surpassed in magnitude by birth and death alone. They are not the passive consequence of external conditions (for example changes in light), but rather are produced *actively* by the human organism. This simple fact alone can make doctors and parents aware that falling asleep should not be induced primarily by external means but rather *must be learned by the child*[1]. – In this process, conditions which differ fundamentally in psychosomatic terms alternate in *rhythmic succession*:

- The waking state, in which sensual perception, consciousness and impulses of the will penetrate the body process to increasingly high degrees and determine its orientation.
- The state of sleep, in which sense perception of the external world, thinking consciousness, active orientation and locomotion are suspended while growth and regeneration processes take the lead.
- Intermediate states in which the soul aspect – in the form of dreaming, somnambulism, etc. – becomes active in the body but still without any direct intervention by the I (no waking consciousness, no self-controlled, fully rememberable consciousness and action).

Evolutionarily speaking, the sleep-wake rhythm evolves in connection with increasing respiration activity (basal metabolism; metabolic rate) and development of warmth (warm-bloodedness; homoiothermy) in higher animals. Whereas ectotherms only demonstrate simply organized phases of rest, highly developed mammals and birds exhibit differentiated, multi-phase sleep processes consisting of so-called REM and non-REM phases. Careful observation and physiological findings indicate that intermediate dreaming states occur in these animals as well [Schmidt and Thews 1995, 152]. The deeper the soul penetrates the body, the more clearly apparent is the necessity to balance the waking state with a corresponding sleeping state. This correlates with previously gained insights into the vital importance of sleep for human beings [Schmidt and Thews 1995,

1 Should this hold for all of us in regard to dying as well? Falling asleep is a matter of vital fatigue and the soul's trust in what supports it. Cf. Girke [2010, 605–612]

152]. From a purely physiological standpoint, this necessity continues to remain completely incomprehensible to date. As opposed to the vital – and measurable – need for fluids and solid food, what constitutes vital core sleep cannot be quantified in ml or kcal; it can only be expressed in terms of time – with relatively large variances. This begs the question as to what occurs in sleep that is so necessary to compensate for the waking state.

Moreover, sleep is a phenomenon of cultural development. In the wild, no deep sleep exists. Wild adult giraffes, which, as full-grown animals, have no natural enemies while in the waking state, sleep less than one hour per day. The lifespan of a wild giraffe is only about 10 years; giraffes living in zoos can live almost three times as long. – *Deep sleep requires the safety of a protected space and trust in the human community which creates such space.* This also illuminates the occurrence of sleep disorders in families in which divorce of the parents is imminent, during and after hospitalization of children, and in other comparable situations. Among adults, the proportion of those in need of treatment for sleep disorders is estimated to be 10 % [Girke 2010, 605]. If one considers that small children learn through imitation and that both the child's temperament and the parents play indisputably significant roles in childhood sleep disorders, it is conceivable that the frequency of sleep disorders requiring treatment is greater among adults than among children. Like it or not, paediatricians who wish to influence sleep disorders or even treat them are always functioning as family doctor.

In bodily terms, sleep is connected with *anabolic* processes, with *growth processes* whereas waking consciousness and active self-locomotion are linked to the dominance of *catabolic* processes. *Deep sleep* is linked to the *impulsation of growth*, REM sleep with *learning processes* (see below). *These two qualities* of sleep are associated with one another, and in infants and small children they are very strongly pronounced in physiological terms. The *ordering function* which sleep provides for normalization of the pulse-breathing quotient during the night is clearly evident; it can compensate in many ways for the bodily effects of "unhealthy" chaotic soul impulses during the day [Roßlenbroich 1994, 21–23; Hildebrandt 1960, 533–615; 1998]. *The rhythm of waking and sleeping stabilizes and orders the entire rhythmical process in human beings.* The basic function of the rhythmical system is to facilitate and organize the interplay of polar forces and functions (for example respiration and circulation, the nervous and the digestive system, etc.) and to balance out the predominance of one-sided qualities [Roßlenbroich 1994, 43]. Ultimately, all psychosomatic connections are conveyed rhythmically; *maintenance or increase of soul and bodily health is determined primarily by the vibrancy and stability of the rhythmical system.* The urgency of this topic shows itself in the current dominance of cardiovascular diseases as well as bronchial asthma and other chronic diseases of the rhythmical system (▸Chap. 6.5).

Great importance is attached to the discovery that REM sleep in particular is connected with learning processes which are of elementary significance for life-long promotion of health, namely *the learning processes of the immune system.* "On the basis of experiments with rats it could be shown that in cases of selective REM suppression, severe immune suppression occurred followed by sepsis. In human beings, complete sleep deprivation leads to death by septicaemia within a period of 14 days at the latest, as is shown by some unfortunately still commonly used methods of torture." [Girke 2010, 610]

Sleep allows the results of soul and spiritual activity performed in the waking state to influence corresponding formative processes of the body: "learning increases the duration of REM sleep and REM sleep is accompanied by an increase in neuronal RNA and DNA synthesis, which is essential for long-term memory." The growth and activity level of plastic synapses [Schmidt and Thews 1995, 153] in the brain are stimulated in the corresponding sleep phases – and one may assume that this holds true for organs like the thymus (▸Chap. 6.3.3.4) and immunological learning processes in comparable ways. These are body-structuring processes which derive their actual shaping principle from I activity, i. e. soul experiences during the day. This is not only true for the brain; the skeletal and muscle growth, for example, essentially follow the form in which they are taxed by the waking human being. "Contrary to previous assumptions, REM sleep primarily plays a role when it comes to learning practical skills." [Girke 2010, 610]. Thus the significance of sleep is expanded; not only does it take strain off the body by releasing it from direct intervention of the soul and spiritual entities (I and astral body) during sleep; it also enables the body to be built up in an individualized way – in accordance with how these higher human aspects, the astral and the I, have acted on the body during waking time. "Thus in regard to sleeping human beings, one cannot speak of mere vegetative activity in the organism. … The difference between sleeping and waking does not lie in alternation between human-animal and vegetative-physical activity. The facts of the matter are completely different." [Steiner and Wegman 1991, 38]. To be sure, when human beings fall asleep the life organization takes the lead; but its formative processes, which are active during sleep, are oriented towards that which was stimulated or induced by soul and spirit-led activity in the waking state, even extending into substance formation: "In the waking human organism, the astral body and I-organization are active themselves, whereas in the sleeping organism their substantial residues are active" [Steiner and Wegman 1991, 39]. This translation of intentional soul and spiritual activity into the (unconscious) formation and alteration of the body is of central significance for human learning and acquisition of skills: only that which has passed "through the night" and extended into the realm of the physical aspect can be truly appropriated by the human being! This not only holds for long-term memory and recollection but also for all kinds of skills. Every pianist has experienced being able to play what was practiced the day before at a level surpassing that of previous performance. Thus small children also often demonstrate new progress and newly acquired skills after waking up in the morning.

What the soul and the human I experience in deep sleep must remain an open question at this point. Nothing contradicts the assumption that the soul and spiritual individuality itself can only achieve direct penetration and guidance of the body for a limited time, that consciously experienced events of the day overtax it, just as the body organization is incapable of enduring persistent wakefulness. On the basis of its own spiritual scientific observation, anthroposophy echoes the assertions made by earlier cultures that sleep enables the soul and the I to regenerate themselves through emergence from the narrow bodily attachment and to move back in the direction of the supersensory, spiritual sphere from which human individuality originates and to which it returns after death [Steiner 1979, 66f., cf. Girke 2010, 608f., including literature].

The rhythm of waking and sleeping presents an elementary challenge for a psychosomatic understanding of the human being. At the same time, what has been expounded here underscores the profound significance which sleep has for child health, development and maturation. Therapeutically speaking, many aspects addressed in this book, from the development of immune regulation in early childhood to hyperactivity and attentiveness disorder, can be strongly influenced by quality of sleep. Treatment of sleep disorders, particularly in early childhood, can have various positive effects on child development, especially since studies show that sleep patterns acquired in early childhood exhibit a large degree of intra-individual constancy. Learning how to sleep is one of the elementary learning processes in early childhood.

7.1.2 Development of sleep during childhood

The sleep duration of newborns, averaging 16 hours out of 24 hours, stands in a ratio of 2:1 to waking phases. At age 3 the ratio is generally 1:1 and by the time adulthood is reached the ratio is exactly the reverse of that of the newborn [Schmidt and Thews 1995, 149]. In the beginning, numerous sleep periods (up to approx. twelve) of relatively short duration are divided up almost evenly across daytime and night-time (polyphasic sleep). It normally takes six to twelve months for the child's night sleep to reach its full extent. Starting with the third week of life, but with significant individual differences, the initial numerous short sleep phases gradually merge into monophasic night sleep differentiated into the various known sleep stages [Kast-Zahn and Morgenroth 1997, 30; Hellbrügge 1965]. From the fourth week of life, a day-night rhythm develops in the warmth organization (measurable by body temperature); from the sixth week of life, a day-night rhythm becomes identifiable on the basis of the pulse rate; various kidney functions begin to exhibit a diurnal rhythm at various times (this development continues until the second year of life), whereas electrical skin resistance, for example, already demonstrates a clear 24-hour periodicity within the first week of life [Roßlenbroich 1994, 114–119].

In scientific investigations as well as in paediatric practice, a *very large range of variation in sleep duration* is found, with extremes between 7 and 20 hours among infants in the first weeks of life, without this being primarily attributable to exogenic factors [Hellbrügge 1965, Hellbrügge et al. 1963, Largo 2001]. However, it is not rare to find similarities to one parent, and in almost every case paedagogical and medical possibilities exist for adjusting the sleep behaviour to the normal development as described above. Establishment of a regular daily rhythm is fundamental for the development of a stable day-night rhythm, particularly in regard to light, feeding and communication with the child.

With the invention of the electric light bulb in the nineteenth century by Edison, who was almost fanatically convinced that human beings sleep too much, human beings became increasingly independent of the natural day-night-rhythm (designated by Webb as the "Edison effect") [Barbely 1984]. The *loss of rhythm* in the work world and decontrol of time structures during leisure time overstrain many young parents confronted with the task of providing their children with the daily routine necessary for ensuring that the maturation processes that takes place during sleep are completed in harmony with the environment. Insecurity, anxiety, irritability, fatigue and irregular, dysfunctional sleep behaviour are characteristic of many adults as well. Shift work involving late and early shifts is particularly problematic. Since *children learn primarily by imitation and actually want to integrate themselves into an order prescribed by adults, it is necessary for these parents to create order and set an example by following it.* Thus in cases of sleep disorders it is of primary importance to call attention to this task while taking the history during consultations, for herein lies an essential key to therapy (▸Chap. 4.4).

If one takes a closer look at a newborn, one will ascertain that his or her apparently peaceful sleep is interrupted by agitation and motion in a wavelike fashion; sometimes sighing is audible followed by a deep, long breath of air and at times respiration is suspended … It almost appears as if the child were perpetuating the uterine contractions of the mother in metamorphized form. – Sleep research has shown that from approximately the sixth month on, when the various sleep stages during night sleep have become differentiated, the consecutive phases of deep and REM sleep are separated from each other by short moments of incomplete awakening. As Kast-Zahn and Morgenroth note, "no child really sleeps through the night" [Kast-Zahn and Morgenroth 1997, 33].

Interplay between soul and body (astral and etheric body) below the level of I-consciousness reflects itself in these phenomena. This also makes the affinity to the birth process, the primary ensoulment of the body in the first breath of air, comprehensible. Evidently the soul acts upon the bodily developmental processes *rhythmically* during the night below the I-level of consciousness; it makes sense to assume that this is of essential importance for processing waking experiences in dreams and for the individualized growth and transformation of organs. *At the same time a possible physiological foundation for sleep disorders lies in the depicted moments of incomplete awakening.* These moments of awakening, which occur from the sixth month of life on, take place at times when problems with sleeping through the night manifest themselves most frequently (for example 21:30–22:30, 1:30, 3:00–4:00). It is known that these points in time play a role for the day-night reversal in various organs (03.00 for the liver-gall bladder rhythm, for example); this seems to be accompanied by a more pronounced intervention of the soul. It is important to convey this knowledge to parents so that they do not react to temporary night time disturbance and brief awakening immediately by taking action on their own part; such interventions emphasize this necessary process as if it were a disorder. *If, however, the parents know about the nature and significance of interplay between body and soul during sleep they are more capable of exercising restraint and being perceptive; in* this way they can provide their child with the atmosphere of peaceful presence and affection necessary for him or her to be able to fall asleep again.

7.1.3 History and diagnosis

To begin with, it is necessary to determine whether the child has a sleep disorder. To do so one must be familiar with what constitutes normal sleep development and its range of variations. Up to 60 % of small children wake up spontaneously as early as 5:00 and up to 90 % wake up spontaneously by 6:00, with this changing considerably in children of school age. It is not rare for parents to depict their child's awakening at 5:00–06:00 as a sleep disorder – a time when a farmer might well open the barn door and a paediatrician might well turn off his alarm clock. Generally speaking, *signs of daytime fatigue* among children and parents are important signs of a sleep disorder which requires therapy. Another indication is found in depictions by parents which suggest that they are taking (increasingly long and frequent) measures to get the child to fall asleep or fall back to sleep. If necessary, a sleep log can clarify the extent of the disorder. Difficulties involving falling asleep or sleeping through the night must be distinguished from the following:

- Agitation day and night (hyperactive children, for example, often exhibit difficulties falling asleep and short sleep – ▸Chap. 7.5). This can possibly involve mutual aggravation of the phenomena but the problem cannot be reduced to the sleep disorder per se.
- So-called parasomnias: pavor nocturnus, nightmares, somnambulism. In diagnostic and therapeutic terms, these are certainly to be viewed as sleep disturbances, also concerning their consequences for daytime activity (see above).

In cases of sleep disorders among infants, a careful *pregnancy history* is necessary (▸Chap. 2.4):

- Was the child already agitated in the womb? Premature contractions, bleeding, tocolysis, emotional and physical stress can create a clear disposition for sleep disorders in early childhood.

Furthermore, questions concerning the child's *birth* (▸Chap. 2.2, ▸Chap. 2.3) are significant (birth trauma, mechanical irritations, delivery).

After addressing such questions, one must clarify when the child started having difficulties falling asleep. Was the child agitated from the very start or did the sleep disorder start to manifest at a later time. The following constitute possible triggers:

- Gastroesophageal reflux (▸Chap. 4.7.1)
- Teething
- Infections
- Vaccinations (▸Chap. 3.5.7), medications
- Changes in diet and dietary intolerances (most of all cow's milk or soy milk), disruption of intestinal symbiosis (particularly Candida, ▸Chap. 4.6)
- Physical and emotional traumata.

Particularly significant factors are *separation anxiety* (▸Chap. 7.2) on the part of the child *and* the parents, family crises, separation of the parents. In such cases one should make a careful attempt in the history to gain a realistic impression without assignment of guilt. It is also important to record the *sleep history of the parents* since the therapy described below must be planned with particular caution if one or both parents suffer from sleep disorders themselves or if the parents' sleeping situation is strained. The doctor should avoid "preaching" about rhythm until he or she is familiar with the real-life rhythms of the family and is thus able to develop approaches for implementing a positive change step by step.

Case study

A ten-year old girl, the youngest of three siblings, is brought in for consultation by her concerned mother because of increasingly pronounced school phobia and fear on her way to school. A separate conversation with the very caring father shows that

- there is a lot of tension in the marriage and the father has slept in another room for quite some time;
- the girl has been sleeping in the parents' bed next to her mother for more than half a year;
- the mother has issued an ultimatum to the father that he must drive their daughter to school every morning due to her fear on the way to school, a demand which he does not necessarily view as appropriate but complies with all the same in order to prevent the situation from escalating.

In a confidential talk with the mother alone – so as to prevent any loss of face – she is asked where the child sleeps. The mother depicts the situation with embarrassment, justifying it by saying she is convinced her fearful daughter needs this attention. As is made clear to her in the consultation, experience shows that in such a case school phobia could probably be cured quite quickly if the child slept alone in her own room (where she slept before the marriage crisis escalated). The mother ultimately agrees to seeing that the child starts sleeping in her own bed again within a period of four weeks. This plan is carried out, as is confirmed at the follow up appointment with the mother and the child 4 weeks later (after asking the child about this matter without any further comment, the doctor praises the child for her courage and self-reliance). After a few weeks the child goes to school every morning with a friend who lives nearby without experiencing any problems.

In children of school age, many disorders are significant: fears which arise in connection with school; conflicts with fellow pupils, parents and siblings as well as previously existing depressive and compulsive-neurotic disorders. Puberty brings about fundamental changes in sleep behaviour, with longer phases of falling asleep and more difficulties falling asleep. *Addictive behaviour* (drugs, video and computer game consumption etc.), adolescence crises, psychiatric disorders etc. can lead to symptomatic sleep disorders among this age group. Generally speaking, *fears* in childhood are often associated with disturbed sleep behaviour; in such cases treatment of the anxiety itself is of primary importance (▸Chap. 7.2).

In terms of differential diagnosis, particularly with difficulties sleeping through the night, *occult inflammation* (otitis, mastoiditis, urinary tract infections) and *malignoma* must be considered as a possibility or ruled out (nocturnal bone pain, for example, in cases of leukaemia and bone tumours, often goes unrecognized for long periods of time). In infancy rickets (▸Chap. 3.2) can manifest itself primarily in the form of a sleep disorder. Night sweats are a guiding symptom of rickets-induced sleep disorders and occult inflammations.

From an *environmental medicine* point of view of, disruptions of the sleeping place (for example through electronic devices and electrical cables, so-called water veins, toxins, etc.) must be ruled out, particularly if the child sleeps much better in other places than he or she does at home or there is a history of such burdens.

7.1.4 Consultation with parents

Wonderfully protected by good forces,
We confidently await what may come.
God is with us in the eve and the morn
And indeed on every new day.

Dietrich Bonhoeffer

The first treatment step consists in *medical consultation,* which – if possible – should convey to both parents insights into the development, the process and importance of sleep for the child. In doing so, the focus is put on the child, who can *learn* how to fall asleep and sleep through the night him or herself. The parents are instructed to stop *"inducing"* the child to fall asleep, *teaching him or her how to fall asleep* instead, i. e. conveying an essential ability to the child who makes it his or her own.

The foundation and prerequisite for treatment is the active and systematic establishment of a *rhythmical daily routine* with *set meal and bed times. The time from 6:00 p. m. on is of particular importance here:* during this time a recurring daily routine should be adhered to. Working mothers or fathers, who often come home late, must learn to integrate themselves into such a routine and not activate the child at inappropriate times, thus preventing the child from being able to fall asleep by him or herself.

An *evening ritual* characterized by responsiveness to the child's soul and a listening ear can facilitate the decisive reversal of endless parental activity into inner attention and serenity. Depending on the child's age this ritual can be carried out in various ways; what is essential is that a moment of open dialogue between the child and the parent engaging with the child occurs. In this moment it becomes possible to perceive the infant lovingly and to calm him or her down, to forgive the older child or give him or her the chance to tell what is occupying his or her thoughts. One can look back at the course of the day together, thus giving the child the opportunity to free himself or herself from tensions and anxieties, rebuilding trust by listening to him or her and speaking a few clarifying words.

Such a regularly recurring evening ritual in childhood can generate a source of emotional and physical strength for a lifetime. In a concluding prayer, the parents can strengthen the child's trust in the world wherein his or her soul approaches while falling asleep. This is the purpose of such a prayer, which corresponds directly with the purpose of sleep (every adult can experience for himself or herself that a genuine prayer spoken beforehand stimulates or facilitates the process of falling asleep as one which emanates from the soul entity and is actively consummated).

The child is laid down in bed, not carried around anymore, not soothed with a pacifier, a bottle or recorded music or a recorded fairy tale. A cuddly blanket or a plain doll, a short (for example pentatonic) lullaby or song played on a children's lyre can have a very calming influence, which can be observed immediately by a change in breathing.

It is important for parents to pay attention to *temperature conditions*. Physiologically speaking, the process of falling asleep is associated with an increased outflow of warmth from the centre to the periphery (this corresponds directly with the relative release of the I from the bodily aspect). On the other hand this means that the child will find it difficult to fall asleep if his or her periphery, arms and legs – and most of all feet! – are too cool and active warmth centralization (stress) or insufficient body temperature keeps the child from being able to warm them up.

Massaging oil into the limbs and back, for example with

- **Mallow oil** Wala or **Lavendula, Ol. aeth. 10 %**[1] Wala/Weleda,

suitable clothing, if possible made of wool, and corresponding blankets or a sleeping bag can aid the child in falling asleep.

7

Every infant and small child is reliant on the parents' perception and care when it comes to regulating his or her own body temperature. Since temperature conditions differ considerably from individual to individual, the doctor's task is primarily to train the *parents' perceptiveness* through instruction and query (▸Chap. 2.2.1). – This fundamental aspect is usually neglected altogether in common parent guidebooks!

- In the case of older children, this aspect is significant as well; in addition to the feet, the *area around the kidneys* is often relatively cool, a condition which can also be accompanied by sleep disorders. In such cases massaging the following into this area of the back has proven beneficial
- **Cuprum met. 0.4 % ointment** Weleda.

Warmth and trust are closely connected. If a child with a sleep disorder is to learn how to go to sleep by himself or herself, then the initial task of the doctor providing consultation

1 In infancy 2–10 %

is to give the parents the necessary reassurance that their child *can* fall asleep by himself or herself and calm himself or herself down. This is the kind of reassurance that parents must convey to their child as he or she falls asleep if they want to change the behaviour. This is only possible with quiet and warmth, not motion and insecurity. Paying attention to the child's body temperature in the evening, administering an oil massage and clothing the child with a truly enveloping garment allow such an atmosphere to be created.

The general principle is that the parents' attention *should be the result of their own initiative and not a reaction* to the child's behaviour. This does not contradict the *principle of awareness* and the necessary *resonance* of parents in regard to the child's needs. It is important for the parents to act out of their own perception of the situation and not to react by responding to the child's signals (perceived as a disturbance) without grasping the situation. The same holds for older children who repeatedly get out of bed in the evening and try time and again to induce the parents into action. The calm, undisturbed, regular evening attention of the parents which has *clear time limitations* is what children really need; this enables both sides to let go of each other afterwards, which is necessary if the child is to learn to fall asleep by himself.

Like the attention given, the end of the evening ritual should be determined by the parents and systematically carried through. It is helpful to have practical and necessary minor tasks to perform (even ones that make a bit of muted noise) afterwards and to go to the child briefly at fixed intervals [Ferber 1985], for example if the child continues to be agitated or cries for longer than 5 to 10 minutes. The child should sense that his parents, father or mother, are present, that they have something else to do now and that they are *confident that he or she will fall asleep by himself or herself,* that his or her restlessness will not affect the steady course of events and that he or she cannot make his or her parents more restless and active. The child should be able to feel like a passenger on board a ship which is held unwaveringly on course by an experienced captain. It is important to point out that the parents will fail if the time between the beginning of the last meal and the child's bedtime is repeatedly and irregularly disturbed by external factors. Whoever goes to the phone during the evening meal or looks at the clock during the evening ritual to see whether time can be provided for it will inevitably fail. It makes sense to establish a time frame and rhythm in such a way that, for example, *the family is not disturbed between 18:00 and 19:30* and children beyond infancy get accustomed to bedtimes which enable the parents to conduct an adult life of their own. An essential prerequisite for treatment of sleep disorders is the current condition of the parents, most of all that of the mother; if she is completely exhausted, *she* needs assistance first before she can address the task of tending to her child again! It must be possible for her to express her aggressions and feelings of guilt for once; on the other hand it is necessary to make her aware that a child with a sleep disorder – which goes unnoticed for quite some time by many mothers – endangers the relationship between the mother and the father considerably.

- Exhaustion on the part of the mother in particular almost always results in increasing disinterest in a lively partnership; more and more is expected of the partner while aggressions towards the child are transferred to him.
- The cooling down of the sexual relationship, which usually occurs, can result in considerable aggression on the part of the father towards the mother and the child. Attention must be paid to these aspects particularly if the parents have a child with a disability,

which is a cause of concern (fear of aspiration, seizures, etc.) that impairs their own nights sleep [Gavidia-Payne and Stoneman 2006].

- The child's sleep disorder becomes quite chronic because the child senses or adopts the subliminal aggression of the parents or reacts to it with increased agitation and insecurity.

The level of parental partnership must be clearly separated from that of the child; the child should not serve as a substitute in an unsatisfying partnership either.

A weekend spent by the parents alone or an evening reserved for the parents once a week without the presence of children often alleviates the situation rapidly; in some cases it helps if the mother spends a few nights elsewhere. The doctor can do a lot to promote the family's stability.

There are remedies available for helping many *exhausted mothers*

- **Neurodoron®** (Kalium Phosphoricum comp.) tab. Weleda
  2 tabs. in the morning and 1 tab. in the afternoon for 4 weeks and longer

and the following medication, recommended by F. Husemann, whom we wish to thank for this, has proven very helpful

- **Strophanthus kombe D4 amp.** Weleda
- **Skorodit D8 amp.** Weleda

intravenously as "first aid" (to be repeated if necessary) [Vademecum 2010, 778]

In cases of extreme *feelings of aggression towards the child* and/or the partner and exhaustion initially

- **Sepia C30 pillules** (various manufacturers)
  7 pillules dissolved in 50 ml water taken in sips over a period of three days

If the mother is not capable of emotionally letting go of the child, if she is suffering from severe anxiety about the child and from sleep disorders of her own, intravenous injections of

- **Cuprum met. praep. D30 amp.** Weleda

taken at relatively large intervals can be a very effective remedy.

On this basis, the process of adjusting the sleeping habits of the child paedagogically can now begin. To do so, a clear agreement must exist between the parents concerning the course to be taken and the role which each is to play in it. *As a rule, the first three nights are the actual hurdle* and the calmer parent with the stronger nerves should take the lead in overcoming it. If the clinician succeeds in putting the initiative and the regulatory framework back into the hands of the parents during this time, many parents are able to remedy the sleep disorder of their child themselves. Recommendations for suitable guidebooks with which the doctor is personally familiar [Kast-Zahn and Morgenroth 2007; sufficient for many parents: Goebel and Glöckler 2008, 503–512, Vagedes and Soldner 2010, 359–363] can constitute important aids.

7.1.5 Medicinal treatment options

Current treatment of sleep disorders in children correctly focuses on parent counselling and paedagogical measures as opposed to medicinal treatment. Specialist literature in child and adolescent psychiatry warns against allopathic sleep-inducing drugs. Steinhausen [2010, 287] recommends Valerian and points out the increasingly common use of *melatonin* today: "Melatonin is viewed as a substance with few side effects although hardly any systematic therapeutic studies on children have been conducted." Hellwig/Otto [2010] puts it another way: "Its use is ruled out for pregnant and nursing women, children and persons suffering from epilepsy or autoimmune diseases." [Hellwig, Otto 2010, 37–10]. In practice, the authors observe increasing use of this hormone for severe sleep disorders. Thus a form of hormonal therapy acts on the core phenomenon addressed here, namely regulation of the sleep-waking rhythm in human beings in which *the pineal gland plays a central role.* It is noteworthy that Rudolf Steiner made a connection between human learning processes associated with sleep (▸Chap. 7.1.1), in particular the formation of (long-term) memory, and his spiritual-scientific research on pineal gland activity (which was still completely unexplored at that time) [see Rohen 2010, 76f.]. The authors view the practice of administering melatonin to children with severe sleep disorders as understandable but fundamentally questionable; it is something which they avoid in their own practice.

On the other hand, enormous relief can be provided in many situations through homoeopathic and anthroposophic medications which are non-toxic and non-addictive, particularly if

- this involves balancing out recognizable *triggers* for a sleep disorder (▸Chap. 7.1.3);
- the *family situation* as a whole or excessive demands which are being put on one or both parents do not allow for sufficient changes to be made in the family;
- *constitutional factors and disorders* on the part of the child contribute to the sleep disorder or perpetuate it.

Ultimately it is worthwhile to inquire in detail about the sleeping behaviour of the child and any sleep changes when diagnosing and treating an illness (the parents are usually surprised when they are asked about this). Especially when it comes to choosing a medicine, this sleep behaviour history can provide valuable clues specific for the indication of the medicine(s) in question.

7.1.5.1 Sleep disorders related to specific triggers

If the history in cases of problems falling asleep and sleeping through the night beginning in early infancy reveals *a birth trauma, a shock immediately after birth* (separation from the mother!) and a probable connection suggests itself, the medicaments listed in ▸Chap. 2.2.2 to ▸Chap. 2.2.4 can be taken into consideration.

Mechanically caused birth traumata with ensuing sleep disorders, often associated with a strong tendency towards *colic attacks*, overstretching and cramps indicate in many cases the administration of

- **Cuprum met. praep. D30 trit.** Weleda
  1 saltsp. in the evening, if need be for several days
  as an initial remedy followed by
- **Chamomilla Cupro culta, Radix eth. Dec. D2 dil./Rh D3 dil.** Weleda
  1–2 drops 2–3 x/d (D2), 3–5 drops 2–3 x/d (Rh D3)

For this patient group, particularly if asymmetries or posture abnormalities in the shoulder-neck region are evident, osteopathic diagnostics and treatment by specially trained therapists could be considered.

As regards sleep apnoeas and breath regulation in sleep ▸Chap. 2.2.2.

- Trauma can trigger sleep disorders at any age. In ▸Chap. 2.2.3 and ▸Chap. 2.4 the interconnections are depicted at length, as is the differentiation of the basic medications listed below:
- **Aconitum e tub. D10–30 pillules** Wala in the evening (D20) 3 pillules for 3 days to 3 weeks or **Opium D30 glob.** or **C30** (from various manufacturers) 3 × 3 pillules at intervals of 6–12 hours each.

Sleep disorders which develop after an automobile accident of the family, for example, can be treated quickly and remedied through administration of Aconit (if need be followed by Argentum/cane sugar – see below). In the case of infants, a connection to previous trauma can often only be surmised, in particular in regard to *pregnancy*. An *amniocentesis*, for example, and the concomitant emotional agitation of the mother prior to and during the intervention and during the period of waiting for the results of the examination can have a long-term negative impact on sleep and can also make it more difficult for the mother to behave appropriately towards the child due to the anxiety which has been produced. In general one can say that *encroachments made by adults on the sheaths and physical boundaries of the child persistently impair his or her trust and thus also the ability to sleep.* This holds for medical interventions (fetal diagnostics, neonatology etc.) as well as for traumatization caused by the familial and later extra-familial environment.

In all these cases remedies which help establish/restore a healthy sleep-waking rhythm can contribute considerably to balancing out disorders. A very effective anthroposophic remedy for this is

- Wala **Amnion Gl D12–30 amp.**
  0.3–0.5 ml in the evening daily or every 2 days.

Generally silver in low potentization or in special pharmaceutically processed form is an effective medicine for these disorders (Chap. 2.2.3), for example

- **Argentum/cane sugar (Rohrzucker) pillules** Wala
  3–7 pillules in the evening daily for approx. 4 weeks.

If as a result of trauma, nocturnal states of restlessness rapidly increase in frequency, intensity and duration and the child makes an "hysterical" impression at night accompanied by a pronounced increase in thirst (which is absent during the day), the following has proved therapeutically effective

- **Bryophyllum Argento cultum D2/Rh D3 dil.** Weleda
  2–5 drops 3 x/d (D2), 5–10 drops 3 x/d (Rh D3) in water.

This preparation is a (diluted) plant extract of bryophyllum, a water hyssop plant indigenous to hot regions. To combat the threat of drying out which poses itself in hot environments, bryophyllum completes part of its assimilation of carbon dioxide at night (a quality it has in common with other so called Crassulacea Acid Metabolism or CAM plants). Normally plants can only do this during daylight hours. In a life-threatening situation (desiccation) this plant has thus partly removed itself from the normal day-night rhythm of the etheric aspect (with the daily accumulation of certain organic acids playing a role here) and exhibits "anti-diuresis" during the day. During daylight it minimizes assimilation processes in which loss of water (loss of life) threatens to occur. This plant is then pharmaceutically fertilized with silver solutions in a process which extends over a period of several years. In the course of this process, traces of the silver are absorbed by the plant and vitally organicized, "potentized". As a result it has a different effect on the human organism because it is processed differently than silver potentized out of an inorganic state; it can exert a direct influence on the life organization of the child (just like iron can be absorbed directly by the human life organization if it is organicized by an animal in a protein complex). At the same time, bryophyllum focuses the effect of the silver – balancing out trauma at the level of the life organization – in the aforesaid direction of a day-night reversal of metabolic activities. This preparation is particularly effective in cases of metabolic activity which is intense but also tends to perpetuate itself – whether due to the person's constitution or period of life (regarding the "hysterical" constitution in the sense of anthroposophic medicine cf. ▸Chap. 6.4.3.6.2, [Vademecum 2010, 241]).

Therapy for problems with falling asleep in connection with baby colics is explained in ▸Chap. 4.4; medicines essential for treatment are:

- **Belladonna Rh D4-6 dil.** Weleda
  Weleda **Oxalis Rh D4 dil.** (alcohol-free)
  3 drops before each meal;
  Belladonna can also be administered less frequently: 1 × 5 drops in the evening

and the various forms of vegetabalized copper:

- **Chamomilla Cupro culta, Tabacum Cupro cultum, Melissa Cupro culta D2/Rh D3 dil.** Weleda
  1–2 drops 2–3 x/d (D2), 3–5 drops 2–3 x/d (Rh D3) (▸Chap. 4.4.4, ◘Tab. 4.1.)

In cases of protracted colic pain in the second trimester after birth in particular due to gastroesophageal reflux, potentized magnesium salts are the most important therapeutic remedy, in particular

- **Magnesit D6 trit.** Weleda/**Magnesium phosphoricum D6-12 pillules**
  1 saltsp. 3 x/d/5 pillules 2–3 x/d (▸Chap. 4.4.4, ◘Tab. 4.2 as well as ▸Chap. 4.7.1).

The latter can also be helpful for treating *dentition-related sleep disorders* (these occur primarily in the form of problems sleeping through the night which peak at around 2:00 – ▸Chap. 3.4.3), and in addition

- **Belladonna/Chamomilla pillules** Wala
  5 pillules each several times a day and
- **Fever and teething supp.** Weleda or **Viburcol® supp.** Heel
- In the opinion of the authors, fever and teething suppositories prove more effective for sleep disorders in connection with inflammatory processes and constitutionally caused states of extreme restlessness, whereas Viburcol® suppositories help most in cases of purely dentition-related, pain-related sleep disorders.

Sleep disorders frequently occur *after vaccinations* (▸Chap. 3.5.7). For therapeutic purposes and as a preventive measure to be taken immediately after vaccination

- **Silicea D30 pillules** (various manufacturers)
  5 pillules as single dosage

may be considered. In cases of vaccination in early infancy with a subsequent sleep disorder, particularly if a new, pathological breathing pattern evidences itself while the child is sleeping

- **Tartarus stibiatus D6 trit.** Weleda
  1 saltsp. 5 x/d

is of great importance! Thuja is less often indicated in comparison to these medicines; it corresponds more to the side effects of vaccinations frequently observed in earlier times after smallpox vaccinations. In cases of severe symptoms (fever, shrill crying at night, for example after a pertussis vaccination) or a persistent disorder after a vaccination, administration of a corresponding nosode, for example

- **Pertussinum C30 pillules** or another corresponding nosode
  5 pillules as single dosage may be considered.

In sleep disorders in infants and small children, *cow's milk intolerance* and *intestinal symbiosis disturbances*, for example involving proliferation of Candida, play a significant role. Diagnostics and therapy are elaborated in ▸Chap. 4.6. Concerning oxyures ▸Chap. 4.9. – This example is also appropriate for showing the limits of purely behavioural approaches to treating sleep disorders.

Toxic exposure, for example caused by *amalgam* in the mother (particularly if she has amalgam fillings and gold crowns in her mouth at the same time, which is not rare!), is very difficult to assess in terms of its diagnostic and therapeutic relevance. The goal cannot be to generate even more anxiety and feelings of guilt in the parents, which in the light of the current environmental situation would be only too easy. States of restlessness and sleep disorders which appear early and are associated *with rashes that are unresponsive to therapy* and which manifest themselves atypically – compared, for instance, to constitution- or allergy-related atopic dermatitis – suggest the possibility of such toxic exposure.

In such cases administration of

- **Hepar sulfuris D6 trit. and Koriander** ∅ Ceres
  1 saltsp. 3 x/d for 6 weeks, 2–5 drops 1 x/d

and interpolation of

- Staufen **silver amalgam D30 pillules**
  5 pillules as single dosage, if need be repeated 1 × week several times.

can alleviate complaints considerably or make them accessible to specific therapies, for example (suitable supplements are zinc and selenium, among other options, each in individual dosages). At the same time promotion of elimination is also to be recommended (stimulation of gall bladder, kidney and intestinal function).

7.1.5.2 Disorders of initating sleep

Falling asleep and waking change the activity of the I in the human organism most profoundly, an insight which is made particularly clear by the change in consciousness and will activity. These manifestations of I activity are inseparably linked to the use and the organization of *phosphorus:* The brain is the organ in the human organism most rich in phosphorus. Energy metabolism in nature and the mineralization of the skeleton is bound to phosphorus. Relatively speaking, no living creature organizes more phosphorus in its organism than the human being does; 1.25 % of an adult's body weight (at 70 kg 875 g!) consists of this element so unique in its behaviour [Simon 2000]. As a chemical element, phosphorus only occurs in pure form on earth through the activity of mankind; in nature it always occurs in the form of phosphate. Whoever has experienced the greenish cool luminescence of white phosphorus at room temperature after some time igniting spontaneously into a hot, orangish-yellow flame (white phosphorus must be stored under water) directly perceives the dynamics and affinity to light which this element possesses and will have a new perspective regarding the question of how the human I and phosphorus correspond to each other.

In terms of constitution, problems falling asleep often have something to do with the I. The soul activity guided by the I is acting on the organism in a one-sided, incomplete manner – in other words, *no complete waking up* to address the "tasks of the day" occurs on the part of the I. This means there is *no bodily exhaustion at the end of the day*. The metabolic process lacks the orientation towards nocturnal regeneration, which springs from the catabolic will activity stimulated by spirit-soul impulses during the day (most visible in the growth of the musculature, which is stimulated and guided by locomotion during the day). In spirit-soul terms a *surplus of activity of an often aimless, errant, dreamy nature* emerges since the proper relation to the body is lacking. Thus the evening turning point in the interplay of body and soul is not reached and a *fear of nightfall and being alone as well as profuse dreaming* are the understandable consequences.

Phosphorus in low potencies is a possible remedy if the I and the astral body do not sufficiently engage with the lower part of the human being, the processes involving metabolism and self-motion upon waking. *Waking proceeds hesitantly* but the child is not unfriendly. The child's sensory perception, concentration, and the will-in-thinking is weak. At school there is a lack of attention; the child "dreams off," engaging only fleetingly with things, and intellectually it exhibits a *rapid exhaustibility* (cf. Acidum phosphoricum as well). At the same time, metabolic activity and limb movement remain feeble, undersupplied, while length growth can occur in spurts (because it is not inhibited by the intervention of the I activity in the will – children also grow during the day!). In the evening these children seek affectionate bodily contact with their parents and love to be massaged – while being very hesitant to make active contact with the world during the day. Sleep itself is long in coming, it is restless and often not deep enough.

- Weleda **Phosphorus D5/Mallow dil.**
  In the morning (!) 5–7 drops (if need be repeated between 3:00 and 4:00 p.m.)

is a very effective remedy in such cases. In weak children with fragile bodies (or in manifestations of sleep disorders after enfeebling illnesses) its effect can be enhanced through administration of

- Wala **Prunuseisen pillules**
  2–3 × daily 5–7 pillules (cf. ▸Chap. 6.5.6.4.3).

Should sleep disorders be accompanied by symptoms or a history of constitutional weakness, these can be balanced out by potentized phosphorus (for example susceptibility to pneumonia – ▸Chap. 5.1.1), Phosphor D6 can be replaced by

- Arcana **Phosphorus LM6 dil.**
  in the morning 3–5 drops.

In the evening it helps to give such children a sweet dessert and some honey [Deterding 1964]; in phosphorus-typical constitutions, the lack of anchoring of the I in the metabolism is reflected in *a need for sugar and unstable blood sugar levels* – physiologically speaking the sugar is incorporated into the metabolism by a phosphorylation process.

Children who develop an animated inner activity as evening approaches, but one which is limited one-sidedly to the realm of the nerves and senses, are to be distinguished from those who suffer from the aforesaid problems with falling asleep [Deterding 1964]. They exhibit a *vivid imagination* and are *wide awake in bed*; this surplus can lead to a development of *intense anxiety* after nightfall and when the child is alone. In the morning they are often overtired and look for an opportunity to sleep during the day, "dozing off" accordingly.

In such cases phosphorus in high potentization is effective when administered in the evening (in this case phosphorus Mallow):

- Weleda **Phosphorus D24/Malva dil.**
  in the evening 5 drops

If a child with such a constitution experiences problems falling asleep *and* sleeping through the night ("cat nap") with frequent waking

- Weleda **Phosphorus/Sulphur D25/25 aa dil.**

is more effective; Sulphur in higher potentization acts specifically on the brief moments of (not fully conscious) waking which stem from the periodic nocturnal activity of the astral body (▸Chap. 7.1.2), and it mutes this to such an extent that no complete waking occurs. If Sulphur is to be administered alone, D12, 1 × in the evening 5 pillules is usually sufficient.

Treatment with Phosphorus D25 in the evening is enhanced by administering

- Weleda **Solutio Ferri comp. D3 dil.**
  in the morning 5–10 drops,

an iron preparation modelled in composition and production method on the stinging nettle (suggestion made by R. Steiner). It counteracts a one-sided "head-oriented" activity of the I and the astral body, anchoring both more strongly in the metabolic region and thus also combating susceptibility to infections [Vademecum 2010, 760f]

The constitutional situations depicted above stand in contrast to the situation in which the soul aspect submerges too far into the bodily realm without sufficient guidance by the I and cannot free itself from this bond in the evening. This constitution has a close affinity to a state that manifests itself physiologically in infants and small children. Such children wake up early in the morning, between 5 and 6 o'clock, are generally in a good mood as long as the appetite, which quickly announces itself, is satisfied (the appetite is a direct reflection of the plunge of the soul aspect into the life processes). Substance assimilation dominates over catabolic, energy releasing activity: such children gain weight quickly and have pudgy, puffy figures (in such children sleep can be impaired by adenoid and tonsillar hypertrophy!), whereas they demonstrate more or less phlegmatic behaviour in regard to self-initiative and locomotion. Thus *a deficit of I-activity* is created here as well, but in a different way than is the case with the aforesaid type. Here the soul aspect in pure form, the primary satisfaction of needs at the animal level, dominates; whereas the development of body warmth, self-initiative and waking consciousness lag behind (as adults one can relate to this condition after a feast day during which one has eaten lots of food and gotten too little exercise). In the evening the I stays shackled to the body because it was given too little shape during the day to let the nocturnal metabolic processes act on their own accord. – *Characteristically, such children experience intense evening anxiety*; as soon as they are able to voice them (starting in the 3rd/4th year of life), they often speak of animals and ghosts. At the same time they exhibit little self-confidence. This all reflects an activity of the astral body, which has become too independent, *"drowning" in the metabolism*. The I must take the lead more forcefully here; for small children, this is more a maturation task than a pathology.

Effective remedies are primarily low potencies of carbonic oyster shell limestone,

- Weleda **Conchae D4–6 trit.**
  in the evening or before bedtime 1 saltspoon

Oysters embody an animal, highly assimilatory activity of the organism, which exhausts itself in formation of protein and its shell while perception and locomotion are increasingly reduced [Simon 2000]. They constitute the pure, regressive counter-image of the soul activity necessary for human beings put in the services of the I, of conscious perception, thinking and will activity.

Oysters have minimal metabolic activity accompanied by minimal development of warmth; a considerable part of the carbon dioxide released during metabolism is not exhaled but rather bound to the calcium out of which they form their shell limestone. Here the adherence of the soul aspect to the substance evidences itself with immediate clarity.

Being able to fall asleep is closely connected to having sufficient thermogenesis during the day (see above) and to the flowing off of warmth via the periphery. It also has a lot to do with free exhalation. From a soul perspective, *falling asleep* constitutes an exhalation process. This is promoted by the administration of *potentized* oyster shell limestone.

If the focus is on an *exhalation disorder* (for example obstructive bronchitis, asthma) – fear *of animals and ghosts* in the dark belong to this level – intermediate potentization might be more effective:

- Weleda **Conchae D12–20 trit.**
  1 saltspoon in the evening

A very characteristic symptom in this context is profuse *sweating on the head while falling asleep*, which is observed in such children. The aforesaid medicament alleviates this rapidly, enabling the astral body to fulfil its task during the day all the way into including catabolism and elimination – instead of having to catch up later in the wrong place. Generally one can say that by administering potentized oyster shell limestone

- Surplus warmth on the head (D20) is “expelled”;
- Exhalation of carbon dioxide (D12, LM6–12) is stimulated in the middle part of the human being;
- Elimination of fluids and solids (tendency towards constipation! – in adults towards formation of kidney stones) in the lower part of the human being can be stimulated (D4–6) and regulated as well (too strong menses) [Husemann 2009, 63–78, Steiner, Wegman 1991, 87f., 93].

In the 2nd seven-year period of life one must pay special attention to problems falling asleep as well as the degree to which the overall development of the rhythmic system is impacted by disorders or developmental crises (for example circulatory regulation disturbances, bronchial hyper-reactivity, inclination towards headaches, emotional instability). Should this be the case the anthroposophic compound

- Wala **Primula comp. pillules**
  3 × daily 5–7 pillules For 4–8 weeks

is suitable for initiating comprehensive stabilization. In this compound, Conchae corresponding to a D10 is potentized in combination with Hyoscyamus, Primula and Onopordon in low potency. If the sleep disorders do not correspond to the aforesaid type of Calcium carbonicum but the condition of the rhythmic system otherwise matches the description, the suitable individual remedy, administered in the evening, can be combined with

- **Cardiodoron mite dil.** Weleda/**Cardiodoron Rh tab.** Weleda
  2–3 × daily 7–12 drops in water/2–3 × 1 tablet

Oysters are very cupriferous animals, which perform the respiratory process, the transport of gas, with the help of a copper-bearing blood pigment. In practice, potentized natural copper carbonate – malachite –is an essential medicament for treatment of problems falling asleep:

- **Malachite D5, D6 trit.** Apotheke an der Weleda
  in the evening 1 saltspoon (if need be alternating with potentized iron in the morning)

Symptomatically speaking it is striking that the children *simply lie awake* in bed without experiencing anxiety, fatigue or imaginative exhilaration; they "simply don't feel like falling asleep." The evening gesture of exhalation in the soul aspect is missing. One gains the impression that they are *emotionally cool*, that they lack the necessary nest warmth; clinically speaking they often show signs of *meteorism, possibly a cool kidney region or sensitivity in the stomach area*. This indicates an abnormal activity of the soul aspect, the astral body in the area of the stomach, pancreas and kidneys. These are the organs which show a pronounced physiological change in function in the course of falling asleep. If their daytime activity persists, the necessary release of the astral aspect (indicated here as the process of exhalation) does not occur.

Malachite, whose effectiveness can be enhanced enormously by application with

- Weleda **Cuprum met. 0.4 % ointment** Weleda and/or Wala **Mallow oil**

is a very valuable remedy for such disorders in the kidney region as well as the epigastrium (depending on the medical finding, local temperature and sensitivity). Further supplementation of this treatment is possible through administration of

- Wala **Cichorium/Pancreas comp. pillules**
  3 × daily 5 pillules (cf. ▸Chap. 6.3.3.2)

At the level of herbal remedies the *alpine anemone, Pulsatilla vulgaris*, has an affinity to the calcium and copper compounds of carbon dioxide. Pulsatilla vulgaris does very well in calcareous sediment soil, which has evolved from the shells of countless molluscs from past warm oceans and which grows its large, pendulous blossoms that are dark violet on the outside and a radiant shade of yellow on the inside, early in the year even before the leaves and stems have developed completely (▸Chap. 6.5.6.11). Later in the year the stems become upright, develop their differentiated foliage and release the light-weight seeds into the wind.

From a therapeutic perspective Pulsatilla plays a particularly important role as a remedy for problems falling asleep before and *in puberty among girls*. Generally speaking these are likeable, nice girls in need of much affection and quick to become teary-eyed. Those who are still young would like to fall asleep to please their parents (or so it seems) but the sandman does not appear! Hours pass before sleep, (and often only light sleep) comes and they do not sleep deeply until morning. Waking up proves difficult and they do not reach their full presence and activity, which extends far, too far, into the night, until early afternoon. In puberty this shift is physiological, particularly if, at the onset of sexual maturity (when the spinal column is not yet completely developed), a certain heaviness with a tendency towards orthostasis, low blood pressure, cool hands and feet (circulation which is too venously pronounced) manifest themselves, making it difficult to wake up.

- **Pulsatilla vulgaris D12 dil./pillules** DHU
  2 × daily 5 drops/7 pillules

stimulates the waking up process, strengthens the exhalation of carbon dioxide (typically patients who require Pulsatilla feel the need for fresh air or an open window) and venous circulation and it gives children and adolescents more emotional stability, connecting them anew with the events of the day.

Individuals who require Pulsatilla as a remedy tend to do more poorly the lower the sun is in the year and the higher the moon rises. – The effect of potentized Pulsatilla used for *problems falling sleep and seasonal depressive moods* can be enhanced by plant extracts of *Hypericum*, which blossoms at the point of the summer solstice and preserves the effect of the summer sunlight in its substance formation to a very high degree.

Very suitable remedies are

- Ceres **Hypericum original mother tincture**/Wala **Hypericum ex herba D2 pillules**
  1–3 × daily 2–5 drops/3–7 pillules daily (careful gradual dosaging, determination of optimal effect)

and prophylactically for external use

- Weleda **Hypericum Flos 25 % Oleum** (back or full-body application)

Datura stramonium, or angel's trumpet is one of the most important remedies for children who cannot fall asleep in the evening; in accordance with the strong toxin production process of this Solanum, the symptoms of children for which this medicament is particularly suitable are of a clearly more *agitated and vehement nature* than are those for whom all previously described medicaments are recommended. The angel's trumpet blooms in the evening and at night with a white, trumpet-shaped blossom of benumbing fragrance which attracts moths. *At night* the blossoms make a sun-following movement(!), they close in the morning and wither immediately after pollination. This clearly shows an intense affinity to the ensouled aspect, the astral aspect "at the wrong time." The plant is very sturdy, forking off in rigid dichotomy with the blossom and fruit positioned right on the fork whereas the two accompanying leaves roam upwards along the two forked stem axes *separately* and unfold "one storey" *above* the blossom. The plant forms stimulating substances (hyoscyamine) as well as dulling ones (scopolamine) and in its toxicity it is thus capable of relaxing the soul aspect of human beings, of wrenching them from the governance of consciousness on the one hand and on the other, from the normal rhythmic bond to corporeality. In the angel's trumpet we encounter a representative of the *Solanaceae trias Belladonna, Hyoscyamus, Stramonium* [Wolff and Stübler 1985], which everyone who wishes to treat psychosomatic disorders in children with potentized medicaments should study in depth (▸Chap. 7.4.4) because they are of eminent therapeutic significance (early on, Hahnemann probably used Stramonium and Belladonna therapeutically as the first remedies in homoeopathicized form, followed by Pulsatilla and Nux vomica) [Seiler 1988].

Stramonium should be considered if the child exhibits *clear agitation and psychic disjunction* in general; during consultation in particular, the child can be very well-behaved, even submissive (already a sign of too weak I guidance of the soul aspect) while on the other hand exhibiting *vehement* – in boys *violent* – outbursts. Behind this lies a *profound fear*, in particular *of the dark* ; such children flatly refuse to let the light be turned off and this is because of an untameable fear! Associated with this is the *fear of being alone, the need for bodily contact* (all this reflects a longing for the I which alone is capable of overcoming the polarization and disjunction tendencies of the animal-unconscious).These are children who get out of bed repeatedly and go to their parents on any number of fanciful pretexts. Inwardly they are under extreme emotional tension which takes control of them and which they feel at the mercy of (older children can articulate this clearly, saying, for example "I do things I don't even want to!"). Their misfortune is that their constitution lends them something wayward, driven, disagreeable; they are a strain upon themselves and upon all others, and no child wishes for peace in bed more than they do! Thus they are confronted from all sides with a constant *conflict,* which makes everything even worse.

In this case, consideration of what medicaments to administer should start by gaining a better understanding of the child and interpreting it in medical terms to the parents. Such children have an *unusual need for movement* which must be accommodated during the day to a strong degree; if one allows them to fidget around while doing homework all afternoon, the evening will inevitably end in a catastrophe. Paedagogically speaking they require strong guidance that is consistent but must not be resentful. The extreme pressure from which such children already suffer should not be aggravated and turned into a vicious circle by the family and the school because otherwise aggressive derailment threatens to occur.

Therapeutic treatment uses

- **Stramonium D12–15 dil./pillules** (various manufacturers)
  in the evening or 2 × daily 5–7 drops/pillules

Apart from its indication for the aforesaid problem of falling asleep, Stramonium is perhaps the most important potentized medicament for treatment of sleepwalking, *somnambulism* [Wolff and Stübler 1985, 26ff.] (less frequently Aconite, Argentite [Vademecum 2010, 107: in the case of dark-haired "low-sulphur children", moon-dependent, after a trauma], opium, phosphorus).

As a medicament Stramonium, like Hyoscyamus, shows a clear affinity to *ADHD* (▸Chap. 7.5) and to epilepsy (cf. ▸Chap. 8.1.5.4). This affinity is shared but in a completely different way with

- **Coffea D12–30 pillules** (various manufacturers),

an additional medicament for children who cannot fall asleep in the evening.[1]

1 Interesting elaborations on homoeopathic medicaments of the Rubiaceae family (Coffea, China, Galium, Ipecacuanha) can be found in the school of K.-J.Müller [2009, 142: Coffea]

7

Everyone who has had coffee has a vague notion of the "remedy picture." Accordingly, children who are helped by Coffea (without having drunk cola or any other caffeinated drink prior to this) experience evening excitation with unusual intellectual and bodily activity. Sensitivity to all external events and influences is typical; pleasant anticipation of approaching events can rob them of their sleep. Thus this is a *restless but positively tinted* picture. Laboratory tests should be done to rule out hyperthyroidism if necessary; in cases of older children and adolescents one should ask about use of stimulants. – A special indication for Coffea is sleeplessness after measles.

In regard to small children it is important to distinguish between the aforesaid remedies and

- **Chamomilla D12–30 pillules** Weleda, **Chamomilla e rad. D20 pillules** Wala
  1–3 × daily 5 pillules

Such children are *oversensitive, truculent, irritable, loud* – the remedy works best in the period between the teething and the defiant stage in the third year of life. Despite, or due to the fact that they are exhausted, they do not stay in bed; instead, they keep wanting to get up and be held by the parents without really being pacified by this. This pathology clearly reflects that behaviour which parental guides discuss extensively when it comes to children with sleep disorders. Such sleep disorders often emerge after colds or teething and during such times parental behaviour sometimes also gets out of sync. Chamomilla is thus a medicament of primarily supportive nature for sleep disorders treatable with behavioural therapy.

The last medicament to be discussed here, which stands at the border between problems falling asleep and problems sleeping through the night, is

- **Causticum D12–D30–C200 pillules** (various manufacturers)
  depending on the potency 2 × 5 pillules daily (D12) or administration of single dosages (higher potencies).

These involve older pre-school and school children who experience no anxiety when alone and have no fear of the dark but who are *afraid of the phase of sleep onset,* and *afraid of the night.* Such children suffer from constitutional melancholy, from *fears and worries,* which can relate to the world, the family, or ill relatives. They feel deep sympathy with other human beings; at the same time they fear aggression because they themselves are extremely *aggression-inhibited* and *they cannot defend themselves* (an important history question). They are driven by idealistic goals early on which cloak resistance against their own aggressions and vital needs; *the ideal of purity has an attraction for them. Motor development is slow and sometimes inhibited* as is the way they present themselves to others; at school they are characterized by quiet *ambition* and they make high demands on themselves.

Such children are *afraid of falling asleep, of losing conscious control* of their own body, their sub-conscious; they are afraid of *worrisome thoughts which accompany falling asleep.* This can induce them to lie awake for long periods of time and as a general rule the parents have no direct influence on this. What is important in this environment is to correct excessive demands on their own performance and that of others; art therapy can be very important for such children (for example painting) with an aim towards helping them gain a new relationship to their own corporeality, to the emotional unconscious.

In addition to problems falling asleep it is particularly characteristic for them to exhibit an inclination towards *nightmares;* in cases of severe, regularly recurring nightmares high potencies of Causticum – and painting therapy – are an important remedy (for remedy picture and casuistics ▸Chap. 6.5.6.11).

7.1.5.3 Disorders of maintaining sleep, combined sleep disorders

The first remedy to consider is banewort, or Belladonna

- **Belladonna D12 dil./pillules** Weleda
  in the evening 5–7 drops/pillules

Generally speaking, such children show fewer problems falling asleep; their sleep disorder more often consists in awakening with a vehement start *before midnight* (typically 1–2 hours after falling asleep or between 10:00 and 11:00 p. m.) with profuse *sweating on the head* (in contrast, sweating on the head while falling asleep is characteristic for Conchae = Calcium carbonicum). Such children make an extremely agitated impression with blood stasis in the head (red face) and *prefer to be calmed down by words (rejection of touch)* – as opposed to children full of fear who require Aconite or Stramonium as a remedy. In cases where the child has a fever and awakens before midnight, pronounced fever deliriums sometimes ensue during which the child is verbally unresponsive; this can startle the parents quite a bit. In the morning "*morning grouchiness*" can be observed (late, ungracious awakening, child does not wish to be addressed); in the evening however, the child appears wide awake and does not seem able to fall asleep before the sun sets (which can be very bothersome in the summer). These are "night owls" with a lively temperament who prefer to participate in the family conversation instead of lying down and going to sleep. What stands in remarkable contrast to the picture painted here is that such children, who appear to be so self-reliant, have a tendency to climb into the parents' bed at night. Administration of Belladonna leads to a disappearance of the sleep disorder before midnight as well as improving the child's awakening in the morning.

If *awakening* in the morning is accompanied *by spasms* it might be advisable to administrate

- **Cinis Belladonnae D6** (Apotheke an der Weleda)
  1 saltspoon in the evening as a supplement to Belladonna

"*Morning grouchiness*" is also characteristic for the remedy picture of *Staphisagria* (grouchiness persists for the entire day – easily offended children who were humiliated early on and have low self-esteem), *Magnesium phos. and carb.* as well as *Nux vomica.* Falling asleep promptly in the evening is characteristic of this remedy but so are untimely awakening at around 3:00 to 4:00 a. m. (liver-gall disorder, poor eating habits, fear of challenges posed by the day to come) with the patient dozing off afterwards, with irritability and unresponsiveness in the morning as a result (▸Chap. 6.6.3.3).

- **Arsenicum album D6–12, LM6–12 dil.** (various manufacturers)
  D6 in the morning, higher potencies in the evening 5 drops

is an essential remedy for problems falling asleep and sleeping through the night for children with a pronounced *neurasthenic constitution* (▸Chap. 6.4.3.6).

This sleep disorder originally derives from *too weak activity of the soul aspect in the metabolic realm* [Deterding 1964, 136], which evidences itself in finicky eating habits, poor digestion and an inclination towards diarrhoea and weak assimilation (among other things, sudden cravings, in particular for easily digestible carbohydrates). Constitutionally speaking, such children usually have a *leptosome physique and dark hair* (Mediterranean type). *Intellectually such children, often highly gifted, tend to exhibit ambitiousness early on.*

The sleep disorders result from these tensions. A fear of being alone and the need for shelter, which can be reliably remedied by having the child lie in the mother's bed, stand at the fore here; then the child falls asleep peacefully. No remedy reflects this characteristic as markedly as Arsenicum album does. The aforesaid disorder often manifests itself through awakening shortly after midnight, sometimes in the form of pronounced pavor nocturnus. In cases of other children with this constition, problems associated with anxiety and the need for shelter can already arise while falling asleep. – Other striking characteristics are nervous agitation, thirst (the child often only drinks small amounts) and the need for warmth – in correspondence to the neurasthenic constitution.

A further medicament to consider in one's differential therapeutics is

- **Aconitum e tub. D20 pillules** Wala
  in the evening 5 pillules

What is also characteristic of this remedy is that pavor nocturnus with awakening accompanied by fits of screaming and anxiety at around midnight can occur (in contrast to Belladonna, speaking with the child does no good; embracing it is the only thing which helps). In the evening there might be quite a struggle before the child goes to bed due to a pronounced fear of the dark.

For the choice of remedy, the *aetiology* is decisive: in the case of Aconitum, it consists in a trauma, paedagogical mistakes (threats which the child is incapable of processing), and emotional duress which cannot be resolved for the child (which is often not discussed). The sleep disorder is the *consequence of an event, not of the child's constitution* (which is quite often exceedingly energetic). In contrast, an indication for Arsenicum album is founded on constitutional one-sidedness.

The effects which Arsenicum album has on sleep disorders can be variously differentiated with *potentized arsenic compounds.*

Should the sleep disorder occur after colds or acute inflammations, in particular of the respiratory tract (e. g. after pneumonia

- **Arsenicum iodatum D6–12 dil.** (various manufacturers)
  2–3 × daily 5 drops

is a very beneficial remedy. Susceptibility to infection, poor appetite (inappetence), fatigue and a weak metabolism can be improved by this remedy long-term.

Should the problems lie in the area of a chronic intestinal disorder with undigested, foul-smelling, diarrhoea-like faeces

- **Olivenit[1] D6 trit., D8–12 dil.** Apotheke an der Weleda
  initially 3 × 1 saltspoons D6, later on for example 2 × 5 drops D12

is recommended. In addition to anxiety while falling asleep, such children often exhibit instances of aggressiveness in their behaviour. The remedy is also very beneficial for spasms in connection with respiration followed by awakening and long and prolonged coughing attacks in the second half of the night (Pertussis; Asthma bronchiale), with D8–12 being indicated. In cases of strong mother fixation and pronounced anxiety in the evening and at night (with indication of a "kidney constitution": formed, tense, more or less cool periphery, slender, sensorially alert, with inclination towards anxiety – cf. [Vademecum 2010, 166]) D30 has also proven to be helpful (in the evening 5 drops).
Should a general developmental crisis manifest itself, in particular in puberty with lack of appetite, anxious feelings of insecurity, problems falling asleep and strongly impaired self-esteem, the iron compound of arsenic

- **Skorodit D10 trit.** Weleda
  in the morning and afternoon 1 saltspoon/7 drops

is an essential remedy which must be accompanied by conversational therapy and if need be art therapy. Diagnostically speaking one should check if there is an iron deficiency.

7.1.5.4 Brief remarks on differential therapeutics

7.1.5.4.1 Normal initiation of sleep with frequent waking during the night:

- **Bryophyllum Argento cultum D2/Rh D3 dil.** Weleda (▸Chap. 7.1.5.1)
  - After trauma,
  - In cases of excessive nocturnal metabolic activity, "hysterical" constitution, moon sensitivity
- **Sulphur D12–30 pillules or Phosphorus/Sulphur D25/25** aa Weleda (▸Chap. 7.1.5.2)
  - "Catnap," awakening at slightest irritation or spontaneous, repeated awakening.
- **Arsenicum album LM12 dil.** Arcana (▸Chap. 6.4.3.6.1)
  - Anxious awakening from midnight on, child only calms down in parents' bed.
- **Thuja e summit. D12–15 pillules** Wala (▸Chap. 4.6)
  - Restless thrashing around in sleep, possibly with awakening
  - pavor nocturnus but with slow, difficult awakening,
  - Chronic or recurrent diseases particularly in cold and wet conditions,
  - possibly jactatio capitis (head rocking).
- **Silicea D12–20 pillules** (various manufacturers, ▸Chap. 6.4.3.6.1)
  - restless sleep,
  - tympanic stomach, digestive insufficiency,
  - very pronounced need for warmth, chronic infections of upper respiratory tract.

1 Natural copper arsenate.

7.1.5.4.2 Children who wake at night and turn night into day:

- **Cypripedium pubescens D6 dil.** (various manufacturers)
  - Are cheerful and happy in this situation.
- **Coffea D12 pillules** (▸Chap. 7.1.5.2)
  - Usually exhibit somewhat "ungracious" behaviour.

7.1.5.4.3 Sleepwalking (somnambulism)

- **Stramonium, Belladonna, Hyoscyamus, Dyskrasite** (Antimony silver), **Argentite, Aconite, Opium**
- **Arg. met. praep. D20 trit.** Weleda
  a saltspoon in the evening during waxing moon,
- **Phosphorus D12 dil.** Weleda
  5 drops in the morning during waning moon

7.1.5.4.4 Rhythmic movement disorder (jactatio capititis)

- **Belladonna, Stramonium, Helleborus, Thuja, Bryophyllum Arg. c.**
- **Apis mell.**
  - Thrashes against the bed with the head.

7.1.5.4.5 Children who sleep in the "knee-elbow position"

- **Medorrhinum, Phosphorus, Lycopodium.**

7.1.5.4.6 Sweating during sleep

- **Conchae**
  - While falling asleep, on the head.
- **Belladonna**
  - One to two hours after falling asleep, on the head.
- **Mercurius solubilis**
  - The entire night, kicks off blankets and tucks himself up alternatingly
  - Foul-smelling discolouring sweat, salivation.
- **Tuberculinum**
  - Strong nocturnal sweat all over the body, must change clothing during the night,
  - Inclination towards recurring, deep respiratory inflammations.
- **Acidum phosphoricum**
  - Sweat on the back with onset in second half of the night

7.2 Anxiety and phobic anxiety disorders

Anxiety is the most intense form of physical constriction

Thomas Fuchs [2000]

The expression "anxiety" is derived etymologically from the Latin angere = to press together, angustus = narrow. The anxious person becomes constricted. Why, where and how does he become constricted? Anxieties "are very common in childhood… After all, the child is constantly forced to expand the horizons of his experience and is in the process exposed to the unknown and, frequently, to fear-inducing experience" [Struck 1989, vol. IV, 45]. Could expansion, the ever widening horizon, be the origin of constriction?

Fear is a *reality of the soul*, a "basic experience known to everyone, the emotional quality of which is discovered up through introspection" [Struck 1989, vol. 4, 44]. Nevertheless no fear exisists without simultaneous expression in a *change in physical functions and life processes, e. g.*:

- *motorically*: in increased tonus and restlessness;
- *changes to the rhythmic system*: breathing, heartbeat and blood pressure;
- *secretions*: in diarrhoea, perspiration and the urge to urinate;
- *vigilance*: Its expression can include over-alertness and sleeplessness, fatigue and an inability to concentrate.

Fear is a psychosomatic reality. It is frequently experienced as constriction in the body, as a state of being thrown back on the constriction of the body. The soul entity is congested into the body. In it the experience of anxiety meets that of pain. Anxious children often experience pain without any discernible somatic trigger; anxiety enhances the experience of pain.

Anxiety can take the form of a clearly object-related *fear* and, on the other hand, with the onset of puberty, assume a free-floating form which appears to emanate from the abyssal depths. It is always possible to find two defining moments of anxiety: constriction, as the congestion of the soul entity in the body (the anxiety is felt literally "in the flesh"!), and, on the other hand, the *feeling of insecurity in the world brought about by the loss of a hitherto supportive sense of familiarity as a result of the expansion of one's own experiential horizons.*

As is evidenced by certain physical changes, which also occur in people in connection with fear and anxiety (see above), it can very confidently be stated that animals too have a fundamental experience of anxiety [Nissen 1989a, 101; Lorenz 1965]. This occurs in particular when the animal becomes estranged from its normal environment, and the unknown situation results in disorientation and an inability to act. Millions of laboratory animals subjected to experimental medical research experience not only pain but also anxiety, a primal, dull, "nameless" anxiety; nameless because the animal never has the opportunity to put a name to its anxiety.

The "basic forms of fear" [Riemann 1975] occurring in childhood demonstrate, however, that anxiety in humans takes on a far more fundamental character than it does in animals. The animal grows into its environment and becomes ever more familiar to it; it develops ever greater similarity to its parents. *Man, however, actively seeks to leave his original environment.* Human development has an inherent predisposition toward questioning integration into the natural order of things (in which the soul of the animal is embedded) and mounting challenges to parents, blood relatives and traditional behaviours; the development of awareness, spiritual horizons and independent thinking is the decisive driver in this process. This leads to the genuine *individuation* of the human being: his ability to think, decide and act differently from his forebears and fellow human beings, to burn old bridges to the world and to follow new paths. *Thus it is that the I itself introduces the human being to the emotional and psychological experience of anxiety.* This phenomenon is demonstrated in the development of every child [Steinhausen 2010, 198].

Thus it is that the "*eight-month anxiety*" or "sense of estrangement" occurs, when, with the onset of teething, the child begins to withdraw from the infantile symbiosis. It is during this period for the first time that the child has a psychological experience of his or her own corporeality as integral and cohesive (body image) and separate from that of his or her mother. The "Leibesraum" or "bodily space" [Fuchs 2000, 97], in which constriction can occur, emerges. At the same time, the connection with the world becomes more sophisticated. A distinction is made between the individuality of the parents, so familiar to the child, and that of other, "strange" people, who, in their physical-psychological movement, do not correspond directly with the child. This experience of contrast leads to the awakening of awareness, the sense of individual existence, the I. As the somewhat older child becomes familiar with this alien individuality and learns to correspond with it psychologically and physically, the anxiety dissipates.

And it is the I that provides the impulse to raise the body from its stable horizontal four-footed posture into the *precarious erectness* which is characteristic of the human[1]. This process puts the child in a situation which generates anxiety: fear of falling, fear of letting go of his mother's hand and taking his first independent steps. As the child learns to inhabit this anxiety, becomes capable of integrating his own upright posture into the space around him and achieves a new balance, his anxiety diminishes.

This makes it easier to understand fear of the dark, the isolation of the small child *(separation anxiety)*: to learn to live in the world separated from the immediately protective cocoon, the tangible experience of the mother's body; to learn to touch, pacify and have confidence in oneself, is an important developmental step. The most profound separation is the act of going to sleep; every form of separation anxiety can result in an inability to go to sleep, in keeping the soul entity firmly fixed in the body.

With his departure from domestic security, the reduction of purely instinctive behaviour and the awakening of awareness, the child becomes conscious of his environment, of nature. This awakening to a more expansive set of horizons is in turn associated with an experience of the world as sinister *(environmental fear*: of animals, thunderstorms, elemental beings, ghosts). This abates through the further development of thought and the child's own practical abilities, but without ever fully disappearing.

Entry into a new community which no longer consists of blood relatives (kindergarten, school) is associated with *socialization anxieties*. Between the ages of 7 and 14, as-yet unknown peers (fellow pupils, children in the street) and authorities (e.g. teachers) are significant sources of anxiety; both psychologically and physically. The child must first find his place, his role in the scheme of things, and familiarize himself with his new, shared

1 On the subject of the upright human posture as the "fundamental phenomenon behind human character", the cause of which cannot be assigned to anything else but which is instead in itself the primary driver of development in evolution and the formation of human character, cf. Vogel [1996, 156], Verhulst [1999, 164ff.]

world. This increasingly becomes the definitive social horizon, a development which spans the entire period between the ages of 7 and 14.

Less attention is paid to prepuberty *internal psychological-physical development.* At the age of about nine, in the midst of childhood [Müller-Wiedemann 1993], there arises the psychological experience, of which the child is only hazily aware, of a boundary which is now being transcended, but whose transcendence means the irrevocable loss of a world into which the child, assuming that he has been allowed to experience normal development, was psychologically integrated, in which he was fully secure and part of a community. By crossing this internal "Rubicon", the river which marks the boundary of this world, the child has the first deep experience of *isolation in the collective*, experiencing himself in a psychologically irreversible manner as different but also as unique in relation to everybody else. This is associated in the unconscious mind with *a new, deeper impingement of individuality into the bodily realm*, right through to the realm of will, of metabolism and limbs. This is revealed through a maximal deceleration, specific to the human being (in contrast to primates), of the speed of growth during childhood development, the reversal of the growth pattern (the growth of the lower limbs, the growth "from below to above" becomes dominant and changes the proportions); the blood sugar and haemoglobin content of the blood increases [Husemann and Wolff 1986, vol. II, 39] and the polarization between the genders begins to take physical shape. The child deepens her possession of her own body, stamps her own mark on it in a more profound way and in this respect also disentangles herself from her parents, the primary formative powers of inheritance.

In about the ninth year a first psychological *awareness* of death, the temporal limit to the body, arises. In developmental psychology terms, it is at this time that "*reality anxieties*", fears of illness and death, on the one hand and wars and natural disasters on the other, begin to manifest. Although the degree to which these fears are suppressed varies widely, they remain constant companions of human existence. It is at this time that suicide first manifests as a possibility.

With the onset of puberty, the *fear of maturation* arises. The young person loses his physical childhood home and develops any of a very wide range of *body-schema-related anxieties*, which, in the extreme case of anorexia nervosa, can take on self-perpetuating and delusional characteristics. "Perceiving the body differently from the way it has hitherto been can really lead to suicide" [Wildermuth 2006, 120]. The all-pervasive *perfectionism* of competitive Western societies has intensified these anxieties: the number of cosmetic operations is increasing, and healthy self-identification with their own physicality is a profound challenge for all adolescents. As is the case with the anxieties considered above, whether or not this challenge is met depends on the child's success in *establishing and deepening relationships*: with its new, different physicality and the associated drives and needs; with peers of the same gender, with whom it is possible to create a field of trust in order to learn how to process the common experiences and fears; and, finally, with young people of the opposite sex. What is encountered here is a new kind of foreignness and unfamiliarity and, at the same time, the elemental drive to overcome these both physically *and psychologically* and to enter into a new, as yet unknown correspondence relationship which, if reduced to the purely physical events, can never succeed. The anxiety associated with this can only be overcome by the "*art* of loving" (Fromm), by means of a newly acquired physical, psychological and spiritual capability. Failure to overcome this anxiety can result in persistent neurotic developmental problems (in the sense of a persistent fear arising on the basis of an inadequately developed capacity to make connections with other people).

In the case of young people approaching adulthood, with the existential separation from the parental home around the eighteenth and nineteenth years, an awareness develops of the possibility and challenge of shaping their own, individual future; *existential anxiety* arises: the dreamlike experience of isolation of the ninth year now grips the vulnerable young person with all its force, manifesting as a fear of failure in life and in social relationships, of illness and death, of helplessness in the face of evil, as a fear of disasters, war and destruction. The frequency of suicides reaches an initial peak, as an expression of loneliness and anxiety, a sense of being thrown back on and isolated in one's own physicality which becomes ever more unbearable. This pressure becomes all the harder to bear when the psychological-spiritual impulse to transcend this constriction, to enter into a new relationship with the Other, society, the world, and nature, reaches its peak. Taking drugs and consuming media provide the psychological illusion of such a connection, which does nothing more than leave behind an even more intense experience of loneliness.

Fear is a companion to human individuation. There is such thing as a *pathological absence of fear* [Husemann and Wolff 1986, vol. II, 39], usually due to attention deficit disorders (e. g. in the case of hyperkinetic children). In paediatric practice, something else needs to be borne in mind: these children "just don't get something". Not only are they devoid of fear, but they are simultaneously incapable of full psychological perception of the situation. Motorically driven children (i. e. children who are more physically active and less motivated by a rich inner life) who struggle to experience *empathy*, the soul entity in others, or *psychological correspondence*, can attract attention, e. g. due to their lack of fear. These children frequently go on to have difficulties in becoming socialized; they do not understand what another person feels, how his behaviour is meant, or what is expected of them in psychological terms. However capable they may be, this is potentially an enormous stumbling block; as adults, such people frequently fall prey to addiction problems (alcohol), failed relationships and so on.

But by what process *is anxiety overcome?* Recognition of the Other, the insight which can give the stranger a name, is merely the first step here. The anxiety will only be overcome in a positive sense if the person manages *to enter into a psychological-physical correspondence, an understanding of the Other, or to go through with and master an initially frightening situation* (the archetypal motif of human cultural development: the test of courage, the ordeal of the soul, such as is encountered, for instance, in Mozart's Magic Flute by Pamina and Tamino). Child and adolescent psychiatrist Matthias Wildermuth characterizes this resolution of the development of anxiety in children and adolescents, corresponding to the experience of Tamino in the world of Sarastro, with the following helpful words: "The last stage, in which anxiety really does become one of the most helpful values of all, would then be one of *awe*, which would involve not just internally experiencing what I must do as a task but having an experience in the deepest recesses of my I that, in the world outside, that which is outside of my self, there is something amazing which I can only approach in a spirit of humility. If such humility and awe becomes possible, anxiety will decrease. Acknowledgement of the Other acquires the character of an *acknowledgement of his spiritual individuality* [Wildermuth 2006, 125].

But why is it that the soul does not feel constricted when correspondence is successful, when action is successful? Access to this is to be found just as much in research into one's own experience as access to anxiety [cf. Fuchs 2000]. In the process, what is revealed in phenomenological terms is that the soul or I *really manages to build a bridge between I and You, Hand and Object;* that, in psychological-spiritual terms, the person is in such moments *not constrained within the limits of his body* but *is really capable of transcending these to reach out to the Other*: The Soul and the I are there where *my feelings and consciousness* are experienced. To think that the soul or the spirit is chained directly to the material is an illusion with far-reaching consequences. The I of the surgeon carrying out an intestinal anastomosis is not present merely in the synapses of his neocortex but also directly in his hand; yes, it succeeds in turning the needle driver and the needle into one of its own organs, it connects this with the body, and its action will succeed to the extent to which it is capable of entering *into this organ* and adapting the actions of the hand to the conditions of this organ. Exactly the same thing happens when it comes to understanding another person. It is sufficient just to follow with full awareness and unbiased thought how, by means of the resonance of one's own body with that of the other person, one's own awareness establishes itself ever more fully in him and experiences his movement increasingly as one's own and begins to correspond with him. This act, this ability to enter afresh and independently *into* the world, *into* the Other, to be able to emotionally feel and understand him, is both a capability and a need of the human soul and its own antidote to anxiety. The sword which made the wound can itself also be used to close it up.

7.2.1 Considerations for parent consultation regarding children's anxieties, fears and phobias

It is generally the parents who report on the anxieties of their children; in the case of childhood anxieties, from a diagnostic point of view it is of crucial importance to get to know *the parents themselves in their own anxieties*, their psychological constitution and the way they behave with the child: "The fate of the childhood anxiety depends to a decisive extent on the behaviour and attitude in the child's surrounding" [Nissen 1989, 156]. Research carried out by A. Freud and D.T. Burlingham in London during German air raids in the Second World War revealed that children up to the age of two only showed fear if the mothers themselves were fearful; "they were otherwise interested, curious and unworried" [Freud 1943]. This underlines the extent to which children in the first seven years, learn by imitation, how intensively they correspond psychologically and physically at this age with their parents – including, and in particular, in the way they deal with anxiety.

For this reason it is necessary in medical terms to make a conscious distinction between the various dimensions which interweave in the genesis of childhood anxieties in order to take the parents seriously as both reporting and affected parties and to learn to separate them from the

- constitutional predisposition of the child to anxiety,
- the child's development and the moments of anxiety connected with it,
- disruptions in physical or psychological development with the resulting anxieties (e.g. specific anxieties in the case of autism or infantile cerebral palsy, etc),
- the anxiety that is brought about by particular trigger moments (which can also be precipitated by children and siblings),
- the induction into anxiety by anxious, under-confident and over-protective parents,

- induced anxiety by psychologically ill (e.g. depressive, psychotic) parents and relations,
- induced anxiety through the exercise of (partially concealed) parental or educational/professional pressure,
- induced anxiety through separation conflicts between the parents, rivalry between attachment figures (e.g. mother/grandmother), (often unstated) family conflicts, through repressed persons or events in the family [Weber 1995],
- "Psychotoxic" [Nissen 1989, 161] injuries to the child – these often start at an early age – through open or concealed hostility to the child.

An important anxiety-triggering moment can arise as early as infancy if the child is unable to integrate his perceptions in respect of his parents, above all his mother, in such a way as to make *unambiguous sense* of them. This can be pathologically conditioned, e.g. in the case of autism; much more frequently, however, the reason is to be found in *contradictory*, psychologically ambivalent behaviour on the part of the parents (which is, it must be said, something that arises in everyone who brings up children if they are over-tired, affected by another conflict or provoked by childish behaviour but making every effort to keep themselves under control). The child will then not be able to correspond – to resonate – without anxiety because he may be receiving totally contradictory signals at the same time. In this case it is urgently necessary to estimate the level of aggression felt by the parents towards the child and to clarify its origin (e.g. also aggression towards the partner, towards oneself) in order to be able to offer helpful counsel.

A further problem that frequently occurs today is the partial *shift of parental tasks and responsibilities onto the child.* This is, for example, the case if a defiantly crying 3½ year old boy is met with words like these: "You're making me sad with all this crying; just tell me what you want, please make your mind up." Very often what arises is a situation in which *the child is overtaxed* in a way inappropriate to his age through being burdened with a responsibility which should only ever be assumed by an adult. Such parental behaviour is not infrequently akin to that of a captain who is trying to negotiate Cape Horn in the face of a brewing storm and asks the passengers which course he should lay in…

Much of what has been mentioned above will not necessarily be reported spontaneously to the doctor, some of it not at all, not even on request (cf. the case in 7.1.3.). What can help with older children is the child's own spontaneous report, which is however usually only delivered late and often only in the absence of the parents, particularly in the case of anxious children.

It can be very helpful to have the children paint pictures when visiting the doctor, e.g. in a quiet place in the practice close to the reception, whilst the medical history is being discussed with the parents (one subject might be "Things I am frightened of", another might be "the family", or "myself" etc. cf. specialized literature).

In the consulting room itself, care must be taken to distinguish between non-verbal and verbal communication; if both parents are present, an important aspect is to observe their behaviour around each other (e.g. the facial expression and posture of the one while the other is speaking). The behaviour of the siblings must also be taken into account; a small age difference (less than 18 months) and the order of age of the siblings (e.g. the second of three children) can be points of reference in the diagnosis of anxiety disorders and depression in childhood.

The question concerning the *use of media* by children (and parents) is of considerable significance in the field of anxiety disorders. It is generally true that the abyss of anxiety opens up as a result of the loss of previous familiarity, and this also includes constraint, limitation, in the life of the child through the expansion of his horizons. *Perceptions of hitherto unknown people, new names and concepts, and unfamiliar actions which overtax the child's processing capacity* encourage the development of childhood fears over and above the extent required for development. *Anything to which the child cannot connect, or that he cannot understand, really emotionally feel or process through action* (e. g. in his own play) can give rise to anxiety. A great many childhood anxieties are nowadays being generated in this way. A classic trigger of anxiety is the television: Watching TV generates impressions in the child's consciousness; it is not, however, amenable to correspondence with the child; it does not respond to the child; it is in reality just appearance (in quite another sense than the fairy tales told by the mother). Unlike a physically talking person, the medium of television has a *laming* effect on the physical movements of the child (right down to the eye movements, which are completely different when the child sees a newsreader than when he looks at his father [Patzlaff 1999]).

But the child will only really *understand* the other person, a perceived process, in a "bodily" sense if he can correspond with the object of perception in a spiritual, psychological and bodily way [Fuchs 2000, 274–284]. This is still possible in the theatre, for instance, in the case of a puppet show, but not in front of the screen. Television encourages the process of gathering information without psychological participation, without bodily involvement. A person who watches a lot of television will have a lot of knowledge but will not get to know anyone or acquire any skills. So he will not learn the capabilities he needs to master his anxiety.

So attentiveness, time and a little luck are required first of all to arrive at an initial diagnostic assessment of the childhood anxieties and their origin, where the extent of the diagnostic clarification is determined by the scope and chronicity of the disorder. It also needs to be taken into account that the reticence of the parents themselves, particularly in the case of a positive relationship of longer standing, can sometimes hinder the clarification of an anxiety situation; in such instances it can in some cases be helpful to involve a neutral colleague before what might be a heavy burden on the child gets overlooked. The therapeutic treatment of childhood anxieties requires not only the *courage to present a truthful diagnosis* but also the art of *involving the parents, helping them understand what is happening and motivating them to take the required therapeutic steps.*

As in the case of sleep disorders (▸Chap. 7.1), one might draw the conclusion that the treatment of childhood anxieties purely belongs to clinical consultation, behavioural and family therapy or, as the case may be, psychotherapy. Such a conclusion would be one-sided. Instead it would be correct to say that the common therapeutic denominator consists in relieving the child of burdens that his capabilities do not allow him to manage: he has to learn to overcome those anxieties which the acquisition of new skills will allow him to master. Important help on this path comes in the form of *art therapies*, such as painting, modelling and music therapy [von der Heide 1997]. These function primarily in a *non-verbal way*, which is a great advantage in childhood; they also promote the disentanglement of the child from his parents and give both sides *more autonomy* and opportunity to change. *The child learns a new form of psychological expression* by means of which he simultaneously develops a new way of relating to the world and acquires new, independent skills for overcoming anxiety.

What value does medicinal treatment have? This question may be answered only on a case-by-case basis, taking the individual situation into account; it is often the case, that the circumstances are anything other than ideal and the possibilities for a change in the behaviour of the parents, family structure or school etc. are limited. The primary role of the doctor is to give the child support and also offer tangible assistance in the event that a treatment which does not involve medication and which might from the point of view of the actual cause be much more fundamentally useful, is not immediately possible or is inadequate in the short term; his first objective is to gain the child's trust, which takes time and can be helped by initial therapeutic successes.

One might otherwise be tempted to say that only homoeopathic-anthroposophic medicines offer a practical and safe perspective on medical therapy for childhood anxieties. If one compares the possibilities offered by conventional pharmacotherapy for anxiety disorders [e.g. Steinhausen 2010, 201], what remains, above all, are selective serotonin reuptake inhibitors (SSRI), which themselves entail a significant risk of side effects, especially in puberty and adolescence. With the possible exception of extreme crisis situations, benzodiazepines should never be used; "the effectiveness of antidepressants in children who refuse to go to school, particularly where separation anxiety is a factor, is in the case of tricyclic antidepressants a matter of considerable controversy." [Steinhausen, l.c.] Anthroposophic and homoeopathic medicines, however, can play a decisive role in the therapy itself, especially in cases where the child's constitution, an age-related maturation process, or trigger situations for which other forms of treatment are either ineffective or of very limited use, are a significant factor (cf. ▸Chap. 7.1.5.1). This applies in the first instance to drugs, which stimulate the organism to change or activate learning processes or promote a new regulatory equilibrium, as is the case with homoeopathic and anthroposophic medicines. A medicinal product of this kind can also help a child to learn new things, overcome hindrances, feel more at ease and freer in his own body and find a new way of approaching his environment. This has been afforded insufficient attention in paediatrics and adolescent psychiatry as yet.

7.2.2 Counselling and non-medicinal therapies

> Overall it can be said that, in the treatment of anxieties, a behavioural therapeutic approach, in which the child learns specific strategies for confronting anxiety-inducing situations, has proved its worth.
>
> F. U. Petermann [2010]

7.2.2.1 Anxiety: birth to age 7

When and by what means does psychological constriction arise, in the child, the mother or the father? Many anxieties have their origin in the parents' past; others, however, arise for the first time in the child, and this is nowadays often the case in association with conception and pregnancy (▸Chap. 2.4). *Maternal anxiety concerning the child* all too frequently threatens to become the *child's own anxiety* [Nissen 1989, 161]. Such anxieties are common: the fear of miscarriage, a disability in the child, a premature birth, a complication; the fear of the new role, in particular when the mother cannot accept her own parents or views them as a bad example; the mother's own inexperience, the ambivalent relationship between parenthood and career, existential financial anxiety: the major significance of maternal anxieties in particular is well documented in the annals of child and adolescent psychiatry, but in practice it is a matter of taking time, listening and offering help before they turn into disproportionate childhood anxieties. In this respect a great deal can be done, for instance, in the context of preventative consultations in the child's first year of life.

But there is above all one "antidote" which is of decisive importance in determining the child's future tendency to anxiety: *Confidence (trust).* The confidence that the child can learn to calm himself if he has previously been shown the requisite care; the confidence that the child can overcome something for himself through his fever and the fever does not have to be immediately taken away; the confidence that he will fall over when learning to walk in a way that will allow him to get up again. Confidence develops out of ability and experience, and a young couple with a newborn child *can* hardly be expected to have both at their disposal in this situation.

For this reason, the paediatrician or general practitioner has a decisive role to play. After all, he potentially has both; what matters is what he passes on to the parents. Many parents, however, experience *medicine itself as a significant source of anxiety.* Every doctor can in this respect ask himself to what extent his practice and he himself are in equilibrium when it comes to dealing with anxiety. A lot of time is spent on excluding disorders: by ultrasound, through genetics, in the context of preventive care, through the provision of information concerning the risks of not taking vitamin D, vitamin K or fluorine or not having the child vaccinated at three, four and six months, if an ear inflammation is not treated with antibiotics, and so on. The reality is that what *the child and his parents can do for themselves does not even feature here!* The only light in the darkness has been the rehabilitation of breastfeeding after so much time was spent in vain on the development of substitutes for it. Only the paediatrician who himself knows where he can trust the child, gives him time to show if he can shake off the infection himself or form his own skeleton, who recognizes and wants to encourage the child's individual possibilities instead of using the schematic generalization of preventive medicine and suppressive drugs to weaken them yet further, is working in harmony with the objective of promoting confidence and learning how to overcome anxieties.

As a general principle, anxieties in the first seven years of life are more strongly influenced by *bodily constitution* and development than is later the case, a fact which must be taken into consideration in discussion with the parents. Many anxieties at this age have their roots in bodily constitution (cf. ▸Chap. 7.2.3, medicinal constitutional therapy); bodily constitution is an important moment for the child's tendency to, and processing of, anxiety. At the same time, attention must be paid to the maturation of *body-centred perception*, the sense of touch, sense of pain and sense of vitality [Steiner 1970], and the perception of movement (proprioception) and balance. Among other things, the oft-cited evening application of oil, use of natural textile fibres, rocking and cradling, but also allowing the child time to raise itself up until crawling has been mastered and the sense of balance has matured, all offer parents an opportunity to contribute to the child's development in this respect. Moreover, in this connection the sense of warmth or the organization of warmth gain special significance (cf. ▸Chap. 2.2.1). *The positive (basic) confidence and trust in one's own physicality* depends very largely on these basal sensory perceptions [Köhler 1994].

It is essential for parents firstly to become aware of the consequences of *learning through imitation*: the underlying principle, that *whatever the child experiences in the family is wor-*

thy of imitation. The important point is that a positive reference is possible and encouraged: e. g. a mealtime ceremony, a beautifully laid table, a conversation about personal experience. Conversation about trouble in the workplace, the cancer of a close relative or the like, on the other hand, is best kept for another context. All that is considered above is the necessary establishment of a regular daily rhythm, the uninterrupted accompaniment in necessary separation situations, with particular reference to going to sleep (▸Chap. 7.1). – The importance of *repetition* in the acquisition of new skills is common knowledge; this applies especially to learning through imitation in childhood. In this way, the evening ritual can involve the repeated negotiation of the fear-inducing situation until the child can deal with it himself. Before every new step, e. g. starting at kindergarten, it is necessary to check whether the preconditions for a further separation from the mother or the parents are satisfied or whether earlier separation anxieties have yet to be overcome. This can always be attempted by gradually building up the negotiation of the separation situation, using a procedure similar to that which has successfully proven its value with sleep disorders [Kast-Zahn 1997]. All this presupposes trust, patient repetition and consistency in parental behaviour.

Alongside the consultation it can be very helpful to the parents, particularly the mother, to create a *moment of inner peace* during the evening and to let the experiences with the child, choosing initially just few experiences, pass in revue before the soul. If possible, one should try to perceive oneself and the child from the outside, as it were from a vantage point adjacent to the scene on which the events were played out. A directly conscious evaluation of the experience should be avoided; instead one can learn to have confidence that practical correctives for the following day will naturally arise from such a review as long as one experiences it in a state of inner calm [Steiner 1993, 22–24]. The regular practice of this exercise over time can generate the strength needed to maintain psychological and emotional equilibrium toward the child, to avoid unnecessary intervention and to gain a direct perception of the potentials and needs of the child.

A regular *exchange between both parents* concerning their experience of the child is also supportive. Although this may very often happen spontaneously, it is frequently fruitless and can even reinforce the problem if the partners trade mutual accusations and blame. It can be helpful to *limit the time for such an exchange, e. g. to a total of 15–20 minutes, and to arrange it so that each parent can describe his or her experience without being interrupted or commented on by the other.* The aim is rather *to learn to accept the other person's experience,* to acknowledge its validity, yes, where possible even to empathize with it, before reporting on one's own experience with the partner now exercising the same empathetic listening. The effects of consistent adherence to this rule can be astounding, even after just a few weeks, both in dealing with the child and at the level of the partner relationship itself.

7.2.2.2 Anxiety: age 7–14

In the period between the 7th and 14th years of life it is very often *psychosomatic complaints*, such as circulation problems or headaches, which drive both parents and child to the doctor. *Bronchial asthma*, an ever more common condition at this age, is also a psychosomatic phenomenon which is accompanied by anxiety and feelings of constriction (cf. ▸Chap. 6.5.1). If childhood atopic eczema either emerges for the first time in the second seven year period, or is exacerbated at this age by school stress and other external triggers, the question should always be asked as to whether there might be an anxiety disorder on the part of the parents (mostly, but not always and not exclusively affecting the mother). Recognising this and the manner in which the child appropriates the anxiety for itself paves the way for dramatic therapeutic successes. For the doctor, the first task is to identify the anxieties and establish their origin. In general, however, it is at this age that the psychological development of the child takes centre stage, corresponding to the bodily maturation of the rhythmic system in all its aspects (respiration, circulation, spine, hormonal organization and others). Thus, for example, an age-related instability in the blood circulation can arise in the context of a growth spurt and quickly subside with medicinal support; on the other hand, any disorder of the rhythmic system may have its primary cause in the soul entity, which at this age must be looked at with particular care.

It is frequently the task of the doctor to diagnose the presence of childhood anxieties and bring them to the attention of the parents; in other cases, however, the child's anxieties are themselves the occasion for the consultation. In this case it is good first of all to listen calmly to the parents and, if possible, not to interrupt them until they have finished their report. After all, this is the attitude, which at the end of the day is to be instilled in the parents themselves: to listen calmly and sympathetically to their child. From the 9th year, however, this presupposes that the parents know that their child feels alone in his anxiety and learn to accept this experience of isolation. *The child must feel that he has permission to feel differently from his parents and that this difference is respected.* Two attitudes above all prevent the child from expressing himself (and force him to retreat even more into his anxiety): *expectations* (e. g. in relation to school, conformity with the teacher etc.) and the *parental fear of anxiety*, the result of which is an immediate urge to drive out of the child the very experience that he is living through as part of his process of developing autonomy.

At this age it is very important for the anxious child to be able to learn to share and express his experience within the family. He has to be able to feel that he is being taken seriously and that his anxiety can be acknowledged by his parents without an immediate loss of psychological equilibrium on their part. In the case of anxious-withdrawn children it can be very helpful if the less anxious parent, who is often the father, goes on a trip for a few days with the child (on foot, by boat or the like), as this can open the floodgates of the soul and simultaneously enhance self-confidence. To give this confidence is the task of the parents, whereas the *direct* contribution they can make to overcoming anxiety (e. g. socialization anxiety at school) is even more limited than it used to be.

Both the doctor and the parents must also try to assess the extent to which the child already has sufficient psychological ability to manage his anxiety. If this ability is insufficiently developed at this age, training in artistic skills takes on particular significance. Artistic activity corresponds to the psychological maturation processes which take place at this age as well as the as yet hazy and semi-conscious experience of the child's own existential situation, of his anxiety. In practice, experience shows that children at this age who have anxiety disorders respond particularly well with long-term effect to appropriate kinds of qualified art therapy. With all children at this age it makes good sense to consult with the parents with a view to promoting their child's artistic development, not least because this gives the child skills which can be of crucial importance in the management of anxiety in the third seven period.

7.2.2.2.1 Typical anxiety disorders in the second seven year period: School phobia

Fear of this separation can arise at and after the "Rubicon age" of the 9th year of life in the form of *school phobia*: Going to school and the task of establishing connections with teachers and peers can make the child anxious because he still feels fully dependent on the symbiotic protection of the connection (above all) with his mother. It is the loss of this familiarity, which has until that point protected the child, that can lead affected children to develop anxieties which urgently require therapy. The predominant constitution as defined by anthroposophic medicine is the large-headed[1] constitution: children who, on the one hand, are intelligent, above average at school and strongly led by the super-I but, on the other, incline to retarded psychological-emotional and anxious-sensitive development [Steinhausen 2010, 203], show little inclination to form connections in their peer group, preferring instead to retain a close connection to their parents. The parents may tend to be overprotective and clingy, but a significant part of the dynamic originates with the child. Care must be taken to distinguish this kind of deep-seated developmental crisis from *school phobia*, which is based on fear of teachers, peers and the pressure to perform, that is, the challenges presented by the new horizon of experience. It is above all crucial that a clear distinction be made from the diagnosis of a "justified" school phobia e.g. in the case of excessive educational demands, serious problems with teachers or assault in or around the school premises. At the same time it is essential to consider that, in the case of school phobia, the reports given by the affected children likewise tend to dwell on the presence of threat at school, yet in these cases an external scrutiny of the medical history usually reveals a well-behaved, performance-oriented child who is, however, poor at establishing contact with others.

- In the case of school phobia, art therapy can be particularly meaningful and helpful. It is not unusual to come across scepticism, primarily on the part of child and parents, in respect of this step (the reasons for this scepticism are manifold). Behind this there lurks the instinctive knowledge that this therapy will result in the loosening of the close, still largely uniform psychological landscape of child and parents. On the other hand, the children can soon flourish psychologically, e.g. in the context of skilfully guided painting therapy, and have their first ever experience of a psychological space which is particular to them.
- Of decisive significance with school phobia[2] is the disclosure to the parents of the true nature of the disorder: "School phobia, and this contradicts the literal meaning of the word 'phobia', is not a fear directed at school: what lies at its heart is a separation anxiety" [Steinhausen 2010, 203]. It therefore follows that a school phobia will escalate at that point of the morning at which the child is supposed to say goodbye to his parents. This therapeutic separation must be actively sought and driven by the parents if the disorder is to be actively overcome. The parents and the child are the decisive "service providers" in the therapy! As, in practice, the prognosis is by no means always favourable for the children, it has been shown to be effective to state this clearly and insistently right from the start:

1 Among the children observed in our own practice, round head shapes dominate until puberty, a head shape with a pronounced forehead, a large head which physically radiates a great deal of heat. The close ties with the mother or parents can also be observed in visits to the consulting room, e.g. when the child sits as close as possible to the parents. [For more on the "large-headed constitution" cf. also Vademecum 2010, 673]

2 What is meant here is the "primary" school phobia, not the kind which can arise after brain tumour operations or other traumatic experiences and which requires different treatment.

- A therapy will succeed only if the parents commit themselves to it
- Every failure makes the conditions for a subsequent attempt less favourable
- Whereas admission to an institution will as a rule overcome the disorder in the short term, after the return to the domestic setting the force of habit will prevail. For this reason, the determination to cut the "umbilical cord", in conjunction with the well-prepared and decisive action of everyone involved, gives rise to the best prospect of success.
- The parents must be prepared for the possibility that their "nice" child may in the context of such a change in behaviour also have tantrums, withdraw socially and demonstrate somatization (headaches and stomach ache, lying in bed etc.) and will have to be "brought back on track" in a sympathetic but consistent manner.

In therapeutic terms, it is a matter of

- Reducing symbiotic behaviours at home which are inappropriate to the child's age
- Avoiding school exemptions, sick notes, therapies in resorts (in the case of "indispositions" the child should be brought to the doctor and, where possible, any sick note should be issued by him alone)
- Making the transition as quickly as possible to a behaviour and style of upbringing, which is consistently focused on regular attendance at school: You're going to school today, and that's that!
- Answering calls from the child on his or her journey to school or from the school itself with the required degree of objective distance
- Furthermore, the following pieces of advice have proved their worth in practice:
- It is helpful for the father to be present and to demonstrate an unambiguous attitude until the child leaves the house
- Reports given by the child which reflect badly on the school or cast it in a threatening light should be investigated by the parents independently of the child (such stories are often driven by anxiety)
- An (appropriate) behaviour-related reward system can have a positive initial effect e.g. if the child goes to school every day in a given week.
- Alongside art therapy, individual and group therapies can also help the child acquire an appropriate level of social competence in respect of his peers [Petermann 2010]
- Another very significant source of help with school phobia, but only in a therapeutic context as outlined here, comes in the form of anthroposophic-homoeopathic medicinal therapy (cf. 7.2.3.2.5)

7

7.2.2.3 Anxiety: age 14–21

During puberty it is often temporarily impossible for the child to express himself to his parents. And the paediatrician, selected by the parent, is seldom the right person to turn to. It can be helpful for the parents experiencing psychological intensification in their child, and in their relationship to him, to call on the help of adult friends of the family with whom the child has a relationship of trust. *Danger arises when the child has no adult point of contact.*

From the paedagogic and therapeutic points of view, treatment in the third septennial, runs in practice into much greater difficulties. On the other hand, however, it becomes possible in direct communication with the adolescent to acknowledge and overcome the anxiety. Considerable reserve is initially required of a doctor if he is to learn about the psychological situation and determine the extent of the anxiety. This can be very varied, free floating, or dark, abyssal and existentially threatening. The adolescent often feels at its mercy and incapable of grasping it. There is very often a negative, fraught and hostile attitude to the past, which correlates closely with the rejection of the adolescent's own physicality. The manifold maturation and existential anxieties have already been described. The power of feeling and the adolescent's own urge for the future are juxtaposed with the powerlessness of his own actions, the external expectations of the performance-oriented consumer society with his own uncertainty and weak sense of self-confidence: He knows a lot already but is capable of little! This above all, is felt experience by the adolescents who spend the ages from 14 to 20 cramming at school (or in front of the computer) without acquiring any competence in art or practical interaction, at an age at which nothing is more urgently required to overcome anxiety. This situation forms the backdrop to the transition, the slide into depressive disorders and symptoms.

As far as diagnosis is concerned, care must be taken not to misdiagnose serious psychiatric disorders, which are strongly accompanied by an anxiety syndrome or initially draw attention to themselves in this form. These disorders are frequently not fully perceived by the family members or are wrongly interpreted, making it essential for the doctor to make his own judgement.

Different approaches to therapeutic treatment are possible. One operates at the *conscious level*: the background to the occurrence of the anxiety and the possible ways of overcoming it can be openly discussed and considered. Taking this approach, the function of the I can be activated to give the soul entity new support and its activity a direction. In the process it is a matter of recognising the adolescent's decisive anxieties and underlying problems and working together to figure out practical steps in life to overcome them. These might concern the way the adolescent relates to friends of both genders, his parents or himself, and the anguish he experiences in those relationships; or the issues might among other things relate to school or work. What is always decisive in the end is that the adolescent takes the initiative and plucks up the courage to take a new step.

In many cases the young person is initially unable to act out of his or her own accord, even in settings involving free creativity. The I is too weak to act creatively; any work done in the context of school or vocational training is accompanied by excessive consumption: of electronic entertainment, substance abuse. Banning these makes almost no difference and is not asked for; the adolescent should instead be encouraged to take the initiative. Involvement in the arts can be of considerable help here[1], e. g. playing music with other young people and, in particular, acting, which offers a wide range of artistic opportunities and also requires the adolescent to consciously work on himself in areas as fundamental as posture and speech.

It is equally important for the adolescent to learn how to be alone, to familiarize himself with silence. In the first instance this presupposes appropriate withdrawal from the family environment, but it also requires a willingness to surrender to the experience of silence without a mobile phone, TV or any other kind of distraction, e. g. by taking a quiet day out in the country. If this skill is not acquired at this age it becomes very difficult to master later in life and it remains a constant source of existential anxiety. It can be a great help if, in the second seven year period, the child's father or mother undertake appropriate activities alone with the child in order to acquaint him with the fulfilling experience of

1 An impressive example of this can be found in the project and film "Rhythm is it"!

silence in the natural world (this is excellently illustrated by Faust's monologue in nature in Part One of Goethe's Faust; Goethe's biography is also sprinkled with exhortations of this kind).

The parents are also significant in the crisis situation in the third septennial. They require the same kind of medical advice as the adolescent himself, albeit at a different time. It now becomes imperative, above all, to listen and accept the psychological situation of the other, to show interest in those things which move the adolescent, to state one's own position without attempting to persuade or directly try to make something happen. Taking the time to listen is often repaid by intense gratitude on the part of the adolescent, whose own self-confidence has been ravaged by anxiety, the time taken to be with him gives him a sense of his own inherent worth. So, at this age, going out for the day or taking a short holiday break with a parent can provide valuable help.

A particularly important relationship for adolescents from broken marriages and adopted families is that with their biological parents. In this instance it can fall to the doctor to do the groundwork to establish this contact and to assist in the processing of this situation. The specific tasks which go with the territory of supporting adopted children, particularly in puberty and adolescence, are unfortunately beyond the scope of this book.

The principal long-term way of overcoming the existential anxiety of the third seven year period, is to enable the adolescent to find an authentic direction in life and to work out his own objectives and ideals. Only then will his I become an effective driving force in the soul entity. At this point it must be noted that, at the age of 18 or 19, an inner experience can spontaneously unfold. 'That's what I want to do, that's what I want to learn, and that's where I want to go'. What is important is to give appropriate guidance to make the adolescent "receptive" to his or her own inner voice and the impulses of his/her own individuality (anyone who is constantly, "plugged into the net", will fail to hear themselves). It is helpful to train the adolescent in the silence and patience required for this experience to arise [cf. Roder 2005, 44–59]. By way of contrast, attempts to give practical advice concerning the most promising career, the right thing to do from the point of view of the parents and the doctor, and so on, can be disastrous.

Adolescence can be considered the decisive phase in the birth of the I; it follows that this period also gives rise to the most deeply felt anxieties. The I is fundamentally and inherently spiritual and requires spiritual nourishment if it is to grow and act. The inner need for ideals is at its strongest at this age, even if what is shown to the world gives rise to a completely different impression. The central, authentic human ideal is intimately connected with the overcoming of anxiety: to act for the good of other people, not for selfish reasons but because the others need it and the adolescent can do it; and to trust that the adolescents needs can be satisfied by other people. Wherever this ideal flourishes, anxiety recedes; where it fails to thrive, anxiety will grow.

At this point a final glance is cast back upon the parents, the therapist or other key adults in the young person's life: at their honesty, their own engagement and dealings with anxiety: "Anxiety depends to a decisive extent on the behaviour and attitude which prevail in one's surroundings" [Struck 1989].

7.2.2.4 Eurythmy therapy

Eurythmy therapy (see appendix ▸Chap. 10) offers an important therapeutic opportunity for children suffering from anxiety. A comparison with the detailed discussion elsewhere on the use of eurythmy therapy in cases of bronchial asthma (▸Chap. 6.5.5.3) sheds light on some key aspects of this therapy: it can

- create the balance required for the development of consciousness through the learning of new, ensouled forms of movement,
- promote a positive and harmonious inner experience of the body, strengthen soul-activity in the body in a targeted manner through eurythmic movements, and
- reinforce the child's self-confidence and loosen inappropriately strong ties to and dependence on the mother.

The most important vocal exercise for children with anxieties is "A", which can be carried out in different ways depending on the individual, e. g. on tiptoe, crouching or with jumps. The "A-H" gestures, when performed in the context of the "reverence-A" exercise, strengthen the different levels of the organization in their protective, enveloping quality. It does children good to thoroughly immerse themselves in the "A" movement until the opening and anxiety-mitigating effect of this exercise becomes a lived experience. Concerning the consonants, important sounds are "L", "M", "N", and "R". Again, "L" and "M" serve to stimulate the development of a balance between inhalation and exhalation and, in the process in general, the transition from one sound exercise to the next is very important (▸Chap. 6.5.5.3). The "M" and, in particular, the "N" serve to counter a depressive tendency to withdraw on the part of the child; the "R" activates the breathing process and connects it intensively with the movement of the spine and the limbs.

The "I" exercise, which is carried out with the neck and head only (in the form of a stretching movement of the neck) is suitable for the activation of the energies of the soul-spiritual individuality, to a certain extent for bringing them more strongly into the child. In the case of anxious children who, as is often the case, *find it difficult to get up in the morning,* intense and repeated stretching in bed will serve a similar purpose. Such children can pat the soles of their feet and, in the case of the tendency to orthostatic dysregulation/grogginess when rising, which occurs in the second septennial, carry out a "U" exercise with their arms whilst sitting on the edge of the bed.

7.2.3 Medicinal treatment options for childhood anxiety disorders

7.2.3.1 Basis for individualized treatment with single-substance medicines

Successful identification of the individually effective potentized medicine depends, in addition to history taking, largely on *the doctor's observation of the child* when they meet and in the latter's interaction with his parents and other children/siblings. In this regard, children with anxiety disorders can be assigned to particular groups, which make it significantly easier to identify the right medicine.

7.2.3.1.1 Quiet, reticent behaviour with fear of unfamiliar people

These children are generally reserved and quiet when they meet the doctor; they are afraid of mockery, making fools of themselves, being *exposed* in front of others (e. g. at kindergarten and school) and are sensitive to every ill-considered, flippant remark made by adults. Their anxiety is primarily conditioned by their constitution and associated with one-sidedness in physical development. They are subject to a more pronounced form of many of the developmentally conditioned childhood anxieties mentioned above (e. g. separation anxiety, environmental anxiety etc.). A doctor's appointment is a typical anxiety trigger for these children because they don't know what to expect and because they are afraid of being exposed as unable to do things they *haven't yet learnt to do*. Their anxiety, their lack of self-confidence arises out of the unconscious perception or feeling of their own lack of maturity.

The most important medicines for this group of children are, on the one hand, potentized calcium carbonate and, on the other, potentized rock crystal:

- **Conchae** and **quartz.**

The type of child who derives profound developmental support from Calcium carbonicum = Conchae (▸Chap. 3.2.5.1) and can by this means reduce his anxiety levels is primarily characterized by *close ties to his mother.* He holds on tightly to her, hides behind her, and would ultimately prefer to stay for longer in the mother's womb as a means of protection from the world (typical of these children is that many of them are born after the expected date of delivery). Such children manifest slow (but consistent!) development, a delayed awakening of consciousness and late development of social contact. It is not unusual for the mother herself to demonstrate traits of the type depicted (conditioned by both constitution and heredity): a somewhat corpulent figure who carries everything she needs in her bags and "sails" into the consulting room in loose and comfortable clothing like a protective ship, taking a while to arrange herself comfortably before sitting down…

The child himself tends to appear young for his age, infantile, with swelling forms, "lymphatic" in the sense of high water content, demonstrating slow ossification (e. g. closure of the fontanelle), a tendency to be catarrhal and a slow transition to an upright posture. The bodily-vital development process is way in advance of the psychological, which always goes hand in hand with the formation and limitation of growth. In this context, such children are often characterized by the delayed onset of active speech (although language comprehension develops normally); the child begins to speak only at the point at which he considers himself able to pass muster without making a fool of himself (the same applies later to oral participation in lessons at school).

Thus it is, that the anxieties these children suffer from are much more apparent to the doctor from their conduct and his diagnosis, whereas the children themselves only later become able to confide in others about their own anxiety. Yes, talking to older children and adults of this constitutional type reveals that they only *slowly become consciously aware* of what triggers their anxiety, but these triggers have long-standing psychological repercussions: e. g. television images showing explicit violence and its effects; scary and unsettling stories (depending on the individual the threshold can be very low here) which cause the child to lie awake at night, even though he may not yet have shown any obvious reaction during the television programme. It is important to ask specific questions about this and, where applicable, not only to administer Calcium carbonicum but also, and most importantly, to alert the parents to the child's sensitivity and encourage them to find an appropriate paedagogical way of dealing with it. *Typical anxieties* of this type of child are:

- Fear of being alone, in the dark, fear of separation from the mother (separation anxiety).
- Fear of (often very particular) animals e. g. dogs, insects, spiders, mice etc. right down to phobias e. g. of ladybugs, even when seen in pictures [Coulter 1989, 100]).
- Fear of violence (natural forces, criminal violence, accidents), including those in stories and the media, of encroachments from the outside world (the child needs the feeling of safety that comes with his own, delimited world, a protective shell to keep the world out in order to feel at ease).

Nocturnal nightmares can reveal similar sources of anxiety.

Particularly with children who have a very pronounced (anabolic) metabolism, the dosage should progress gradually from low to higher potencies. This is in line with the fact that the cause is to be found less in a pathology than in a delayed development, which is in turn due to a relative preponderance of the metabolism. The authors have found the following to be effective

- **Conchae D6–12 trit.** Weleda, **LM6–12 dil.** Arcana
  1 Saltspoon 1–3 x/d or 5 gtt. 1–2 x/d, administered for approx. 3–6 weeks, depending on the case

This remedy is supported by a rigorously observed evening ritual; an evening prayer spoken in a state of calm concentration has a particularly calming and confidence-building effect on the young soul and can compensate for the after-effects of experiences from daily life. Further impulses for the development of consciousness can be derived from essential oils (e. g. rosemary, Hypericum and thyme, as a foot or full bath, rubbed into the legs or ribcage [thyme] or the back [Hypericum]. With this therapeutic process, one may observe the formation of the body (discernible also in a sharp reduction of often excessive perspiration, in ossification, the erectness of the back, the facial features), a reduction in susceptibility to infection and the tendency to the production of catarrh (and, in some cases, in hypertrophy of the adenoid and tonsils), more intensive pneumatization (i. e. improved formation of the air-filled cavities as an expression of more pronounced soul-entity-forming activity ▸Chap. 5.1.2), an opening up and a burgeoning feeling of security in relation to the outside world, coupled with a reduction in levels of anxiety.

- **Quartz D20 trit.** Weleda, **pillules** Wala
  1 saltsp. or, alternatively, 5 pillules, in the morning

While, in the case of Calcium carbonicum, the constitutional problem consists, physiologically speaking, in a preponderance of metabolism which needs to be more strongly taken hold of and formed by the breathing process, the issue with the type of child we are about to describe, the "Quartz (silicea) child" (▸Chap. 3.2.2.2) is a polar imbalance which gives rise to anxieties: a one-sided dominance of the head pole, of the development of the nerve-sense system in the case of weak up-building metabolism and insufficient warmth generation.

On entry into the consulting room it becomes apparent that such a child sticks less closely to the mother. Instead he tries to get her to leave with him, to drag her to the back of the room (likewise quietly). Physically speaking, the child appears immature, as if born prematurely (which, with this type, is indeed more frequently the case), with a tendency to be underweight, delicate, with translucent skin and a pronounced head pole. His eyes are wakeful but cautious, and clear. Weak warmth generation, the tendency to cool down too much, is directly apparent, as is a lack of vitality.

What is striking here is *the fear of* (physical and psychological) *contact, the "thin skin"*. Any encroachment onto the child's territory can directly result in the transformation of his inner anxiety into a panic, which nothing can pacify (a well-known example is the extreme fear of needles and sharp objects which can in practice lead to scenes of correspondingly extreme behaviour). What is manifesting here is deep-seated fear rather than mere truculence and anger in response to an incursion from outside (which in medicinal terms would speak for the use of Chamomilla or Nux vomica), the child *cannot help himself*; his lack of vitality prevents him from *being flexible*.

The one-sided preponderance of sensory processes in the case of insufficient warmth generation manifests in *hypersensitivity* [Steiner, Wegman 1991, 77ff.], above all in respect of noise and sudden sounds, cold and draughts and with regard to anything out of the ordinary. Psychologically speaking, such children are very much more alert than the Calc. carb. type described above, as well as being cooler and more objective; they are also slow yet consistent in their development and need more time in the early years at school e. g. to learn to read or do maths. The cause in this case is not the slow development of awareness arising out of excessive metabolism, as is the case with the Calcium carbonicum type; instead it has to do with the lack of metabolic dynamism, which slows down the psycho-physiological processes.

In social behaviour, children of the Silicea type are characterized by the fact that it takes them a long time to establish emotional contact with other children, associated with difficulties in their psychological ability to resonate (their psychological life is marked by an ever-objective coolness of the sort to be found in rock crystal). They don't want to be noticed but do in spite of their difficulties want to get involved wherever possible: thus it is that they quietly and unobtrusively practise (e. g. sport, an instrument, any kind of skill) before daring to try it out in public. Panic can be triggered by anything that does not work (e. g. if the sum doesn't add up) or is (as yet) too much for their level of ability. Whilst the Calcium carbonicum type will then retreat into his shell, digging his heels in and refusing to take part, Silicea children work themselves up into a frenzy in which they cannot calm themselves down. They will find no rest within themselves for as long as the connection with the physical processes of digestion and metabolism remains too weak. They lack the internal psychological space, which can only be formed out of this connection.

Therapeutically speaking, when potentized silicon dioxide is being administered it can be seen that the warmth conditions within the child undergo a significant change: the susceptibility to the cold, cold sweat on the head and characteristic, foul-smelling sweat on the feet all diminish (by way of contrast, the Conchae type is characterized by warm perspiration, in particular at the back of the head, and by damp hands and feet.) The chronic tendency to catarrh in the winter is reduced, leading to an improvement in pneumatization derived from the increased generation of warmth, above all in the middle ear and sinuses (▸Chap. 5.1.2); the result is a positive effect on appetite and growth. Anxiety recedes in inverse proportion to burgeoning energy and vitality.

Once quartz or conchae have been administered, the administration of medium potency Ferrum phosphoricum or Ferrum arsenicosum can consolidate the therapy. e. g.

- **Skorodit** (= Ferrum arsenicosum naturale) **D10 trit.** Weleda:
  1 saltsp. 1 x/d in the morning for 6 weeks

This remedy is used to promote self-confidence and the connection of the soul and I organization with the physical and its penetration. Scorodite is of key significance in childhood anxieties in cases where the *anxiety is caused by lack of self-confidence arising out of delayed psycho-physical maturation.*

For girls who appear pallid and withdrawn, who develop little "bite" in the upper digestive system and generally have little appetite and who tend to develop iron deficiency and anemia between 9 and12 years of age,

- **Ferrum pomatum D1 dil.** Weleda
  10 gtt. 1–2 x/d

is a very suitable and highly effective remedy which also improves iron resorption. Suitable for the continuation of this therapy is

- **Ferrum hydroxydatum 5 % trit.** Weleda, **50 % trit.** Apotheke an der Weleda [Engel 2006]
  ¼–½ tsp daily before the main meal (▸Chap. 7.2.4, incl. Case study)

7.2.3.1.2 Loud or restless-anxious behaviour

Reviewing the medicines, which come into consideration for these children, generally reveals strikingly high degrees of *toxicity* of the initial substances. The children themselves suffer from anxiety not because their development is retarded but above all because frightening experiences and mistakes in their education are disrupting the interplay between the physical and the psychological (like a toxin).

- **Aconitum e tub. D20 pillules** Wala, **LM12 dil.** Arcana
  5 pillules or 5 gtt. x/d – often preferentially to be administered in the evening

(▸Chap. 7.1.5.1) – in the case of shocking experiences in the distant past, where applicable, higher potentization (C200).

A very characteristic indicator for this remedy is the behaviour of the child in cases where a noisy fight between mother and child ensues before they have even come through the door. Both are exhausted; the child is completely beside himself with wide, staring eyes: An expression of sudden, unmanageable anxiety, of fear and shock – and at the same time of robust and vital strength. In cases where anxiety suddenly erupts with elemental force, Aconitum is the most important and also the most effective medicinal product.

The *origin of the anxiety* here is not the constitution but an experience: a shock, a scare, an acute injury which has befallen the child; a pain or an illness (e. g. with shortness of breath) which overwhelms the child's soul entity and cannot be processed. The long-lasting effect, which even results in physical changes, of such traumatic experiences in childhood are nowadays widely known and acknowledged as a result of work carried out in the field of pain therapy [Nickel and Egle 1999, 20]. In many cases, however, the child does not initially have a memory of the trigger event; yet the body, the juvenile life organization, retains a memory of it, which can be triggered or recalled in situations and result in an upsurge of anxiety akin to a panic attack.

Triggers of anxiety, alongside visits to the doctor, can be taking an elevator or using the subway, being in a crowd, waking up in the night (typically around midnight) and any experience which recapitulates the original trauma. Characteristic symptoms, alongside the elemental anxiety, are always an *intense yet vital restlessness* and the *suddenness* of the complaint.

When the description of the remedy is taken into account, the *toxic effect* of the alkaloid toxin in Aconitum napellus is remarkable. It develops quickly, like a violent assault [Stübler 1986, 17–36] and is brought about by the effect of Aconitum, which, "forcibly increases the sodium permeability of the cell membrane and strongly impedes physiological repolarization." *In this way, aconite poisoning precipitates a storm of excitation which can abruptly result in paralysis:* "If, as a result of a massive aconitine impact, repolarization should deteriorate sharply, no more action potentials can be formed. The nerve cell suddenly 'falls silent'" [Stübler and Krug 1987, vol. 3, 598]. The primary effect is on the nervous system, followed by cardiovascular regulation, the heart, the blood vessels and kidney function: Aconitum is both a neuro and a cardiotoxin. Aconitum has a peracute toxic effect, Arsenicum album has a toxic effect on the human life organization that is both acute and chronic, and in both cases intoxication is closely associated with deep-seated and unrelenting anxiety [Lewin 1992, 185 (arsenic), 602 (aconite)].

- **Arsenicum album D12–C30 pillules** (var. manufacturers.), **LM12** dil. Arcana
  5 pillules/5 gtt. in the evening

This medicine is appropriate for children who, as in the preceding case, attract the attention of the doctor during the consultation with their anxious truculence and restlessness. At the same time, however, they appear a great deal less energetic and vital; their anxiety causes them to cling to their mother (and at night they can often only be soothed in the parental bed, into which they slip between midnight and 3 AM and where they then sleep happily through until morning). In the daytime they are characterized by high levels of restlessness and impatience with a tendency to tire easily, ambition (and avarice), a fastidious attention to detail and pedantry (in their area of interest). Their hypochondriac sensitivity can manifest in the exhaustive detail in which they report on the extent and origin of small injuries. Anxieties occur

- when they are alone; if those people who serve to satisfy their need for security (family, friends) are not well
- as fear of intruders (they typically reassure themselves several times before going to bed that there are no strangers in the room),
- as fear of evil (against which there is no defence), of loss
- as compulsive perfectionism, the compulsion to control
- as fear of illness, loss of control
- as pavor nocturnus (▸Chap. 7.1).

The soul entity of these children is restless and tense; in physical terms they are deficient in vital warmth, and their need for contact is also a need for warmth. The anxiety is caused in part by an imbalance in their neurasthenic constitution (▸Chap. 6.4.3.6.1). A signifi-

7

cant primary cause, however, is to be found in the expectations of the parents and their own anxieties, just as imperceptible chronic intoxication has a corruptive effect on the psychophysical harmony of the child (cf. chronic arsenic intoxication). Therapeutically speaking, for school-age children artistic therapies (particularly painting therapy) are a very effective means of supplementing and consolidating medicinal treatment.

Aconitum and Arsenicum album relate to childhood anxieties that can have grave consequences right into adult life if not treated properly (e.g. the development of chronic anxieties or pain syndromes in the former case and neurotic disorders in the latter). All the more important in all cases is the clarification of possible causes of anxiety and the continuation of therapy until sustainable success has been achieved. By way of contrast, the anxiety situation presented in the following is of more limited character; here, *it is more the case that the child is frightened by his environment*, than that the anxiety itself has a permanently traumatising character for the child.

- **Belladonna Rh D10–20 dil.** Weleda
  5 gtt. 1–2 x/d

Characteristic of this are violent *attacks of agitation*; one prototype of what is meant here is the delirium brought about by fever (up to and including febrile convulsions). Here, what the child experiences subjectively are fear-inducing and delusionally exaggerated fantasies e.g. of ghosts and animals. Atropa belladona is also one of the most important medicinal products to counteract fear of dogs, on the other hand, such children, when in the grip of attacks of rage and anxiety, can themselves bite or hit bystanders (including their siblings). The experience in medical practice is that it is easier to quiet a child in the grip of such an attack by talking calmly to him in words or arguments which he can understand rather than by physical contact: "it's possible to negotiate". Anxiety is triggered by situations in which one unwittingly gets too close to the child but also by the vivid imagination of such children.

It is crucial to make a *distinction* between such children and others who

- fundamentally do not want to be examined and put up implacable resistance until the examination is over without being psychologically damaged in the process (in homoeopathic-constitutional terms one thinks of Antimonium crudum or Antimonite)
- as a result of deep-seated psychological hurt, experience any approach by the doctor as *going too far* (and do not forget the doctor if he simply uses force) an important indicator for Natrium muriaticum.

7.2.3.2 Medicinal treatment for specific forms of childhood anxiety

One of the most important and specific anxiety disorders is associated with *going to sleep*. This has already been expounded in detail in ▸Chap. 7.1.5.2. In this connection, two constitutional medicines with far-reaching effects, which are significant in the treatment of childhood anxieties have also been considered in detail.

- **Phosphorus** and **Causticum.**

We therefore merely refer the reader to them here and dispense with a separate presentation. The differential therapy of *Pavor nocturnus* has also been presented in ▸Chap. 7.1.5.3

and ▸Chap. 7.1.5.4. Intimately associated with anxieties experienced when falling asleep are the fears of being alone and of the dark presented in the following.

7.2.3.2.1 Fears of being alone and of the dark

- *Aconitum* is effective here if the trigger of the condition was a shock, especially an experience of unexpected abandonment: e. g. if the child woke up in the night and found that, unbeknown to him, his parents were not in the house.
- *Arsenicum album, Phosphorus, Calcium carbonicum* and *Stramonium* also continue to feature prominently and have already been presented.
- *Pulsatilla* or *Lycopodium* can also be considered for differential therapy in cases of overly strong *attachment to the mother* (Pulsatilla is used more with girls and Lycopodium with boys).

7.2.3.2.2 Fear of illness and death

- Calcium carbonicum or Phosphorus can be considered in the case of constitutionally conditioned anxiety,
- *Aconitum* or *Arsenicum album* in the case of *fear of death as a symptom of an illness* (e. g. Aconitum in pseudocroup, also as a follow-up treatment, or Arsenicum album in the case of bronchial asthma; cf. the corresponding sections).
- *Aurum met. praep.* in the case of *thoughts of death* or fear of death in the context of developmental crises or depression (▸Chap. 7.2.3.3).

7.2.3.2.3 Abnormal lack of fear

If a noticeable *absence of anxieties* (in the sense of a psychological weakness in perception coupled with the one-sided dominance of the will) is established, two constitutional medicinal products may be considered:

- **Sulphur LM6–12 dil.** Arcana
  5 gtt. x/d in the morning

in the case of full-blooded, inquisitive, headstrong and open children who seem unacquainted with fear and always want to be the centre of attention (have an urge to prove themselves);

- **Calcium fluoratum = Fluorite D12 trit.** Weleda
  1 saltsp. x/d in the morning

in the case of children who behave in a *psychologically unmoved* manner, who show no compassion, have thin lips, a slim build and weak connective tissue, although they can spend all their time eating. With this constitution, there is a particularly obvious deficit in psychological perception.

7.2.3.2.4 Exams and anticipation anxiety

- **Gelsemium D30 pillules** (var. manufacturers)
  5 pillules 1 x/d in the evening 3–5 days before start of the exam

is appropriate if the child feels *paralysed sitting the examination*: The limbs go on strike and start to tremble (pseudoparalysis) and the ability to think is lost ("*blackout*"); this can be associated with nervous diarrhoea. On the day of the examination

- **Aurum/Valeriana comp. pillules** Wala
  7–10 pillules in the morning, repeat at the start of the examination

This medicine is also effective by itself in cases without particular characteristics (tried-and-tested information from clinical experience provided by M. Sommer). Generally suitable for anxiety in association with circulatory disorders and nausea. E.g. before and during travel and on long-distance flights and *fear of flying*, in each case administer up to 7–10 pillules 5 x/d. A highly proven medicine for chronically sick children waiting for stressful medical procedures/visits to a clinic (e.g. a spinal tap administered to children with cancer): on the evening of the day before 7–10 pillules, on the day itself up to 5–10 pillules per hour. [cf. Vademecum 2010, 185]

- **Argentum nitricum D30 pillules – C200** (var. manufacturers): dosage (D30) as with Gelsemium; D200
  5 pillules in the morning of the day of examination

is more appropriate in the case of *nervous and restless children* who are prone to the fear that they won't have enough time; such children are likewise prone to nervous diarrhoea (both nervous and digestion processes are accelerated). In the examination they easily flounder and make unnecessary mistakes due to pressure of time. At the same time they experience a pronounced urge to eat sweets (unstable blood glucose level). **Tip:** give them something sweet when they are doing their schoolwork.

- **Anacardium D30 pillules** (var. manufacturers)
  Dosage same as Gelsemium.

What predominates here is deterioration on an empty stomach, e.g. if the child has to wait a long time for an exam; the child or adolescent has a feeling of emptiness or heaviness in his head and demonstrates *sudden lapses of memory*. Both blood pressure and the blood glucose level are unstable (tendency to hypotension and hypoglycaemia). In constitutional terms, the right medicine in this case is frequently sulphur. It is not unusual for the child to have a problematic relationship with his father.

During the exam,

- **Strophanthus Kombe e sem. D6 pillules** Wala
  5 pillules per hour

is the most effective treatment; it can generally be administered in cases of *examination stress*. Many people are helped by being allowed taking something sweet into the exam [Vademecum 2010, 778].

Generally advisable in cases of inability to concentrate in children: e.g. four weeks before the exam-administration of

- **Helleborus niger LM6 dil.** Arcana/**D6–12 pillules**/d Wala
  5 gtt./5 pillules in the morning

in cases of exam fear, supplemented by the above mentioned medicine shortly before and during the examination. Potentized black hellebore not only promotes the ability to concentrate but also stabilizes the ability not to lose control when confronted with sudden demands. [Vademecum 2010, 477–481]

With regard to the great variety of possible anxieties, which relate to specific trigger moments (e.g. thunderstorms, certain animals, heights, enclosed spaces etc.), the homoeopathic repertoire (e.g. Kent; Synthesis; RADAR) can be of value for differential therapy.

7.2.3.2.5 School anxieties, school phobia

The most important medicinal product for school phobia (cf. Chap 7.2.2.3.) is

- **Ambra grisea C12 pillules** Gudjons
  5–7 pillules 1–2 x/d for 4–12 weeks

In several cases of school phobia this has proved itself to the authors to be a fast-acting and strikingly effective medicine, which can be prescribed almost from the point of diagnosis.

Ambra grisea is a medicine advised by homoeopathic circles for preferential use with shy girls, who feel *inhibited and overwhelmed in larger groups of peers.* D. Grandgeorge worked out that, diagnostically speaking, an early transition from the symbiotic child in nappies to the child who independently does her "number twos" in the potty can present a serious problem [Grandgeorge 2004, 32]. It is a helpful medicine in cases of *psychogenic constipation* at this age [Vademecum 2010, 61]. He later characterized the principal symptom in the words of a patient as follows: "People eat me up" [l. c.], which is reminiscent of the common motif in fairy tales, e. g. of the wolf and the seven little goats.

Children affected by this are often excluded from group situations. Girls can, for instance, be teased by other girls acting in a socially aggressive manner. They almost feel as though they are about to stop breathing. The physical side of the pathology is characterized by symptoms of the upper and lower respiratory tract. Grandgeorge relates a devastating example: A mother organized a surprise third birthday party for her daughter (at a sensitive phase in toilet training). Thereafter the child developed therapy-resistant asthma attacks, which could last for several days. Her favourite game with her little sister was "Playing wolf" ("I'm going to eat you up"). Grandgeorge was able to cure this girl at the age of 7 only by administering Ambra grisea. This is an excellent example of how homoeopathy can cure conditions and shed light on correlations.

In constitutional terms, an important background medicine is

- **Calcium carbonicum** (cf. above, ▶Chap. 7.2.3.2.1)

Furthermore, in the context of *fear of school*, the following can also be considered:

Children who suffer from abdominal pain or the like on Sunday night or Monday morning during their years at school often respond positively to

- **Calcium phosphoricum D12 pillules dil.** (var. manufacturers)/**C12 pillules** Gudjons
  5–7 pillules/gtt.

Should the effect prove insufficient, a composition of Apatite, Aurum and Stannum is often more effective:

- **Stannum comp. trit.** Weleda
  1 saltsp. 2 x/d

Fear of school in connection with weakness, tendency to chronic rhinitis and school headache and thirst:

- **Acidum phosphoricum D12–30 pillules dil.**
  5 pillules 1–2 x/d

In the case of fear of school associated with grief, depressive imbalance:

- **Aurum/Apis regina comp. pillules** Wala
  7 pillules 3 x/d

This composition, which contains, among other things, Acidum phosphoricum, Hypericum and Aurum chloratum in a (jointly) potentized form, is a tried-and-tested and very broadly effective medicine [Vademecum 2010, 165].

7.2.3.3 Anxieties related to developmental crises from age 7–14 and age 14–21

Anxieties which are originally connected with *individuation* itself can be treated medicinally in particular with potentized gold,

- **Aurum met. praep. D6–30 trit.** Weleda

The link between gold and human individuation becomes apparent by virtue of its particular cultural significance, associated not just with the rarity of this metal but, in particular, with its qualities. Gold can more readily be kept pure under terrestrial conditions than any other metal: it is a metal with a soft, warm sheen, similar to the sun in colouration, which, whilst extremely rare, can be found in nature in its pure form. It is specifically heavier than almost any other natural element and can at the same time be more finely hammered and drawn out to make wire than any other metal: it possesses gravity and lightness in equal measure. In its pure metal properties, lustre, plasticity, capacity for alloy formation and conductivity, it demonstrates some of the properties of fluid (water, too, has lightness and gravity in equal proportion); on the other hand, it represents an extremely stable terrestrial element. Since time immemorial, man has seen in it a symbolic expression of his own individuality, which combines and expresses an "ever liquid" versatile being in an earthly body. Yet individuation is the way to appropriate this body and form it into a physical expression of one's own being without falling victim to the terrestrial laws governing what one has become and losing one's versatility.

Therapeutically speaking it has been shown that potentized gold can exert a strong effect on the evolving individuality which is only just starting to take possession of the body, especially if the child or adolescent is experiencing bodily constriction, and physicality, which has already suffered being too heavy. Appropriately potentized gold promotes the process by which the individuality begins to anchor itself bodily in metabolism and limbs, up to and including acts of will, and starts to act out of this position, to build its own bridges to the world. From the age of nine to the end of adolescence, Aurum remains the most important and comprehensive remedy for the treatment of anxiety, especially the existential anxiety suffered by young people [for a homoeopathic differentiation of Aurum-salts, cf. Wulfsberg 2001]

With regard to *potentization*, the following aspect can be key:

- **Aurum met. praep. D6 trit.** Weleda
  3 × 1 saltsp. x/d

is suitable for curbing an excessive development of will which is, at the same time, insufficiently amenable to conscious control (a manically exaggerated sense of self-importance and hyperactivity). With these patients, the problem is usually *an overly autonomous primary dynamic in the metabolic-limb pole.* The principal constitutional remedy in such cases is often

- **Sulphur LM6–12 dil.** Arcana
  5 gtt. 1 x/d

which can alternately be administered as a complementary remedy. These patients tend to be characterized by a (pathological) lack of fear (▸Chap. 7.2.3.2.5).

- **Aurum met. praep. D10–15 trit.** Weleda
  1 saltsp. 1–2 x/d

primarily affects the child's rhythmic organization, chest, breathing, cardiovascular events and spine.

Psychosomatically speaking, anxieties are most closely related to this central region of the human body, which, in developmental terms, is in the foreground between the ages of 7 to 14. Accordingly, this degree of potency of Aurum met. works best in the case of anxieties associated *with feelings of trepidation, shallowness of breath, abnormal heart sensations and circulatory dysregulation, as well as postural disorders* (in this latter case, Stannum comp. could also come under consideration; see below). The effect can be roughly described as follows: administering the medicine imparts a sense of buoyancy and lightness, the child is better able to get over past illnesses and losses, self-confidence is reinforced and the child establishes a new equilibrium in the centre of his being. Therapeutic experience and close observation must be drawn on to decide on the exact level of potency and period of administration of the medicine; for the inexperienced practitioner we initially recommend D12 as the level of potency.

The use of gold is complemented by the following plant-based composite

- **Cardiodoron gtt.** Weleda/**Cardiodoron Rh tab.** Weleda (Onopordon)
  7–15 gtt./3 × ½ – 1 tab. 2–3 x/d (it is recommended to decide on the dosage on a case-by-case basis)

This medicine has a comprehensively harmonizing and stabilising effect on the child's rhythmic system, which is still in the process of formation [Weckenmann 1982], e.g. in the case of orthostatic problems, palpitations, the tendency to faint, and mood swings brought about by anxiety. [Vademecum 2010, 273]

In the case of a tendency to orthostasis, *stabbing pain* in the chest wall and general anxiety, therapeutic efficacy has been established for the administration of

- **Cralonin gtt.** Heel
  2 × 15–20 gtt. in water prior to lying down and to getting up, over the course of 1–2 months (contains Spigelia, which is a tried-and-tested remedy for this form of chest

wall pain, generally described as "pain to the heart", with its characteristic Punctum maximum in the direction of the left thoracic side[1]).

More powerful than this plant-based remedy as a complement to gold is the effect of potentized meteoric iron,

- **Ferrum sidereum D6–10–20 trit./D 20 tab.** Weleda
  3–5 x/d; up to hrly in acute cases (Vademecum).

Here, one has the unique special case that iron (in the form of nickel-cobalt alloy) appears in refined form on the Earth. This iron is of directly cosmic origin. The element iron occurs here in a *form which, in qualitative terms, is second only* to gold; no metal testifies more eloquently to the very real connection between the Earth and the cosmos, to the connection between light and matter, than meteoric iron. In the human organism, the ability to absorb iron and to turn it into a catalyst of mitochondrial energy metabolism (cytochrome) and of respiratory events is crucial for the development of the individual will, the person's own development of warmth and consciousness (as an inner development of light). Iron is elevated here to the level of organization of the human I, allowing the effective development of the non-terrestrial, spiritual individuality of the person in the terrestrial, physical organism. This event can be stimulated by potentized meteoric iron and thus contribute to the overcoming of fears.

In therapeutic practice, low potencies have especially proven themselves in the case of low self-esteem, of undefined anxieties, right through to panic attacks [Vademecum 2010, 437] in association with impairment of the will:

- **Ferrum sidereum D6 trit.** Weleda

Administered several times a day, a saltsp. can have a simultaneously *calming* and activating effect, where, in allopathic medicine, thoughts might turn to tranquilizers, which are, however, addictive and enhance passivity.

- **Ferrum sidereum D10**

is in most cases the most suitable complement to medium-high potencies of Aurum, it counteracts frequent disruptions to, and irregularities in, the drive in teenagers and, at the same time, promotes the alertness and clear delineation of consciousness. This effect is enhanced with higher potentization.

- **Ferrum sidereum D20 trit.** and **tab.** Weleda
  e.g. 1 tab. 1 x/d

This has proven especially effective in children and adolescents with *low self-confidence* conjoined with *excessive motor activity and restlessness.*

- **Aurum D10/Ferrum sidereum D10 aa amp.** Weleda
  1 ampoule **s.c.** or per os

represents a very effective composition of both metals as a treatment for anxieties (e.g. exam nerves, fear of crowds etc.) and depressive disorders which have their origin in a lack of self-esteem and self-confidence.

1 No less a person than Bernard Lown ("The Lost Art of Healing") makes use of the distinction between retrosternal pain – pain inside the left front of the chest wall as the first distinguishing clinical indication of grave symptoms in the heart – and mainly psychosomatically conditioned pain in the region of the left wall of the thorax.

- **Stannum comp. trit.** Weleda
  1–2 saltsp. daily

also contains Aurum in D12 in combination with Stannum met. D15 and Apatite D6. The use of this is indicated when the anxiety disorder threatens *to leave its impression in the sphere of the rhythmic system and to penetrate right into the physical*, in particular in the area of the spinal column. It is also effective in the case of chronic pain in the abdomen and head associated with anxiety and states of psychophysical tension [Vademecum 2010, 766].

In the case of this pathology, the use of craniosacral therapy generally provides evidence of significant disruptions to the function of the craniosacral system (which can be assigned to the human rhythmic system) [Upledger and Vredevoogd 2000, 319, 401]. This form of therapy, when carried out with sufficient expertise, nowadays accordingly offers a useful complementary therapeutic approach; therapeutic procedures in anthroposophic medicine which take this further are rhythmic massage, rhythmic oil applications (rhythmische Einreibungen) and eurythmy therapy. Stannum comp. promotes and stabilizes the formation of erect posture in the area of the spinal column, which comes from the centre, from the rhythmic system, and which takes place in particular between the 11th and the 15th year.

A suitable complementary plant-based medicine is

- **Bambusa[1] e nodo D6 pillules** Wala
  1–2 x/d

In conclusion we would draw the reader's attention to treatment using high potencies of Aurum, which is appropriate in the case of severe anxieties, experienced as directly existential (up to and including mortal fear and *suicidal thoughts*), such as occur in particular in the teenage years and in association with depression:

- **Aurum met. praep. D30 trit.**
  1 saltsp. daily – 2 × 1 saltsp. weekly in the morning

As a complementary plant-based remedy for anxiety and depressiveness, Hypericum, or St. John's Wort, should be considered, either in phytotherapeutic doses or in combination with gold as a vegetabilized metal,

- **Hypericum Auro cultum D2, Rh D3 dil.** Weleda:
  5–10 (D2)/7–20 gtt. 3 x/d (Rh D3),

is indicated in the case of low self-confidence, incipient slight inhibition of the thinking faculty, (the psychological ability to communicate and take initiative).

7.2.4 Children with poor self-image and low self-esteem

In practice this aspect is especially significant at preschool and school age; it must at the same time be said that many more boys than girls are presented for treatment of this problem. The intention here is to give some brief therapeutic suggestions.

1 The idea of using bamboo as a medicine to stimulate the development of an erect posture in the area of the spinal column can essentially be attributed to G. Husemann [1965]. Cf. also Schuster [1996].

7

As a basic therapy, the following is suitable:

- **Hypericum Auro cultum D2, Rh D3 dil.** Weleda
  3 × 5–10 (D2)/7–20 gtt. x/d (Rh D3)

In individual cases, the following may be considered as therapies:

- **Arsenicum album D30** or **C30 pillules** (various manufacturers)
  5 pillules in the morning
- **Ferrum sidereum D20 tab.** Weleda
  1–2 tab. in the afternoon

in the case of introverted boys with a neurasthenic constitution, intelligent children with "*pale ambition*", who find it hard to make connections in social situations and are subject to teasing. These problems are reinforced by a not uncommon tendency to send children, whose psychological maturity trails in the wake of their development of intelligence, to school before they are ready.

- **Phosphorus LM6 dil.** Arcana
  5 gtt. in the morning

in the case of fast-growing boys whose *growth is excessive* and who show a wide range of talents, including artistic ability, but who have little stability, experience difficulties in the fullness of their talents with the development of structure and awareness of goals and therefore readily experience their social environment as confusing and inhibiting. The administration of the remedy improves self-esteem and resistance and has a positive effect on the strong tendency to distraction experienced by such children.

- **Quartz D20 trit.** Weleda, **pillules** Wala
  1 saltsp./5 pillules in the morning

is, by way of contrast, helpful in the case of children (boys and girls) who make slow (but steady) progress in growth and psychological maturation and have *a highly structured psyche but are lacking in light and quickly reach the limit of their powers*. This makes such children relatively inflexible in social situations; they tire easily, are shy and need sufficient peace and quiet and opportunities to withdraw. Physical changes and minor health complaints trigger worry and anxiety; the connection to the parents is usually very strong even in the face of a strong sense of self and need for autonomy. Promptly administered constitutional medication can help these children open up to their peers and more readily accept their own physical maturation process, which in itself can compensate for a constitution which is one-sidedly dominated by the head pole.

- **Calcium phosphoricum C12–30 pillules** Gudjons
  5 pillules in the morning 1 x/d or 1–2 x/w

is an important medicine which is more suitable for girls if the symptom identified by Jan Scholten [1993, 91] can be determined by means of a sensitive history: "*The worst thing is when other people think I'm stupid.*" Criticism of their prowess at school affects these children very strongly. They ascribe a disproportionate importance to learning and success at school: such children continually feel weighed down by their own exaggerated sense of what has to be done, associated with a deep-seated emotional insecurity and fear of failure to live up to these demands. In this way, psychological energies are withdrawn to a striking extent from their physical function during infantile and adolescent development and instead directed outwards, manifesting in the need to travel and learn. What is striking in practice is a constant inner, *dissatisfaction, frequent headaches and, in adolescence, lumbosacral pain syndromes* during and after intellectual exertion. There is a tendency to idiopathic scoliosis (cf. 9.3.3): It is in the spine as a central organ of the rhythmic system that the psychological cleft which develops in these children tends to express itself. In the case of back pain, the following is suitable as a follow-up remedy:

- **Stannum comp. trit.** Weleda
  ¼ tsp. in the morning
- **Magnesite D6 trit.** Weleda, **D12–20 dil.** Apotheke an der Weleda, given in increasing potencies,

is useful for boys whose lack of self-esteem is not initially very pronounced. Most *boys of short stature, who also tend to be thin*, come across as aggressive, prickly, and ambitious. They conceal their shyness and lack of self-esteem, further amplified by the lack of physical stature which is of such importance to boys, behind a front reminiscent of a dogged defensive player in a game of football. They have a strong *dislike of breakfast*, and are evening people. "The mere sight of the doctor triggers a wild scream of terror which nothing is able to appease". [Stübler 1969]

- **Pulsatilla D12–30 dil./pillules** DHU
  5–7 gtt. or 5 pillules in the evening
- **Neurodoron® (Kalium Phosphoricum comp.) tab.** Weleda
  1–2 tab. in the morning

are helpful medicines in the case of *shy boys* who give the impression of being soft *and are strongly attached to their mothers*, who suffer from anxiety and feelings of failure and struggle to concentrate for long enough periods at school. The gold and iron components of **Neurodoron®** (Kalium Phosphoricum comp.) tab. Weleda strengthen the insufficiently aggressive male side (it is not uncommon for the father to show a weakness in this area himself or to be rarely present in the child's life), while the higher Pulsatilla potency in the evening has the effect of relaxing the overly close ties to the mother and diminishing the associated anxieties.

- **Ferrum hydroxydatum 5 %** Weleda/**50 % trit.** Apotheke an der Weleda
  ¼–½ tsp. immediately before eating (morning or noon)

represents a deeply effective remedy, in particular for girls who suffer from shyness and a lack of self-esteem and demonstrate a tendency to iron deficiency. Physical symptoms often include a tendency to recurrent infections of the respiratory and urinary tracts and pallor of the skin; psychologically there is an inclination to put the demands of others before their own needs and an inability to defend themselves appropriately against insults and attacks. Resistance is weakened. (For more on the production of this very effective iron preparation, specific to anthroposophic therapy, cf. Angel [2006]).

Case study

A fourteen year old patient has been undergoing treatment for eight years for recurrent uncomplicated urinary tract infections. The treatment has only been partially successful, as a foul-smelling bacteriuria (E. coli) is still present in the urine along with leukocytosis and nitrite. The faecal smell of the urine decreases in the course of the therapy, yet the bacteriuria remains in spite of various complementary medical treatments. No antibiotic therapy.

The girl is an only-child, demonstrates low levels of self-esteem, is introverted and has dyscalculia. Her complexion is pale. She often comes back dispirited from school, above all from math lessons in which she is frequently told that she needs to do more, even though she consistently applies herself to learning and has coaching in her spare time. ½ teaspoon per day of Ferrum hydroxydatum 50 % is then prescribed, a total of 100 g. Then, for the first time, several urine samples show no pathological findings; six weeks after cessation of therapy only a trace of protein is detectable in the morning urine. The greatest success for the prescriber, however, was the story which the girl told her mother at lunch one day during treatment: The mathematics teacher had made her so cross that day that she had stood up and gone up to him in front of all her classmates and given him a piece of her mind!

7.3 Depressive disorders

20 % of all young people have experienced depression by the age of 18.

H. C. Steinhausen [2010]

7.3.1 Aspects of diagnosis

The *diagnosis* of depressive disorders in childhood requires, apart from the history and the inspection, most of all a careful observation of the child's behaviour. Thereby, depressive disorders can generally manifest themselves as rather *regressive or else emphatically aggressive* (!). From his own investigations, G. Nissen reports: "The depressive girls displayed a *Cinderella-Syndrome*, they predominantly behaved in a passive, quiet and inhibited way, they were prone to mood swings and to brooding … The depressive boys … behaved like: "aggressive and isolated outsiders" [Nissen 1989b, 166]. In general, a knowledge of the *age-specific symptoms* is necessary; they can be subdivided [Leitlinien zur Diagnostik 2000, 66] into

- Infancy, up to 3 years of age:
  - sad-expressionless face, decreased desire to play,
  - sleep disorders, heightened irritability,
  - eating disorders, delayed corporeal-psychological development,
  - Self-stimulating behaviour (e. g. excessive thumb-sucking),
- Pre-school age, up to 7 years, during the course of which the following depressive symptoms become more clearly observable:
  - lacking ability to be happy,

  - introverted or aggressive behavioural disorders,
  - contact disorders when in groups, inhibited (or contact-addicted) behaviour,
  - abnormal, mostly inhibited movement behaviour,
  - poverty of verbal and nonverbal expression, retardation e. g. in childlike drawings,
  - nocturnal anxieties and nightmares,
  - enuresis, encopresis,
- School-age, during the course of which particular attention has to be paid to:
  - Accounts of sadness, suicidal ideations (especially upon enquiry; if necessary one-to-one conversation with the child),
  - inferiority feelings, social withdrawal tendencies,
  - scholastic impairment of performance (in comparison with the individual ability),
  - strong tenseness, especially cervical, tensed-up/inhibited motions,
  - head and stomach aches,
- puberty and adolescence: here the symptoms of depression approach the picture familiar with adults.

During the history, it is necessary to enquire about

- depressions or psychosis of the parents and grand-parents,
- position and age difference of the siblings and their spontaneous behaviour (e. g. an outgoing or gifted 3rd child, which is especially loved by the parents, can constitute a traumatic strain for the 2nd child),
- experience of loss (especially parental separation, death of close relatives, loss of home),
- sleep disorders and anxieties,
- excessive auto-aggressive or auto-stimulating actions,
- violence and dependency in the family,
- Mental overload through parental or scholastic expectations exceeding the maturity or ability of the child.

Hurtful early-childhood experiences are most significant (this already applies to the partially unconscious rejection of the child during pregnancy or to motherly depressions during the early phase of childhood [Freud 1993]) and *losses* (cf. ▸Chap. 2) as well as *hereditary (constitutional)* strains. The most important phenomenon is the disordered, inhibited, *impoverished kinesis*: facial expression, gestures, expression including written and pictorial articulation, stereotypy, muscular tenseness, a depressed/tensed-up posture. *Emotionally,* the children feel unloved, unsecured, bad and inferior" [Nissen 1989b].

In light of the fact that syndromes of depression, to a considerable degree, go back to constitutional and early-childhood causes, a carefully individualized approach in childhood, which takes into consideration the potential constitutional change through acute illnesses, the effects of potentized medicaments, the resources available in the family as well as the possibilities available today though artistic therapies and psychotherapy, possesses a unique, lasting chance concerning the treatment of depression, which is not given at any later point in time. The paediatrician and general practitioner have to be conscious of this responsibility.

At this point we would like to refer to the 4th lecture of the "Heilpädagogischer Kurs" (Curative Education Course) by R. Steiner [Steiner 1995, 66–75] for a deepening of the understanding of childhood depression and its treatment through therapies based on therapeutic-artistic paedagogy.

7.3.2 Options for medicinal treatment

The following medicine has a universal therapeutic role for the treatment of syndromes of depression, especially after *early-childhood experience of loss* (extreme premature birth, loss of a parental attachment, separation through hospital stays, loss of security through severe generalized skin infections in infancy, or similar things):

- **Amnion Gl D30 amp.** Wala
  1 x/day – every 2 days ½ ampoule per os, given predominantly in the evenings
  acute 1 ampoule i.v. (if indicated, mixed with 1 ampoule Cuprum met. praep. D30 ampoule Weleda, see below)

It may also be given as a supportive medicine following sexual abuse and traumatizing experiences of violence during early childhood. This anthroposophic medicine [Schad 1982, Vademecum 2010, 65f] is a potentized preparation made from an (animal) *embryonic organ,* which proceeds from the originally ectodermic sheath, 'the skin', clear and tender, which covers the embryo in utero, the initial hull of the human embryo, which is lost, or shed, at birth (cf. ▸Chap. 6.4.3.6.1).

The impact of the medicament can often be observed in striking immediacy: The feeling of not being loved and forlornness is eased, and a feeling of being warmed-through sets in (Amnion is very rich in silicic acid), the vital build-up processes are intensified.

As metallic medicine, copper in its potentized form is often suited at the start of a therapy:

- **Cuprum met. praep. D6–10 trit.** Weleda
  1–3 x/day 1 saltsp. (to be administered esp. in the evening)

promotes a relaxation, a more harmonic combination of the soul with the metabolic processes. In high potentization

- **Cuprum met. praep. D20–30 trit.** Weleda
  1–2 x/week 1 saltsp. in the evenings (D30), daily in the evenings (D20)

is indicated, if the *motherly aggressions* or *ambivalences* or the *loss of the mother* are of importance for the depressive disorder. The same holds true in the case of death of close relatives of the family.

Possibly the most important homoeopathic medicine with a lasting effect against childhood depressive disorders is

- **Natrium muriaticum LM6–12 dil. Arcana, C30–200 pillules** (various manufacturers).
  daily 5 gtt. or as single doses (1–3 × 3–5 pillules or 5 pillules dissolved in water administered over 3 days),

It is most predominantly indicated for girls, and has been portrayed in detail in this book several times (▸Chap. 6.4.3.6.3, case report ▸Chap. 2.4).

Natrium muriaticum is made from table salt by way of potentizing. It is a clear, rectangularly (cubically) crystallizing substance, which, in its dissolved form, is of utmost importance for all excitation processes of the animal and human organism. As salt, sodium chloride allows conservation of perishable food, among other things, which equals a drying process, through salting, living substance is taken out of the circle of life (which is bound to water) and, mummified so to speak. Here, something of the pathogenesis of depressive disorders becomes visible: A trauma, a loss, or a one-sided constitution can result in *expe-*

riences not getting processed and thereby not being resolved again in the course of development; instead they are preserved in a sort of *pathologic memory.* The balance between vital self-change and physical-invariable structures is tipped in favour of the latter (this is still recognizable in the childhood drawings of patients with depressive disorders, which often appear rigid and edgy, lifeless).

The guiding symptomatology for the prescription of Natrium muriaticum may be summed up as follows:

- reduced assimilation activity, little appetite, constipation tendency, slow growth, predisposition for iron deficiency anaemia,
- hunger for salt and sweets,
- emotional grief, which does not undergo a process of transformation, which cannot be forgotten (e. g. loss or rejection by the parents), which leads to emotional withdrawal and implies a deep-seated shock that impacts right down into a person's constitution.
- deterioration of the state of health, *in springtime*, in direct *sunlight* (headaches).

This commonly known leading symptom illustrates once again just how much depression is opposed to *the life-processes*, which are given new impulses in spring-time and depend on the sunlight.

- strong tendency towards *atopic dermatitis, bronchial asthma and pollinosis* (Spitz [1946] already pointed out the connections between early-childhood eczemas and "psycho-toxic" disorders),
- often migraine or lasting predisposition for headaches during school-age.

In practice it can be observed that this medicine has a higher than average indication for *only-children,* especially when they themselves, the father or other circumstances of life in connection with the child, have led to *grave disappointments of the mother*. The same holds true for children of ambitious mothers.

In their behaviour, the children often appear precocious, socially excessively dutiful and responsible during school-age (and later), while at the same time having a marked oversensitivity, being easily hurt. In their grief they have a tendency for withdrawal, and weeping alone in their rooms. Consolation only aggravates things at this point; they are emotionally unable to accept help. Especially at school-age, these tendencies are opposed by the possibility of abrupt hysterical outbursts, accompanied by tears (just as table salt is, in principle, dissolvable at any given time, becoming that which mediates excitation!). According to our own experience, this medicine can also have a powerful effect in depressive boys, especially when a strong maternal attachment, an inner-family experience of loss, or motherly depressions are of importance for the case.

In the course of adolescence this can manifest itself as an inability of opening up inwardly (and bodily) towards a partner of the opposite sex, due to the oversensitivity towards disappointments. Natrium muriaticum is an important medicine when adolescents (mostly women) are unable to overcome their love sickness, and cannot process what they have experienced. The root causes of this behaviour are mostly temporally situated in childhood experiences and the person's constitution, which only emphasizes the importance of starting treatment early.

- **Causticum D12 dil. – C30–200 pillules** (various manufacturers)
  5 drops/day or single doses (as described for Natr. mur.)

is comparable to Natrium muriaticum in its spectrum of effectiveness when used against syndromes of depression.

The extraction of the base substance of the homoeopathic medicines is preceded by a *long process of devitalization* (the authors are indebted to M. Sommer for key information): On the one hand, burnt marble is used in the production; marble comes into being from sedimented chalk shells (of marine molluscs), which are subjected to high pressure and heating through tectonic processes and as a result of this get trans-crystallized and compacted as marble. On the other hand, beech wood ash is used for the production, which also entails the long way from the substance production in the green leaf of the beech tree, over wood formation, up to its combustion. From these substances, a distillate is made (the motive of purity is also of central importance for the understanding of Causticum), which is subsequently potentized.

The homoeopathic proving has been delineated in great detail in ▸Chap. 6.5.6.11 and ▸Chap. 7.1.5.2. It shall now be summarized with regard to the aspects of interest here:

- strikingly early *sensibility, strong compassion,* intensively radiant personality,
- inability to defend oneself, suppression of own aggressive impulses,
- strong fear of loss of control, while falling asleep, of animals (e. g. dogs),
- intellectual *ambition*, obsessive need to master any given situation through exact control,
- nocturnal, recurring *nightmares* (important lead-symptom for childhood depressions),
- enuresis nocturna,
- inhibited physical contact.

In the history, either a primary disposition of the child in the sense of the described leading symptoms may be found, or a lasting grief, e. g. resulting from early experience of violence. Often, significant *movement inhibitions* are characteristic:

- learning to walk late, orthopaedic disorders of the lower extremities (hip dysplasia, clubfoot deformity, or similar symptoms),
- stuttering when excited, coercion to clear one's throat, bronchial asthma through suppressed emotions,
- inhibitions of facial expression, in which suppressed aggression is seen.

(Later on, rheumatic complaints, cervical spine and lumbar syndromes, diseases with restrictions of movement and paralysis are extraordinarily characteristic for this medicine).

The medicine of Causticum illustrates that depressive developments are invariably coupled *with the loss of vitality and free physical motility*. This can be an important starting point for non-medical therapies.

The positive effects of the administration of medicine manifest themselves not only via the reduction of anxieties and nightmares, the emotional and corporeal inhibitions, but coupled with that, via a significantly increasing demarcation against others and the expression of aggressive impulses. It is important to influence the family and school environments in such a way that they will not react to this with disappointment and repression, but with understanding! Because precisely the splitting off and suppression of aggression (which is originally bound to the motility potential of the extremities) leads to the increasing depressivity, anxiety and paralysis of the patients; the potentized medicine releases these forces once again, making them positively available to the child.

In close relation to the aforementioned medicines are the indications for

- **Staphisagria LM6–12 dil.** Arcana, **D30–C200 pillules.**
  5 gtt./day or as single doses (as described for Natr. mur.)

Root causes of childhood depression are here

- humiliations,
- experiences of abuse,
- deep seated *disappointment through family-members*, whose actions overwhelm the child, without it having the possibility to defend itself (this also holds true regarding siblings).

Often, the child has a difficult position in the family system ("scapegoat", "Cinderella"), which becomes especially well observed when the whole family comes to the medical appointments. The grumpy expressionless facial expression, the often somewhat plump figure (these children eat more, when they suffer from grief) and bad temperedness are also not attractive for the medical practitioner. Hidden below this mask, there is a large quantity of emotional sensitivity and a very low, hurt, self-esteem: "*Sensibility, inhibition and vulnerability* are very apparent. Every now and then, the child might have phases with *outbursts of emotions and rage.*" [Morrison 1995, 632]. Staphisagria is a central medicine for depressive disorders of *adopted* (and often early traumatized) *children*.

Suppressed rage, possibly a traumatized sexual development, pose psycho-dynamically essential problems in these cases. *Premature tooth decay*, which is known to be a lead symptom of Staphisagria, appears like a symbol for that. In the teeth, the aggressive potential of the organism culminates physically; inhibitions of aggression can promote tooth decay or periodontitis. The well known healing promoting effect for *cuts* (D12), important for all operations, is connected to the described image, which is related to external (corporeal and emotional) injuries.

Staphisagria (just like the complementary agent Causticum) may lead the suppressed or pent up aggression to burst through (esp. against the perpetrators of the humiliations). Generally, though, along with the depressivity, the dull inhibition wanes, and the child is able to face his environment with more self confidence and realize its own potential for development.

- **Lycopodium LM6, D15–30–200 pillules.** (various manufacturers)
  daily 3–5 gtt./pillules or (D30–200) single doses

is a constitutionally effective medicine for use against depressive developments during early childhood, if the *inhibition of vitality* is of utmost priority. It is predominantly boys who are affected, mostly with a strikingly close attachment to their mother (and, accordingly, motherly concern).

Indeed it is often *motherly anxiety about the child (especially concerning possible failure to thrive),* which leads to consulting the medical doctor. Leading phenomena in the symptoms include:

- *lack of appetite* and failure to thrive (the child is hungry, but satisfied after a few morsels),
- the *insufficiency of digestion* coupled with meteorism, underweight, constipation tendency, food hypersensitivity,
- a striking dryness (of the skin, in connection with the constipation).

The impression is of an *inhibition of the life-processes,* of an *overly physical organism.* At the same time, the children often possess well-shaped heads, a keen intellect, but the forces of their emotional intellectual individuality do not make connection with the metabolism, which becomes visible in their weak digestion (▸Chap. 4.5). *Emotionally* a low self esteem is the consequence; these children also *avoid* situations that would call on their extremities and their *body bound aggressive potential.* On the other hand, they may behave verbally in a *tyrannical and egocentric* way, where they feel safe (especially in the family). As professions, they prefer sedentary occupations: nowadays especially work on the computer (which, in turn, reduces their vitality even further).

Lycopodium can be therapeutically effective in many cases, in which the *primary* background of a depressive development lies in a weak connection of the emotional intellectual individuality with the (sluggish) activity of metabolic and motor system. Regarding the family, attention has to be paid to a separation from the mother, above all, and to sufficient physical and social activity.

- **Lac caninum D30–D60–C200 pillules.** (various manufacturers)
  single doses

is an important single agent against depressive disorders, if the symptoms described further down occur. The authors owe the essential points for the understanding of the indication of this agent in conjunction with depressive disorders to J. Gnaiger [Gnaiger 1990, 1991].

Lac caninum is indicated, if

- the motherly role/the *child's relationship to the mother is divided between multiple (two in most cases) female persons of attachment* (classic case: the mother and a grandmother),
- the child has the (often unconscious) sentiment of not knowing to whom it belongs (especially girls are concerned),
- as often found in such constellations, one of the adult persons of attachment suffers from a guilty conscience or depression, which are adopted by the child.

Corporeally this corresponds to the odd symptom of inflammations (especially of the tonsils) *changing the sides of the body* repeatedly (e. g. from left to right and vice versa).

Psychologically there is a depressivity, which remains hidden for a long time, even to the child himself, which finds its expression in many anxieties, sleep onset insomnia, insecurities with regard to concentration and memory as well as the above mentioned corporeal symptomatology (in this context, this may even lead to restrictive rheumatic illnesses).

Therapeutically, apart from the administration of medicaments, systemic family therapy is of primary importance.

- **Pulsatilla D12–30 dil.** (various manufacturers)
  2 × daily 5 drops/single doses

is especially indicated with girls suffering from strong attachment to their mothers.

Depressive syndromes usually only develop starting with school age, but for the most part

- in puberty
- seasonally, in the dark winter time

With these patients, the depression runs *in phases* on principle, even though it can be accentuated now and then. The child or adolescent shows gratitude in these cases, if attention is bestowed on her (which easily triggers tears). There is a strong yearning for nature, for fresh air and sunlight and at the same time, an abnormal dependency on nature, which as a consequence can lead to seasonal depression during the cold and dark seasons. Likewise, there is a strong yearning for empathy, comfort and affection, up to strongly developed jealousy and precisely this dependency can lead to depressive disgruntlements (which can take on a subliminally demanding character towards the social surroundings, and support is sought after by the patient) during the crisis of adolescence, the emancipation and the process of independence. Physically, the patients generally show a robust vitality; but with a certain venous congestion, up to a tendency for fainting: a fragility that is dependent upon the current hormonal situation, nutrition (worsened through heavy, fatty foods), and external thermal conditions. *The dependency on external nature, on the changes in the digestive system and the menstruation cycle, and on the emotional attention by others* is the lead motive, which indicates the application of Pulsatilla in potentized state. The *moods, and the symptoms change* (like seasons, weather phases); the emotional condition is unstable and fragile (and thereby reminiscent of the large, hanging, violet Pulsatilla blossom, swaying in the springtime wind).

The therapeutic goal must be to lead the patient towards more independence, *to reinforce her self organization:* potentized preparations of iron and phosphorus (Ferrum sidereum, phosphoricum) are important complementary measures to Pulsatilla (▸Chap. 7.2.3.3).

For the patients themselves it is important to pay attention to sufficient light exposure (planning of vacations, rubbing oil into the skin (Einreibung) or oil dispersion baths with oleum hypericum in the winter part of the year, if necessary a couple of solarium visits during mid winter time).

The pathology of Pulsatilla indicates strongly, just how much the human being owes his or her inner uprightness and independence, versus the interplay of external (and internal) nature, to his or her *potential of inner "light-production"* [Steiner 1976, 216]. This is most apparent in the realization of the inner consciousness, but at the same time organically, up to the human posture, which in comparison with the animal kingdom is unique and to be understood in such a way, that the uprightness is the expression of internalized light dynamics [Verhulst 1999, 164–223].

These dynamics, which proceed from the very nature of the human being, can be medicinally reinforced through

- **Phosphor LM6/D10–12 dil.** (various manufacturers)
  5 drops in the mornings

which, apart from its purely homoeopathically justified indication, generally promotes the corporeally focussed activity of the self-organization in the sense of reinforced "light-production" (be careful, if this process is already going to excess). Through this, depressive disgruntlements, but also an increased vulnerability against infections and corporeal fragility, can be countered, especially during the dingy season.

On the plant level, this therapeutic principle finds its equivalent in the application of *Hypericum,* which even blossoms in mid summer and produces photosensibilizing substances [Kaul 2000, 175], among other things. Scientific studies are confirming [Kaul 2000, 150], that Hypericum extracts show a comparable therapeutic effect on seasonal depressions as the light therapy used for this purpose. In potentized states, the positive effect on reaction to pain after preceding trauma is known. – *Oil dispersion baths with Hypericum oil* possess at the same time a positively stimulating effect on the thermal organization (the same holds true for the repeatedly mentioned Malva oil Wala, which contains some Hypericum).

This examination shows that the reception and effect of *solar powers* does not only play a role for the vitality of plants, but also for the human being. In depressions, this process is disrupted: the eyes of the patient "do not shine anymore", his extremities (the basic shape of which is radial) do not move freely, his orientation towards the outer world is inhibited, but the same holds true for his inner vitality. R. Steiner pointed out, that the human *internalization of solar powers* in connection with the development of the life-organization takes place over the course of the first seven years of life [Steiner 1984, 56], and that sensual experiences in this time have immediate effects upon the forming (or deforming) of the body. He points out in clear words, that the I quality, the moral "in the gesture" of the adult in this phase, is crucial for the determination of what part of his actions are transferred into the child's body! The paedagogy and paediatric treatment of the child, being able to receive and absorb natural and human solar powers during the course of his first seven years of life allows, to a certain extent, *prophylaxis of depressive illnesses.*

An important enhancement of the therapeutic possibilities against *seasonal winter depression*, as a speedily effective alternative to the light-therapy, originates from our Dutch colleague Ernst Ellis and has been applied many times both in the practice of the authors and of others, with success:

- **Hepar-Magnesium[1] D10 amp. 10 ml** Weleda Switzerland (!)
  1 × weekly 10 ml in ratio (ca. 3 injections per winter season) [Vademecum 2010, 483f]. The acquisition of the ampoules takes several weeks, so it might make sense to keep a few of them in stock for acute treatments.

These aphoristic explanations give a larger picture of *gold,* the sun related quality and therapeutic application in potentized state, which has already been described in

1 Made from collectively potentized organ preparations of the liver, magnesium hydroxyde and honey

▸Chap. 7.2.3.3 in detail. Gold constitutes a central and harmonizingly effective medicine in the treatment of childhood anxieties and depressive syndromes.

The potency indicated in most cases of the paediatric practice is

- **Aurum met. praep. D12 trit.** Weleda
  daily 1–2 × 1 saltsp.

In connection with milder or early depressive disgruntlements,

- **Hypericum Auro cultum D2 dil.** Weleda
  3 × 7–20 drops daily

as a plant-based preparation, tinged with a gold solution, is therapeutically applicable. The application of potentized gold can be supplemented most of all by Cardiodoron drops Weleda (▸Chap. 7.2.3.3).

Gold and Hypericum preparations can also be effective against depressive disorders with *aggressive* symptoms; other medicines for aggressive behavioural disorders are discussed in the subsequent section.

In the practice of the authors, the most important *composition agent* for use against depressive disorders, especially at school age (9–14 year-olds), is

- **Aurum/Apis regina comp. pillules** Wala
  3 × 5–7–10 pillules daily

The Aurum chloratum = muriaticum processed in the above mentioned composition is positioned regarding its effect in between Aurum met. and Natrium muriaticum [Morrison 1995, 107; Wulfsberg 2001], and is particularly suited for the treatment of childhood depression at this age; the Hypericum contained in this composition supplements the effect of Aurum and improves (acting together with Acidum phosphoricum) the concentration ability [Vademecum 2010, 165f].

This medicine can also be considered for *depression related enuresis nocturna* (along with Causticum and Staphisagria, inter alia); it can be given in alternation with an individually indicated single agent.

Of utmost importance in conjunction with syndromes of depression is a *body-focussed* diagnosis (drawings of the child can be helpful to discover the locations of potential physical injuries) and, if necessary, treatment. (For example, sometimes the child can barely manage a tender touch, or rejects it.) Specific body regions may be excluded or distorted in self-portraits. The expression of a disrupted emotional-corporeal integration, which can still be made up for through appropriate therapies, may be visible. This aspect is of particular importance in cases of abuse and for extremely premature children.

7.3.3 Eurythmy therapy and non-medicinal therapies

By way of introduction, *rhythmical massage therapy* according to Wegman/Hauschka fulfils the children's need for an empathetic, understanding and tender touch; as a back massage, it can re-establish a point of reference and trust into the back space, which is often amiss or disrupted in the case of depressive disorders. Diagnostically, attention has to be paid to tenseness and congestion of tissue or hypotonic areas. Conspicuous oversensitivity to touch points towards primary sensory disruptions and/or traumatic experiences; traumas of the mother during pregnancy are also of importance here. Cold areas of the skin may be hinting at organ malfunctions and are as a principle of therapeutic relevance. *Hypericum* is also effective in the form of Hypericum-oil for massages and *Einreibung* (a rhythmic medicated body rub) of depressive children, especially in the darker season.

Eurythmy therapy is often a good succession to rhythmical massage. For depressive children the vowel "I" (here the German "I" is meant, which sounds like the "ee" in "see") is of great importance, through which the child is able to realize the internal experience of light, of a light ray going right through the child: "I" promotes an internalization of the soul-spiritual powers, which effect uprightness, the power of the human self, of individual personality. Exercises with the vowel "E", (as it sounds in the word "ex") which include a crossing of arms or legs while focussing on the crossing point, help to corporeally internalize these forces of individuality, all the way down into an invigoration of metabolic and physical activity. In terms of consonants, the sounds of "L" (stimulation of life-organization), "M" (promotion of exhalation, easing congestions), "N" and "R" (▸Chap. 7.2.2.4) are effective. The sound of "N" can stimulate the attention of children, which is usually disrupted in conjunction with depressive disorders. In the exercise of three-fold stepping (for older children and youth), a disruption shows itself with depressive children, especially of the first phase (lifting), whereas anxiety-centred disorders reveal themselves in the second phase (carrying), to which special attention should be paid.

Artistic therapy (painting and clay-modelling) based on the concepts of anthroposophic artistic therapy has a very lasting effect on depressive children. Independent of the home environment and family context, this therapy provides the child with a very far-reaching, non-verbal way of expression, independently of its artistic abilities and know-how, because it starts from elementary, very simple assumptions. Suppressed emotional-corporeal experiences resurface and can be processed, new emotional experiences, which thus far had been largely out of reach for the child, become possible, e. g. through the change of colour moods, transformation of plastic shapes and other things. If an adequately qualified therapist is available, this form of therapy is, according to the experience of the authors working with depressed children, often superior to other alternatives (such as game, behavioural, or conversational therapy); nevertheless, this decision has to be taken individually for each single case.

7.4 Aggressive behaviour disorders

"Thus, should you be seeking to learn in what manner the will of the world is revealed in the outer body parts, you should study arms and legs, hands and feet. Should you be seeking to learn how the intelligence of the world reveals itself, then you should study the head with regard to the skull... the nature of the human head and the nature of the human extremities are antithetical..."

R. Steiner [1919]

7.4.1 Towards an understanding of aggressive and hyperkinetic behaviour disorders

It is striking that depressive-emotional problems with inhibited motor function are clearly more frequent in girls than in boys, while the opposite is true for aggressive and hyperkinetic disorders. According to the KiGGS child health survey, the gender ratio with ADHD in the pubertal age range is approx. 1:4 [Huss et al. 2008]. This also affects delinquency statistics: 95 % of all prison inmates are male! It is worth paying closer attention to these simple and impressive facts. R. Steiner suggested considering the polarity between head and extremities (which again repeats the proportion of 1:4) to a comparative analysis considering different aspects. In the process of which, attention will be primarily drawn to the spherical, *internally centralized* character of the head (especially and foremost of the human head) [Steiner, 1992, 156]. In contrast to this is the radiating shape of the extremities, finding its vanishing point and also its "centre" point in the sphere, at infinity. From a morphological perspective, sphere and line constitute polar opposite principles (a purely visual presentation of these principles is drawn by teachers and pupils on the first day of grade one in Waldorf/Steiner schools). In nature they appear in their purest form as light ray and drop (or one might say, they appear in fire and water).

The sphere of the human head forms a reposing bony shell inside of which the brain, surrounded by cerebrospinal fluid, is held in a resting, almost weightless position (Archimedean principle). Repose and concentration are clearly recognizable by the shape itself. In contrast, the musculature of the limbs extends outwards, with development of strength and mobility dictating the appearance.

A simple comparative observation shows clearly that, morphologically speaking, the male gender shows an emphasis on the limbs (including the shape and name designation of the male sex organ; in German "Glied" means penis, and "Gliedmaßen" means limbs), which is to say that the male gender is associated with a more pronounced formation of the limbs while the female stature accentuates spherical forms. During pregnancy the embryo in utero takes on a position which likens that of the brain in the skull (with amniotic fluid and cerebrospinal fluid even having an almost identical composition). *The female stature emphasizes repose and internalization,* having an affinity to the life principle of water, whereas *the male constitution* accentuates *the principle of the limbs, extroverted development of strength and mobility* [for a detailed discussion of this aspect see Husemann 2009, 171–186]

This corresponds to the observation that girls and women are more susceptible to strong "tendencies toward internalization" which can even develop into depressive withdrawal and inhibition of aggression, whereas one central developmental motif for boys and men lies in learning to control the activity and impulsivity of the will which issues from their limbs. This also explains why for the latter *paedagogical guidance* (even including behavioural therapy for aggressive disorders) plays such an essential role and is most effective when provided by a *male person of reference* who acts in a self-controlled manner himself. In rural, pre-industrial societies in which the sons were primarily raised by their fathers, the activity of the limbs was shaped by learning how to perform physical tasks and acquiring, physical dexterity and self-control (for example while hunting). Considerably fewer problems occurred involving hyperkinetic disorders than in present day sons whose fathers are not involved in raising them due to their professional work or due to divorce and have little opportunity to engage in purposeful limb activity in daily life. The social causes of aggressive behavioural disorders lie for the most part “in a dysfunctional, disorganized family structure. Usually a familial hierarchy based on approval is missing or no binding rules and responsibilities exist” [Nissen 1989c, 117]. This often coincides with a *dysfunctional fatherly position*, due to illness, addiction or behavioural disorders of the father, absence of the father or other causes. In a standard work on child and adolescent psychiatry [Steinhausen 2010] the key word “father” is found only once in the index: under the item “father-daughter incest.” This does not do justice to the dimension and organization of the father-child-relationship in terms of child and adolescent psychiatry, particularly concerning the development of sons.

In the sense of these observations, ordered movement, and impulse-controlled behaviour, can be viewed as the *result of interdynamics*: the head and the limbs, perception and impulsivity, *female and male qualities*. These must collaborate if free and socially acceptable behaviour is to be made possible. Such dynamics are primarily *learned* through the *interaction of father and mother*, whose presence and clear understanding of roles shapes the development of the child’s physical activity and aggressive behaviour to a decisive degree.

Diagnostically and therapeutically it is necessary to pay particular attention to such relationships in addition to the disorders caused by the child’s constitution. In cases of aggressive and hyperkinetic disorders, the father should be especially included and he should intensify his paedagogical engagement. Television and computer consumption (particularly depictions of violence in films and so-called “computer games” which have nothing to do with genuine play) have an unfavourable effect [Spitzer 2005, 155–206]; an important aspect of this is that they contain no purposeful, ensouled movement of the limbs but deactivate it instead. *The potential of the limbs can only be trained through purposeful use and practice.* In modern-day classrooms this hardly ever occurs. Competitive sports are only suitable for this to a limited extent; high-performance sport mechanizes movements and fails to lead to a penetration and formation of the soul in the intended sense. Performing purposeful tasks in nature and engaging in artistic activities is a different case altogether (the effect which active pursuit of music has in reducing violence has been empirically proven).

7.4.2 Differential diagnosis indications

For diagnostic assessment of aggressive and antisocial behaviour in kindergarten and school age children, the followed aspects are worth noting [Guidelines for diagnostics 2000, 237ff.]:

- pregnancy history (infections, alcohol and medicaments, serious psychosocial duress),
- previous illnesses, for example epilepsy, encephalitis etc.,

- food and medication allergies, drugs,
- indications of an emotional disorder (▸Chap. 7.2, ▸Chap. 7.3), in particular trauma, experiences of loss,
- learning disorders, in particular dyslexia, chronic overload situations,
- hyperkinetic or attention deficit disorder,
- psychotic developments.

In each case, cause-related observation and treatment can contribute to an improvement of symptoms and modified, more appropriate interaction with the child. It is important to differentiate acute causative aspects which are primarily found in aggressive behavioural disorders in connection with

- constitutional conditions or
- disturbances of family structure.

For both aspects, a thorough individual and family history is important, which includes addressing the issue of similar disorders in earlier generations or close blood relatives. It is important to know whether the child has normal friendships or lives in social isolation and whether the behavioural disorder manifests itself primarily in the family or outside the family sphere. Reports made by third parties, in particular schools and kindergartens, are diagnostically significant. After all, it is important to assess the degree of self-endangerment or endangerment of others and the possibility of delinquency.

7.4.3 General treatment indications

It should first be mentioned, that here is an important therapeutic opportunity in the treatment of accompanying disorders or triggers of the aggressive behaviour, such as a reading and spelling weakness or excessive demands of the child at school. A targeted and consistent intervention in the family is essential if the child has accompanying emotional disorders. The child must be able to sustain positive relationships with authority figures (including men if possible) as well as to peers. Schools for children with special needs, day schools for children with behavioural problems, and, for more dysfunctional families or maternal stress due to separation, a boarding school that effectively relieves the family situation can provide the child with necessary security, guidance and support. Within the context of outpatient treatment, these opportunities should not be taken into consideration too late. They are always preferable to a purely suppressive drug therapy.

The medicinal therapies noted under ▸Chap. 7.4.4 may provide a lasting impact on constitutional causes of behavioural disorders in childhood and may to this extent be a form of therapy that addresses the roots of the problems. This is more applicable for potentized medicines than for low-potency neuroleptics, antidepressants, anticonvulsants, lithium, or stimulants (the latter prescribed for Attention Deficit Hyperactivity Disorder), which tend to show symptom suppressing effects without constitutional change. On the other hand, each medicinal therapy can be a bridge and support until other forms of therapy provide sufficient effectiveness.

7.4.4 Options for medicinal treatment with potentized single-substance medicines

The main *plant-derived* medicines for the treatment of aggressive behaviour problems originate from the family of the *nightshades (Solanaceae). Botanically,* these plants often show *divisions or polarization* (especially impressive in this respect are the shoots in *datura stramonium*, thorn-apple). A complex architecture exists in these plants, in which the ratio of *flower and leaf* is *intersected and shifted* relative to the normal arrangement of, for example, a crowfoot. This is very clearly seen in the example of the deadly nightshade which has each of its flowers *underneath* a leaf, always in partial shade. *Toxicologically,* these plants produce *alkaloid poisons* which have a strong toxic effect on humans, while many animal species tolerate them well. Interestingly, ingesting these poisons often results in *agitation, sensory hallucinations* and *delirious states* in which *animal figures* appear or the behaviour of those having ingested the poison becomes animal related (i. e. barking, biting).

With *Belladonna* the *central exciting* effect is in the foreground while in contrast *Hyoscyamus* (containing up to 40 % scopolamine in its alkaloids contents) is more absorbing, dulling and at the same time emotionally disinhibiting. The effect of *Datura stramonium* (like the plant form) is in itself very polar and can vary greatly from dampening analgesic to arousing. Accordingly, Belladonna and Stramonium have been indicated for homoeopathic use, i. e. high fever (hyperergic states), while this is not true for Hyoscyamus. A summary of leading symptoms for aggressive behaviour disorders is found in ◘ Tab. 7.1.

All three medicaments can be indicated for epilepsy. In general, middle potencies are recommended (D12, 15, 20 or LM6–12), which must be administered over relatively long periods of time before any change in the organism occurs.

An important medicament for adolescents with

- psychomotoric delay, autistic disorder,
- aggressive and most of all
- autoaggressive states of excitation,

which has proved effective in anthroposophic special needs education as well as in the authors' practice is

- **Hyoscyamus/Valeriana dil./amp.** Weleda
  3 × daily 15–20 drops/only as required 1–3 × weekly 1 ampoule s.c.

Constitutionally speaking, a very effective remedy for lack of impulse control, high levels of activity and a strong dependency of behaviour on metabolic activity is

- **Sulphur D12 (–200) pillules, LM6–12 dil.** (various manufacturers)
  daily 5 pillules/drops or individual dosages.

Children whose constitutions respond positively to this remedy show the following characteristics:

- predominantly *male*,
- often poor posture,

Tab. 7.1 Leading symptoms of aggressive behaviour disorders.

Belladonna	Hyoscyamus	Stramonium
Verbal aggression biting in early childhood	Emotional disorders: jealousy, suspicion, depressiveness	Sudden physically aggressivity, and on the other hand severe anxiety
In the case of psychoorganic disorders, autoaggressive actions (hitting, self-biting)	Inconsiderate but not brutal, socially unrestrained (e. g. hits mother during consultation!) at home possibly frequent masturbation	Ambivalent behaviour (compliant/aggressive)
Sturdy constitution, usually intelligent	Can be talkative; attention disorder, agitation partial impairment of performance occurs frequently, constitution tends to be pale, child does not run high fevers	Bad friend: angers others, uncontrolled violence; fear of being alone, most of all fear of the dark
In cases of fever delirium and states of agitation which end as abruptly as they begin	Tendency towards developing tics, hiccup (singultus), agitation,	Tendency towards stuttering, spasms of the respiratory tract
No information	History of neurological deficits or sequelae (for example after epilepsy in early childhood)	Cannot look others in the eye, schizoid personality, danger of psychotic developments
General exacerbation after falling asleep	Exacerbation after lying down	Exacerbation in the dark

- full lips, must eat a lot at frequent intervals, mostly sweet things, show *aggression when hungry* (particularly important for school-age children: such children must eat their breaktime snack!).
- "*surplus energy*, indestructible will to live (resiliency factor), seeks out as much life as possible" [Stübler 1969] – beginning in early childhood, even in the doctor's office.

Clinically speaking a tendency towards hypoglycaemia often manifests itself in the second seven years, associated with cravings for sweet things (which can create a vicious circle). Administration of medicaments almost always effects clear improvement and stabilization in this respect

- The need to be the *centre of attention*: bragging, with tendency towards being verbally aggressive (sometimes with instances of massive derailment), insuppressible urge to talk, constantly interrupts others.
- Poor emotional perception of others, who are often steamrollered by the child's behaviour without the child being aware of this (emotional egocentricity) – the child's own will impulses assert themselves in a disorganized way.
- There is disorder in regard to the child's belongings, clothing, behaviour, knowledge, self-portrayals, but with a rich store of memories, various possessions whose value the child is unable to assess.

- Unbounded-expansive behaviour in relation to age as well: such young people resent not being treated like adults. During adolescence a strong sexual desire can lead to behavioural anomalies.

Through the sulphur treatment these children begin to gain ownership of their actual potential, of their as such, large capacity for achievement. They become more orderly, less reliant on food, start tidying up and watching out for their appearance and, as friendly, "practical idealists" they show the positive side of their constitution.

Thus potentized sulphur counteracts a metabolism which takes on a life of its own like outer nature, contributing to a *consolidation of the child's life organization as the basis of the will to live.* In contrast, therapy involving potentized plant and snake *poisons* has a stronger, more immediate effect on the *emotional organization of the child.*

Apart from Solanaceae, two animal medicaments play a particularly important role here, first of all:

- **Lachesis D12 dil., D30–200 pillules** (various manufacturers)
  1–2 × 5 drops daily/individual dosages.

Lachesis is indicated in cases of

- jealousy, envy, intense feelings of hatred,
- inability to accept a subordinate role, a strong *need for domination*,
- strong tendency towards being socially *possessive*, on the other hand capable of heedlessly abandoning a friend of yesterday,
- *inability to tolerate harmony*, has an unerring instinct for knowing how to hurt others emotionally: *emotionally aggressive,*
- intensive sexual energy and associated with this pronounced aggravation of behavioural anomalies,
- generating social unrest, discord, "poisons the atmosphere."

Such children are often brought in for consultation because they are experienced as *no longer bearable in the social context*, be it in the family, the school class or some other type of community.

In principle, the depicted character traits emerge primarily in the context of maturation crises during puberty. In connection with deeply rooted aggressive behavioural disorders, Lachesis can be highly effective in all phases of childhood and youth. Apart from constitutional causes, the family structure should be examined carefully. What status does the child have? What type of emotional dynamics takes place among siblings and between parents? It is not uncommon to find concurrence of a high degree of inner (constitutionally determined) and external (psychosocial) tension which has led to the dynamics described. Administration of medicaments should always be accompanied by consultation with the parents concerning how to deal with the child and as the case may be, his or her siblings.

- **Tarantula hispanica D12–30 pillules** (various manufacturers)
  1–2 × 5 pillules daily/individual dosages

is another medicinal animal preparation.

This is indicated in cases of

- pronounced hyperactivity,
- morally (lies, cheating) and physically destructive behaviour.

In such children and adolescents, constitutional factors play a large role. A strong metabolically and sexually determined drive dynamic manifests itself in early childhood in the form of clearly hyperactive behaviour.

R. Steiner gave important advice concerning the treatment of aggressive behaviour disorders with *cruel behaviour* on the part of the child (originally in connection with epileptic disorders, ▸Chap. 8.1), recommending therapeutic use of potentized *lead* [Walter 1987, 112]. When administered in a suitable pharmaceutical preparation, lead counteracts destructive activity of the astral body which uncouples itself from the I organization [Steiner and Wegman 1977, 126f.]. It is also cited by R. Steiner in connection with disorders of instinctive behaviour and addiction. In summary one can say that potentized preparations consisting of lead, lead salts and lead-honey-sugar-compounds strengthen guidance by the I in response to one-sided destructive impulses of the will (and thus in this connection fostering the guidance of movement from the head) [Selawry 1985, 385].

Therapeutically the authors' view is that preferential consideration should be given to

- **Plumbum mellitum D20 trit.** Weleda
  1 saltsp. daily.

And in addition

- **Cichorium Plumbo cultum D2 dil.** Weleda (cf. the following section 7.5) [Vademecum 2010, 318] and
- **Minium D4–6 trit.** Apotheke an der Weleda [Vademecum 2010, 598]

In cases of addictive behaviour.

In addition one might also mention

- **Anacardium D30 pillules** (various manufacturers): single dosages

The difficulties involved are reminiscent of those treated with Sulphur (aggressive behaviour highly dependent on food intake) and Stramonium (pronounced anxieties, feelings of inferiority which can develop into physically aggressive behaviour); the causes of such disorders are possibly traumatising family circumstances and abuse in early childhood.

- **Hepar Sulfuris LM6–12 dil.** Arcana
  daily 5 drops.

In such patients, hypersensitivity and a lack of life warmth are coupled with aggression extending as far as violent and pyromaniac impulses (at the same time anxieties and dreams about fire). A high degree of inner tension persists (similar to the substance Hepar Sulfuris, which emerges from lime and sulphur through application of heat and degrades spontaneously); ambition and claim to leadership contrast with a high measure of physical susceptibility which is ignored whenever possible. Inclinations towards biting others are observed; school age boys who are affected do not always try to avoid physical confrontations. In physical terms, these patients suffer from sensitivity to cold and frequent inflammation of the throat (tonsillitis, stenosing laryngitis).

7.5 Attention deficit disorder with and without hyperactivity (ADHD/ADD)

His violent temperament causes us much distress, though he is so funny and often so tender and loving. Then come complaints from top and bottom and left and right ... Hermann has pushed my child! – Hermann has smashed the glass! Hermann is throwing stones at the neighbour's children!... Just hearing someone mention the name of Hermann causes me to fear what may have happened ... again.

Hermann Hesse's mother at the beginning of his kindergarten days

It would be so humiliating for us, but I am seriously considering whether we should not give him to an asylum. We are too nervous, too weak for him, the whole house is not disciplined and ordered enough. He seems to be gifted in all manners: he observes the moon and the clouds, fantasizes at length on the harmonium, draws wonderfully with pen and pencil, sings rather well when so inclined and never lacks a rhyme...

H. Hesse's father as he was reaching school-age[1]

7.5.1 Who is hyperactive?

„The passionate boy was later, after various other strokes of genius and aberrations, to tackle the suffering of life in strict discipline, and has, if not a hero, become a man." This is how the narrative on Hermann Heilner in "Beneath the Wheel" (1906) ends; an autobiographical report of a 15 year-old, who, like the Nobel prize winning Hesse, breaks out of his evangelical-theological seminary at Maulbronn into an unquiet, changing life that is painful and creative, both for himself and for others.

When the book of the 29-year old Hermann Hesse appeared, he had been living for 2 years as a freelance writer. During World War I he worked for prisoners of war, he reminds his patriotically minded German colleague of Schiller's words in Beethoven's Ninth Symphony: friends, not these tones! – and attends to prisoners of war. His novel "Demian" (1919) is the first work of German literature that foresees the collapse of the imperial-authoritarian order and gives a voice to the dawn of a new Era – while the German elite need a further 26 years to realize this. The contrast between spirit and nature, Apollo and Dionysus, "Narcissus and Goldmund" was created by him at the peak of his career, "the search for a harmonious balance essentially determined his literary work" [Brockhaus, 2006]. That a German (Swiss citizen since 1923) would be awarded the 1946 Nobel Prize in Literature for his life's work was not foreseeable in 1883 in Calw, nor in 1892 in Maulbronn, nor even in 1946.

His mother, daughter of a missionary and Indologist soon noted how unusual her son was. "He gives the angels work to protect him, because he is too quick and too powerful" she noted already when he was 9 months old. Her notes contain remarkably clear descriptions of hyperactive behaviour, emotional and intellectual talents and the experience of her own insufficiency, which many parents of hyperactive children know. At only 20 months a broken arm had to be set, and the above-quoted words of the father, as Hesse

1 The authors thank his colleague Hartmut Horn, a Child and Youth Psychiatrist, for pointing to these quotes and would like to take this opportunity to thank him for his ideas on this topic.

was 6 ½ years old, bear witness to impressive awareness of the situation as well as to the individuality of the boy.

In its spectrum from Siddhartha and Steppenwolf to Narcissus and Goldmund, Hesse's work focuses on the struggle to find a centre, mediation, harmonization, which often comes in two polar representations, as in Hans Giebenrath and Heilner in "Beneath the Wheel". Life, individualization, is the task of creating a centre, a balance in this polarity. In his last great work, "The Glass Bead Game" (1943) Hesse depicts several biographies of the same individuality – a unique phenomenon in the history of German literature. He thus calls on the perspective of reincarnation in the struggle to achieve harmonization and individualization that on the one hand is the fabric of our individuality and on the other hand the root of stress and disease. – The pressure to adapt found in paedagogical institutions is strongly criticized in "Beneath the Wheel", and in the 60 s of the 20th century, Hesse was especially popular. Historically, his diagnosis of the Wilhelmine world was certainly right, and the world would be a different place had more individuals understood how to not be perfectly functional.

Yet you feel the sincerity and authenticity in the words of his parents: the birth pains of a human individuality, the inability of a hyperactive child to regulate himself, result in a pain and helplessness in his social environment that have their own truth and validity. In the end it is about a third element that, arising between polarities, brings about that which is really human. It is about becoming oneself, bearing polarities in one's own expectations and demands. The interaction of adaptation and individualization is something other than "bend early, he who wants to be a sickle." Above all it is about first perceiving, who this "difficult child" is, who is urging to be born out of childhood and yet needs sheathing and support, even though he is "difficult". The accompaniment of hyperactive children whose attentiveness, social behaviour and motor skills are often unusual is a "midwifing" challenge requiring a good perception of the unborn individuality, of the parents and surroundings.

7.5.1.1 ADHD and adaptation

The term "Attention Deficit Hyperactivity Disorder" (ADHD) includes

- Inattentiveness and increased distractibility (= ADD)
- low impulse control, reduced self-inhibition (inhibition) capabilities in the areas of thought and behaviour, as well as, optionally
- increased urge to move, motor hyperactivity (= ADHD).

"These symptoms" – see above – "are pervasive and interfere with the individual's ability to function under normal circumstances" [Nelson 2003, 107]. "Pervasive" means that there is a "dominant" behavioural disorder manifesting in various situations; "normal circumstances" means "western lifestyle" settings (family, kindergarten, school). What "to function" means in today's adult "normal" world has been expressed in a child and adolescent psychiatry review on ADHD by Schmidt, Meuser and Momsen in the following manner: "The hyperkinetic disorder is primarily a disorder of impulse control. While we all usually consider before an action whether it is appropriate for the moment, adequate or correct (sic), in these patients" – children, actually – "the impulse shoots through before reflection and leads to action that may in the aftermath be regretted or lead to unpleasant results" [Schmidt et al. 2003, 184].

7

The concept of "shooting through" aptly characterizes the central problem in the ADHD symptom complex:

- impulses from motor function and metabolism: movement impulses, metabolically dependent instinctual impulses
- sensory input from the environment, spontaneous ideas
- are not brought into harmony with the social environment, with the feelings and needs of others. Rules, which are the internalized content of a bond with adult caregivers, develop no regulatory power. Whether the child is distracted by "bouncing from impression to impression" or whether out of an inner urge he performs meaningless, even destructive acts, the child lacks the inhibiting inner reflection into which attachment, especially to the parents, could blend. The same ability which, unimpressed by the splendour of the Empire or the cheers of the masses, recognized the criminal intent of the Wilhelmian military that used a targeted grenade shot at the steeple of Verdun to herald the planned killing of a million young men in a battle of attrition, the same authenticity and independence which distinguished Hermann Hesse as an adult from his contemporary elite of German professors can, in the situation of childhood, lead to extraordinary difficulties. People with ADHD function especially well where normal rules and laws lead to ruin or are suspended.

Returning to the above definition of the "normal case" of controlled thought and action, it is striking that it is based on the control of the will by reflection and thus on the dominance of control. This reflects exactly the dominant thought and behaviour of high-tech Western industrial societies. It does not correspond to an artistic and creative style of thinking that is marked by an intense openness to new ideas emerging in the present. Man as an artist, and as inventor, is characterized by an ability to break free from the safe calculus of rational goal-oriented action (one can really speak of a "risky" style of thought and behaviour in this context!). In another way, reflection and control rarely correspond to the leisure and parenting style of adults relating, for example, to food, alcohol and tobacco – and parental use of alcohol and nicotine, especially in pregnancy, has been demonstrated to favour the symptoms that medicine diagnoses as ADHD in children.

The problem with the above definition based on the dichotomy of intention and reflection, is that it bypasses the *level of the heart* as a decisive level of mediation. "The brain – a relationship organ" [Fuchs, 2008] does not work as a control in the frontal lobe without the whole person feeling involved. "For the living, for the soul as well as for the spiritual, relationality is *constitutive*: the living relationship with the environment, the emotional relationship with others, the intentional relation to the contents of mental acts, the relationship to the past and future" [Fuchs, 2008, 289]. The key to the "dysfunction of neural networks" [Steinhausen 2010, 146] most likely lies *between* the parties, between the individuals involved and their relationships which, in early childhood, form the body in a more decisive way than at any other period of life. What today is explored epigenetically, the physical consequences of events and lifestyle in pregnancy and infancy, reflects a reality in which the child meets his parents and his environment, physically, emotionally and spiritually. "For me he is too powerful," wrote Hermann Hesse's mother, as Hermann was 9 months old. In these words, Hermann Hesse is still present.

"In the words of the other I hear his thoughts. Grasping his hand, I give *him* a hand. Through the look in his eyes I see *himself*. We are not dreams of our brains, but incarnate people" [Fuchs, 2008, 298]. In the available scientific research and data, *the emotional rela-*

tionship level, not just the neural inhibition level, is often found to be affected in hyperactive children. Maybe the central goal of a sustainable and effective therapy and the prognostically decisive quality are to be found in the (delayed) maturation of this emotional relationship level.

From the authors' point of view, the social behaviour, the quality of relationships that the child and parents experience and exercise together in the early years (in a "pre-reflective" life period of the child) is a decisive quality regarding ADHD, both pathogenetically as well as in terms of "co-morbidity". Empirically proven influencing factors (see below) are all present in this life period and act on children and parents with great power. There are many indications that "partner conflicts, mental health of the parents, educational deficits and disorders of the parent-child relationship" [Steinhausen 2002, 95] strongly affect – and may disturb – attention, impulse control, and activity behaviour of children. All these influences are rarely subject to the paradigm of deliberate, well-planned and adequately reflected actions!

If one searches for the origin of the adaptation ideal that is socially and educationally followed and called for in western industrialized countries, one finds it not in the world of the soul, but in that of *technology.* Accident-free driving of a car, launching an aircraft, carrying out an operation, virtually every professional activity within a society based on modern technology requires a style of behaviour that is characterized by

- focused attention (suppressing awareness of the environment as a whole in favour of more accurate, visually-driven attention to individual processes),
- planned action that is *focused on a future outcome*
- relinquishing whole body motion in favour of partial precision movements, particularly in the control of machines.

The same applies to economic necessities relating to technology. This style pervades the education of children, such as the presently dominant requirements for pupils, or the management and treatment of patients and thus also of hyperactive and inattentive children: medical, educational and social norms are moulded into technical standards and are implemented in the form of "management" and "self-management". "To function under normal circumstances" is thus *a historically relative criterion* and was not only so in the Maulbronn monastery.

7

In the above-mentioned review article, Schmidt, Meuser and Momsen quote a remarkable forecast by Rudolf Steiner in 1920, the founding year of anthroposophic medicine:

> "... Man is not merely an intellect: he has sensations, he has feelings. The latter have to put up with what comes from technology, from the machines.
> A different feeling from what I have just described ensues. I spoke of the feeling of deprived longing, of yearning deprivation. In contrast, that which the soul synthesizes in the subconscious out of technology (...) that reacts, comes up into consciousness as thoughts, ideas, but it comes up as something that is similar to fear. And in addition to the yearning deprivation that will be seen coming up in school children in the coming years and decades, a vague, but no less lively fear of life will appear. This fear will translate into nervousness, into a fidgety, nervous nature. I mean this literally." [Steiner 1920; cited by Schmidt et al. 2003]

At this point it becomes apparent that *technologically induced changes in consciousness* can also be experienced psychologically as *alienation* from life, as *imprisonment* in predetermined inherent necessities, as the *loss* of both one's soul experience of the present and any possible individual spontaneity. At a time when the concept of neuronal impulse control is in full swing and prescribing stimulants has become standard therapy, leading neurobiologists such as Gerhard Roth hold this view of the true nature of human behavioural control: "The statement 'What made the decision was not I but the brain' seems correct to me." [Roth 2004, 77 – cited in Fuchs 2008]. Today this school of thought is the underlying conviction dominating most academic psychiatric circles. The real subject is not the human individuality but the brain and its neuronal networks. What meaning is reserved for human consciousness in this case? "Characteristics of specific brain processes that the brain provides for itself in order to orient itself in its own incredible complexity"? [Roth 1994, 276] What reality corresponds to our will? Who guides – or ought to guide – my activity? As early as 1988, Blakemore [The Mind Machine, 272] formulated it like this: "The sense of will is an invention of the brain." Hyperactive behaviour becomes an error in the functioning of the brain, which has become the heir of our soul, of our existence as a subject and as a human being [Fuchs 2008, 77–86]. Perhaps hyperactivity is an expression of lack of fuel in this system and must be balanced out, either endogenously or exogenously. The brains of prescribing physicians induce them to provide what the brains of their patients need....

Hermann Hesse's parents did not figure him out – in contrast to Gerhard Roth, Thomas Metzinger and other opinion leaders, who are already imagining a national conservation area for human free will, since they believe their science has pulled the carpet out from under it. The operant conviction among modern neurobiologists is that in reality, the brain acts before we become aware of it, and from this perspective the hyperactive child is in good company. "To function under normal circumstances": Are paediatricians becoming service stations for brains, fuelling them with the prescriptions their guidelines endorse while therapists adjust all the sensors and maintain the electronics of a neuronal machine? Those who pursue these ideas to their logical conclusion are not so much independent professionals as managers in scientific-industrial complexes.

But we can also look at it in a very different way: The human brain makes a unique degree of freedom available to us [Fuchs 2008, 86]. It does not shape itself; to the contrary, it is more open than any other neurological system. Open to whatever befalls us and to whomever we meet, and perhaps even to whoever we may be. In critical times, how important the fundamental convictions that guide human beings become. Specifically in dealing with the subject of ADHD and those affected by it, it can be helpful to return to Parsifal's question, born not out of reflection and will but out of compassion: *Who are you? What do you need for your development? And how can we establish a good connection to you?*

7.5.1.2 ADHD – A Sign of Talent?

Curative educator Henning Köhler [2002] contrasts the problems and abilities of children who can become socially conspicuous today due to hyperactivity, impulsivity, or attention deficits. (◘ Tab. 7.2)

Tab. 7.2 Abilities of children with conspicuous behaviour such as hyperactivity, impulsivity, or attention deficits.

Problem	Abilities
Compulsive, driven, motor deficits	Motor skills often highly developed ("kinaesthetic intelligence" [Gardner 1994])
distractibility	Wide-ranging interest in the world
Short attention span	Panoramic vision: rapid perception and intense attention for this brief period of time
Poor listening ability, inadequate auditory perceptual processing and connection to the space behind	Visually dominated and forward-oriented perceptual style
Impulsivity	Great flexibility and receptivity to new things
Claim to leadership is often pronounced in relationship with peers and adults	Longing for authentic authority, personal leadership abilities not uncommon

Winston Churchill was an impressive example of this. Son of a father that can be suspected to have had ADHD and who had precious little time or attention for the boy, Churchill displayed all the signs of an attention disorder at school. He made progress in learning only when motivated by personal interest. Throughout his life, he was most energetic in confrontational situations. In 1940, after an already very eventful political career and seemingly against all reason, he led Great Britain into an initially almost hopeless-seeming confrontation with Germany and accepted national bankruptcy in consequence (which all "normally functioning" British politicians had been attempting to avoid). Churchill, who had the longest and most successful political career in British history, was also awarded the Nobel Prize for literature in 1953 (seven years after Hermann Hesse) for his monumental literary work and was also known for his extensive artistic activity as a painter in his old age.

Another example is the successful inventor *Thomas Alva Edison*, who registered over a thousand patents and was always working on several inventions at the same time. He viewed sleep as a waste of time and revolutionized the life and sleeping habits of his contemporaries and successors with the invention of the incandescent light bulb. A complete failure in school, he left home at age twelve and initially eked out a living by doing odd jobs. – How would he be diagnosed and – if applicable – treated today? Would anyone immediately recognize and foster this "difficult" boy's talents?

In literature, Astrid Lindgren has shed light on the subject of ADHD from many perspectives in the character of *Emil of Lönneberga*: his strenuous character traits, his parents' suffering but also their profound understanding, the lack of understanding of his fellow citizens, who wanted to buy him a one-way ticket to America (his mother threw all the money they collected out the window) – and finally his later career as city council president.

In view of these facts, the definition coined by ADHD expert C. Neuhaus is extremely problematic: "As soon as unusual behaviour has no positive effects but constantly creates problems for the person involved, it is no longer a manifestation of creativity but of disturbance" [Neuhaus 2000, 66]. Ever since the days of the Pharisees, "constant problems" have depended not only on those who purportedly cause them but also on those who carry the social responsibility of reacting negatively to unusual behaviour, recognizing the splinters in the eyes of others but not the beam in their own eyes.

Any definition of ADHD, therefore, *must also test the one who defines what counts as normal.* This dimension eludes most scientific medical literature because *natural sciences dominate* the education of modern physicians. Still, there is no "standard value" that clearly delineates ADHD as a disorder or disease from the broad stream of possibilities in child development. Rather, diagnosis is based primarily on the activity of *understanding* children's behaviour, which is underlined by the fact that there is *no scientific test that establishes a diagnosis of ADHD.* "The diagnosis is deduced from the *patient's life story.*" [Leitlinien 2003, R7, 3]. Even questionnaires are of very limited value, and guidelines place less value on extensive psychological testing than on "negative evaluations of intellectual ability and attention in school by teachers and in their school reports; examining the contents of the child's backpack and schoolbooks (tidiness, sequencing, handwriting, organization) provides indications of disorders in visual-motor coordination (writing), attentiveness (errors due to oversights), dyslexia, and dysgraphia." Clearly, however, these criteria are assessed according to the *child's adaptation* to the terms and conditions of the modern nuclear family, the modern kindergarten (25 children, noise levels around 85 dB), and modern education with all its expectations of educational performance. In this case, the term "disorder" is vastly different from the concept of illness that is applied in cases of meningitis or even mental retardation or psychosis.

This viewpoint was especially emphatically confirmed by a 2010 study that agreed with the conclusions of studies conducted since the mid 1960 s in the US and other industrialized nations (including Germany). As early as the 1980 s, the findings of these studies led some states of the US to increase the mandatory school enrollment age after having decreased it earlier. Early school enrollment was shown to correlate with increased rates of suicide in 20-year-olds [Uphoff, Gilmore 2003]:

The chance of being treated with stimulants in grades 5 and 8 is only *half as great* among children who are *the oldest in their class* as in the youngest in the class at age of enrollment. [Elder 2010]. In this study, 8.4 % of the youngest and 5.1 % of the oldest were diagnosed with ADHD.

R. Largo talks about "fit" as a decisive process in human socialization. Against the backdrop of such experiences, the "misfit" (as Largo calls it) between a child and the institution to which he/she is meant to adapt needs to be understood and addressed as a two-sided problem. In ADHD, in any case, the question of school readiness acquires greater significance and should be decided responsibly, independent of locally applicable regulations.

7.5.1.3 Age, gender, relationships, social class: genetic or epigenetic?

It is worth noting that far more boys than girls are diagnosed with ADHD: The proportion of boys to girls ranges from 3:1 to 9:1! [Steinhausen 2010, 140] For ADD without hyperactivity, a proportion of 2:1 is assumed, although without the hyperactivity factor, "the validity of the ADD type is problematic" [Steinhausen]; that is, the transition to "normal" can no longer be determined with validity. – On the other hand, ADHD is considered *genetically determined* to a considerable extent. Several recent studies indicate inheritability rates of approximately 80 percent – based on studies of twins *without the typical preponderance of male ADHD!* [Cf. Schmidt et al. 2003, 186] This finding conflicts with what we observe in practice. – The pathogenetic genetic effects are supposedly based primarily on a disturbance in dopamine metabolism and in some cases on additional neurotransmitter disturbances in the brain, which cause susceptibility in the children affected; however, this hypothesis also offers no explanation for gender differences in the prevalence of ADHD. Thus an *obvious contradiction exists* between genetics and neurobiology on the one hand – that is, the scientifically comprehensible aspect – and the phenomena observed in educational and clinical settings with regard to the *unequal distribution of ADHD between boys and girls!* And there are also other factors such as socioeconomic ones that do not fit into this picture, not to mention the observable differences between the oldest and the youngest in a school class.

Anthropological and anthroposophic aspects of the gender issue have already been presented in ▸Chap. 7.4.1. In *historical* and *social* terms, how children grow up in societies with Western lifestyles is characterized today by a multitude of factors, including:

- Modern media and the PC, which have caused very significant declines in activity levels, in the alternation between speaking and listening, and in shared play and family rituals (such as meals).
- For the most part, both girls *and* boys are now raised *primarily by women* (mothers, kindergarten teachers, and most elementary school teachers).
- Children experience their fathers only during their free time, during weekend visits every two weeks (if the parents are separated) or not at all.[1]
- Due to the mechanization of household tasks and travel, children experience physical activity ever less frequently as a *meaningful need.*
- Boys in particular experience only seldom "typically male" movement activities that require physical strength and endurance, and then as (arbitrary) athletic activities rather than as socially useful, valuable, structured work.
- *Free space* to develop impulsivity, independent movement, and changing levels of attentiveness as offered by *nature* and unscheduled time is disappearing increasingly.
- Although child and adolescent psychiatry speaks of "neuronal network disorders... specific to children with hyperkinetic disorder" [Steinhausen 146] and genetic factors are assumed to be the probable cause, epigenetic characteristics acquired in the course of early physical development (which is heavily influenced by a child's experience of relationships) are another possibility. There is no known hereditary basis for the male-female ratio of ADHD cases, with 3–9 times more boys than girls affected by hyperactive behaviours worldwide.
- Instead, recent studies confirm that the risk of ADHD is 2.2 times less likely in children who grow up with their biological *father* present (At least on the epigenetic level, the father's presence seems to be a protective factor) [Schneider, Eisenberg 2006].

1 A study by Streeck-Fischer and Fricke [2007, cited in Neraal, Wildermuth 2008] was able to determine that among 30 children for whom insurance claims for psychotherapy had been submitted, 18 fathers were not present in their lives due to death or separation, 4 were frequently absent, 3 were "in a difficult position", and one was chronically ill.

- It is quite apparent that boys need role models and caregivers who share their "problem" of being male. Any woman will realize that there are certain things her daughter can effectively learn, experience, and share only with her, in particular anything to do with her experience of her own body. But feelings, relationships, and preferred and least favourite activities are most different in children of school age – the age of gender polarization – which is also when hyperactivity becomes especially socially problematic and is most likely to be treated.
- As a general rule, genetic disorders do not to correlate with income levels – a fact known to any paediatrician who deals with children with Down syndrome or cystic fibrosis. Is ADHD a hereditary disease? In the US, children from families with incomes below the 20th percentile and above the 80th percentile are at increased risk of ADHD (2.2 times and 1.5 times, respectively), while in Germany the risk of ADHD is *2.8 times greater in children from poor families* than in families with higher incomes [KiGGS Huss 2008].
- For children in the US who attend village schools, the risk of ADHD is almost 6 times lower, and the teacher's ethnicity also affects ADHD risk [Schneider, Eisenberg l. c.].

In addition to the social realities, "head starts" in life also play a significant role in ADHD genesis, not only with regard to school enrollment but also much earlier: In Norway, 27 percent of premature babies [Ulvund et al (in Norwegian), cited by Neraal 2008, 69] with birth weights under 1.5 kg displayed symptoms of ADHD at a follow-up examination at age 8 or 9. Carers of extreme preemies (born in weeks 24–28 of gestation) are familiar with the major problems many of these children have in the first few years of school, independent of IQ.

Early separation of a newborn and mother is a well-known risk factor that corresponds exactly to the animal experimental model used by researchers at the Max Planck Institute for Psychiatry in Munich to demonstrate the epigenetic development and fixation of lifelong disturbances in stress regulation [Murgatroyd 2009]: The animals were exposed to *"early life stress"* (the title of the paper) consisting of daily separation from the mother for several hours. Infant regulatory disorders are very likely to persist in the form of ADHD behaviours. In one study [Wolke et al. 2002], a group of children treated for regulatory disorders as infants was reexamined at age 8, revealing ADHD symptoms in 19 percent. Infant regulatory disorders are also associated with parental stress (cf. ▸Chap. 4), especially marital conflicts and maternal psychological stress. The *aberrant sensory development* (e. g., hypersensitivity to sounds, touch) described by Frey [2005] as an essential consideration in prescribing homoeopathic medications for ADHD appears in many children treated for regulatory disorders in infancy. Unstable attachments in early childhood, critical or hostile interfamilial interactions (e. g., between the parents), and maternal alternation between anxious and anxiety-triggering behaviour all favour disorganized attachment behaviour in children, which is associated with increased prevalence of ADHD [Neraal, Wildermuth 2008, 59–87].

Summarizing the findings of these and many additional studies results in the following picture:

- *Early childhood* seems to play a central role in the problem of ADHD, especially with regard to the environment and relationships in which the child grows up. With regard to bodily development and epigenesis, this period of life has already been shown to be of considerable significance to the capacity for self-regulation. One epigenetic animal study, famous in this context and conducted by the Max Planck Institute for Psychiatry (!) in Munich, was able to demonstrate that *"early life stress"* can have life-long negative consequences for the capacity for self-regulation.

- *The capacity for self-regulation and social competency are closely related:* 40 to 90 percent of children with an ADHD diagnosis display profound *disorders in social behaviour* [Steinhausen 2010, 141]; the "most common comorbidity in ADHD is of ADHD with a disturbance in social behaviour" [Kain 2008]. The ability to communicate empathetically with other people is not a purely cerebral faculty but a breathing, feeling ability based in the human rhythmic system. In a broader sense, this system encompasses all human (self-)regulatory capabilities, that is, any ability to actively *mediate between polarities* and form a meaningful whole. This is the quality that Hermann Hesse struggled to achieve throughout his life, giving artistic expression to the struggle in his writing. *ADHD correlates with an immaturity, weakness, or disorder of the child's rhythmic system; any salutogenic therapy can and should tackle the problem on this level* [1]
- The role of the constitutional factor, *the child's temperament,* is uncontested. Undoubtedly, Hermann Hesse's early childhood is also an expression of his temperament. From the perspective of the anthroposophic study of the human being, the child's temperament is of great importance in education. Rudolf Steiner draws a direct connection between temperament and the quality of the child's life organization, i. e., the character of the child's ether body [Steiner 1975, 143]. Ultimately, this is also the level where the epigenetic processes of early childhood are localized. On this level, the sexes are as different as they are on the physical level [for a thorough discussion, see Husemann 2009, 171–186]. Temperament and sexual polarity, therefore, always need educational, diagnostic, and therapeutic attention.
- Ultimately, the question is, what role is played by the *abilities and weaknesses* of the child's soul-spiritual individuality? How do Hermann Hesse's ADHD characteristics, as described by his parents, relate to the author of "Beneath the Wheel" and "Siddhartha"?

Here, a paediatrics devoted to the individual is called upon to engage all responsible parties – parents, carers, teachers, activists in politics and in the field of prophylactic medicine – in *how we can reshape children's surroundings so that the problem of ADHD becomes less widespread and acute.* – In this respect, H. Köhler's book "War Michel aus Lönneberga aufmerksamkeitsgestört?" [Did Emil of Lönneberga have ADHD? 2nd German edition 2002] points to many concrete and practically tested options that not only lead to successful "ADD management" in the sense of an adaptive strategy but also take the *unique abilities and strengths* of the affected children seriously and allow them to bear fruit.

1 The authors thank Matthias Girke for his important suggestions on this point.

7.5.2 Diagnostic aspects

"We compile a thorough, very detailed biographical and family case history. From the very beginning, we place special value on describing not only the child's weaknesses but especially his strengths."

H. Köhler [2002, 196]

7.5.2.1 Case history

All authors agree on the *great diagnostic importance* of an extensive, uninterrupted (!) conversation with the child's parents (both of them, if at all possible!) in compiling the case history. – In practice, this purpose can be served by:

- Asking the parents to write a free-form *letter* to the physician, to include any background information that seems important to them, a few observations about the child, a description of the family's living situation, any illnesses and therapies the child has had, and any comments by other people (relatives, day-care providers, teachers).

The advantage of this format is that it eliminates any time pressure, and any forgotten items can be added later. For the parents, it is an opportunity to concentrate and to compile and evaluate their recollections. Without being inhibited by the child's presence, they can also express their own feelings of stress. If the letter is handwritten, the physician also gains an additional important impression of the parent who did the writing. At the same time, an important part of the case history is already documented, thus taking pressure off the actual conversation. In addition, we recommend:

- separating the case history compilation from actually meeting the child.

It is important in any case, also in paediatric or general medical practice, to schedule *enough time* for this conversation. Due to the need for *creative diagnosis and deciding on therapies, one hour* is generally required for the initial consultation when ADHD is suspected, regardless of the normal medical fee schedule.

Independent of the patient's age, the first crucial question to ask is about the *first seven years of life.* Symptoms indicative of a disorder that requires treatment *may* include:

- In infancy:
  - Long-standing, recurring symptoms that suggest *over-tiredness* in the infant: protracted crying, motor agitation, irritability, difficulty falling asleep, difficult to calm down.
  - Infant care is strenuous and unsettling for the parents; disturbed development of a *satisfying emotional child-parent attachment*
- In early childhood:
  - *Temporal dissociation* acquiring speech, motor development, and toilet training, for example: striking earliness or lateness of individual developmental steps, e.g. in fine-motor coordination, in understanding language, etc.
  - *Driven, restless motor activity,* little endurance (usually with a few important exceptions!); frequent *unpredictable* changes in activity; enjoys risky activities, increased risk of accidents.

  - *Easily distracted* by sensory impressions: "lives entirely in his surroundings," moves instantly from sensory impressions to activity.
  - Children are *socially "difficult,"* "barge in" impulsively, lack interest in listening (except when you tell them stories one-on-one); frequent *rule-breaking, early and inappropriate need for guidance,* in spite of defiant demands for autonomy. Due to these behaviours, the child and his/her nuclear family may become *socially isolated;* siblings become enemies or victims; attachments to family members and friends are disturbed (this symptom in particular also illustrates that the reverse is also true, of course: for example, separation of the parents, loss of a beloved family member, etc. can lead to disturbances in attention and behaviour).
  - Situation-dependent *intensification of these problems, especially in kindergarten:* Most kindergartens today are an especially inappropriate setting for children with hyperactive tendencies and attention deficits. They do better in kindergartens that work with small groups of children and emphasize outdoor activities in nature.
  - At this point it is also important to ask about *allergies and sensitivities* and to compile a thorough case history of eating habits, digestion (dysbiosis/fungal infections?). Is abnormal behaviour worse after eating certain foods or better after dietary changes?

It has already been pointed out in ▸Chap. 7.5.1 that these negatives generally occur in tandem with *unique talents* and "improved behaviour." For example, gymnastic talent may be evident at an early age (many ADHD children have a special liking for circuses and playing circus), as may skills in climbing, creative talents, etc.

In general, any attention deficit with hyperactivity can be recognized through careful compilation of a case study and observation of the child during the medical examination at age five (in Germany this is called the U9; the 9th preventive examination). Almost without exception, a holistic therapeutic approach without stimulants constitutes adequate treatment at this point in time.

- The symptoms associated with ADHD in school-age children are well-known:
  - Distractibility, forgetfulness, carelessness, lack of persistence especially with regard to least favourite schoolwork and chores; disruptive, impulsive, rule-breaking social behaviour
  - Conspicuously poor handwriting, difficulties in reading and writing
  - Constant, over-hasty talking
  - Emotional fragility and low self-esteem; outsider role in contrast to mental ability

Once again, it is worth noting that boys who impress their mothers, teachers, and classmates as extremely hyperactive can spend long, quiet hours fishing with their fathers, and that in anxiety-provoking emergency situations (e.g., during a house fire), these children can do the right thing with astounding aplomb and presence of mind and later have excellent recall of the details!

- Indicators to consider in *adolescence* are:
  - Dropping out of school early or repeatedly
  - Social isolation, constant conflicts with others, few or no friends
  - Attraction to risky types of sports, risky driving, etc.
  - Constant need for distraction; inner restlessness

Drug issues, addiction-like media and computer game dependency, and socially stressful experience with age peers become increasingly important.

Today, when we emphasize the dangers untreated ADHD poses to adolescents and adults, this says as much about our society as it does about the affected individuals who live in it. In this connection, it is important to realize that only a real *understanding of the difficulties and specific talents of these individuals,* not suppressive therapeutic models such as stimulants, will change their increasingly being ostracized. Because stimulant therapy is generally not controllable in adolescents, it is essential to set the therapeutic goal of encouraging and treating these children and adolescents and to integrate them into appropriate contexts so that they can remain or become independent of daily tablet intake during this phase of life.

In compiling the *family case history,* the following questions are of primary importance:

- The course of the pregnancy and birth (▸Chap. 2.4)

A *quick* or *difficult* birth or *intubation* after birth, among other factors, can lead to lasting *cranio-cervical transition disorders* and must be effectively counteracted through appropriate therapy (see below). Along with the classical US homoeopaths Ullmann and Reichenberg-Ullmann, the authors have also observed that "the thoughts and feelings parents experience immediately prior to conception and during pregnancy can have a direct effect on the child's condition" [Reichenberg-Ullmann 2002, 115]. Research findings on early regulatory disorders [Papousek 2004] and their persistence in school-age children [Wolke et al. 2002] confirm the importance of this viewpoint. The medications listed in ▸Chap. 2.4 are therefore of great therapeutic significance; the impressive case histories the authors of "Ritalin Free Kids" [2nd German edition 2002] offer as proof of the efficacy of homoeopathically potentized medications include this dimension.

- *Toxin loads* (esp. nicotine, alcohol, prescription medications, and other drugs)

The importance of these factors is now generally acknowledged. To a certain degree, therapies can compensate for toxin loads, especially during the first seven years of life. Possible therapies include exercises to be practiced at home, lifestyle changes, and (to a certain extent) homoeopathic and anthroposophic medicines.

- *Parents' and grandparents' constitutions*

In the course of discussing and diagnosing their child's ADHD, many parents become aware for the first time that they themselves display the same character traits (or did as children) that they are now struggling to cope with in their children. This insight often makes it possible for parents:

- To gain a new understanding of how the child is feeling
- To relax about the situation somewhat, since many parents ultimately experienced something positive in their lives as a result of their own difficulties; many do not want to be "completely normal"
- To recognize a therapeutic opportunity, because changes that result from the parent's learning and making changes in their own behaviour *are often most effective*

A psychiatric study of children and adolescents by A. M. Sant'Unione and Matthias Wildermuth entitled "Therapy of hyperkinetic syndrome including its sub-forms (ADD, ADHD, hyperkinetic disturbance of social behaviour) and accompanying comorbid disturbances in the social-psychiatric practice" [2007], presents 30 thorough case studies and has the advantage of dealing with the subject from the authentic perspective of actual practice. The study makes it clear that *the paradigm of genetically determined paediatric disorders of brain metabolism is not sufficient for understanding any of these individual case histories* – let alone for prescribing therapy. The authors have had the same experience in their practice. The case history that follows, taken from the above-mentioned study, may serve as an example that clarifies the work that is involved for *parents dealing with ADHD in their children:*

Case Study

[Sant'Unione and Wildermuth 2007] At the time of the initial consultation, the boy was eight years old and living with his mother, an older mentally handicapped brother, and another brother two years younger than himself. His father had been separated from the family for about two years and visited his sons only on an irregular basis. His mother was employed and had high expectations of herself and her sons, especially in terms of academic performance and housework. The consultation took place on the recommendation of the boy's paediatrician, who had already made a diagnosis of ADHD and had been prescribing methylphenidate (Ritalin) for two years but now questioned whether medication was the best or only treatment option. The medication had only temporarily improved the boy's abnormal behaviours in school. His standing in the class was poor; he was not liked and was sometimes disruptive, out of control, or aggressive. His academic performance was poor, especially in language skills, and he was often laughed at when he had to read aloud because he had not really learned to read. At home he was defiant, did not listen to his mother, quarrelled a lot with his siblings, didn't do his homework, told lies, and was almost incapable of occupying himself. Any attempts to play with him were disastrous because he responded to any form of losing with fits of rage. He was always on the go and so restless he was "driving his mother crazy." It became obvious that the mother was very regimented and rather rigid in her dealings with the children, especially the patient.

With regard to his early childhood, it is worth mentioning that although he was the second child, he was soon forced into a quasi-parental role due to his older brother's mental retardation, and his mother later saw him as a partner substitute. His mother had "kicked his father out" because he had hit her repeatedly, forced her to have sex, and tried to kill her in the boy's presence. Talking about it made her so upset that she broke down in tears, unable to hide the panicky fear that still gripped her. She had escaped with her life by a hair's breadth, and the boy had tried to help her. Nonetheless, she said that she had noticed that the boy was still fond of his father, which is why she had wanted him to stay in contact with the children. In further conversations with the boy, it became obvious that although on the one hand he loathed his father, he still sought out contact with him and felt abandoned by him. He craved his father's approval but at the same time was afraid of being identified or equated with him. It helped that in the course of therapy, his mother was able to tell him the positive things that had attracted her to his father and the good qualities he had demonstrated in their relationship before he began beating her. For a while, she had been very fond of him. She also conceded that in spite of his erratic behaviour toward her, he had always behaved properly with the children. She had never been afraid of leaving the children alone with him, which made her all the more regretful that he was so unreliable about staying in touch with the children.

Later, when she was in a new relationship and her new partner moved in with the family, the boy was initially hostile to his stepfather due to his libidinous connection to his mother – he didn't want any man to get close to her. Another contributing factor was certainly the fact that he feared renewed attacks on his mother. He was especially afraid of his own violent fantasies and aggressive action. Eventually his aggression toward his mother completely receded and was redirected elsewhere. His mother's high expectations of her son also moderated. The boy dealt with his conflict of self-esteem playfully projecting his anxiety about failure, about "being no good," onto the therapist, whom he made fun of and attempted to demoralize whenever he made a mistake, no matter how small.

His mother gradually grew able to perceive the boy's distress and to release him from his role as quasi-parent and partner substitute. She resigned herself to his poor spelling and refrained from blaming it entirely on malicious intent and laziness on his part. At the boy's own initiative, contacts with his father became ever less frequent. He did not demonize his father, but arrived at a compromise between desire and reality that worked for him. In this context, he was then able to accept his stepfather as a substitute father, although with a certain distance. He was very clear, for example, that the name "Dad" was reserved for his biological father. As the course of therapy drew to a close, he had successfully completed fourth grade and his mother had enrolled him in the middle school (Hauptschule) that he had chosen for himself. He put up with the one-hour bus ride without complaint. Six months after conclusion of therapy, a prearranged consultation to review his development took place. Meanwhile, he had become integrated into the class and was well-regarded by his classmates. He had friends, his grades were satisfactory, and his mother was proud to report that she had heard very positive things about him in his parent-teacher conferences. She seemed to have given up the spectre of her son, like his biological father, becoming a "monster" or "tormentor" to her. She trusted him and saw him as a child, not as a partner substitute. Both mother and son were able to leave their sadness about the past in the therapy room. A year after the psychotherapy sessions ended, the situation remained stable and no further treatment was needed. A decisive factor seemed to be that the boy's mother had been able to develop empathy for her son's feelings and to give up her bitterness toward him.

The following points, in particular, are ones the paediatrician should emphasize in the parents' case history and in working with them:

- How do the parents interact with each other?
- On what points do they disagree?
- How do they differ in their responses to the child's behaviour?

It is also important to get a picture of the following points:

- Is the father absent, unavailable to the child, or reserved in his relationship to the child?
- The father sees child-rearing as exclusively the mother's job
- The child's father was not raised by or had bad experiences with his own father
- The father competes with the child for the mother's attention
- The mother has difficulty relating to men, bonds closely with the child as a substitute parent or substitute partner, and rejects the child's father
- The mother discriminates against the son who reminds her of his father
- The father's and/or mother's behaviour toward the child is impulsive or erratic
- The father's and/or mother's communication with the child is ambivalent toward the child (e. g., verbal vs. nonverbal communication)
- The child experiences triangulation (the development from a you-me to you-me-him/her relationships) as punishment and rejects it; triangulation has not been achieved (especially relevant beginning with age 5)
- The child does not live up to parental expectations, is aware of it and depressed by it and reacts with restlessness and aggression
- Having a child is traumatic for the mother or father
- Mother interprets outside suggestions as a failure on her part
- Mother and/or father lack confidence in their parenting style
- Parents lack self-confidence and attempt to compensate with excessive, controlling attention

It is not uncommon for parents to develop a new understanding of each other on the basis of insight into their own attention span and impulsivity. Even severe disappointments and separations can be handled better when care is taken to involve the parents in the treatment of a difficult child and to help them develop the awareness that more careful attention and mastering their own impulsivity (if necessary, by giving up a drug habit) will help their child and spare him similar disappointments and painful experiences. (For more on advising parents, ▸Chap. 7.5.3).

Finally, reports from the child's kindergarten and school are important, including (if needed) a face-to-face consultation with the parents and the child's class teacher. The therapist should personally inspect the child's school notebooks and early drawings.

7.5.2.2 Examination and differential diagnosis

The written case history (parents' letter) and conversation with the parents takes much of the pressure off the examination appointment. For the physician, the purpose of that appointment should always be to perceive and experience the child directly, whether by engaging him/her in conversation, playing a game together, or at least engaging in wordless dialogue through gestures. A physical examination appropriate to the child's tolerance is also an important component of this appointment. Often, *constitutional traits* are revealed by *first impressions* of the child's appearance and behaviour as he/she answers. It is important to find out how the child engages in dialogue. How does he establish eye contact, and how long does he maintain it? What does she notice in the exam room? How much interest does he show in people and things, and how quickly does his attention wander? – Is conversation possible *if you listen intently to the child?* Behavioural assessment of preschoolers should focus on attention span, impulsivity, and movement patterns. (Here, too, an attempt should be made to coax the child out of her shell by playing together.) School-age children with ADHD problems are often precocious in their ability to assess their own situation and may make quite profound statements about it if an open-ended, unpressured conversational setting can be provided for them. Not infrequently, to the surprise of all involved, hidden pressures or interests surface, which if they are then taken into account allow important progress to be made. – As a first step, compiling the case history and examining the child should *clarify the diagnosis:*

- Does the child present with a *hyperactivity disorder* that requires treatment according to the defining criteria of ADHD?
- Are their grounds for suspecting an *attention deficit disorder* (ADD) *without* hyperactive behaviour?

First of all, *differential diagnosis* should distinguish between:

- *reactive behavioural* disorders due to pressures on the child from:
  - Family (parents' problems in raising and relating to the child; inappropriate expectations; problems in the parents' relationship; pressures due to problems with siblings or close relatives; unspoken, stress-inducing "family secrets")
  - Kindergarten or school (excessive expectations, personality conflicts with a difficult teacher, etc.)

Next, it is important to identify or rule out:

- *depressive disorders* (▸Chap. 7.3), which are definitely compatible with hyperactive behaviour in boys and in most cases compromise attention span (sometimes severely).

Also important in this connection are:

- Peripheral and central *hearing impairments* must always be ruled out!
- Autistic spectrum disorders or (very infrequently) psychoses;
- Endocrine disorders (especially thyroid and adrenal).

In the process of diagnosing ADHD/ADD, it is important to figure out which of these factors may be triggering or contributing to the disorder:

- vegetative regulatory disorder; circulatory hypotension

Constitutional weakness of the rhythmic system may be evident in:

- Changes in skin colour or uneven distribution of body warmth
- Orthostatic dysregulation and arterial hypotension (low blood pressure); a significantly skewed pulse-respiratory quotient
- Perspiration and posture
- In fluctuating blood sugar levels; tendency toward hypoglycaemic episodes of ravenous hunger, increased restlessness and aggression, especially in the morning (during school hours!)

...and is especially significant in the second seven-year period. The child's *iron metabolism* is an interesting factor in this connection. *At this age, there is a positive correlation between tissue iron levels (ferritin) and the ability to regulate the rhythmic system.* Konofal [2004] was able to confirm a significant *connection between ADHD and low ferritin* (▸Chap. 7.5.3.6). This discovery points to the underlying problem in ADHD: to what extent does the "higher human being," the I and astral body, manage to control, regulate, and guide the dynamics of the metabolism and limbs, of natural, constitutional impulsivity? The most important metal in this process in the body is iron. Its assimilation by and concentration in the organism (Hb, ferritin) increase significantly in healthy children, starting around age nine.

- Cranio-cervical transition disorders

Beginning at birth, disorders in the cranio-cervical system can contribute significantly to ADHD-like symptoms. Diagnosing it becomes very important in late infancy, with significant diagnostic and therapeutic repercussions. Special attention should be paid to asymmetries and functional disorders of the jaw and to interactions among the upper and lower jaw, the cervical spine, and the cranio-cervical transition area, and to alternate tensing and slackening of the back and abdominal muscles. The medical history often reports excessive crying at an early age along with sleep disorders and severe restlessness already in infancy; the birth history (emergency C-section, very rapid delivery, positional anomalies, etc.) is also informative.

- Specific developmental delays

Specific developmental delays may be noted during preventive care appointments (especially yearly appointments at 3, 4 and 5 years of age and the school enrollment examination). Activities may include observing the child while:

- Playing catch, walking downstairs, doing jumping jacks, etc.
- Balancing, standing and hopping on one leg
- Painting a picture; handling toys and items in the office
- Monitoring verbal understanding, listening ability, and active use of language
- Testing specific pre-writing or writing skills
- Responding spontaneously during a conversation with the parents
- Telling a story; establishing contact with others (or not)

These observations are complemented by the developmental case history and later testing, as needed – cf. Baumann [2006]. Fundamentally important – also in terms of differential diagnosis – are tests of the child's *intelligence* and special aptitudes, and a consideration of the appropriateness of the demands of the child's environment (low expectations or excessive demands). In this connection, terms such as "highly gifted" are not necessarily helpful, because in reality these children suffer from major *discrepancies* – for example, between their mathematical/logical thinking and their "emotional intelligence," or between their artistic gifts and their reading and writing ability.

Whether supplemental testing by a specialist in child or adolescent psychiatry, a paediatric audiological examination, allergy testing including an assessment of the gut flora, endocrinological testing, or an EEG is needed to confirm the differential diagnosis must be determined on an individual basis.

In the process of diagnosis and in introducing therapy, the objectives are:

- *First*, for the child to experience a comprehensive appreciation in the paediatrician's or family doctor's office, as described above, and to make an initial diagnosis.
- To explain the findings and consequences in detail after the diagnostic process is complete and to agree on a therapeutic approach together. The child should be included in a way that makes him feel that he is being helped and supported: "The personal connection is the actual therapy" [Köhler].
- To consult with *all of the adults involved with the child* during a common consultation. This practice has proved valuable. In particular, the conversation should include the parents, the child-care provider or teacher, the child's therapist or curative educator, and the physician responsible for the diagnosis. (For more information on the principle of "protective circles", cf. [Köhler 2002, 236–238]). A conversation of this sort can achieve a comprehensive perception of the child with all his weaknesses and talents. Diagnoses, goals, and responsibilities can be discussed and explained. It is not uncommon for the participants to experience that a conversation that places the child in its centre and strives to perceive him as fully as possible has an immediate effect on the child, who is not even present, as well as on all of the participants. In retrospect, it may prove to be the most important step therapeutically, uniting parents and educators, physician and therapists, into a meaningful, effective whole and a foundation that supports their common efforts.

7.5.3 Treatment

7.5.3.1 Constitutional, social and situational factors[1]

Therapeutically, much depends on whether a specific classification of the child's disorder can be achieved, hence being able to arrive at a purposeful, *curatively oriented* form of treatment.

From the perspective of the *threefold organization* and the fundamental guidance of patients one can start by differentiating:

- Children with *hypersensitivity of the senses, i. e.* "emotionally sore" children, possibly children with early trauma, who are immediately run out of control by external stimuli and inducements, and who improve in states of quiet and envelopment. Treatment for forms of shock is often indicated. Extremely prematurely born children often fall into this group. These patients predominantly have a delicate physique, and partial impairment of performance occurs frequently (independent of intelligence). They find it easiest to integrate themselves into small groups; they require individual attention for a long time and suffer from rejection by other children, against whom they are not capable of defending themselves. The weight of expectations is particularly detrimental for such children.
- Children with *impulsive drivenness* manifesting a strong desire for movement which easily gets out of hand and impacts on others before the child's consciousness can grasp what his own limbs are doing. Inner drive, tension and temperament make it difficult for these children to stop this disturbing behaviour. In such patients, the body tends to be relatively sturdy and the body warmth is quite strong. Such children try to dominate in a group and can profit from well-guided groups which they do not succeed in throw-

1 The authors wish to thank M.Girke for valuable suggestions.

ing off balance. These children improve through movement, male caretakers and tasks which are purposeful and demand exertion and courage. Thus they require tasks which are suited to their disposition and do not aim towards early intellectualization. Medicaments which regulate the metabolism are helpful, as are foods which help regulate the metabolism. There is no great need for emotional closeness like in the first-mentioned group of hypersensitive children. Male guidance and communication style suits such children better, even the girls.

- Children who primarily have relationship problems with older and same-age children, are highly stressed by ambivalent-uncertain relationships and parental conflicts, children with a strong tendency towards jealousy, sometimes in cases where siblings are close in age, often benefit from social change which creates more distance while offering safety and guidance at the same time. It is important to guide the family as a whole in such a way as to promote authenticity and more stable bonding as well as boundaries. Otherwise all interpersonal relationships run the risk of being "poisoned."

7.5.3.2 Stimulants

Treatment with stimulants (e.g. Ritalin®) as it prevails today has a symptomatic effect – which can be very beneficial in certain situations. This holds in particular for situations in which societal pressure to adapt is very pronounced, familial and therapeutic resources are exhausted and the patient is cooperatively integrated into a therapeutic framework. Then stimulants can counteract social isolation and persistent failure, reducing dependency on the parents, boosting self-confidence and opening up new perspectives for the individual's future life in the process. Approximately one out of four children who are viewed as affected by this disorder does not respond to stimulants or shows a negative reaction to them. Therapy involving stimulants alone cannot open up a path towards *recovery*, i.e. salutogenesis, in child development.

Current stimulants therapy claims to provide *substitution treatment* for the metabolism of the central nervous system. The claim made in this form – unlike treatment of diabetes with insulin – continues to remain a hypothesis. Generally speaking, every type of substitution can impair the balance and weaken the autonomous development of the child's metabolism. During or even before adolescence this treatment, which calls for regular intake of pills and medical monitoring, often leads to massive self-doubt and inappropriate use of the administered substances. – The question is whether stimulants still actually play the role of an *acute treatment* if the child remains unreachable, highly impaired in her concentration and socially isolated or unbearable despite all measures.

Careful observation reveals that stimulants themselves also exert a *suppressive* effect on many children. This is true for the emotional area, the area of original creativity in the human being. Whereas the ability to concentrate on one thing can be enhanced, those affected notice that their creativity and the colourfulness of their soul suffers. The *suppressive effect on the appetite*, and at higher dosages the frequently observed *disorders of weight gain* and thus of the child's life organization are well-known. The sense of *thirst* can be impaired too, and in blood tests threshold values for creatinine and uric acid are frequently found. In adolescence reversible cardiac arrhythmias, sometimes accompanied by ventricular arrhythmias, have been observed which disappear if the medicament is discontinued. It is always recommendable to refrain from taking stimulants on weekends and during holiday times if possible, even if recommendations to this effect are contradictory.

One preparation aligned to the anthroposophic approach to therapy has proven specifically beneficial for children and adolescents who are undergoing stimulants therapy. This remedy is proving to be an equalizing factor, especially for the frequent side effects of stimulants. Even without stimulant medication, positive therapeutic experiences in treatment of ADHD have been made with this preparation, which also stimulates anabolic protein metabolism: Organum quadruplex.

- **Organum quadruplex amp.** Wala
  2 × weekly – 1 × daily 1 ampoule per os

Experience has shown that it is better to administer it in the evening if the focus is on the side effects of stimulant treatment because its own effect can unfold better in this case. For constitutional disorders it can be taken in the morning.

The guiding idea for this widely effective medicament is initially stimulation of the life organization of vital organs. Liver, heart and kidney activity is perceptibly affected by stimulants therapy (careful observation reveals influence on lung activity as well, from which appetite issues, ▸Chap. 5). In this way "[Organum quadruplex] facilitates individualized organ formation in child development and thus also a freeing up of the spirit-soul aspect for social learning and communication processes" [Vademecum 2010, 633] since it is not physically bound to such a high degree any more (exhausting itself herein). The medicament is constitutionally effective in children who are strongly influenced by the metabolic area, who appear "too dense" and possibly have difficulties resonating deeply with others, do not sweat sufficiently, have dense skin and sturdy hair, are insensitive to pain and at the same time easily distractible and socially incapable of entering into deep relationships. It can also be administered to good effect to counterbalance toxic side effects of stimulants, in particular where anorectic tendencies play a role, but also in cases of children with other types of constitution (cf. 7.5.3.1.)[1]. It is usually advisable to prescribe it for long periods of time.

Many affected children generally seem to have problems *managing their own anabolic metabolism*, which is directly related to unconscious dynamics of impulses and the will. It is no coincidence that stimulants unfold a suppressive effect here, subduing a part of these dynamics. The organ preparation in question was originally developed to generate a stimulating effect on "insufficient formation of the highly differentiated and individualized protein substance" [Vogel 1994, 607]. – This brings to mind the current discussion on ADHD, which focuses on the notion that it constitutes a lack of highly differentiated protein substances (catecholamine metabolism) necessary for impulse control and that stimulant treatment is viewed as substitutive. From a therapeutic perspective the objective conclusion from this can be to give *regulative and stimulating impulses for the protein metabolism*. The Organum quadruplex preparation provides a general possibility for doing so and the constitutionally effective medicaments listed below (e.g., Calcium carbonicum) allow for individualized and long-term modes of therapy.

The more therapy focuses on helping the child or adolescent recover in his or her development (salutogenesis) rather than aiming to manage a disorder, the more stimulants acquire the status of acute medication which cannot be avoided in some cases – particu-

1 Proven to be beneficial for children in the context of chemotherapy as well, for ex. 1 × daily – 3 × a week 1 ampoule per os, in the afternoon or evening.

larly when diagnosis is made at a late date – but which must be viewed as an unsatisfactory therapeutic option long-term.

7.5.3.3 General views on treatment

The first and already therapeutically relevant step is an exact *clarification of the medical diagnosis*, which facilitates an understanding of the child, with all his or her weaknesses and strengths. In this way, a new interest in the child as an individuality is awakened, as an individual who is still in the process of manifestation, and who still has something startling to unveil. The purpose of this is to understand how the child experiences important life situations and reference persons, and what the child can and cannot (yet) do.

The second step consists of *paedagogic counselling* of the parents, but also – in an appropriate way – of the teachers and caregivers involved (cf. the concept of the protective circle). Today, there is excellent literature on this subject; reference should be made, once again, to H. Köhler [1994, 2002] and the work of Schmidt et al. [2003]. Parent handbooks are very helpful for practical everyday advice, e.g. Neuhaus [2007], and also, Aust and Hammer [2001]. However much their ideas may differ; there are broad areas of agreement when dealing with the children concerned. As regards the question of *the PC and electronic entertainment* the works of R. Patzlaff [2000] are fundamental; the parent handbook by Goebel and Glöckler [2008] give numerous references to literature on this subject, as do Vagedes, Soldner [2010, 372–379].

What is important is the establishment of *authentic* paedagogic relationships; so that parental relationship crises or financial difficulties, among other things, can be made conscious, in order to be dealt with separately and not played out through the child. Briefly, the following points should be mentioned here:

- Positivity: only positive reinforcement brings about lasting paedagogic development. This knowledge is so indisputable and simple, but educational reality contradicts it. This point takes on a special meaning with children who have an attention deficit disorder. Tried and tested are the following:
  - The use of point systems do deal with most important "hotspots": For example, starts homework himself/herself – 1 point; one homework task completed – 1 point; all homework tasks completed (not necessarily error-free!) – 1 point; reward every week, when approx. ⅔ (70 %) of possible score is attained. The reward should be agreed upon beforehand.
  - There should be praise every day! It is always possible to find something to praise. Three times a day is better!
  - With dyslexic children, underline every correct word in their composition in green, and do this with every task where performance is mixed (Fight the red pen! Green has right of way!)
- *Coherence:* The parenting style should be as clear and consistent to the child as possible. Small "duties" bind the child into the family. *To be told to do only one thing at a time* (instead of five things, which cannot be carried out) enables a child to settle and consistently grasp what is required (coherence). Make sure that the child is paying attention; before you speak (establish eye contact, exude calm).
- *Live social rules.* For example, during conversations at the table, let a kitchen spoon be passed around as a "speakers-rod". Whoever holds the rod may speak and may not be interrupted. The consequences for breaking the rules should be established beforehand and adhered to.

- *Closeness and distance:* with tactfulness and consistency one must ensure that the child achieves age-appropriate autonomy in the family context. Healthy nine-year-olds should not spend the night in their mother's bed, children of divorced parents are entitled to clear regulations which are not misused by the parents as a means of putting pressure on each other, and anxieties of the mother in particular must be taken seriously but they often regulate themselves by creating appropriate distance between mother and child. The child must learn to respect the autonomous lives of the adults.
- For every forms of attention deficit *nutrition consultation* focusing on the individual plays an important role.

The third step consists in assessing whether the child is adequately challenged at kindergarten, school or, as the case may be, the day care centre. Often changes are called for here regarding group size, individual possibilities for fostering the child as well as the amount of time the child spends in the institution. Thus an all-day school with qualified afternoon care can be a decisive source of relief for the family. The authors have observed time and again that children (starting at age 10 or so) who have massive hyperkinetic disorders and exceedingly strained family situations have developed exceptionally well by spending several years in a boarding school whose special needs education is oriented to Waldorf paedagogy without any stimulant therapy at all. In such cases the task is to convince a cost bearer to cover the fees. – In any case, affected children quickly convey whether they are really benefitting from the change or not and in the case of a positive change they are willing to accept many inconveniences. – For the consulting physician it is important to be familiar with what various schools and care facilities in the vicinity have to offer.

Dependent on the preceding steps, the therapeutic procedure in the narrower sense may be formulated, in which anthroposophic and homoeopathic medicines play an important role. They do not act in a substitutive or suppressive manner as do stimulants; when properly individually selected, they promote learning processes of the organism. They stimulate maturation of the living order of processes and forces within the child, manifested in growth and function of the organs, but also in the formation and function of memory. These medicines do not work solely on the nervous system, but on the whole organism. Precisely the *relation* of the nerve-sense system to the metabolic and limb pole and the compensatory integration of these polarities in the middle, rhythmic system and therefore at the heart level is the problem in attention and impulse control disorders, and usually also in social behaviour disorders [see Pohl 2002, Schmidt et al. 2003]. In principle, the duration of taking these medicines depends on how long the child takes until he has completed – and learned to stabilize – the learning and maturation step that the medicine is meant to stimulate. Some widely indicated composition medicines require a long treatment period (several months) while potentized individual agents are administered depending on the activity and potency level for weeks to months, or as a single dose. Reichenberg-Ullman produced an impressive publication on classical homoeopathic treatment of ADHD [2002]. With regards to anthroposophic medicine, a series of case reports has been published by Saverne [2002] and a review by Schmidt et al. [2003]. Another important step is a study by Hamre, Witt et al., showing that anthroposophic medical treatment of 61 children with ADHD in a primary care setting was effective according to generally accepted standards [Hamre, 2010].

A scientifically important publication, which simultaneously represents a major step forward in the *homoeopathic treatment of children with attention deficit disorder with and without hyperactivity* stems from Heiner Frei [2005]. In a first step Frei precisely describes a methodical procedure and careful evaluation that enabled him to double the effectiveness of his treatment.

Especially important is his understanding that prescribing single doses of high potencies is clearly inferior to prescribing LM or Q potencies daily or every two days (starting with Q3!). The authors wish to explicitly confirm this experience; daily administration of anthroposophic medicines is also usually necessary in children diagnosed with ADD/ADHD.

Taking a further step, in a placebo-controlled double-blind cross-over study with 62 children (55 boys, 7 girls!), Frei was able to show the following:

- Homoeopathic therapy is significantly superior to placebo ($p = 0.0479$).
- For the children treated homoeopathically, the degree of improvement, measured using the Conners Global Index, averaged out at 55 %, thus lying slightly above the average improvement achieved with methylphenydate.
- 75 % of the treated children adjusted "so well that they needed no other medication and were well-integrated into family and school life" [Frei 2005, 158].

In his publication Frei depicts his procedures for diagnosis and therapy very precisely and comprehensibly. From an anthroposophic standpoint it is noteworthy that for Frei *precise assessment of disorders of the senses* among children affected proved to be a particularly reliable basis for arriving at the appropriate medication. For purposes of repertorization he emphasizes:

- Aversion to touch
- Exacerbation by strained sight, hypersensitivity to light
- Hypersensitivity to noise, does not tolerate noise *of other children* well
- Hypersensitivity to smells

At this point one should make note of the positive results of *smelling therapy for children with ADHD-symptoms* achieved by B. Kraker von Schwarzenfeld [2005]. Clear improvement through differentiated smelling exercises with 14 different natural smells was observed, indicating the connection between the frontal lobe and the olfactory system. An important observation is that "intensification of smell ... can also eliminate feelings of exhaustion," which are typical for many children who have ADHD. R. Steiner points out the connection between the olfactory sense and inner emotional experience [Steiner 2005, 26] – something everyone is familiar with from their own childhood. Nothing calls childhood memories to mind as strongly as re-encounters with smells which were experienced intensely from an emotional perspective back then. *The study supports the thesis that through intensively differentiated experiences of smell, conscious processing of sensory experiences, activation of the frontal lobe in central perception and regulation of motion is promoted* (cf. ▸Chap. 6.6.1). Medicaments which contain potentized lead, primarily in vegetabilized form, counteract hypersensitivity to smells while at the same time promoting formation of consciousness in connection with the olfactory sense [Vademecum 2010, 318] and are beneficial for sensorily hypersensitive children with autistic disorders (**Cichorium Plumbo cultum Rh D3 dil, Plumbum silicicum D10–20 Trit.** Weleda [Schmidt 2007]) as well.

In this context one should consider how much experience of smell children with a "Western lifestyle" have contrasted with children living in natural rural life surroundings under different hygienic conditions! This could indicate the benefit of paedagogical measures which give restless children with attention deficits the chance to experience and perceive nature intensively and in a highly differentiated way, particularly in the first seven-year period. Kindergartens which make excursions outdoors, in the woods and to similar places on a regular basis are particularly well-suited for this.

- Decisive factors for choice of remedies are improvement or exacerbation of ADHD symptoms in response to heat and cold, whereby many children display a longing for sheathing protection.
- Exacerbation through writing (cramped, tiring, slow) was identified by Frei as the most reliable motor symptom in differential therapy: Writing encompasses eye-hand-coordination, stable lateralization, development of fine motor skills and thus also quality of motor development, which is often disturbed or delayed in the cases of such children.

Another important insight gained by Frei is that *Calcium carbonicum Hahnemanni* is the most frequently indicated medicament for ADD/ADHD cited in his study! This is surprising at first since no one would immediately associate oyster shell with hyperactivity and socially problematic attention disorders. What is particularly striking about the oyster is the retrogression of its senses in the course of its lifetime; the weak sensory perception of its environment accompanied by very vital metabolic activity! – At second glance Frei's observation points to an essential aspect of the clinical picture of "Attentiveness disorder," namely *overly autonomous metabolic processes far-removed from consciousness.* Oysters fend off all influences of sensory perception, of consciousness with their shell while at the same time containing a highly vital protein. – Human beings must conduct their metabolic life in the reverse fashion and, through synthesis of neurotransmitters, for example, build up highly differentiated substances from protein precursors (tyrosine) in order to promote consciousness [cf. Steiner, Wegman 1991, 87f.]. *In anthroposophic anthropology, the difficulty of penetrating the body's own vital metabolic impulses* and expressing these adequately rather than simply living them characterizes the *hysterical constitution*, which is found in many children with attentiveness disorders. Sulphur and Calcium carbonicum (the former more so in cases of hyperactivity, the latter more so where there is none) are excellent constitutional medicaments in this context. *The regressively accentuated delay of development* which is not infrequently found in children with attention deficit disorder is also characteristic of Calcium carbonicum. (Concerning details of and Conchae/Calcium carb. consult 6.4.3.6.2.)

In cases of ADD and ADHD, *non-medicinal therapy must* always be considered in a differentiated way. These include:

- special needs education, play and exercise therapy,
- eurythmy therapy and rhythmical massage therapy according to Wegman/Hauschka,
- rhythm as group therapy for pre-school and elementary-school age children,
- craniosacral therapy,
- therapeutic clay modelling (less frequently therapeutic painting, speech formation and music therapy),
- ergotherapy, in connection with breathing therapy exercises,
- therapeutic circus work (the list must remain incomplete here)

These therapies have the advantage that children *acquire new skills* or overcome bodily impediments (through craniosacral therapy and rhythmical massage therapy) so that real steps towards recovery can be made. For this reason these therapy forms should come *before* using stimulants. On the other hand, an already initiated stimulant treatment should not simply be discontinued. In this case the aim must be to introduce supplementary non-medicinal therapy and to reduce or discontinue the use of stimulants afterwards within the measure of what is possible. To begin with, it is particularly important to interrupt stimulant treatment on weekends and during holiday periods. – Depending on the child's age it is also important to involve the child in the assessment of the therapy from the very start. *Many school children can evaluate the effectiveness of the treatment very well themselves.*

In clinical practice, the authors have found that *food supplements* showed a positive effect in many of the affected children, at least subjectively. There are some indications that a dose of magnesium can have a particularly positive effect in cases of restlessness, sleep disorders, tics, and ataxia (in the area of the extremities); the positive effects of taking fatty acids such as Omega 3 and Omega 6 for better functioning of the nervous system, improved attention and concentration have been discussed at length (please also refer to ▸Chap. 4). Finally laboratory tests reveal low to insufficient zinc levels in many patients, which, like any other deficiencies, not only depends on a balanced nutrition, but also on the digestive capacities of each child. The authors noted positive experiences for many children using one supplement: Esprico®, which contains all of the previously mentioned substances (made from fish oil and evening primrose, 2 × 2 capsules or 1 sachet a day).

It is the experience of the authors that stimulants seem to be inevitable in many cases if there is no differentiated handling of both anthroposophic medicine and homoeopathic remedies. Since currently there are only a few systematic reviews based on personal therapeutic experiences, this form of therapy will be the main focus in the following text.

7.5.3.4 Medication for attention deficit and hyperactivity disorder (ADHD)

A constitutional predisposition for hyperactive, impulsive behaviour with attention deficit disorder (ADHD) is clearly referenced to the *masculine gender*, although it does occur on rare occasions in girls too. A family history is not rare (father, male ancestors) and a development of this disorder can often be traced back through the previous generations. Hyperactive behaviour is constitutionally more likely if there is a "short circuit" between environmental stimuli and personal action, a lack of control (and lead) on the part of the head when moving the limbs (the movement coordination of many of these children is not suitable to their age). *Embryologically, it is noteworthy that the regulatory connection between the nervous system and the musculature is not hierarchically created by the nervous system, but is actually due to the fact that the organism (and thus a not explicitly named middle realm between muscle and nerve!) simultaneously brings the structures of the central nervous system and the muscle blasteme to "mate"* [Christ 1990, 859].

The primary effect of nerve cells on muscle cells is *inhibition* (observable in embryos when the nerve fibre reaches the muscle cell and grows into it – the fibrillating movement occurring until then is interrupted for the first time), whereas *movement* represents the original "mode" of every muscle cell. – If one recognizes the central nervous system for what it really is, namely as a *mirroring organ* necessary for guiding the movements of the body, and the limb system for what it actually is, namely as a system which primarily and predominantly develops of its own accord [Christ 1990, 839] and which, together with the digestion and metabolic processes, represents the primary human *will formation organ*, then the *mediation task* becomes clear which human beings are confronted with in their development. The female and male sexes differ most clearly in the areas of body and limb development – but an explanation suggested by brain metabolism (dopamine hypothesis) throws no light on the gender-specific manifestation of hyperactivity (▸Chap. 7.4). – Successful performance of the depicted mediation task is in fact not a process which takes place *within* the nervous system but rather one which depends on the *rhythmic system which mediates between the nervous and the limb systems* and the soul-related processes connected with them (respiration, circulation, vertebral function and craniosacral rhythm) [cf. Pohl 2002, 296f.]. The task is to create one's own personal congruence between movement and consciousness.

7.5.3.4.1 Strengthening the centre – composite aurum medicines for ADHD and ADD

In regard to this task the therapeutic focus lies on the *rhythmic system of the child*. Indeed, the authors along with others (A. Schmidt, U. Momsen i. a.) ascertain that anthroposophic medicaments which contain potentized *gold* are particularly important and effective for children with attentiveness disorder and hyperactivity. They stimulate the inner ability to mediate between the polarity of impulse and perception, will and reflection, Thou and I, and to delay the "onslaught" of sensory impressions, associative thoughts and stimuli for action in such a way that the child can balance and regulate its relationship to itself and the world (formulated as a goal which is to be approached as well and as much as possible).

The following medicaments which play a central role here in the practice of the authors are:

- **Aurum/Stibium/Hyoscyamus pillules** Wala/**Aurum/Hyoscyamus comp. dil.** Weleda
  2–3 × daily 7–12 pillules./3 × daily 10–15 gtt. in the case of:
  - hyperactive-impulsive,
  - simultaneously aggressive,
  - rivalry-prone children who often get embroiled in physical confrontations.

The Vademecum of Anthroposophic Medicines formulates the guiding principle as follows: "Shielding and strengthening the rhythmic system in the case of disordered metabolic impulses from below or, as the case may be, from the physical into the psyche." [Vademecum 2010, 172] It is suitable primarily for impulsive, hyperactive children, but also for children who have primary difficulties in the emotional sphere itself and are prone to rivalry, jealousy and aggression.

This medicinal product is one of the "early therapeutic compounds created on the basis of an anthroposophic view of the human being by the circle of doctors at the Klinisch-Therapeutisches Institut founded by Dr. Ita Wegman" (created in the form used here in 1935); the aim was to create a medicinal product to stimulate the rhythmic system and overcome a "tendency to one-sidedness" in both the nervous and sensory system and the system of metabolism and limbs [Vogel 1994, 171]. Gold, antimony and extracts of henbane are for this purpose jointly potentized to form a new whole. In the process, the gold component (equivalent to a D10 in finished medicinal products) addresses the cardiovascular system, provides spiritual support for wakefulness in everyday consciousness and – as has been shown by a wealth of clinical experience – has a particularly beneficial effect in situations in which the child has too little experience of his father. Antimony (D8) has a structuring effect on metabolic processes (it can, for instance, promote healthy blood coagulation) as well as on the life of the mind (this has also been tried and tested in psychiatry in situations where the conscious mind is flooded in a no-longer-controllable manner by a chaos-inducing mass of intrusive contents of consciousness). In the potency employed (equivalent to a D5), Hyoscyamus (▸Chap. 7.4) works to counteract the manifestation in movement of instinctive impulses and promotes the development of the rhythmic system (cf. both the toxicity and the strictly rhythmic structure of this Solanacea!). – The drug has a mildly anti-depressive component which is very helpful for many of these children. – This therapy stimulates the rhythmic system, and many children and families feel this to be of significant help. At the same time the physician gains time that may be needed to get to know the child and parents better and plan the further therapeutic steps and conversations.

- **Aurum comp. pillules** Wala/**Myrrha comp. D10 (D8–30) dil.** Weleda
  1–3 × daily 5 pillules/5–8 drops (D10)

are more suitable for children with polar-type ADHD (cf. 7.5.3.1):

- Fearful, insecure, emotionally unstable
- Made easily irritable by sensory impressions, sensorily hypersensitive
- Made easily irritable in children's play groups, social change
- Become distraught easily
- Partial learning disability, psychomotorically delayed development (might only affect certain areas with other areas being quite well developed)
- Autistic disorders, predominantly in the sense of a lack of central coherence (conflation of sensory perceptions, comprehension of what is perceived), in regard to understanding what is meant (what can be expressed with gestures as an intended meaning, for example[1])

Responses to administration of this medicament developed by a work group led by the pioneer of anthroposophic special needs education Karl König [highly recommended: Engel, König, Wiedemann 2007 with case histories] in a special needs educational context are often quite clear; the children become more centred, have a better inner stability, the warmth organism is strengthened. ([K. König] repeatedly observed high-fever crises with the onset of medication, and this promoted development). An impressive case history on a prematurely born child (25th gestation week, among other things with a grade III infant respiratory distress syndrome, and a grade II intracerebral haemorrhage) which involved prescribing an increasing and decreasing potency series was published by Hessenbruch [2007]. This case shows how this mutually potentized medicament consisting of gold, olibanum and myrrh can also *preventatively* promote psychomotoric development and the formation of inner coherence in regard to processing sensory perceptions (which is a great problem for children born extremely prematurely) during the first year of life.

Whereas gold unfolds a different effectiveness in regard to hyperexcitability and depressiveness depending on the degree of potentization (cf. ▸Chap. 7.2.3.3), myrrh and frankincense (olibanum), as precious plant resins [Kunz 2009], enhance the gold in its mood-lifting, expanding effect and its constringent, hyperactivity-subduing effect: "Whereas myrrh tends to form a contracted, barren thornbush, frankincense trees have

1 It helps these children a lot if their parents are taught how to acquire an easily comprehensible ("Italian type of") gesture language. For such childen irony is profoundly hurtful and incomprehensible.

the appearance of energetic trees whose branches spread out towards the sky, with the blossoms appearing to create sprays of foam on the periphery. Whereas myrrh, as a tanning essence, has a formative and stabilising effect (for example on sore gums), frankincense, when heated over glowing coals so that it smelts and evaporates, dissipates the soul..." [Sommer 2007]. The manufacture of Myrrha comp. S is described very clearly in an article by W. Engel. [Engel 2007a]

The authors attach central, universal importance to this genuinely anthroposophic remedy for treatment of the group of children characterized above and deem it to be of much wider, more universal application than is described in the original publication by König, Engel and Wiedemann. This publication primarily made reference to psychoses in early childhood, autistic children with severe contact disorder and delayed speech development [cf. commentary by Schmidt, 2007]. Myrrha comp. and Myrrha comp. D8/Belladonna, Radix D10 as cited below do indeed continue to constitute important basic remedies for these children. Their hyperactivity is more the result of an onslaught of sensory perceptions, unprocessed impressions than it is a form of disorganized and rampant vitality urging outwards or upwards. Thus it is often a reaction to stimuli which are still "indigestible" for the child and which cannot be passed through the centre and "forgotten." This remedy can also prove very valuable in cases of attentiveness disorder where no hyperactivity is involved; it strengthens I presence.

The authors have a preference for these pillules (which contain Aurum in D7) in cases where there is no or only moderate hyperactivity, where the indication primarily relates to sensory disorders, and at the beginning of therapy. In cases of more pronounced erethism, Karl König and his colleagues [Engel 2007, 553] recommend higher potentizations of Myrrha comp., descending potencies when the primary aim is to reduce hyperactivity in the limbs and increasing potencies if the primary aim is to strengthen the functions of the senses. In the case of Myrrha comp., D10 is well-suited for treatments that remain at the same potentization level for longer periods of time.

- **Myrrha comp. D8/Belladonna, Radix D10 dil.** Weleda[1]
  1–3 × daily 5–8 drops

This medicament, which additionally contains a medium potentization of Belladonna, is closely related to Myrrha comp. Weleda. Children who benefit from this medicament tend to be more or less sturdy, pasty, have a more pronounced body warmth but also exhibit unbridled impulsivity. It is specifically suitable in cases where attentiveness deficit and impulsivity *are part of a more comprehensive developmental disorder requiring special needs educational treatment*. Specific symptoms which indicate this remedy are:

- speech development disorder (▸Chap. 7.8),
- delay of psychomotoric development,
- emotionally instable frame of mind, difficulties establishing contact with same-aged children,
- *metabolism-accentuated constitution* in the sense of anthroposophic anthropology.

1 The authors wish to thank M. Winkler, the president of the Dutch Anthroposophic Physicians' Association, for valuable reports on positive experiences treating ADHS with this medicament on a wide scale.

The dosages must be carefully individualized; the medicament may not be taken for too long because this might exacerbate the condition.

In alternation with Myrrha comp. D8/Belladonna, Radix D10 dil. a suitable remedy for delayed development in children with a metabolism-accentuated, energetic constitution can be administered, for example **Apis regina comp.** (marked delay in speech development), **Bryophyllum Argento cultum** (hypersensitive, thin-skinned, energetic, agitation in the evening), **Calcium carbonicum LM6–12** (regressive bond with parents, alternation between impulsive-disruptive behaviour towards same-aged children and passive-orally fixated behaviour in the family).

Additional medicaments with potentized gold/vegetabilized gold which can be considered particularly in cases of ADD without hyperactivity and which are characterized in more detail later on are:

- **Neurodoron® (Kalium Phosphoricum comp.) tab.** Weleda **Hypericum Auro cultum D2, Rh D3 dil.** Weleda
  a lack of energy characterizes its indication; in the case of Neurodoron® in combination with iron and calcium phosphate the focus is on controlling the metabolism; in the case of Hypericum Auro cultum the "inner light" of the soul plays a more central role.
- **Aurum/Apis regina comp. pillules** Wala
  3 × daily 5–7 pillules
  can be a helpful remedy particularly for *depressive moods, emotional duress and experiences of loss, developmental crises* (thus also in cases of reactive attentiveness disorders in reaction to separation of parents, for example). When prescribing this remedy the age of the child indicates the choice of remedy: the 9th year of life and the following years [Vademecum 2010, 165].

7.5.3.4.2 Single-substance medicines for children with ADHD and ADD

As *individual remedies* for further *individualization of treatment,* the author's experience has shown the following medicaments to be beneficial most of all. Frequently used potencies are listed; in individual cases a higher or lower potentization might prove effective if the result is unsatisfactory but the remedy is suitable.

Constitutionally effective medicaments can stimulate this process in the child and have a harmonizing influence. In the following a selection of key remedies will be described and depicted briefly in ◘ Tab. 7.3. (In the case of children with partial performance disorders it is impossible to avoid overlapping between the remedies listed below and those named in ▸Chap. 7.5.3.4.)

- **Sulphur D12 pillules** (various manufacturers), **LM6–12 dil.** Arcana 1 × daily beginning with 1 pillules/drop and increasing to 5 pillules/drops daily if possible
  Discontinue use in cases of clear reactions or administer less frequently or in weakened form by dilution in water (▸Chap. 6.4.3.6.2).

Tab. 7.3 Overview of medicinal therapy for attention deficit disorder and hyperactive behaviour.

Sulphur	Dominance of metabolism, egocentricity, curiosity, vitality
Hepar sulfuris	Aggressive, dominant behaviour, fits of rage. High susceptibility to colds and purulent inflammation
Magnesite (Mg carbonicum)	Irritable-aggressive pre-school children, frequent screaming, small and skinny, tendency towards stomach colics, restless sleep especially in infants
Belladonna	Strong consciousness, uncontrolled emotional impulses
Hyoscyamus	Hyperactivity in cases of epilepsy, jealousy, clear emotional disorder
Stramonium	Torn between anxiety and aggression, strong mood swings. Vital metabolism
Veratrum	Hyperexcitability and vegetative instability in regard to circulation and digestion (renal-adrenal-weakness); hyperactivity and intellectual disability, obtrusive
Mercurius	Hard to grasp, restless, hasty in all actions, susceptibility to purulence
Bryophyllum Mercurio cultum	Hard to grasp, restless, has difficulties falling asleep
Bryophyllum Argento cultum	Thin-skinned, effusive tendency, fear of failure with secondary aggression, sleep disorder
Acidum nitricum	Aggressive, antagonistic, deceitful. No moral scruples. Inflammation along border between skin and mucosa
Argentum nitricum	Haste and drivenness, craving for sweets, strong need for movement outdoors
Tarantula	Massive, destructive hyperactivity, untameable desire for movement
Tuberculinum	Insolent, disobedient, provocatively destructive, highly intelligent, artistically gifted, enjoys travelling, susceptibility to allergies of the respiratory and urinary tracts
Medorrhinum	Allergies, susceptibility to infections, passionate extreme behaviour, partial performance disorder
Agaricus	Tics, hyperactivity, slight impairment of CNS
Zincum, Zincum valerianicum	Partial performance disorder, agitation, easily distracted, impairment of CNS

Characteristics of children who benefit from administration of this medicament are:

- male gender
- more or less slender physique, distinctly *poor posture*
- intelligent but lazy; keen on discussion and dispute; gain a lot from instruction even though they talk a lot and make a disinterested impression
- socially egocentric, make hurtful remarks, alienate others by their behaviour while being emotionally naive and gullible (such children are actually not difficult to understand)
- handwriting is practically illegible; written materials are in disarray, have grease spots, etc.; such children are unable (and unwilling) to keep their things in order; many things get ruined (materials are used up at great rate!)
- typically exhibit unbearable behaviour when hungry; condition improves immediately after the child has eaten; also craving for sweets (which decreases considerably after medicament is taken)
- tendency towards hypoglycaemic phases in second septennial with clear aggravation of behavioural problems in late morning (at around 11 O'clock)

The history often shows an *abundance of allergies* and a *subsiding respiratory infection previously treated with antibiotics*; one should also watch out for *imbalance of enteric flora* (Candidiasis!). Such children benefit a lot from symbiosis control and adjustment of diet accordingly. A substantial breakfast – ideally on the basis of oats – has a positive effect not only on this constitution. The medicament develops a regulative effect on metabolic dynamics which essentially shows a disposition towards 'running down' the centre through an overabundance of energy. "Sul-fur" means "sun-carrier;" is yellow and is a completely combustible mineral. Thus in such sun children every structure is in danger of dissolving in a dynamic of heat. Potentized sulphur can help the light shine in such children.

- **Hepar Sulfuris LM6, 12 dil.** Arcana
  daily 3–5 drops in the morning

In accordance with the inner tension of the (spontaneously degrading) primary substance, "liver of lime," which is made of lime and sulphur synthesized under heat (a compound made of two polar primary substances), this medicament is suitable for children with

- a high degree of inner tension (primarily boys);
- desire to dominate, aggressivity, bursts of rage;
- high susceptibility to catching colds, intolerance of cold, sleep closely wrapped up in blankets (in contrast to sulphur);
- susceptibility to purulent inflammations of the skin, in the nose and sinuses, the tonsils and the bronchia.
- It is the key remedy in cases of amalgam contamination (D6).
- Constitutional weakness of the centre, lack of sustained warmth, threat of a breakdown into polarities characterize the constitution of such children.

- **Magnesite D6 trit.** Weleda, **D12–20 dil.** Apotheke an der Weleda
  3 × daily 1 saltsp., 1 × daily in the evening 3–5 drops

7

is an important constitutionally effective medicament especially for children *of kindergarten and preschool age*. Like Sulphur it primarily stimulates the life organization, the etheric body of the child. Magnesite is also preferentially suitable for boys. – Such children are strong-willed while at the same time stand out for *bodily and emotional assimilation problems*. The life organization of such children appears to be inhibited and insufficiently developed in its coherence; weak trophics can manifest itself in dry skin, for example [cf. Vademecum 2010, 557]. In this context one might mention that magnesium is of decisive importance for assimilation of sunlight in living organisms (chlorophyll), thus constituting an element which is central to the formation of self-reliant life organization, i. e. the capacity for growth and assimilation. Key symptoms for use of this medicament are:

- *short stature,* skinniness (in particular in the first septennial),
- inability to eat anything in the morning, not until 9 or 10 o'clock,
- dislike of most vegetables (green vegetables!),
- crabby, unruly, irritable, hypersensitive,
- combative, scream a lot: "It is a kind of rehearsed yelling…the appearance of the physician triggers wild, fearful screaming which cannot be allayed." [Stübler 1969]
- susceptibility to *stomach colics*, sour smelling diarrhoea (cf. ▸Chap. 4.4.4),
- often restless sleep, scream a lot at night as well as during infancy, tendency towards growth pains.

Such children often suffer from a frequency of *family quarrels*. In cases of *school-age girls* who are emotionally afflicted by distress in the family and are possibly afflicted with allergies and weak digestion, **Magnesium chloratum (muriaticum) LM6** can be helpful.

- **Belladonna Rh D20 dil.** Weleda
  1 × daily 5 drops

This medicament, like Hyoscyamus and Stramonium, is one of the remedies also indicated for aggressive behaviour disorders (cf. ▸Chap. 7.4). In connection with ADHD the following traits are characteristic:

- *early awakening of consciousness*, listens during consultation with the physician, it is possible to converse with the child – intelligent children,
- the child becomes aware of his inclination towards lack of self-control early on but without acquiring the ability to take control as a result,
- the child has an inclination towards fits of rage (such children suddenly develop high fever in cases of acute infection!!) accompanied by biting (in particular small children), hitting and also autoaggressive actions – such children often come down with illnesses very suddenly; pain often takes the form of acute colics,
- such children hate to be touched, particularly on the head; they cannot tolerate any kind of poultice, compress or anything else which is confining,
- they develop fear of storms, dogs (– a fear of being attacked the way they attack others!), water and the dark.

As much as such children reject physical affection, poultices, loving attention etc. *during the day* it is not uncommon for them to climb into the bed of their parents after waking up in a sweat one to two hours after falling asleep; when the life organization expands upwards during sleep and the soul aspect disengages, a crisis occurs resulting in a need for support.

The soul aspect of such children does not connect harmoniously with the child's own body and his surroundings but rather appears like a demon which attacks suddenly, vehemently and in ambush-style (in accordance with the poisoning process of Belladonna); such children are carried off by it without being able to guide the process. Belladonna is an important, constitutionally effective remedy in such cases. – It is a mistake to prescribe Belladonna only in cases of acute disease.

- **Stramonium D12 pillules** (various manufacturers)
  daily 1–2 × 5 pillules

What is characteristic for the indication of this medicament can be observed in the very first encounter with the child (as follows):

- In the consulting room the child usually behaves in a conformist way; *eye contact, i. e., direct encounter is avoided*, the child is evasive, apparently insecure and anxious; it might *stutter*; acute illness can be severe, leading to spasms of the respiratory tract.
- There are reports of anxiety manifesting itself at home in the evening (most of all, the need for a source of light while falling asleep and the fear of being alone are conspicuous).
- In contrast to this, *sudden, abrupt* aggressivity can erupt which, like Belladonna, can be quite severe – the child is relatively unaware of this, however, with its conforming side having no awareness of the unrestrained aggressive side. A split reminiscent of that characterizing Dr. Jekill and Mr. Hyde makes itself apparent; the nerve-sense system and the metabolic-limb system *dissociate.*
- Attention is impaired to a much higher degree than is the case with Belladonna.

In this quite difficult situation, Stramonium is a very effective remedy. Here the hyperactivity corresponds to an individual, emotionally unpenetrated part of the metabolic-limb organization of the "lower human being." A complementary relationship to Sulphur exists.

In cases of ADHD, the authors use *Hyoscyamus* essentially as a component of the compound Aurum/Stibium/Hyoscyamus elucidated at the beginning of this chapter; this separate remedy (Rh D6 dil. Weleda) plays a special role for *children with epilepsy who develop symptoms reminiscent of ADHD* (cf. ▸Chap. 8.1). In a number of cases the combination of Hyoscyamus D6 and Stramonium D12 has been successful as well, administered during and also after seizures stopped.

- **Veratrum e rad. D12–30 pillules** Wala
  1 × daily 5 pillules or individual dosages.

This is another important individual remedy which is extracted from an indigenous poisonous plant. The striking feature of this Liliacee is that the blossom transforms from a dingy white into a shade of green and is barely distinguishable from the foliage (the blossoms are relatively inconspicuous), whereas the, for a member of the lily family, strong root is permeated with a strong poisonous process which can induce a collapse of the human metabolism.

In patients one observes a profound weakness of the rhythmic system and metabolic organization (cf. the *hypotonic-vegetatively instable* type). They do not feel stably anchored in their own body, their circulation and their metabolism and they try to compensate for this by constant driveness and limb movement. It is striking that such children exhibit an exuberant, excessive gesture of affection in that they

- have the desire to grasp, touch, embrace and kiss everything,
- have an inward feeling of nervousness and drivenness,
- have a strong preference for eating *sour things* (which stimulate soul activity in the digestive process),
- have a strong urge to move but exhibit a disposition towards cool extremities and also peripheral cyanosis,
- like to eat cold things ("The symptom of cold is characteristic for all effects of Veratrum," says J. T. Kent at the beginning of his description),
- suffer from severe stomach colics, vomiting and diarrhoea and in the case of girls dysmenorrhoea – always accompanied by weak circulation and cold – which make clear that the organization of the soul aspect, the astral body, does not "feel at home" in this area, not being able to connect in a positive manner with the metabolic-limb organization. The remedy can be very valuable for hyperactive, intellectually disabled children. One strange, characteristic symptom can be observed: when excited such children have the tendency to *spit on others*. This is a figurative expression of the aforementioned strong oral fixation coupled with a reduced capacity for articulation on the part of such children.

- When treating such children, external application should focus particularly on the kidneys; kidney rhythmical Einreibung using
- **Copper ointment red** Wala or **Cuprum met. 0.4 % ointment** Weleda in the evening,
- is recommended to promote relaxation and a more harmonious interplay of body and soul in the circulation and the metabolism.
- In cases of acute shock or a history thereof, rhythmical Einreibung of the kidneys or upper abdomen with
- **Oxalis 30 % ointment** Weleda is recommended [Vademecum 2010, 638f. with casuistics].

As metallic remedies for treating ADHD the following are first line recommendations:

- **Mercurius vivus/solubilis D12 trit.** Weleda/**pillules** DHU:
  daily 1–2 × 1 saltsp./5 pillules, possible higher potentization as well.

Potentized mercury is helpful for children with pronounced hyperactivity who

- exhibit incomprehensible behaviour,
- *avoid all rules,* always "wiggling through,"
- are susceptible to purulent inflammation,
- exhibit pronounced hyperactivity.

Here one sometimes gains the impression that the rhythmic system has taken on a life of its own with the organism as a whole failing to develop force. The calming, guiding function of the nerve-sense system does not take hold; *everything happens too fast*, including speech (compare R. Steiner's characterization in the course on eurythmy therapy [1981,

16]). At night incomplete disengagement of the soul aspect from the body manifests itself in the form of sweating; the anabolic processes of the nerve-sense system remain incomplete as well, which leads to *chronic absent-mindedness.*

Where difficulties falling asleep – or compulsive fears – are observed as well, one might consider administering a vegetabilized form of mercury alternatively or supplementarily:

- **Bryophyllum Mercurio cultum D2** or **Rh D3 dil.** Weleda
  2 × daily 7–10 drops
- **Bryophyllum Argento cultum D2, Rh D3 dil.** Weleda
  2–3 × 5–7 drops (D2)/2–3 × 10–15 drops (Rh D3)

is a basic remedy for hyperactive children with attention deficit who have an hysterical and at the same time metabolically accentuated, hypersensitive constitution.

Conspicuous characteristics of such children can be [Vademecum 2010, 241]:

- thin skin, thin hair, hypersensitivity to pain,
- vital constitution in regard to metabolism
- inclination to "effusiveness": sweat on hands and feet, body odour,
- enuresis nocturna
- very dependent on their environment in terms of behaviour; quick to lose their own thread,
- inclination towards sleep disorders at night, exceptional thirst at night (cf. ▸Chap. 7.1.5.3), moon-dependent
- fear of failure, inhibition of fear of failure, sudden panic attacks.

The remedy can have a positive constitutional influence on the "thin-skinned" nature of such children. The "overly childlike" behaviour and nature of these children (and with it an essentially positive prognosis) constitutes an indication for prescription of silver salts. Children who require this medicament often exhibit quite vital metabolic activity and accordingly pronounced impulsivity but it is not very individualized or penetrated by the soul aspect, thus leading a life of its own. The time-tested supplement (Wispler) – ▸Chap. 7.5.3.2 – is:

- **Organum quadruplex amp.** Wala
  1–3 × weekly 1 drinking ampoule

The ratio here aims towards allowing the remedy to stimulate the "influence of protein," the intervention of the higher members in the metabolism so as to help the child guide his impulsive life of the will more successfully.

Nitric acid is one of the most aggressive, oxydating acids which even affects silver, a precious metal, having the capacity to turn it into a salt, silver nitrate (in combination with hydrochloric acid, as "aqua regia," silver nitrate can even attack gold; cf. Aurum muriaticum). Potentized nitric acid,

- **Acidum nitricum C30–200 pillules, LM6–18 dil.** (diverse manufacturers)
  in individual dosages (pillules), daily – 3 × weekly 3–5 drops

is an important remedy for children who

- are principally and *unrelentingly antagonistic*, immune to rules, unwilling to integrate themselves into the social order,
- attempt to set the tone,
- evade all institutional frameworks and find ways of missing school whenever they can (during holidays they are more agreeable),
- exhibit social behaviour which is difficult and deceitful and most of all blatantly aggressive[1] – the aggressive nature of acid is called to mind here!
- are fascinated by fire (acids, as hydrogen donors, also come to mind here) – this holds for Hepar sulfuris as well, which is also indicated for children with a high potential for aggression,
- have one-sided food preferences: extremely fatty, sweet, salty, spicy foods (preference for extremes),
- have bodily susceptibility to inflammations, fissures along the skin-mucosa boundaries, in particular in the mouth and the anus.
- (This remedy is a major, highly effective remedy for treatment of anal fissures even in gentle, amiable individuals. The "anal" nature of this symptom corresponds to the *significance of power* for such children. Their bodily pathology is focused on the transition from the inside to the outside. Problems occur where the child should let go of the inside and subject himself to external laws – in the intestine the opposite occurs; the external world is robbed of its own nature and subjected to the body's own laws completely. The rhythm of defecation, as a rhythm of keeping and letting go, is sometimes painfully disturbed.

For treating this, potentized silver nitrate

- **Argentum nitricum LM12 dil.** Arcana
  daily 5 drops

is indicated when the focus is on the nerve-sense-system and this system does not develop any calming and regulating effect on the organism itself, generating *undirected catabolic tension* instead. In such cases one observes that:

- the child always feels rushed and restless,
- it loves exercise in the fresh air, external cooling, sports
- it suffers from nervous, strained anticipation, which can also cause diarrhoea,
- it attempts to achieve a balance by eating sugary and salty foods but this only exacerbates the nervousness even more (fluctuating blood sugar level).
- emotionally such children are much more amiable than are those who correspond to the Acidum-nitricum picture.

In cases of very severe and destructive forms of hyperactive behaviour one might consider

- **Tarantula hispanica LM12 dil.** Arcana, **C12–200 pillules** (various manufacturers)
  daily 5 drops or individual dosages.

1 "He can't be a Nitricum acidum case; for that he is too nice!" (Morrison [1995,479])

This homoeopathic medicament is extracted from the Spanish tarantula, a poisonous spider; it has an excitatory effect on the rhythmic system and is suitable for girls and boys with pronounced constitutional ADHD. Such children have a sturdy appearance, have energy in abundance and can ignore inner and outer restraints with self-abandonment, this being a trait which already exhibits itself clearly in the consulting room:

- they like to dance and climb,
- they sometimes behave in a *deceitful* and also mendacious manner, stealing and destroying objects,
- they always demand attention,
- rebukes are clearly useless and leave no impression on the child,
- notably, some are afraid of spiders or insects,
- stuttering and asthma can occur.
- here a clear dominance of the metabolic-limb system can be observed whereas the rhythmic system shows clear weaknesses. This medicament is also suitable for children with ADHD *and* asthma bronchiale, just like Hepar Sulfuris, for example, and the following homoeopathic nosode:

- **Tuberculinum Koch (alt) LM6–12 dil.** Arcana, **C30–200 pillules**
  daily 3–5 drops or individual dosages.

It is indispensible for treatment of hyperactive children. Physically one frequently observes (cf. ▸Chap. 5) a *chronic vulnerability of the respiratory tract*, most of all in the tympanum and the lungs (susceptibility to pneumonia, asthma bronchiale); concerning the behaviour of such children key traits are:

- *provocative destructiveness*: no valuable object is safe from such children; they can unscrupulously smash a beautiful vase to pieces before the very eyes of the owner, ruin the toy of a friend or even their own favourite play things in order to achieve the desired effect,
- punishments have absolutely no effect,
- they exhibit a high intelligence, frequently coupled with an artistic disposition,
- they cannot stay in the same place for very long; they love to travel,
- they dominate their family with their behaviour,
- food and lack of appetite are instruments of power for them [Stübler 1969].
- Lack of appetite is constitutionally determined and corresponds to a susceptibility to chronic-inflammatory infections of the lungs and respiratory tract (cf. ▸Chap. 6.5). For such children this also becomes an instrument of power vis-a-vis anxious, weak mothers. Supplementary medicaments for this constitutional lack of appetite are **Abrotanum Urtinktur – D6** Apotheke an der Weleda and **Rose iron/Graphite pillules** Wala, which can both supplement treatment with Tuberculinum. As a mild, finely differentiated bitter plant, Abrotanum has a greater effect on the digestive system whereas Rose iron/Graphite has a greater effect on chronic susceptibility to inflammation of the lungs (cf. ▸Chap. 6.4.3.6.2).

In comparison to children for whom Tarantula hisp. is well-suited, these children make a more adept, controlled, deliberate impression; they can deceive adults whereas the tarantula typically succumbs to its own impulses in an unconcerned fashion. As a nosode,

- **Medorrhinum LM6–12, C30–200 pillules**
  daily 3–5 drops or individual dosages.

corresponds to the condition of *an unregulated dynamic of the metabolic life, of unconscious impulses of the will, which are acted out in an extreme fashion.* The extreme disorder of the metabolic life and the immune system has an affinity to Sulphur. Such children are conspicuous very early on [cf. Herscu 1993, 134–189; Gnaiger 2002; Grandgeorge 2004, 125]. They:

- sometimes appear very energetic and passionate in their behaviour;
- experience restlessness which makes them inclined to hit and perform other aggressive and autoaggressive actions (in the case of small children nail biting, in the case of adolescents possibly self-induced cuts with razor blades!);
- exhibit an *extremely fluctuating emotional picture*; injure those they love; lapse into shy-depressive-introverted states but only to appear devilish again,
- have a susceptibility to recurrent inflammations of all orifices from birth on and suffer from unusually *persistent nappy (diaper) rash,*
- have a very characteristic preference for sleeping in the *knee-elbow position* as infants; love to sleep on their stomach,
- are highly susceptible to allergies, which improve notably by the sea,
- exhibit early disorders in their motor and cognitive development in the sense of delayed development, "minimal cerebral dysfunctions" of memory and the ability to concentrate,
- have difficulties learning how to read and write.

- **Agaricus musc. D10–30 dil.** Apotheke an der Weleda/pillules (various manufacturers)
  1 × daily 5 drops/pillules or individual dosages.

is extracted from the fly amanita, which is used as an intoxicating drug in many places. Here ADHD-similar traits manifest themselves. As a potentized remedy Agaricus can be considered especially in cases of

- tics (cf. ▸Chap. 7.9): these are sometimes accompanied by ADHD but sometimes also result from stimulants therapy,
- reckless, impulsive-volatile but in principle benevolent behaviour,
- such children have the desire to do good,
- during fits of rage they sometimes develop enormous powers.

The case history sometimes shows *pre-existing defects of the nervous system* (in such cases Agaricus played a major therapeutic role for R. Steiner); such children also give the clinical impression of having a *neurological inhibition deficit.*

- **Zincum met. praep. D10–20 dil.** Apotheke an der Weleda
  daily 5 drops in the afternoon – evening.
- **Zincum valerianicum D6(–30) dil.** Apotheke an der Weleda

Possibly also external application in the form of

- **Zincum met. 0.1% ungt.** Apotheke an der Weleda on the forehead in the morning (generally effective for concentration disorders in school-age children!)

Potentized zinc and Zincum valerianicum play a therapeutic role primarily when *the formation of the nervous system has been compromised, for example by extremely premature birth or convulsion disorder* and partial performance disorders are clearly pronounced (cf. 7.5.3.1)

Such children:

- are very easily distractible, fidgety and restless,
- have a tendency to spasms and at night to head-nodding,
- have a *weak memory* and unsure judgment, which makes them appear fearful,
- often also exhibit psychomotoric retardation,
- experience periods of hyperexcitability alternating with stupurous inactivity,
- often make mistakes when speaking and writing,
- exhibit restless-legs-syndrome (Zincum valerianicum D6 is indicated here), in particular in the evening while lying in bed.

Potentized phosphorus is *not* used by the authors for children with pronounced hyperactivity since this remedy often has a highly exacerbating effect on ADD + H; in cases where attention deficit without hyperactivity prevails (see below) this is not the case.

For hyperactive children it is generally helpful to give them the following in the evening before they go to sleep:

- A footbath with one capful **Lavender bath milk** Weleda

The child sits in the warm bathroom, if possible alone with one parent, on a warm surface. The child's feet are immersed halfway up the calves in water at body temperature with legs covered for 10 minutes. Such baths have a very relaxing effect and are sleep-inducive, giving the child a positive feeling of acceptance, love and care at night which allows him to forget worries and frustrating experiences.

7.5.3.5 Eurythmy therapy for children with attention-deficit disorders with hyperactivity

It is striking that hyperactive children *like to do eurythmy therapy exercises* and often experience these as helpful. In Waldorf schools it is possible to receive eurythmy therapy during the school day. Eurythmy therapy is preferably done in the middle of the morning, *initially preferably daily*, and less frequently later. For children who do not attend Waldorf School, efforts should be made to have the child practicing at home *every day of the week*. To achieve therapeutic effects, daily practice is as important as it is for learning a musical instrument. eurythmy therapy is a **centrally acting instrument** of self-help for children with ADHD! Prior to initiating therapy, careful consultation between physician and therapist is important. The therapist should radiate confidence, joy of movement and also some willingness to experiment. The authors have had very good experience with male eurythmy therapists in this indication.

Hyperactive children often appear to be without "sheathing"; they seem exposed to their environment without the ability to inwardly come to rest and feel comfortable within themselves. A first step in this direction can be achieved by stimulating the rhythmic system with the *contraction and expansion exercises*. The "U" and the "A" can be added as basic *vocal exercises*. The "U" can first be done up "to the stars", and then come back down to approximately heart-level, from where the "A" can radiate forwards and upwards: feelings thereby become inwardly lighter and more luminous; the "A" promotes the connection of the soul with the body, the internalization of the soul-spiritual individuality.

The first eurythmy therapy exercise ever described by R. Steiner refers to children who become "increasingly fidgety" until the teacher does not know how to deal with them anymore [Steiner 1981, 16]. Here Steiner recommends a specially performed "A"-exercise, the so-called "Fidget-Iamb" (Zappel-Jambus) [cf. Steiner, l. c.]. – *Consonantally the* "B" conveys boundary and containment, control of nervousness and motor agitation. For the patient it can be helpful to imagine being surrounded by a "blue armour." The "B" can be reinforced by continuing with a "P;" another supplement which plays a central role in cases of aggressive, injurious behaviour is "S."

A sound sequence suitable for children with distinctively hyperkinetic behaviour is "M-N-B-P-A-U."

It is important and has proved beneficial to offer eurythmy therapy to the *parents* as well. It has been shown that this makes it easier for parents to maintain their composure towards such children and avoid becoming the uncontrolled image of their "little tyrants." Among the exercises suitable for this are "I steadfastly place myself in my existence" („Standhaft stelle ich mich ins Dasein") and "I think speech" („Ich denke die Rede"). These must be carefully rehearsed together with a trained eurythmy therapist and performed daily. This only takes a few minutes time and the effectiveness of doing these exercises is experienced immediately; it radiates into family life as well.

7.5.3.6 Medication for attention and concentration disorders without hyperactivity (ADD), diminished performance and learning difficulties

7.5.3.6.1 Definition and basic treatment

In this section the authors will compile various indications which are often difficult to distinguish in practice. – In the simple notion of ADD without hyperactivity we find *an overlapping of brain function disorders in early childhood, specific learning disorders and attention deficit disorders in the narrower sense of the word*. Diagnostically the concept is inadequate and requires individual concretization. Regarding the ratio of boys to girls, varying figures are cited but in practice both genders are affected to the same degree – in stark contrast to hyperkinetic syndrome. The roots of attention and concentration deficit can lie in

- *constitutionally* delayed development,
- *seasonally* declining concentration in connection with light deficiency,
- disorders of the senses and the nervous system (classic "partial performance disorders" or learning disabilities),
- drive disorders, disorders in the life of the will,
- *excessive strain* caused by school or the family situation (external misjudgement of developmental needs of the child), e. g. premature school enrollment

and in all significant aspects of differential diagnosis listed in ▸Chap. 7.5.2. What matters here is whether the abnormality is persistent rather than occurring reactively. Excessive strain at school can manifest itself relatively acutely after a change of school, for example. And a severe loss such as the death of a parent or divorce of the parents can induce depressive "ADD."

Children born prematurely, before the 32nd week of pregnancy, often manifest a picture of inconsistent performance of the nerve-sense system which defies systematic classification; they have manifold difficulties integrating and processing perceptions but they also often exhibit a shortened attention span in terms of their metabolism (cf. ▸Chap. 7.5.3.1, ▸Chap. 2.3.2.1).

In the following, therapy options *involving anthroposophic and homoeopathic medicaments* which are in part little known will be depicted in detail; otherwise it must suffice to make reference to relevant publications.

As basic therapy for children who suffer from attention and concentration disorders, the anthroposophic compound developed by K. Magerstädt is suitable:

- **Neurodoron®** (Kalium Phosphoricum comp.) tab. Weleda:
  in the morning 1–2 tablets, at midday 1 tablet before lunch.

The phosphorus potassium in this compound shows an effect relationship to the liver-gall system; in the morning it opens up the metabolism for the catabolic processes (connected to phosphates) necessary for the activity of consciousness, for the "inner formation of light".

This medicament is indicated for all children who

- exhibit a "*lack of energy*" in regard to attention and thought processes and who are quickly exhausted by mental activity and "tune out,"
- are not sufficiently awake in the morning,
- appear to be *exhausted* in encounters with the physician due to persistent problems,
- develop *headaches* and *thinking barriers* during relatively long periods of mental exertion.
- show symptoms especially during spurts of growth, which are associated with reduced ability to concentrate and circulatory problems

Like Aurum/Stibium/Hyoscyamus it contains Aurum met. praep. D10, thus unfolding a mild anti-depressant and energizing effect (see above) and it contains a deeply potentized iron-quartz preparation (corresponding to Bidor® by Weleda) which stimulates incorporation of iron into digestion and metabolism, thus having an indirect energizing effect. – The medicament has a broad effect, is reliable and is excellently suited as an *initial medicament* for treatment. It is also specifically indicated when the *father is felt to be missing*.

For some of these children a supplementary effect is provided by the *organ preparation*

- **Glandulae suprarenalis comp. pillules** Wala in the morning and at midday 5–10 pillules.

This medicament primarily stimulates the adrenal function and the day phase of liver metabolism (compare children with vegetative instability and circulation hypotony) and is suitable for initial treatment as well.

A general therapy option for children with simple ADD without hyperactivity is deep potencies of Coffea, a plant that itself in caffeine synthesizes a substance with stimulating effect.

- **Coffea D3 or D4 dil.** (diverse manufacturers)
  daily in the morning and at midday/in the afternoon 2 × 5–10 drops

can lead to clear improvement of attention and concentration in such children without them manifesting the undesired medication effects sometimes caused by substantial administration of stimulants. This treatment is also based on a stimulating, non-substitutive-substantial principle of application.

If there is a history of *disorders of the nervous system* (for example after brain haemorrhage, epilepsy in early childhood, etc.) with partial performance disorders lying behind the ADD symptomology, then the comprehensive effect which Arnica has on the nervous system can be generally beneficial, most of all applied as an **oil dispersion bath according to Junge** (www.jungebad.com)

- **Arnica e flor W 5 % Oleum Wala:** 3–5 ml/full bath

(cf. ▸Chap. 2). For this indication, internal use aimed at stimulating a further maturation of the nervous system is most effective using potentized dosages of

- **Arnica e pl. tota D10–30 pillules** Wala
  daily 5–2 × weekly 5 pillules in the morning,
- **Hypophysis/Stannum pillules** Wala
  daily 5 pillules in the morning,
- **Amnion Gl. D30 amp.** Wala
  daily 0.5 ml – 2 × weekly 1 ml in the evening.

If such children appear to be "too weak to think by themselves" and process what they perceive, Arnica can be replaced by

- **Calcium silicicum comp. D6 dil.** Apotheke an der Weleda
  3 × daily 5 drops,

a mineral compound which also contains elements of Arnica, reinforces the effect of Arnica and allows it to have a longer-lasting effect.

7.5.3.6.2 Individually indicated medicines for attention deficit disorders (ADD), diminished performance and learning difficulties

- **Helleborus niger[1] D6–12 pillules/amp.** Wala, **LM6 dil.** Arcana
  daily 5 drops or 1–2 × daily 5 pillules

is a medicament specifically used to treat ADD [Soldner 2010, Ziller 2005]. It is noteworthy that the Christmas rose, which blossoms *in winter*, forms high concentrations of beta-ecdyson in its roots, this being a substance which plays a role as a *metamorphosis inductor* in ensouled organisms (in hormonally effective, fine concentrations), for example for the metamorphosis from caterpillar to butterfly. Helleborus niger is indicated *if the*

1 Special Issue 6/2010 of the journal "Der Merkurstab," which is dedicated entirely to Helleborus niger (including a pediatric contribution with case studies provided by the author) can help give you a comprehensive picture of this remedy which is central to treatment of attention deficit and concentration disorders.

nervous system has not developed as an instrument of consciousness to a sufficient degree (disorder in organ development and organ metamorphosis):

- Such children appear absent-minded, "as if they were in outer space," but some also manifest emotional hyperexcitability, quickly losing control (cf. ▸Chap. 7.5.3.1).
- The remedy is suitable (compare opium) for treatment after early shock experiences which the child is often incapable of remembering.
- During the winter in particular a (seasonal) depressive disorder might manifest itself with symptoms being exacerbated from the pre-Christmas season until February (the blossoming period of the Christmas rose!) and improving clearly from April on
- *Sensory perceptions are insufficiently processed* (central sensory processing disorders)
- Intelligence can be but is not necessarily impaired, also *as a result of inflammatory and traumatic diseases of the CNS.*
- There is no hyperactivity but symptoms are exacerbated by anticipatory tension (for example exam anxiety).
- The child's memory performance is weak; such children find it difficult to commit things to memory.

This picture can be contrasted with the following type of child:

- *intellectually bright* but with a more or less
- frail and nimble disposition and a sanguine temperament
- and *an empathic* nature (even with over keen senses), often
- artistically gifted, at the same time easily distractible, with a sense for beauty, images, colours (such children often have beautiful eyes themselves). They sometimes have trouble grasping mathematical tasks, for example, which have little appeal and enticement for their soul. Their soul life is strongly guided by feeling experiences
- develop attention and concentration problems primarily in the *dark season*
- more susceptible to infections during this period, especially in the respiratory tract
- they are slender and often grow tall quickly. The well-known disposition towards nose bleeding and bruising shows symbolically the tendency of such patients to flow out in the mid-rhythmic system and to be touched by their surroundings.
- Physically they are on the one hand conspicuously *ticklish and sensitive to touch* but on the other hand they love being massaged and enjoy cuddling with the parent of the opposite sex; during adolescence they develop quite lively sexuality, which is also an expression of their constant need for contact (thus Acidum phosphoricum, phosphorus ash, is a major medicament for lovesickness)
- in groups they are initially shy but then enjoy being the centre of attention, which they achieve playfully and theatrically, not by pure force. *Emotional contact plays a major role for phosphorus.*
- They love putting on a show, at the doctor's office as well, developing quite a bit of charisma in doing so[1]. They feel like something special (and every human being is indeed, in his or her ensouled and enspirited individuality, something special!). In accordance with this they are ambitious and wish to do well at school.
- On the other hand they sometimes quickly develop *vivid fears*; the dark, storms, being alone make them afraid and during adolescence fears of death can occur, usually

1 J.W. von Goethe combines many traits of phosphorus.

during the phase of detachment from the family, with whom they feel a lively sense of connectedness [Hee, Förster 2008, 131–135]

- **Phosphorus LM6 dil.** Arcana/**D8–12 dil.** Weleda/**C30 pillules**
  in the morning starting with 1–2 drops daily and increasing to 5 drops daily if no agitation sets in. Higher potencies in individual dosages

is a medicament with very strong constitutional effect. Phosphorus gives such children more presence of mind and susceptibility to infections decreases. This treatment can be supplemented by rhythmical Einreibungen on the back or oil dispersion baths using Hypericum oil in the evening during the dark season.

Exacerbation during the dark season is a key symptom which plays a major role not only for homoeopathic, but also for phytotherapeutic and anthroposophic selection of medication. Sunlight quite clearly has an activating effect on the sensory life of the child; it is well-known that lack of sunlight – most clearly observed in hibernation – can induce emotional and mental activity to disengage from its bodily anchorage and the regulation of metabolism and motion. This is also well-known from the picture of seasonal depression (which is particularly typical for girls and women) (cf. ▸Chap. 3.2). "Sadness" is an emotional symptom found with significant frequency in children with ADD and ADHD; it should not be interpreted as only being reactive. Apart from encouraging activities outdoors, which improves any form of attention disorder, medicinal therapy can play a crucial role here. A key medicinal plant in this context is Hypericum perforatum, St John's wort, whose phytotherapeutic effect on children with depression and vegetative complaints is proven [Hübner and Kirste 2001]. St John's wort blossoms in mid-summer; its red oil shows a photosensitizing effect (in this context, Hypericum oil is well-suited for oil dispersion baths and rhythmical Einreibungen in the winter half year). Hypericum can be viewed as "*herbal phosphorus.*"

In cases of

- depressive behavioural disorders,
- attention deficit and decline of school performance in late autumn and the Christmas season
- but also constitutionally for the type of children with attention deficit and weakness of the nerve-sense system as described (▸Chap. 7.5.3.1)

in particular light-rhythmicized anthroposophic Hypericum preparations as deep potencies.

The authors have found the following to be beneficial:

- **Hypericum Auro cultum D2, Rh D3 dil.** Weleda
  3 × 10–15 drops Rh D3 (alcohol-free), 3 × 7–12 drops D2

It can be used quite universally. In a very subtle way it promotes a gold effectivity potentized by the plant itself, thus also enhancing stabilization of the child's sense of self-worth and its emotional presence. The rhythmic system, the capacity for centering, is reinforced. If the effect proves insufficient D2 can be prescribed (contains alcohol); another very beneficial effect can be obtained using a preparation by Wala treated with rhythmic light and warmth.

- **Hypericum ex herba D2 pillules** Wala
  2–3 × 5–10 pillules daily.

It is almost always possible to use these preparations to achieve what phytotherapeutic ones do; on the other hand they are sometimes tolerated better than phytotherapeutic medicaments and show a considerably more sustainable effect.

Another very effective medicament is

- **Hypericum Urtinktur** Ceres
  1–3 × 2–5 drops diluted in water, only increase dosages very gradually! Determine optimal individual effect!

Especially amongst girls a certain type of child with a slightly phlegmatic disposition can be observed, who goes into *"hibernation mode"* during the cold season. These children also tend to have *seasonally reinforced attention and concentration issues through the lack of light.* – They prefer sitting in front of the TV-set and eating, and they enjoy the bodily movement in the water, which gives them buoyancy (*they love visits to the public pool*); all in all they exhibit a rather slow, but steady development. Given the contemporary school conditions, these children may stand out, especially by

- being mentally absent and dreaming,
- forgetting homework, not comprehending or noting given tasks,
- appearing heavy and sluggish in their movements,
- requiring lots of time for each task, having problems with getting started.

In the warm seasons they are clearly more active and more in the open air, and they develop more intellectual activity and flexibility. They feel right at home on the beaches of the Adriatic or in Spain during summertime. Often, one of the parents remembers having similar tendencies or still exhibits a certain sluggishness and phlegmatic temperament. Nevertheless, the continuity of their development (their health!) is always apparent in these children; their problem consists in the adaptation to their environment and certain seasonal conditions. The etheric body, the life organization of these children is soundly developed, whereas their soul-spiritual part is slowly, but mostly continuously, "*taking hold*" of the body (a process assisted by the sun). In wintertime they often develop catarrhs, which is more a testimony to the overpowering watery-vitality than a weakness of any real concern.

The development of those who grow up as immigrant children with mothers who do not speak the language of their new environment well and timidly withdraw into the family circle can be critically impaired. Timely intervention designed to break through the regressive vicious circle can be necessary in order to prevent severe delay in development.

An effective medicament for treating such conditions is

- **Calcium carbonicum LM6 dil.** Arcana: 1–3 (!) x daily 5 drops

As an indication for this medicament, which is important and effective for treating children with attention deficit Frei [2005] emphasizes:

- hypersensitivity to light exacerbated by *strained vision*. Such children (and often their mothers as well) attempt to "close their eyes" to external demands and challenging situations (like oysters, whose organs of perception regress in the course of their life) – they *do not want to look at things*!

- hypersensitivity to alien noise and smells.
- pronounced exacerbation, *cramps and exhaustion while writing.*
- reduced sense of taste, "always adds seasoning to foods at the table."

Behaviour towards warmth must be observed in a differentiated manner. Often such children are slightly overweight and *they quickly break into a sweat on exertion* with there being reports of such children "needing to uncover themselves" and quickly feeling "too hot." On the other hand such children like a warm and cosy atmosphere and they dress more warmly than do children with a Sulphur constitution, for example. This corresponds to their love of southern climes and sunny beaches. Thus the physician must ask about the relationship to light and warmth in a differentiated fashion. A feeling of being too hot can be induced by movement, glaring light, TV and PCs, yet such children generally like sun and warmth (cf. ▸Chap. 3.2.2.1).

- **Equisetum limosum – Rubellit D6 dil.** Apotheke an der Weleda
  1 × daily in the morning 5–7 drops

is an important medicament that combines potentized red tourmaline (=Rubellit [Vademecum 2010, 729]) in D12 with filigree horsetail knotgrass.

Potentized tourmaline – the tourmaline can integrate 46 chemical elements into its unique structure – shows a deep relationship to the organization of the human I. In its many varieties, the mineral itself represents the entire colour spectrum; here use is made of the red variety. The medicament is indicated in cases where the focus lies on a *weakness of I organization*: affected children

- make a slightly sad and depressed impression
- have great difficulty initiating tasks, "getting into gear," "developing a desire"
- concentrating on the task at hand
- suffer from exam anxiety
- This medicament strengthens the presence of the I. The practice of the authors has proven it to be a profound medicament the significance of which places it alongside the Aurum compounds. Its effectiveness can be assessed within 4 weeks.

- **Rubellite D12–30 amp.** Weleda
  1 ampoule as individual dosage s.c./i.v.

Can prove effective for acute crisis situations during adolescence in which

- The self-relationship of the patient, his relationship to his own biography, needs to be strengthened in cases of acute panic, disorientation and identity crises
- In cases of acute exam anxiety coupled with a history of severe identity crisis and lack of self-assurance
- D12 for cases of pronounced symptomology involving metabolism, sweating, anxiety; D30 for patients with pronounced rational orientation with strain exerted by the super-I.

- **Carcinosinum C30, C200 pillules** (various manufacturers) in individual dosages.

This is an indication for *severe disorder and weakness of the rhythmic system* (the medicament can prove extremely beneficial for extremely severe difficulties falling asleep). Due to an *ambitious achievement orientation* coupled with *a weakness in regard to the ability to reach goals through one's own effort (often adopted unconsciously from the environment) the child traps itself, the result being rising frustration.*

Conspicuous are:

- profound restlessness and lack of concentration connected with,
- pronounced *frustration* and a lack of "*get-up*" which is difficult to break through,
- such children work hard but without achieving satisfactory results; they ultimately stop doing their schoolwork,
- such children find it difficult to occupy themselves, need social contact to be active, place great store by "making it" in the peer group and like to travel.

If the weakness of memory exhibited by the child with attention deficit is the result of disinterest – the child does not wish to be attentive to the appropriate degree and does not remember things even if he were capable of doing so, then

- **Cuprum sulfuricum D6 dil.** Apotheke an der Weleda
  3 × daily 5 drops

can help the child become more open and at the same time more relaxed.
Clearly strong-willed but at the same time mentally lazy children can be stimulated to increase their attentiveness and mental structure through administration of

- **Stibium met. praep. D6 trit.** Weleda
  3 × 1 saltsp.,
- **Sulphur D12 trit.** Weleda
  in the morning in addition 1 saltsp.,
- **Stibium met. 0.4 % ointment** Weleda
  in the morning massage 1 small-pea-size amount onto the forehead.
- **Acidum phosphoricum D12 pillules** (various manufacturers)
  in the morning and as required at midday 5 pillules

is indicated for children who *become cognitively exhausted quickly.* headaches and thirst after school are key symptoms of this constitution. During adolescence such patients can be afflicted by lovesickness (C30). Such children have a tendency to develop allergic, in part perennial rhinitis (cf. ▶Chap. 6.7), which results in further impairment of their attention and concentration.
Children who have difficulties with *arithmetic and logical thinking* but otherwise – for example in regard to reading and writing – have no difficulties benefit from treatment with potentized natural phosphorus (lime apatite) and zinc:

- **Apatite D12 trit.** Weleda
  in the mornings 1 saltsp. and
- **Stannum met. praep. D12 trit.** Weleda
  in the evenings 1 saltsp. as well as
- **Stannum met. 0.4 % ointment** Weleda
  in the morning a small-pea-size amount massaged into the forehead.

A profoundly effective metallic medicament used for stimulating differentiated thinking processes is potentized antimony-silver, *dyscrasite*. The key aspect was already described in constitutional respect in 7.5.3.1: an attention deficit disorder manifests itself which results from poor processing of sensory impressions, i.e., weakness of the synthesizing activity in the central nervous system which integrates various sensory impressions. "The metabolic forces in the nerve-sense system are not sufficiently active (mental capacity, power to synthesize sensory impressions)." [Vademecum 2010, 398].

- **Dyscrasite D30 dil.** Apotheke an der Weleda
  in the evening 5 drops

are indicated in cases of children

- who have attention deficit and poor cognitive capacity
- who behave in a clumsy and undifferentiated way in terms of fine motor skills.

Such children profit greatly from learning how to play an instrument such as the flute, which also supports intellectual maturation (important in 2nd septennial). –
Attention disorders after chemotherapy (most frequent sequelae in paediatric oncology!) can be positively influenced by increasing potencies of **Dyscrasite (D6 trit.** Weleda, **D10–30 dil.** Apotheke an der Weleda); this medicament must be taken over long periods of time.
In contrast, lead

- **Plumbum met. praep. D10 trit.** Weleda
  in the morning 1 saltsp. daily

is indicated in cases of

- macrocephalic, sometimes somewhat hydrocephalic-appearing and at the same time more or less slender children,
- who are delayed in terms of cognitive development,
- appear slowed down,
- often exhibit delayed success of toilet training,
- find it very difficult to catch up on delays in development.

It should be administered at intervals of 4–6 weeks in alternation with copper or, for example sulphur. This medicament has gained in importance for the authors; it clearly strengthens I presence and the ability to set boundaries. [Vademecum 2010, 673]

7.5.3.7 Children with craniocervical junction abnormalities

7.5.3.7.1 Pathogenetic connections

Osteopathy and cranio-sacral therapy as therapeutic directions have pointed out that the junction from the rear base of the skull to the spine in humans is very sensitive and often susceptible to interferences [Upledger and Vredevoogd 2000, 116–187]. Liem [2010, 665] currently defines hyperactivity and learning disorders during childhood as indications for the need of an osteopathic treatment in the cranio-sacral area. In this regard it has to be taken into account that the bony skull and the spine, both derived from the notochord, form an oscillating unity, a *system of more or less mobile bony structures*. In newborn and infants, this capacity for oscillation and vibration in the area of the craniocervical junction is exposed to extreme strains (in particular through birth) and may in many cases be pathologically deformed by vertebral body shifts, by disorders concerning the normal mobility of the vertebra joints or by constitutional disorders [Upledger and Vredevoogd

2000, 304–309]. Scientific studies have also found evidence to suggest that this area is particularly susceptible to interferences in the first six months of life– SIDS-syndrome (which occurs more frequently in the prone position, i. e. when the head is strongly rotated to the side) may also be related to this in certain cases [Deeg et al. 1998]. – The blood flow to the brain depends to a considerable extent on the vertebral arteries. These in turn can be considerably irritated through distorted balance, vertebral body shifts as well as flexibility disorders in the area of the upper cervical spine/base of skull.

Embryologically, B. Christ [1990, 831] defines "*the cervico occipital junction area as a "vital centre for humans"*. The first embryonic vessels are to be found here, the regulation of breathing and circulation is located in this area, central formation processes of the rhythmic system occur here; including the septation and crossing of the outflow tract of the heart as well as the development of the intramural nervous system in the gastrointestinal tract, which allows for peristalsis. – This indicates that the spine and especially the cranio-cervical junction should be conceived as a part of the rhythmic system: disorders of the spine, of blood flow, eventually of breathing regulation and of motor function interact here directly with each other!

The breathing rhythm has an *integrative effect* in particular, which continues in the rhythm of the cerebrospinal fluid flow. Cerebrospinal fluid contact neurons have recently been detected which perceive this flow in the brain ventricles in ways similar to those in which the sensory cells of the inner ear perceive the flow of endolymph. "The cerebrospinal fluid wave becomes a likeness of the inner ear wave" [Husemann 2010, 90]. Here one can begin to grasp something which was discussed at the beginning of this chapter, namely that the integration of sensory and bodily experience in rhythmic, sentient processes is of central importance for the inner experience of emotion and consciousness in human beings. *The central nervous system, the spinal cord and the brain are embedded in a rhythmic system by the rhythmics of the spinal column and the interplay of respiration and cerebrospinal fluid circulation which at the same time surrounds the central nervous system – amnion-like*[1] *– with a protective cavity of fluid and propulsion (this being indispensible for its function, as the cerebrospinal fluid hypotension syndrome in children with a ventriculo-peritoneal shunt shows).* A. Husemann (l. c.) has explored how important proper functioning of this system is for human experience of self.

Clinically speaking, in disorders of the cranio-cervical transition one finds limitations of rotation, palpable asymmetries in the uppermost transverse processes of the cervical interbody and asymmetries of the shoulder girdle; a mixed picture of tension in the cervical musculature on the one hand and on the other a relatively high degree of muscle hypotony in the segments of the spinal column below can occur, as can disorders in the tone of the muscles of facial expression and in the position of the jaw. The diagnosis is confirmed ex juvantibus if the behaviour of the patient receiving corresponding treatment of the spinal column shows clear, abrupt improvement, with him manifesting a sense of well-being in his own body.

In the case of such disorders a *dissociation between head and body* occurs which requires more extensive examinations with respect to the aspects of anthroposophic anthropology characterized in ▸Chap. 7.4.1. It leads to a condition in which the forces whose effect issues from the head pole and form the body out of the soul- and spirit-deter-

1 Cerebrospinal fluid and amnion fluid are almost identical in composition; the cerebrospinal fluid system evolves as a pinch-off of the amnion, as intraembryonal amnion so to speak.

mined individuality of the child do not succeed in becoming fully effective, i.e., fail to extend completely into the limbs. The primary forces of will which take effect in the limbs develop a misfit to the impulses issuing from the head pole; they do not integrate themselves properly into the child's organism. This constitutes itself in the first septennial in such a fashion that limb-metabolic organization is forced to adapt itself to the impulses forming the child's individuality whose effect issues from the head.

7.5.3.7.2 Treatment options

The treatment should only be performed by trained osteopaths or therapists with a cranio-sacral training. Specific experience with children is indispensible. Intervals between treatments should be at least one to two weeks. As a rule, positive effects clearly manifest themselves within this period of time.

Treatment can be enhanced and stabilized by administration of the following medicaments:

- **Amnion Gl D15–30 amp.** Wala
  in the evening daily – 3 × weekly 0.5 ml per os, in particular during the first year of life, after disorders in pregnancy and problems arising during the birth process (cf. ▸Chap. 2).
- **Disci comp. cum. Argento pillules** Wala
  daily 2 × 3–5 pillules for 3–6 weeks
- **Hypericum D12 dil./pillules** Weleda/DHU
  daily 2 × 3–5 drops followed by
- **Stannum met. praep. D20 trit.** Weleda
  in the morning 1 saltsp. for 4–6 weeks as stabilizing therapy.
- *In cases of traumatization of cervical vertebrae and of the cranio-cervical transition* (whiplash) a combination of Disci comp. c. Argento (contains Arnica D19) with the little known but extremely effective medicament for this indication, namely
- **Tulipa e planta tota D6 amp.** Wala
  daily ½ – 1 ampoule per os for 1–2 weeks [Vademecum 2010, 808]

has proven to be highly reliable therapeutically. For every case history it is necessary to ask about physical traumata and in particular traumata of the back and the cervical vertebrae because many fail to report spontaneously on such events.

For purposes of *early diagnostics and therapy,* cranio-sacral therapy and osteopathy play a major role especially in connection with ADHD but also in cases of children with a neonatologically problematic case history. It is impressive to see time and again how, as a result of treatment, infants who had previously exhibited such classic early symptoms as long periods of screaming, motor agitation, eating and sleeping disorders and bad temper became more relaxed and calmer, being able to establish a day-night rhythm and an eating rhythm much better as well as becoming more harmonious in terms of motor development.

7.5.3.8 Children with autonomic lability and labile hypotonic circulation

This group of children attracts the attention of the physician primarily due to the *instability of their rhythmic system*:

- fluctuating, situation- and position-dependent disorders of warmth distribution with varying paleness,
- cool-sweaty extremities, vegetatively caused sweating, dermographism,
- susceptibility to stomach aches, varying indefinable paraesthesia, later on headaches (tension headaches or migraine-type headaches),
- not infrequently whining-anxious moods with a lack of basic trust,
- nervousness.

Such frequently observed symptoms sometimes worsen considerably around the ninth year of life, during a growth spurt and during the detachment phase in adolescence, leading to manifest attention disorders. Disorders of the cranio-cervical transition can exacerbate these symptoms considerably (see above). As a rule, attention and concentration are inconsistently impaired; among those who tend to develop a higher degree of motor agitation the impression can arise that they stimulate themselves motorically all the time in order to achieve sufficient body toning (in cases of pronounced hyperkinetic symptomology cf. ▸Chap. 7.5.3.2, for example Veratrum album).

As basic therapy the following is suitable for such children:

- **Cardiodoron mite dil.** Weleda/**Cardiodoron Rh tab.** Weleda
  daily 3 × 5–15 drops/3 × 1 tab.

Cardiodoron unfolds a comprehensively stimulating effect on the rhythmic system and should not be misconstrued as a "heart medicament." Thus there is a broad and significant indication for it especially in the second septennial since the formation of the human rhythmic system essentially occurs during this period (lungs, cardiovascular system, spinal column). –

In cases of schoolchildren whose ADD symptomology is connected with a *too weak intervention of the soul aspect in kidney function and circulation* and who have a tendency towards cardiovascular hypotony, lack of drive, poor capacity to concentrate and poor memory retention and develop depressive moods

- **Ginseng, eth. Decoct D1 dil.** Weleda
  2 × 5(–10) drops daily

is a specifically effective medicament (the authors wish to thank B. Brandl for substantial information; [Vademecum 2010, 467]).

Ginseng roots contain steroid saponines (Helleborus niger, for example, contains similar substances in similar ways). In substantial dosages this medicinal plant, valued in Eastern Asia since time immemorial, stimulates the activity of the sentient organization in the area of the renal-adrenal system. This causes a toning of hypotonic circulation and strengthens alertness, waking consciousness, inner warmth distribution and thus vigilance and the concentration span in the process.

Approximately half of the children, most of all those with a combined weakness of the cardiovascular system and digestion, benefit clearly if the following organ preparation

- **Glandulae suprarenales comp. pillules** Wala
  3 × daily 5–10 pillules

is combined with one of the abovementioned herbal remedies.

The most important *metallic* medicaments for children of the type described above is potentized *iron*. In this context it is interesting that Konofal [2004] succeeded in showing that on average, children with ADHD had considerably lower ferritin levels than the control group; 84 % of children with ADHD had ferritin levels which were 18 % below the norm value calculated on the basis of the control group. *Low ferritin levels correlated with more severe ADHD symptoms and more pronounced cognitive deficiencies.*

In this context, a medicament used by anthroposophic therapy appears to be especially suitable for children affected from age 9 on, in particular if they

- exhibit inhibited behaviour at school or in groups
- have a tendency to shiver
- suffer from fatigue, the feeling of being overstrained by school, affective lability
- have low ferritin levels, rhagades of mucous membranes and paleness which indicate poor iron metabolism
- exhibit attention and concentration disorders.

Hyperactivity is less characteristic for the indication of this medicament:

- **Ferrum hydroxydatum 5%** Weleda/**50%** special manufacture, Apotheke an der Weleda
  daily 1/4 – 1/2 tsp. before meals.

From the 9th year of life on the authors prefer administration of the 50 % preparation, which is considerably more effective.

The effect of this medicament originating with R. Steiner and depicted in a highly differentiated way by Engel [2006] in his writings on the manufacture of pharmaceutical products originally aimed at "strengthening the emotional capacity." Most of all, patients report that they feel less at the mercy of their moods. In many cases the authors observed increases in ferritin levels after administration of the medicament but without the undesired side effects often observed in use of allopathic medicines. The main effect of the medicament is to stabilize circulation, reduce affect lability, improve the emotional capacity to concentrate and ultimately to reduce vulnerability of skin-mucosa boundaries, i. e., the bodily boundaries, this also being viewed as a physical expression of an improved ability to set boundaries.

Cases in which the symptomology corresponds to the depiction above usually involve boys whose development during the second septennial tends to be inhibited; if they appear to be "too soft" the following is indicated:

- **Ferrum met. praep. D6–12 trit.** Weleda
  in the morning 1 saltsp.

For children and youths whose problems arise in the context of a growth spurt (they grow too fast and mentally "nothing works") an extract of blackthorn blossoms and shoot tips, produced and potentized together with ferric oxide (cf. ▸Chap. 6.5.6.4.3), has a very beneficial and time-tested effect:

- Prunuseisen **(blackthorn-iron) pillules** Wala
  3 × daily 7–10 pillules

If the child is weakened, for example by previous illnesses or emotional duress, has a tendency towards hypotony and latent depressivity the compound consisting of Prunuseisen combined with Levico water and Hypericum is more effective (cf. ▸Chap. 6.5.6.4.3); [Vademecum 2010, 544 regarding the guiding idea]

- **Levico comp. pillules** Wala
  2–3 × daily 5–10 pillules

A widely indicated medicament for cardiovascular hypotony, attention deficit and poor capacity to concentrate is

- **Scorodite circulation pillules (Skorodit Kreislauf glob.)** Wala
  2–3 × daily 10 pillules, administered primarily in the morning and at midday.

This compound is based on scorodite, arsenic-acid iron, and is supplemented by Veratrum album and Prunus spinosa (blackthorn). It is primarily helpful during puberty and adolescence, especially if there is a need for a medicament with a quick toning-strengthening effect. The patients appear sluggish, feeble and hypotonic but not dismissive or aggressive.

- **Cralonin Heel drops**
  2 × 20 drops daily for schoolchildren

have, as a hawthorn extract, a harmonizing and stabilizing effect on cardiovascular circulation. For susceptibility to orthostasis it is effective as well as for anxiety and sharp pain sensations in the chest which have no specific cause and occur relatively frequently at this age.

Helpful non-medicinal therapy options consist of rhythmical massage therapy and eurythmy therapy [Köhler 1994, 34–56] (in this order).

In this context, where the therapeutic effect on the *rhythmic system* is emphasized, one can generally point out the importance of

- giving the child clear guidance and structuring the day rhythmically, especially in the morning and evening hours (cf. ▸Chap. 7.1),
- lots of exercise (in all kinds of weather) and guided physical activity (involvement of children in housework and gardening, horseback riding, etc.).

Köhler [2002, 200f.] makes further suggestions.

7.5.3.9 Food intolerances

In many publications Egger [2000] succeeded in showing that an "oligoantigen" diet could improve the behaviour of some hyperkinetic children considerably. Hypersensitivity to certain foods, in particular sugar, colourants, preservatives and foods rich in phosphates varies from case to case. In regard to colourants and sodium benzoate, an influence on hyperactive behaviour has been clinically proven. [McCann 2007]. Usually there is no development of allergies in the classic sense but rather of an intolerance ("an idiosyncrasy"), which often remains undetected for a long time and can only be revealed when the major intolerable foods are systematically left out and then reintroduced on a trial basis in the course of an exclusion diet. Thus one begins with a basic diet which is sure to be tolerated, adding foods previously eaten step by step according to a prescribed plan in order to detect intolerances. *In general, sugar and food additives often result in exacerbation.* At the same time it is not uncommon for there to be a craving for intolerable foods.

In the experience of the authors it is important to determine whether a pronounced intestinal Candida mycosis exists. If it proves possible to rectify the situation in accordance with the principles laid down in ▸Chap. 4.6 in cooperation with the child (diet, rhythmic eating with fasting periods) and the family (everyone eats "more healthily"), i. e. by employing a large amount of will power (!) and suitable medicaments, then many children exhibit a much clearer mental and emotional presence, show less addictive behaviour, for example less craving of intolerable foods, and have healthier instincts and improved attention as a result! From an anthroposophic perspective O. Wolff [1993] commented on this aspect extensively; in the works of R. Steiner [1976, 15th and 16th lecture, in particular 294] one finds immediately relevant indications. In general, reference must be made to the diagnostic and therapeutic illucidations to be found in Section 6.3. From an anthroposophic perspective one should note the significance of spleen activity in regard to complete assimilation of nutriment by the human organism. What R. Steiner [Steiner 1999, 294] describes about this organ activity in its significance and pathology is strikingly similar to what has been observed in hyperkinetic children regarding food intolerances as well as craving for sweets and intolerable foods. This aspect can prove therapeutically beneficial (see below).

In practice one can deal with this group of patients as follows:

- Each patient's individually tolerable diet is determined by precise case history, exclusion diet, diet consultation; this takes effort but it is indispensible for affected children. The general rule is that the positive effect must be experienceable for parents, teachers and the child!
- Stool diagnostics (enteric flora, pancreas function) and symbiosis control, if necessary antifungal treatment.
- Medicinal therapy which especially affects the breakdown of nutrients, the boundary function of the intestinal mucosa, liver and pancreas.

- **Sulphur LM6 dil.** Arcana
  5 drops in the morning daily

often has a quick stabilizing effect on sugar metabolism particularly in cases of fluctuations in blood sugar levels with typical sudden cravings for sweets and corresponding worsening of behaviour!

- **Cichorium/Pancreas comp. pillules** Wala/amp. Wala
  3 × 7 pillules/1 drinking ampoule daily

In general, potentized antimony promotes structuring in hyperkinetic children; the organ preparation Pancreas has a positive effect on digestion as well as on regulation of blood sugar.

- **Lycopodium comp. pillules** Wala
  3 × 5–7 pillules

is indicated especially if toxic exposure plays a role in the course of the ailment, bowel movement is irregular (perhaps with a tendency towards constipation) and fluctuates in colour, and metabolically induced adynamia and exhaustion occur.

- **Spleen (=Lien) Gl D6** or **Spleen/Plumbum amp.** Wala
  for food intolerances 3 × weekly 1 ampoule per os

helps strengthen spleen function and the immune system associated with intestinal mucosa (to which the spleen has a close connection in terms of developmental history).

- Spleen rhythmical Einreibungen with **Oxalis 10 % ointment** Weleda, **Plumbum met. 0.1 % ointment** Weleda – possibly in alternation with **Cuprum met. 0.4 % ointment** Weleda.

Afternoon rest with application of a warm liver poultice (for example using yarrow tea) has a beneficial effect on the entire function of digestion and metabolism, enhanced by

- **Hepatodoron (known as Fragaria/Vitis in some countries) tab.** Weleda
  2 × 1 tab. daily after lunch and dinner; most effective when chewed but the taste of dried wine leaves takes some getting used to

This basic medicament for liver, and in particular, sugar metabolism is particularly suitable for phlegmatic children who are tired and sluggish in the morning and have a tendency to simply "tune out" during morning classes [Vademecum 2010, 489].

7

7.6 Affective respiratory spasms

7.6.1 Symptoms and pathogenesis

This is a paroxysm that, once started, follows its own pattern. The children respond to certain emotions with great agitation and loud cries, which give way to a cessation of breathing (this is likely to be a spasm of the glottis, followed by apnoea [Strunk 1989a, 217]). They "cry themselves out of their body" rapidly developing cyanosis – the spasm then usually dissolves after a (seemingly endless) ¼ to ½ minute caught in inspiration; in rare cases it can lead to a grand mal-like exacerbation.

The *triggers* are usually certain situations in the domestic setting – the symptoms almost always subside spontaneously with a change of environment! The event is *age-dependent*: it occurs from the age 6 months up to the end of the 3rd year of life, and disappears spontaneously at this age at the latest. It is not etiologically related to epilepsy; there are phenomenological correlates with stenosing laryngitis (pseudo-croup), which occurs at the same age and also represents a paroxysmal event whose symptoms is most common in the larynx.

The symptoms themselves are a paroxysmal spasm of the respiratory region, triggered by certain emotions and with a tendency to recur (in the sense of a certain conditioning). These symptoms refer to the astral body, to the *soul-organization of the child as pathogenetically decisive level.* The age-related development also shows that here the *immaturity* of the soul is important. We refer here also to the section on stenosing laryngitis (▸Chap. 5.1.4). – Breath holding spells develop in a phase in which the child, ending lactation, has the task of loosening the deep relationship with the mother in order to build differentiated social relationships to the family (▸Chap. 7.2, 8-month anxiety, separation anxiety). It will take until the end of the terrible twos before the interaction between "I" and "you" stabilizes – differentiated into the various relationships with mother, father and siblings. Parallel to this, the soul is anchoring itself in the body via pneumatization – a process that is accentuated in childhood illnesses and respiratory infections (▸Chap. 5). In the 4th to 5th year of age a physiological stabilization of the rhythmic system occurs: a stable interplay develops between respiration and circulation, between air and fluid organism.

The soul, the astral body shows its effect in the body through the construction of opposites, polarities that find their primordial expression in inspiration and expiration: the modulation of breathing mirrors all emotions and inner movements of the soul, such as excitement or pain. In principle this can always lead to a spasmodic paralysis if these opposites short-circuit instead of being guided by a higher rhythmical order and of harmoniously flowing into one another as for example in inhaling and exhaling. The latter ability stabilizes in the child usually only in the 3rd to 5th year of age – noticeable in breath and movement, but also in social behaviour (able to play in groups, to temporarily detach from the mother, etc.). Social and organism-related maturation of the soul organization occur simultaneously!

On the other hand, failures of this development process, especially in the 3rd to 5th year of age, can cause persistent disturbances in the respiratory organization such as asthma or stuttering – disorders in which somatic and social aspects are entangled (whereby developmental issues in the relationship with the parents, especially with the mother, are of particular importance). – Breath holding spells represent a less profound development disorder that nevertheless may indicate a fundamental *instability in the child's soul organization in relation to developmental problems in the child's family and social relationships.*

Affected children are often emotionally very sensitive and *vulnerable.* On the other hand, they often bond particularly strongly with the mother and show *jealous* behaviour (e.g. towards a sibling). They seem overwhelmed by the task of having to reconcile being *emotionally impulsive* and demanding on the one hand and being very sensitive on the other hand; they are under a high tension that they cannot easily express and thereby resolve. – This can be accentuated by the adult's attitudes, especially by that of the mother: lack of sensitivity to the emotional needs of the child, abrupt intervention in the child's activities as well internal tension on the part of the mother often call out the first attack, which in turn exacerbates the parent's tension.

7.6.2 Treatment

The first aim of a consultation with the parents is to explain the background and good prognosis of the disease. It is important that the parents learn to perceive the child before engaging with it. Loving observation, emotional care and a smooth transition to actions in order not to overwhelm the emotional capabilities of the child are required – and parents often need some guidance in this regard.

On the other hand it is important to learn calm and purposeful distancing from the child's impulsivity, to set a framework of action. This is only possible if the parent gains some distance to themselves in moments of inner peace and, from this inner space, are able to take an outside view on certain situations such as conflicts with the child. This can be done as an exercise in the evening before going to sleep. For children with breath holding spells (but also for children who stutter, recurrent pseudo-croup or asthma) it is important that the disease *does not lead to the child claiming all attention at all times.* – Rather, attention should be given to the child *when it is not sick*: the child's soul organization is nurtured by emotional closeness in which own impulses are initially held back in order to tune into the child.

Suitable medicinal treatment

- **Ignatia D12 dil./pillules.** (various manufacturers)
  2 x/day. 3–5 gtt./5 pillules for 3–4 weeks.

Ignatius bean is a "thornless climbing shrub that climbs up to the highest tops of the trees with its compressed hook-shaped, woody vines" [Madaus 1979, 1606]. As Loganiacee it is related to Nux vomica and contains the toxins brucine and strychnine. The plant lacks its own uprightness: it hooks itself into a tree to find the way to the top. – This self-entanglement is found in the homoeopathic drug proving again as a tendency for disappointment and injury to lead to spasms, tics and convulsions (to get caught in oneself). On the other hand, the patient is liable in a paradoxical way to cling to the person who induces the injury or disappointment – and whose emotional support is, at the same time, needed or requested. The behaviour thus always has a contradictory character: hysterical-demonstrative, seizure-like symptoms in an otherwise loving and sensible child.

Ignatia is effective in the following conditions, amongst others

- Tics,
- hyperventilation tetany,
- psychogenic (tickle-)cough,
- (suppressed) jealousy.

If the efficacy of Ignatia D12 is insufficient, D30 can be given (it also has to be repeated several times). The treatment can be introduced or supplemented by the administration of

- **Cuprum met. praep. D20 trit./dil.** Weleda:
  5 gtt./1 saltsp evenings.

Tab. 7.4 Selection of medicaments on the basis of emotional impulses.

Lachesis D12–200	Hyoscyamus D12–30	Ignatia D12–30
openly aggressive, hurtful jealousy	Mistrustful-destructive provoking behaviour	"silent" jealousy caused by hypersensitivity and injury
Extremely impulsive behaviour which fluctuates between hatred and possessive desire	malicious actions which are dangerous for smaller, weaker children!	Very controlled for long periods of time, makes a kind and reasonable impression but is often very vulnerable close mother bond, has difficulties accepting siblings in particular (typically a single child with a close mother bond)
Generally very energetic	Jealousy can manifest itself physically in migraines, asthma	
Strong sexual energy, possessive	obscene-exhibitionistic	Emotional immaturity, otherwise inconspicuous children

7.7 Treatment indications for childhood jealousy

Paediatric physicians quite frequently encounter jealousy as a factor in psychosomatic disorders. In addition to advising parents, potentized medicaments can provide valuable benefit. – What guides the selection of medication is the way in which emotional impulses inhabited by compulsive-body-bound desire express themselves (cf. Tab. 7.4).

A very effective medicament (in the sense of anthroposophic anthropology) for treating hysterical behaviour disorders is *Bryophyllum*. This medicament primarily strengthens the coherence and vitality of the child's life organization, muting any excessive release of emotional-compulsive impulses in the process.

Bryophyllum is contained in the compound

- **Ignatia comp. pillules** Wala
  2–3 × 5–7 pillules daily

in combination with Lachesis and Ignatia. This has proven therapeutically beneficial in many cases of jealousy in which silent desperation is coupled with aggressive impulses. As an individual medicament Bryophyllum is indicated in combination with silver (as vegetabilized metal) for jealousy in cases where a shocking event has triggered the emotional disorder:

- **Bryophyllum Argento cultum D2 dil.** Weleda
  2–3 × 5–10 drops daily

7.8 Stuttering

7.8.1 Insight into the disorder

In general, stuttering develops and becomes chronic between the 3rd and 5th year of life, emerging only rarely after the first septennial; in cases of severe physical and emotional trauma or shock it can also occur in adults, however [Strunk 1989b, 210]. It involves an *inhibition* of movement (cf. ▸Chap. 7.3, depressive syndromes) which increases with the *awareness of the inhibition* (whereas batterism, which can also occur at this age, improves if the person is encouraged to speak quietly and control his speech). If one views the family constellations most frequently found among stuttering children the following characteristics can be described [Strunk 1989b, 210]:

- In 40 to 60 % of the cases one of the parents (boys and men are affected two to ten times more often than girls and women) has a similar history of stuttering (the person affected usually suffers from emotional insecurity him- or herself).
- Frequently the other parent (usually the mother, sometimes also a successful, more authoritarian father) does not give the child a chance to speak, often interrupts the child out of her or his own vigour and impulsivity, and after the stuttering has set in, out of anxiety, concern, and an ever increasing not-being-able-to-listen.

In the child, such family circumstances trigger different, partly contradictory psychological reactions:

- The child feels misunderstood, does not get a chance to speak, and therefore feels patronized and humiliated.
- The child feels insecure, her self-confidence and self-esteem are impaired, and she develops fears of doing something wrong.
- On the other hand, the child also develops an accumulation of unexpressed impulses, which leads to a congestion of suppressed aggression, which in turn can further impede the child's stream of speech.

In this way, a doctor will often observe a sad-depressed general mood in the affected children. Physically, there is a profound disturbance of the rhythmic system – the prognosis of the natural course is not very favourable (persistence into adulthood in about 30 to 60 % of the cases [Steinhausen 2010, 178]). A certain "over intellectualization" is often found, a conscious inhibition of exhalation (▸Chap. 6.5, Asthmatic bronchitis), which can settle deep in the life organization of the respiratory tract. This in turn loses its natural vitality. – An impairment of the life organization in the region of the respiratory organs within the first seven years of life favours the development of *compulsions* (persistent emotional tightness), which is in fact frequently observable in stuttering children.

Shock events also have a similar effect: They induce a form of pathological body memory, in which the traumatized organ region, in a rough or even only in a fine-structured physically unobservable manner, is deformed and devitalized (every new formation of memory is based on fine "sal" processes – a solidifying, "crystallising", "salt-forming" process – inside vital structures). In the first 7 years of life, children are especially susceptible in this respect because their organs are just being formed and in the process, even pure emotional perceptions have a direct impact on the process of bodily organ formation (so that when later recalling the first 7 years of life, trauma-victims often cannot discern whether they were physically or psychologically traumatized).

A consequence of the stuttering is that the child is at the centre of the parents', especially the mother's, attention. This usually has a negative effect on the symptoms, since parental expectations, admonitions and coaxing only intensify the problem, which often already existed prior to the stuttering. But on the other hand, the child experiences what it is like to be the centre of attention, experiences his power over the attention of his parents. Moreover, children who stutter often withdraw increasingly into the family for fear of being mocked, etc. by strangers. – Similar to bronchial asthma, domination towards parents and siblings can arise indirectly: now they are paying attention to the child, now they have to learn to hold back, etc. – In this way, the deep contradiction, which the child experiences emotionally, can continue to increase in the behaviour. With one part of her psyche, the child can even actively retain the stuttering. – This applies even more when the child "makes" the stuttering himself, to use an expression by Viktor von Weizsäcker (▸Chap. 6.5.1). If the patient's own control of his own speech is eliminated, the stuttering disappears [Strunk 1989b, 211]! The doctor must always remain cognisant of this if hassled by the parents and the child with the question of when the stuttering will finally stop!

7.8.2 Medicinal treatment

It is important that treatment begins *as early as possible.* The *conditions under which the stuttering developed* can also best be observed at this stage. If triggers or contributing circumstances are found, therapy can address them first. The most important are:

7.8.2.1 Shock

- **Aconitum D20 pillules** Wala, **LM12 dil.** Arcana, in cases of events in the remote past **C30–200 pillules**
  daily 5 pillules/3–5 drops, higher potencies in individual dosages

is indicated if the shock experience triggers anxieties or the child is clearly affected by problems with anxiety. Such children are under enormous strain, develop a clear awareness of the disorder and develop a fear of speaking in the course of the affliction (group 3 according to Steinhausen [2010, 177]).

- **Opium D30 pillules** (various manufacturers)
  1 × weekly 5 pillules

in cases where anxiety is absent.

7.8.2.2 Delayed speech development

A considerable number of stuttering children (about one third) suffer from delayed speech and language development with signs of brain damage in early childhood (e. g. pathological EEG, elektronystagmography) from which, for the most part gradually, stuttering can evolve (group 2 according to Steinhausen [2000]).

In such cases the following is indicated:

- **Myrrha comp. D8/Belladonna, Radix D10 dil.** aa. Weleda (cf. extensive treatment of this in ▸Chap. 7.5.3.4.1)
  1–3 × daily 5 drops

alternating every 14 days with

- **Apis regina comp. pillules** Wala
  2–3 × daily 5–7 pillules

7.8.2.3 Disturbance of self-consciousness, development of the neurotic personality.

- **Aurum met. praep. D12 trit.** Weleda
  1–2 × daily 1 saltsp.

in combination/alternation with a potentized iron preparation, for example Ferrum sidereum D6–10 is indicated; the authors usually prescribe

- **Skorodit D10 trit.** Weleda, **D12–20 dil.** Apotheke an der Weleda
  1–2 × daily 1 saltsp., 5 drops

As a supplement in clear cases of compulsive symptoms

- **Cinis Tabaci D6 trit.** Weleda
  1–2 × daily 1 saltsp.

can be given. In cases of weak personality forces, depressivity and inner lack of light

- **Phosphorus LM6 dil.** Arcana
  5 drops daily in the morning

prove beneficial. For internal use the following medicament is generally of importance:

- **Stramonium D12 dil./pillules** DHU
  daily 1–2 × 5 drops/5–7 pillules

Stramonium is the *most important herbal single-plant medicament* for stuttering (▸Chap. 7.4.4). Morphologically, the plant especially emphasizes *dividedness,* even within the nightshade family. This finds its expression right down to the produced toxins, which have both excitatory and inhibitory effects. – Stramonium is indicated against stuttering, if

- highly shocking events were experienced,
- pronounced fears (especially alone, in the darkness, of animals) are present,
- possibly if neurological illnesses, injuries, vaccination side-effects preceded the stuttering,
- the fears are faced by a strong, sometimes violently impulsive out-bursts (therefore, there is also a high tonus when stuttering),
- there are possibly tic-disorders,
- stuttering quite predominantly occurs in the first syllable (e. g. "a … a … lways").

In addition to stramonium, but far more rarely, as a further Solanaceae

- **Belladonna Rh D10 dil.** Weleda
  2 × daily 5–7 gtt.

can be considered therapeutically (can be well combined with Aurum met.).
stuttering in connection with high excitement levels and possible tic-disorders can be an indication for

- **Agaricus D10-12-20 dil.** Weleda Pharmacy
  1–2 × daily 5 gtt.

Agaricus is a very important single-plant medicament that is particularly indicated in cases with pre-existing neurological damage.
Externally, daily application of ointment on the back between the shoulder blades has been useful, with

- **Cuprum/Nicotiana comp. ungt.** Wala, possibly alternating with
- Pyrite 5 % : Equisetum arvense 10 % aa ointment Weleda Pharmacy

7.8.3 Non-medicinal therapies

In cases of generally delayed speech and language development, traumatizing birth, accidents involving injury to the head and the spinal column or other similar findings (cf. ▸Chap. 7.5) *cranio-sacral therapy* can be very beneficial at the beginning of treatment, especially in the area of the cranio-cervical transition.

In general *rhythmical massage therapy* is an important form of treatment in order to re-balance deformations of the rhythmic system. It is indicated in most cases of stuttering. – The same holds for therapeutic application of *rhythmics*. Differentiated *eurythmy therapy* is preferable to the breathing exercises often used in such cases.

Vocalically the sequence "A–E–I–O–U" [cf. Steiner 1987, 134; Kirchner-Bockholt 1997, 69] is recommended here. It is advantageous for the child to say (– _ _ – _ _ – _ _) using a dactylic rhythm with the vowel always being spoken on the long syllable (**A** _ _ **E** _ _ **I** _ _); one should have the child walk forwards while moving from "A" to "E" and finally to "I" and then have him *turn around* and articulate "I", "O" and "U" in the same rhythm while walking in the opposite direction – in other words, with the child never walking backwards. *Consonantally* the sound sequence "D–F–G–K–H" is suitable; one should note which sounds make the child stutter the most. By incorporating speech with the bodily movements to which it was originally linked, eurythmy therapy can have an immediate influence on speech flow. – Such exercises can be followed by choric recitation and singing.

The basis of therapy remains *consultation with the parents and the affected child himself* (allowing the child to "have a say" constitutes a guiding goal of treatment which should also become a reality in the consultation (!)). A conscious effort should be made to involve the child in the conversation and not "spare" it. Today, speech therapy for stuttering is also focused to a considerable degree on working with the parents. Close cooperation and conferring is necessary in some cases.

If the child suffers from strong tensions, tendencies towards depressivity and anxiety, *therapeutic painting* sometimes plays an important therapeutic role.

7.9 Tic disorders, nail biting

7.9.1 Tics

Tics appear most often in the second half of the first seven years of life (see also oral fluency disorders). They are often associated with attention and concentration disorders (ADD) and hyperactivity disorders (ADHD, ▸Chap. 7.5). Phobias and depressive disorders are also more frequent in children with tics (▸Chap. 7.2 and 7.3). This should be taken into consideration from an anamnestic, diagnostic and therapeutic point of view. At the age at which the soul organization, the astral body are released from the parental sheath and are completely internalized by the child, at the age of puberty and adolescence, ticks frequently increase, only to disappear completely quite often in early adult life – a sign of the regulating influence of the I organization. Family tensions can intensify tics; successful separation from the parental home, but also liberation from tensions in the parental home bring calm. In this respect, the whole family context must be kept in mind. Tics often have an unconscious "hysteric"-demonstrative character, they can be frequently regulated and suppressed by the I, which underscores the generally benign nature of the tics during childhood and young age but is also important for counselling and therapy.

From a therapeutic point of view, a medicinal therapy has often proven to be effective when at the same time the environment and the interaction with the child are integrated in the therapy (see stuttering, ▸Chap. 7.8). Eurythmy therapy can assist in regulating and practicing tension and release, which is a problem for the affected child (Dopamin-D2 receptor blockers can often effectively suppress the tics). Many children and adolescents learn to apprehend the tics and suppress them, for example, by a countermovement or muscular strain opposing the tic. Especially in the case of family tensions and symbiotic-ambivalent relationships of the child, the authors recommend art therapy, e. g. anthroposophic painting therapy which here has a relaxation effect in the broadest sense and can strengthen the autonomy of child and adolescent.[1]

From a homoeopathic and anthroposophic perspective therapy focuses on:

- **Agaricus D12 dil.** Apotheke an der Weleda/various manufacturers
  1–2 × daily 5–7 drops is the key medicament for tics.

A suitable homoeopathic compound is

- **Agaricus olpx. dil.** Madaus
  Several times a day 7–15 drops
- **Hyoscyamus D10 pillules** Wala
  1–2 × daily 5 pillules,

In cases of swallowing spasms, involuntary movements of the pharynx, hiccups and similar symptoms – cf. ▸Chap. 7.4 and ▸Chap. 7.6.

- **Ignatia D12–30 pillules** (various manufacturers)

for tics, sorrow and the factors depicted in ▸Chap. 7.6.

- **Arsenicum album LM12 dil.** Arcana, **D30 pillules** Wala
  in the evening 5 drops/pillules

In cases of extreme nervousness and anxiety; cf. extensive treatment in ▸Chap. 6.4.3.6.1. For tics a balance between the copper side (tension, cramps which do not easily resolve during the night) and the iron side (being able to control and regulate metabolism and movement on the basis of the I) is salutogenetically important. In these terms it is important to effectively support constitutional transposition by promoting incarnation and healthy toning in the morning with

- **Skorodit D6–10 trit.** Weleda
  1 saltsp. in the morning and

on the other hand promote relaxation and distribution of warmth in the evening using a copper preparation. For the evening one can consider prescribing, for example **Cuprum aceticum D6–12** (cf. ▸Chap. 6.5.6.3.3) in cases of tendency towards cramps and ambivalent relationship to the mother or **Melissa Cupro culta D2 dil.** Weleda in cases of emotional tension, depressive moods, poor heat formation and susceptibility to spasms [cf. Guiding Ideas Vademecum 2010, 576].

When administered substantially as well as in potentized form the metal *zinc* can bring about a clear improvement of symptoms.

As a form of non-medicinal treatment *eurythmy therapy* should above all be taken into consideration.

1 The authors thank their colleague A. Schmidt, a specialist for paediatric and adolescent psychiatry, for valuable suggestions.

7

7.9.2 Nail biting (onychophagia)

In regard to this frequent phenomenon in childhood, treatment with potentized silver and phosphorus alternating at intervals of two weeks has proven therapeutically beneficial. Treatment is oriented towards the moon rhythm, which shows itself to be the universally basic rhythm of the interplay of soul and body, of astral body and etheric body (see its importance for the reproductive process of ensouled organism, success of cures etc. [Hildebrandt et al. 1998, 18f.]). Promoting the harmony of the interplay between soul and body while guiding the I organization is the goal of the time-tested therapies listed below:

- **Argentum met. praep. D12 trit.** Weleda
  1 saltsp. in the morning during waxing moon
- **Phosphorus D12 dil.** Weleda
  5 drops in the evening during waning moon.

In cases of very restless, impulsive children who chew their nails, additional strengthening of the rhythmic system, the bodily basis for feeling, is necessary. In this context it is helpful to administer as a supplement

- **Aurum/Stibium/Hyoscyamus pillules** Wala (cf. ▸Chap. 7.5.3.2)
  1–2 × daily 7–10 pillules

7.10 Treatment perspectives on childhood migraines and tension headaches

7.10.1 Parameters for medicinal treatment

Treating these afflictions with potentized remedies is usually very effective in children. In additional to diagnostic exclusion of a tumour, for example, it is initially indispensible for this therapy to establish the necessary preconditions for successful medicinal treatment by a thorough anamnesis and counselling.

7.10.1.1 Nutrition

Omission of *chocolate* and cocoa products, hazelnuts, hard cheese, drinks which contain caffeine and quinine (for example cola) as well as foods which are known not to be tolerated. Reduction of sugar consumption (in cases of therapy resistance stool tests, bowel treatment as appropriate). (Caution is recommended in regard to colourants, preservatives and flavour enhancers). Drinking sufficient amounts of water during the day is essential.

Strict avoidance of cigarettes and drugs (in cases of adolescents).

7.10.1.2 Rhythm

Ensuring a regular day-night rhythm (prevention of exhaustion), a regular eating schedule (avoidance of hypoglycaemia in the mornings, strain on digestion in the evening) and regular, ample exercise is important.

Targeted questions are: time spent at computer, in front of television, etc.; if necessary, set up a framework for such activities.

7.10.1.3 Sleeping place

Strain caused by strong alternating current fields, geopathic influences etc. must be determined and eliminated (by putting the bed in a different place, mains isolation, no electronic devices near the bed).

Emotional distress as well as overstrain at school constitute important factors and require careful diagnostics and consultation including school consultation and if necessary art therapy.

In terms of differential diagnostics, migraine differs from tension headaches in regard to sudden onset, accompanying vegetative symptoms and frequent occurrence in the family but with one-sidedness (hemicrania), for example, not being as clearly pronounced as it sometimes is in adults.

It is essential to differentiate and if necessary treat the *cervico-occipital transition,* the dysfunction of which can seriously impair intracranial circulation.

7.10.2 Medication options

In cases of migraine in children the therapy described by H. Imhäuser [2000] using

- **Digitalis purpurea D4–6 dil.** Apotheke an der Weleda
  2 × 5 drops over a period of 3–12 months (!) has proven exceptionally effective.

F. Husemann [2009, 31–52]] has depicted the manifold relationships between Digitalis purpurea and the rhythmic system in terms of Goethean natural history and anthroposophic anthropology. In this dosage Digitalis stabilizes the rhythmic system and thus also the vascular system.

It constitutes a system-related, *non-individualized* therapy. – The following preparation was developed by R. Steiner [Steiner, Wegman 1991, 128f.]:

- **Kephalodoron (called Bidor in UK) 0.1 %, 5 % tab.** Weleda
  in concentrated form the original substance, made of ferrous sulphate and quartz processed with wine and honey [Engel 2006], as
- **Ferrum-Quartz caps. D6–12 trit.** Weleda
  also potentized under this name.

7

This medicament is effective for classic migraine as well as abdominal migraine and even tension headaches, in particular in cases of

- Weakness/undersupply of iron metabolism, iron deficiency
- exacerbation in the course of the day, as evening approaches
- exertion at school and physical exertion (in clear cases of school headache **Neurodoron®** (Kalium Phosphoricum comp.) tab. Weleda can be considered, cf. ▸Chap. 7.5.3.6.1).
- paleness, weak heat organization with sun being poorly tolerated

The dosage found by the authors to be most effective is

- in the morning individual dosages should be administered, with the strongest well-tolerated substantial dosage being chosen, before the 9th year of life 0.1 %, thereafter 5 %, for adolescents with an iron deficiency 1 cps. Ferrum-Quartz
- at midday Ferrum-Quartz D6 and in the evening D12, 1 saltsp. each, (or only in the evening 1 saltsp. D12)

(see extensive discussion of indications for Kephalodoron/Ferrum-Quartz (**Kephalodoron is called Bidor in UK**)in childhood in: Vademecum 2010, 522–523).

A medicament developed out of this is

- **Ferrum/Sulphur comp. pillules** Wala
  in the morning and afternoon 10 pillules

This preparation contains iron, and quartz in mutually potentized form (Sulphur D5, Ferrum D7, Quartz D19) and in kindergarten- and school-aged children it serves to strengthen the rhythmic system. It is particularly effective when several of the symptoms listed below occur as well:

- motor agitation,
- fluctuations in blood sugar and blood pressure,
- exertion-induced asthma bronchiale and
- migraine attacks;

This medicament is indicated more frequently for boys.

It must be taken over a relatively long period of time, in some cases followed by Ferrum sidereum (which also contains traces of phosphorus) or Vivianite.

- **Spigelia D12 dil.** (various manufacturers)
  1–2 × 5 drops

is an important herbal medicament for *one-sided, in particular left-sided* migraine (for right-sided migraine Belladonna, for one, is indicated). Symptoms are mostly accompanied by *heart sensations* and *anxiety*. Patients exhibit a high level of bodily and mental differentiation while also showing insecurity. For cases of precordial fright in adolescents and adults (pain in the region of the left nipple) it proves very reliable – this condition primarily affects men.

- **Natrium muriaticum LM6–12, D12–200 dil./pillules** (various manufacturers)
  daily 5 drops in the morning, higher potencies as individual dosages

is indicated for school-age children suffering from migraine and tension headaches (cf. ▸Chap. 7.3.2).

"The key [homoeopathic] remedy for migraine and headache in general" [Morrison 1999, 32].

It is effective for school-age girls who appear to be too serious and intent for their age (particularly at the beginning of puberty) even when hardly any constitutional symptoms indicating this medicament are present. One almost always finds *exacerbation of headaches in direct sunlight,* during the warm season, when eyes are strained, when stress is put on the cranio-cervical transition by tension and trauma of the cervical spine occurs but also during long hikes. – Migraine attacks are often initially accompanied by impaired vision.

During the daytime there is a worsening of complaints between 10 a.m. and 3 p.m. when the sun is highest.

- **Acidum phosphoricum D12 dil.** (various manufacturers)
  1–2 × 5–7 drops and
- **Aurum/Apis regina comp. pillules** Wala
  2–3 × 7–10 pillules

are indicated in cases of *school headaches* and headaches after mental exertion and are reliably effective treatments for this.

- **Solum pillules** Wala
  for acute cases hourly or more often 5–10 pillules, for longer periods of time 2–3 × 7 pillules

is an anthroposophic compound originally developed by Dr. R. Jensen for treatment of *sensitivity to changes in the weather.*
It has generally proven beneficial for headaches in connection with changes in the weather, onset of migraine headaches and also for long-term prevention of migraine attacks [Vademecum 2010, 757]
In severe cases of adolescent patients

- **Solum 10 ml amp.** Wala
  10 ml i.v. as effective treatment of acute attacks can be considered.

In cases of *migraine accompagnée* the authors have discovered empirically that a combination of

- **Secale olpx dil.** Madaus and
- **Cyclamen olpx dil.** Madaus
  is astonishingly effective.

Substantial administration of *magnesium* in sufficiently high dosages has proven beneficial in many cases.

7.11 Enuresis nocturna

7.11.1 Pathogenesis as the starting point for treatment

In connection with his depiction of tuberculosis, R. Steiner discusses in fundamental terms the nature of the *elimination activity* of the human organism: “One must, however, in order to appreciate this matter completely, know a bit about the close inward connection which all elimination processes … have with what otherwise encompasses emotional and mental activity. The synthesising processes … are merely the foundation of the unconscious. That which corresponds to the waking, conscious, emotional-organic activities involves excretion processes in all realms.” Using the example of the role played by night sweat for tuberculosis R. Steiner describes a *dissociation* of bodily excretion activity on the one hand and emotional and mental activity on the other. As he proposes, this is founded on the fact that “the upper” aspect – the soul and spirit forces of formation and consciousness which issue from the head pole and induce bodily catabolic processes – and “the lower” aspect, to which the anabolic processes of metabolism as well as the organs which perform excretion activity belong – do not have the proper interrelationship: “Because the upper aspect does not have the proper interrelationship with the lower aspect something is saved up for the night when the organism gets a respite from its mental-emotional activity" [Steiner 1999, 47].

This aspect illuminates various phenomena of enuresis nocturna:

7.11.1.1 Delayed maturing process

Bed-wetting is defined as several involuntary night-time urinations per week from the age of five [Steinhausen 2012, 273]. Up until the age of 12 the symptoms will spontaneously disappear each year in just under a seventh of affected children. It is evident that bed-wetting represents a maturation delay rather than a medical condition. – Physiologically the first seven-year period of life is characterized by a *permeating of the body by the soul and spirit, starting from the head downwards.* The development of directed movement in an infant, for example, starts with the eyes and head, proceeds with the arms and finally reaches the legs and feet. The same applies to the development of uprightness. At the same time the pure anabolic-assimilating processes decrease, which is expressed in the decreasing growth rate. The conscious regulation of bowel movement is developed in this process, at a pace that is individual and, especially, *constitutional.* Paedagogical mistakes – such as toilet training at the wrong phase of development with psychologically inhibiting methods – can strongly increase bed-wetting. Conversely, the maturing process is encouraged through relevant behavioural therapy measures. These are based on paedagogical precepts [Steinhausen 2012, 278]:

- Appropriate age (the child should be at least six years old for a Doctor-led behaviour-therapy)
- No more use of nappies (diapers)
- Positive cooperation from child *and* parents
- The genetic aspect

A family history of bed-wetting is a known factor, "only a third develop the symptoms… without affected relatives" [Steinhausen 2010, 276]. *Biologically*, especially physically, the child is a descendent of its parents (unlike its soul-spiritual individuality). The speed with which the soul-spiritual individuality of the child can permeate the body seems to also depend on the bodily conditions.

7.11.1.2 Hormonal aspect

In endocrine control of renal excretion activity the interrelationship between the upper and the lower organism referred to by R. Steiner becomes vivid at once. This is usually regulated by a *day-night rhythm* (cf. ▸Chap. 7.1), which develops early on in the first septennial. It normally leads to a situation in which emotional-conscious activity of the individual is focused on the day, thus running parallel to renal excretion activity (the connection between urination and nervousness is familiar to everyone). In contrast, anabolic processes – the ones related to plant growth – predominate during the night and are accompanied by a strong reduction of excretion. This rhythm is regulated in part with the help of the *pituitary gland as overarching, central control organ.* By virtue of its very shape and location this organ shows that it is involved in the interrelationship between "upper" and "lower", consciousness-related and anabolic processes; it lies *below* the brain, consists of two different complexes (coming from "above" and "below" respectively) and as an endocrine organ it is located in the *middle* between the hypothalamus (as the intracerebral control region) and the so-called peripheral effectors in the organism.

In many children nocturnal enuresis is related to an immaturity of the rhythmic system, especially the day/night rhythm that on the one hand is expressed in a belated awakening („Arousal-Dysfunction" [Moll et al. 1999]) and on the other hand in an inadequately formed circadian rhythm of anti diuretic hormone secretion. – Because in the second year of life the emphasis is on the ripening of the rhythmic system [Husemann and Wolff 1986, 36–44], it becomes understandable that at that time a high rate of spontaneous healing can be observed. – A treatment with hormone analogues (DDVAP) is a purely symptomatic substitution that can, if at all, be justified as a short term solution (for a school trip, for example): The relapse rate after discontinuation is about 100 % [Moll et al. 1999], the treatment is not without risk (electrolyte fluctuations) and, like any hormone replacement during childhood development, disturbs maturing. There are, in the author's opinion, no indications for prescribing the tricyclic antidepressant Imipramin. The effects of DDVAP and Imipramin "do not outlast the discontinuation of the medication" [Steinhausen 2010, 280].

7.11.1.3 Delayed pneumatization

Many children with nocturnal enuresis show a disturbed inhalation (adenoid or tonsil hypertrophy, relapsing and chronic rhinitis, breathing through the mouth and adenoid facial features). W. Holtzapfel [1995, 47] has pointed out this correlation, often found clinically as a concurrence of symptoms. The paediatrician will often find that enuresis increases or decreases parallel to impediments, particularly of nasal breathing. This is related to the influx of forming catabolic forces into the organism through the breathing process, the pneumatization (▸Chap. 5.1.2). This connection highlights that a maturation delay in the upper region of the child related to the astral body (compare also the function of the pituitary gland!) induced a respective weakness in the lower region of the child, because in the first seven years of life the forming of the "lower" region is dependent on the forming of the "upper" region. A very important therapy in this context is eurythmy therapy.

7.11.1.4 Soul-psychological disorders

The anthroposophic study of man clearly shows how the part of the soul connected to the body – which expresses itself particularly through the breathing, the inner (endocrine) secretion and the secretion directed outwards – on the one hand and the emotional, conscious soul-experiences on the other hand are connected to the same entity (the astral body). – Relatively undisputed is the correlation between certain forms of (especially secondary) nocturnal enuresis, with *psychosocial and family stress* (for example divorce of the parents, shocking experiences, etc.). Many children with nocturnal enuresis, moreover, show psychological anomalies that should be valued more as expressions of one-sided constitutional conditions and less as psychopathology. An important harmonization can be obtained by a therapy with potentized medicines, for example. – In any case, *secondary psychological stress* caused by the nocturnal enuresis itself must also be taken into account. Because these stresses are very dependent on the handling of the disorder, the interpretation of the disorder conveyed by the doctor to the parents is of paramount importance: what positive perspectives can he impart to the child?

7.11.2 Treatment

The necessary differential diagnostics are assumed to be known. – Behavioural measures cannot be presented here in detail (see scientific literature). The authors observe that for *motivated the school age children wake-up devices are very likely to succeed*, often already after 2–3 weeks – and, in the absence of further pathology (such as disorders in pneumatization and of the upper respiratory tract; mental disorders), these devices are also recommended and used in the authors' practice. This is consistent with the general therapeutic experience, according to which this therapy shows the highest cure rate [Steinhausen 2010, 278], even though it is just a device-based behavioural conditioning therapy. It is crucial that the procedure is explained to the child and that the child wants the therapy. In the author's opinion, such a "therapeutic contract" between doctor, child and parents legitimates the use of such a mechanical technique (in the same way that an alarm clock is allowed for school age children). Age is important (>6 years) and a favourable moment (not close to large celebrations or exciting events), so that the conditioned learning effect can consolidate itself.

Paedagogical advice is given, for example, by parent guidebooks [Goebel and Glöckler 2008, 515–519]; those interested will find a discussion of eurythmy therapy in more advanced works [Kirchner-Bockholt 1991, 154–157]. Eurythmy therapy has the capacity to increase the creative activity of the soul aspect in the bodily realm to a particular degree, for example when enuresis is accompanied by adenoids, tonsil hypertrophy and dysfunctional pneumatization. Through – therapeutically guided – eurythmic movement the child actively limits lymphatic vegetation in the upper human being and the excretion processes in the lower human being.

In terms of eurythmy therapy, the *sound "F"* is a specifically effective sound for enuresis if it is articulated in the corresponding fashion (accompanied by a leap) [cf. Kirchner-Bockholt 1997, 154–157]. It promotes maturation of the child's organism in the area of the efferent urinary passages. In order to understand the effect of this sound it is helpful to imagine that the child's physical body grows during this process while the life organization and the soul organization contract (thus the life organization exerts a pulling effect on the growing body, as it were!). In many cases of enuresis such contraction (which is a day, i. e. waking-up process) is delayed. This can for example have constitutional causes. Dysfunctional inhalation caused by adenoids can have an inhibitive effect here and difficult emotional situations can hinder this inner consolidation process, the "coalescence of body and soul" in the child, as well. – Thus it is all the more important to induce a child to engage in activity, to make movements himself which allow his development and maturation to proceed!

If *emotional duress* plays a role for the symptomology of enuresis the vocal *"I" can be of supplementary benefit as a vocalic exercise* (cf. ▸Chap. 7.3.3). For a discussion of eurythmy therapy in cases of dysfunctional pneumatization cf. ▸Chap. 5.1.2.6.

The "F"-exercise is primarily supplemented by the sound "B," which helps the child envelope and isolate himself better and which supports the contraction process characterized above. "B" and "P" both have a specific stimulating effect on the emotionally regulatory activity in the kidney-bladder region. – And lastly, when treating children with enuresis nocturna it is always important to *direct one's attention to the back* from the perspective of eurythmy therapy (observing posture, warmth distribution, tension and muscle tone disorders).

In the following, recommendations on external and internal use of remedies can be made but this always only constitutes one aspect of therapy. The depicted medicaments have no substitutive effect limited to the application but rather exert a *maturation-inducing, stimulating* effect on the child's organism.

7.11.2.1 External applications

- Brief cool showers or ablutions on lower abdomen
  stimulate I activity is this area via warmth organization. They should have a stimulating effect but not be emotionally injurious and be administered accordingly.
- Inunctions on the insides of the thighs and possibly in the lumbosacral region with **Hypericum Flos 25 % oil** Weleda, **ex herba 5 %** oil Wala
  stimulate light forces in this area. – Through combined stimulation of warmth and light forces via the skin (and thus also the nerve-sense system!) the astral body and the I are anchored in the corresponding organ region more strongly. The "sense of life" [Soesman 1995, 13–40] is stimulated which forms in the first septennial.
- Bladder compresses (warmed) overnight with **Eucalyptus Oleum 10 %** Wala
  have a comprehensive warming and slightly toning effect on the bladder region. They are particularly appropriate in cases of a susceptibility to a dysfunction of the bladder wall muscles, in cases of a susceptibility to cystitis and in general in children prone to hypothermia. The latter should also be followed by warmth treatment of the calves and foot soles in the evenings, for example, by rubbing with
- **Cuprum met. 0.4 % ointment** Weleda.

Hypothermia and abnormalities of warmth distribution in the lower organs and the kidney region do not only impair the therapeutic process: they themselves constitute a finding that needs treatment!

7.11.2.2 Internal medication

7.11.2.2.1 Initial treatment

The aim of this treatment is to achieve an *order and maturation* of the organism through which the astral and etheric body of the child connect better. – Potentized sulphur is primarily taken into consideration if the dysfunction has more to do with the vital constitution of the child; in the event that the cause has more to do with irregularities in the soul organization, of the astral body, Tuberculin is an important, constitutionally effective medicine.

- **Sulphur D6 trit.** Weleda, frequently **LM6 dil.** Arcana: 1 Saltsp. 3 x/day or 1 × 3–5 gtt./day in the morning

has a generally vitalizing and ordering effect on the life organization so that the latter is inclined to take up impulses of the soul.

Long years of homoeopathic experience have shown that patients are more concerned about cleanliness and orderliness in their surroundings than before – they develop a clearer perception, a more alert sense for that which involves vital processes (including their own excretions). Sulphur is indicated at the beginning of therapy especially for children whose life organization has been impaired and weakened by previously administered suppressive medicaments and the like (D6), but also for children with excessive, uncontrolled vitality and limb activity (LM6).

- **Tuberculinum (Koch) LM6–12 dil.** Arcana/**C200 pillules** Gudjons
  is a very valuable modulating medicament which corresponds directly to the constitutional situation described by R. Steiner [1999, 41] in the passage quoted at the beginning of this section; thus functional disorders of activity in the lower organism result from the upper organism not being strong enough in its correspondence to really grasp the lower one in its entirety." The soul aspect is not effective enough in its bond with the body; it is "too active spiritually," which can lead to neurasthenic weakness of the lower human organization.

Symptomatically conspicuous are:

- chronic recurrent inflammatory disorders of the respiratory tract (including allergic inflammations), for example recurrent otitis, bronchitis, recurrent tonsillitis and susceptibility towards asthma,
- inflammation can also occur in the urinary tract, most of all following respiratory infections,
- behaviours such as restlessness, fluctuating concentration, emotional imbalance,
- weakness of warmth organization, susceptibility to cold.

7.11.2.2.2 Further treatment

One must primarily differentiate three lines of treatment focusing on:

- disturbance of day-night rhythms,
- delayed pneumatization, bodily constitution
- psychosomatic disorders.

Immaturity and *disturbance of the day-night rhythm* (which can even lead, in extreme cases, to a reversal of rhythm in regard to urination) constitutes an indication for therapy using *Equisetum* (cf. ▸Chap. 6.3.3.3). The form of the Equisetum plant, which is completely reduced to the stem principle (related to light), and the siliceous content of this plant (in opal form) attest directly to its relation to formative processes; its habitat and growing conditions attest to its relation to the watery element and its capacity for organization and the relatively high sulphur content attest to its relation to vital-anabolic life processes. – The affinity to the kidneys and urination is generally known; the relationship to enuresis nocturna is also documented in the homoeopathic repertorium; R. Steiner [1980, 21] describes the relationship between Equisetum and the kidneys in terms of spiritual science.

It is therapeutically beneficial to strengthen the activity of the kidneys in the morning hours by administering Equisetum which has been roasted and then potentized together with and to then accentuate the silica-related formative side by a specially rhythmicized and subsequently potentized horsetail preparation:

- **Equisetum cum Sulfure tostum D6 trit.** Weleda
  in the morning and at midday 1 saltsp.,
- **Equisetum ex herba D15 pillules** Wala
  in the evening 5–7 pillules.

Another key medicament in this context is

- **Bryophyllum Argento cultum D2/Rh D3 dil.** Weleda
  primarily in the evening 5–7 drops (D2)/10–15 drops (Rh D3).

This medicament is indicated for children with "hysterical constitution" as described by anthroposophic anthropology. The *outflowing, insufficiently delimited nature of such children* manifests itself in enuresis nocturna and nocturnal sleep disorders with anxiety. Such children react strongly to stimuli and impulses in their surroundings, have a tendency towards restlessness and weepiness, are afflicted with anxiety and have a close mother bond. Shock experiences can be a significant factor in their medical history (cf. ▸Chap. 2.2.3).

Children with delayed pneumatization, respond best to rhythmical Einreibungen with

- **Oleum Salviae 10 %** (cf. ▸Chap. 5.1.3.3)

These stimulate the soul organization – the astral body – to penetrate the "lower organization" more strongly, at the same time enabling the decrease of the adenoids. They are particularly recommended for this form of enuresis (see above 7.11.1.3).

Internally, these children respond to potentized calcium salts, particularly against the background of constitutionally induced (partial) developmental delays:

- **Calcium iodatum D12 pillules** (various producers)

in case of thin, thirsty, erethistic children with adenoids;

- **Calcium phosphoricum D12 pillules** (various producers)

in case of rather skinny, anorectic, dissatisfied children (see remarks about Tuberculinum above!) with tonsil hyperplasia.

- **Conchae D6-12-20 trit.** Weleda:

in case of anxious, calm, slowly developing children susceptible to the cold, chronic rhinitis, with a propensity to adenoids, (soft) lymphe node swelling.

In case of children with *psychosomatic conspicuities* or disorders, there are primarily two potentized drugs that come into consideration: Causticum and Sepia.

- **Sepia D12, LM6–12 dil.** (various producers)
  1–2 × 5 gtt. per day

is advised in case of lively children who show a whiny hypersensitivity (noli me tangere!) combined with apparently aggressive traits. They enjoy being active, like to dance and often occupy the centre stage. In their case, an inner tension can be sensed, which is also quite often the case with the mother, who feels herself divided in ambivalence between her wish for professional activity and the strongly felt obligation of her role as a mother.

- **Causticum D12 dil.** (various producers)
  5 gtt. every evening or 2 × 5 gtt. per day.

is effective in the case of introverted, sensitive, mentally restrained children, who may radiate restrained sadness (▸Chap. 7.2).

- **Aurum/Apis regina comp. pillules** Wala
  1–3 x/d 7 pillules

has a reassuring and elucidative effect in case of anxious, depressive, mentally strained children. For these children, it can also be very effective in case of enuresis nocturna.

Sepia and Causticum are complimentary to each other and may be needed successively in the course of the treatment. Thus, they affect different layers of the child's soul-physical dynamics which only become apparent in the course of the treatment.

The *organization of the family evening* plays a therapeutically significant role for children suffering from enuresis nocturna, especially when psychosomatic disorders are in the background. A stable temporal order after approx. 6 p. m. constitutes a basis that has a direct regulative effect on the life organization during childhood. The presence and inner devotion of mother *and father* at that time is particularly important: the evening should be arranged in such a way that it offers the *opportunity for a harmonization of the soul.* If external influences (telephone, video and computer games) are kept away at this time, the family can evolve their own connection. The joint dinner, a game, a story, but also the parents' listening, when the child expresses something about what is happening in its soul – all this can help the child to mature psychologically and to find more harmony.

7.12 Diurnal enuresis

The treatment of this problem, which mostly occurs among boys at preschool age, is not easy. Today we diagnostically speak of "functional urinary incontinence", including

- urge incontinence (pollakisuria, decreased bladder capacity, use of holding manoeuvres)
- urinary incontinence with voiding postponement (the child continues his or her activity without interruption until urination spontaneously starts).
- detruser-sphincter dyscoordination (urodynamic disturbances) [Steinhausen 2010, 273]

From a holistic point of view the affected children frequently exhibited difficulties integrating adequately into their peer group, while having close, but for both sides ambivalent, parental bonds. The child cannot stabilize himself psychologically between regressive desires (diurnal enuresis is physiological for the infant) and an aggressive desire for autonomy and power over others. A mature play with these extremes is not yet successful. – The effectiveness of therapy with anticholingerics is often not particularly convincing. It does not really address the context described.

- **Digitalis purpurea D6 dil.** Apotheke an der Weleda
  3 × daily 5 drops administered over relatively long periods of time (months)

In potentized form, Digitalis is an important medicament for promoting maturation of the rhythmic system and thus also emotional development (cf. ▸Chap. 7.10.2).

Sufficient presence of the father plays a key role here, but the father must have achieved sufficient autonomy in regard to his wife/partner and to his mother (!) while at the same time training his child through transparent guidance to accept rules and develop age- and gender-appropriate activities.

It is also important for the parents to make sure the child carries out all steps to be taken after enuresis such as changing clothes, washing themselves and cleaning up, performing these tasks alone but in the presence of the parents, thus ensuring that the child is alert and responsible during the process which initially occurs semi-consciously.

Finally, one can infer from remarks made by R. Steiner on bladder function [Steiner 1999, 178] that it is helpful for the parents to encourage the child to chew and digest carefully and to take age-appropriate hikes in the mountains with the child in their free time.

These promote the maturation of the soul aspect through exposure to light in the mountain landscape and changed respiration.

Detrusor-sphincter-dyscoordination is an indication for eurythmy therapy (cf. 7.11.).

Casuistic

An eight-year-old boy with Down's syndrome who suffered a stroke at the age of one, battled with in part life-threatening laryngitis accompanied by acute hypoxaemia in his 2nd and 3rd year of life, exhibited a very pronounced mental disability in the framework of Down's syndrome, manifested impulsive and aggressive behaviour and was hardly able to communicate. When about to start school, this boy developed therapy-resistant (and due to the odour it caused very objectionable) enuresis diurna. From a homoeopathic perspective one could speak of a "luetic," destructive miasma here; from the perspective of anthroposophic medicine one could speak of a severe disorder of the rhythmic system (stroke, stenosing laryngitis, but also enuresis diurna). In this case administration of potentized fluoric acid,

- **Acidum fluoricum C12 pillules** Gudjons
  daily 5 pillules in the morning,

proved beneficial; it is the only Grade 3 (Grades 1 to 3 display increasing "fit" or effectiveness of the medicament) medicament among the seven medicaments listed in the Synthesis Repertorium for "Urinating – involuntary – during the day." The reason for the selection of this medicament was the relationship of the chemical nature of fluoric acid to the pathology of this patient: fluoric acid is the most aggressive chemical substance known; it has a penetratingly destructive effect, even on glass containers and it transforms everything it attacks into insoluble fluorine salts. This substance, as well as its homoeopathic proving picture, is materially-destructive in nature. In the human being, that which is the hardest, the most substantially aggressive – dental enamel – is formed by the organization of fluoric forces. – In the case of the depicted patient the potentized fluoric acid was able to relieve the internally and externally excessive, aggressive dynamics to the point that the enuresis diurna disappeared and the patient's entire behaviour, his capacity to learn and communicate, changed for the better. The health of the boy has become very stable. It was necessary for him to take the medication for over a year.

References for Chapter 7

(every reference marked with a ▪ Bullet point indicates the English translation of the reference above it)

Affolter, F.: Wahrnehmung, Wirklichkeit und Sprache. 8. Aufl. Neckar-Verlag, Villingen-Schwenningen 1997.

Aust-Claus, E., P.-M. Hammer: Das ADS-Buch. 5. Aufl. Oberstebrink, Ratingen 2001.

Baumann, T.: Atlas der Entwicklungsdiagnostik. Thieme, Stuttgart 2.Aufl. 2006.

Barbely, A.: Das Geheimnis des Schlafs. DVA, Stuttgart 1984; zit. nach Heimann 1989, 216.

Blakemore, C.: The mind machine. BBC Publications, London 1988.

Christ, B.: Entwicklung der craniocervicalen Übergangsregion: In: Humanembryologie. Hinrichsen, V. (Hrsg.). Springer Verlag, Berlin 1990.

Coulter, C.: Porträts homöopathischer Arzneimittel, Bd. 1, 2. Aufl. Haug Verlag, Heidelberg 1989.

7

Deeg et al.: Ist der plötzliche Kindstod Folge einer lageabhängigen Minderperfusion des Hirnstammes? MSchr. f. Kinderheilk. **146**, 597–602 (1998).
Deterding, E.: Diagnostik und Therapie der Schlafstörungen (II). Beitr. zu einer Erw. d. Heilk. **17**, 135 (1964).
Egger, J.: Möglichkeiten von Diätbehandlungen bei hyperkinetischen Störungen. In: Hyperkinetische Störungen bei Kindern, Jugendlichen und Erwachsenen. Steinhausen, H. C. (Hrsg.). Kohlhammer, Stuttgart 1. Aufl. 1995, 2. Aufl. 2000.
Egle, U. T., C. Derra, W. A. Nix, R. Schwab: Spezielle Schmerztherapie. Schattauer, Stuttgart 1999.
Elder, T.: The importance of relative standards in ADHDdiagnoses: Evidence based on exact birth dates. Journal of Health Economics **29,** 641–656.
Endres, K.-P., W. Schad: Biologie des Mondes. S. Hirzel Verlag, Stuttgart 1997.
Engel, W.: Gold im Zusammenklang mit Weihrauch und Myrrhe in der Arzneimittelherstellung. Der Merkurstab **60,** 517–521 (2007a).
Engel, W.: Eisen, Wein und Essig – zur Herstellung von Kephalodoron und Ferrum hydroxydatum. Der Merkurstab **59** (2006).
Engel, H. H., König, K., Müller-Wiedemann, H.: Über schwere Kontaktstörungen im Kindesalter und deren Behandlung mit der Substanz Thalamos.
Ferber, R.: Solve our child's sleep problems. Simon & Schuster, New York 1985.
Frei, H.: Die homöopathische Behandlung von Kindern mit ADS/ADHS. Haug Verlag, Heidelberg 2005.
Freud, A., D. T. Burlingham: Infants without families. Int. Univ. Press, New York 1943.
Freud, A.: Wege und Irrwege in der Kinderentwicklung. Klett-Cotta, Stuttgart 1993; zit. nach Nissen 1989b.
Fuchs, T.: Leib, Raum, Person. Klett-Cotta, Stuttgart 2000.
Fuchs, T.: Das Gehirn – ein Beziehungsorgan. Kohlhammer, Stuttgart 2008.
Gavidia-Payne, S., Stoneman, Z.: Marital adjustment in families of young children with disabilities: associations with daily hassles and problem-focused coping. Am J Ment Retard **111**, 1–14 [2006].
Girke, M.: Innere Medizin. Salumed, Berlin 2010.
- English translation in progress at this time – Ed.
Gnaiger, J.: Lac caninum. In: Doc. Homoeop. **10**, 99–118. Maudrich Verlag, Wien 1990.
Gnaiger, J.: Angst, Sehnsucht und Unvermögen bei Lac caninum. In: Doc. Homoeop. **11**, 171–186. Maudrich Verlag, Wien 1991 (und Vortrag Köln 1991 zur Verl. des S.-Hahnemann-Preises).
Gnaiger, J.: Medorrhinum – eine Arznei für "moderne Kinder". Allg. Homöopath. Ztg. **247**, 91–100 (2002).
Goebel, W., M. Glöckler: Kindersprechstunde. 17. Aufl. Urachhaus, Stuttgart 2008.
- Gloeckler, M., Goebel, W.: A guide to child health. Floris Books, Edinburgh 2003.
Grandgeorge, D.: Homöopathische Arzneimittelbilder in der Kinderheilkunde. 2. Aufl. Sonntag Verlag, Regensburg 2004.
Hamre, H. J., Witt, C. et al.: Anthroposophic therapy for attention deficit hyperactivity: a two-year prospective study in outpatients. Int J General Medicine **3**, 239–253 (2010).
Hee, H., Foerster, G.: Homöopathische Behandlung von Jugendlichen Haug Verlag, Stuttgart 2008.
Heide, P. von der: Therapie mit geistig-seelischen Mitteln. Verlag am Goetheanum, Dornach 1997.
Heimann, R.: Der Rhythmus und seine Bedeutung für die Heilpädagogik. Urachhaus, Stuttgart 1989.
Hellbrügge, T., J. Lange, J. Rutenfranz, K. Stehr: Über das Entstehen einer 24-Stunden-Periodik physiologischer Funktionen im Säuglingsalter. Fortschr. Med. **81**, 19–26 (1963).
Hellbrügge, T.: Zeitliche Strukturen in der kindlichen Entwicklung. MSchr. f. Kinderheilk. **113**, 252–263 (1965).

Hellwig/Otto: Arzneimittel. Wissenschaftliche Verlagsgesellschaft, Stuttgart, 11. Auflage 2010.

Herscu, P.: Die homöopathische Behandlung der Kinder. Kai Kröger Verlag, Groß Wittensee 1993.

- Hercsu, P. The homeopathic treatment of children: pediatric constitutional types. North Atlantic Books, Berkeley, C. A. 1991.

Hildebrandt, G.: Die rhythmische Funktionsordnung von Puls und Atmung. Zschr. f. angewandte Bäder- und Klimaheilk. 7, 533–615 (1960).

Hildebrandt, G., M. Moser, M. Lehofer: Chronobiologie und Chronomedizin. Hippokrates, Stuttgart 1998.

Holtzapfel, W.: Seelenpflegebedürftige Kinder. 5. Aufl. Verlag am Goetheanum, Arelsheim 1995.

- Holtzapfel, W.: Children's destinies : the three directions of human development. Mercury Press, Spring Valley, N. Y. c1977; 1981. This is the English publication of Seelenpflegebedürftige Kinder, vol. 1. Vol. 2 of Dr. Holtzapfel's work was published in English as: Children with a difference. Lanthorn Press, East Grinstead, England 1995.

Hübner, W. D., T. Kirste: Experience with St. John's Worth (Hypericum perforatum) in children under 12 years with symptoms of depression and psychovegetative disturbances. Phytother. Res. **15**, 367–370 (2001).

Husemann, A.: Der hörende Mensch und die Wirklichkeit der Musik. Verlag Freies Geistesleben, Stuttgart 2010.

Husemann, F.: Digitalis purpurea und die Herzbewegung. Der Merkurstab **2**, 39–48 (1985); **3**, 80–85 (1985).

Husemann, F.: Anthroposophische Medizin. Verlag am Goetheanum, Dornach 2009.

Husemann, F., O. Wolff: Das Bild des Menschen als Grundlage der Heilkunst. 4. Aufl. Verlag Freies Geistesleben, Stuttgart 1991.

- Huseman, F. Wolff, O.: The Anthroposophical approach to medicine: v. 1, 2. Steiner Books, Great Barrington, M. A. 1983, v.3 Mercury Press, Spring Valley, N. Y. 2003.

Husemann, F., O. Wolff: Das Bild des Menschen als Grundlage der Heilkunst. Bd. II. Verlag Freies Geistesleben, Stuttgart 4. Aufl. 1986, 6. Aufl. 2000.

- Huseman, F. Wolff, O.: The Anthroposophical approach to medicine: v. 1, 2. Steiner Books, Great Barrington, M. A. 1983, v.3 Mercury Press, Spring Valley, N. Y. 2003.

Husemann, G.: Die Dynamik der Aufrichtekraft. Beitr. z. Erw. d. Heilk. **2**, 46–51 (1965).

Huss, M. et al.: How often are German children and adolescents diagnosed with ADHD? Prevalence based on the judgment of health care professionals: results of the German health and examination survey (KiGGS). Eur Child Adolec Psychiatry [Suppl 1] (2008).

Imhäuser, H.: Homöopathie in der Kinderheilkunde. 12. Aufl. Haug Verlag, Heidelberg 2000.

Jan et al.: Sleep Hygiene for Children with Neurodevelopmental Disabilities. Paediatrics **122,** 1343–1350 (2008).

Kain, W. et al.: Komorbidität bei ADHS. MSchr Kinderheilk **156,** 757–767 (2008).

Kast-Zahn, A., H. Morgenroth: Erfahrungen und praktische Hinweise für den Umgang mit Schlafproblemen im Säuglings- und Kindesalter. Der Kinderarzt **26/1**, 46–52; **26/2**, 204–212 (1995).

Kast-Zahn, A., H. Morgenroth: Jedes Kind kann schlafen lernen. 4. Aufl. Oberstebrink, Ratingen 1997; Gräfe & Unzer, 1. Aufl. 2007.

Kaul, R.: Johanniskraut. Wissenschaftliche Verlagsgesellschaft, Stuttgart 2000.

Kirchner-Bockholt, M.: Grundelemente der Heileurythmie. Verlag am Goetheanum 3. Aufl. 1991, 4. Aufl. 1997.

- Kirchner-Bockholt, M.: Fundamental principles of curative eurythmy. Rudolf Steiner Press, London 1977.

Köhler, H.: Von ängstlichen, traurigen und unruhigen Kindern. Verlag Freies Geistesleben, Stuttgart 2. Aufl. 1994, 4. Aufl. 1997.
Köhler, H.: War Michel aus Lönneberga aufmerksamkeitsgestört? Verlag Freies Geistesleben, Stuttgart 2002.
Konofal, E. et al.: Iron deficiency in children with attention-deficit/Hyperactivity disorder. Arch. Pediatr. Adolesc. Med. **115**, 1113–1115 (2004).
Kraenz et al.: Häufigkeit und Belastungsfaktoren bei Schlafstörungen im Einschulungsalter. Praxis der Kinderpsychologie und Kinderpsychiatrie **53**, 3–18 (2004).
Kraker von Schwarzenfeld, B.: Riech doch mal! Erfahrungen mit einer Riechtherapie bei Kindern mit ADHS-Konstellation. Medizinisch-Pädagogische Konferenz **35**, 46–57 (2005).
Kummer, K. R.: Hyperaktives Verhalten im Kindesalter. Erziehungskunst **9**, 872–884 (1992).
Kunz, C.: Von edlen Baumharzen. Der Merkurstab **62**, 152–158 (2009).
Largo, R.: Babyjahre. Piper, München, Zürich 2001.
Leitlinien zur Diagnostik und Therapie von psychischen Störungen im Säuglings-, Kindes- und Jugendalter. Deutscher Ärzte Verlag, Köln 2003.
Lehmkuhl, G., Wiater, A. et al.: Schlafstörungen im Einschulungsalter – Ursachen und Auswirkungen. Deutsches Ärzteblatt **105**, 809–814.
Lewin, L.: Gifte und Vergiftungen. 6. Aufl. Haug Verlag, Heidelberg 1992.
Liem, T.: Kraniosakrale Osteopathie. 5. Aufl., Hippokrates Stuttgart 2010.
Lorenz, K.: Über tierisches und menschliches Verhalten. Piper, München 1965.
Madaus: Lehrbuch der biologischen Heilmittel, Bd. 2. Olms Verlag, Hildesheim 1979, 1999a.
McCann, D. et al.: Food additives and hyperactive behaviour in 3-year-old and 8/9 year-old children in the community: a randomised, double-blinded, placebo-controlled trial: Lancet **370**, 1560–1567 (2007).
Moll, G., A. Rothenberger: Neurobiologische Grundlagen. Ein pathophysiologisches Erklärungsmodell der ADHD. Kinderärztliche Praxis (2001), Sonderheft "Unaufmerksam und hyperaktiv", 9–15.
Moll, G. H., M. Wicker, A. Rothenberger: Zentralnervöse Regulationsmechanismen bei isolierter Enuresis nocturna. MSchr. Kinderheilk. **147**, 90–98 (1999).
Morrison, R.: Handbuch der homöopathischen Leitsymptome. Kai Kröger Verlag, Groß Wittensee 1995.
Morrison, R.: Handbuch der Pathologie zur homöopathischen Differentialdiagnose. Kai Kröger Verlag, Groß Wittensee 1999.
Murgatroyd, C. et al.: Dynamic DNA methylation programs persistent adverse effects of earla-life stress. Nature neuroscience, published online doi:10.1038/nn.2436 (2009).
Müller, K.-J.: Materia Medica Müller 2.0. Selbstverlag K.-J.Müller, Zweibrücken, 2009.
Müller-Wiedemann, H.: Mitte der Kindheit. Verlag Freies Geistesleben, Stuttgart 4. Aufl. 1993, 5. Aufl. 1999.
Nelson textbook of paediatrics. 17th ed. W. B. Saunders, Philadelphia 2003.
Neraal, T., Wildermuth, M. (Hg): ADHS. Symptome verstehen – Beziehungen verändern. Psychosozial Verlag, Gießen 2008.
Neuhaus, C.: Hyperaktive Jugendliche und ihre Probleme. Urania-Ravensburger, Berlin 2000.
Neuhaus, C.: Das hyperaktive Kind und seine Probleme. Urania-Ravensburger, Berlin 1999.
Neuhaus, C.: ADHS bei Kindern, Jugendlichen und Erwachsenen. Kohlhammer, Stuttgart 2007.
Nickel, R., U. T. Egle: Therapie somatoformer Schmerzstörungen. Schattauer, Stuttgart 1999.
Nissen, G.: Angstsyndrom. In: Kinder- und Jugendpsychiatrie. Eggers, G., R. Lempp, G. Nissen, P. Strunk (Hrsg.). 5. Aufl. Springer Verlag, Berlin 1989a.

Nissen, G.: Depressionssyndrom. In: Kinder- und Jugendpsychiatrie. Eggers, G., R. Lempp, G. Nissen, P. Strunk (Hrsg.). 5. Aufl. Springer Verlag, Berlin 1989b.

Nissen, G.: Aggressivität. In: Kinder- und Jugendpsychiatrie. Eggers, G., R. Lempp, G. Nissen, P. Strunk (Hrsg.). 5. Aufl. Springer Verlag, Berlin 1989c.

Pädagogische Forschungsstelle beim Bund der Freien Waldorfschulen Stuttgart (Hrsg.): Studienmaterial der Waldorfkindergärten: die zwölf Sinne des Menschen. 4. Aufl. Stuttgart 1993.

Palmstierna P. et al.: Parent perceptions of child sleep: a study of 10.000 Swedish children. Acta paediatrica **97,** 1631–1639.

Papousek, M., M. Schieche, H. Wurmser: Regulationsstörungen der frühen Kindheit. Huber Verlag, Bern 2004.

Patzlaff, R.: Kindheit verstummt. Sonderdruck aus: Erziehungskunst **63** (7/8), 7 (1999).

Patzlaff, R.: Der gefrorene Blick. Die physiologische Wirkung des Fernsehens und die Entwicklung des Kindes. Verlag Freies Geistesleben, Stuttgart 2000.

Petermann, F. und U.: Schulangst. MSchr Kinderheilkunde **158,** 391–400.

Pohl, W.: Das Aufmerksamkeitsdefizitsyndrom menschenkundlich betrachtet. Der Merkurstab **55,** 294–298 (2002).

Reichenberg-Ullmann, J., R. Ullmann: Ritalin. 2. Aufl. Michaelsverlag, Peiting 2002.

Riemann, F.: Grundformen der Angst. Reinhardt, München, 31. Aufl. 1999.

Roemer, F., M. Sommer: Zur Bedeutung der potenzierten Organpräparate in der anthroposophischen Therapierichtung. Der Merkurstab, Sonderheft Organpräparate, **51,** 4 (1999).

Roder, F.: Mondknoten im Lebenslauf. Verlag Freies Geistesleben, Stuttgart 2005.

Rohen, J.W: Eine funktionelle und spirituelle Anthropologie. Verlag Freies Geistesleben, Stuttgart 2010.

Roßlenbroich, B.: Die rhythmische Organisation des Menschen. Verlag Freies Geistesleben, Stuttgart 1994.

Roth, G.: Worüber dürfen Hirnforscher reden – und in welcher Weise? Deutsche Zeitschrift für Philosophie **5,** 691–705 (2004).

Roth, G.: Erkenntnis und Realität. Das reale Gehirn und seine Wirklichkeit. In: S. J. Schmidt (Hg): Der Diskurs des radikalen Konstruktivismus. Suhrkamp, Frankfurt/M. 1994.

Sant'Unione, A. M., M. Wildermuth: Zur Therapie des Hyperkinetischen Syndroms inkl. seiner Unterformen (ADS, ADHS, hyperkinetische Störung des Sozialverhaltens). Forum für Kinder- und Jugendpsychiatrie **17** (2,3) 2007.

Schad, W.: Die Vorgeburtlichkeit des Menschen. Der Entwicklungsgedanke in der Embryologie. Verlag Freies Geistesleben, Stuttgart 1982.

Schmidt, R. F., G. Thews: Physiologie des Menschen. 26. Aufl. Springer Verlag, Berlin 1995.

Schmidt, A., M. Meusers, U. Momsen: Wo ein Wille ist, aber kein Weg – Aufmerksamkeitsdefizitsyndrom mit und ohne Hyperaktivität. Der Merkurstab **56,** 181–195 (2003).

Schmidt, A.: Vorwort, Der Merkurstab **60,** 531–532 (2007).

Schneider, H., Eisenberg, D.: Who receives a diagnosis of attention-deficit/hyperacivity disorder in the United States elementary school population? Paediatrics **117,** e601–609.

Scholten, J: Homöopathie und Minerale. Stichting Alonnissos, Utrecht 1993.

Schuster, B.: Bambus. Kent Gesellschaft 1996.

Seiler, H.: Die Entwicklung von Samuel Hahnemanns ärztlicher Praxis. Haug Verlag, Heidelberg 1988.

Selawry, A.: Metall-Funktionstypen in Psychologie und Medizin. Haug Verlag, Heidelberg 1. Aufl. 1985, 2. Aufl. 1991.

7

Simon, L.: Grundzüge einer anthroposophischen Behandlung der chronischen Polyarthritis. Weleda Korrbl. f. Ärzte **149**, 36–95 (2000).

Soesman, A.: Die zwölf Sinne. Verlag Freies Geistesleben, Stuttgart 1. Aufl. 1995, 4. Aufl. 2000.

- Soeman, A.: The twelve senses. Hawthorn Press, Stroud, U. K. 1990.

Soldner, G.: Helleborus niger. Der Merkurstab **63,** 508–517 (2010).

Sommer, M.: Vorwort. Der Merkurstab **60,** 529–530 (2007).

Spitz, R. A.: Anaclitic depression. An enquiry into the genesis of psychiatric conditions in early childhood. Psychoanal. Study Child **2**, 313–342 (1946).

Spitzer, M.: Vorsicht, Bildschirm! 2. Aufl. Klett Verlag, Stuttgart 2005.

Steiner, R.: Wie erlangt man Erkenntnisse höherer Welten? Rudolf Steiner Verlag, Dornach 24. Aufl. 1993.

- Steiner, R.: Knowledge of the higher worlds : how is it achieved? GA (complete works) 010. Rudolf Steiner Press, London 2004.

Steiner, R.: Die Theosophie des Rosenkreuzers. 7. Aufl. Rudolf Steiner Verlag, Dornach 1985.

- Steiner, R.: Rosicrucian wisdom: an introduction: fourteen lectures given in Munich between 22 May and 6 June 1907. Rudolf Steiner Press, London 2000.

Steiner, R.: Allgemeine Menschenkunde als Grundlage der Pädagogik. Rudolf Steiner Verlag, Dornach Taschenbuchausg. 9. Aufl. 1992.

- Steiner, R.: Study of man: general education course : fourteen lectures given in Stuttgart between 21 August and 5 September 1919. GA (complete works) 293. Rudolf Steiner Press, London 2004. See also: Steiner, R.: Foundations of human experience. GA (complete works) 293. Anthroposophic Press, Hudson, N. Y. 1996.

Steiner, R.: Das Zusammenwirken von Ärzten und Seelsorgern. Pastoralmedizinischer Kurs. Rudolf Steiner Verlag, Dornach 3. Aufl. 1984, 4. Aufl. 1994.

- Steiner, R.: Pastoral medicine: the collegial working of doctors and priests: eleven lectures delivered in Dornach in September of 1924. GA (complete works) 318. Anthroposophic Press, Hudson, N. Y. 1987. Also published as: Broken vessels: the spiritual structure of human frailty. Anthroposophic Press, Great Barrington, M. A. 2003.

Steiner, R.: Die Geheimwissenschaft im Umriss. Gesamtausgabe Bd. 13, Taschenbuchausgabe. Rudolf Steiner Verlag, Dornach Taschenbuchausg. 1. Aufl. 1972, 30. Aufl. 1989.

- Steiner, R.: An outline of esoteric science. GA (complete works) 013. Anthroposophic Press, Hudson, N. Y. 1997. Also pubilshed as: An outline of occult science. GA (complete works 013. Anthroposophic Press, Spring Valley, N. Y. 1972.

Steiner, R.: Heilpädagogischer Kurs. Rudolf Steiner Verlag, Dornach, 8. Aufl. 1995.

- Steiner, R.: Education for special needs: the curative education course; twelve lectures for doctors and teachers given at Dornach between 25 June and 7 July 1924. GA (complete works) 317. Rudolf Steiner Press, London 1998.

Steiner, R.: Meditative Betrachtungen und Anleitungen zur Vertiefung der Heilkunst. Rudolf Steiner Verlag, Dornach 2. Aufl. 1980, 3. Aufl. 1987.

- Steiner, R.: Course for young doctors: meditative contemplations and instructions for deepening the art of healing: lectures for physicians and medical students. GA (complete works) 316. Mercury Press, Spring Valley, N. Y. 1994.

Steiner, R.: Geisteswissenschaft und Medizin. Rudolf Steiner Verlag, Dornach 5. Aufl. 1976, 7. Aufl. 1999.

Steiner, R.: Introduction to anthroposophical medicine. GA (complete works) 312. SteinerBooks, Great Barrington, M. A. 1999.

Steiner, R., I. Wegman: Grundlegendes zu einer Erweiterung der Heilkunst nach geisteswissenschaftlichen Erkenntnissen. Rudolf Steiner Verlag, Dornach, 7th ed. 1991.

- Steiner, R., I. Wegman: Fundamentals of therapy : an extension of the art of healing through spiritual-scientific knowledge. GA (complete works) 027. Mercury Press, Spring Valley, N.Y. 1999. Also available as: Extending practical medicine: fundamental principles based on the science of the spirit. Rudolf Steiner Press, London 1996.

Steiner, R: Die zwölf Sinne im Zusammenhang mit Imagination, Inspiration und Intuition. Taschenbuchausgabe. Rudolf Steiner Verlag Dornach (2005).

Steiner, R.: Konferenzen mit den Lehrern der Freien Waldorfschule in Stuttgart 1919–324. I. Band Rudolf Steiner Verlag, Dornach 1975.

- Steiner, R.: Faculty meetings with Rudolf Steiner : 1919–1924; volumes 1 and 2. GA (complete works) 300a,b,c. Anthroposophic Press, Hudson, N.Y. 1998.

Steinhausen, H.C.: Psychische Störungen bei Kindern und Jugendlichen. 7. Aufl. Urban & Schwarzenberg, München 2010.

Streeck-Fischer, A., Fricke, B.: Lieber unruhig sein als in einem tiefen, dunklen Loch eingesperrt." ADHS aus psychodynamischer Sicht. Praxis der Kinderpsychologie und Kinderpsychiatrie **56**, 277–299 (2007).

Struck, P.: Zwangs- und Angstsyndrome. In: Pädiatrie in Klinik und Praxis. Bachmann, K.-D., H. Ewerbeck, E. Kleihauer, E. Rossi, G. Stadler (Hrsg.). Thieme Verlag, Stuttgart, 2. Aufl. 1989.

Strunk, P.: Respiratorische Affektkrämpfe. In: Kinder- und Jugendpsychiatrie. Eggers, G., R. Lempp, G. Nissen, P. Strunk (Hrsg.). 5. Aufl. Springer Verlag, Berlin 1989a.

Strunk, P.: Stottern. In: Kinder- und Jugendpsychiatrie. Eggers, G., R. Lempp, G. Nissen, P. Strunk (Hrsg.). 5. Aufl. Springer Verlag, Berlin 1989b.

Stübler, M., E. Krug (Hrsg.): Leesers Lehrbuch der Homöopathie. 3. Aufl. Haug Verlag, Heidelberg 1987.

Stübler, M.: Das homöopathische Arzneimittelbild von Aconitum napellus. In: Stübler, M., D. Wolff: Die Hahnenfußgewächse (Ranunculaceen), Quadrivium, Lahnstein 1986.

Stübler, M.: Das schwierige Kind. Acta Homoeopathica **13**(5), 1969.

Uphoff, J.K., Gilmore, J.: Einschulungsalter – Wie viele Schüler sind leistungsbereit? Medizinisch-pädagogische Konferen **26**, 25–32 (2003).

Upledger, J.E., J.D. Vredevoogd: Lehrbuch der CranioSacralen Therapie. 4. Aufl. Haug Verlag, Heidelberg 2000.

Vademecum Anthroposophische Arzneimittel. 2.Aufl. Der Merkurstab **63**, Supplement (2010).

- Vademecum of anthroposophic medicines, CD format. Medical Section of the School of Spiritual Science, Dornach, Switzerland 2009.

Vagedes, J., Soldner, G.: Das Kindergesundheitsbuch. Gräfe & Unzer, München, 3.Aufl. 2010.

Verhulst, J.: Der Erstgeborene. Mensch und höhere Tiere in der Evolution. Verlag Freies Geistesleben, Stuttgart 1999.

Vogel, H.H.: Organ der Ich-Organisation. Natur Mensch Medizin, Bad Boll 1996.

Vogel, H.H.: Wege der Heilmittelfindung. Natur Mensch Medizin, Bad Boll 1994.

- Vogel, H.-H.: Finding remedies: spiritual knowledge of man and naure; a contribution toward understanding anthroposophic remedies, based on the example of the Wala remedy compositions. V 1, 2 Natur-Mensch-Medizin, Bad Boll 1994.

Walter, H.: Abnormitäten der geistig-seelischen Entwicklung in ihren Krankheitserscheinungen und deren Behandlungsmöglichkeiten. Natura Verlag, Arlesheim 1987.

Weber, G. (Hrsg.): Zweierlei Glück. 7. Aufl. Auer, Heidelberg 1995.

Weckenmann, M.: Cardiodoron – eine kasuistische Betrachtung. Beitr. Z. Erw. d. Heilk. **1**, 26–38 (1982).

Wieland, W.: Medizin als praktische Wissenschaft – Die Frage nach ihrem Menschenbild. In: M.Girke/J.-D. Hoppe et al.: Medizin und Menschenbild. Deutscher Ärzte-Verlag, Köln 2006.

Wildermuth, M: Angstentstehung und -bewältigung im Säuglings-, Kindes- und Jugendalter. Mayer Verlag, Stuttgart 2006.

Wolff, O.: Das hyperkinetische Syndrom. Der Merkurstab **46**, 1–8 (1993).

Wolff, O., M. Stübler: Die Nachtschattengewächse. Quadrivium, Lahnstein 1985.

Wolke, R. et al.: Persistent Infant Crying and Hyperactivity Problems in Middle Childhood. Paediatrics **109**, 1054–1060.

Wulfsberg, T.: Gold. Aurum-Salze in der Homöopathie. Urban & Fischer, München 2001.

Zabern v., B.: Das Dilemma der Stimulanzienbehandlung unruhiger Kinder. Der Merkurstab **55**, 84–87 (2002).

Zabern v., B.: Kompendium der ärztlichen Behandlung seelenpflegebedürftiger Kinder, Jugendlicher und Erwachsener. Erfahrungen und Hinweise aus der anthroposophischen Therapie. Medizinische Sektion am Goetheanum, Dornach (Schweiz) 2002.

Ziller, H.: Wohin des Wegs, schwarze Nieswurz? In: Swoboda, F. (Hg.): Documenta homoeopathica **25**, Maudrich Verlag Wien (2005).

8 Neurological disorders

The representation of this paediatrically very comprehensive and important field is restricted to a few, selected clinical pictures. The focus hereby is on those aspects which can extend an understanding of the diagnosis and, above all, the treatment possibilities of the affected children through anthroposophic medicine and homoeopathy.

8.1 Epilepsy

Something is basically required which would need greater vigilance and attention; such vigilance, such attention is not achieved. Instead, the pendulum swings to the other extreme ... Instead of walking there is falling, instead of action there is convulsion, instead of clarity there is blackout ...

If we further consider that children – particularly infants – have a much greater susceptibility for convulsions than adults, then we will be led to an even greater extent to look at the whole convulsive event as something which affects the whole of humanity ... that we are all 'susceptible', as it were

Karl König

8.1.1 General insight into the illness

The anthroposophical doctor and teacher of children with special needs Karl König [1984, 98, 128, 134] left a fundamental account of epilepsy, which he wrote in the last years of his life. In it he quotes from a work by P. Vogel [1961], published in *Der Nervenarzt*, who wrote that Raphael "created a magnificent picture at the end of his short life in which he combined and related to one another two consecutive stories from the gospels. In its lower half, the painting depicts the presentation of the epileptic boy to the disciples and above, like in a transcendental space, the transfiguration of Jesus. The painting has been given the name 'The Transfiguration'". The textbook on epilepsy by Lennox [1960] depicts the lower part of the picture. "... it will not derogate from the recognition due to Lennox and his work if, through the fragment of the painting which he uses as the guiding principle for his work, we allow ourselves from time to time to be reminded of the larger, more complete picture and place our scientific questions under its signature." Who today remembers or, indeed, looks for the whole painting?

Epilepsy occurs relatively most frequently in childhood: 50 % of all patients suffering from epilepsy are under 16 years old, 75 % of all epilepsies manifest before the age of 18. Four percent of all children have at least one cerebral seizure in the course of childhood. Epileptic attacks can occur in each person as a consequence of *acute changes of the inner equilibrium and external, physical traumatization*, e.g. through hypoglycaemia or, in the first septennium, following an acute rise in temperature, birth traumas or accidents. People whose body has a *hereditary and genetic* disposition (this group of people is approx. ten times larger than the group of people with the manifest condition) appear particularly "prone".

The guiding symptom of epilepsy is the *seizure*. Paroxysmal diseases are not restricted to neurological disorders: bronchial asthma, for example, is a classic disease with a paroxysmal course. Paroxysmal phenomena cannot be observed in the sphere of the purely vegetative life (e.g. in bamboo) whereas higher animals can also display paroxysmal seizures. *Seizures are fundamentally connected with the soul organization* (as it is in reality at work in the body and encapsulated in the term astral body) and are *an expression of body-related activity.*

If we look at cerebral seizures to their full extent, we can objectively and introspectively observe three complexes of symptoms:

- mental trauma-like feelings which impose themselves (aura[1]),
- the independent activity of the motor functions (partial or generalized) with a tendency to lose erectness,
- restriction or loss of consciousness.

Any doctor who observes this without bias will note that these phenomena of an epileptic seizure trigger *profound shock* in the people nearby (the behaviour of patient relatives can often not be understood without the fact that the seizure at first triggers a *sustained shock* in the parents for example). An epileptic seizure was and is *profoundly unsettling.* A "dehumanization" comes to expression in it, but also a great, tempest-like power [König 1984].

An epileptic seizure deprives a person of his or her consciousness, free sentient ability, erectness, freedom of movement – and yet is an expression of a soul-related activity. This fact highlights the necessity of differentiating the animalistic soul layer of existence, the astral body which humans and animals have in common, from the human I-organization and to grasp it in concrete terms [Steiner 1985, 42–60].

A further aspect which is important in this context becomes clear through the *situations* in which epileptic seizures occur: one aspect relates to the *sleeping-waking rhythm* (seizure on awakening, on going to sleep, from out of sleep) which can continue to be of importance for the classification and prognosis of seizures, as well as to certain *activities* and *mental agitation* or tensions (an aspect which is particularly important with regard to adolescents and adults, while it is of importance for small children in the form of family tensions). In the medical history, a trauma largely erased from memory and only remembered with some help[2] can – as in almost all paroxysmal diseases – be of importance.

The initial aspect referred to by Rudolf Steiner in connection with epilepsy, particularly in childhood, relates to the sleeping rhythm: "Take the connection between the physical body and the etheric body to begin with. It is maintained throughout life, from conception, the embryonic state, until death because it continues through all the sleeping states. In contrast, the connection with the astral body and I-organization is interrupted each

1 Cf. in this connection also König's aspect of displacement [1984, 107]: feeling "rises to the head" while the limbs begin to jerk and beat regularly as would happen physiologically in the movement of the heart, the rhythmical system.

2 Cf. the excellent case study of W. Rimpau [1999].

time we sleep" [Steiner 1985, 43]. Epileptic seizures reveal the fragility of the interaction between soul and body.

All the aspects we have mentioned so far can be simply summarized by saying that epileptic seizures are connected with a failure of the body-related activity of the soul entity, of the astral body. As the soul organization only forms the body into an "instrument of the soul" (W. Bühler) between birth and the end of adolescence, and the body *must first be appropriated by the soul* during childhood, it is easy to understand that the body-related activity of the soul entity is more prone to disorders during this phase. This perspective also explains that *physical obstacles to soul activity* related to birth trauma or genetic circumstances elevate the risk of seizure (bodily physical defects do not necessarily reduce the corresponding soul potential but, on the contrary, frequently produce a relative surplus of soul dynamics in relation to the possibilities of physical incarnation – something which many parents of children with disabilities clearly perceive in their children). Every trauma can disrupt the interaction between soul and body for a sustained period (▸Chap. 6.5).

Each awakening contains a birth event in so far as the soul thereby passes over into the active use of the body. The moments at which the soul connects with or separates from direct body-related activity represent particularly vulnerable times in the interaction between the soul and the body (like the moments of take-off and landing); it is no surprise that they play a special role in the occurrence of seizures. Seizures further occur cumulatively when there is increased activity in the soul entity (agitation or developmental steps in the organism) – thus childhood epilepsies occur cumulatively or get worse particularly at specific developmental "milestones" (e.g. during puberty).

But such interaction between the body and soul in humans is *not an end in itself* in two respects. On the one hand, from the outset the soul entity in humans serves a higher organizational level, a higher component of their being, namely the *human I* as an entity with real action (I-organization). Erectness, language and thinking represent *qualitative differences between humans and animals* which are connected with this relationship between the astral body and I. Every epileptic seizure turns this relationship into its opposite – that is a key aspect both of its pathology and its shocking effect on others: the activity of the astral body (the acute seizure is a hyperergic state) makes itself independent of the I-organization and the specifically human aspect of the soul activity is lost in the seizure: "A person not used to these states *is shocked by the dehumanization which takes place before our eyes*" [König 1984, 103]. That leads directly to the essential goal in any treatment of epilepsy: the *regulating power of the I over the soul organization* must be strengthened.[1] *Physiologically* it happens through development above all in adolescence itself (with a decrease in the epileptic frequency); the relationship between the I and the soul organization can only come to full expression in the adolescent and adult (cf. the effectiveness of behavioural therapeutic measures at this age). This aspect represents a significant goal extending as far as the use of potentized medicines which act at this level.

1 But we should also always bear in mind the shock and anxiety which the experience of a seizure triggers in the parents. Much in the behaviour of parents of children suffering from seizures is due to the completely unexpected shock when the first seizure occurs; this must be addressed by the doctor to avoid a reactive, anxiety-fuelled reinforcement of a psychological one-sidedness in the bond between child and parents so that the power of the I-organization can be strengthened. This aspect, too, is depicted in Raphael's painting. Christ not only heals the epileptic boy, he also gives support to the shocked adults and agitated disciples in their encounter with this event and its demonic action.

But human beings do not only awaken in order for their soul to work in the body but *they awaken to grasp the world perceptually and actively with their body* [Steiner 1985, 44]: in perception, thinking and independent action *they always go beyond themselves – otherwise they do not acquire consciousness.* From this perspective it is significant that it is also the I-organization which takes the lead when the human being fully awakens. As children learn to walk erect and imitate their mother in speech, they endeavour to unite their I with the world in the way they take hold of the environment. This path into the world is fundamentally different from that of the animals. They awaken into a closed Gestaltkreis (circular Gestalt process) [Viktor von Weizsäcker 1973] with their specialized bodily organization which precisely does not allow for consciousness. From a human perspective, animals awaken incompletely (into a comparatively dreamy state): they are governed by their organs – human beings govern their organs (Goethe). Epilepsy is connected with a disorder of the latter ability.

Complete awakening is particularly dependent on *equilibriums:* in erect posture itself, in the warmth organization, at the level of neurophysiological excitation. The brain, the inner ear are not only connected physiologically with thinking consciousness but equally with the perception and regulation of such equilibriums. Disorders of this organ particularly affect the connection between the I and the world as much as the control and regulation of the interaction between the soul and body by the I. Rudolf Steiner succinctly summarizes the associated impairment of the human soul and spiritual individuality in the context of his description of epilepsy: "To achieve consciousness requires that we get away" (from the simple connection with the organism to the connection with the outside world). "We acquire consciousness when we have broken through. If we have only entered" (the body, the organs) "we wake up; if we break through we acquire consciousness." If we remain "stuck in it", then "sleep, which is healthy unconsciousness, carries over into pathological unconsciousness, i. e. the human being wakes up but does not obtain consciousness" [Steiner 1985, 50].

So it is only when we look at the *intentional dynamic* of the human soul (which can sometimes be greater in the child with serious disabilities than in a so-called normal child!) in *relation to the impaired physical body* (which is undoubtedly a significant condition for epileptic diseases) that the term "seizure" (in the sense of an *increased, unsuccessful effort; in German, "Krampf" is the word used for both, epileptic convulsions and cramps)* acquires meaning[1]. On this basis parents and the other people affected can also obtain a new understanding of the disorder: now we can understand, for example, why the time when we wake up (in the morning or during the night) represent a particularly vulnerable phase for the patient, why children injured at birth are subsequently at greater risk of seizures just at the time when they embark on a developmental step – but also that following a phase of increased seizures there can be clear developmental progress *connected with the intentional activity of the child's individuality working under more difficult bodily conditions.* Every therapeutic effort should be made to smoothen the path of the latter without thereby placing even bigger obstacles in its way. Against this background, the allopathic

1 Rudolf Steiner refers to this dynamic being dammed up at the "surface" of the impaired organs (either the brain or another organ which could also lead to a reflexive functional disorder in brain activity) – something which corresponds remarkably with current research which, up to and including pharmacology, has its focus on research into the pathological processes at the cell membranes: "Else it is an empty concept when we speak of seizures if we are unaware that the astral body and I-organization ... are squashed up at the surface. They cannot get out, are pushing outwards and are held back" [Steiner 1985, 51].

anticonvulsant therapy is a particular balancing act in which it should always be examined whether it really creates or maintains space for the I or whether it restricts the activity of the I (and also the vitality of the life organization) to such an extent that the damage is greater than the benefit.

Against the background set out above, the composition of the gospel which underlies Raphael's painting can become clearer: epilepsy, the "sacred disease" (Hippocrates), was not just seen by humanity far into the modern age as a sinister phenomenon, testifying to the tempestuous incursion of demonic forces into human nature – it was also experienced as the expression of a soul whose potential could not be managed by its own body [Madeleyn 1990, 370]. In the violence of the seizure, the soul might also have heard the voice of the gods! Readers at the end of the nineteenth century found in Dostoyevsky the writer who – before the advent of depth psychology – most intensely depicts the soul and spiritual drama of the human being in wrestling with his or her unconscious drives and physical conditions. In the epileptic Prince Myshkin he wanted to describe humanness appearing in his time in its purest form – and called his novel "The Idiot". "But in the epileptic the day side is brighter and the shadow side is darker; it is the case that, in the polarities between which all human beings find themselves, the epileptic is positioned with much greater potentials of his or her existence" [König 1984, 102].

8.1.2 Diagnostic aspects

Age, anamnesis and a clinical neurological examination allow for a very precise diagnosis as early as in the paediatric surgery. The classification of epilepsy following instrumental diagnosis (EEG, sleep deprivation EEG, MRT and similar), which does not succeed satisfactorily in every case, solves only part of the problem of diagnosis.

The following questions should be addressed:

8.1.2.1 Triggers, accompanying circumstances

The seizure classification often has little or only generalized things to say in that respect; certain pathological EEG findings also occur in phenomenologically healthy people. The question is *always* important: what preceded the first seizures in particular, what were the existing circumstances? The latter can be a cause in themselves or reinforce preexisting stresses, leading to seizures. Important are

- disorders during pregnancy; prenatal developmental disorders/diseases,
- injuries, e. g. birth trauma,
- brain damage in early childhood, e. g. inflammation-related,
- vaccination (▸Chap. 3.5.7.2.4, incl. case study).

Exact classification of epilepsy can never replace the search for the concrete triggers.

- Psychologically tense family situation through relationship problems or excessive stress at work.

These triggers can be found relatively frequently. Even if they are recognized, the readiness to do something about them is relatively small in many cases. The rigidity, the inflexible continuation of the parental behaviour which has produced this tense atmosphere can eventually drive the child into a corner in its psychological development – these triggering moments play an important role above all in *newly manifesting epilepsies beyond the age of nine* – but even in infancy a clear influence of parental tension on the child's seizure activity can be seen in individual cases. Of significance from the second septennium are above all

- anxiety of the child or adolescent about social/school demands/overload incl. parental expectations,
- undigested or suppressed shock experiences [Rimpau 1999],
- detachment problems, crises of puberty and adolescence.

It is important not to confuse these *triggers* with the *consequences* of epileptic seizures, which can call forth strong anxiety and shock-related *secondary* overprotective behaviours of the parents with the corresponding emotional disorders in the child.

- Disorders of spinal column function, the craniocervical junction, depth of respiration and breathing rhythm,
- Circulatory and blood sugar regulation problems,
- Food intolerances,
- Abnormal sensory hypersensitivity (above all light, but also smells and other things),
- Abnormal sensitivity to the moon and weather,
- Preceding medicines, particularly suppressive ones, anaesthesia,
- Environmental pollution (poisoning, pollution of the sleeping place and other things).

8.1.2.2 Rhythm in daily life

This is of crucial importance for the interaction of the soul and body in childhood.

- Sleeping behaviour and irregularities, fatigue,
- Abnormalities in the waking up process (there is frequently a long interval between waking up and "really being present and responsive") and in going to sleep,
- Irregularities in or displacement of the eating rhythm,
- Rhythm disorders through tense school and training situations,
- Stimulants, drug use.

In this connection we can enquire about media consumption and, as appropriate, time spent in front of the computer (lack of sleep, the consumption of stimulants and excessive activity at the computer can trigger seizures, as can flickering in discotheques and similar places).

8.1.2.3 Nutritional habits

In view of food intolerances (these are the foods which are sometimes consumed with particular addiction!), blood sugar disorders (failure to eat breakfast, consumption of sweets) and also malnutrition (e. g. vitamin B_{12} deficiency in children of rigorous long-term vegetarians), a detailed anamnesis is always to be recommended.

8.1.3 Extending treatment options

Antiepileptic drugs probably do not influence epilepsy course; they merely suppress seizures.

A. Geerts et al. [2010]

The treatment of children suffering from epilepsy is currently almost wholly the domain of allopathic anticonvulsant therapy. The meta-analysis quoted above of a 15-year follow-up study from the Netherlands of children with newly occurred epilepsy shows that after 15 years 70 % of the affected children were in remission for least five years. On the other hand, it also shows that the course can worsen again for a long time after a remission. As indisputably effective as anticonvulsants can be in everyday clinical use, the authors advocate the following hypothesis in agreement with some earlier studies: "We think that treatment does not seem to have a major impact on the outcome of epilepsy. In our opinion the natural course of epilepsy better explains our results..." [Geerts 2010, 7, see also the literature quoted there]. They even emphasize that also untreated seizures can spontaneously enter remission. Even in a comparatively well treatable group of seizures, such as absence epilepsy, it has been shown in more recent studies that the standard treatment with Ethosuximid (which is statistically slightly superior to Valproat) leads to an absence of seizures in barely 60 % of the treated children after 20 weeks, with Lamotrigin it is just 29 %. Attentiveness disorders occurred in 49 % of children treated with Valproat (Lamotrigin 24 %, which speaks in favour of the latter) [arznei-telegramm (2010)].

Arzneimitteltelegramm concluded in 2005: "Immediate anticonvulsant treatment after one or a few initial epileptic seizures [does] not influence the long-term prognosis of epilepsy. Neither do the data show any differences in view of complications such as status epilepticus or injuries or mortality. Immediate anticonvulsant treatment is often accompanied by unwanted side effects... The question when to start an epileptic treatment must continue to be decided on the basis of an individual risk-benefit assessment. In a decision against immediate treatment no disadvantage arises to the patient according to the new data." [arznei-telegramm 2005]. As these data and statements are very far removed from the convictions prevalent in practice and, on the other hand, represent an encouragement for everyone individually to seek the appropriate treatment path for the affected children and come to a joint decision with the parents, they are given voice here in the detailed quotes.

Anticonvulsant therapy frequently shows measurable toxic side effects (elevated transaminases, thrombopenia and others). This *impairment of the childhood life organization* can be a sufficient motivation in itself to seek *complementary* treatment which is directed less at the brain than, for example, at the liver, kidneys, intestine and bone marrow, i. e. at the large organs which are responsible for vitalization and detoxification processes.

Allopathic anticonvulsants can have a *psychologically* liberating effect and release great developmental potentials of the child which were inhibited by the seizures and threatened to exhaust themselves. That fact should be expressly emphasized here. On the other hand, emotional disorders of a depressive or also aggressive or agitated kind can occur as the result of anticonvulsant treatment; an alienation and passivation of the soul entity might also be determined ("that is no longer my child", "that is no longer me"). *Potential mental development* might in part be irreversibly impaired (e. g. the development of the intelligence in long-term phenobarbital treatment in infancy). This forces us to keep assessing the treatment in accordance with the perspective set out in ▶Chap. 8.1.1 and not just to use the ideal of freedom from seizures as a guide – the latter need not necessarily always correspond with the optimization of long-term treatment success.

With regards to homoeopathy, various authors from Stauffer [1998, 766–774] through H. Imhäuser [2000] to R. Morrison [1999, 847–863] have emphasized that the treatment with potentized medicines is very difficult, protracted and often unsuccessful. This contrasts with encouraging work e. g. by Lorz [2004] and impressive sustained treatment successes in individual cases (cf. the case study by H. Imhäuser [2000], for example). Homoeopathic single preparations – thus also the experience of the authors – which very precisely represent the simile of the case can often initially make the disease worse in epileptic children. This must be taken into account when providing the parents with information and also with regard to the administration of the medicine and the management of the patient.

Case study

A ten-year-old boy, dark haired, macrocephalic, introverted, age-appropriate development, is presented for the first time after a total of three generalized seizures in the awakening phase. Stress at school resulting from the change to an academic secondary school (pressure of selection in the fourth primary school class) has created clear tension in the capable and somewhat ambitious pupil. A certain restrained anxiety is noticeable. He is the eldest; has a younger brother and a little sister came along after a large interval. No pathology in the EEG; empty family anamnesis. – Belladonna (D15), indicated for epilepsy on awakening remains without effect; there continue to be major tonic-clonic seizures at intervals of two to four weeks with unconsciousness and wetting directly after (early) awakening.

The parents are still reluctant to agree to the administration of valproic acid; from a medical perspective, the attempt to stimulate the organism to regulate itself appears reasonable as the seizures are restricted to a manageable situation and a florid risk to the development of the child is not yet given. At this point Causticum in D200 is prescribed. After the first administration (in the evening) of 3 pillules, there are three major seizures during the night at intervals of one to two hours. Any further intervention is carefully avoided; the child remains at home for three days. Then no more seizures for a year. One more seizure in the morning after awakening in a very pronounced situation of overload. Causticum was repeated, this time without any aggravating effect. Since then (follow-up observation 8½ years) no more seizures.

From an anthroposophical perspective, R. Madeleyn [1990] has presented a detailed account of the possibilities and limits of a supplementary and/or alternative treatment of childhood epilepsy with anthroposophical and homoeopathic medicines. This study – which takes a stance on all important forms of epilepsy in childhood, analyses the clinical treatment results of 125 children and sets out the approach of anthroposophical epilepsy diagnosis and treatment, including case reports – has not been equalled to date. In the diagnosis of the children (and the neuropaediatric qualification of the author) it also meets the fundamental requirements which need to be met with regard to comparability with so-called conventional medical standards (which is not given in the older literature). We can only make reference to this account here. The collaboration with the neuropaediatric outpatient department and the inpatient treatment opportunities at the Filderklinik in Stuttgart under the direction of R. Madeleyn have become a valuable help for the authors in the outpatient treatment of children suffering from epilepsy.

There is increasing scientific literature on *self-regulation in epilepsy* which grows in importance in adolescence (particularly in seizures with preceding aura) and which particularly highlights the prospect of a *cure* through *the activation of the I (Ego) within the soul* (cf. the case study from Rimpau [1999] quoted above and the references there). It is important to point out in this context that the homoeopathic and anthroposophic directions of therapy do not primarily develop a suppressive action but rather have a stimulating and harmonizing effect on the physical, soul and spiritual activity of the patient himself or herself; they do not work directly as active substances but indirectly through the *response which they call forth in the organism* (▸Chap. 1.2).

The therapeutic concerns of the patient and parents should be clarified at the start of the treatment: do they only want an accompanying treatment alongside an already existing anticonvulsant therapy, for example because of feared side effects or side effects which have already occurred, or is the seizure itself the focus? It is important under all circumstances to communicate very clearly about diagnosis and the *therapeutic goal.* Here it is important to work out a *realistic prognosis* and to *investigate the expectations.* This is relevant in order for the necessary therapeutic distance to be acquired which makes it possible to include the patient and his or her family in the therapeutic activity. Paediatrically it is a matter of understanding *the child itself in its individuality.* This is perhaps also the deepest expectation which the parents bring along.

A *pre-existing anticonvulsant therapy* should, to begin with, *not be changed* as far as possible if this can be justified with regard to possible side effects and the treatment is reasonable under common standards. Contact, as relevant, with the neuropaediatrician who treated the patient previously or is still treating him or her is absolutely necessary and should be open and trusting. It is necessary with pre-treated patients – which most are today – to assess the possibilities and reciprocal effects of a supplementary treatment beforehand. But it is almost always possible, despite pre-existing allopathic medication, to achieve an effect with supplementary medicines if they are properly applied, i. e. a reduction in the frequency, seriousness and duration of seizures and the associated findings. *Only once this has happened can a reduction of the anticonvulsant therapy be cautiously initiated.*

In *patients without pre-existing treatment*, the doctor bears a particularly great responsibility. In all cases he or she must protect the child against the consequences of dogmatically unrealistic misjudgements of the parents and must not turn into their tool. The possible risk to the patient must be set out clearly and realistically (but not in a way that creates anxiety). If there is a basis of trust, such cases can, on the other hand, lead to a particularly impressive course of treatment. The possibility must be given at all times to keep querying the treatment path to be pursued if there is a lack of success.

Epilepsy treatment is always a long-term task; short-term success is deceptive. As with bronchial asthma, it has proved worthwhile to set out a *timeframe* from the beginning (which here always extends over several years) and to discuss it clearly. Seizures trigger deep-seated *anxieties;* as in all paroxysmal diseases, the *ability to contact the doctor* (i. e. the availability of doctor) is imperative to build up the necessary *trust.*

General rules of behaviour, particularly the establishment of a *stable life rhythm* (waking-sleeping, meals, etc.), represent a necessary framework for treatment; they are generally familiar (but too often are communicated to the patient in a cold or anxiety-creating way). In this field, too, *building trust that there is room for manoeuvre* is required: what the child is allowed to do, what rules the child has to keep and where the child is deliberately granted some latitude, even if there is a small residual risk, must be precisely discussed. The *secondary complications of over-protective behaviour* are generally familiar today; the explanation at the beginning of this chapter (▸Chap. 8.1.1) sets out even more clearly that a *weakening of the I and its initiative through actions fixated on fear, particularly of the parents, can reinforce the pathogenesis.* With recovery in mind, the child or young person must know what latitude her or she has and be allowed to use it.

Acquiring *a new attitude* with awareness of our own anxieties, of unresolved tensions and of the expectations we bring along without thinking can open up a new path for the child and ourselves – a path in which the focus can shift from suppressing the seizure to releasing the potential of the soul entity which comes to expression in it.

Anthroposophically and *homoeopathically extended treatment* is primarily guided by four aspects:

- the symptoms incl. the neuropaediatric classification of the seizures,
- the age and associated constitutional situation of the child,
- the causes and associated circumstances which trigger a seizure,
- reference to the associated functional organic disorders, not just of the brain but also other organs (particularly liver and kidneys).

The authors were able to observe impressive therapeutic results, particularly in children who could not be satisfactorily managed with any medical treatment (allopathic or anthroposophic-homoeopathic), with a *ketogenic diet* [Hartman 2007]. Baumeister [2002, 2003] has published studies of his own on this subject; our own experiences relate primarily to patients which were treated jointly with R. Madeleyn (Filderklinik Stuttgart) who has been successfully using this form of treatment – known for the last 80 years – for epilepsy for a considerable period of time. We see a particular indication to use this diet, which is complex but has few side effects when successful, if *metabolic causes of the epilepsy* are suspected (even if the metabolic defect cannot be clearly classified). This accords with the assumption that the diet works partly through circumventing impaired metabolic pathways [Baumeister 2003, 79]. A further research field is represented by serious myoclonic-astatic epilepsies occurring “out of the blue” at the age of three and four, possibly starting after an infection or vaccination. Here the question arises as to (auto?) *immunologically determined* pathogenic processes. Here too this diet has shown itself to be very effective in individual cases as a component of treatment. It should fundamentally be considered in good time as an option if there is *therapeutic resistance*, particularly in view of the lack of toxicity – although the ketogenic diet can also have unwanted side effects.

8.1.4 Eurythmy therapy

Eurythmy therapy forms an important treatment possibility in childhood seizures, not just in relation to the illness but also in the sense of actively promoting the child’s development (salutogenesis). It must be prescribed very individually. *Of the vowels,* the sounds “A” and “E” are of particular importance; the “A” in the sense that the activity of the soul entity re-establishes its connection with the physical processes to a greater extent (in the sense of an awakening process), the “E” in that the activity of the I-organization is reinforced in its guiding action on the life processes. Carried out accordingly, the “E” movement (a crossing movement of arms/legs which can be strengthened through bringing them into contact at the point where they cross and feeling this contact point) can also inhibit individual seizures so that it makes sense to show the parents how they can do the movement with the child, as necessary.

The sound "B" strengthens the development of the soul envelope and the separation from the stimuli of the environment, something which is of importance above all when seizures are triggered by specific sensory stimuli or psychological influences (e. g. photosensitivity). "B" has a specific relationship with those soul and physical processes which are connected with the kidney organization (▸Chap. 7.11). Here it should be observed that the renal and adrenal organization works not just in an exocrine but also in an endocrine way – the first embryonic hormonally active substances can be shown to exist in the kidneys. The renal and adrenal organization takes a leading role in respect of ensouling the organism, the interaction of the soul and life organization (cf. also the physiology of awakening). "B" is an important sound for children giving a restless, driven impression.

The sound "M" supports the regulation of the respiratory rhythm in connection with epilepsy and also the rhythm of the anabolism and catabolism of the hepatic organization (supplemented as "L" – "M"). Here it should be taken into consideration that children treated with conventional anticonvulsants almost always display a hepatic metabolic burden.

The sounds "G" and "K" have a profound effect in epilepsy. Superficially they have a beneficial effect on intestinal peristalsis (every constipation makes epilepsy worse – a change of diet and an enema to begin with can be helpful, as appropriate). Biliary secretion is supported in the same context (which is partly negatively affected by anticonvulsants and is relevant as a detoxification process). But "G" and "K" also have a supporting effect on the inner metabolic processes in that they stimulate the physical structural development of the organism. That is very important in connection with childhood epilepsy [cf. Kirchner-Bockholt 1997, 137–140].

8.1.5 Anthroposophic and homoeopathic medicines for childhood epilepsy – an overview

Set out below is an overview of the medicines used, followed by treatment possibilities for childhood epilepsy structured by age. It is based on the practical experience of the authors in epilepsy treatment with anthroposophic and homoeopathic medicines, as complementary and as stand-alone treatment. These observations can only serve as suggestions for the doctor's own course of action; familiarity with the Materia medica, knowledge and experience in the field of epilepsy and individual familiarity with the patient are the indispensable conditions for a responsible treatment.

8

8.1.5.1 Metals

The three most important metallic medicines are *copper, lead and silver.* The administration of copper acts directly on the *interaction between the soul and the life entity, the astral body and etheric body*; lead acts primarily on *reinforcing the I-organization* with regard to the astral body, while silver has a supporting and *regulating action on the life organization*, the etheric body, in various organic regions.

- **Cuprum met. praep. D6–20 trit./30 amp.** Weleda
  acutely 1 ampoule s.c./i.v., 1 saltsp. per os/d. in the evening

It is recommended in most cases to start with a lower potency (D6).

This medicine

- opens the path for the soul organization, the astral body, to become active in the life organization, and
- at the same time vitalizes the anabolic activity of the life organization, the etheric body, in the organs in a way that is related to the astral body so that
- the release of the soul entity in the evening and during the night from the body and its (daytime) activity is supported (▸Chap. 6.5.6.3.3).

Ensouled life is not possible without copper. Potentized copper counters congestion of the soul entity in the organism during the day and the soul entity being unable to release itself from the body during the night.

Guiding symptoms which should make us think of copper in the treatment of epilepsy (▸Chap. 2.2.4) are:

- status post preeclampsia, *placental hypoperfusion,*
- status post asphyxia, following intracranial bleeding in premature babies and newborns, during and after newborn seizures (▸Chap. 2.2.4),
- nightly seizures, cyanosis during seizure,
- focal or, as relevant, secondary generalized seizures, aura (stomach sensations, nausea, acoustic aura, visual disturbance are typical before the seizure),
- epilepsy in connection with the female cycle.

Cuprum aceticum D6 dil. Weleda, *LM6* can be more effective in *focal* seizures with *symptoms moving* from outside to inside, from below upwards. Very important to supplement and deepen the copper treatment in childhood epilepsy is the administration of *vegetabilized copper: Chamomilla Cupro culta D2 dil.* Weleda (▸Chap. 8.1.5.4).

- **Plumbum mellitum D20 trit.** Weleda
  1 saltsp./d in the morning

supports the activity of the I-organization emanating from the head if the latter is primarily too weak. The astral entity then makes itself relatively independent which is reflected in an (incomplete) catabolism, a bogging down of the soul impulses and the corresponding tendency to develop seizures (later tendency for sclerosis) [Steiner and Wegman 1977, 126f.]. Potentized lead can make children with epilepsy more awake, more present and accessible in their individuality.

- **Plumbum met. praep. D20 amp.** Weleda
  1 ampoule s.c. 2–3 fingerbreadths below the naval

is an effective medicine in the experience of the authors for generalized seizures occurring mostly at night and can produce a reduction in seizures with *acute* rapidity, including if an anticonvulsant therapy remains without success. The injection fundamentally represent a possibility of emergency treatment for therapy resistant generalized seizures. The injections should be administered as needed and not repeated too frequently. For children with psychomotor impairment and seizures who accord with the above characteristic the medicine can also be alternated with **Helleborus niger D12 amp.** Wala (also as an injection s.c.).

In general, it is beneficial to give potentized lead *after Cuprum*; its action requires a better penetration of the astral body into the life organization; and the administration of Plumbum in turn guide the Cuprum effect towards the I-organization.

Madeleyn [1990, 375f.] summarizes Rudolf Steiner's statements on Plumbum in the treatment of epilepsy in the following sentence: "We can see something in lead which comprehensively *supports the awakening processes*." It is suitable above all for epileptic children who generally, but particularly after and between their seizures, *show difficulties* in awaking fully; who with *retardation* and psychological restriction cling *enechetically* to details and have difficulty in seeing the wider picture, the essence (corresponding to the I) [cf. König 1984, 123]. The seizures occur above all following or out of deep *sleep*.

An important aspect of the action of lead is also the indication for *neurodegenerative* diseases (e. g. tuberous cerebral sclerosis), particularly if they are associated with calcification [Madeleyn 1990, 376]. Then potentized lead carbonate (cerussite) and pharmaceutically produced lead silicate (Plumbum silicicum) should also be considered, depending on the constitution of the child:

- **Cerussit D20 amp.** Weleda/**D20 dil.** Apotheke an der Weleda **Plumbum silicicum D10–30 trit./amp.** Weleda
  5 gtt. or 1 saltsp. 1 x/d/1 amp. s.c. 1–2 x/wk

supplemented particularly by Viscum, Vespa and Nicotiana Tabacum (medicine for scarring degenerative remodelling processes in the central nervous system). **Helleborus niger D6-12** can support the development of these children, improve vigilance and have a regulating effect on psychological excitability.

The lead therapy should, in principle, be an *interval therapy* (intervals of four to six [up to eight] weeks each), injections should not be repeated too frequently without an intermediate medicine being given. In alternation, copper can be given again, for example as **Cuprum sulfuricum D6-12 dil.** (▸Chap. 6.5.6.3.3) to support the assimilation of the soul and spiritual impulses into the metabolic sphere. Lead should in general *not* be given to infants and small children with birth trauma-related epilepsy (cf. Cuprum, Argentum, Arnica in this respect).

Potentized silver may be considered particularly for epilepsies which have their origin in early childhood.

- **Argentum met. praep. D20 trit.** Weleda
  1 saltsp. in the evening, together with
- **Amnion Gl D30 amp.** Wala
  0.3–0.5 ml per os in the evening

is indicated primarily in the first septennium for organic brain disorders with *reduced vitality* in this organic sphere.

This is more frequently the case in, for example,

- epilepsy in extremely premature babies (e. g. status post hypoxaemia, leukomalacia),
- status post encephalitis,
- microcephaly (following cerebral damage in early childhood),
- following vaccination damage.

A further characteristic symptom for a silver indication in epilepsy is a pronounced *lunar phase dependency of the epilepsy*

In this case it has often proved beneficial to administer *Argentum met. praep. D6* Weleda 1 saltsp. in the evening with a waxing moon, *Phosphorus D6-12 dil.* 3–5 gtt. in the morning with a waning moon. Madeleyn [1990, 380] has published a case study on this. In a pronounced *deterioration at new moon Quarz* and in specific *deterioration at full moon Conchae* (= Calcium carbonicum) should additionally be considered.

In the treatment of epilepsy, silver treatment can be applied as vegetabilized silver through a medicinal plant fertilized with silver and cultivated specifically in that way over several years in the form of *Bryophyllum Argento cultum D2, Rh D3 dil.* Weleda (▸Chap. 8.1.5.4).

Also well suited for supplementing the silver treatment of cerebral damage are *organ preparations* of the mainly affected cerebral regions [Sonderheft Organpräparate, Merkurstab 1999, 7]. There are also proven preparations, above all

- **Cerebrum comp. A pillules** Wala
  5–7 pillules in the evening,

for disorders affecting the region of the eye and the visual pathway and

- **Cerebrum comp. B pillules** Wala
  5–7 pillules in the evening,

if the hearing, the sense of balance and the region of the posterior cranial fossa are also affected.

Potentized silver and silver sulphide should be considered if there is a generalized retarded development of the child with weak assimilation, slow growth and a weak metabolism.

With the latter perspective in mind, if the digestive and metabolic region is underdeveloped as well as the brain, the administration of *silver* for a longer period in rising potency (D6-20) is to be recommended.

Here silver sulphide

- **Argentit D4-6 trit.** Weleda
  1 saltsp. 3 x/d can be given to begin with.

Underweight, weak anabolism, "low-sulphur" constitution (dark hair, weak warmth organization, thin, dry skin, constitutionally low vitality in the metabolic sphere, sleep disturbance), but also an *allopathic medicinal burden*, particularly in former premature babies, indicate the administration of this medicine which directs the action of the sulphur into the region of the digestion on the one hand and the central nervous system on the other (cf. in this context, which is also relevant for epilepsy, also ▸Chap. 4)

In puberty, silver (*Argentum met. praep. D20*) has a regulating effect on the sexual sphere which is of considerable significance with regard to epilepsy – cf. Bufo, Agaricus, Arum maculatum, Hyoscyamus.

- In *restless children who appear driven* and have a weak anabolism, potentized silver nitrate can have a better effect
- **Argentum nitricum D15 dil.** (various manufacturers), **LM12 dil.** Arcana (▸Chap. 7.5.3.2).

We can additionally still refer to *zinc,* with which the authors only have little – although positive – therapeutic experience (for example in otherwise treatment-resistant seizures resulting from non-classifiable metabolic defects). "In the treatment with Zincum, it is above all the impression of a disorder relating to the inner release of light with a certain "dullness" during contact and a simultaneous feeling that there is great inner potential whose appearance has been inhibited which indicates this medicine" [Sommer 1999]. Zinc is an important metallic medicine for the *consequences of medicinal suppression,* connective tissue defects and metabolic defects and the consequences of injuries and vaccination; it supplements the above metals in a complementary fashion (▸Chap. 7.5.3.4.2).

8.1.5.2 Single-substance mineral medicines

Quarz (Silicea), *Conchae* (Calcium carbonicum) and *Sulphur* as well as the synthetically produced mineral composition *Causticum* should be primarily considered here. All these medicines have already been presented in detail elsewhere.

As mineral medicines, they have a profound, sustained *constitutional* effect.

- **Quarz D20 pillules** Wala/**trit.** Weleda
  5 pillules/1 saltsp. 1 x/d

intensifies the I activity in the warmth organization and thus addresses the necessary stimulation of the child's soul and physical development from out of the I-organization in a particularly profound way [cf. Steiner and Wegman 1991, 76–80].

Quarz promotes the assimilation of sun forces in the child's life organization particularly in the first septennium which forms the basis for the ability of the soul and spiritual individuality to work in the organism. The impulses moving from the head pole to the organism – at the etheric level these are light and warmth forces [Steiner 2001, 28–36] – are strengthened and the metabolic and limb organism is formed more strongly and warmed through [cf. Leitgedanke Vademecum 2010, 700]. Quarz counters a "blockage at the surface of the organ" [Steiner and Wegman 1991, 77; cf. Lennox 1960].

Indications specifically suggesting the use of Quarz in the treatment of epilepsy are

- *premature birth*, neurasthenic constitution (▸Chap. 6.4.3.6.1),
- early childhood *cerebral lesions also resulting from epilepsy*, pathological remodelling processes and *scarring,*
- *sensory hypersensitivity*, particularly to noise,
- *weak warmth generation*, worsens when cold, at new moon,
- failure to thrive, delayed physical development,
- consequences of vaccination: Quarz is the most important medicine if *vaccination* has triggered or worsened the epilepsy, (▸Chap. 3.5.7.1).

The administration of Quarz in potentized form is important in *night seizures,* to counter inhibiting remodelling processes in the central nervous system and to "clear the way" as much as possible for the effectiveness of the I-organization.

- **Conchae D5–20 trit.** Weleda, **Calcium carbonicum D30–200 pillules** (various manufacturers), **LM6–12 dil. Arcana**
  1 saltsp./3–5 gtt. 1–2 x/d each; high potencies in rare individual doses

is indicated, in contrast, for hypertrophic metabolic processes with too much vitality which produces too much resistance to the formative soul impulses and make awakening difficult. This corresponds to a deterioration of the condition at full moon which has a stimulating effect on fluid-bound life processes.

Conchae in low to medium potentization contributes to the coherence and stabilization of the life organization if vitality in the metabolic sphere is either too strong or damaged so that the rest of the organism is properly nourished and, on the other hand, excretion (particularly of the intestine) occurs in the right measure (observe the *deterioration of many epilepsies with constipation,* which should make us consider Conchae and Argentum, among other things, along with dietetic measures).

An important composite medicine in this connection is

- **Conchae comp.[1] pillules/amp.** Wala
  5–10 pillules 1–3 x/d or ½ ampoule per os 1–2 x/d

which contributes significantly to the harmonization of intestinal function and stabilization of vitality – also during and after the administration of anticonvulsants. Together with Conchae D4 it also contains: Agaricus D6, Argentum met. D4, hart's tongue fern, worm fern and bracken in D2, jointly potentized by one level).

A general indication for Conchae is *congested* and *blocked* vitality which is insufficiently penetrated and developed by the astral body and I-organization or excreted or given form at the right location: constipation with undiminished appetite, sweating on the head with delayed ossification, rapid weight gain with sluggish motor development indicate that something is wrong. A *delayed teething process and epilepsies which manifest or worsen during this phase* fall within the range of indications: Conchae drives teething forwards and also has a decongesting effect.

In the course of its life, the oyster's soul entity increasingly withdraws, into the development of the shell, in giving up mobility and in the regression of the sense organs: an image of increasing regression with the tonic closure of the shell being the only remaining motor ability. Conchae can be very effective when *the soul entity anxiously withdraws and is dammed up on the inside* because the child feels overwhelmed by school and parental expectations, something which may be reinforced through perceived slights, frightening experiences (▸Chap. 7.2) and similar things – that is when epilepsy starts. This can be a primary generalized epilepsy or one with preceding aura: in that case the "aura feeling" starts in the epigastrium and rises upwards. In these cases LM potencies or higher potencies of Conchae are indicated (cf. also the treatment possibilities described in ▸Chap. 7.2 for anxieties in the second septennium). They stimulate the I-organization to counter an "oyster development", a psychological withdrawal, and to open the path for the soul to the outside.

1 Agaricus comp. Weleda corresponds to Conchae comp; the potentization is a little higher

- **Sulphur LM6–12 dil.** Arcana, **D6–20 trit.** Weleda
  1 × 5 gtt., 1–2 × 1 saltsp. daily–2 x/wk.

has an ordering effect on the metabolic sphere (▶Chap. 7.5.3.2, ▶Chap. 6.4.3.6.2).

Indications for this medicine can be

- metabolic imbalances, ravenous appetite for sweet things, strongly fluctuating blood sugar level, seizures if there are longer gaps between food,
- uncontrolled *impulsiveness*, particularly in boys during puberty and adolescence (then sometimes also strong sexual drives),
- *toxic or suppressed consequences of allopathic medicines*, restlessness and aggressiveness during/after anticonvulsants have been given,
- deterioration through external heat, in summer.

It is often only the ordering effect of Sulphur which enables the individuality to become active again in the will and concentration.

- **Causticum D12, 30, 200 pillules** (various manufacturers), **C12–200** Gudjons
  5 pillules D12 daily in the evening or single doses

represents a synthetically produced distillate from burnt marble, beech wood ash and sulphuric acid (▶Chap. 7.1.5.2, ▶Chap. 6.5.6.11).

This is a very effective medicine for *epilepsies which start in the second half of childhood.* The key issue here is soul development: sensitivity and empathy, possible traumatization in early childhood or early *grief, anxieties* about the demands of others and *high demands of oneself, pent up aggression* cause a blockage in the soul which is related to the picture which was drawn for Calcium carbonicum in its indication in the second septennium. The pronounced sensitivity, the empathy also with regard to the unjust treatment of others, grief which is silently and quietly borne, the tension between pent up aggression and striving to perform, as well as the physically slim and not so plump-looking body shape allow for a clear differentiation. D12 can already be very effective but then has to be given for a long time. The seizures occur particularly *after awaking* and during the morning. A specific symptom which should be looked out for is (temporary) states of paralysis associated with the seizure.

8

8.1.5.3 Animal medicines

The following animal medicines are of particular importance in the treatment of epilepsy: *Apis regina* and *Apis mellifica, Vespa crabro* and *Bufo rana.* The action of these medicines is directly evident from their position in nature and the organism.

8.1.5.3.1 Apis regina

Apis regina, a potentized preparation of the queen bee, comes from a sphere of animal life which is *related purely to warmth and light.* Bees live in the sphere of the plant's flower, related to astral animal life – and that is what they live for (cf. the way that bees support plant growth). Bees embody a soul activity which is associated with light and warmth and wholly in harmony with life. Their honey has a stimulating effect on human sensory activity and consciousness (in small doses in the morning, while larger quantities of honey promote sleep at night). The ability of a bee colony to organize warmth is unique in the insect world and is remarkably close to the human warmth organization. That represents a model for the interaction of the various components of the human being (I, astral body, etheric body).

"The queen bee, as a single animal, represents the visible centre of the bee colony. In its 'body-oriented' activity ... it integrates the communal life of the colony through the hormone-like queen substance. Potentized medicines of the queen bee (Apis regina) are beneficial ...[when there is] a lack of integration of the various sense perceptions into conscious understanding and its expression in language and movement, e.g. psychomotor developmental delays and partial impairment of performance, after intracranial brain haemorrhage in premature babies or complex delays in language development." [Leitgedanke zu Apis mell./Apis regina Vademecum 2010, 92]. These disorders occur with relative frequency in children with predominantly focal and multifocal and possibly generalized secondary seizures. Constitutionally they also correspond to the picture of children with attention deficit disorders and a lack of integration of the nervous and sensory system as set out in ▸Chap. 7.5.3.1.

The queen bee preparation, Apis regina, stimulates the integrating forces of the I, the light and warmth forces working from the top downwards, so that they become active in the body and give orientation and uplift to the soul entity. The preparation has a vitalizing, consciousness-enhancing effect particularly also in *cerebrally impaired children.*

For the latter the composition with a brain stem organ preparation has proved particularly effective:

- **Apis regina comp. pillules** Wala
  5 pillules 1–2 x/d.

This is an important medicine to counter the negative consequences of a steroid pulse or ACTH therapy in children treated with anticonvulsants. Language development disorders are a further important field of indication (▸Chap. 7.8.2).

8.1.5.3.2 Apis mellifica

Apis mellifica, a potentized medicine of the normal (virgin female) worker bee, is particularly indicated for *suddenly occurring serious epileptic courses in which there is a suspicion of an autoimmune process.* Such an assumption appears justified for example in children who, *after an infection or vaccination,* develop a *serious, rapidly progredient* myoclonic-astatic epilepsy *which does not respond to anticonvulsants (except corticosteroids and ACTH)* from full health: here the authors were able to achieve therapeutic success in collaboration with R. Madeleyn in which *Apis mell. D30 – administered daily over a number of years – and a temporary ketogenic diet,* particularly at the start of the treatment, were the key medicines (after the failure of all anticonvulsant treatment attempts and in place of ACTH therapy).

There are positive experiences with the preparation

- **Apis ex animale Gl D30 amp.** Wala
  0.3–0.5 ml per os 1 x/d.

8.1.5.3.3 Vespa crabro

- **Vespa crabro Gl D8 amp.** Wala, **D6 dil.** Weleda
  5–7 gtt./0.3–0.5 ml per os 1 x/d

is generally indicated for *connective tissue remodelling processes* and scarring, supplemented primarily with

- **Tabacum Rh D10 dil.** Weleda/**Nicotiana e fol. D10 pillules** Wala
  5–7 gtt./pillules 1 x/d.

The hornet, a colony-forming insect like the bee, does, however, display a completely different character in that it lives off (rotting) fruit and animal food, the colony dies in the cold (only the queen survives the winter) and the paper-like rustling hornets' nest is much closer to the earth in character than the honeycomb (of wild bees). Hornets have just as much of a relationship with death and decay as they do with the air. They thus assumes an intermediate position in the classification set out here. They counter the organ structure becoming "too physical" so that the astral body, the air-related soul organization can no longer act in it.

8.1.5.3.4 Bufo rana

- **Bufo D6–30 dil.** Apotheke an der Weleda, **D12–200 pillules** (various manufacturers)
  in individual dosage

This medicine embodies a polar principle to the preparations set out above; it is applied accordingly not in the sense of a "model" but primarily as a simile in the homoeopathic sense [Stübler and Krug 1987, Tierstoffe, 160–178].

Its long-known effectiveness in epilepsy can be understood[1] if we look at the toad of which the poison glands are used to make the medicine: an animal that lives in humid darkness at ground level, the polar opposite of the bee!

Accordingly the medicine works particularly well in children whose equilibrium between metabolic pole and nervous and sensory pole has been displaced above all through *cerebral damage* in such a way that *impetuousness* and *sexual impulses* primarily determine behaviour while mentally consciousness often lags and has something dull about it. At school age these children may go to bed early to masturbate there for a longer period before going to sleep; in infancy the sexual tinge may, however, be absent with the focus on a *hyperkinetic obtrusive behavioural disorder* (cf. also Veratrum album ▸Chap. 7.5.3.4.2 which similarly displays the connection with humid coldness).

1 Cf. also the impressive casuistic account by Geukens [1989, 401–426] which describes the homoeopathic guiding symptoms of Bufo in epilepsy in very vivid terms.

Case study

A three-year-old boy with Lennox-Gastaut syndrome suffers from up to 30 brief myoclonic-astatic seizures per day. Clonazepam, Phenytoin and Valproat, given simultaneously, cannot change either the massively pathological EEG or the clinical symptoms. The cause of the disorder is an extremely premature birth with peri-postnatal hypoxia-related brain damage, third level intracranial brain haemorrhage with a shunt. There is clear psychomotor retardation, very much delayed language development, and slight spastic disparesis – which does not hinder the child in its uninterrupted compulsion to move. Behaviour appears completely without boundaries with little modulation. The mother reports that the child likes to have baths and has never had a seizure while doing so. Furthermore, the child never eats or drinks anything hot (something which does not change for many years).

After an initial administration of Cuprum met., the child was given Bufo rana in ascending order of potency over several weeks. After no initial and then minor success, the administration of the medicine in D200, 5 pillules dissolved in 50 ml of water, 1 tsp. 3 x/d (!), produces a rapid reduction in seizures to approx. 5 per day; in the further course, which at first extends over approx. two months in which 1 tsp./d continues to be given, the seizures disappear completely. The EEG diagnosis remains strongly pathological in the whole follow-up observation period (7 years). In that period there were only three seizures associated with the disease or as the result of stent failure. It was possible to stop Bufo after about 18 months. Clonazepam had been stopped relatively quickly at the beginning, Phenytoin incrementally in the course of the first year of treatment. In view of the EEG diagnosis, the collaborating neuropaediatrician could never quite decide to stop Valproat completely, which continues to be given at a low therapeutic level by the parents. The massive pre-existing anticonvulsant medication is probably the reason for the necessity of giving a very high potency with such frequent repetition (cf. the case discussed previously with a single administration of Causticum in a child without premedication).

As his seizures reduced, the boy himself showed a very clear improvement in his psychomotor and, above all, psychosocial development; when he was seven it was possible to send him to a school for physically disabled children with learning difficulties.

Rudolf Steiner [1985, 44–53] himself pointed out that in epilepsy treatment the *relationship of the child to the elements* was very important. The one-sided relationship of the patient with coldness and humidity led the way in this case (not the homoeopathic repertory). The boy was "at home" in these elements – like the toad is. In the bath he could be almost harmonious – but he was unable to take the step out of this amphibian world, and did not succeed in making it "to shore" like the prince who was transformed into a frog.

8.1.5.4 Plant-based medicines

These can be ordered in an initial overview into

- *the Compositae* as the most highly developed flowering plants with a strong "model" character (cf. the colony forming insects): Arnica, Chamomilla, Taraxacum, Absinthium, Artemisia, which strengthen the leading role of the I with regard to the astral element,

- *the Solanaceae* as highly developed toxic plants (▸Chap. 7.4): Belladonna, Hyoscyamus, Stramonium, Nicotiana, which form nitrogen containing alkaloids in their roots and as potentized medicines relieve the organism of the burden of a one-sidedly dominant astral body and have a relaxing action,
- *the Umbelliferae* as plants strongly connected with the air which can contribute to integrating soul impulses better into the life organization: Levisticum, Cicuta virosa,
- *the "autumn and winter flowering"* [Steiner 1976, 249–256] *toxic plants* Viscum album, Helleborus niger, which in their emancipation from outer warmth have a strong effect on the I-organization, the human warmth organization and its potential for cerebral reorganization, e. g. following brain damage in early childhood, BNS epilepsy,
- *fungi and ferns* for physical damage and etheric weakening of the nervous system, e. g. epilepsies after pre- and peripartum brain damage: Agaricus muscarius, ferns (cf. Conchae comp., ▸Chap. 8.1.5.2).

The *vegetabilized metals,* i. e. medicinal plants which are treated with metal fertilizer over several years and thereby "potentize", dynamize and transmit in both a fine and sustained way the effect of the metal, are of particular importance in anthroposophical paediatrics:

- Bryophyllum Argento cultum, Chamomilla Cupro culta, Chelidonium Ferro cultum and Taraxacum Stanno cultum are the most important of these medicines for the treatment of epilepsy.

Of the Compositae, the authors particularly use

- **Arnica planta tota D12–30, Arnica (=radix1) Rh D6–20 dil.** Weleda/**Rh D30 amp., e flor 20 % Essenz** Wala/Weleda

This medicinal plant is particularly indicated for *cerebral damage in early childhood* (▸Chap. 2). In the epilepsy treatment of children with such injuries (particularly premature babies with status post intracranial haemorrhage), it can be given internally at the beginning in deep potentization, if the lesion lies further in the past in D20–30, (A. planta tota acutely, subsequently Arnica = A. radix). The *external application of the essence as a bath* can be very effective (cf. case study in Madeleyn [1990, 382]) (this treatment would have been possible also in the above case treated with Bufo). Arnica as a Compositae also has an *ordering and vitalizing* effect on the nervous system, particularly if traumatic influences caused the lesion. Anyone who lets their soul be affected by the power of this bright yellow Compositae, which flowers in high summer on wet upland meadows up to the tree line, defying storms and cold surges, and which produces its stem from a subterranean highly ordered perennial rhizome, will be able to understand the healing effect of Arnica as directly as that of the bee.

- **Chamomilla Cupro culta D2 dil.** Weleda, **Rh D3 dil.** Weleda
  2–5 gtt. 3 x/d in the first year of life, then in accordance with age 3–7 gtt. 3–5 x/d
  (Dosage related to D2 which mostly is clearly more effective in this indication)

1 "Arnica" (e. g. Weleda, DHU) corresponds to Arnica rhizome with roots.

This preparation represent an important basic medicine above all in infants and small children with epilepsy (▸Chap. 2.2.4).

- Birth traumas in the previous medical history,
- restlessness and general susceptibility for seizures,
- "spasms" of the infant which cannot be clearly assigned with rolling eyes and grimacing,
- gastrointestinal disorders with colicky pain and sour diarrhoea which
- gets worse during teething
- should make us think of this medicine which has a deeply relaxing and harmonizing effect particularly in the first two years of life. This medicine applies the therapeutic action of copper in a fine but sustained way (▸Chap. 8.1.5.1: indications of copper).

Artemisia vulgaris (typical: conspicuous agitation before the seizure as a sign of impaired metabolic processes) and *Absinthium* (▸Chap. 6.6.3.1) are valuable epilepsy medicines in deeper potencies if there is a functional weakness in the region of the *liver/gall bladder and pancreas* with corresponding disorders of awakening and drive, but also of digestion (▸Chap. 4). This can often still be reinforced or triggered through allopathic anticonvulsant therapy.

A very effective composite medicine for the treatment and prophylaxis of hepatotoxic side effects and disorders of the digestion in the upper gastro-intestinal tract through anticonvulsants (phenobarbital, phenytoin and others) is

- **Gentiana Magen globuli (Stomach remedy)** Wala (▸Chap. 4.6)
  5–10 pillules 1–3 x/d

which together with Absinthium contains Taraxacum as another Compositae [Vademecum 2010, 463]. With the correct indication, the reversal of the dulled consciousness and an improvement in drive are evident.

Taraxacum, the dandelion, can also be specifically treated with zinc solutions. After a process lasting several years, in which the plant integrates traces of the metal in its life organization, a stable plant-metal preparation is obtained in the form of an alcohol-free, rhythmically carried out fermentation:

- **Taraxacum Stanno cultum Rh D3 dil.** Weleda
  5–12 gtt. 2–3 x/d (alcohol-free) before or also after meals.

This medicine has proved itself above all as medication to accompany *treatment using valproic acid, the side effects of which were very clearly reduced.* But independent therapeutic effects on the seizure are also evident. The primary target location of this medicine lies in the metabolic sphere (liver/gall bladder activity). Here it should be observed that in the central nervous system the metabolism is linked and interwoven in many respects with the liver as the centre of the metabolism in the upper abdomen. The medicine is particularly valuable in connection with greater celandine treated with iron fertilizer:

- **Chelidonium Ferro cultum Rh D3 dil.** Weleda
  5–7 gtt. 2–3 x/d before or also after meals

for those children who under anticonvulsant treatment are clearly impaired in the presence of their will in thinking and action, *e.g. strongly dropping school performance*. They can show an impressive improvement in their intellectual development and independent activity through the administration of this medicine (over the long term).

The most important Solanaceae in the treatment of epilepsy are Belladonna and Hyoscyamus:

- **Belladonna D20 dil./Rh dil.** Weleda
  5 gtt. in the afternoon

is particularly indicated for children who, while otherwise well developing(!), get into states of "hypertonicity" at the level the soul organization which is dammed up in the life organization. Hyperergy occurs in the head and neck region (detectable by the overheating in this region, sweat, cerebrally elevated agitation) in dissociation with the body and (initially often cool) extremities.

A classic sign of this situation is *awakening epilepsy and febrile seizures*. Children often feel better after a seizure; the seizures mostly do not damage development (as has meanwhile been shown for febrile seizures ▸Chap. 5.4.3).

The action of Cuprum (which supports the movement of the impulses emanating from the head into the body and limbs) above all complements Belladonna. Belladonna has a very wide action in childhood epilepsy; here it has been the experience of the authors in recent years that the *effectiveness can often be enhanced* through the additional administration of

- **Cinis Belladonnae D6 trit.** Apotheke an der Weleda
  1 saltsp. 1–3 x/d

One particular indication for Cinis Belladonnae is if the child suffers convulsions after going to sleep and on awakening, including convulsions which need not correlate with EEG changes.

8

An important medicine above all for *epilepsies in the first septennium* is

- **Belladonna/Chamomilla pillules** Wala
  3–5 pillules 3–5 x/d

The subterranean parts (roots) of these two medicinal plants are processed in low potentization and this is done – in accordance with the Wala procedure – with the addition of the respective plant ash. The medicine has a primarily relaxing effect on the autonomic nervous system of the abdomen and the smooth muscles of its hollow organs and is an important medicine during the teething phase. But beyond that it is an important basic medicine for the treatment of epilepsy in childhood with a clearly calming effect on the central nervous system (cf. also the close interplay of the intestine-related enteric nervous system (ENS) and the central nervous system (CNS), ▸Chap. 4). Interaction between the gastro-intestinal tract and seizure activity can often be clinically observed in children with epilepsy (e.g. in constipation).

- **Hyoscyamus Rh D6–3 dil.** Weleda
  5–8 gtt. 2–3 x/d

is, in contrast, indicated above all in epilepsies which occur as part of already impaired development. A weakness of the rhythmical system with outbreaks of impulsiveness is characteristic.

The seizures frequently develop against the background of lesser or greater cerebral disorders; there is a relative dominance of the metabolic region and sexual sphere which is why low potencies are indicated. Accordingly there is often an aura with dizziness, for example; obscene behaviours, sudden ravenous hunger and other prodromes point to impulses of the metabolic pole breaking through which cannot be compensated by the rhythmical system if the sensory and nervous system has been damaged or weakened, leading to further disorders of the nervous and sensory system. Impulsiveness and hyperactivity can continue even with successful epilepsy treatment.

Physically, such children are often pale and thin; eye contact is often difficult and there are frequently lasting emotional disorders (▸Chap. 7.4) with strong jealousy and destructive behaviour. The seizures with Belladonna are sudden, violent and generalized; Hyoscyamus, in contrast, is indicated *also in partial* seizures, restricted to the facial area for example, or psychomotor seizures. Effective for *rolandic epilepsy* with Bryophyllum Argento cultum [Madeleyn]. Viscum album has a very complementary effect in the case of pre-existing cerebral damage. With Hyoscyamus the *emotional disorder* is always of importance; this can have a significant cause in the family environment.

- **Stramonium D12 pillules** DHU
  5–7 pillules 1–3 x/d.

as a Solanaceae is particularly suitable for *restless and hyperactive, also aggressive and, on the other hand, anxious* children, preferentially male. Some aspects of development are delayed, more strongly impaired than for Belladonna, but less than is typical for Hyoscyamus. It is a characteristics feature that the child in many respects has *two very contradictory sides which he or she cannot reconcile himself of herself*, just as the plant itself is characterized by a dichotomy throughout (in contrast to Hyoscyamus and Belladonna (▸Chap. 7.4.4). In collaboration with R. Madeleyn, the authors were able to observe impressive results in two cases using the combination of Hyoscyamus D6 and Stramonium D12 which led to a complete cure of the epilepsy in children of kindergarten age (approx. age 4) *with pronounced myoclonic-astatic epilepsy, ADHD and partial impairment of performance* (particularly of motor functions), in which anticonvulsants could either be completely waived or all anticonvulsants had previously shown themselves to be ineffective. The – already effective – treatment with Hyoscyamus and Stramonium rapidly and sustainably (3 years follow-up observation) took effect in the latter case in combination with a ketogenic diet.

The anthroposophical doctor Armin Alles [2009] took up Rudolf Steiner's and Ita Wegman's reference to *Levisticum* in epilepsy and, in order to obtain the "rubber-like substance" of the plant [Steiner and Wegman 1991, 83], used a preparation produced by Weleda Switzerland which the authors have also used:

- **Levisticum, Folium D3 trit.** Weleda Switzerland
  1 saltsp. 3–5 x/d

Levisticum has a fundamental effect on the shaping and "aeration" of the rhythmical system of respiration and circulation as exemplified in the way it supports pneumatization of the middle ear. In epilepsy the medicine can be helpful if the *rhythmical system of the child displays noticeable symptoms of a disorder* and the energy of the astral body is too much used up while the maturation of the nervous system receives too few impulses. This medicine is indicated in children with

- disorders of the sleeping-waking rhythm, starting out of sleep with throwing up of arms and legs,
- conspicuous tachycardia and/or other pulse irregularities,
- startled reactions to noise and light
- a slowing down or cessation of psychomotor development.

An important, botanically heterogeneous group of medicinal plants for epilepsy treatment are the plants which Rudolf Steiner originally referred to in the context of cancer treatment: plants which flower in the autumn and winter. These develop a certain *"stubbornness"* with regard to the cosmic formative forces which lie in the seasons – as is the case in epilepsy due to focal or multifocal damage to the central nervous system (e. g. BNS epilepsy) which becomes an obstacle to the body-bound activity of the soul and spiritual entity.

- **Viscum Mali D2-6 amp.** Wala, **D2–5 dil.** Weleda
  Viscum Pini D6–15 pillules Wala
  5 pillules, 5–8 gtt., 1–3 x/d, 0.5–1 ml s.c. 1–3 x/wk

was already used by Paracelsus in epilepsy [Madaus 1979, vol. 3, 2836]. As a composition, the following has repeatedly shown itself to work in epilepsies in the first septennium which have been difficult to influence:

- **Viscum comp. pillules/amp.** Wala

contains poplar mistletoe in D5 and Belladonna root in D11 jointly potentized by one level (in practice that means D6/12).

8

Rudolf Steiner recommended treatment with Viscum for epilepsy patients; more recently Madeleyn [1990, 376] has worked out its application in greater detail. He describes its action in these words: "The aim of treating the carcinoma with mistletoe is to surround the former with an envelope of warmth and dissolve it. We can similarly see its action as a releasing, dissolving one when organs harden in a way that prevents the body from being properly taken hold of in the awakening process, creating a disposition for epileptic seizures."

The action of mistletoe is directed at the *warmth organization* and thus the *activation of the I-organization* in relation to the organic regions which cannot be normally structured and thus ensouled by the life organization. The mistletoe itself does not follow the course of the year and forms an embryonic spherical form whose leaves above and below are not differentiated. It represents the precise opposite of the child's development in the first septennium. Correspondingly the mistletoe avoids the effect of the sun in the summer by staying in the shadow of the host tree and blossoms when the sun is lowest and the moon highest (cf. the frequent moon phase dependency of epilepsy patients).

The relatively strong dose required for the application of mistletoe in epilepsy is intended to stimulate the I activity by provoking a *reaction* to the mistletoe. It is therefore logical to increase the dosage in such a way that this provocation occurs (cf. Madeleyn [1990, 376]). The reorganization in the sphere of the damaged organ areas can be stimulated by means of such artificially raised I activity.

Tuberous sclerosis represents a classic case for the indication of mistletoe therapy; there are encouraging single case reports.

- **Helleborus niger LM6 dil.** Arcana, **D6–12 pillules** Wala
  5 gtt., 1–2 × 5 pillules/d

is indicated above all for peri-postnatal or post-inflammatory and also epilepsy-related brain damage. [Vademecum 2010, 477].

The effect of the Christmas rose is directed primarily at the differentiation of the *etheric element* originating with the astral body which is obstructed in its flow by physical destruction and blockages. Renal and adrenal activity is stimulated (also relevant for epilepsies treated with steroids). Helleborus niger in potentized form significantly supports the vital functions of the brain, the *vigilance* and helps the patient to be involved in and perceive the surroundings to a greater extent. *Silver*[1] *in potentized form* has a complementary effect (▸Chap. 8.1.5.1). The medicinal plant Bryophyllum is very important in this connection, particularly as

- **Bryophyllum Argento cultum D2/Rh D3 dil.** Weleda
  3–7 gtt. (D2)/5–12 gtt. (Rh D3) 3 x/d

This medicine is indicated in children with a "hysterical constitution" as defined in the anthroposophical understanding of the human being [Vademecum 2010, 241]. They react too strongly to stimuli and impulses from the environment, tend to be restless, to cry and sweat on the hands and feet, suffer from anxieties and display a close bond with the mother. Because they are so "thin skinned", these children can also appear impulsive and aggressive in excessively demanding social situations (secondary!), which is due to a pronounced sensitivity; it clearly improves on administration of this medicine. The outflowing nature of the child with its lack of boundaries is also revealed in the nocturnal enuresis and sleep disturbance with anxieties during the night. Deterioration at full moon is also an indication for silver treatment and Bryophyllum.

The action of Bryophyllum Argento cultum is calming on the one hand and anabolically helpful on the other. Bryophyllum Argento cultum is specifically indicated for *rolandic epilepsy in combination with Hyoscyamus* (proven experience of R. Madeleyn, but in the author's experience there was, however, not always a response to the treatment).

1 The relationship with Plumbum met. praep. in epilepsies is also dealt with above under ▸Chap. 8.1.5.1).

With very great restlessness and anxiety

- **Bryophyllum 50% trit.** Weleda
  1/4 tsp. several times/d, increase dose as required

can have a stronger effect.

- **Agaricus muscarius (= Amanita muscaria), D4–12 dil.** Apotheke an der Weleda

is indicated for epilepsy patients whose behaviour is clearly characterized by a preponderance of the metabolic pole with motor restlessness and impulsiveness (cf. also ▸Chap. 7.9, ▸Chap. 7.5).

Guiding perspectives for giving Agaricus are:

- frequently small partial or generalized seizures: absences; benign focal seizures,
- motor restlessness, myoclonic twitches,
- emotional agitation, hysterical symptoms, active sexual impetuousness,
- possible genetic or focal previous cerebral burden/damage,
- deterioration of the neurological symptoms through cold [Lorz 2004, 769].

Hyoscyamus, Sulphur, Cuprum, Bufo and others have a complementary action. Cf. also Conchae comp. (▸Chap. 8.1.5.2).

8.1.6 Treatment

The treatment of an epileptic child can give rise to the same feeling in the doctor which probably also filled the disciples at the foot of Mount Tabor as they stood before the epileptic boy: this illness is bigger than its therapist, this child gives us an inkling of a soul presence which is greater than what can incarnate in the normality of human existence.

Hence the treatment of epilepsy is beyond a stringent classification; that becomes as clear in every meeting with neuropaediatricians as it does in the anthroposophic and homoeopathic literature.

Accordingly we can only make tentative therapeutic suggestions – experience arising from many attempts to assist a person to make their way through rocky terrain which is sometimes successful, constantly has to be interrupted due to adverse conditions, requires many detours, and challenges our strength and patience.

8.1.6.1 Epilepsy: birth to age 7

A *widely applicable basic therapy in epilepsy* at this age includes the administration of

- **Belladonna Rh D20 dil.** Weleda
  (alternatively in BNS epilepsy **Viscum comp.** Wala)

together with

- **Belladonna/Chamomilla pillules** Wala and
- **Chamomilla Cupro culta, Radix D2 dil.** Weleda

in the dosage specified in ▸Chap. 8.1.5.4. Each of the specified preparations brings a different aspect in various potencies of Belladonna or Chamomilla to bear which is why giving them together is more effective.

Birth trauma-related epilepsies with manifestation in infancy can be treated with

- **Arnica D20–200 pillules,**
- **Cuprum met. praep. D20 trit.** Weleda,
- **Apis regina comp. pillules** Wala,

and as a basic medicine with

- **Chamomilla Cupro culta D2** or Rh D3 dil. Weleda.

The following can be very effective in all forms of epilepsy with peri-/postnatally acquired cerebral damage:

- Baths with **Arnica Essenz/Lotion (20 %)** Wala/Weleda, 1 ml/bath

In *BNS epilepsy* (and associated forms of Lennox-Gastaut syndrome) [cf. Madeleyn 1990], *mistletoe therapy* with oral or also parenteral application is indicated (▸Chap. 8.1.5). The dose can be increased until a clear reaction becomes apparent. The following are a possibility

- **Viscum Mali D5** (and lower) **dil.** Weleda – later it may be appropriate to move to **Viscum Pini D5–15 pillules** Wala or **Viscum comp.** pillules Wala,
- **Apis regina comp. pillules** Wala
- **Arnica D20/Arnica baths.**

Apis regina comp. also has a favourable supporting effect in steroid pulse therapy and ACTH treatment.

With BNS epilepsy the metabolic pole does not receive the necessary impulses and structure from the soul organization; the following has a balancing, and thus also anticonvulsant effect in this respect

- **Hyoscyamus D3–6 Rh dil.** Weleda,
- **Agaricus D4–12 dil.** Apotheke an der Weleda.

In many cases, also following allopathic treatment, the following has a consolidating effect on the formation of the life organization in the metabolic pole and the connection of the soul entity with the body in this sphere

- **Conchae comp. pillules** Wala.

Bufo rana is not indicated in this connection until infancy (cf. the case study in ▸Chap. 8.1.5.3).

An anticonvulsant effective metallic medicine to be considered for children with previous cerebral damage at this age is

- **Cuprum met. praep. D20 trit.** Weleda.

With its harmonizing effect, it is located in the middle between the primarily cerebrally acting medicines and the medicines which are active in the metabolic pole. Cuprum also counters irregularities in perfusion and vascular spasms which are induced by lesions of the craniocervical junction and can cause seizures.

Very important as part of infant epilepsy treatment is also the treatment of *complications arising from seizures.* In this respect

- **Argentum met. praep. D20 trit**. Weleda,
- **Helleborus niger D3-12, LM6** (various manufacturers.)
- **Apis regina comp**. Wala,
- **Cerebrum comp. A/B (pillules/amp.)** Wala

are of great importance. These medicines stimulate the life organization in the sphere of the nervous system, support the development of consciousness and stimulate potentials of possible neuronal reorganization.

States with pronounced *connective tissue-related remodelling and* scarring of the brain should make us think of

- **Arnica D20–30** Weleda – **Arnica D200** DHU,
- **Tabacum Weleda/Nicotiana e fol. Wala D10-20,**
- **Quarz** D20,
- **Agaricus** D6, D12.

Epilepsies in the first septennium occurring without detectable previous damage of the brain *in a primary generalized* form, can be treated in the form of a basic therapy with

- **Plumbum mell. D20 trit.** Weleda in the morning,
- **Belladonna D20 dil.** Weleda in the afternoon,
- **Quarz D20 trit.** Weleda in the evening.

The guiding force of the I-organization is strengthened, a blockage of the astral element in the sphere of the head is countered and the permeability of the organ surfaces for soul and spiritual impulses is positively supported.

In all cases where the epilepsy in early childhood is associated with *erethism and aggressiveness,* the following is suitable

- **Chamomilla e rad. D20 pillules** Wala

as a supplement for the Cuprum treatment.

In the treatment of *rolandic epilepsy,* R. Madeleyn has found the administration of the following to work

- **Bryophyllum Argento cultum Rh** D3 Weleda,
- **Hyoscyamus Rh** D6 Weleda.

8

8.1.6.2 Epilepsy: age 7 to 14

At this age the aspect of the threefold structure of the human organism is of particular importance: driving forces and growth forces increasingly develop in the metabolic and limb sphere and the beginnings of sexual development must increasingly be taken hold of in the middle of the second septennium by the soul and spiritual individuality of the child and brought under their control. If the first septennium is under the guidance of the formative forces and impulses coming from the head, a dialectic between the nervous and sensory pole and the metabolic pole develops in the second septennium in which the rhythmical system matures and the balance of these forces must gradually be achieved through the respiration, blood circulation and spinal column.

Epilepsies which occur newly at this age are often connected with the immaturity and overload of the rhythmical system which is reflected in the cerebral seizure. Inner and outer obstacles and stresses of *soul development acquire a corresponding importance.* On the other hand, this means that epilepsies at this age therefore often have a better prognosis, a more symptomatic and temporary character, something which should be taken into account with regard to any aggressive treatment. Parents and therapists are particularly called upon here to look at the development of the child from the perspective of the harmony between soul and body and how it can be supported therapeutically, which is often not done in any purely pharmacologically oriented suppression of seizures. That can potentially lead to greater problems later on than would arise from the seizures themselves.

A *basic therapy* for epilepsies in the second septennium, which is of importance for example in each absence epilepsy (also when medicated with anticonvulsants!) because it supports the maturation of the rhythmical system, is

- **Cardiodoron mite gtt./Cardiodoron Rh tab.** Weleda, or
- **Primula comp. pillules** Wala
  particularly for maturation crises of the soul entity (age nine), stresses, experiences of loss (family separation, moving), depression, combined with
- **Aurum met. praep. D10–12 trit.** Weleda (▸Chap. 7.2.3.3).

Children with *absence epilepsy* require help in several respects:

- **Agaricus D12 dil.** Apotheke an der Weleda, in the morning
- **Arum maculatum D3 dil.** DHU, possibly together with **Conchae comp. pillules** Wala in the afternoon,
- **Sulphur D12 pillules.** Wala/**trit.** Weleda in the evening

order, form and limit the metabolic dynamic which puts the child under pressure. If compulsive sexually tinged behaviours occur, the triad

- **Bufo rana D12–30** DHU,
- **Hyoscyamus Rh D6–15** Weleda
- **Argentum met. praep. D12–20** Weleda, **Argentit D12–20 trit.** Apotheke an der Weleda

should be considered.

Pronounced *emotional disorders* and epilepsy are an indication, among other things, for the use of the single medicine

- **Hyoscyamus Rh D6 dil.** Weleda-**C30 pillules** Gudjons

(▸Chap. 7.4).

A *greater psychological blockage* with inhibited expressiveness but without an advanced psychopathology in the sense of a problem arising as part of *delayed psychological maturation* indicates in particular

- **Conchae D12–30 trit.** Weleda, **LM6–12** dil. Arcana or also high potencies.

- Causticum (▸Chap. 8.1.5) and Calcium phosphoricum should be differentiated with regard to treatment; in the latter case the inner psychological inhibition is associated with restlessness, dissatisfaction, head and stomach aches.

The *nervous and sensory pole* is primarily addressed by treatment with

- **Belladonna Rh D20** Weleda

which is indicated specifically for greater *photosensitivity*. If there is a grand mal risk one thing to be considered is

- **Plumbum silicicum D10–30 trit.** Weleda

in combination with Belladonna.

Eurythmy therapy is very important in the second septennium to develop the rhythmical system, as are the *artistic therapies* (including anthroposophical speech therapy) to harmonize psychological development. If there are major tensions, disorders in the region of the spinal column, traumatizing experiences in early childhood and pronounced disharmonies in the warmth organization (hyperthermia – hypothermia), *rhythmical massage therapy* is a treatment which can open new paths for the soul.

In school children with epilepsy who develop *learning and memory disorders*, the administration of the following organ preparation has proved itself effective (e. g. 1 drinking ampoule 2 x/wk)

- **Hippocampus Gl D15 amp.** Wala [Vademecum 2010, 493]

8.1.6.3 Epilepsy: age 14 to 21

Epilepsies in the transition to the third septennium may be connected with development or disorders, inhibitions of the will forces and sexuality. The crisis of adolescence (▸Chap. 7.2), the full awakening to start creating an independent connection between the I and the world is the subject of these years and thus also a cause of their pathology.

The *impulsive petit mal*, a form of awakening epilepsy typical for this age, is connected with the above context: the uncontrollable jerking of the limbs is the physical expression of the struggle for independence and control of the will. Together with the question of the life rhythm, constitutional and family-related disorders of the drive and of independence are partly responsible for triggering the seizures.

Therapeutically, the Solanaceae and sulphur are indicated here:

- **Belladonna Rh D20 dil.** Weleda,
- **Sulphur D20 trit.** Weleda,
- **Stramonium D12 pillules** DHU.

The following triad is generally effective for supporting consciousness, the inner development of light and the control of the metabolism in epilepsies

- **Belladonna D20 Rh dil.** Weleda in the morning,
- **Carbo Betulae D20 trit.** Weleda in the afternoon,
- **Sulphur D20 dil.** Weleda in the evening.

8.1.6.4 Considering the organs in epilepsy treatment

Starting from the age of three or four, and on reaching the third septennium at the latest, *functional organic disorders* (which can become evident both psychologically and somatically) grow increasingly important in relation to the treatment of the epileptic event: these disorders can represent an important obstacle preventing the astral body and I activity from fully taking hold of the body and turning it into the tool (Greek: organon) of their connection with the world. R. Treichler [1979, 14–27] has dealt with this aspect of epilepsy (particularly in adults) in detail.

The organic relationship with the *brain*, which is the almost exclusive focus of conventional medicine, represents a reductionism in its exclusivity which is still connected with the Cartesian concept that the human soul is only connected with the pineal gland and the rest of the organism is a robot controlled from there (Descartes, *Passions de l'âme, traité de l'homme*). If, in contrast, we can accept and perceive that the I and soul organization are just as much present and active in the heart and hands as in the limbic system, then inhibitions of organ function *everywhere* in the organism acquire a possible pathogenic meaning when looking at epilepsy, as *indeed the totality of the organism's physical processes are reflected in the brain* (and can accordingly lead to disorders there).

The most important organic relationship with regard to the treatment of childhood epilepsies is with the *gastro-intestinal tract.* The wall of the gastro-intestinal tract is the most enervated organ outside the central nervous system (enteric nervous system, ENS, ▸Chap. 4.1). Researchers today refer to a "constant dialogue" between both nervous systems which possess approximately the same mass. The importance of *constipation* in epilepsies has already been addressed. The authors refer in this context to two published case histories in which serious epilepsies (myoclonic-astatic epilepsy and Lennox-Gastaut syndrome) at preschool age were healed with the help of homoeopathic and anthroposophic medicines: in both cases an constipation or a "defecation aura" was the guiding symptom for the authors [Black 1992, Husemann 2009, 97–98] in their choice of medicines (in the second case Nux vomica, in the first Lycopodium). Both cases show that the perspectives on the development of the digestive tract developed in ▸Chap. 4, including the treatment possibilities set out there, represent an important basis for epilepsy treatment.

Guiding symptoms in connection with *disorders of the hepatobiliary system, pancreas function* and the *digestive tract* are:

- constipation tendency, especially preceding the seizure,
- thirst for cold drinks, peculiar food preferences, e. g. for cold food only,
- bloated appearance, slightly pyknic bearing,
- changing stool colour,
- maldigestion symptoms
- increase in the above disorders of the somatic function and of behaviour in connection with anticonvulsants and antibiotics (which particularly burden the hepatobiliary system).
- changing drive, depressively inhibited will activity, tendency for sadness ("without reason"),
- choleric angry outbursts (in contrast to the nervous but cooler appearing irritability connected with the kidneys),
- obstinate and stubborn behaviours, phlegmatic (choleric) in temperament,

The following medicines may be considered for therapy in connection with childhood epilepsy (cf. in detail ▸Chap. 6.3.3.2):

To stimulate hepatobiliary function and detoxification of a pre-existing, specifically anticonvulsant medicinal burden

- **Gentiana Magen globuli (Stomach remedy)** Wala (above all if there is slight nausea – contains low potency of Nux vomica which should also be considered as an individual medicine, cf. ▸Chap. 6.5.6.11).
- **Lycopodium comp. pillules Wala** (particularly if there is dulled consciousness, changing stool colour, constipation; Lycopodium can also be considered as an individual medicine, ▸Chap. 6.3.3.2),
- **Liv 52 Ayurveda** 1–3 × 1 dragée (coated tablet) if there are strong intoxication manifestations.

The most important metallic medicine in the liver disorders-epilepsy link is zinc, e. g. as

- **Arandisit** (a zinc mineral) **D12 trit.** Apotheke an der Weleda/**D15 amp.** Weleda [Vademecum 2010, 99] or in vegetabilized form as
- **Taraxacum Stanno cultum Rh D3 dil.** Weleda

in connection with

- **Hepar GI D4–6 amp.** Wala.

The most important mineral medicine is

- **Sulphur D6, LM6 dil.** (various manufacturers).

Important herbal medicines in connection with hepatobiliary function are

- **Cichorium Stanno cultum Rh D3 dil.** Weleda
- **Taraxacum e pl. tota D3 pillules** Wala.

A medicine which is indicated above all for functional gall bladder disorders (D6) and simultaneously has a very profound effect on *traumatic skull and brain injury following an accident* (during and after symptomatic transitory psychotic syndrome; use high potencies, D30–200) is

- **Natrium sulfuricum D6–200 pillules, LM6–12 dil.** Arcana

Externally, embrocations with

- **Stannum met. 0.4 % ointment** Weleda

and warm liver compresses/wraps with yarrow tea are effective.

A further important organic relationship is with the *kidneys*, whereby there are close connections with the endocrine system, particularly the *adrenal gland*. The action of the astral body in the region of the digestion and metabolism on the one hand, the awakening of consciousness on the other, are essentially linked with the function of kidneys and adrenal gland.

Indicative symptoms for therapeutically relevant disorders in this sphere can be:

- nervous restlessness, easily agitated,
- particularly after early shock experiences (shock experiences noticeably lead to changes in and, potentially, serious disorders of kidney function),
- decrease in excretory functions before the seizure (sometimes followed afterwards by a flood of urine),
- disorders of the depth of respiration (no abdominal breathing), susceptibility for asthma in a neurasthenic constitution, migraine with visual disorders and tension (▸Chap. 7.10.2, Natrium muriaticum),

- reduced appetite, fussy (impaired stomach function and susceptibility for spasms in the digestive tract),
- disorders of the blood pressure regulation,
- lack of internal warmth, but also no sensation of warmth.

Therapeutically the most important medicine is *copper*, externally as embrocation in the region of the organ or internally in the possible combination with the homologous organ preparation:

- **Cuprum met. 0.4%/Tabacum D6** ointment Weleda
- **Renes/Cuprum amp.** Wala (per os), e.g. 2 x/wk
- **Cuprum met. praep. D20 trit.** Weleda, together with **Renes Gl D8 amp.** Wala (per os).

With strong, aggressively tinged agitation:

- **Chamomilla (Radix) Cupro culta D2 dil.** Weleda
- **Chamomilla e rad. D20 pillules** Wala, in combination with Cuprum and Renes,
- **Equisetum arvense D3 dil.** Weleda/**pillules** Wala.

With pronounced *neurasthenia, hypothermia, cerebral (e.g. birth-related) pre-existing damage*

- **Dioptas D20 amp.** Weleda (nat. copper silicate).

In *circulatory hypotonia:*

- **Glandulae suprarenales comp. pillules** Wala,

in combination with

- **Nierentonikum (kidney tonic)** Wala, (this must be carefully gradually dosed! 1–3 tsp./d).

The birch charcoal already mentioned also has a strong connection with the kidneys,

- **Carbo Betulae D20 trit.** Weleda,

strengthening the formative-catabolic, internally light-releasing activity of the astral body under the control of the I which is connected with kidney function in human beings [Steiner 1976, 216].

The *genital tract* lies in proximity to the kidney organization. The former is comparatively important with regard to epilepsy, particularly if the *child's sexual inhibition,* which originates in the head pole (including the epiphyseal function), is weakened because of cerebral disorders. Together with directly sexually tinged actions and fantasies, an extreme compulsion to move, overexcitability and destructive aggression indicate disorders in this organic sphere.

The lengthy inhibition of sexuality is a basic prerequisite for the uniquely long childhood of humans, in comparison to the primates for example, but this is what enables the spiritual individuality of the human being to take hold of the body, to acquire freedom. The medicines to be considered in this connection have already been referred to[1] (Agaricus, Bufo rana, Hyoscyamus, Argentum, Arum maculatum).

1 In addition, the administration (per os) of Epiphysis D6 amp. Wala can have a positive regulating effect.

8.2 Movement and sensory development disorders

The child connects actively with other people and the world through perception and movement. The central importance of the sense organs in this development is revealed by the child's organism itself: thus all the parts of the labyrinth of the inner ear "have already acquired their final form and size at birth" [Rauber and Kopsch 1987b, 608] and the olfactory mucosa initially still reaches up over the middle concha in the foetal period [Rauber and Kopsch 1987a, 136]. In other words, the sense organs speed far ahead in growth and maturity in embryonic and early childhood development. The small child does not mature physiologically in such a way that the stimuli from the external world produce automatic responses; maturation ensues through the *interplay* of the perception of the other person and his or her own movement, which in turn has an effect on the other person. Every newborn child carries the impulse within himself or herself to initiate and maintain up such interplay – at no age, on the other hand, do the sensory experiences intervene in the physical and soul development of the human being more deeply than in the first years of life [Steiner 1969, 120–137].

Modern thinking, based as it is on the one-sided deterministic connection between cause and effect, finds it difficult consciously to follow such an interplay in which I and you *simultaneously* encounter, move and change one another: every mother tries to organize her actions in such a way that there is a *positive resonance* of soul and body with the child. Conversely the child tries to achieve a similar thing, be it through imitation or through the impulsive expression of vital needs. The simultaneous reciprocal transformation of everyone involved does not follow any causal laws but is an expression of *active human correspondence* as described by, among others, F. Schiller [e.g. 1966, 445–520], M. Buber [1997] and currently Th. Fuchs (▸Chap. 1) [2000, 244–251; 2008] as a qualitatively independent, dynamic causative principle in human development. It is the causal principle at work in art, in the experience of art.

Every obstacle to perception and independent movement disrupts this correspondence. It is both a physical and soul experience; and the far-reaching consequences of a hearing disorder or cerebral palsy, but also just delayed or absent left-right lateralization [Rodriguez 2010] can only be judged if both aspects, the development of the body and the development of the soul and spirit are taken into account in equal measure. A strong connection develops in hearing to the rear space hidden to the eye, and to that which in things and humans lies behind superficial appearances; the left side has a stronger connection to the emotions, but also to the past, the right side, accordingly, to the will and the future. Every delay, every impairment of childhood development in this area thus requires a diagnosis which takes account of all levels and seeks the corresponding balance. A detailed account would go far beyond the scope intended here, which is restricted to suggestions from the experience of the authors which have therapeutically proved themselves with regard to specific disorders as a supplement to what is generally familiar.

The *preventive medical checkups,* but also every other consultation, offers the opportunity to observe the correspondence of the child with the mother, the father and, in addition, the examiner:

- How does the child move his or her head? Is this movement flowing or inhibited?
- How does the child move his or her eyes? Does he or she register his or her human opposite? Does his or her look slide past people and things or can it linger? Are eye movement and head movement in harmony?

- Does the hand display play between opening and closing, in the movement of the fingers, or is its movement inhibited?
- How does the child drink? How is the movement of the head and torso connected in the neck region?
- How is facial expression developing, how transparent is it to the child's inner life?
- What diversity and modulation do the sounds show, how does the child react to language, music, sounds, light?

All of these things reveal activity of the soul in the living entity – just as the movement of air acts on the water and sets it in motion, so the child's soul organization takes hold of the body – and nothing is more necessary for that than the encounter with his or her equally ensouled, living counterpart.

This is where the key diagnostic questions take their starting point: is there an age-appropriate free *resonance from the child* in the encounter or do the mother or examiner have to struggle to establish it? Where is the *correspondence* in perception/movement *not possible and where is it impaired?*

This perspective is significantly more comprehensive than a fixation on reflexes and so-called developmental "milestones", even if it assumes a knowledge of these milestones as cornerstones of the child's age-appropriate scope. Above all, this perspective allows us to take the parents seriously in a comprehensive way and include them: because they can tell us from their experience how the interaction of the child with the surroundings is developing; and they feel that their concerns are understood when a childhood disorder means that there is a struggle to achieve correspondence.

The doctor is dependent on the parental experience. The key thing is to make sure that during the consultation an awareness can arise through the questioning and observing attitude of the doctor as to what the child and parents are experiencing.

8.2.1 Infantile cerebral palsy

The little limping girl

The girl smiles: "Wait,
I'll go and get the crutches!"

Sun and roses. The swaying
and fresh avenue of trees throws
pure green light. Noise
of birds. New north-east winds.
The girl smiles: "Wait,
I'll go and get the crutches!"

A heaven made of dreams and silk
penetrates as far as the heart.
The children, in white, come,
play, sweat and shout:
"...ruuun!"
The girl smiles: "Wait,
I'll go and get the crutches!"

Her eyes shine. Her leg hangs
twisted and strange.
Her shoulder hurts. She gasps for air,
leaning against some alders, sits down,
laughs and cries and laughs: "Wait,
I'll go and get the crutches!"

But the birds don't wait;
nor do the children! Spring
errs. The festival belongs to those
who run and fly ...
The girl smiles: "Wait,
I'll go and get the crutches."

J. R. Jiménez

8.2.1.1 Differentiation of levels of disease manifestation

Children with infantile cerebral palsy experience space and the movement and perception of their own body "differently": thus in spastic palsy the relationship between top and bottom (paralysis of the legs, e.g. following periventricular leukomalacia in premature babies), left and right (spastic hemiparesis, e.g. following ischaemic infarction of the contralateral capsula interna region) or primarily the relationship between forward and rear space (tetraplegia) can be affected in that spastic tetraplegia is associated with the loss of the ability to develop a stable and relaxing relationship between the back and the bed or matt on which the back is lying: a particularly profound loss for the child, for his or her movement and experience [cf. K. König 1984, 34]. The external loss of space has its counterpart in a corresponding impairment of inner bodily perception.

Spasticity as an active paralysing event is not just the result of a physical defect: it develops to the extent that *the soul entity attempts to immerse itself in the body and thereby enter into a relationship with the world* (▸Chap. 8.1). The injury-related weakness of the life organization impairs the necessary interplay between arousal and inhibition, contraction and relaxation and leads to a *one-sided dominance of contraction and hypersensitivity* in the muscles and the structures of the spinal cord associated with motor functions. A muscular imbalance between agonist and antagonist frequently arises [Schröder 2009.1122]. The absence of relaxation and mostly one-sided contraction of the muscles threatens to lead to increasing physical deformation of the skeleton and joints and thus to an ever greater loss of freedom of movement. It is important to understand that here it is the *own soul organization of the child which has a deforming effect on the physical body because its impulses cannot be transformed into "fluid" (!) movements through the life organization;* thus muscles and joints threaten to become "fixed". Rudolf Steiner describes this state such that "the etheric body atrophies and the astral body gains direct influence over the physical body without the mediation of the etheric body" [Steiner and Wegman 1977, 109].

Therapeutically it is a matter of:

- Supporting as far as possible the child's damaged life organization e. g. with potentized medicine, balneotherapy, rhythmical massage therapy and eurythmy therapy. Craniosacral therapy also acts on this sphere.
- Psychologically providing the child with a *positive experience of space and his or her own body through movement* and stimulating a healthy progression of movements e. g. through the corresponding neurophysiologically-based physiotherapy, ergotherapy, conductive support and much else. The authors would like particularly to point out that accompaniment with music (e. g. lyre) and singing can help to address the soul entity of the child.
- Helping the individuality to get out of its isolated and unstable situation and identify with its own physicality and environment, to experience successful correspondence through own movement. The experience of upright posture and language is of particular importance for the individuality.
- Countering physical deformation and offering movement and communicative assistance.

Allopathically, the attempt is made today to weaken the one-sidedly dominant agonists with *botulinum toxin* in order to balance the polar active muscle groups by therapeutically mobilising the antagonists (in an integrated approach). Here the one-sidedly tensed muscle is paralysed with the toxins, i. e. its vitality is further depressed: "In terms of the fine structure, a neurogenic atrophy of about 30 % of the muscle fibres in a BoNT/A-injected muscle with signs of regeneration could be observed in test person A [= biopsy of a healthy test person treated with botulinus] 12 months after the injection. In summary we can say: the one-time injection of a standard dose of BoNT/A [botulinus toxin] in healthy adults was still evident by MRT two years after the injection. This is contradicted by the effects mostly wearing off after 3–6 months" [Schröder 2009, 1125]. As much as one can understand the desire to improve the balance and play of the patient's muscles, this path must continue to be viewed with reservations as regards the long-term consequences. Adverse loss of tone if an excessive dose is applied and other side effects can also be problematical.

8.2.1.2 Medicinal treatment options

8.2.1.2.1 Standard treatment for cerebral palsy-related muscular spasticity and muscular disbalance: Plantago Primula cum Hyoscyamo

The most important innovation in the field of anthroposophic medicine for the treatment of children and young people with cerebral palsy is seen by the authors in the introduction by Markus Sommer of

- **Plantago Primula cum Hyoscyamo amp.** Weleda
  ½–1 ampoule s.c. 1 x/wk-1 x/d depending on effectiveness and need; in infants and small children also 0.3–0.5 ml per os 1 x/d

as the standard treatment for neurogenic muscular spasticity in response to a key reference and report from the brothers Hessenbruch, therapeutically very experienced anthroposophical medical colleagues from Remstal in Schwäbisch Gmünd [Vademecum 2010, 663–665]. The medicine has also proved its value for example in the treatment of Friedreich's ataxia and other genetically-related spastic syndromes.
The response to the application of this medicine can mostly be judged with the first injection, sometimes as soon as after one hour. If three injections remain without effect, there is no sense in further repetitions.

The injection of this medicine by the authors has proved effective in many cases of children and young people with muscular spasticity. It can relax the spasticity without showing any of the side effects of botulinus toxin and positively influence the balance between hypo- and hypertension in the muscles. The authors were also able to gather positive experiences with the administration per os in infants and small children. A detailed rationale for the medicine, which is similar to Cardiodoron® and thus oriented towards the rhythmization and development of balance in the rhythmical system (here in the muscular system between agonist and antagonist), is provided by Markus Sommer [2009] and explains in detail the medicinal plants Onopordon (thistle), Plantago (buckthorn) and Hyoscyamus. The injection is stressful; yet the authors have experienced, for example, that young people with hemiparesis themselves repeatedly ask for it. The injection interval varies a great deal; sometimes injections at an interval of several weeks are found helpful. At the beginning, and if there is a weak response, injections several times a week are to be recommended. For the authors, Plantago Primula cum Hyoscyamo is a regulatory, non-toxic medicine that offers an effective alternative to the standard treatment with botulinum toxin.

8

8.2.1.2.2 Therapeutic accompaniment of children with cerebral palsy

Infantile cerebral palsy mostly develops as the result of *difficulties in the process of birth.* That is why the medicinal treatment possibilities set out under ▸Chap. 2.2.2 to ▸Chap. 2.2.4 and ▸Chap. 2.4 are very significant. Most important are:

- **Cuprum met. praep. D20–30 trit./amp.** Weleda
- **Arnica e pl. tota D6–30 pillules** Wala.

In this phase the greatest possibilities exist for medicinally influencing the supply and reorganization of impaired organ areas.

The potentized, embryonic organ preparation indicated in this phase is above all

- **Amnion Gl D8–30 amp.** Wala

Here two aspects stand in the foreground:

- *Too early loss of enveloping protection* in premature babies, experiences of shock and loss of maternal security as the result of asphyxia and similar things as well as the subsequent medical interventions [Vademecum 2010, 65].
- *Injuries in the sphere of the sensory and nervous system.* The organ preparation Amnion stimulates the life organization in this area; as an embryonic and extra-embryonic ectoderm, Amnion has a clear relationship with it (this action originally was the reason for producing the preparation).

The authors have had positive experiences in carrying out a follow-up treatment with the following medicine for 3–6 months after birth trauma

- **Chamomilla Cupro culta, Radix eth. Dec. D2 dil./Rh D3 dil.** Weleda
  1–2 gtt. (D2) 2–3 x/d, 3–5 gtt. (Rh D3) 2–3 x/d

which combines the calming action of chamomile with the relaxing effect of copper in a very suitable form for infants (▸Chap. 2.2.4, ▸Chap. 8.1).

In the first six months of life, the development of infantile cerebral palsy mostly enters a phase with few symptoms which is characterized less by spasticity than by *muscle hypotonia*. The birth anamnesis and the already recognizable disorders in the movements of the child are important diagnostic indicators.

In premature babies with serious brain haemorrhage (ICH III and IV) who develop clinical signs of a manifest cerebral palsy, the neonatologically very experienced anthroposophical paediatrician Bernd Ulrich [2000] reports impressive experiences with the administration of

- **Aurum met. praep. D20 trit./amp.** Weleda
- **Arnica e pl. tota D30 pillules/amp.** Wala,
- **Hypothalamus Gl D20 amp.** Wala,

jointly administered in individual dosage.

The aim is "to avoid a hardening process in the sphere of the extremities (will organs)." Here the gold has a balancing effect on the "equilibrium between the spiritual impulse to incarnate and the material development of the body" which is interrupted by the traumatizing premature birth. The reason for the Hypothalamus organ preparation is the bleeding-related lesion, for Arnica the brain haemorrhage. Ulrich describes an impressive case study which shows – with x-ray documentation – the stabilization through the above treatment (in this case supplemented by rhythmical massage therapy) of a neurogenic subluxation of the right hip in a former premature baby born in the twenty-sixth week of pregnancy with grade IV intra cerebral haemorrhage (ICH) on the left.

We can confirm these experiences. A child with schizencephaly, for example, also reacted positively in his development to the administration of Hypothalamus and Aurum (and Plantago Primula c. Hyoscyamo from the start of the spasticity).

Other medicines to consider are:

Internally: vegetabilized copper (cf. ▸Chap. 4.4.4 on differential therapy in early childhood)

- **Tabacum Cupro cultum Rh** or **D3 dil.** Weleda
  3 gtt. before each meal, for paleness and periodic colic tendency, or
- **Melissa Cupro culta Rh D3 dil.** Weleda
  3 gtt. before each meal, for gentle children with weak vitality and cold extremities and
- **Arnica e pl. tota D10–12 pillules.** Wala
  2–3 pillules/d.

Externally:

- **Primula Muskelnähröl (muscle oil)** Wala alternating with
- **Rust e flora. 10 % Ol.**
  as embrocation or as part of rhythmical massage therapy primarily of the back in craniocaudal direction.

In this connection the simultaneous administration of

Helleborus niger D6–12 is also often of benefit (▸Chap. 7.5.3.6, ▸Chap. 8.1.5.4).

In the transition to spasticity, which often manifests itself in the second third of the first year of life, the following is an important medicine – particularly in spasticity affecting the legs – together with **Plantago Primula cum Hyoscyamo amp.** Weleda, already discussed above

- **Lathyrus sativus D6 pillules/dil.** DHU

the effect of which can be judged within a short time.

M. Sommer [1998] has drawn up a detailed explanation of the therapeutic rationale in his comprehensive, basic account of Lathyrus sativus – which can be used at all ages for spastic paresis. In a small pilot group at the children's polyclinic of Munich Technical University, seven of ten treated children showed a positive influence on the spasticity. On the other hand the authors also experienced a temporary increase in muscle tone in rare individual cases; then Lathyrus sativus (also in other potencies) is of no benefit. (Alternatively, **Cuprum aceticum comp. amp.** Wala, can be considered.)

As *organ preparations*, the following deserve primary consideration:

- **Hypothalamus Gl D15–30 amp.** Wala
  0.3–0.5 ml per os 2–3 x/wk

for s/p intracranial brain haemorrhage (see above) to stimulate the vitality and function of the correspondingly impaired organ area (cf. also Cerebrum comp. A and B, see below).

- **Hypophysis/Stannum pillules** Wala
  3–5 pillules/d

to stimulate the impulses for the child's whole life organization (pituitary gland) coming from the head pole and the reorganization in the region of the nervous system itself (Stannum) [Vademecum 2010, 505]

- **Agaricus D12 pillules** DHU/**dil.** Apotheke an der Weleda
  3–5 pillules/d

supports the latter aspect.

This medicine should always be considered when, as a result of injuries of the nervous system, movement disorders up to and including convulsions occur and when a blockage and chaotic activity of the child's movement impulses as a result of a vital disorder of the motor functions can be detected.

As an external application or as an oil dispersion bath (www.jungebad.com) – effective in patients with cerebral palsy to vitalize and strengthen the warmth organization – the following should be considered, among other things:

- **Lavandula 10 % Ol.** Wala,/Weleda
  to stimulate vitality and as an anticonvulsant, e. g. alternating with
- **Rosa e flor. 10 %** Wala.

It is important from a therapeutic point of view to take account of other perceptual disorders accompanying the movement disorder.

If in this respect *vision*, the relationship to light, to forward space, predominates,

- **Cerebrum comp. A cum Auro comp. pillules** Wala
  1 × 3–5 pillules/d

should be considered. If *hearing and the sense of balance*, the relationship with backward space, predominates, then accordingly

- **Cerebrum comp. B cum Auro comp. pillules** Wala.

This preparation should be given at intervals (two to four weeks).
An effective help for delayed, inhibited language development is the administration of

- **Myrrha comp. D8/Belladonna, Radix D10 dil.** Weleda
  3–5 gtt. 1–3 x/d

in 14-day alternation with

- **Apis regina comp. pillules** Wala
  3–5 pillules 2 x/d

K. König, who developed Myrrha comp. D8/Belladonna, Radix D10 dil., already pointed out that it was necessary to *give it at intervals* (▸Chap. 7.5.3.2). The practice of the authors has shown that in this respect Apis regina comp. has a specific complementary effect (a brainstem organ preparation is potentized together with Apis regina in the preparation of the medicine, ▸Chap. 8.1.5.3). Both medicines can be used for all language development disorders due to cerebral lesion in early childhood (e. g. also following meningoencephalitis and others). The craniocervical junction is fundamentally of particular importance in all language development disorders; this area should always be carefully investigated and, if necessary, included in treatment.

Beyond what has already been explained, the authors can make no additional generalizing statements with regard to *athetoid* cerebral palsy.

8.2.2 Treatment indications for constitutional motor development disorders

Delays in motor development are often observed in practice; in many cases that is not an expression of a pathology but a constitutional one-sidedness.

If metabolic assimilation predominates, i. e. if the life organization dominates over the development of the soul's initiative in movement, supporting medicinal treatment with

- **Calcium carbonicum LM6 dil.** Arcana
  3 gtt., possibly 2 × 3 gtt./d; later LM12, as necessary, 1 × 2–3 gtt.

should be considered even if no catarrhal infections, middle ear inflammations etc. occur.

There is fundamentally a good prognosis for these children; they mostly typically like lying on their back with a tendency for hyperopia, are psychologically contented, and detach themselves more slowly than others from the mother's lap to start coming to terms with the earth.

These contrast with children with general developmental delays who give an immature or underdeveloped impression both psychologically and with regard to vitality, develop little warmth, have sensory hypersensitivity and are easily irritated.

These children are supported by the administration of silicic acid-containing substances, e. g. the relevant grasses:

- **Bambusa e nodo D3-6-10 pillules** Wala
  3–5 pillules in the morning or
- **Triticum comp. I amp.** Wala.
  0.3 ml per os in the morning
  This medicine is made of wheat and a brainstem organ preparation which are potentized jointly; it is intended to support the "reorganization of the integrative structures of the nervous system in the joint action of the life and physical organization" (approved indication).

If cerebral lesion is suspected, the following has a complementary effect

- **Apis regina comp. pillules** Wala
  3–5 pillules in the afternoon.

Oil embrocations on the back and limbs are externally indicated with

- **Primula Muskelnähröl** (muscle oil) Wala.

Intellectually awake, psychologically disharmonious children with bad appetite and a clear deficiency of vitality in the metabolic and limb system can react very positively in their development to the administration of

- **Natrium muriaticum LM6 dil.** Arcana
  3–5 gtt. in the morning

(In these cases the symptoms represent an early form of a depressive disorder.

Human warmth and affection from the people who are bringing the child up and the action of light on the organism are of general importance for the child who is obtaining upright posture. The oil embrocations, which realize an intensive form of affection and warmth treatment, should be seen in this light.

If there is a delay in obtaining upright posture, the action of light can be intensified medicinally through the administration of

- **Phosphorus LM6 dil.** Arcana
  1–3 gtt./d in the morning and
- **Ferrum sidereum D20 trit.** Weleda
  1 saltsp. in the afternoon

With these medicines a significant improvement in obtaining upright posture could also be achieved in children with cerebral functional disorders; their administration is only of relevance where it is possible to achieve upright posture and the child is already attempting to do so.

8.2.3 Sight disorders

8.2.4 Hyperopia and myopia

Hyperopia in early childhood is less of a disorder than a delay in development. The characteristics set out in ▸Chap. 8.2.2 for the Calcium carbonicum type often apply to these children.

Accordingly

- **Conchae D10–12–20 trit.** Weleda
  1 saltsp. 1 x/d.

is most likely to be medicinally indicated.

During the course it should be carefully observed how the child unites with the world and where he or she anxiously withdraws into himself or herself to avoid a direct encounter (which is entailed in acute vision).

Medicinally it can make sense in these cases to follow the treatment with calcium carbonate with iron preparations, e.g.

- **Meteoreisen pillules** Wala
  5 pillules 1–2 x/d

and in pronounced anxieties

- **Skorodit D10 trit.** Weleda
  1 saltsp. in the morning.

Children with *myopia*, in contrast, often have a more delicate physique and are relatively awake in their head; but their spiritual and soul individuality is too little connected with the body in its activity, the living developmental processes require stronger formative support.

- **Atropa Belladonna e rad. D20 pillules** Wala
  3–5 pillules/d

has the effect of letting the formative forces of the astral body flow more strongly into the physical growth processes.
As a complement,

- **Levico comp. pillules** Wala
  5 pillules 2 x/d.

can be given. In children with a strongly dolichocephalic head shape, particularly myopic premature babies, the specified treatment is supplemented with

- **Hypophysis/Stannum pillules** Wala
  5 pillules 1 x/d.

The following individual mineral preparations should be primarily considered:

- **Phosphor D10–12 pillules, LM6 dil.** and
- **Quarz D20 pillules** Wala,

which, depending on the constitutional circumstances, can be administered differentially or also in sequence.

These medicines can intensify the action of light on the physical formative forces (just as, on the other hand, it is known today that reading without sufficient light, for example, can trigger a pathological growth stimulus of the eyeball with the corresponding increase in myopia).

Organ preparations are important above all in cases where, for example in an extremely premature birth, lesions or weakness of vitality have occurred in the sphere of the visual organ (retina, optic nerve and other structures of the central nervous system).

In general, the following is suitable as a much proven composite medicine

- **Cerebrum comp. A glob. velati** Wala
  5 pillules 1–2 x/d

This medicine should be given over a longer period (several months to one year).

Educationally, a guiding aspect during the course is to expand the scope of view of the myopic children above all by creating a more intensive connection between them and nature (and thereby also engaging the soul entity more intensively in the life entity). Conversely, the hypermetropic child should learn to become more centred in himself or herself and to concentrate e. g. by introducing him or her deliberately to reading.

An exceptionally valuable and effective form of therapy is *eye eurythmy therapy* developed by the anthroposophical doctor I. Knauer. A significant visual normalization can be achieved both in hyperopia and myopia as well as in strabismus if the child does the appropriate intensive exercises at kindergarten and school age. That clearly illustrates the extent to which the development of vision is not just dependent on the physical circumstances but also on the connection between the soul of the child and his or her physical development and environment. The trend for eye glasses since the twentieth century combined with a one-sided and intellectually accentuated ("shortsighted") strain on the eyes is very clear, hence the proportion of students in Korea and Taiwan wearing glasses has grown to over 90 % today. Such a maldevelopment can only be balanced if the child learns to unite himself or herself actively just as much with what is alive as with the world of abstract thinking.

8.2.5 Esotropia (convergent strabismus)

A differentiated diagnostic and therapeutic account is not possible here. Medicinal treatment is also possible alongside the normal treatment and eye eurythmy therapy.

Apart from the treatment with Conchae for the type described in ▸Chap. 8.2.3.1 (hyperopia), the long term (up to two years) administration of the following medicines has proved its worth in the practice of the authors

- **Conchae D12,**
- **Argentum met. praep. D12**
- **Magnesium phosphoricum D6 dil.** Apotheke an der Weleda aa ad 60.0 ml
  5 gtt. 3 x/d

as well as massaging the following daily into the temple region

- **Equisetum 10 %**
- **Tabacum 1 %**
- **ungt. aa** ad 50.0 g Apotheke an der Weleda.

The following should be specifically considered as a potentized organ preparation

- **Nervus abducens Gl D8 amp.** Wala
  0.3 ml/d in the morning per os or 2 × 1 drinking ampoule/wk

for which there have been favourable therapeutic experiences in individual cases.

8.2.6 Hearing disorders

The most frequent hearing disorder in childhood is related to disorders of the pneumatization (▸Chap. 5.1.2). Inner ear and central hearing disorders represent an invasive disorder for the psychological development of the child: the relationship with depth, with the space behind and the spoken word is disrupted which can have a very negative effect on the development of *trust* in the world and other people. Diagnostic and technical therapeutic possibilities for hearing disorders in early childhood are currently undergoing an impressive development. Alongside early recognition, the paediatrician and general practitioner above all have the task of providing general support and rehabilitation. Social integration, the promotion of contact and trust, is of central importance.

Medicinally, there is restricted therapeutic help:

- **Cerebrum comp. B glob. velati** Wala
  5–7 pillules/d

is suitable as a general composite organ preparation given over a longer period; depending on the cause of the hearing disorder, specific organ preparations can be given individually (Cochlea, Nervus statoacusticus, etc.).

Gold should be considered above all as a metallic medicine:

- **Aurum met. praep. D12 trit.** Weleda
  1 saltsp./d or
- **Hypericum Auro cultum D2 dil.** Weleda
  3 × 5–7 gtt./d

As an external application, an ointment base might be massaged into the mastoid, into which 1 %

- **Plumbum silicicum D6–10 trit.** Weleda

has been incorporated.

Motor restlessness, outbursts of aggression and disruption of social integration in children with hearing disorders can also be improved by the treatment of the hepatobiliary region, e. g. with

- **Thenardit (= Nat. sulf. nat.) D6 dil.** Apotheke an der Weleda./**Natrium sulfuricum D12–30 pillules** (various manufacturers)
  5 gtt. 1–3 x/d or 5 pillules 1–2 x/d
- **Taraxacum Stanno cultum D2/Rh D3 dil.** Weleda
  7–10 gtt. 1–3 x/d

References for Chapter 8

(every reference marked with a ■ Bullet point indicates the English translation of the reference above it)

Alles, A.: Erlebnisse, Erfahrungen, Fragen bei Epilepsiebehandlung mit Levisticum, Folium D2 und D3. Der Merkurstab **62**, 631–632 (2009).

Baumeister, F. A., G. M. Liebhaber, E. Riemann, K. Gempel: Die ketogene Diät, Renaissance einer vergessenen Therapie: Grundlagen, Indikationen und Effektivität. Kinder- und Jugendmagazin 3, 76–86 (2003).

Baumeister, F. A., G. M. Liebhaber, E. Riemann: Efficacy of the ketogenic diet for the treatment of refractory epilepsy in children. Neuropediatrics **33**, A 23 (2002).

Buber, M.: Das dialogische Prinzip. 8. Aufl. Lambert-Schneider, Heidelberg 1997.

Fuchs, T.: Leib, Raum, Person. Klett-Cotta, Stuttgart 2000.

Fuchs, T.: Das Gehirn – ein Beziehungsorgan. Kohlhammer, Stuttgart 2008.

Geerts, A. et al.: Course and outcome of childhood epilepsy: A 15-year follow-up of the Dutch Study of Epilepsy in Childhood. Epilepsia, published online doi.:10.1111/j.1528–1167.2010.02546.x (2010).

Geukens, A.: Homöopathische Praxis, Bd. II. Hechtel 1989 (zu beziehen über U. Burgdorf – Verlag für homöopathische Literatur).

Hartman, A. L. et al.: Theneuropharmacology of the ketogenic diet. Pediatr Neurology **36,** 281–292 (2007).

Husemann, F.: Anthroposophische Medizin. Verlag am Goetheanum, Dornach 2009.

Imhäuser, H.: Homöopathie in der Kinderheilkunde. 12. Aufl. Haug Verlag, Heidelberg 2000.

König, K.: Heilpädagogische Diagnostik. 2. Aufl. Verlag am Goetheanum, Arlesheim 1984.

König, K.: Being human : diagnosis in curative education. Anthroposophic Press, Hudson, N. Y. 1989.

Lennox, W. G.: Epilepsy and related disorders. Boston 1960; zit. nach König 1984.

Lorz, Th.: Krampfanfälle und Epilepsie. In: Homöopathie in der Kinder- und Jugendmedizin. Pfeiffer, Drescher, Hirte (Hrsg.): Urban & Fischer, München 2004.

Madaus: Lehrbuch der biologischen Heilmittel, Bd. 2. Olms Verlag, Hildesheim 1979, 1999a.

Madaus: Lehrbuch der biologischen Heilmittel, Bd. 3. Olms Verlag, Hildesheim 1979, 1999b.

Madeleyn, R.: Behandlung der Epilepsie bei Kindern. Der Merkurstab **43** (6), 369–384 (1990).

Matthes, A.: Epilepsien. 6. Aufl. Thieme Verlag, Stuttgart 1999.

Merkurstab, Der: Sonderheft Organpräparate 1999.

Morrison, R.: Handbuch der Pathologie zur homöopathischen Differentialdiagnose. Kai Kröger Verlag, Groß Wittensee 1999.

Rauber, A., F. Kopsch: Anatomie des Menschen, Bd. II Innere Organe. Leonhardt, H., G. Töndury, K. Zilles (Hrsg.). Thieme Verlag, Stuttgart 1987a.

Rauber, A., F. Kopsch: Anatomie des Menschen, Bd. III Nervensystem, Sinnesorgane. Leonhardt, H., G. Töndury, K. Zilles (Hrsg.). Thieme Verlag, Stuttgart 1987b.

Rimpau, W.: Selbstkontrolle bei Epilepsie. Erinnerungsspuren in der Therapie einer Epilepsiekranken. In: Krankengeschichte. Biographie – Geschichte – Dokumentation. Beiträge zur medizinischen Anthropologie Bd. 2. Janz, D. (Hrsg.). Königshausen & Neumann, Würzburg 1999.

Rodriguez, A. et al.: Mixed-Handedness is linked to Mental Health Problems in Children and Adolszents. Pediatrics, published onlien doi: 10.1542/peds.2009–1165 (2010).

Schiller, F. von: Über die ästhetische Erziehung des Menschen. In einer Reihe von Briefen. Werke in drei Bänden. Hauser, München 1966.

Schröder, A. S. et al.: Botulinumtoxin als Teil einer integrierten Behandlung. Update 2009. MSchr Kinderheilk **157,** 1120–1127 (2009).

Schwarz, R.: Myoklonisch-astatische Epilepsie bei einem Vorschulkind. Beitr z Erw der Heilk **45**, 6–8 (1992).

Simon, L.: Grundzüge einer anthroposophischen Behandlung der chronischen Polyarthritis. Weleda Korr.blätter Sonderheft (Rheumatologie) 2000..

Sommer, M.: Lathyrus sativus und spastische Parese. Der Merkurstab **51** (2), 74–84 (1998).

Sommer, M.: Plantago Primula cum Hyoscyamo – ein fast vergessenes Arzneimittel bei Muskelkrankheiten.

Sommer, M.: Zink – Versuch einer Annäherung. Der Merkurstab **52** (1), 18–23 (1999).

Stauffer, K.: Homöotherapie. Faks. d. Ausgabe von 1924. Sonntag Verlag, Regensburg 1998.

Steiner, R.: Die gesunde Entwicklung des Leiblich-Physischen als Grundlage der freien Entfaltung des Seelisch-Geistigen. 3. Aufl. Rudolf Steiner Verlag, Dornach 1969.

- Steiner, R.: Soul economy and Waldorf education. GA (complete works) 303. Anthroposophic Press/Rudolf Steiner Press, Spring Valley, N. Y./London 1986.

Steiner, R.: Geisteswissenschaftliche Gesichtspunkte zur Therapie. Rudolf Steiner Verlag, Dornach.5.Aufl. 2001.

- Steiner, R.: Anthroposophical spiritual science and medical therapy: second medical course, nine lectures to physicians and medical students, Dornach, April 11–18, 1921. GA (complete works) 313. Mercury Press, Spring Valley, N. Y. 1991.

Steiner, R.: Heilpädagogischer Kurs. Rudolf Steiner Verlag, Dornach 7. Aufl. 1985, 8. Aufl. 1995.

- Steiner, R.: Education for special needs: the curative education course; twelve lectures for doctors and teachers given at Dornach between 25 June and 7 July 1924. GA (complete works) 317. Rudolf Steiner Press, London 1998.

Steiner, R.: Geisteswissenschaft und Medizin. Rudolf Steiner Verlag, Dornach 5. Aufl. 1976, 7. Aufl. 1999.

- Steiner, R.: Introduction to anthroposophical medicine. GA (complete works) 312. SteinerBooks, Great Barrington, M. A. 1999.

Steiner, R., I. Wegman: Grundlegendes zu einer Erweiterung der Heilkunst nach geisteswissenschaftlichen Erkenntnissen. Rudolf Steiner Verlag, Dornach 5. Aufl. 1977, 7. Aufl. 1991.

- Steiner, R., I. Wegman: Fundamentals of therapy : an extension of the art of healing through spiritual-scientific knowledge. GA (complete works) 027. Mercury Press, Spring Valley, N. Y.1999. Also available as: Extending practical medicine: fundamental principles based on the science of the spirit. Rudolf Steiner Press, London 1996.

Steinhausen, H. C.: Psychische Störungen bei Kindern und Jugendlichen. 3. Aufl. Urban & Schwarzenberg 1996, 4. Aufl. Urban & Fischer, München 2000.

Stübler, M., E. Krug (Hrsg.): Leesers Lehrbuch der Homöopathie. Bd. 5 Tierstoffe. 3. Aufl. Haug Verlag, Heidelberg 1987.

Treichler, R.: Vom Wesen der Epilepsie. Verlag Freies Geistesleben, Stuttgart 2. Aufl 1979, 3. Aufl. 1991.

Ulrich, B: Anregung der Sinne bei einem Frühgeborenen. Der Merkurstab **53,** 261–262 (2000).

Vademecum Anthroposophische Arzneimittel. 2.Aufl. Der Merkurstab **63**, Supplement (2010).

- Vademecum of anthroposophic medicines, CD format. Medical Section of the School of Spiritual Science, Dornach, Switzerland 2009

Verhulst, J.: Der Erstgeborene. Mensch und höhere Tiere in der Evolution. Verlag Freies Geistesleben, Stuttgart 1999.

Vogel, P.: Von der Selbstwahrnehmung der Epilepsie. Der Nervenarzt **32**, 438 (1961); zit. nach König 1984.

Weizsäcker, V. v.: Der Gestaltkreis. Suhrkamp Verlag (stw 18), FfM. 1973.

9 Disorders and constitutional aspects of growth and morphogenesis

"... if one traces the dynamic aspect in the structure of the human skeleton one can say: we do not find this in any other realm of the earth; forces appear here which we ... cannot find if we merely take into account the forces which exist outside of the human being."

R. Steiner

In childhood development, acquisition of an upright posture is a fundamental milestone; for the first time the child "stands on his own feet"; in his self-acquired upright posture, which he only adopts during waking hours, his individuality takes on an immediate bodily presence. – Human uprightness is not the expression of specialization, of adjustment to external conditions; it represents a consummate equilibrium of the forces active in the formation of the human gestalt. R. Steiner [1999, 29] compares it to the results of a parallelogram of forces: the head's spherical shape, the brain, which almost floats in the buoyancy of the liquor cerebrospinalis, "the entire human head constitutes a reproduction of the cosmos." This forms a contrast to the long bones, particularly those of the lower extremities, which the human being can position directly in his axis of gravity, thereby relieving his musculature.

These extremes are mediated by the spinal column as the bony central organ of the middle human being, the rhythmic system [cf. Sommer 2003], with the form of the vertebral bodies representing a "balance between the cosmic and the terrestrial" [Steiner 1980, 47]. In healthy human beings the spinal column mediates, in rhythmic oscillation, "between flexion and extension on the one hand and between lightness and heaviness on the other" [Vogel 1996, 165]. The formation of the primordial spinal column, the Notochord, establishes the future central body axis and in its interaction with the ectoderm it triggers the individuation of the embryo: "For the first time the germ material is directed towards a future bodily gestalt. The formation of a notochord also determines that *one* individual will evolve out of the germ developed up to this point" [Hinrichsen 1990, 113]. Hence from the very start, the spinal column is an "organ of I-organization" [Vogel 1996].

In its organizational activity the I aims to balance out forces and create the equilibrium of forces which is a necessary pre-condition for non-predetermined learning, play and free human action. – For this reason the human being does not acquire uprightness instinctively but rather individually through imitative learning, in the presence of upright human beings.

If one looks at the emerging gestalt of the child from the perspective of the aspect alluded to here, new possibilities for more intense encounter and perception can arise (cf. also ▸Chap. 9.7, Epilogue):

- The bodily gestalt is not simply an expression of genetically determined "programmes" but rather of formative forces which are related to those found in animals while at the same time differing from these qualitatively in terms of the way they are oriented and guided: the presence of human individuality *in the formation of the body, the body as an expression of the person,* becomes experienceable.
- Restraining the physical gestalt and leaving it open in its universally predisposed original form is a fundamental necessity for human morphogenesis; e. g. it is essential to restrain the growth of the intermaxillary bones (to prevent snout formation) and to leave open the fontanelles (to allow for postpartal growth of the telencephalon). This should be taken into consideration in cases of intervention on the part of the physician such as vitamin D prophylaxis and administration of fluoride (▸Chap. 3.2, ▸Chap. 3.4). On the other hand, the formation of the human skeleton is dependent on sufficient absorption of sunlight and active self-locomotion. This should also be taken into account since today many children do not get enough outdoor exercise, in particular school children during growth spurts in puberty. One frequently finds pronounced vitamin-D deficiencies in this age group (▸Chap. 3.2.2); this is confirmed by the author's experience.
- Such restraint makes it possible for the universal original form to mature (which human beings preserve in the form of their five-star, non-specialized hands) [Verhulst 1999, 133–149]) on a level reached nowhere in the animal kingdom while maintaining their general, non-specialized character, the human telencephalon being an excellent example of this. This also holds for the naked skin covered with sweat glands which lend the human being the singular capacity to regulate warmth freely [Verhulst 1999, 332–334].
- Grasping these connections, promotes respect for the child's individuality concretely, in a "bodily" way. Increased caution is exercised in regard to dietary measures and preventative interventions which accelerate bodily maturation and the like but which have a tendency to de-individualize the child in the process.

His childlike nature, is what distinguishes the human being fundamentally from members of the animal kingdom; no other comparably ensouled creature experiences such a time span of immaturity which is put at the disposal of learning and progressive individualized body formation. Even in adulthood, human beings do not stop being children insofar as they do not let themselves be fixed to the behaviour of their predecessors in terms of their actions, perceptions and thoughts, remaining flexible and able to learn instead. Upright posture, an actively realized equilibrium between "above" and "below," is the immediate expression of a free capacity for development.

Here the importance of growth and gestalt formation in the child becomes evident. In the following, only brief mention can be made of this area from a therapeutic perspective. In general one should emphasize at this point that it is not merely a matter of improving or eliminating disorders but rather of perceiving the *development of the child's gestalt in a new way so as to gain an understanding of it.* This will promote the insight that no isolated correction or therapy of the physical body can be undertaken without this having repercussions and consequences for the individuality of the child, which takes effect here. The therapeutic goal, the orientation of treatment cannot be an abstract, ideal body image, a norm or a mean value; instead, the focus must lie on a kind of bodily development which the child can identify himself with, which allows him to form his own individual expression.

9.1 Growth, stature and proportion

In the 5th lecture of his course for physicians held in 1920, R. Steiner emphasizes how "important knowledge of the entire human being is, even for treatment of the most special cases." The first aspect he mentions is age, for as he says, "therapy is highly dependent on the age of the patient." The second aspect he names as one to be taken into consideration in cases of disease is growth. Steiner says: "One should always carefully observe the growth of the patient in question, whether he is short and compact or tall and lanky, and it is very important to learn from this … which forces that which we call the human etheric body holds. … And this must be considered if one wants to recognize the relationship between the human being and his remedies" [Steiner 1999, 97]. Later in the same lecture Steiner refers to Calcium carbonicum and Phosphorus as medicaments, thereby bringing the aspect of growth and constitution discussed at the beginning of this chapter into relation to constitutionally effective remedies.

9.1.1 Shape of the head and constitution

How can we grasp the child's body? In cases of infants and small children a concrete possibility, after cautious observations have been made in connection with the physical examination, is to take the child's head between your hands and palpate it to feel how its spherical curvature is formed. In this way one can perceive such conditions as a premature attack of gravitation in the wrong place, for example, premature mineral-lifeless formation in a microcephalic child or a child with a large, sweaty head and large fontanelles which makes the impression of having excessive vitality and warmth in his head. Such children often calm down through touch.

This can already reveal preventative-therapeutic aspects. One can ask oneself: *does the child require vitalization,* more lightness and warmth *or should warmth and vitality be released from the head* and pass over into the movement of the limbs? (▸Chap. 3.2.3, Prophylaxis of rickets) In the former case the nerve-sense system and the skeleton threaten to unfold and develop too fast; therefore risking to remain incomplete ("small-headed" constitution [Matthiolius 1989]). Such children exhibit early closure of the fontanelles, motoric development occurs at a fast pace, the head appears older than the child's biographical age, the appetite is quite moderate and fluctuating, and such children often seem agitated and fidgety during the day. Later on they exhibit an inclination towards the analytical (one might be reminded of an Excel table in this context). As a means of harmonization one might consider the following:

- in terms of diet an ample amount of leafy vegetables and home-made desserts after meals
- in terms of body care sufficient warmth, a footbath and oil application in the evening; after lunch, if it proves beneficial, a warm yarrow liver compress (enabling a rest time for the necessary anabolic processes to take place), and head coverings sufficient to keep the head warm.
- in terms of the physician's care administration of silver compounds [cf. Vademecum 2010, 114], sulphur baths and calcium phosphate.

In the latter case, which involves "large-headed" children, there is a risk of the necessary formative-anabolic processes being delayed by excessive metabolic activity. Such children have heads with a relatively large circumference which are somewhat pear-shaped and their fontanelles remain open for a long time. Their movements are rather cumbersome; they prefer to lie on their back at first, observing the world. Their faces make them look younger than they actually are and they tend towards fantasizing (and are imaginative). Later on they tend to think synthetically, in terms of entireties, having difficulties with analytic thought, and in this vein sometimes with arithmetic. Abstract thinking develops quite slowly; the imaginative life is very vital. In such children feverish illnesses are often accompanied by febrile convulsions and also meningeal irritations and inflammations the roots of which lie in excessive vitality dammed up in the head. For such children

- medicinally: treatment with Apis mellifera, Belladonna, Bryonia and Calcium carbonicum can prove beneficial; for constitutional prophylaxis in cases of delayed development and poor I-presence, potentized lead [cf. Vademecum 2010] can be administered, followed by potentized copper and Conchae, oyster shell calcium (the oyster is one of the most copper-rich animals there is).
- paedagogically: bodily care consisting of cool face washes in the morning help to alleviate the sluggish waking-up process.
- dietary: root vegetables and sufficient amounts of salt are helpful.

A well-formed, spherical forehead (and frontal brain lobe) is important for the development of a harmonious, individualized process of thinking [Steiner 1982, 193]; a receding forehead is sometimes accompanied later on by difficulties with concentrating on thoughts and grasping ideas which are not directly related to objects; a narrow forehead is often accompanied constitutionally by agitation and in some cases a short attention span. Such seemingly archaic considerations correlate with our current knowledge of how the frontal brain lobe functions, however, as well as with the insights of craniosacral therapy concerning the significance of free mobility and the possibilities which the skull bones have to unfold while the head is still growing. It can also be that the head of the infant or small child is already very well-formed and quite well-proportioned but all in all relatively small, this being accompanied by weakness of the digestive system and the metabolism, slow thriving and a small or quickly satisfied appetite. In such cases constitutional treatment should focus on Silicea and Lycopodium as potentized medicaments (prophylactic and therapeutic) and in cases of quite high degrees of agitation and extroverted behaviour Calcium phosphoricum (▸Chap. 3.2).

In the first septennial the formation of a harmonious body shape can be promoted and supported to a considerable degree therapeutically. In cases of narrow and longish heads or such that are a bit constricted in the area of the temporal lobe and those with a narrow or receding forehead or ones with one-sided, posturally caused deformities the following

- **Stannum met. 0.4% ointment** Weleda daily pea-size amount applied locally and rubbed in [Vademecum 2010, 707] and
- **Hypophysis/Stannum pillules** Wala
  1 × daily 5 pillules [Vademecum 2010, 505]

over a sufficient length of time (several months) can prove beneficial in additional to individual constitutional remedies.

Tab. 9.1 The face as an expression of the constitution.

	Propulsive-accelerated development	Retarded, slowly progressing development
Relatively large, pronounced forehead, cerebral type	Phosphorus	Quartz
Very expressive, high middle face, respiratory type	Arsenicum album	Causticum
Pronounced mouth region and chin area, digestive type	Sulphur	Calcium carbonicum
Muscular-motoric type	Iodum, iodine salts, Fluorite = Calc. fluor.	Zincum met., Kieserite = Magnesium sulph.

9.1.2 The threefold organization of the face as an expression of constitution

N. Glas [1934] and B. Lievegoed [1984] have published studies on the proportions of the face in relation to temperament and constitution which are valuable in diagnostic-therapeutic and paedagogical terms. They premise their work on the specifically human *threefold* organization *of the face* into forehead (nervous system), middle face (respiratory system) and mouth-lower-jaw region (metabolic system). Depending on which region dominates proportionally (relative to the average for age) one can distinguish between types with a "cerebral," a "respiratory" and a "digestive" emphasis. Lievegoed, building on the works of Sigaud in the early 20th century, characterizes a fourth, muscular-motoric type in which none of the facial regions is particularly pronounced and motoric development is often predominant [Lievegoed 1984, 28–30]. This typology can already be applied for infants and it offers valuable prophylactic-therapeutic indications for young school-age children (7th to 9th year of life) in particular. It is refined by another aspect, namely the distinction which is made between an accelerated-"propulsive" and a decelerated-"retarded" developmental dynamic (but with the term "retarded" not being used in a pathological sense).

As an orientation for grasping the relationship between remedy and constitution one can consult the comparison outlined in Tab. 9.1 as a cautious approach to this aspect (the medicaments listed here are used as examples only and cited purely in terms of the constitutional aspect).

Although this list follows a homoeopathic simile principle, other approaches towards dealing with constitutional imbalances are possible, for example promotion of qualities which are lacking. Here one should pay particular attention to harmonizing effects produced by the organism itself which simultaneously constitute an emotional-bodily foundation and an expression of the *emotional life*: *the rhythmic system, respiration* (▸Chap. 5.2). Promoting this area is an important task of modern paediatric practice, also in prophylactic terms, since environmental conditions often prove unfavourable for harmonious respiration, and blood circulation and for an upright posture capable of oscillation.

Rhythmical massage therapy, rhythmical applications of oils and ointments, a corresponding paedagogical approach to the child and artistic activities (singing, working with colours, etc.) are valuable measures which can be taken.

The following anthroposophic compounds are medicaments which promote the rhythmic system in childhood:

For children whose development is generally slow and introverted

- **Primula comp. pillules** Wala
  2–3 × daily 5–7 pillules (contains Conchae = Calcium carb. D9)

For more extroverted, restless children (▶Chap. 7.5.3.4).

- **Aurum/Stibium/Hyoscyamus pillules**
  Wala: 2–3 × daily 5–7 pillules.

For school-age children

- **Cardiodoron mite dil./Cardiodoron Rh tab.** Weleda
  2–3 × daily 5–12 drops/2–3 × daily ½–1 tablet

is an important remedy which strengthens the child's centre (▶Chap. 7.2). These medicaments, in particular the last two, are also indicated for pronounced irregularities in blood pressure and pulse during the second septennial.

For school children who exhibit anxiety and insecurity one can also consider administering

- **Hypericum Auro cultum D2 dil.** Weleda
  3 × 7 drops
- **Ferrum ustum comp. trit.** Weleda
  2 × daily 1 large saltspoon in the morning and at noon

or another potentized iron compound, e. g. (**Ferrum sidereum D6** or **Scorodite D6–10 trit.** Weleda (= Ferrum arsenicosum).

9.1.3 Short stature and tall stature

Apart from having genetic and constitutional causes, *microsomia* in children sometimes involves causes which can be influenced therapeutically, most of all a *weakness of the liver-gall system*, a relative predominance of the physical body over the life organization, the etheric body, in this region.

In cases of such organ weakness

- **Lycopodium D12 (–C200) pillules** (various manufacturers), **LM6 dil.** Arcana
  1 × daily 5 pillules/drops or individual dosages of higher potencies is an important constitutional remedy.

Lycopodium works better if its administration is preceded or accompanied by a medication which has an immediate vitalizing effect (for. ex. **Sulphur, Argentite D6 trit.** Weleda (▶Chap. 8.1.5) or external applications (for. ex. warm yarrow liver compresses).

Medicines which especially stimulate liver metabolism and biliary are

- **Kieserite D4–6 dil.** Weleda (= Magnesium sulf. nat.)
  3 × daily 5 pillules or 3–7 drops
- **Taraxacum e pl. tota D3 pillules** Wala
  daily 2–3 × 3–5 pillules

The following organ compound has a universally vitalizing effect on protein synthesis:

- **Organum quadruplex amp.** Wala
  eg 2–3 × weekly 1 drinking ampoule (▸Chap. 7.5.3).

A further possible factor in microsomia is a disorder in impulsation of growth issuing from the head and proceeding in the craniocaudal direction. For diagnostics the cranio-cervical transition should be examined and treated manually if necessary (e. g. using craniosacral therapy).

It might also prove possible to stimulate growth in such cases by administering the following remedies in alternation, for three weeks each (▸Chap. 10.5):

- **Epiphysis/Plumbum pillules** Wala
  1–3 × 5 pillules daily and
- **Hypophysis/Stannum pillules** Wala
  3 × 5 pillules daily

In cases of children with microsomia who exhibit mentally delayed development, the most important constitutional remedy is

- **Barium carbonicum D12–LM6–LM12** (various manufacturers)
  daily 1 × 5 pillules/drops, administered over a relatively long period of time.

Therapy involving growth hormone has established itself in paediatric practice to a large extent. This holds for the practice of the authors as well. One can definitely ascertain that a lack of growth hormones in the classic sense cannot be influenced by homoeopathic or anthroposophic remedies any more than a lack of insulin can in cases of Diabetes mellitus. In such cases growth hormone therapy is unquestionably indicated. The authors have never observed any side effects except for when ambitious increases in dosages are given, which can impede the child's emotional-spiritual individuality in its bodily penetration. Hormone substitution therapy calls for sound judgement and experience, as is the case for all forms of endocrinological substitution therapy.

Children born extremely prematurely/SGA [Small for Gestational Age] infants with insufficient catch-up growth and pronounced microsomia at age 4 may also benefit from growth hormone therapy. This holds especially for promotion of thorax and lung growth, which can contribute to pulmonary stabilization and a strengthening of the child's centre. For such children, making use of the aforementioned therapy options during infancy and early childhood is of crucial importance and can even make it possible to dispense with hormone substitution. As important as it is to ward off commercial penetration of this field, the paths which therapeutic options for growth hormone substitution have opened up in paediatric medicine are significant.

Generally speaking *macrosomia* can become a concern addressed in the consulting room from a patient's 9th year of life and onwards, particularly if there is no clear genetic disposition (height of parents), the gestalt does not make a harmonious appearance and the child has entered the phase of growth acceleration in puberty. Movements now become quite gangly and insecure due to an increased awareness of them; in the course of distal-to-proximal growth spurts, distortions frequently occur. Acceleration of growth and average increase in body size correlate with the child's diet. As regards youths living in Western industrialized countries, the physician might be reminded of grain which grows tall quickly after being treated with artificial mineral fertilizer (containing such elements as potassium salts, nitrogen and phosphates) but which snaps easily in stormy weather as a result. Agriculturally speaking this is "counteracted" by applying stalk-shortening substances; for treating growth processes in children, another way must be found to achieve a harmonious measure.

A diet not too rich in protein and fat is beneficial; it should include regular portions of millet or barley if possible. An additional grain which is beneficial in this context is amaranth. A sufficient amount of minerals, most of all silicic acid and magnesium in vitally organized form is necessary whereas "overfeeding" the metabolism with high-calorie, industrially processed foods such as potato chips, sweets etc. acts like an artificial fertilizer on the child's growth.

Medication and eurythmy therapy stimulate the effectiveness of the I-organization in the area of the metabolism and the limbs, which shapes growth processes, gives contours and sets limits. Between the ages of nine and twelve a physiological intensification of I activity in the area of the metabolism sets ins (▸Chap. 7.2); this manifests itself, and can be stimulated, in the digestive activity of the organs in the upper abdomen, the gall bladder and the pancreas, and in the will initiative of the child.

For treatment of one-sided excessive macrosomia the authors focus on the following medicines:

- **Prunuseisen pillules** Wala
  2 × daily 7–10 pillules;
  as a plant remedy the original substance of which contains traces of the iron oxide haematite (▸Chap. 6.5.6.4.3).
- **Bambusa e nodo D6 pillules** Wala
  1–3 × daily 5 pillules;
  as a plant remedy with high concentrations of silicic acid which is also the plant with the closest association to elastic-oscillating uprightness [cf. Schuster 1996]
- **Calcium phosphoricum D12 pillules/dil.** (various manufacturers)
  1–2 × daily 5 pillules/drops
  is an important calcium salt (alongside apatite, which it is related to) for treating cases of disharmoniously accelerated growth of the spinal column. Children affected by this tend to be restless, unsatisfied, have a moderate, fluctuating appetite and a tendency to get headaches at school. The remedy can be supplemented by an iron preparation in the evening and the morning, e.g. **Vivianite** (= Ferrum phos. nat.) **D6 trit.** Weleda, 1 saltspoon (▸Chap. 6.5.6.3.2) or **Kephalodoron (Bidor) 5 % tab.** Weleda, 1 in the morning (cf. ▸Chap. 7.10) with excellent results if a tendency towards iron deficiency and recurrent headaches is observed. Iron preparations strengthen the effectiveness of the I in the metabolism and thus the capacity for regulation of length growth.

Tab. 9.2 Potentized remedies for disorders of growth and skeleton development in children.

Disorder	Remedy
Joints * cannot be completely stretched out, swelling connective tissue turgor, pudgy body shapes, tendency towards varization in the knees	Conchae or Calcium carbonicum
Joints cannot be completely stretched out, normal turgor, slender, especially in the neck area, early spurts of length growth, tendency towards valgisation in the knees	Apatite, Calcium phosphoricum
Joints overstretchable, pronounced connective tissue weakness, translucent veins, dry skin	Fluorite, Calcium fluoratum

* determined by examination of elbows and knee joints in particular

9.1.4 Connective tissue and joints

The general elasticity of the connective tissue and joint mobility indicate which potentized remedy should be administered preferentially for disorders of growth and the development of the skeleton in children. In keeping with an observation made by the Swiss homoeopath A. Voegeli, the distinction made in Tab. 9.2 has been verified over the course of many years. It is an aspect of great practical importance which is necessary for determining constitutional therapy.

9.2 Skeletal deformities of lower extremities

9.2.1 Foot deformities

In cases of *clubfoot* emphasis is placed on paediatric orthopaedic therapy.

Such therapy can be supplemented by daily rhythmical Einreibung of the affected areas using

- **Stannum met. 0.4 % ointment.** Weleda

and internal administration of

- **Stannum met. praep. D12 trit.** Weleda
  1 × daily 1 saltspoon and
- **Bambusa e nodo D6 pillules** Wala
  1 × daily 5 pillules

Despite increasingly optimized orthopaedic treatment techniques, the patient must be cared for emotionally in a sensitive way. In this as well as in a physical sense, eurythmy therapy constitutes a very beneficial form of treatment. Positive experiences have also been made with Feldenkrais therapy, for example.

In cases of *pidgeon toe* one should also consider supplementing osteopathic or chiropractic treatment with the aforementioned Stannum ointment application.

9.2.2 Malalignment of the knee joint

For Genu varum

- **Conchae D12 trit.** Weleda
  daily 1 saltspoon

and for Genu valgum

- **Calcium phos. D12 pillules** (various manufacturers)
  daily 1 × 5 pillules

is indicated; a complementary effect is achieved by

- **Hypophysis/Stannum pillules** Wala
  daily 5 pillules

Physiotherapy and eurythmy therapy in combination with the aforementioned remedies can lead to a lasting improvement of the leg position in the first septennial.

In cases of connective tissue weakness, "flail joints," especially around the knee joint – and in connection with psychomotoric retardation as well – therapy involving

- **Fluorite D4 trit.** Weleda
  1 saltspoon in the morning
- **Fluorite D10 trit.** Weleda
  1 saltspoon in the evening

have often proven to be effective. Therapy must continue for 6–12 months.

9.2.3 Congenital hip joint dysplasia

Thanks to ultrasound imaging, early and precise diagnostics are possible (and should not be neglected in routine check-ups). Orthopaedic treatment can be effectively supplemented by the following types of therapy and the scope of orthopaedic interventions can be reduced as a result.

For external use, alternating application of

- **Stannum met. 0.4 % ointment.** Weleda
  in the morning a pea-size amount and
- **Cuprum met. praep. 0.4 % ointment.** Weleda
  in the evening a pea-sized amount rubbed into the hip area over a sufficiently long period of time are indicated.

For internal use therapeutic preference is given to calcium phosphate [Steiner 2003, 49] with best effects achieved in combination with Stannum and in alternation with the organ compound of the pituitary gland which is indicated for all types of congenital skeleton deformation, namely:

- **Apatite/Stannum trit.** Weleda
  daily 1–2 saltspoons in alternation with
- **Hypophysis/Stannum pillules** Wala
  daily 5 pillules

In more severe cases, *eurythmy therapy* is effective even for very young children (the authors have observed use of this in some cases of severe hip joint dysplasia). – In cases of pronounced dysplasia, administration of the homologous organ compound

- **Articulatio coxae serial package I amp.** Wala
  3 × weekly 0.5 ml per os can be administered early on, alternating the potentization rhythmically between D5 and D8 with each new ampoule.

9.3 Disorders of the spinal region

9.3.1 Hyperlordosis ("Hollow back")

For children with poor posture and bulged stomach who otherwise tend to be skinny and develop poor digestive activity it is recommendable to proceed therapeutically as follows

- **Quartz D20 pillules** Wala
  in the morning daily 5 pillules,

to strengthen the formative forces which issue from the head pole and the activity of the I-organization in the middle (rhythmical) and lower (metabolic-motoric) human being, especially in the connective tissue and digestive activity.
Complementary use can be made of a compound which stimulates digestive activity in the upper abdomen, thus strengthening uprightness "from below." Suitable medicines, among others, are

- **Lycopodium comp. pillules** Wala
  3 × daily 5 pillules (▸Chap. 6.3.3.2) in cases of primarily disturbed or too weak liver-gall-activity

or

- **Cichorium/Pancreas comp. pillules** Wala
  3 × daily 5–7 pillules (▸Chap. 6.3.3.2) if the focus lies more on influencing the function of the stomach, the duodenum and the pancreas. The effect of this medicament can be augmented in regard to the liver-gall-system by simultaneous administration of
- **Taraxacum Stanno cultum Rh D3 dil.** Weleda
  3 × daily 5–10 drops

9.3.2 Postural weakness

Diagnostics of functional disorders in the back region are an important part of the physical examination of school-age children in particular. One should watch out for vestibular disorders, disorders in left-right, up-down and front-back orientation, which are primarily controlled by the spinal column as a rhythmic organ. This should include the lower extremities and the pelvis on the one hand, and the craniocervical transition on the other. It is important to note any cases of jaw malposition and anomalies: the proportions of upper and lower jaw very clearly show the relationship between the "upper" and the "lower" human being. In the second septennial, the upper and lower jaw often fail to interlock or align properly, a condition which should not be viewed exclusively as a case for the orthodontist. In fact osteopathic/chiropractic or craniosacral therapy of the craniocervical transition, physiotherapy and eurythmy therapy of asymmetries and postural abnormalities in the back often constitute the foundation for a positive correction of jaw development, which might possibly spare the child tooth extractions or braces, for example. For this reason it is important to pay attention to all of these aspects in the context of check-ups at age 5, for example, so as to work with the child and help him shape his gestalt.

In the long-term it is advisable in practice to form a collaborative team of paediatricians, orthodontists and therapists. Then the second septennial can be used to accompany the child and help him find *his own centre, his own balance* in the areas of the spinal column and natural dentition. Thus a *self-formed set of teeth* can stand at the end of this development rather than the attempt to fixate what are actually dynamically moveable teeth into calculated positions.

Manual therapies (osteopathy/chiropractice/craniosacral therapy) and rhythmical massage therapy as developed by M. Hauschka as well as *movement therapies* which build on these approaches, (physiotherapy exercises, Bothmer gymnastics, eurythmy therapy [Titze 1999]) provide the basis for therapy.

In the experience of the authors the following medicines are indicated for poor posture:

- **Bambusa e nodo D6 pillules** Wala
  daily 1–2 × 5 pillules [cf. extensive discussion by Schuster 1996]

in alternation with

- **Equisetum/Stannum pillules** Wala
  daily 1× 5–7 pillules

These two medicines influence and stimulate the organism's own fomative forces in the area of the spinal column. As far as diet goes, their effectiveness is supported by small portions of millet, oats or barley eaten daily. Wheatgrass juice can also prove beneficial in this connection.

In cases of children whose soul aspect is distracted towards the outside due to external circumstances, emotional sensitivity or empathy and who develop a bodily weakness in uprightness, inner light forces,

- **Phosphorus LM6 dil.** Arcana
  daily 3–5 drops in the morning

can intensify the abovementioned therapy, particularly in the winter months.

For external use paravertebral rhythmical Einreibungen moving from up to down can be applied for poor posture, alternating between

- **Plumbum met. 0.1 % ointment.** Weleda and
- **Mallow oil** Wala.

Moreover, deeper-seated imbalances in the back raise the therapeutic question as to which individually determined constitutional remedies might be effective. The four most important ones, which are described extensively in this book, are

- **Quartz** or **Silicea**,
- **Sulphur**,
- **Calcium phosphoricum**,
- **Conchae** or **Calcium carbonicum**.

(▶Chap. 3.2.5; ▶Chap. 6.4.3.6)

9.3.3 Idiopathic scoliosis and Scheuermann's disease (osteochondrosis)

In the second septennial the soul organization of the child develops into an autonomous entity. The fundamental characteristic of the soul aspect is that it exists in *polarities*. In the second septennial the male/female polarity evolves into a psychological and physical reality; at the same time other polarities of human organization unfold as well, which manifest themselves for one in growth itself (craniocaudally oriented growth is confronted by a caudiocranial growth impulse, and during the growth spurt in puberty the centre, in particular the spinal column, begins to lead in terms of growth [Verhulst 1999, 93–102]).

Pathologically one-sided formative forces can interfere with the task of mediating between opposing formative principles of the human organism to create a stable rhythmic system. Idiopathic scoliosis, which develops in the second septennial (as opposed to secondary and infantile forms), and Morbus Scheuermann, two conditions contrasted in ◘ Tab. 9.3, are expressions of such a pathology, which is connected with the maturation of the astral body.

Patients with scoliosis frequently exhibit a prematurely accelerated growth spurt. The disease constitutes a physical one-sided accentuation of the *lordosis, the mark of highly moveable spinal column segments* (cervical spine and lumbar spine), allowing these to encroach upon the actually kyphosing thoracic spine, i. e. appearing in "the wrong place." The higher up the scoliosis is, the worse the prognosis is: "A high thoracic spine scoliosis can hardly be treated with a corset, the torsion produces quite a pronounced rib hump and the condition often requires surgery" [Hübner 2003, 301]. Due to the fact that it is practically painless, scoliosis calls less attention to itself than Morbus Scheuermann does although the former can lead to much more severe deformations. The symmetry and uprightness of the spinal column, which are an expression of the forces of the upper human being (cf. anatomy of the head), are dissolved "from below," fostering distortions and asymmetries (see anatomy of the abdominal cavity) which are typical of the metabolism. Within the spinal column itself, the anterior part located in proximity to the metabolism rushes ahead of the posterior part, which is connected with the central nervous system. Depth of respiration decreases. This constitutes a manifold imbalance of the rhythmic system in which the forces of the lower human being are not sufficiently formed, limited in their growth and oriented by the upper pole.

The typical female constitution is predisposed to this to a stronger degree than the male constitution. – One can frequently observe in practice that the relative weakness of the formative forces of the upper human being has a cause which is found in girls in their second septennial more often than in boys: *emotional distress, depressive moods* can lead to

Tab. 9.3 Comparison of idiopathic scoliosis and Morbus Scheuermann.

Idiopathic adolescent scoliosis	Morbus Scheuermann
Primarily girls	Primarily boys
Primarily thoracic, almost always painless	Primarily lumbar, the most frequent cause of backaches in adolescents [Hefti 1997, 161]
"One could also speak of a rotational lordosis rather than scoliosis" [Hefti 1997, 71] (pathological rotation)	Marked by fixation of the kyphosis [Hefti 1997, 96] (flat back ("pathological extension")
Aetiological imbalance between ecto- and mesodermal structures, vertebrae growth (ventral) and the dorsal parts of the spinal column [Hefti 1997, 71], the spinal chord (front – back); imbalance of the spinal column/musculature, disorder of matrix function (collagen tissue [Hübner 1999]) with ensuing torsion (left – right)	Aetiological imbalance between spinal disc (high inner pressure of the Nucl. pulposus) and cartilaginous ring apophysis as growth zone of the vertebral bodies [Hefti 1997, 95] (above – below)

a withdrawal of the I and the astral body from body-bound tasks in the lower human being and allow it to become excessive (in other cases a primary predomination of the metabolic-limb-pole can be observed). Such distress and inner withdrawal are sometimes difficult to identify since the child is often not aware of them or only becomes aware of them while dreaming, and the kinds of behaviour which issue from the social aspect and vital metabolic processes sometimes conceal the person's emotional situation as well.

In any case *early detection* of the disease and the disturbed equilibrium of forces which lie behind it are of enormous importance. Then orthopaedic measures can be coupled with medicines, rhythmical massage therapy, physiotherapy and in particular specific eurthymy therapy [Titze 1999], and if necessary the emotional-spiritual situation of the child can be addressed and modified as well.

For cases of skeleton deformation, external applications can generally be considered:

- **Tabacum 1 % ointment** specially manufactured by Apotheke an der Weleda
  a pea-sized amount daily rubbed in paravertrebrally on the affected segments of the spinal column.

The tobacco plant unites a strong vitality with toxin production which affects the soul aspect (cf. discussion of toxic production in Solanacae in ▸Chap. 7) and can have a stimulating effect on the equilibrium between the astral and the etheric body when applied properly and in beneficial dosages.

This medicament can be supplemented by rhythmical Einreibungen using

- **Stannum 0.4 % ointment.** Weleda and
- **Mallow oil** Wala
  the warming effect of which activates the I-organization in the corresponding area.

Generally speaking it is important to harmonize the connection between inner light forces, which orient the spinal column to uprightness, and growth-promoting life forces (upper and lower etheric forces), this being all the more difficult the more advanced the pubertal growth spurt.

For internal use

- **Stannum comp. trit.** Weleda:
  1–2 × daily
  is a basic compound remedy (cf. ▸Chap. 7 as well). In addition to the potentized gold and tin in the apatite it contains a mineral (natural calcium fluorine phosphate) which is important for such patients. [Vademecum 2010, 766]

From a constitutional perspective the most frequently suitable single remedy is

- **Calcium phosphoricum C12 pillules** Gudjons, **LM6–18 dil.** Arcana
  1 × daily – 2 × weekly 5 pillules in the morning, 1 × daily – 2 × weekly 5 drops (cf. case study as well).

This remedy is primarily indicated for girls who constantly compare themselves to others and worry a lot about how they are judged by others, particularly in regard to their intellectual capacity and performance. They are very critical of other people. What is also striking is their constant *dissatisfaction and anxiety.* They tend to get *stomach aches and headaches* (especially after school), eat very little when under emotional duress and often do not fall asleep until late at night due to their inner tension (and anticipatory tension). They invest a lot of energy into studying, depriving their body of energy needed to build it up. Their emotional constitution is very vulnerable; disappointments and emotionally taxing experiences affect them deeply and can foster deforming tendencies in the area of the spinal column (concerning the importance of muscle tone for scoliosis and M. Scheuermann cf. Hübner [2003], whom the authors are also indebted to for the case study below). They are usually slender and experience fast growth spurts.

In the past years, the authors have gathered positive experience with a mixture of potentized organ preparations which have a positive effect on the coherence of ligaments and vertebral bodies:

- **Ligamentum longitudinale anterius Gl D8 amp.** Wala,
  Ligamentum longitudinale posterius Gl D8 amp. Wala,
  Disci intervertebrales (feti) Gl D8 amp. Wala,
  Bambusa e nodo D6 amp. Wala,
  Hypophysis/Stannum amp. Wala,
  aa ad 5 ml, daily in the morning 0.7 ml. (mixture keeps for several days if kept in a closed syringe).

For diseases of the spinal column occurring during adolescence which are accompanied by deformations the compound

- **Disci comp. c. Nicotiana pillules** Wala
  1 × daily 10–3 × daily 7 pillules
  has been developed for this specific organ focus. It constitutes a basic therapy primarily for M. Scheuermann (see below) [Vogel 1994, 375–379] but also for scoliosis, especially when muscular tension or pain occurs in the paravertebral region (see above).

If the focus is more on weakness of the rhythmic system and a depressive emotional situation

- **Disci comp. c. Auro pillules** Wala
  1–2 × daily 7 pillules

can be considered. As concerns the rhythmic system as a whole (respiration, circulation and spinal column) where physically deforming disorders are involved

- **Aurum/Cardiodoron comp. dil.** Weleda
  2 × daily 10 drops

is a remedy with a harmonizing-strengthening effect.

Emotional distress can be grasped profoundly and treated by

- consultation with the physician, possibly without the parents,
- art therapies, in cases of scoliosis through sculpture, painting and speech therapy,
- single potentized remedies (▸Chap. 7.3).

Orthopaedically, treating patients suffering from idiopathic scoliosis is a demanding task. In progressive cases, timely use of a brace is necessary.

The limiting-formative power of the I-organization in the metabolic realm can be strengthened through medicines, among others iron preparations and other medicines which activate gall bladder and pancreatic activity (see above). – Suitable types of physiotherapy are indispensable when treating scoliosis. – Eurythmy therapy, which has developed scoliosis-specific types of exercises, for example forming the sound "L," plays a major role in stimulating self-healing powers in cases of idiopathic scoliosis. The following case study developed by the anthroposophic orthopaedist M. Hübner, which is reprinted here, depicts an exemplary case.

Case study

Treatment of the patient, now 12 years old, began in 1995. She exhibited a pronounced developmental delay; she could not sit up unsupported until she was 13 months old and did not walk until she was almost 2. Suspicion of rickets was not confirmed. At age 5 a slight left-convex lumbar scoliosis was diagnosed, with a conspicuous asymmetrical rotational ability of both hips with 90° flexion accompanied by restriction of inner rotation on the right side. The child was very thin, also thin-skinned, had a poor appetite, still wet her bed at age 5 and suffered from severe anxiety. Treatment began using eurythmy therapy involving exercises typically employed to treat scoliosis – "L," "I" and rod exercises. In 1996 the hips showed a bilaterally equal rotational capacity; now eurythmy therapy focused on lots of "A" exercises. Medicinal treatment using rose iron/graphite. From 1997 on regular alternation between physiotherapy and eurythmy therapy. In 1998 administration of Calcium phosphoricum LM18, after which the mother reported an improvement of the child's ability to straighten herself up. "In 1999, on the basis of a 3-D measurement and radiological monitoring, the scoliosis angle showed a progression from 21 to 32° according to Copp as compared to 1995. Now a Charleston-Bending corset was fitted which did not cause the child any problems while sleeping." – This corset is only worn at night and is suitable for lower thoracic spine and upper lumbar spine scolioses. "In the same year, a certain consolidation of the constitution in the sense of strengthening and weight gain was observed. In 2000 a clear improvement of the scoliosis was ascertained on the basis of stereography as well as in clinical terms; this was confirmed in 2001 and again in 2002. Last examination: 4th November 2002: height 159 cm, weight 37 kg, expected final height 167 cm. Physically and emotionally the child has clearly become more stable. Previous anxieties have been overcome and no abnormalities have been observed at school" [Hübner 2003, 301].

Morbus Scheuermann has a polar relation to idiopathic scoliosis. A flat back, rigid, kyphotic spinal column segments, loss of vital, dynamic movement in a painfully fixated posture show a relative predominance of the upper human being in this disease. The kyphosis is accentuated and pushes downwards into the region of what constitutes, physiologically speaking, the flexible, lordotic lumbar spine. Kyphoses form relatively inflexible segments of the axial skeleton; in addition to the thoracic spine these include the sacrum and the occipital bone, which evolves embryonically from the Notochord, the primordial the spinal column [Christ 1990, 831]. In the kyphotic extremes of the axial skeleton there is a physiological tendency of the vertebral bodies to fuse, creating an immoveable bone formation reminiscent of the head.

Thus in cases of Morbus Scheuermann there is a clear predominance of the head pole "in the wrong place," i. e. in a region where vitality and self-development of the will (culminating in active and dynamic straightening up) should predominate.

It is known that a "persistently hyperkyphotic posture" leads to "increased pressure in the ventral parts of the spinal column", thus fostering the development of M. Scheuermann. "Although there is only little scientific data to confirm this, it is nevertheless clear *that emotional factors play an important role in the development of M. Scheuermann.* Those afflicted are often youths who show a submissive bearing under the impression of a very dominant parent, do not dare contradict the parent and exhibit a poorly developed personality" [Hefti 1997, 95]. *High-performance sport fosters the disease* (as is the case with so many other orthopaedic clinical pictures).

In therapeutic terms it is important here to help the youth gain more autonomy, develop emotionally animated movement and strengthen his self-confidence. In acute cases osteopathic treatment and rhythmical massage therapy can prove very effective in alleviating pain and improving mobility. At the same time the youth receives emotional attention and his back is vitalized, both of which are experienced with a great degree of gratitude.

For *external applications* one might also consider administering

- **Tabacum 1 % ointment.** Weleda,
- **Stannum met. 0.4 % ointment** Weleda,
- **Mallow oil** Wala

which all stimulate and regulate rhythmic processes in the spinal column and strengthen them in terms of the I-organization.

Pathogenetically speaking the Nucleus pulposus, as the vestige of the embryonal Notochord, plays an important role in the disease process. – Today we know that the disc core, which is under turgor pressure, contains substances which can cause severe pain even in very small traces (for example in cases of prolapsed vertebral disc this is often much more serious than the physical compression of the spinal nerves). Cases of M. Scheuermann also constitute a type of vertebral disc prolapse but such that is directed vertically into the vertebral bodies. It is becoming increasingly clear today that growth-related weakening of the ring apophysis only causes part of the imbalance because from adolescence until age 40 the turgor of the Nucleus pulposus itself increases.

This is the rationale behind the application of Disci preparations in anthroposophic medicine, which unfold an organotropic effect directed towards this region. For treatment of M. Scheuermann, fundamentally one can also consider

- **Disci comp. c. Nicotiana pillules** Wala
  2 × daily 10–3 × 7 pillules

which is also affective in alleviating pain.
For cases involving more intense, acute pain in the lumbar spine

- **Disci/Rhus tox. comp. amp.** Wala
  i.c./s.c. or 3 × daily ½ ampoule per os

can be administered; for further stabilization

- **Disci comp. c. Stanno pillules** Wala
  1–2 × daily 10 pillules

is well-suited. As long as severe pain persists, higher potencies of lead silicate (recommended by M. Hübner [1999, 18]),

- **Plumbum silicicum D20–30 trit.** Weleda
  up to 2 × daily 1 saltspoon (for acute symptoms)

can be administered to relieve the lower human being from forces of the disease process which foster formation of head forces and have a paralyzing effect (and thus fixate consciousness in the state of pain) For consolidation and strengthening of the personality in the will life it is suitable to continue therapy with

- **Calcium silicicum comp. D6 dil.** Apotheke an der Weleda
  3 × daily 7 drops

From the depicted, comparative view of this disease and the individual circumstances of individual patients, further therapeutic aspects can be developed (▸Chap. 7.2.3.3).

9.4 Aseptic bone necroses

9.4.1 Perthe's disease (juvenile osteochondrosis of femure head)

This disease most frequently afflicts boys between the 5th and 7th year of life [Schmitt et al. 2000]. Those afflicted strike the physician as having an untameable compulsion to move (concerning the following see discussions in Chap 7.4 and 7.5). Rest and motion, head and limb poles are not balanced; in individual cases tensions in the family can, like the constitution, aggravate the disharmony.

On the femoral head itself the "blood supply, which originally issues from three vessels," is sometimes reduced to "one vessel at the age of six" [Hübner 1999, 14]. "Recently, blood clotting disorders in the sense of thrombophilia were found in 75 % of diseased children" [Schmitt et al. 2000]. In the meantime, an epidemiological relationship between M. Perthes and an increased incidence of cardiovascular diseases has been proven [Hailer 2010], which confirms the crucial role which the vascular aspect plays in the emergence of the disease. "In addition, external inducements such as microtraumatization, for example," can have a triggering effect.

Pathology research has thus developed the notion that the femoral head, which is cut off from the blood circulation in the case of Perthe's disease, falls out of the life nexus. Clinical observations of patients have shown a pre-existing *dynamic of limb movement* which takes on a life of its own. In bodily-emotional terms this contrasts with a weakness of the rhythmic system, of the emotional centre: family conflicts, jealousy among siblings, tensions and insecurities in social interaction and in some cases weak development of rotation during infancy can be observed here. Therapeutically much attention should be devoted to strengthening the centre; the disease itself forces the child to restrain movement for some time and internalize himself more intensely; this is an opportunity which should be taken advantage of. As a joint the hip joint itself is part of the rhythmic system. The mobility of the limbs and the repose of the pelvis collide with each other, as do the growth dynamic of the longest human long bone and the spherical rounding of the femoral head, which corresponds to the formation of the head in terms of its shape and dynamics of formation and is already developed to a large degree (like the head) at this age, whereas the femur continues to grow until the person reaches maturity.

The disease emerges during a period of time in which the life organization reaches a certain independence of the forces of heredity (a process which manifests itself in the onset of second dentition). The femoral head itself receives its shape from a reduction of vital-dissolving life processes as represented by the blood. In the case of Perthes, the "clotting process" which forms the bone threatens to go too far – as an inner process opposed to one which radiates into the environment, taking all its vitality with it.

Therapeutically it is important to create a warming-vitalizing sheath around the diseased joint. This can be done with evening rhythmical Einreibungen in the hip region using

- **Cuprum met. 0.4% ointment.** Weleda,

while re-organization of the form is stimulated by

- **Stannum met. 0.4% ointment.** Weleda,

applied in the morning.

In the passage quoted at the beginning of this chapter, R. Steiner draws a connection between calcium phosphate and the cosmic-spheric tendency of skeleton formation on the one hand and between carbonic calcium and consolidation of the gravitation-absorbing long bones on the other [Steiner 1980, 47].

Thus the authors treat Perthe's disease *internally* in accordance with this, administering

- **Apatite/Stannum trit.** Weleda
  1–2 × daily 1 saltspoon

supplemented by

- **Hypophysis/Stannum pillules** Wala
  1–2 × daily 5 pillules

and

- **Articulatio coxae serial package III amp.** Wala
  (D5–30 in decreasing potenties and then increasing potencies with the next serial package) 2 × weekly 1 ampoule per os. Later serial package I (D5–8) can be administered.

A constitutional remedy is

- **Sulphur LM6 dil.** Arcana
  daily in the morning 5 drops

which has a calming, regulative effect on the metabolism, thus strengthening the life organization in the metabolic area, which finds itself in a period of instable transition. Afterwards

- **Phosphorus LM6 dil.** Arcana
  in cautious dosages, beginning with 1 drop daily is possibly indicated.

In cases of more severe familial tension, also in view of possible circulation disorders,

- **Lachesis D12 dil.** Weleda
  1–2 × daily 5 drops
  is possibly indicated instead of phosphorus. This remedy can be administered for relatively long periods of time if it proves to be constitutionally suitable.

Experiences with this treatment have been generally satisfactory as far as organ findings are concerned as well as in terms of the general condition of the child in question.

It is important for such children to find more repose (the disease itself seems to want to achieve this); every acute joint affliction indicates a possible lack of inner quietude (this holds for almost all sport-related joint lesions, for example).

9.4.2 Excursus: transient synovitis

Transient synovitis sometimes constitutes the onset of Perthe's disease. For this reason careful observation is diagnostically indicated.

Very good therapeutic results can be obtained by treatment using

- **Apatite/Stannum trit.** Weleda
  2–3 × daily 1 saltspoon and
- **Bryonia D12 pillules** Wala
  2–4 × daily 5 pillules

or with

- **Bryonia/Stannum pillules** Wala
  starting with hourly dosages; after clear improvement 4–5 × daily 5 pillules [Vademecum 2010, 236]

In cases of severe symptoms or suspicion of onset of Perthe's disease, this treatment can be supplemented by the organ preparations

- **Articulatio coxae Gl D15 amp.** Wala
  2 × weekly one drinking ampoule

9.4.3 Köhler's disease I

Good experiences have been made with external alternating use of

- **Cuprum met. 0.4 % ointment** Weleda in the evening and
- **Stannum met. 0.4 % ointment** in the morning

as well as internal use of

- **Apatite/Stannum trit.** Weleda and
- **Hypophysis/Stannum pillules** Wala

as described for treatment of Perthe's disease.

9.4.4 Schlatter-Osgood disease (juvenile osteochondrosis of tibial tubercle)

A similar therapy can be used but without application of Cuprum met. ointment:

- **Apatite/Stannum trit.** Weleda
  in the morning 1 saltspoon
- **Stannum met. 0.4 % ointment.** Weleda
  in the morning a pea-sized amount rubbed in
- **Hypophysis/Stannum pillules** Wala
  in the evening 5 pillules

9.5 Retropatellar pain syndrome ("Chondropathia patellae")

Anterior knee pain is often found in youths during growth spurts in puberty who engage in intensive sports activities. The pain typically gets worse while crouching down and climbing stairs. Apart from abstaining from sports for approx. four weeks and wearing a knee bandage, the administration of the following proves effective:

- **Cartilago comp. pillules** Wala
  2, at onset 3 × 10 pillules over six weeks. The treatment can be repeated if necessary.

9.6 Osteogenesis imperfecta (brittle bone disease)

Although this disease is very rare and can be subdivided into various sub-types, the therapeutic approach used by the authors, based on many years of comparatively very satisfying experience, will be outlined here in brief.

Pathogenetically speaking this involves a dysfunction of the osteoblasts which manifests itself primarily in a disorder of collagen production. No polymerized collagen can be formed; "histologically speaking one finds thin bone trabeculae and reduced bone substance" [Hefti 1997, 661]. This primarily constitutes a *dysfunction of the bone matrix* accompanied by more or less pronounced osteoporosis (deficiency in deposition of calcium salts). It will not be possible to discuss the various sub-types, progressions and co-existing extra-osseous symptoms here.

Clinically the focus lies on:

- fractures and bending of the long bones in particular due to a lack of pressure resistance and tensile strength
- scoliotic deformations of the spinal column.

The *area of the diaphysis,* which carries most of the weight in human beings (in animals the musculature generally carries a larger proportion of it), is affected to a particular degree. – From the explanations on the importance of calcium phosphate and carbonate for the development of the human skeleton given by R. Steiner [1980, 49] and cited here several times, it follows that

- *calcium carbonate* plays a synthesizing role for those *segments of the skeleton* which are *vulnerable to "earthly forces"*. This certainly holds to the utmost for the diaphysis of the long bones. This is the rationale behind stimulating integration of calcium salts into the bone structures in the area of the diaphysis through administration of potentized calcium carbonate.
- calcium phosphate plays a synthesizing role for the spherical, head-like parts of the skeleton the shape of which are of "cosmic origin"
- *silica is closely related to the mesenchymal matrix* (▸Chap. 3.5) and periosteal formation (in this area incorporation of calcium salt is preceded by an increase in silica concentration). Since the defect of osteogenesis imperfecta primarily lies in the matrix area (which pervades the entire organism and consolidates it, which is why the disease also has extra-osseous symptoms) this is the basis for the rationale behind using potentized silicea preparations; in connection with collagen formation, its effect can be intensified through iron; in connection with incorporation of calcium salts, its effect can also be intensified through lead compounds.

Treatment primarily involves the following medicines:

- **Calcium carbonicum LM6,** later **LM12 dil.** Arcana
  daily 5 drops in the morning

and simultaneously

- **Conchae/Quercus comp. S trit.** Weleda
  1–3 × daily 1 saltspoon.

The guiding idea of this medication was to intensify the effect of calcium carbonate by the oak bark mixed in with this preparation, which mainly contains calcium salts permeated with tannins, and Stannum met., which is also added to this preparation in D10. In skeleton formation Stannum stimulates vigorous plasticization of the skeleton's shape during skeletal formation through the life organization in combination with soul and I-organization.

The disease picture is such that children affected must tolerate considerable restrictions of physical activity. Cheerfulness and exuberance are muted in their development.

In this situation potentized meteoric iron and phosphorus are very helpful, which are contained in

- **Meteoreisen pillules** Wala
  1–3 × daily 5–7 pillules

and potentized together with Quartz in D12. Quartz in medium potency, constitutes the central potentized remedy for the extracellular matrix and complements Calcium carbonicum in its effect.
Low potencies of lead can intensify the effect of Calcium carbonicum, for example in the form of lead carbonate,

- **Cerussit D6 trit.** Apotheke an der Weleda
  1–3 × daily 1 saltspoon.

Especially in cases of strong bone deflections and spinal column deformations

- **Hypophysis/Stannum pillules** Wala
  1–3 × daily 5 pillules is indicated. [Vademecum 2010, 505]

Other preparations which might be considered are:

- **Periosteum Gl D8 amp.** Wala,
- **Parathyreoidea/Aurum amp.** Wala, among others.

Simultaneous *eurythmy therapy* intensifies the effect of medicinal therapy enormously. If deformations have already occurred – which is usually the case – consonantal exercises are indicated; later other exercises can follow.

Case study

A 6-year-old girl comes to the surgery for her first consultation in a wheelchair. The parents report that she had been afflicted with blue sclerae since birth although development was initially inconspicuous. Her length growth had been in the lower normal range. In her 4th year of life the first fracture occurred, a thigh fracture incurred by a "harmless" fall; on the basis of the x-rays the orthopaedist diagnosed osteogenesis imperfecta. According to the quite undifferentiated classification used back then (in 1974), it was a form of the Lobstein type with autosomal dominant succession.
After this first fracture, other fractures of the upper and lower extremities followed despite the extreme caution which was taken and sometimes due to slightest occurrences. The child could hardly move around freely anymore; every risk was avoided if possible. Up to the time of her first consultation, 14 fractures had occurred, most of them caused by the excessive callus formation which is typical for this disease, with the healing process being accompanied by changes in the form of the bone. The joints could be overstretched. The general aspect was that of a child who was too small and whose bone structure was deformed. The child's skin was thin, delicate, translucent. Her coarse strength was highly reduced but she exhibited good fine motor skills. Her head was freely moveable. The treatment so far had been Vitamin C and D in high dosages.
Treatment began which took a total of eight years; individual modifications in the therapy cannot be reported here in detail.
To begin with, so as to support the uprightness of the girl

- **Apatite/Phosphorus comp. K dil.** Weleda (contains Ferrum sid. D20): 10 drops in the morning were administered.

Potentized calcium carbonate was administered in the form of

- **Conchae/Quercus comp. S trit.** Weleda
  in the evening 1 pea-sized amount.

The effect of the Conchae was intensified by administration of lead carbonate in the form of

- **Cerussit D6 trit.** Weleda
  for 3 weeks 3 × 1 saltspoon followed by a 3-week intermission.
- **Hypophysis D6 dil.** Weleda, later **Hypophysis/Stannum pillules** Wala
  2 × 5 drops daily or 2 × 5 pillules

were used repeatedly to treat the bone deformation. Later, treatment using Hypophysis D6 and Epiphysis D6 in alternation followed.

At intervals the therapy was intensified by administration of

- **Cinis ossis D6 trit.** Weleda,

and injections of

- **Gl. parathyreoidea D4 amp.** Wala (corresponding to potentiation Gl D6 today),
- **Stannum met. praep. D12 amp.** Weleda,
- **Periosteum D4 amp.** Wala (corresponding to Gl D6 today),
- **Quartz D12 amp.** Wala.

At the same time eurythmy therapy was performed on a regular basis, starting with the consonants "K-D-M-N-S-L" and vocals "A-I-E," later using the series "L-A-O-M." Shortly after treatment began one could observe an increase in the girl's confidence while walking; the musculature and the ligaments became more taut and the deformations in the places where fractures had occurred earlier decreased again over the course of time. 6 years later a fall from a height of one and a half metres only caused a small fracture of a vertebral body. – At age 14 it was possible to end treatment. At the last follow-up examination when the patient was 20 years old she exhibited a normal gait. She goes skiing and horseback riding, enjoys good health and has successfully completed her secondary school leaving exam [Stellmann 1985].

9.7 Epilogue: specifics of human morphogenesis in comparison to animal morphogenesis

"The skeleton is the physical image of I-organization."

R. Steiner[1]

In his first lecture for physicians marking the foundation of anthroposophic medicine, R. Steiner compared the human gestalt with that of higher mammals, especially primates, in detail. He pointed out that in the case of the gorilla, for example, what started out as a comparatively human-like gestalt took on specifically animal-like features in the course of growth characterized by protrusion of the viscerocranium, which increasingly extends beyond the neurocranium (while the foramen magnum moves out of its central lower position into a position tilted backwards). In accordance with this, powerful spinous pro-

1 Cf. [R. Steiner 1999, 30] and [R. Steiner and I. Wegman 1991, 43].

cesses develop on the cervical spine of the gorilla, serving as insertion points for strong postural muscles designed to hold up the head of the animal, which bears forward in the adult and whose lower jaw can no longer be raised above the shoulders [Verhulst 1999, 192]. "... thus you cannot get around concluding that in human beings an upthrusting gesture opposes these forces ... For you see, these forces have to be there, the forces which oppose those which form the gestalt of the gorilla" [Steiner 1999, 28].

In the most extensive work on this observation by R. Steiner to date, J. Verhulst [1999], taking into account the 500 or so new empirical studies in this area, has worked out the specifics of human gestalt formation in comparison to that of higher mammals. Apart from incorporating aspects of anthroposophy, he bases his investigation on research conducted by the Dutch anatomist L. Bolk, who was appointed professor at the University of Amsterdam in 1898 at age 32. In the 32 years of research which followed, Bolk developed his empirically founded terminology which allowed him to determine more clearly the specifics of human morphogenesis compared to that of the animal gestalt. Verhulst depicts these in his book, documenting them by numerous additional bodies of evidence.

What holds for all primates is that they "differ from other mammals through the fact that they have few specializations and remain much closer to an undifferentiated form than animals of other mammal orders do. In primates we find no hoofs, wings, trunks, horns, etc." [Verhulst 1999, 37]. "Primates are the least specialized mammals and human beings are the least specialized primates of all," being "specialized at being non-specialized." [Verhulst 1999, 40]. "Human gestalt features are distributed among various primates in an amazing way. This suggests that the human shape approximates the *original* primate anlage to a high degree. ... In human beings the original pattern is preserved best. The human being is the most primitive primate" [Verhulst 1999, 50].

Bolk designates this provocative aspect as the *principle of fetalization:* in morphogenesis, the human being succeeds in preserving features which he originally shared with many mammals, for example, but which were increasingly abandoned by the others in favour of irreversible specializations. Thus the embryo of a wild boar originally has a five-star hand which is transformed into a claw in utero (a fact which M. Sommer [1999, 46] showed using impressively dyed specimens and whom the authors are indebted to for essential information). The same holds for naked skin, the naked forehead and the position of the neurocranium placed vertically above the viscerocranium, for example, which newborn chimpanzees also possess but which they lose in the course of childhood. [Verhulst 1999, 263–268] Newborn chimpanzees still exhibit the architecture of the head which is clearly oriented towards an upright position[1], and which is only abandoned *secondarily* in favour of the horizontal axis typical of animals (snout in front of neurocranium, foramen ovale in the back of the cranium instead of at its basis). In contrast, human beings actively prevent the upper jaw from protruding in that the intermaxillary bones which grow dynamically outwards in various directions in animals are overgrown and enclosed by the maxilla, being prevented from further (snout-forming) growth early on [Verhulst 1999, 301–306]. This is the reason why it took so long for people (Goethe, among others) to discover that the human being actually has an Os incisivum– for this can only be seen from the back side of the jaw. The enclosure of the intermaxillary bones and prevention of their growth also constitutes an important *prerequisite for the emergence of the faculty of speech,* which is fulfilled at the same time. Many other retardation processes

1 Cf. the photographs taken by Naef in the 1930's in Kipp [1980, 40]

in human gestalt formation prove purposeful in connection with language as well: "Human *speech* proves to be the centre around which the entire spectrum of retardation effects group themselves like a well-planned overall scheme" [Verhulst 1999, 379].

In comparison to animal growth, human growth is marked by a qualitatively unique power of restraint which Bolk has recognized as the capacity to preserve originally common fetal features of gestalt. What emerges by virtue of this power can be designated according to the terminology developed by Bolk as the appearance of "Type I": an archaic, universal, non-specialized gestalt which forms the basis for all higher animal development. Morphologically speaking, the human being reveals a basic form verifiable evolutionarily long before the appearance of the hominids, but a form which simultaneously represents "what is specifically human" in many respects! Thus the human hand can be derived from the skeletons of primitive reptilian hands on the basis of the same principles of growth and retardation of form [Verhulst 1999, 216], and the same holds for many other features of gestalt.

This contrasts with an opposed dynamic; human beings realize the primary basic plan for higher animal development in the farthest-reaching way, fulfilling in this way the possibilities for universal formation which lie therein, for example in the emergence of the telencephalon, maximum increase in possibilities for heat regulation through generalized development of sweat glands and much more, but especially through the achievement of uprightness. In doing so, the human being achieves a biomechanical balance which "by far exceeds that of any other animal." Human beings are the only ones who can liberate their musculature from the task of overcoming gravitation completely in an upright position: "Human beings consume only 7 percent more oxygen while standing than they do while lying down" [Verhulst 1999, 168]. In this way respiration is relieved from having to support muscle activity and warmth regulation (as opposed to, for example, a panting dog) – this being another important prerequisite for the human faculty of speech and the expression of a qualitatively different immersion of the soul into the body and connection of the soul with the body to that of animals. Due to the relatively far-reaching perfection of his universal anlage, the human being can return from any special situation and activity to a condition of balance in repose. The vestibular organ appears like a symbol for this: "When a human being adopts his normal position, the axis of gravity of the body runs through the atlas joint and the centre of gravity in the head." It "intersects ... the line connecting the two vestibular organs ... in the middle" [Verhulst 1999, 181]. In dogs this is not the case, for example; due to this position on the upper end of the axis of gravity, human beings can perceive any deviation from upright carriage organically in an optimal position.

Human beings bring to realization what was originally predisposed in the evolution of ensouled organisms and consummate it in the universal, freedom-enabling form of the human body. This is made possible by virtue of the powers inherent in the I-organization which "instruct the organs" – whereas animals "are instructed by their organs" (Goethe) – and thereby prevent the predominance of any organ or particular specialization. In the human gestalt the original "formal cause," the "entelechy" (Aristotle) of the evolution of ensouled life appears, and at the same time the human being becomes capable of expressing his origin in words.

References for Chapter 9

(every reference marked with a ■ Bullet point indicates the English translation of the reference above it)

Christ, B.: Enwicklung der craniocervicalen Übergangsregion. In: Humanembryologie. Hinrichsen, K. V. (ed.). Springer Verlag, Berlin 1990.

Glas, N.: Die Formensprache des Gesichts. Vienna – Leipzig 1934.

Hailer, Y. D. et al.: Legg-Calve-Perthes disease and risks for cardiovascular diseases and blood diseases. Pediatrics **125**, e1308–1315 (2010).

Hefti, F.: Kinderorthopädie in der Praxis. Springer Verlag, Berlin 1997.

Hinrichsen, K. V. (ed.): Humanembryologie. Springer Verlag, Berlin 1990.

Hübner, M.: Dysplasien: Skelettreifungsstörungen und Fehlwachstum in Kindheit und Jugend. Weleda Korr.bl. **147**, 16 (1999).

Hübner, M.: Die Wirbelsäule und ihre Erkrankungen in verschiedenen Lebensaltern. Der Merkurstab **56**, 300–305 (2003).

Kipp, F. A.: Die Evolution des Menschen im Hinblick auf seine lange Jugendzeit. Verlag Freies Geistesleben, Stuttgart 1980, 2nd ed. 1991.

Lievegoed, B.: Heilpädagogische Betrachtung. Edition Bingenheim 1984, Verlag Freies Geistesleben, Stuttgart 1995.

Matthiolius, H.: Das großköpfige und das kleinköpfige Kind. Beitr z Erw d Heilk **42**, 1–5 (1989).

Schmitt, S. et al.: Morbus Perthes. päd. praxis **57**, 488 (2000).

Schuster, B.: Bambus. Homöopathische Prüfung und Verifizierung. Kent Gesellschaft, Kronberg 1996.

Sommer, M.: Gezielte organotrope Therapie des Karzinompatienten. Der Merkurstab, Sonderheft Organpräparate (1999).

Sommer, M., G. Soldner: Die menschliche Wirbelsäule. Der Merkurstab **56**, 260–269 (2003).

Steiner, R.: Meditative Betrachtungen und Anleitungen zur Vertiefung der Heilkunst. Rudolf Steiner Verlag, Dornach 4th ed. 2003.

■ Steiner, R.: Course for young doctors: meditative contemplations and instructions for deepening the art of healing: lectures for physicians and medical students. GA (complete works) 316. Mercury Press, Spring Valley, N. Y. 1994.

Steiner, R.: Allgemeine Menschenkunde als Grundlage der Pädagogik. Gesamtausgabe vol. 293 Rudolf Steiner Verlag, Dornach 3rd ed. 1982.

■ Steiner, R.: Study of man: general education course : fourteen lectures given in Stuttgart between 21 August and 5 September 1919. GA (complete works) 293. Rudolf Steiner Press, London 2004. See also: Steiner, R.: Foundations of human experience. GA (complete works) 293. Anthroposophic Press, Hudson, N. Y. 1996.

Steiner, R.: Geisteswissenschaft und Medizin. Rudolf Steiner Verlag, Dornach, 7th ed. 1999.

■ Steiner, R.: Introduction to anthroposophical medicine. GA (complete works) 312. SteinerBooks, Great Barrington, M. A. 1999.

Steiner, R., I. Wegman: Grundlegendes zu einer Erweiterung der Heilkunst nach geisteswissenschaftlichen Erkenntnissen. Rudolf Steiner Verlag, Dornach, 7th ed. 1991.

■ Steiner, R., I. Wegman: Fundamentals of therapy: an extension of the art of healing through spiritual-scientific knowledge. GA (complete works) 027. Mercury Press, Spring Valley, N. Y. 1999. Also available as: Extending practical medicine: fundamental principles based on the science of the spirit. Rudolf Steiner Press, London 1996.

Stellmann, H. M.: Ein Fall von Osteogenesis imperfecta. Beiträge z. Erw. d. Heilk. **38** (2), 37–39 (1985)..

Titze, O.: Heil-Eurythmie bei Haltungsschäden. Weleda Korr.bl. **147**, 25–26 (1999).

Vademecum Anthroposophische Arzneimittel. 2.Aufl. Der Merkurstab **63**, Supplement (2010).

- Vademecum of anthroposophic medicines, CD format. Medical Section of the School of Spiritual Science, Dornach, Switzerland 2009

Verhulst, J.: Der Erstgeborene. Mensch und höhere Tiere in der Evolution. Verlag Freies Geistesleben, Stuttgart 1999.

Vogel, H. H.: Organe der Ich-Organisation. Natur Mensch Medizin, Bad Boll 1996.

Vogel, H. H., Wege der Heilmittelfindung. Natur Mensch Medizin, Bad Boll 1994.

Vogel, H.-H.: Finding remedies: spiritual knowledge of man and naure; a contribution toward understanding anthroposophic remedies, based on the example of the Wala remedy compositions. V 1, 2 Natur-Mensch-Medizin, Bad Boll 1994.

10 Extending treatment options for specific diseases

This chapter provides brief descriptions of the authors' clinical experience with particular illnesses.

10.1 Childhood cardiac disease – complementary treatment

10.1.1 Congential heart defects – options for and value of complementary medical treatment

Congenital cardiovascular anomalies are a domain of paediatric diagnosis and heart surgery. Surgical correction is now typically successful, even with hypoplastic left heart syndrome. Many years of experience have convinced the authors that there is a real need for complementary medical treatment both preoperatively and postoperatively, as in the following case study.

Case study

A six-month-old infant was seen with a heart murmur first noted at 4 weeks of age. The boy had been cyanotic with crying since birth, but otherwise was developing normally. Echocardiography showed pulmonary atresia with ventricular septal defect (VSD), moderately hypoplastic pulmonary vessels with an extensive high-degree stenosis in the outflow to the left pulmonary artery, a secundum atrial septal defect, and vascular anomalies (small persistent left upper vena cava and aortopulmonary collaterals.) A Blalock-Taussig stunt was first done from the left subclavian to the left pulmonary artery. Oxygen saturation in room air was 85–90 %, sometimes down to 80 %. Weight after recovery from operation was 4.4 kg and excessive sweating when breastfeeding every two to three hours (sign of heart failure) was noted. His parents reported that he was alert and vigorous, but even at this first visit the boy was irritable (he later developed major breath-holding spells) and had watery rhinitis and diarrhoea. After weaning at the age of 6 months, he failed to thrive further with his weight just 4.8 kg.

A major improvement was achieved with:

- **Arsenicum album C30**

Stools were more formed, restlessness decreased, and weight, having been static for several weeks, now increased by 50–100 g/week.

- **Crataegus e fol. et fruct. D2 pillules.** Wala,
- **Prunuseisen pillules** Wala (▸Chap. 10.1.2

were then given to stabilize. Additionally, because the child had frequent respiratory infections and poor appetite,

- **mare's milk** (▸Chap. 2.3.2.2)

was introduced, with appropriate fortifications. Appetite improved, infections regressed, sleep normalized, and at 10 months his weight was 5.85 kg. The Blalock-Taussig shunt was reoperated at 11 months, when he reached 9–10 kg body weight, considered necessary for surgical correction to be a possibility. However, cor pulmonale slowed his weight gain from the 10th to the 13th month. The boy was now crawling actively and pulling himself up to stand. Watery rhinitis recurred (in the summer) and he was still overly excitable.

- **Arsenicum album C200** 3 times 3 pillules in 12 h

was given in high dosage for the first time. Six weeks later he had weight gain of 500 g, and after 10 weeks a total of 900 g; the boy was happy, walking independently, and sleeping peacefully. Selenium supplementation due to a deficiency was started. Arsenicum album C200 was repeated a number of times when weight gain slowed or infection occurred. An intercurrent problem with going to sleep was treated with Phosphorus D25 (▸Chap. 7.1) At 23 months, weighing 8.75 kg, he had corrective surgery: VSD patch occlusive connection of right ventricle with pulmonary arteries using pulmonary homograft, ASD occlusion, widening outflow of left pulmonary artery with patch. The surgery was uncomplicated and recovery rapid with resolution of heart failure symptoms, including cyanosis. At age 4½ the boy could exercise normally, weighed 15.4 kg, and had good ventricular function bilaterally with volume increased in the right ventricle. Recurrent respiratory tract infections in upper and lower tract responded to treatment with potentized medicines.

This brief case study demonstrates the outstanding achievements of heart surgeons and paediatric cardiologists, which have become commonplace in paediatrics. However, complementary approaches can contribute to the improved outcome of surgery and resolution of *heart failure*, which in congenital cardiac anomalies is *due to blood flow anomalies and obstruction*.

The heart develops in conjunction with the flowing blood. Lancelets, a primitive fish, have no heart structure; instead, purely venous blood exists anterior to the gills, with oxygenated, arterialized blood then flowing from the gills through the body without any additional "pump"(for full details on the evolution of the heart, see Rohen [2000, 197–212]). Investigations on zebra fish hearts have shown that vascular endothelial cells perceive blood flow, conduct it, and so regulate the growth of vessels and cardiac structures. Experimental flow manipulation in embryonic fish hearts leads to dramatic malformations of the inflow and outflow tracts and cardiac loop development [Hove 2003.] Cardiac anomalies often remain latent in the embryonic period – e.g. one of the two ventricles may be practically missing as in tricuspid atresia or hypoplastic left heart syndrome, with circulation nevertheless adequate, as both chambers are "set in parallel." At the same time oxygen tension is low and the embryonic heart is relatively large (7.6 g/kg body weight) with a high proportion of non-contractile elements. The functions of the human heart only develop fully when pulmonary respiration starts; the pumping volume of the left ventricle doubles [Bernuth 2003, 1117], with the relative weight of the heart reduced by half (to 3.8 g/kg) in the first three months of life in healthy infants [Rohen 2000, 211]. Only then does the heart develop its independent movement (parallel to movement developing in lungs and limbs at birth) in close connection with the flowing blood. The heart performs a number of functions:

- sensory
- rhythm-inducing
- movement-inducing.

The atria, especially the right, are of prime importance for the *sensory function* of the heart. They are polar opposite to pumping function which is located mainly in the ventricles, especially the left ventricle after birth [Girke 2010, 179–181]. *Expansion* as the blood flows in is essential for the sensory function of the heart. It stimulates the heart, giving the blood impetus in the systole and bringing it to a congested halt at the end of the diastole – the heart thereby acting as a receptive sense organ. The heart responds to this expansion by secreting the natriuretic peptide (already active in the embryonic period) and by adaptation, starting from the sinus node, of heart rate and cardiac output to the needs of the organism. "It is altogether a basic quality of this marvellous organ that it always only reflects peripheral processes – always seeking, 'selflessly', "to optimize the functions of the system as a whole" [Rohen 2000, 198]. Determination of B-type Natiuretic Peptide levels, a hormone governed by the sensory function of the atria, provides a simple and prognostically relevant means of assessing heart failure.

Congenital cardiac anomalies interfere with this regulation, which normally serves the interaction of heart and organism. Aldosterone, the opponent of the natriuretic peptide, is of considerable importance; in contrast to natriuetic peptide, aldosterone is only produced in appreciable amounts after birth in the glomerular zone of the adrenal cortex. Sodium chloride retention increases the circulating volume, the cardiac preload, increasing pressure on the heart, which increases wall stress, and finally leads to stasis. The latter disproves the "pump theory", since there has never been a pump on which the whole circulation in a system depends and by which a decrease in performance leads to stasis *before* the pump. The very fact that central venous pressure rises in right heart failure proves that the periphery of the circulation (an *open*, living vascular system permeable to fluids) shapes the system [Lauboeck 1999], with healthy blood circulation depending on a *correspondence* between myocardium and organ periphery. The afterload also increases, mainly under the influence of hormones from kidneys and adrenals. In heart failure the heart is under permanent pressure and stress from neurohormonal regulation, so it progressively loses its perception and regulation. One can sense this pathology in the children whose restlessness, increased sweating, sleep disorders and anxieties all indicate that the psyche cannot relate harmoniously to the body. The astral body and I cannot separate as needed for sleep, but instead intervene in a one-sided, sympathetic way that is progressively destructive.

The heart develops an intermittent pulse in its *rhythm-inducing function*. The original heart movement in evolution was peristaltis, like the intestinal. No pump theory satisfactorily explains the more profound meaning of this rhythm given to the blood, the reversal of flow in the (mainly left) ventricle. A more thorough study shows that the intervention of the psyche with the body is always rhythmic (day/night, inhalation/exhalation, etc.) and that the complexity and full development of the rhythmic system in the animal world accompanies intensification of soul processes. The configuration of cardiac movement, the rhythm of systole and diastole, reflects the need for ensouled movement, which has its archetype in inhalation and exhalation. The significance of linking pulse and respiration in the ratio of pulse rate to respiratory rate points to the interaction between mental processes directly linked to the breath and the movement of the heart. This is in line with the fact that the human heart, still immature before birth, only becomes fully functional and formed with the onset of respiration at birth.

With reference to heart failure in congenital cardiac anomalies, one sees *tachycardiac acceleration* of the heart rate *with decreasing variability* of heart rhythm. The heart – looking at it from a musician's point of view – no longer comes to rest. In health, the resting state of sleep reveals the ideal pulse-breath ratio for the given age [Hildebrandt, 1999]; normalization of the ratio at rest and the swinging variability of the heart rhythm have been found to be important indicators of cardiac health (also for the prognosis after MI in adults). *The heart's state of health is reflected in its rhythms.*

The idea of a pump is questionable when it comes to the *propulsive function* of the myocardium. The action of the heart in the flowing blood leads to a comprehensive reversal of *the organism's spatial dimensions*, entering into new rhythms induced by the heart. This quality of heart movement evolved through many intermediate stages. In embryonic development, the atria, originally inferior, move upwards, and the originally superior ventricular parts come to be below; the left heart supplies the organism (its actions normally with right-sided emphasis) with arterialized blood, while the right heart is more receptive by nature. The efferent vessels finally go from front to back, while the orientation of the moving organism is from back to front. The movements of the heart create an inner balance between the dominant spatial orientation of the organism at any given time [Rohen 2000, 188ff.]. The cardiac anomalies seen resemble the evolutionary stages in the phylogenesis of the heart (e. g. ventricular septal defect, mixed arteriovenous blood in many instances, etc.). When the heart cannot give the blood the movement configuration which the human being needs, abnormal flow resistances develop (e. g. valvular abnormalities, stenosis, etc.).

Three-dimensional nuclear magnetic imaging (MRI) of human intracardial blood flow [Kilner 1993] shows that in healthy subjects myocardial functions and blood flow are different from any mechanical pump. The heart can only be understood as an organ *placed in an existing flow system*. It causes stasis, reversal of flow, pulsating "quantization" of the original blood flow, taking it to a new level of flow and movement – in interaction with the peripheral arteriolar resistance and organ-specific regulation, primarily regulated by the kidney and adrenal gland.

Congenital cardiac anomalies interfere with this flow configuration, forcing the heart into the function of a mere pump which is increasingly subject to excessive demand by abnormal resistance in valves and vessels, arteriovenous shunts, etc. *The paradigm of the heart as a pump is most likely to apply to a diseased heart* that is increasingly losing its healthy powers of perception and rhythmic regulation, turning into muscle under increasing strain. On the other hand, this also explains why children in heart failure – as in the above case study – will frequently have *failure to thrive, which* for children with anomalous pulmonary venous flow may be their only symptom. Severe cardiac anomalies may cause a marked increase in body temperature due to the enormous effort required of the heart, similar to competitive sport. This is also a reason why the children require increased vitamin and trace element supplementation.

Complementary treatment can support paediatric cardiology and heart surgery by:

- reducing anxiety, stress, eating and sleeping disorders and balancing excesses of the sympathetic nervous system,
- supporting the rhythmic system, mainly of the heart,
- protecting the myocardium from destructive metabolic processes.

10.1.2 Medicinal treatment

10.1.2.1 Medicines and trace element substitution for supporting myocardial function

Extracts of hawthorn in phytotherapeutic or rhythmically potentized form are a valuable basic medicament for this treatment goal. The efficacy of hawthorn (*Crataegus*) in heart failure has also been demonstrated in clinical trials. It does not depend on a single active principle; different parts of the plant (leaves, flowers and fruit) produce or contain different proportions of the substances that contribute to the Crataegus action for patients in heart failure [Weiss 1999]. Extracts of hawthorn appear to protect the vital organization, above all of heart and lung, against excessive oxidative attack and to stabilize, calm, and improve cardiac function. Crataegus is also effective in treating chronic destructive inflammation of the lung, as in cystic fibrosis.

For infants and children under 3 years of age the authors preferably use

- **Crataegus e fol. et fruct. D2 pillules** Wala
  3–5 pillules 3 times daily.

If the result is not adequate,

- **Crataegus Tr.** Weleda (made from leaves and fruit, like the Wala product, and different from purely phytotherapeutic extracts)
  5–7 drops twice daily

For older children

- **Crataegus tab.** Weleda (Switzerland) – again made from leaves and fruit – or **Crataegutt® 80**
  1 tablet twice daily.

No side effects or toxicity have been observed, so the usual contraindication statement for children under 12 due to lack of clinical trials seems unwarranted.

The treatment is complemented by giving potentized *blackthorn shoots* processed using a special fermentation process with rhythmic exposure to warmth, sunlight, and added iron oxide (haematite) to a stabilized extract which is then potentized to the D3 (pillules) or D6.

- **Prunuseisen** (Prunus spinosa ferm. cum ferro) **pillules** Wala/**amp.** Wala
  infants 3 × 2 or 3 pillules 3 times, young children up to 5 pillules daily.

From the second year onwards, this may be replaced with

- **Levico comp. pillules** Wala
  3–5 pillules 3 times/day; school children: 7 pillules 3 times/day.
  In acute situations, like heart failure,) daily s.c. injections of the ampoule may be even more effective.

Levico comp. contains Prunuseisen, Levico water (▸Chap. 6.5.5.1.4) and Hypericum. The components are each potentized to the D2 and then together taken one stage further in the manufacturing process, so that the preparation is really in the D3.

Prunuseisen is effective in treating hypotensive states of weakness and supports cardiac function, especially for enlarged hearts under myocardial stress. Crataegus and Prunus are two basic medicines in anthroposophic medicine when there is need to stimulate the vital organization in the region of the heart and lungs. Levico comp., being in a lower potency and including the potentized metal, acts more strongly than Prunuseisen alone. It is suitable not so much for infants but for children who are a bit older. The Hypericum component has a calming, antidepressant effect which may be significant in treating chronic heart conditions.

Potentized organ preparations offer major support with congenital cardiac anomalies, above all in the first seven years of life. This form of treatment is often misunderstood by allopathic colleagues, but the authors have frequently seen impressive results with these preparations (see also ▸Chap. 10.9).

Case study

Years before, an older brother had died of hypoplastic left heart syndrome 13 weeks after birth. Now his ten-day-old brother was emergently admitted with clinical signs of decompensated heart failure and with the closure of the ductus arteriosus. Examination showed coarctation of the aorta, a hypoplastic aortic arch, and a small perimembranous ventricular septal defect. An emergency operation was done, but the stenosis could not be satisfactorily corrected, and postoperative resuscitation became necessary. The difference in pressure between upper and lower extremities was marked and persistent, and the left ventricle developed a concentric hypertrophy. The surgeon's prognosis was that a second intervention would be necessary in 3–6 months.

This was the situation when – for the first time in the clinic's history – we were able to treat an inpatient receiving postoperative care:

- **Crataegus e fol. et fruct. D2,**
- **Prunuseisen,** as stated above and
- **potentized Organ preparations** (Arcus aortae, Aorta thoracica, Cor sinistrum, Septum interventriculare ampoule Wala in D4–6 = today Gl D6–8),

As a rule 0.5 ml of each organ preparation was given 2 or 3 times a week by mouth. With the treatment, which was continued for a number of years, development was more or less normal (constitutionally a bit slow,) as expected from the parents' own developmental history. At the age of one, the cardiologist reported that "inspite of the somewhat unsatisfactory operative result, the condition seems to be acceptable. The child is thriving, with no signs of heart failure, and in my opinion a further surgical intervention does not seem indicated for the time being." Propanolol 5 mg twice/day, was prescribed by the cardiologist. Now, seventeen years later, the boy has had no further surgery, and his general development has been satisfactory, aside from legasthenia and mild fine motor concerns. Various other anthroposophic and homoeopathic medicines were prescribed over the years, but he currently needs no medication. The young man is now training as an electrician and is running a Boy Scout troop.

The significance of potentized organ preparations for cardiovascular anomalies in the early years is above all:

- an impulse to support the final maturing of organ structures and
- support of growth and function of specifically affected organs, above all the ventricles.

10

Unfortunately, excessive and bureaucratic requirements as well as small numbers of patients, means that many of the organ preparations previously available are no longer in existence (e.g. Arcus aortae, Cor sinistrum). It is no longer possible to make subtle differentiation in treatment, which, on the other hand, makes it easier to decide on treatment.

- The most important preparation to treat cardiac anomalies is **Cor Gl amp.** Wala.
  Low potencies are particularly suitable when the myocardium is under stress (Gl D5–8, Series I,) and Gl D30 for myocardial disorders due to myocarditis (esp. if chronic,) twice a week in either case, more frequently in individual cases, always 0.5–1 ml by mouth.

The preparations available for conditions affecting the main arteries – coarctation of the aorta, hypoplastic pulmonary artery, etc. – are

- **Aorta Gl**
- **Arteria pulmonalis Gl amp.** Wala

as well as organ preparations of the various heart valves and atrioventricular conduction tissue (**Fasciculus atrioventricularis amp.** Wala) and both endocardium and pericardium.

Most important in treating childhood heart disease in general is an *adequate supply of trace elements and vitamins.* Treating a girl with a history of severe myocarditis, which had led to a milder chronic condition with eosinophilia, normal myocardial biopsy persistent mitral insufficiency, partial loss of ventricular function and a distinctly enlarged heart on x-ray, the authors diagnosed a selenium deficiency. The correlation between selenium deficiency and damage to the myocardium has long been known, especially in China, but is still not given enough attention. Selenium and coenzyme Q10 substitution resulted in definite stabilization for the girl.

Above all supplementation of

- Selenium (aiming at normal serum levels of 60–100 µg/L),
- B vitamins (above all B_1, B_2, aiming at high normal levels,)
- Coenzyme Q 10 (ubiquinone), 10–30 mg/day),
- Magnesium

has repeatedly resulted in remarkable clinical improvement in childhood heart diseases involving either the right or left heart, with measurable reduction in ventricle size and improved myocardial function.

10.1.2.2 Medicines to stimulate the rhythmic system

The most important medicament to stimulate rhythmic function in the heart in the authors' practice is

- **Cardiodoron/Cardiodoron mite drops** Weleda: according to age
  1 drop 3 times or 3 drops mite for infants;

Alcohol-free alternative:

- **Cardiodoron Rh tab.** Weleda
  ⅓ tablet 3 times/day or ½ tablet twice/day

From the second year of life, about 1 drop/year/dose; from the 5th to the 7th year, dose is established individually.

Originally proposed by R. Steiner, Cardiodoron contains extracts from the flowers of cowslip (*Primula veris*) and scotch thistle (*Onopordon acanthium*), with 1 %/0.1 % (mite)/9.2 % (tablets) of *Hyoscyamus* and regulates the rhythmic functions of the heart. It brings together the polar opposites of scotch thistle and cowslip, just as the heart mediates polar opposite needs between head pole and metabolic pole. The small amount of *Hyoscyamus* is the extract of a poisonous plant which directly stimulates the astral body, which is primarily active in respiration. M. Weckenmann did years of research with trials and questionnaires [see above all Weckenmann 1973, 1986] and was able to show that the medicament has a positive, regulative action on the pulse/breath ratio, on mild arrhythmias, and for longterm use in heart failure. Similar studies with Cardiodoron on healthy subjects were published by the cardiologist Kuemmell [Kuemmel and Bettermann 1996.)
Cardiodoron Rh tab., Cardiodoron or Cardiodoron mite drops, which are milder, containing 10 % less *Hyoscyamus*, help in infancy to counteract one-sided, usually tachycardic, changes in rhythm and generally stabilize the interaction of body and soul. Following cardiac surgery, for example on the AV channel in children with the Down syndrome, the medicament helps with stabilization. Supraventricular arrhythmias in the newborn have also responded to Cardiodoron (Cardiodoron mite, 3 times 3 drops).[1]

10.1.2.3 Medicines for tempering anxiety and stress and failure to thrive in children with chronic cardiac disease

For the last seven years, the authors have seen benefit in children with congenital cardiac anomalies and chronic heart disease who received single remedies in divided doses – sometimes at intervals of weeks or months – of

- **Arsenicum** album C30 or **C200 pillules** Gudjons
  3 pillules at 12 hour intervals 3 times, in either dose.

(Start with the C30 and if there is a noticeable positive response change to the higher potency – see case study in ▸Chap. 10.1)
Meanwhile, positive results have been seen in treating schoolchildren with heart failure, dilated cardiomyopathy, and chronic myocarditis following treatment with:

- **Levico** stark (strong) water,
  5–12 drops once/day in the mornings;
  apart from bivalent iron this also contains traces of arsenic and copper [Gasperi 2008].
  In Germany **Levico D1 dil.** Weleda is available [see Levico *Vademecum* 2010, 541].

Indications for this treatment were:

- *treatment-resistant failure to thrive* of cardiac origin and catabolic metabolism,
- inadequate nutritional and fluid intake,
- myocardial hypertrophy, partly limited ventricular function,

1 R. Schwarz's case of a newborn infant with second or third-degree AV block presented in 3rd edition of this book was reviewed by Dr B. Nagel, a paediatric cardiologist. Unlike the physicians who had treated the child he interpreted the ECG as blocked, intermittent SVES. It is worth noting that with Cardiodoron mite, 3 times 3 drops, this infant with initial heart rate reductions of down to 30/min had a normal ECG at 5 months, and that in view of the good clinical condition on Cardiodoron the parents decided against the proposed pacemaker implantation.

- *Anxiety and restlessness, problems sleeping through night* (▸Chap. 7.1.5.3)
- tendency to frequent catarrhal respiratory tract infections, asthma or obstructive bronchitis (see case study ▸Chap. 10.1.1)

Patient and prescriber were often surprised at how effective this single medicament proved to be.

From a letter sent by parents

Three yearold patient, coarctation of the aorta, status post surgical correction, aortic valve stenosis with low-grade aortic valve insufficiency, dystrophy, delayed speech and motor development and marked restlessness, recurrent otitis media; foster child.

"You have achieved the actual miracle for our son. With Arsenicum album, our son was finally able to learn to eat, grew calmer and was able to stay with us. None of the physicians at the hospital and university hospital have been able to help us more. He was about to be given a gastrostomy tube."

L. Gerlach has stated in a review that arsenic is a vital trace element. "In animal experiments, an arsenic-free diet stopped growth and increased perinatal mortality, especially due to dilated cardiomyopathy. The biological role of arsenic is connected with metabolization of sulphur-containing amino acids." In contrast, internal respiration is interrupted with arsenic poisoning, exactly at the intersection of anabolism and catabolism with respiration. "Physiologically, arsenic has now been shown to play "a key role in the energy metabolism of myocardial cells and for the enterohepatic circulation of bile salts""[Gerlach 1998, 135f.]. This defines exactly what arsenic in homoeopathic potency is meant to stimulate – internal respiration especially in the sphere of the heart, the interplay of anabolism and catabolism, and improvement in nutrition (including the breaking down of fats, which depends on the enterohepatic circulation of bile salts).

In our practice we have had repeated evidence that cardiac function improved following prescription of potentized Arsenicum album. It appears to encourage the process of *concentration* which normally occurs after birth and involves a decrease in relative heart size with increasing myocardial function (see under 10.1). This process depends largely on the stimulant action of the thyroid [v. Bernuth 2003, 1117]. Arsenic levels are particularly high in the human thyroid. Potentized Arsenicum album encourages the soul to intervene in a breathing way directed towards the living body, with *anxiety, nervousness, sleep disorders and restlessness decreasing at the same time*. This action of potentized arsenic is known from the homoeopathic literature.

R. Steiner gave a highly differentiated description of the relationship of arsenic to the functions of the astral body, the human soul organization [Steiner 1984, 81–5]. He also gave detailed consideration to the connection between astral body and thyroid (Steiner 1991, 121). According to him, potentized Arsenicum album facilitates engagement of the soul in the living body to counteract "proliferation of physical and etheric processes"– one may think of ventricular hypertrophy with reduced contractile function – "enabling the spiritual in us to regain dominion in our body"[Gerlach 1998, 139] to reduce persistent stress in the organism.

Finally, potentized gold in form of:

- **Aurum met. praep. D10–12 trit.** Weleda once/day is of major importance in treating heart conditions [Girke 2010, 193]" Gold acts on the human heart" [Steiner 1993, 57]. In the present context, it is not so much indicated for treatment in the initial stages, but helps with long-term stabilization (see detailed discussion of this medicinal agent in ▸Chap. 7.2.3.3).

The action is enhanced in children with cardiac anomalies and chronic heart disease by potentizing the gold together with an organ preparation of the heart,

- **Aurum D10/Cor D4 aa amp.** Weleda or
- **Cor/Aurum I amp.** Wala
  once/day – twice/week ½–1 ampoule per os
- This combination along with **Cardiodoron Rh** (Cordiodoron in the USA) tab. Weleda (and generally coenzyme Q10) has proved useful as basic medication for Down syndrome and also for complex, inoperablecongenital cardiac anomalies.

10.2 Idiopathic thrombocytopenic purpura (ITP)

In cases of acute platelet dysfunction, crises and intense developmental demands on the *psyche* or the family must be detected as well as infectious triggers. These easily escape notice if history-taking is superficial. In conventional medicine, the results of clinical studies have recently made the approach to treatment more conservative, so it is difficult to assess spontaneous evolution in the individual case. "The evidence increasingly suggests that primary standard treatment of ITP is of little clinical value, although it does often result in a rapid rise of thrombocytes. … Escalation of treatment must be avoided on principle in childhood ITP. The side effects of the many medicines used to treat ITP can risk morbidity and even mortality. Clinical research is needed to explore other treatment aims and not only the most rapid increase in thrombocytes possible" [Kuehne and Imbach 2006, 538].

In anthroposophic and homoeopathic medicine the elements of group V (now group 15) of the periodic system are noticeably to the fore: phosphorus – arsenic – antimony. All three clearly relate to conditions with a tendency to haemorrhage.

- **Phosphorus LM6 dil.** Arcana
  5 drops daily in the mornings

Phosphorus is generally recommended as the first choice, especially for constitutionally sensitive, slender children who are easily upset and anxious, but this constitution is not always a necessary prerequisite for this medication. Signs indicative of phosphorus are:

- respiratory tract infections in the darker months of the year,
- biographical situations calling for increased intervention of the I or self, for instance in the ninth year of life or the twelfth, with the demands overwhelming the child,
- persistent susceptibility to infection and an inability to overcome infections fully (▸Chap. 7.1.5.2, ▸Chap. 7.5.3.6.2).

- **Arsenicum album D30–C200 pillules**
  3 pillules up to 3 times/day for days or even weeks.

Arsenicum album can be extraordinarily effective in treatment-resistant situations. In many situations the action is specific for abnormal thrombocyte counts and functions not only with ITP, but also with Wiskott-Aldrich syndrome. It must be given in high potency and for a sufficiently long period.

Arsenic symptoms in terms of classical homoeopathy may be almost completely absent.

- Typical infections are above all recurrent otitis; remarkably shiny lips are a rare hallmark.
- Physical death, particularly deaths in the family and cancer is in the background for the child's soul [see Grandgeorge 2004, 43–45;] also the dying nature of late autumn.
- The antimony preparations used in anthroposophic medicine directly address the I organization's activities in the living body. The blood coagulation status, a sensitive state of balance between dissolution and solidification, is determined by the I organization (▸Chap. 3.3) Many experienced anthroposophical colleagues, among them Reinhard Schwarz (Graz, Austria) and Alfred Laengler/Christoph Tautz (Herdecke, Germany), have found the treatment generally effective with ITP. The method given here is partly based on important suggestions from them.

- **Stibium met. prep. D6 (10 ml) amp.** Weleda: initially as a short-term infusion [Vademecum 2010, 773]

Followed by

- **Antimonit D6 trit.** Weleda
  a good pinch 3 times/day

Combined with an organ einreibung (medicated rub) of the spleenwith

- **Stibium met. 0.4 % ointment** Weleda

And administration of

- **Cichorium 5 % pillules** Wala
  5 pillules 3 times/day

And of the organ preparations

- **Thrombozyten Gl D30 amp.** Wala
  initially 1 ampoule s.c. once/day, 2nd week 3 times/wk, 3rd week twice/wk, from 4th week once/wk. In courses for 2–4 years [*Vademecum* 2010, 798]. The advantage of injection is that action is more reliable and direct on the rhythmic system.

The above discussion of phosphorus and arsenic suggests that children with ITP show some weakness in maintaining immunological boundaries. In pathological terms this is reflected indestruction of thrombocytes. The guiding principles for prescribing antimony are:

- The *ratio of "self" to "foreign"* has been upset at the organic level, the catabolic activity of the higher levels of existence (I and astral organization) exhausts itself in the wrong place in an autoaggression process, generally triggered by infections.

- In this situation the aim is to stimulate and regulate splenic function using the above-mentioned antimony preparations and Cichorium. It is also important with ITP to pay careful attention to the aspects of splenic function considered in ▸Chap. 6.3.3.4.
- Antimonite has a direct stimulatory effect on thrombocyte production, mainly in conjunction with the organ preparation, an aspect which can be helpful in treatment of children with tumours during chemotherapy.

Lachesis is indicated particularly when there are profound mental and emotional problems in the background.

- **Lachesis D12 dil.** Weleda
  5–7 drops twice/day.

Case study

A two-year-old boy developed acute ITP with thrombocytes between 7000 and 19000/mm^3. Immunoglobulins and steroids given i.v. did not change the symptoms. The condition persisted with thrombocytes repeatedly below 10000/mm^3, petechiae, and sometimes prolonged epistaxis. Following attempts at treatment with phosphorus, Apis mell., thrombocyte organ preparations (GI D30) were all to no avail. Crotalus horr. D12 was effective in treating protracted epistaxis.

Mentally and emotionally the boy impressed his physician as unhappy and driven. His relationship with his older sister was uneasy, his mother was in mental and emotional turmoil, and his father was always reticent, so that the marital crisis was not apparent for some time. When the condition persisted for more than 6 months, haematologists were considering splenectomy. It was then decided to give Lachesis D12, 5 drops twice/day, as a single medicament. The thrombocyte count rose to 70000/mm^3 within a fortnight, and never again went below 30000, even with infection. Continuing Lachesis, the count rose to the lower normal range within a year. The symptoms disappeared completely once the parents had separated and have not recurred in 12 years of follow-up.

The coagulation system (including the vascular endothelium) may be seen as the *middle system of the blood*, characterized by constant near coagulation and dissolution, in rhythmic processes that are directly connected with the psyche, similar to respiration and cardiac function. The authors are indebted for this view to Broder v. Laue [1995] who followed up suggestions relating to physiology made by R. Steiner [1978, 133f.]. It is presented here because it illuminates the individual genesis of coagulation disorders and endothelial function disorders. This is also important with vasculitic processes, such as Henoch-Schoenlein purpura. Respiration and cardiac function directly show mental and emotional processes in their modulations, and coagulation changes similarly relate to such processes.

10.3 Henoch-Schoenlein purpura

10.3.1 Clinical picture and constitutional illness disposition

Henoch-Schoenlein purpura is the most common form of vasculitis in children. *Conventional treatment is symptomatic and* not the best choice for initial treatment. Steroids, may lead to serious side effects, such as masking symptoms of intestinal perforation. To prevent renal involvement, "the use of glucocorticoids cannot at present be recommended" [Weller 2007, 89]. Although minor involvement of the kidneys is common, severe Henoch-Schoenlein nephritis is rare but can be life-threatening for 1–5 % of cases with terminal kidney failure [Weller, l.c]. Microhaematuria develops frequently and may linger after acute symptoms have gone.

From the conventional medical point of view, the causes of the disease are idiopathic. "The children are well then suddenly ill, a recent mild respiratory tract infection is often reported" [Weller, 81]. But the picture is very different from a holistic point of view because the physician recognizes a particular type of child, who is intensely affected in the rhythmic sphere by inner experiences. The knowledge, especially of children's constitutions, developed at the end of ▸ Chap. 10.2, is fundamental. *These patients are often slender, sensitive and overly attached to their family.* Infections, anxieties, concern for others (especially family members,) and crises in mental and emotional maturation may play a role, especially during the dark seasons. Tonsillitis, which may be streptococcal, often precedes onset as an early sign that the child is not quite managing to cope with inner experiences and needs to rest (▸ Chap. 5.2 and ▸ Chap. 5.3.4). Additionally, there is often an exceptionally close bond between mother and child. Anxieties for the child often emerge on gentle enquiry. The relationship is symbiotic, with the child's readiness for close emotional bonds interacting with the mother's frequently over-protective attitude. The situation may become critical for the child when events in the family environment, the child's own biographical maturation and demands (particularly the 'Rubicon' crisis in the 9th year, ▸ Chap. 7.2) or the mother's return to work make "cutting the cord" inevitable. The fruit of the illness may be a gain in autonomy for both parent and child, provided the illness is properly recognized and adequately treated.

Case study

A four-year-old girl, her mother's first child was born after a normal pregnancy followed by a difficult parturition and Caesarean birth. The girl cried frequently in the first 3 months of life, and her mother did not find it easy to calm her. She thought that the birth had been difficult and that breast-feeding was inadequate. The child did not take solids for almost 3 years, but only drank from the bottle. Two years later a little brother was born. The girl had hexavalent (Sixfold) and MMR vaccinations and in her 4th year was twice vaccinated against Lymes disease. Repeated attacks of croup in her 2nd year were treated with steroids. She had no acute febrile illnesses. Mother said the child was lovable, very sensitive, empathetic, but also difficult to control "when she got herself into a state." The child's father, a dermatologist, was very concerned about his daughter.

Six weeks before the first consultation, the child had a URI and sore throat. Henoch-Schoenlein purpura then developed 4 or 5 days later, typically evolving from hands and feet towards the centre. Antibiotics were given empirically for streptococci and steroids for the purpura just four days before Christmas. As soon as the antibiotics and steroids had been discontinued, the family went to a chalet at 1 000 metres above sea level in the mountains followed by the child's immediate return to kindergarten. Another URI with barking cough was treated with a cough suppressant at night and symptomatic medication. Three days later she had severe abdominal pain, limp, andrecurrence of purpura with painful, swollen ankles bilaterally. Her father had immediately given corticosteroids, 10 mg of prednisolone by mouth for 2 days, with no definite response.

Steroid discontinuation was then advised andthe girl was treated with Formica D1 baths every other day and Apis D30/Pulsatilla D30 by mouth (3 pillules 2 x/day). After one week all skin and joint symptoms resolved. The nature of the disease was discussed with the parents. Following an adequate period of rest, the child was reintroduced to her usual activities gradually and family travel was limited. The father sat in the Formica baths with the girl. He had from youth suffered a treatment-resistant lichen planus. To his amazement, the stressful pruritus he had suffered for years improved dramatically. Encouraged by this, he then took the baths twice a week, resulting in resolution of all skin changes and no recurrence more than a year later (*Vademecum* 2010, 448).

This case study shows the following:

- It confirms the constitution described above and the close parental bond.
- Social and school transitions for children so closely connected with their mothers is very strenuous for the children, with behavioural reactions common. Sibling relations also are demanding for these children. Family incidents touch them deeply and they fear insufficient attention. The immune system is not infrequently immature; vaccinations or long-term medication (e. g. anticonvulsives) may play a role as stress factors.

In ▸Chap. 3.5.1 reference was made to the publication by Watanabe [2010] noting a paediatric nephrologist's report of 4 children between the ages of 5 and 7, who all developed acute Henoch-Schoenlein purpura one day after an H1N1 Influenza vaccinationin 2009. He also refers to another 7 cases reported in the literature. Five of the total of 11 affected children had a preceding history of immunological diseases, including Henoch-Schönlein purpura, drug reactions, and food allergies. One child developed terminal renal failure and one chronic glomerulonephritis. This demonstrates that Henoch-Schoenlein purpura is not always idiopathic, and that the influenza vaccine, in this age group, may provoke the development of purpura and its vast range of complications. This is an entirely different situation from "spontaneous" Henoch-Schoenlein purpura, which, in our view, is constitutional in origin.

- The families we observed generally had no understanding of the child's need to rest. In the above case, the pre-holiday conventional medical intervention, the family trip on conclusion of treatment, and prompt return to school showed no respect for a time to recover. Adequate rest in familiar surroundings is a necessity for the child, though excessive parental anxiety will be counterproductive.
- It is vital to have *rest*, not bed rest, but quiet and release from all outside activities and obligations until the symptoms have completely subsided. Only then should there be

gradual return to everyday life. Children with this constitution do not seek peace and quiet, but clamor for social contact and activities, so active coaching will be needed!

- The basic aetiology of Hennoch-Schoenlein Purpura is that the I organization has weakened powers to actively form and individualize the body. Mentally and emotionally the child lives too much in his surroundings, with I and astral body powerfully pulled to the outside. Mobility, kindergarten and school all can increase this tendency. At the same time, lack of sunlight further decreases the formative forces. Histology shows leukocytoclastic vasculitis, which ascends from feet and hands. Oedema of the intestinal wall causes severe colicky pain, and increased kidney permeability to iron-containing erythrocytes and protein. This clearly is the signature of an inflammatory, destructive process making itself independent in the organization of metabolism and limbs. Iron is reduced and cannot be maintained. Typically the children are under nine years old at onset, or have just come to the 9-year crisis ("Crossing the Rubicon" see above).

Case vignette

A 9½-year old boy had a recurrence of his Henoch-Schoenlein purpura three days after Christmas. First onset at age seven, directly connected with starting school. He is slender, blond, sensitive and described as an 'anxious observer' on his report card. But, when not the centre of attention, he teases his peers mercilessly. He is close to his mother, but his father is rather choleric. Six weeks before Christmas, his beloved grandmother, who lives nearby, had a severe stroke. She returned from rehabilitation a few days before Christmas and now needs nursing care. The boy's mother, working half days, took on that care with her two sisters.

- In early childhood, before the ninth year, I organization activity comes solely from the head pole; after this it unites more strongly with the metabolic pole (see a fuller discussion of this in section 7.2). The crisis of the disease may also be seen as the need for the individual soul and spirit to start to separate from close parental care and to penetrate his or her own metabolism and limbs, home of the will. Treatment would consist in strengthening I organization activity in the cardiovascular system and anchoring the astral body more strongly in the kidney and digestive tract. Adequate counselling of the parents will be needed to ideally encourage a gradual release of the child from the close bond with the mother while more actively involving the father or other adults.

Another case study, concerning a girl aged 10, kindly made available to the authors by Renate Karutz, will further illustrate these points:

A 10-year-old girl was brought to us as an emergency and the parents gave the following history:

The girl, an only child, had been given intensive attention from birth, but was always nervous, wide awake and delicate. At almost three years of age, she got lost during a farm holiday and was found by strangers. Since then her nervousness had increased and she always wanted to keep her mother within sight. At the age of 6, she developed an influenza-type infection and Henoch-Schoenlein purpura. The symptoms had disappeared after 14 days, with no treatment given. There were two self-limited recurrences in the next year. An allergic reaction to an insect bite was followed by severe gastroenteritis and a further bout of Henoch-Scoenlein purpura. After 4 weeks of persistent symptoms, including violent colicky pain, loss of appetite, weight loss and hematochezia, she was admitted to a paediatric university hospital.

Strict bed rest, parenteral feeding, and antibiotics brought no improvement. Rapid improvement occurred after Prednisolone 2 mg/kg/day was given i.v., so the the steroid was stopped and she was discharged home. Two days later, she became somnolent. Cerebral oedema due to the Henoch-Schoenlein purpura was suspected, but it proved to be an iatrogenic adrenal crisis. Steroids were therefore given again. The parents then searched for an alternative form of medical treatment. While still on low dose steroids, she had another recurrence of Hennoch-Schoenlein purpura, which improved rapidly. Steroids were discontinued, but several weeks later, she had febrile tonsillitis and otitis media. For the first time, she was treated without antibiotics, and had no subsequent Henoch-Schoenlein purpura.

She was symptom-free for over a year until she suffered an influenza-type infection with otitis media, which was treated with antibiotics and antipyretics because homoeopathic treatment did not succeed. She then had another recurrence of Hennoch-Schoenlein Purpura with serious symptoms and slow recovery. Two months later, she had another influenza-type infection, which within five days triggered severe joint swelling with intense pain on movement and touch, fever to 40 °C, sore throat, otalgia, petechiae on feet and buttocks and intermittent abdominal pain. Urinalysis remained unremarkable. In the light of their previous experience, the parents refused antibiotics.

On examination at our first consultation, she was a very pale, tall, slender girl, in poor condition with numerous petechiae on the lower extremities, erythematous tonsils, and bulging tympanic membranes. She had diffuse back and leg pain on touch and movement.

She had no improvement by the next day following intake of Apis/Belladonna cum Mercurio pillules Wala and Levisticum Rh D3 dil. On urging from the primary paediatrician, who was concerned about her significantly elevated Anti-Streptolysin O (ASO) titre and leukocytosis, amoxillin was given. She had dramatic deterioration in the hours that followed, with unbearable abdominal and back pain. The next morning, she had more petechiae and painful, palpable forehead and back swellings as well as severe anxiety, restlessness, and sleeplessness.

In this situation a change to Phosphorus D20 and Apis mell D20 dil., 5 drops twice/day each, resulted in improvement within a few hours. At the next visit, five days later, she had no appreciable disease. The following week, her mother spoke of perceptible changes in her with more confidence, new self-awareness, initiative at home and energy for school again. This was the first time that the mother could hope for no further recurrences of the Henoch-Schoenlein purpura, as the girl had taken a definite step forward in her development, something she had not seen previously when the symptoms had abated.

Rationale of treatment: Apis mell., an animal substance, acts primarily on the etheric organism. It stimulates the life organization to take in the powers of the astral body and I more strongly. The life organization's functions are directly linked to organizing the fluid principle in the living body. With Apis, the life organization can be stimulated to reabsorb fluid that has collected in connective tissues outside the capillaries back into the blood stream. The same applies to exudative processes in the region of the middle ear.

Phosphorus, a mineral, acts primarily on the I organization. Weakness of the I organization is evident in emotional instability, anxiety, excessive dependency, or extreme sensitivity combined with a weak will. This weakness creates an imbalance in the life organization, which is evident in one-sided active growth, marked weakness and exhaustion, or a tendency to develop oedematous inflammation which dissolves organ boundaries. Phosphorus primarily holds the I closer to the body, freeing the individual to be outwardly active again. With the I and astral body more strongly connected with the lower human being, an excessively awake, stressed neurosensory system will be calmed.

Our patient improved for the following six months of summer. But in September, following a mild infection of the upper respiratory tract, she had another, very mild recurrence of Henoch-Schoenlein purpura. When given Phosphorus D30, 5 drops twice/day for a week, the girl was symptom-free although microhaematuria was demonstrable for the first time, initially intermittent, later almost continuous, but asymptomatic and with no progression. Severe otitis media and tonsillitis in early March resolved without antibiotics with only a few days of petechiae. Her microhaematuria persisted, so next we planned to prescribe a suitable medicament, start painting therapy, and implement prophylaxis against infection in the winter months.

10.3.2 Treatment

10.3.2.1 Phosphorus and formica

The authors have been able to consolidate their treatment for Henoch-Schoenlein purpura into a paradigm concept which is effective even in difficult presentations. A communication from Godhart Husemann, who in 28 years of paedriatic practice had seen excellent outcomes with Formica baths, proved most helpful. In one difficult case this treatment tipped the scales for us.

A 10-year-old boy with longtime complex focal epilepsy and with gastric aura (nausea) had needed oxcarbazepine inspite of homoeopathic and anthroposophical adjuvant treatment. He was a slender, playful child, closely attached to his mother, who had intense conflicts with his teenage brothers. After an acute febrile infection, massive Henoch-Schoenlein purpura developed with proteinuria, swollen joints, severe abdominal pain and extensive skin changes involving his extremities and back. The author, consulted 3½ weeks after onset, decided to wean the anticonvulsant. Treatment with all the oral medicines mentioned stabilized the evolution, with a regression of nephritis; however, over the next four months, the purpura recurred with any strain or stress, even sibling rivalry. The author then learned of the treatment with Formica baths, which were added to the treatment regimen. Within 3 weeks the purpura was gone completely and urine normalized. Remarkably, after the Formica baths, neither purpura nor complex focal seizures occurred after discontinuation of the oxcarbazepine during two year follow-up.

To understand the rationale for the highly effective treatment with Formica baths, we have to consider the words of Rudolf Steiner based on his research into the functions of the human I organization. He referred to this unconscious structure as the "I scaffolding." "When you try and bring Formica in very high dilution close to the human being ... you encounter a consolidation ... of this scaffolding, so that it is filled with I quality" (R. Steiner [1999, 228]). To understand this it is helpful to consider the activity in an ant heap. Of all insects, ants establish the most complex and coherent communities, which may cover areas of many kilometres in the woods. They function there as an "immune system", daily inspecting and cleansing the bark of the trees, and through their activities and their formation of formic acid, they make the decomposing matter in the woodland soil available again for plant growth. We might speak of a central digestive and immune system of the woods (the "dying of woods" has to do with ants withdrawing from damaged woodlands.) "The ants actively fight parasitic life and effect the loosening, aeration, and warming through of the soil" [from the key principles of Formica, *Vademecum* 2010, 446]. In the summer months, the ant population is able to establish a uniform warmth system in the nest, completely renewing all nest material in about a month. In human beings, the use of Formica can trigger "the ordering intervention of the I organization" to be stimulated. "The metabolism is orientated towards the maintenance and building up of the human form and healthy warmth throughout the organism" [Vademecum, l. c.] Henoch-Schoenlein purpura with its necrotizing and leucocytoclastic vasculitis, is a destructive form of inflammation in the vascular sphere of the lower human being, the limbs, intestines, and kidneys. External application of Formica and internal use of potentized Phosphorus activates the I organization to transform destructive inflammation into a constructive process. (For more on the physiology of inflammation and Phosphorus in anthroposophic medicine, see Girke [2010, 115–123]). The basic treatment therefore is as follows:

- **Formica D1 dil.** Weleda
  20 drops to a full bath, 20 min. (ideally between 9 and 10 a.m., so that treatment coincides with the I's incarnating movements). Followed by 30 minutes rest. Initially alternate days, then less often.
- **Phosphorus LM6 Arcana, D20 dil.** Weleda
  5 drops daily in the mornings.

10.3.2.2 Pulsatilla and Apis

At the level of the soul and astral, the medicinal plant which matches this type of patient is *Pulsatilla vulgaris*. This member of the buttercup family flowers in early spring, before the new grass sprouts, producing impressive purple flowers that are a radiant yellow inside. The temperature inside the flower may be up to 10 °C above the ambient temperature due to absorption of sunlight, enclosure of air in the calyx, and catabolic processes. This allows for early flowering when the air is still cool. The finely divided leaves and corolla are covered in fine hairs and highly sensitive in character. The flower sways in the wind and shows a very different soul quality when upright and open than when it bends down to the ground. Insects buzz and land, indicating a close connection with ensouled life and the astral. The vegetative element is still minimal at this time and delicate. Clinically this corresponds to the manner of patients with Henoch-Schoenlein purpura in meeting the physician: intense, yet only partly incarnated, distracted, yet stuck in their body. Moods are flighty and impressionable. Pulsatilla in higher potency is a key plant-based medicament when the mother-child bond is too tight.

A medicament from the animal world that has proved effective with Henoch-Schoenlein purpura is Apis mellifica given by mouth (see Vademecum, 91f.). The relationship to community-forming insects has been described above for Formica. Apis mellifica is a proven homoeopathic and anthroposophic medicine for acute inflammatory conditions in the lower human being: vasculitis where walls and boundaries become too permeable, in hypersensitive constitutions with overreactivity, and to temperature control, unable to maintain needed warmth. The beehive with its stable temperature, regular hexagonal wax cells, and the bees' intuitive sense of order and orientation is the therapeutic picture of what this constitution most needs. Giving Apis D30 and Pulsatilla D30 together once daily has been helpful for acute, autoimmune processes.

Finally, the authors have found potentized organ preparations in high potency effective in treating acute rheumatic conditions. Organ preparations of arterial vessels, kidneys, and affected joints have repeatedly proved their value in acute situations.

- **Pulsatilla D30 pillules. DHU/dil.** Apotheke an der Weleda
  5 pillules once/day, evenings
- **Apis ex animale Gl D30 amp.** Wala/**pillules** Weleda
  0.5 ml once/day by mouth/5 pillules, may be taken together with Pulsatilla in the evenings
- **Renes Gl D30 amp., Arteriae Gl D30 amp.** Wala
  as required, ½–1 ampoule orally every 2 or 3 weeks, where indicated also homologous organ preparations, above all from ankle region (Articulatio talocruralis, Articulatio subtalaris).
- **Aurum/Equisetum I pillules** Wala
  5–7 pillules in the mornings for 3–9 months

serve in cases where the kidneys are initially involved to stabilize children with Henoch-Schoenlein purpura during the months that follow the illness and to strengthen the "presence of I, their ability to be independent." The authors have been impressed with the gold and horsetail combination, which prevents "the heart dropping into one's boots (kidneys), " so that the child is able to develop a centre of warmth in the middle [see basic principles in 1st lecture R. Steiner gave for medical students and physicians; 1987, 20f.].

The above medical treatment must be combined with insight into the child's constitutional disposition and counselling the family to maintain rest until acute symptoms are gone, and only then to gradually resume everyday activities. This is an approach to treatment which in the authors' practical experience is both effective and free from potential side effects. A particularly satisfying aspect is that the disease is no longer "random" and provides an opportunity to initiate healthy changes for the entire family.

10.4 Cystic fibrosis

In Cystic fibrosis normal *secretion* of sweat, tracheobronchial secretions, biliary and pancreatic functions is disrupted, resulting in too much salt in the sweat and viscid secretions. Catabolism and assimilation of foods, especially warmth-bearing fats, is reduced and requires continuinal support. Secretory and respiratory processes suffer from increasing deformation of physical organs, mainly the lung, but also the pancreas and the hepatobiliary system. The guiding principle for treatment is to support the life organization with dietary measures, enzyme supplementation, and with appropriate anthroposophic and homoeopathic medicines. This paves the way for possibilities of stimulating respiratory and secretory processes directly with medication.

Rich experience over many years in complementary treatment of children with CF enables us to say that even in advanced cases, these treatment methods can achieve significant improvement in the disease course and in the patient's sense of well being. It is also possible to reduce the length and extent of long-term antibiotic treatment. In the authors' view, daily prophylactic antibiotic treatment at all stages is not advisable; however, when antibiotics are indicated, they must be given consistently. Enzyme and vitamin supplementation as required, mucolysis and physiotherapy, optimal nutrition, and sufficient active movement are required in every case.

The complementary treatment which is probably the most successful is *climatotherapy*, now also accepted at our university hospitals. It is remarkable how much the symptoms of the disease can improve in a *warm, sunny climate close to the sea*. For the patients this move on reaching adulthood gives a *long-term prospect of life and helps more than any* additional medicines. From early infancy, climatotherapy is one of the most important measures, especially at the beginning and end of the cold, wet winter months, always so stressful for the patients. The same applies to wet summer months with subnormal temperatures. Here, too, the indication for intensive antibiotic treatment should be handled in a liberal way. Advice should be given about the type of holiday needed. *It is important to stimulate the combined action of light and warmth with the life organization.* This can best by stimulated by a *sea climate* with light and warmth, optimally *near the equator.*

Medicinally this goal is strengthened by iodine compounds. Iodine was first isolated as an element from seaweed on the Atlantic coast of France in 1811. It accumulates in enormous amounts by bladderwrack, though the exact process is not yet known. In the natural world iodine is maximally present in the zone of transition from water to land-and this mirrors the physiological function of iodine. The metamorphosis of tadpoles into frogs that have lungs and limbs depends on thyroxine, and therefore on iodine [see Girke 2010, 375–7]. Iodine stimulates the move from water to land in animal life, not only for amphibians, but also for all higher vertebrates. Lung develops as the metamorphosis of part of the foregut. Cystic fibrosis is characterized as incipient "regression of the lung" to an "intestine-like" state of inflammation with viscid secretion, chronic inflammation, and bacterial involvement (▸Chap. 6.5). Clinically, low potencies of the iodine compounds listed below can counteract this tendency.

- **Sulphur iod. D4–6 dil.** (various manuf.),
- **Stannum iod. D6 tab.** (various manuf.),
- **Kalium iod. D6–12 dil.** (various manuf.).

10

The iodine component stimulates the light-filled formative, cleansing, and catabolic activity of the astral body in the metabolism. Sulphur, tin, and potassium support and order the life organization activity and its main organ, the liver. Clinically, they act on the digestion, the function of the epigastric organs, and decrease inflammation and harmful bacteria in the respiratory tract. It is recommended to give one of the three medicines for one or several months and then pause or make a change.

- **Echinacea/Mercurius comp. supp.** for children. Wala
  1 suppository twice/day
  has proved particularly effective as standard treatment for all respiratory infections, especially URIs and prevention of inflammation in the lower respiratory tract in the winter months for children with cystic fibrosis. This treatment is particularly important as the nose and paranasal sinuses are major foci for chronic respiratory tract inflammation in patients with Cystic fibrosis. More than any other potentized medicine they help to reduce the need for antiobiotics for children with CF.
  The treatment is effectively complemented with cinnabar.
- **Zinnober D6 tab.** Weleda and **Myristica sebifera comp. pillules** Wala (see. ▸Chap. 5.1.2).

Agents for pulmonary treatment and prevention are, among others,

- **Pulmo/Vivianit comp. amp.** Wala
  once or twice/day (4 times for infections) 0.5 ml by mouth/(alternatively) once or twice/day 0.5–1.0 ml inhaled with saline solution for tendency of inflammation of lower respiratory tract (bronchitis, bronchopneumonia)
- **Pulmo/Tartarus stib. II amp.** Wala
  acute, 1 ml s.c./i.v., twice/day ½–1 ampoule orally, or inhaled with saline solution if mainly viscid phlegm.
- **Ferrum phosphoricum D6 tab.** Weleda, or
  Ferrum sidereum D6 trit. Weleda,
  Phosphor LM6 dil. Arcana (phosphorus) and
  Tartarus stibiatus comp. Weleda (Tartarus stib. D6, Quarz D12)
  1–3 times/day, especially if given in the mornings are suitable for stabilizing the patient's pulmonary situation. An alternative is the proven composition
- **Meteoreisen pillules/amp.** Wala (meteoric iron)
  twice/day 5–7 pillules morning/afternoon, for children with acute influenza-type viral infections initially 1 ampoule i.v.

During and after every acute infection one of the above-mentioned medicines should be given together with the indicated nosode (note culture results), for example:

- **Bac. Pyocyaneus (= Pseudomonas) D6–10 dil.** Staufen® or
- **Sanukehl® Pseu D6**
  5 drops once or twice/day

Other nosodes to be considered are Staphylococcus aureus, Haemophilus influenzae, Aspergillus, etc. Subcutaneous injection in the D30 repeated three times has been efficacious in individual cases, with improved well being and cultures. With acute and severe pulmonary infections, particularly in schoolchildren, injections of

- **Argentum D30/Echinacea D6 amp.** Weleda
  1 ampoule s.c./i.v. proved effective. May be complemented (mixed injection) by
- **Pulmo/Vivianit comp. amp.** Wala

and/or

- **Lachesis e ven. D30 amp.** Wala/Weleda

Crataegus preparations can be helpful for the cardiopulmonary system, especially from school age onwards, e. g.

- **Crataegus tab.** Weleda[1] (Switzerland)
  2 tablets once or twice daily

Apart from the well-known action on the cardiovascular system, high flavonoid levels are helpful with the chronic destructive pulmonary processes.

Sea buckthorn, *Hippophae rhamnoides*, concentrates warmth and light qualities to a remarkable degree in its bright orange berries and the seeds within them. This member of the oleaster family is rich in fat and water soluble vitamins, so extracts and low potencies of sea buckthorn are valuable medicinal agents for children with cystic fibrosis, especially in the winter months. It has also proved helpful for other children susceptible to infection. B. Fersch [2004] described the medicinal plant and its indication in children susceptible to infection. A possible dietetic measure is to give:

- Sanddorn-Ursaft (sea-buckthorn pure Juice) (Weleda),
  e. g. 1 tsp. daily in juice expressed from 1 orange. In our experience this treatment is more effective in combination with an appropriate potentized medicine.

Digestive function is further stimulated by giving

- **Cichorium/Pancreas comp. pillules** Wala
  5–7 pillules 2 or 3 times/day,
- **Natrium sulfuricum D6 pillules** DHU/**Thenardit D6 dil.** Weleda (= Natrium sulf. naturale (see. ▸Chap. 6.5.6.6.1),

and from school age, Curcuma preparations, well proven as

- **Chelidonium/Curcuma comp. tab.** Weleda Switzerland
  1 tablet 2 or 3 times/day [*Vademecum* 2010, 305.]
- **Luvos Heilerde ultra** (medicinal clay)

can be beneficial for the gastrointestinal tract; and for gastroduodenal symptoms or diarrhoea

- **Bolus alba comp. Pulvis** Wala
  is recommended,
  1 tsp. in either case Bolus alba comp. dissolved in water; although many children refuse anise, even masked with honey; however, it is worthwhile.

1 In the author's experience the most effective Crataegus preparation.

- Microbiologic therapy to control infections (▸Chap. 4.6) is required frequently, sometimes for extended periods, depending on cultures, and previous antibiotic treatment. With cystic fibrosis, the diet must not only provide calories, but also beneficial intestinal flora (lactic-fermented vegetables, sour milk products, etc.). Whole milk may need to be restricted if nasal congestion is exacerbated.

This has only reviewed the most frequent CF treatments; hopefully, as experience increases the choices will become more individualized and extended. The importance of intense sunlight, vitamin D supplementation, and monitoring Vitamin D levels is particularly important (▸Chap. 3.2).

10.5 Undescended testicle

In paediatric practice, physicians are often confronted with the problem of management of undescended testicles. Knowledge of standard treatment is assumed [DGKJ, Leitlinien 2010, 36]. "So far it has been noted that surgically moving the testis to the scrotum does not remove the increased risk of malignancy" [l. c., 12; Mathers 2009]. Reduced fertility is the primary concern. The authors are sceptical about hormonal treatment. The guidelines refer to the argument against hormonal therapy due to possible inflammation and induction of apoptosis, but fail to refer to the deep-reaching effect of hormonal therapy on the sentient organization, the astral body, especially at an age when physiologic development may be shifted due to hormone therapy. Since the guidelines state that hormonal therapy is only indicated in the first year of life [DGKJ, Leitlinien 2010, 36], the authors prefer surgery, if intervention is required. They agree with R. Madeleyn that attempts to treat bilateral cryptorchidism homoeopathically or anthroposophically have been unsuccessful.

The following recommendations refer to retractile testis in paediatric surgery [*Definition Leitlinie* 36, 1–3].

Over many years we were able to develop a treatment that gives satisfactory results. The treatment outlined below is given for three months after making the diagnosis, then a follow-up examination is made. If there is mobilization or descent, the treatment is continued until a satisfactorily stable result is achieved. If the condition has not changed or the testis is not palpable, the child must be referred to a paediatric surgeon. The child's age determines how much time a physician can allow for conservative treatment, since the current standard dictates that treatment should start early in the 1st year of life. If an older child presents with retractile testis, time is also an option, since the treatment goal of complete descent by the first birthday is impossible (however, this option needs careful consideration as it may be considered culpable in some countries).

Medically, to stimulate craniocaudal maturation one first gives:

- **Epiphysis/Plumbum pillules** Wala
  3–5 pillules 3 times/day for three weeks.

Phylogenetically the pineal gland is a sense organ for the cosmic light and warmth streaming into the earth. Governing processes of the I flow via the pineal gland, including the day and night rhythm and gonadal growth. The function of the human pineal gland may be seen as enriching light and warmth qualities with inner impulses from the I.

The treatment prepares for activation of the pineal gland [*Vademecum* 2010, 503–5], which then sends impulses for the life organization. After three weeks, follow with

- **Hypophysis (pituitary gland)/Stannum pillules** Wala
  5 pillules 3 times/day

And treatment then continues, alternating every three weeks. To stimulate astral body activity in the lower human being, which is directly connected with all maturational processes in the genital region, treatment is combined with administration of potentized copper arsenate

- **Olivenit D8 dil.** Apotheke an der Weleda
  3–5 drops twice/day

Considering in particular the maturational processes in the testis in the first year of life, it is advisable to give the following in addition when cryptorchidism is diagnosed early.

- **Testes/Argentum amp.** Wala

3 times/wk by mouth at the treatment stage where Hypophysis/Stannum and Olivenit are given. This may also be continued for stabilization once the primary treatment has been concluded. In the first 6 months of life, it may also be given as inductive monotherapy. Parents need to be told that the warning on the package, not to give it under the age of 12, is routine and has nothing to do with any real risk in using the medicament.

10.6 Phimosis, penile adhesion, labial adhesion

Taking up a suggestion by their dermatological colleague, L. Jachens, good resolution of boys' mild to medium phimosis and with simple foreskin adhesions occur with regular external applications of:

- **Polygonatum 5 % ointment** Weleda
  Once/dayevenings; for maintenance twice/week.

The original indication for this ointment made with an extract of Solomon's seal is to soften scars and keloids. Applied regularly, gently retracting the foreskin after the bath in the evening, it is often effective in avoiding surgery [Soldner 2005]. A number of anthroposophical paediatricians have confirmed the reliability of this treatment.

For inflammation and irritation of the foreskin, a hot-water extract of arnica and chamomile may be used externally:

- **Arnikamill ointment**

Polygonatum 5 % ointment may also be used for labial adhesions. After using it for 3 or 4 weeks, one can carefully attempt to separate the adhering labia with a blunt instrument, a cotton-tipped applicator, or the mother may be able to do so after the bath. Often these will spontaneous resolve by age seven (and can therefore also just be left alone).

10.7 Acne vulgaris

10.7.1 Acne from an anthroposophical perspective, problems related to conventional treatment

Acne vulgaris develops in the *third seven-year period* for most young people, reaching a peak between the ages of 16 and 18 (▸Chap. 6.4.1). Fats collect in the subcutis, sebum production increases, and seborrhoea due to keratinisation of sebaceous gland ducts will occur. Remarkably, this tendency develops mainly in the *upper human being*, in the region of face, shoulders, upper back and neck below the throat. At the time, the sexual organs are maturing in the *lower human being*, the *organism of metabolism and limbs*, as well as the musculature in the extremities, completing longitudinal growth. Internal *secretion of hormones* leading to changes in metabolism and *outward-directed skin secretion* indicate that the activity of the *astral body activity has changed and is more fully present.*

The young person is in a difficult period of transition when bonds to adults, especially parents and teachers, are loosening, yet bonding with contemporaries is still uncertain. The authority of adults no longer rules the teen's will activity, but the I forces are not yet fully and consistently available. Great uncertainty prevails with a desire to expand and avidly explore combined with self doubt, vulnerability, disappointment, and embarrassment. This congested, unstable situation is reflected in the way the organism deals with fats, which are in a sense the warmth and will potential in the human organism. Simultaneously fat production increases but in the wrong place (the skin of the upper human being), in the wrong degree (causing seborrhoea) and in poor fat excretion (development of comedones). "The cause of acne thus lies in the internal metabolism below; the processes in the skin are merely external effects from above" [Jachens 2004, 256].

When young people have acne, the situation is that the organism is not completely consuming fats and instead creates a "valve" for itself in the skin. If we consider that 98.5 % of all energy is stored in fats in the healthy body, we may speak of the dammed-up sebum as "parasitic heat foci" in the skin. These have an "inherent tendency to get inflamed, "as Rudolf Steiner and Ita Wegman put it in their fundamental discussion of fat metabolism, which is as true for acne as it is for atherosclerotic plaques (Steiner and Wegman 1991, 59f.). In the case of acne, the "origin of such foci must be sought in the body's tendency to produce more fat than the I organization needs for internal warmth" [l. c.]. When about age 21, the I is "born" and comes fully into existence, acne has usually regressed.

The observant physician may note that acne improves when the young person is fully connected to his individuality, actively unfolding his will. Acne patients often still have inhibitions, self-consciousness, and reserve about intimate relationships, with tendencies towards procrastination, avoidance, and awkwardness. Often the bond with the parents is still too close or there are other unresolved obstacles to a "full birth of the I", in the crisis in the 18th year, the first moon node [Roder 2005.]

Clinically it is helpful, especially in severe cases, to provide for adequate physical activity to create a balance, including plentiful physical work in the open air.

With reference to the organs involved, it is most important to address I activity in the liver and bile in a differentiated way [see Jachens, l. c.]. It is always impressive to see how this will not only improve acne, but harmonize and encourage the will activity of the young person.

At this point, brief reference may be made to the problems of conventional treatment for acne. Indirectly this accurately confirms the above anthroposophical views.

- Up to 80 % of propionibacterium are now resistant to topical *erythromycin and clindamycin*. Metabolism of these causes further stress and promotes both allergies and antibiotic resistance.
- "Oral retinoids are the gold standard in treating *hyperkeratosis and seborrhoea* systemically" [Maerker-Stromer and Hoeger 2005, 25]. The side effects of this "gold standard" are worth noting. *Hyperlipidaemia* and *elevated transaminases* indicate drug-induced toxicity for liver and fat metabolism and deposition of lipids in arterial endothelium, dangerously displacing excess fats to the inner organism. (Are atherosclerotic plaques meant to take the place of acne?) At the same time, the skin and mucosa become dry due to lack of fats in the epidermis, which reflects the disorder in the central metabolic organs (▸Chap. 6.4 and the section on epidermal fat metabolism there).
- Retinoids are also *teratogenic*, so that *girls must be given contraceptives*. This is a therapeutic diversion of the maturational step taken by the youthful organism. Contraceptives impose further stress on liver metabolism, often clinically evident in increased susceptibility to infection. More subtle observation frequently notes a disruption of I presence in the unfolding of the will.
- The risks to which conventional medicine exposes these patients – usually without complete information – are remarkable. "Minocycline, widely used to treat acne in the past, is today recommended as a second choice because of unexpected side effects of fulminant pancreatitis and liver failure" [Maerker-Stromer and Hoeger, l. c.]. Anyone who takes acne treatment which risks fatal liver damage should consider if this is the right approach. Its toxicity points to a phenomenon known in the anthroposophical view of the human being – the significance of the hepatobiliary system for the development of the human will and the role of human fat metabolism.
- Instead of mere suppression of skin changes, we must first realize that acne constitutes a "relief phenomenon" as part of the adolescent maturational crisis. Our aim in the light of this understanding should be treatment which will strengthen the will, the patient's hepatobiliary function, and self-confidence. Through validation, not suppression, of the patient's own intentions, this approach will support the "birth of the I."

10.7.2 Anthroposophical and homoeopathic treatment of acne vulgaris

> "A major environmental factor with acne is the diet in the western life style. ... These acne-free populations do not consume milk and dairy produce or carbohydrates with high glycaemic index"
>
> B. Melnik [2010]

The case study which follows illustrates the far-reaching possibilities for treatment even of severe acne using the above treatment.

A neurasthenic young man, who was treated successfully for acne between 13 and 15 years of age. He was considered gifted academically and musically, as a performance pianist. He felt both internal pressure and ambition. He had little connection with natural world and preferred spending time in his room to the outdoors. He could hardly be persuaded to help in the garden, so there was little exposure to sunlight. His father suffered from scarring nodulocystic acne; his mother seemed dominant, chatty, and always accompanied him to visits while his acne was florid.
History included previous unsuccessful university dermatologic treatment with benzoyl peroxide, oral and external antibiotics, and external treinoin; oral retinoids had not yet been prescribed. He suffered rapid exacerbations of severe acne vulgaris with comedones and scarring, acne conglobata, and extensive scars. The face was mainly affected, especially the forehead, and also the shoulders, below the throat, and the back of neck. His acne was better by the sea and in the sun. There had been no unusual events or serious illnesses.
Initially, topical conventional treatment was complemented, the aim being to avoid topical antibiotics, while continuing benzoyl peroxide. The patient was relatively satisfied with the new topical treatment using

- **Aknewasser** Wala and **Akne-Waschcreme** Hauschka daily

and several times weekly an application of

- **Gesichtsmaske** Wala (facemask) and **Gesichtsdampfbad** Wala (facial steam bath).

Among other things these products contain Tropaeolum (nasturtium). Used externally and orally often proved effective in treating inflammatory changes with bacterial infection Angocin tablets and Tropaeolum alcea drops are available for oral use).
Natrium muriaticum was first given by mouth, with no effect. Moderate improvement was achieved by starting Arsenum iodatum (ambitious, thin, highly neurasthenic, does not feel the cold), Kalium iodatum, and Argentum/Quarz Wala. Intestinal dysbiosis/candidiasis was treated and in conjunction with this Gentiana Magenglobuli (stomach pillules) Wala were given. Dietary changes brought no improvement, which is not surprising with a distinctly neurasthenic constitution. Since no substantial progress had been made in the two years of previous benzoyl peroxide treatment this was stopped. Conventional dermatologists were seen for acute episodes while on holiday, with courses of topical antibiotics, but never again oral.
Now, at 15 years old, treatment was changed to a proven anhroposophical therapy to primarily stimulate and strengthen intervention of the individual spirit, the I, in hepatobiliary metabolism. The rationale may be briefly formulated as follows:

- His one-sided dominance in the head, upper extremities, and in fine motor functions. His scrawny, skinny build indicated the lack of muscle and physique for his age.
- He was not developing age-appropriate will engagement (biliary function), as shown by his avoidance of physical work, sport and even leisure activities with his contemporaries ("stay-at-home").
- Heat was inappropriately held in the upper human being, and not developed in the lower human being.
- The iron process seemed too weak, with his I not intervening sufficiently in the liver and gallbladder region.

Treatment involved

- **Choleodoron** Weleda
  12 drops 3 times/day

This medicament is based on two "sulphuric", coloured roots/rhizomes: *Chelidonium majus*, greater celandine, a member of the poppy family, with an orange, sharp-tasting latex rich in alkaloids present throughout and similar to bile, and also *Curcuma*, a basic Asian curry seasoning. Both substances activate and medicinally regulate bile secretion (the action of coloured roots acts on the bile, see also *Berberis)*. A purifying effect is also connected with this. Choleodoron has a noticeably stabilizing effect on drive in adolescents [see *Vademecum* 2010, 308].

- **Hepatodoron tab.** Weleda
  1 tablet 3 times/day, to chew.

This is based on two different leaves – grape and strawberry. The extraordinary performance of the grapevine in carbohydrate metabolism is generally known. This preparation, which like Choleodoron originated with R. Steiner, comprehensively stimulates liver function and sugar metabolism, which is the foundation for consciousness and will. Organically, the preparation may also treat constipation, which is important in acne care.

- **Legalon 140** Madaus
  1 capsule twice/day.

Made from the oily seed of milk thistle (see also **Carduus marianus caps.** Weleda,) act powerfully on the liver, particularly in fat metabolism and due to toxic damage from earlier long-term conventional treatment.
Even two years after his last visit, the patient notes aggravation of his acne whenever he runs out of one of these medicines.

- **Ferrum phos. D6 tab.** Weleda
  1 tablet 3 times/day before meals (potentized iron phosphate, obtained from siderite which is converted to ferrum sesquichlor, then to ferrum phos., which stimulates both weak I activity directly and the iron process in the metabolic system [see Jachens 2004, 256].

With this treatment, quite typical for acne, complete success was achieved in a few weeks. What matters is if the treatment serves the patient's individual nature and not how original the physician is in writing the prescription. Subsequently, the boy has been coming without his mother and also helps in the garden. Follow-up at 30 months showed the inflammatory acne healed, although with old scars remain. Neither the special diet nor the benzoyl peroxide is still necessary. Continued anthroposophical medication is needed, especially due to the history of inheritance. His mother's handwritten note said, "I wish to thank you most sincerely for the treatment you found to improve and, indeed, to cure the acne."

10.7.2.1 Nutrition

The significance of diet in acne has been established in epidemiological studies of populations whose diet is dairy-free and does not contain carbohydrates with high glycaemic index. Acne prevalence is related to the level of daily milk consumption (Adebamowo 2005). Milk contains growth hormone factors, especially IGF-1, which survive all processing and lead to "metabolic decompensation, with the clinical picture of acne" [Melnik 2010, 116]. The relative insulin resistance during the growth spurt at puberty favours the

Tab. 10.1 Foods effects on acne vulgaris [Melnik 2010]

Foods to be avoided	Preferred foods
Milk and dairy products, such as yoghurt, whey, soft cheeses, whey albumin concentrates	raw foods, fruit, vegetables, blue berry fruits, soya products, tomatoes
chocolate, sweets, crisps, cornflakes	wholemeal bread, muesli with soya milk, homecooking, no fast foods
white bread, white rice, wheat noodles	sea fish like salmon, walnut oil, linseed oil, olive oil
lard, liver sausage, egg yolk	linseed sauerkraut, raw, in small amounts; fermented vegetables
sugared soft drinks	Water and tea without sugar, ideally green tea
smoking	no smoking!
frequent in-between meals	complete fast for several hours
lack of exercise, excess weight	sporting activities, meaningful physical work

influence of insulinotropic growth factor signals in milk. In casein, IGF-1 is particularly able to survive digestion in the gastrointestinal canal and act as a foreign hormone in the organism. Homogenized milk passes more rapidly through the stomach than non-homogenized milk, so it is deleterious.

Poor consumption of raw foods, accompanied by overconsumption of chips, crisps, chocolate and sweets is the best recipe for more acne vulgaris. "It has been shown that by *adding 200 ml of milk to a meal* with low glycaemic index, the insulin response was 300 % greater than with a typical meal with high glycaemic index and no added milk." Milk with cocoa increase insulinaemia by a further 45 % compared to milk with strawberry flavour, (which is not meant as a recommendation!)

Concerning the glycaemic index:

- the level of processing of high carbohydrate foods directly influences blood sugar levels (crisps > mashed potato > unpeeled potatoes);
- 'al dente' raises blood sugar less than noodles cooked till soft;
- roughage slows down the release of carbohydrates – wholemeal bread raises blood sugar less than white bread;
- fats and proteins can delay the emptying of the stomach and thus reduce the influence of carbohydrates on blood sugar.[1]

Finally, the western diet leads to significant elevation of pro-inflammatory omega-6 fatty acids, seven times higher in the diet today (relative to omega-3 fatty acids) than is physiologically wholesome. This creates additional readiness to develop inflammation. If we consider that these metabolic processes have consequences not only for pimples, but also

1 The authors are indebted to Johannes von Lorentz for dietetic information.

for the health of the vascular endothelium (plaque development), it is justifiable to take acne seriously as a 'metabolic signal' and to counsel young people about optimal nutrition. The following may be helpful with treatment.

In chronic cases it is important to get a stool analysis and if necessary restore normal intestinal flora (▸Chap. 4).

10.7.2.2 Medicinal treatment

Basic treatment by mouth:

- **Choleodoron** Weleda
  10–15 drops 2 or 3 times/day
  Given after meals as a rule, e.g. for symptoms of fat intolerance. If there is a constitutional primary weakness of biliary function, as with the patient presented above, administration before meals can be even more effective. Important above all if seborhoea is severe. Alternatively,
- **Akne-Kapseln** Wala
  1 capsule in the mornings, 2 at night. More effective before meals, gentler after meals. May trigger primary aggravation if antibiotics taken earlier, in which case start at a low dose, increasing slowly. Dose adjustment may be needed, since some patients need 2 capsules twice daily. Broad-spectrum medicament and alternative to Choleodoron in cases where treatment is not constitutional. Also encourages elimination, may improve mild habitual chronic constipation.[1]
- **Hepatodoron tab.** Weleda
  in milder cases 2 or 3 tablets to be chewed at bedtime, otherwise 1 three times daily
- Milk thistle preparations **Legalon 140**, or **Carduus marianus caps.** Weleda:
  1 or 2 capsules 2 or 3 times/day. Basic medication! Especially in severe cases, previously on allopathic treatment, male patients.
- **Menodoron drops** Weleda
  15 drops 2 or 3 times/day

for young women with irregular menses and/or premenstrual aggravation of acne.

Basic external applications

Daily, morning and evening,

- **Gesichtswaschcreme** Dr Hauschka
  mix with some warm water (2 or 3 cm of the cream) and apply; rinse off with lukewarm water.

Follow with

- **Akne Gesichtswasser** Wala
  applied on cotton wool or using hands.

May be complemented with a little **Gesichtsöl** Dr Hauschka (face oil) applied in the mornings.

1 The authors are indebted to F. Roemer for practical dosage suggestions. The results achieved with Acne-capsules depend greatly on an individually tolerated and adequately intensive dosage.

Twice a week

- **Akne Gesichtsdampfbad** (Acne facial steam bath) Wala. 2 tbsp./0.5 L of hot water, apply for 10 min.

Follow with

- **Akne Gesichtsmaske** (Acne facial mask) Wala. Mix 2 tsp. to a paste with 1 tsp. water, apply for 15 min.

Rinse off and apply Akne Gesichtswasser Wala. Many patients say they find the face mask and facial steam bath to be effective external applications. Where resources are limited or compliance is low, the authors concentrate on these care products for external application. If indicated, cosmetic acne care by trained personnel.

As complementary and individualized treatment by mouth,

- **Ferrum met. praep. D6 trit.** Weleda [*Vademecum* 2010, 430]/**Ferrum phos. D6 tab.** Weleda
  A good pinch daily in the mornings of Ferrum met. praep./1 tablet Ferrum phos.
  Especially for young males who seem inhibited (see case record) but it must be given chronically, slow but deep acting.
- **Glandulae suprarenales comp.** Wala,
  7–10 pillules in the morningssupports the action of Ferrum met., esp. with lack of drive or morning grogginess, since action regulates bile and adrenals.

Halogen compounds are particularly important with acne. In full strength they provoke acne, but in potency they help to cure it (see also ▸Chap. 6.7). With iodate salts, restlessness tends to be a key symptom; with sodium chlorate (= muriaticum) there is inner tension and ambivalence.

- **Arsenum iodatum D6–12 dil.** (various manuf.)
  7 drops 2 or 3 times/day
  Best for intelligent, restless, but rapidly exhausted patients; tendency to chronic allergic rhinitis; ambitious; pressure from parental expectations is often great.
- **Iodum D12 dil.** (various manuf.)
  5–7 drops twice/day.
  Best for nervous, skinny child with large cervical lymph nodes and tonsils, unstable thyroid function. Impression may be that the patient is consuming himself (even if there is no manifest hyperthyroidism.) Often with heat-intolerance.
- **Sulphur iodatum D6–12 dil.** (various manuf.)
  7 drops 3 or 3 times/day
  Best for restless, nervous young people, poor appetite, changing stools, poor posture, susceptibility to infection.
- **Natrium chloratum (= muriaticum) LM6 dil.** Arcana
  5 drops once/day, mornings
  Acne in the region of the forehead, hairline; patients have notably prominent foreheads; great predilection for chocolate, preserved meats, salt; do not tolerate sun well (headaches); very fond of music; not infrequently inhibited, emotionally ambivalent in puberty (▸Chap. 6.4.3.6.3)

Other recommended single homoeopathic medicines:

- **Sepia D12–30, LM6–12** (various manuf.)
  dosage individual

Premenstrual acne, baby acne, and acne during pregnancy; hyperandrogenous acne of women; periods usually late and scanty; tendency to develop herpes; better after intense physical effort such as jogging, dancing; generally dark-haired (▸Chap. 6.4.3.6.3)

- **Graphit D12–30 trit.** Weleda: a good pinch once or twice/day

Phlegmatic patients; soft, impure skin; like "dry Calcium carbonicum" (▸Chap. 6.4.3.6.2)

- **Hepar sulfuris D6–12 trit.** Weleda
  a good pinch 2 or 3 times/day

tendency to develop furuncles, angular cheilitis; indicated mainly for toxic factors (e.g. amalgam); mentally vehement and dissatisfied, susceptible to colds, recurrent sore throats; indicated when acne develops and gets worse in combination with sinusitis.

- **Bovista C12–30 glob.** (single doses) Gudjons
  acne after and due to cosmetics.

Using the kind of treatment demonstrated here, it is possible in the vast majority of cases to avoid the standard treatment for acne vulgaris which is a stress for the organism, and simultaneously support maturation in the 3rd seven-year period. It is important to balance stress with appropriate physical and social activities.

10.8 Skin, hair and nails – further disorders and clinical pictures

10.8.1 Warts, verrucae, molluscum contagiosum

Susceptibility to warts is typical for children because they are open to the world, who live in imitation, and are not yet able to develop boundaries through their I, as is typical of adults. Animals have specialized epidermal structures such as fur, feathers or scales that largely define their warmth organization. Children with atopy are particularly susceptible, their epidermis lacking adequate skin barrier protection (▸Chap. 6.4.1) These children may be more difficult to treat and need highly individual medication based on their constitution.

Below are typical medicines that prove effective in most cases:

10.8.1.1 Verrucae

The following has frequencly proved effective in treating plantar warts.

- **Antimonit D6 trit.** Weleda
  a good pinch 3 times/day

In conjunction with

- **Ferrum picrinicum D6 dil.** DHU
  5 drops 3 times orally.

Externally – apart from creating dry conditions permitting the skin to "breathe" with suitable shoes and change of socks –

- **Bismutum-Stibium ointment** Weleda
  massage in twice/day.

It is always important to keep the feet warm. This is accomplished by wearing suitable indoor shoes, meals and drinks providing adequate warmth (also meat for children who are cool or anaemic), and by rosemary footbaths or massage.

The creation of warmth can be supported, if necessary, by treatment with

- **Melissa Cupro culta Rh D3 dil.** Weleda
  10–15 drops 2 or 3 times/day, and
- **Cuprum met. 0.4% ointment** Weleda
  massage into lower legs and feet at night.

Amazingly effective in support of warmth is to place an ivy leaf (Hedera helix) in the sock, *covering the affected part of the sole.* The authors hypothesize that the appreciable iodine content of the plant plays a role in its efficacy.

10.8.1.2 Verrucae vulgaris (common warts)

An indication shared by the most important medicines is weakness of defense from environmental influences, causing warts to proliferate.

- **Thuja e summit. D6–12 pillules** Wala
  5 pillules twice/day

The indication for should be established individually. The children are generally susceptible to infection, tend to have eczema and asthma, and are insecure and restless. Digestion and creation of inner warmth are inadequate (see Chap. 6.4.3.6.5). Thuja is also the single most important medicine for molluscum contagiosum (▸Chap. 10.8.1.3). The child with a dry, weakened skin barrier is susceptible to molluscum when exposed to damp environments, such as bathing together with an affected sib, or by auto-innoculation due to scratching. Another characteristic of Thuja is that the individual tolerates the warts, spreading foreign life in his own sphere. However, Thuja should not be considered to be the sole treatment for warts. It is most effective if there is a profound constitutional weakness in setting the boundary between self and the outside. Consider how people seek to define their personal space with a Thuja hedge. The warts grow rampantly and large, and may be soft and fleshy, thriving on atopic, weakened, cool skin areas in children who are constitutionally low in iron.

- **Causticum D12 dil./pillules** DHU, **C12 pillules** Gudjons
  5 drops or pillules twice/day in each case.

The typical indication for Causticum is the *inhibition of aggression, the introvert nature combined with powerful empathy and a sense of fairness.* With Thuja, the creation of warmth by the I in metabolism is inhibited, allowing the ether body to become dominant and leads to a hysterical constitution. With Causticum, the constitution is markedly neurasthenic, but lively mentally and emotionally, but exhausts itself intellectually and does not live enough in the limbs. Children with this constitution are prone to infections and to *warts in the peripheral region of their hands and feet.* Warts close to the fingernails are a well-known indication for Causticum. Gait tends to be slightly clumsy and inhibited (opposite of Thuja), all showing the dominance of the head pole with reserve, inwardness, and profound sensitivity. The warts may accordingly be harder and more cornified, though the wart's appearance alone does not permit reliable prescribing.

- **Dulcamara D12 dil./pillules** DHU
  5–7 drops/pillules twice/day

The characteristic sign is lack of adjustment to rapid temperature changes from warm to cold and to damp cold; a tendency to develop atopic, itching eczemas and asthma as well as cystitis if chilled rapidly or in damp cold. For instance, aggravation after a bicycle excursion along a river bank on a September evening is typical. In contrast to the closely related picture of Thuja, the plant itself scrambles on the ground, with its leaves often partly eaten. The psyche lacks support from the I, from inner warmth and stable uprightness, but also shows definite sensitivity. The warts are located more often on the fingers and areas close to the nails, as with Causticum, but have a smoother surface and are less healthy appearing than is typical of Thuja. Dulcamara thus holds a middle position between Thuja and Causticum and does not enter as deeply into the constitution.

- **Antimonit D6 trit.** Weleda
  a good pinch 3 times.

This agent is above all suitable for warts with distinctly cornified, hard surfaces. As with flat warts, prior treatment may be applied with salicylic acid plasters (Guttaplast, always for 48 h) and using a pumice stone after every treatment to abrade the cornified layer.

Application of
- **Polygonatum 5 % ointment** Weleda (▸ Chap. 10.6)

for several days will soften and smooth the wart surface, making it accessible to treatment with
- **Bismutum-Stibium ointment** Weleda
  massage in twice/day

Is also suitable as basic treatment with common warts and molluscum contagiosum.

10.8.1.3 Molluscum contagiosum
Reference has been made in the preceding section to the risk of infection when sharing a bath and in swimming pools, and to the marked prevalence of children with atopic skin. Massive disseminated lesions may develop in early childhood. The authors do not advise conventional dermatological treatment since thorough search will, in every case reveal among potentized medicines, the key that will stimulate the child's organism to rid itself of the molluscum. This is a brief summaryof the most frequently indicated medications.

- Potentized autologous blood according to Imhaeuser (▸ Chap. 6.3.3.4)
  starting with the C5, daily or alternate days 3–5 drops for 3 weeks, followed by C7 (3 times/wk) for 4 weeks, C9 (twice/wk) for 6 weeks and C12 (once or twice/wk) for 6 weeks, preferably in the mornings.

If carefully prepared, glycerol may be used instead of alcohol for preservation, and the preparation will in many cases prove highly effective. Also the remedy has a positive effect on the atopic child's weak resistance and tendency to allergies. This is generally recommended as first treatment.

Multiple molluscum contagiosum with dry, atopic skin or atopic dermatitis will as a rule respond well to treatment with:

- **Fluorit D12 trit.** Weleda/**Calcium fluoratum C12 pillules.** Gudjons 1.5 g
  a good pinch twice/day/5 pillules once/day.

This has now become the standard treatment for this dermatologically frustrating problem. Clear regression of the molluscum usually occurs within 4 to 6 weeks. The treatment may be given as first treatment on this indication, with no other measures required.

- **Thuja e summit. D12 pillules** Wala, Thuja Argento culta Rh D3 dil. Weleda:
  5 pillules/day and 5–10 drops 2 or 3 times/day respectively

is the most important single medicament for molluscum contagiosum (▸Chap. 10.8.1.2). It is also suitable as an external application in form of

- **Thuja Essenz** Wala/Weleda:
  dab on molluscum once/day.

Otherwise, if these treatments do not give results, a careful search is indicated for the constitutional medicine.

10.8.2 Onychia (nail bed inflammation, panaritium)

Infection of periungual tissues of the big toes is seen especially in boys during puberty. They still lack some of the quality of iron to hold their own in the world of action. In this phase of active growth, the organism's boundaries in the nail region do not yet have adequate powers of resistance. In addition, there is the down-to-earth fact that young people often cut their own toenails, usually incorrectly rounding edges rather than straight across. Specific advice is essential.

The basic constitutional treatment to prevent recurrence is potentized iron.

- **Ferrum met. praep. D6 trit.** Weleda
  1/4 level tsp/day, mornings, for a sufficiently long period [see *Vademecum* 2010, 430].

Adequate immobilization is an important aspect of treating infections of periungual tissue and paronychia. Many failures are due to ignoring the need for rest, especially with today's relentless pressure never to miss school or any activity. It is far better to have the child rest a few days than to risk onychoplasty, which offers no protection against recurrence anyway. If the toes are involved, tight and athletic shoes must not be worn. Sugar should be avoided, as with any acute inflammation.

Effective external applications are

- Cool compresses with **Retterspitz äußerlich** (undiluted)[1] while elevating and resting the limb and/or

bathing in **hard soap** solution, followed by dressing with

- **Ilon Abszess ointment** (Paronychium) or
- **Mercurialis 10 % ointment** Weleda if inflammation is limited to periungual tissues.

Suitable for internal treatment are

- **Pyrogenium C30 pillules**
  to initiate treatment for paronychium 5 pillules once.
- **Belladonna D6 dil.** Weleda/**Rh D6 dil.** Weleda
  for throbbing pain 50 drops/½ glass of water in sips over 12–24 h

or, more generally applicable,

- **Apis Belladonna cum Mercurio pillules** Wala or **Erysidoron 1** Weleda
  5 pillules/5–10 drops at first stage of inflammation (redness, no pus)
- **Hepar sulfuris D12 trit.** Weleda/**pillules** DHU
  if purulent, a good pinch/5 pillules 3–5 times/day complemented with
- **Calendula D3 amp.** Wala
  ½ ampoule orally 2 or 3 times/day.

For children with relevant disposition (susceptible to infection-triggered asthma, weak bile production, irritability)

- **Natrium sulfuricum D12 pillules** DHU (various manuf.)
  7 pillules twice/day may support this.

10.8.3 Head lice

Infestation of children with head lice has increased in paediatric practice. In a fundamental review, M. Sommer [1994] pointed out that the usual treatment with pyrethrins has potential neurotoxic side effects. Infectious Diseases Prof. Haustein, Leipzig, has stated, with regard to InfectoPedicul® that "permethrin is the most toxic agent for insects (lice and nits) and the least toxic for humans", but we must examine this viewpoint. Prof. Mueller-Mohnsen [1994] has gathered extensive material on the toxicity of pyrethrum and pyrethroids.

In contrast to the medicinal agents generally used for head lice, there have been methods and non-toxic medicines of proven value for centuries that provide safe treatment of this annoying parasitic infestation (see Sommer 1994, 2002].

Once the infestation has been diagnosed (usually in the occipital region), careful daily removal of nits using a nit comb and thorough laundering of hats, soft toys, hairbands, combs is a necessity; cutting the hair is sometimes necessary.

Effective and safe is

- **Neem-Shampoo Trifolio M**, applied on the 1st, 3rd and 8th day (⅓ of pack at a time).

Neem extracts have been used for centuries in India against parasites; various constituents of the plant inhibit chitin synthesis. It is "an insect-specific biocide – i.e. an insecticide

1 English website: www.retterspitz.de/en

that merits the name" [Mueller-Mohnsen 1994]. Although Neem is non-toxic for humans, the lice do not die immediately but are unable to reproduce. Extra effort in haircare for about 8–10 days is required. The authors continue to prefer Neem to Nyda L, dimeticone. The advantage of Nyda L, now widely used and far more acceptable than pyrethrum products, is its rapid availability. However, Neem is more effective.

Unfortunately some children are highly susceptible and will have a recurrence as soon as another affected child is near them. Here it is advisable to massage a few drops of essential oils[1] into the hair, especially before going to school, so that a faint and unpleasant smell is evident.

10.8.4 Disorders of nail and hair growth disorders

The configuration of the organism is defined from the outside in nails and hair [Steiner and Wegman 1991, ▸Chap. XIV, 76]. Synthesis of these boundaries requires nourishment for the skin from the digestive tract via metabolism and circulation, a process in which hair and nails are developed. The essential substance for developing hair and nails, "where vital tissue is devitalized" [l. c.] is silica. Hypersensitivity, brittleness, dysplasia all indicate a local deficiency or abnormal processing of silica. Distribution or secondary silica deficiency can also be present. "Distribution of localized silica activity over the whole organism can be achieved with a course of sulphur treatment, for example" [Steiner/Wegman Chap. 1, 70 in English edition]. The nourishment of the skin is dependent on healthy digestion and on processes that may be stimulated by sulphur in subtle doses. Hair demonstrates, as is immediately evident when hair is burning, the importance of sulphur-mediated protein synthesis extending to the periphery. Hair that is thin or falls out easily, will often indicate disorders of intestinal function and metabolism. While digestion and metabolism are guided by the I and astral body, disorders of thyroid function demonstrate the consequences which abnormal intervention of the astral body can have in guiding metabolism both in the digestion (diarrhoea, chronic constipation) and in the hair (hair loss). Intervention of I and astral body in the digestive process is mainly strengthened with iron. Stinging nettle acts in a similarly, stimulating the I's intervention in metabolism. Interestingly, nettles have high sulphur levels and show vigorous growth while also developing a perfect silica organism in the leaf's peripheral stinging hairs, which are like finely ground injection needles.

- **Ferrum ustum comp. trit.** Weleda
  A generous pinch 3 times/day.
- **Ferrum silicicum comp. pillules** Wala
  5–7 pillules 3 times/day

These anthroposophic compound medicines contain nontronite iron silicate, aniseed and hammer scale (also called, anvil dross, this synthetic magnetite contains both Fe^{2+} and Fe^{3+} ions and is sometimes formulated as $FeO \cdot Fe_2O$) as well as stinging nettle extracts in low potencies. These medicaments prove effective in children who show weaknesses in silica absorption and distribution. Their appetite is poor, they tend to be easily exhausted, and their nails are weak and fragile. Ferritin levels tend to be low or reduced. One should also think of this medicament if the scalp is pruritic.

1 Oil of cloves, rosemary, eucalyptus and lavender are among those suitable.

- **Solutio Siliceae comp. D6 dil.** Weleda
  5–10 drops 3 times/day
  is a basic form of medication for disorders of the silica organism.

The guiding principle in composing this mineral complex and its complicated synthesis, is to deepen the action of silica and sulphur-rich *Equisetum arvense* (▸Chap. 6.3.3.3), Silica and sulphur are processed with calcium, sedum, and potassium carbonate in a soluble complex for Solutio Siliceae.

The product is indicated especially for dysplastic nails which develop in an irregular or incomplete way; whereas, Ferrum silicicum comp. or Ferrum ustum comp. are indicated for constitutional or short-term weakness of nails.

10.9 Rheumatoid arthritis during childhood and rheumatic spectrum disorders

10.9.1 Individualized paediatrics and rheumatic spectrum disorders

The way in which rheumatoid arthritis is discussed in textbooks on paediatrics notably says that

- the origin of the disease is not known [Wagner, Dannecker 2007, 67],
- treatment is symptomatic, and that
- immediate treatment to rapidly eliminate the inflammation in the joints [Joseph 2010].

In view of this, the term "juvenile idiopathic arthritis" or "juvenile arthritis" is now used. Out of this background, the question of personal history, aetiology, and pathogenesis is often only investigated superficially. Reviewing our twenty-five years of experience with 45 children, the emotional and biographical aspect and its role in pathogenesis has not been elucidated. The following findings demonstrate the importance of comprehensive diagnosis and treatment. In this patient-centered approach, the term "idiopathic arthritis" becomes inappropriate and may deaden the physician's acumen and attitude. A wide field for research is now opened offering better understanding of these children and their parents, as well as treatments that both stabilize the disease and restore health. Our experience is as follows:

- Children with rheumatic diseases often have a *highly individual, characteristic history*. Reviewing 35 case records we find common characteristics, *which have* now been prospectively confirmed in new patients. Awareness of this knowledge during the initial interview increases rapport and may initiate a therapeutic response.
- Using the biographical history as the basis for treatment with anthroposophical and homoeopathic medicines, about one third of all children with rheumatic diseases had longterm remission, and often, cure.
- *The percentage is more than twice as high for the ANA-positive oligo arthritis, usually of little* girls in the first nine years of life. A comparatively simple method of treatment can be taught which allows for a high level of certainty. In the authors' opinion this may compete and surpass immunosuppressives, like Methotrexate, without their side effect profile. If patients respond to the treatment, which can be assessed after 3 or 4 months,

a good long-term outcome can be expected. Even the uveitis, which is common, has had thoroughly positive results in individuals cases.

- In a subset of the cases, the characteristic symptoms allow us to find the indicated medicines. However, homoeopathic and anthroposophic treatment is not very promising unless such a history is also considered.
- To be honest, it has to be said that in about half of our patients with JRA (excluding ANA-positive oligoarthritis) only a conventional approach including *immunosuppressive, such as MTX and, etanercept,* proved effective. However, adjuvant medicines for these children can be supportive and reduce side effects.
- The potential for treatment with anthroposophic and homoeopathic medicines is much greater before the 9th year. The author is emphatic in treating these older children immediately and thoroughly with conventional drugs, to reduce rapid joint destruction. But there can also be milder flares in this age-group that will respond to the proposed treatments.

In those children for whom anthroposophic or homoeopathic medicine contributed to a clear improvement or remission, a specific potentized remedy usually was more effective than a composite preparation. Among the effective anthroposophic and homoeopathic preparations, there are clear groupings according to the *age of the children.*

- *Potentized organ preparations* used in anthroposophic medicine *are crucial treatment in the first seven to nine years of life.* The efficacy of these organ preparations is often greater than that of classic homoeopathic medicines for these youngsters. *In our practice, the treatment has brought a "therapeutic revolution" in the treatment of ANA-positive pauciarticular (oligo) arthritis.* Being animal-based, potentized organ preparations have a direct effect on the ether body, the child's vital organization, which forms in the first seven to nine years of life. Their prescription for rheumatoid arthritis in young children is based on the simple principle of homology and, in our experience, it is important to prescribe homologous organ preparations in the D30, typically they are effective orally at 0.5–1.0 mL/dose. Following a careful examination and considering the child's age, it will be easy to prescribe appropriately. The case studies given below illustrate this approach. ◘ Tab. 10.2 lists these useful preparations.
- Use ampoules in the D30 by Wala to treat *ANA-positive oligoarthritis,* and any more difficult, extended oligoarthritis. Administer per os in the first 9 years of life, usually 0.5–1.0 mL on an empty stomach after waking up in the morning daily, at the acute stage maximally; for maintenance twice weekly. It is advisable to continue at that potency level for years.
- Classic homoeopathic animal-based medicines: Lac caninum, Lachesis, Apis mellifica, etc. are also very effective in first 7-year period.
- Classic constitutional homoeopathic medicines are important for lasting success in the second half of childhood; those based on plants or minerals are most useful between 7 and 14 years of age. The child's soul aspect must be included for correct prescription and for true healing. This is not easy to "see", and prescribing these medicines calls for careful listening and synthesis on the part of the physician. Insight based on history, examination, careful comparison of different medicines, and inwardly "hearing" which animal, plant, or mineral substance is indicated will inspire a successful prescription.

Tab. 10.2 Potentized organ preparations in the treatment of rheumatoid arthritis

Articulatio radiocarpea	wrist
Articulatio genus	knee joint
Articulatio talocruralis	talocrural joint
Articulatio subtalaris	subtalar joint
Articulatio coxae	hip joint
Articulatio temporomandibularis	temporomandibular joint
Articulatio sacroiliaca	sacroiliac joint
Articulatio humeri	shoulder joint
Articulatio cubiti	elbow joint
Articulationes intervertebrales cervicales	upper cervical spine
unfortunately no preparation is available for the interphalangeal joints	
Cutis feti	skin, effective with circumscribed scleroderma

Diet with rheumatoid arthritis

- Thanks to the paediatric rheumatologist J. v. Lorentz and our own experience (see. ▸Chap. 4.7.1, Coeliac disease), we understand additional important therapeutic aspects of diet for children with juvenile rheumatoid arthritis. Asymptomatic and unrecognized gluten intolerance has repeatedly proved to be present in synovitis and uveitis (Case study ▸Chap. 4.7.1). In these cases, and with some other conditions such as multifocal aseptic osteomyelitis, compliance with the coeliac diet largely cured the arthritis. Children and young people benefit from having a diet that is as minimally pro-inflammatory as possible, as outlined in ▸Chap. 10.7. The "Western lifestyle" has caused increases in Th1-mediated, autoimmune chronic inflammatory conditions, especially diabetes, coeliac disease, Crohn's disease and juvenile arthritis (▸Chap. 4.1). In juvenile arthritis, even if celiac disease is not documented, a limited gluten-free diet trial may improve symptoms. Otherwise it is advisable to eat a diet low in gluten, using older grains that have not been bred for higher gluten levels as have all modern wheat varieties used in the conventional food industry. For example consuming more spelt, rye, oats, millet (gluten-free and rich in iron and minerals) amaranth, and buckwheat can be efficacious. We also encourage wild and line-caught sea fish, such as pollack. Let us refer again, as discussed in the chapter on atopic dermatitis (▸Chap. 6.4) to the value of vegetable oils obtained from plants grown in cool regions. Cold-pressed linseed, sunflower, and hemp oils all have an ideal ratio of omega-6 to omega-3 fatty acids. Quality nuts, linseed, and sunflower seeds also help children to create adequate internal warmth, which is vital for transforming chronic, cool and autoimmune inflammation. Tab. 10.2 in ▸Chap. 10.7 shows the foods to be avoided.

10

10.9.2 Anthroposophical perspective on juvenile rheumatoid arthritis

Children with rheumatic complaints often make a deep impression in the physician's memory. When well they may seem radiant, "like light", but they also show a unilateral tendency in the psyche. The soul principle, *the astral body, often seems exaggerated* and their extreme sensitivity [Simon 2005a, 3–1] warns the physician to be patient in establishing trust and rapport. The doctor's relationship to these children is unique and intense, with a bilateral potential for hurt. *Emotions are strong*, even if this is not always articulated. These children, most of whom are girls, may feel marked jealousy. Tact and empathy are required to explore the background of the psyche of the child, the parents and the siblings.

Remarkably, we are in most cases dealing with an *afebrile minimally febrile intermittent inflammation*, predominantly affecting girls. These disease phenomena suggest the predominance of the child's astral body: the male-female polarity, the afebrile progression in bouts, but then also the main symptoms of the *pain and limitation of movement*, the *dreaded breaking down of hyaline joint cartilage*, the destructive chronic inflammation, and the *loss of form*. One-sidedly progressive destructive processes point to one-sided destructive activity of the astral body, i. e. of the soul entity at work in the body. The astral body's lack of regulation by the I results inTh1dominationand dysfunction of T-regulatory lymphocytes, which cascades into further disintegration of the immune system (▸Chap. 6.1).

These phenomena reflect the importance of soul qualities in juvenile arthritis and classification according to age shows us a further relationship to the child's soul and spirit. The most important threshold is once again the *9th year* (see Horneff und Wahn 2005, 64.5)

- Oligoarthritis in the first 7 years, *affecting mainly girls* (50 % of all cases)
- late, enthesitis-associated arthritis after the 9th year, predominantly *affecting boys* (15–20 %);
- polyarthritis in childhood, rheumatoid factor-negative, evoking severe arthritis in only 10 % of cases,
- Rheumatoid factor-positive polyarthritis, – polyarthritis after the 9th year, 10 % of all cases; serious in half of the patients [see Horneff and Wahn 2005, 64.5].

In the 9th year, children go through a critical developmental process of individualization (▸Chap. 7.2, they "cross the Rubicon River") as they grow aware of the mortality of their parents and of themselves, the development of their own inner independence, their dawning awareness of their own unique soul and knowing new moments of lonely isolation. Their strong bond to their parents changes, and relationships with peers assume more importance. At the same time, pubertal sexual maturation begins, dividing the genders and triggering thelarche for some girls. A new human form is created as the configuration of growth radically shifts, leading to gawky limbs, lower trunk, and lower face while the upper human being, dominant in the first seven years, grows more slowly [Verhulst 1999, 82–93]. It is evident that the soul and I organization connect more strongly with the metabolism and limbs than previously. The presentation of rheumatic diseases also changes at this age. The classification of juvenile arthritis shows the importance of biography.

Here the question arises as to what goes on in the inner life of a child who develops a rheumatic condition in childhood. Rudolf Steiner's anthroposophic research and the resulting view of human nature offer insight into the disease. The authors are indebted to Armin Husemann for valuable impulses to expand our understanding.

- In the first years of life and up to the 9th year, the most essential inner activity of children is to imitate the world around them. "Imitation" does not mean the conscious imitation practised by adults, but an unconscious and immediate resonance involving the whole living body. Because of the strong bond with the parents, their every action, inner mood and care for the child is reflected in the child's gestures, speech and attitude. Their actions are normally imitated most intensely and become physical through the child's own inner activity. The sense of sight is of crucial significance in the process of imitation – "children turn into what they see." [A. Husemann.]
- In infancy and the early years, the body is still very pliable. Imitation actually develops the body and impresses its mark on it, not only in developing the brain, but in the whole living body. This connection is increasingly studied in epigenetics (▸Chap. 1.1, ▸Chap. 6.1). The young child's body resonates in its development with the mental and moral sentience and actions of the parents. The children reflect in their vital processes, all that happens and can be felt around them. This means that the higher level of existence, the souls of adult caregivers, influences the next lower level of existence, the child's vital organization, [1] to create both illness and health.
- Normally the child's own initiative in soul and spirit, his will, present in his metabolic and limb organs, matures around the ninth year of life allowing the child to break through mere imitation to develop conscious insight into their own experience. This means that child awakens to their own perception. Parallel to this new "resistance" to imitation, the child produces the second dentition, casting off the merely inherited milk teeth and replacing them with their own teeth. The configuration of the permanent teeth, developed entirely after birth, reflects the child's individual nature and biography [see Husemann 1996, 49].
- At the same time, the direct influence of sensory perceptions on the child's bodily nature distinctly wanes. However, many phenomena experienced between the 9th and 12th years, are experienced much more consciously, often painfully. For instance, a loss of love between parents, which would have gone unnoticed when younger, now causes pangs; a distant look in mother's eye now hurts deeply. A number of our patients presented with severe crises in their illness around the 9th year of life.

Analysis of cases where arthritis onset was before the 12th year shows that family relationships and needs must be understood and are key to individual diagnosis and treatment. Mother, father, siblings, and grandparents all affect the child's soul. The primary question is what the children had seen in their mother and father during the pregnancy and after birth. Both the case studies below, as well as all other cases analyzed, demonstrate that during this crucial age before the fifth birthday at the latest, the circumstances of the child's conception and birth involved a shock for the parents. These difficult parental experiences of seemingly insurmountable obstacles, impossible demands,

1 "Here we come upon a law of education ... It is that in the world any level of existence in human nature, whatever its origin, is influenced by the one immediately above it, which can only take effect in this way. ... What does this mean? When you realize that a child's ether body is stunted in some way, you have to configure your own astral body so that it can influence the child's ether body and correct this." [Steiner 1995, 33]

unbearable pain, or shame, froze their sense of equilibrium and made it impossible to fully welcome the child. The specific aspect for rheumatic diseases is the mother's experience of self, the pain she experienced due to the the child's arrival. This creates paralysing ambivalence in her relationship to the child, though this secret cannot be uttered or recognized, which makes it all the more powerful. The child "sees" the inner experiences of the parents with his whole body. This perception and its bodily imitation by the child create the seed for the painful, paralysing disease to come. In the cases we have observed these experiences were still present in their full intensity, still active in the souls of the parents – and also in the child's bodily imitation.

The history-taking must be completely free of accusation or guilt. The parents, especially the mother, need to be given the opportunity to become aware of their own experiences in a loving and respectful way that enables them to recall these painful experiences, work through them, accept, and then, let go. It may be helpful to involve a skilled therapist, but often simply taking the history with empathy and adequate time is therapeutic and can have far-reaching benefits.

In a second meditative step, the physician must recognize, weigh, and judge which events in the history are more closely connected with the child's illness, thus broadening the paediatric rheumatologic diagnosis. Struggling to grasp the interplay of the child's constitution and current symptoms, may open the way to deeper treatment that harmonizes the child's own forces.

Rheumatoid arthritis typically attacks joints, tendons, and related connective tissue structures robbing the child of his unbridled power to express inner experience outwardly in active movement. Joints reveal the soul's activity in building the living body and in the capacity for movement, which human beings share with animals. Plants are only touched by movement from outside, in their form, colour and the stirrings of their flowers. The inner principle of the soul is movement and polarization, developing and releasing intention in movement. If guidance from the I is not sufficiently developed, the soul organization threatens to separate and self destruct. Understanding polarity as the inner nature of the soul sphere permits deeper insight into how the look in the child's eye and joint mobility relate and reflect one another.

Comparing joint and eye (◘ Tab. 10.3) we find a comparison which generally characterizes the relationship between the head and limbs. The eyes correspond to a ball-and-socket joint in their degree of mobility, permitting precise and essentially weightless rotating movements in the sphere of the head while the joints enable rotating movements, both one dimensional and multidensional, in the limbs.

Eye and joint are polar opposites in the upper and lower human being. They are the places of greatest mobility in their particular location, but are organized in a divergent way for different purposes. With our joints, we are mobile within gravity and able to overcome it as the forces of gravity are linear and directed towards the centre of the earth. With our eyes, human beings see the light of the sun, which is linear from cosmos to earth.

A remarkable phenonemon in paediatric rheumatology is that the most important, most common and most feared complication of idiopathic juvenile rheumatoid arthritis during the 'imitation age' specifically affects the eye. Rheumatic uveitis or iridocyclitis, threatens active mobility in the 'heart' of the eye where it regulates the relationship to light, just as arthritis threatens the child's joints and ability to overcome earth's gravity in

Tab. 10.3 Eyes and joints as polar opposites in the upper and lower human being

Eye	Joint
Eye socket immovable part of the external skeleton in the bony skull	Joint partly (hip, jaw, atlanto-occipital joints) or wholly mobile part of the inner skeleton
Aqueous humour inside	Synovial fluid between and around the articulating bones (outside)
Musculature inside the bony socket	Musculature outside the articulating bone surfaces
Instrument of conscious visual perception and (re)cognition (opening our eyes is the moment of awakening)	Instrument of will in movement ('sleeps' when healthy)

movement. The anthroposophic view understands that rheumatic diseases in childhood are connected with early loss of resonance between parents and child, of the 'development of joints' between mother and child, mother and father. The physician's first task is to coach the parents to open their eyes and help them to release their traumatic experiences. At the same time, it is important to avoid further trauma due to memories which cannot yet be healed. The second task will be to free the child from the consequences of this imitation, to achieve inner balance mentally and immunologically, and to see the world "in a new light." Unconsciously, the child with arthritis gets frozen like Lot's wife, stuck on unwanted impressions inescapably transmitted by family. Child and mother, child and parents created this situation together, caught in a web of destiny, unable to break free. The organs which are physiologically able to bring about release are the tear glands in the eye; oddly enough people would go blind if tears were not produced all the time and would become frozen in their souls, if unable to weep. Put in poetic terms, we may pick up on the analysis of asthma made by the great psychosomatic specialist Viktor von Weizsaecker (▸Chap. 6.5), and say that in rheumatic inflammation we have a "dissolving in tears" scene in the joint, with the synovia taking on the function of the tear glands and with a joint effusion collecting tears that are shed in the wrong time and place [Simon 2005a].

Rheumatic inflammation in children leads to a painful bodily awakening, in locations and organs that should really serve movement while being in a "state of sleep." Rheumatic children live with "having to do without and having to regain" their own movement. Competent physical therapy is essential to successful rehabilitation. Accepting and overcoming the rheumatic disease can strengthen the child's individual nature in the long term, something we see in many of these patients. This is a profound and meaningful dimension to these destiny-shaping conditions for both the child and the parents.

10.9.3 Disease type as mirrored by the case history – case reports

10.9.3.1 Systemic course of illness, Still's syndrome

Just under a seventh of all cases of juvenile idiopathic arthritis take the form of *Still's disease*, a systemic form *manifesting before the fifth year of life. It is febrile, with exanthema, and affects both genders with equal frequency*. The condition triggers hepatosplenomegaly, lymphadenopathy, and frequently, a massive and destructive arthritis. Amyloidosis may lead to kidney failure. Fevers and the equal prevalence of girls and boys being are signs of the pathological involvement of the I organization. The child has difficulties receiving the parental substance, which leaves something indigestible and foreign, and sculping his or her individuality. This alienation from the inherited body is not genetic, but at a soul level of experience.

With Still's disease, we see primarily the working of the I organization. In fever the I organization attempts to destroy anything perceived to be foreign within the child's body. Childhood infectious illness balances this process and typically follows a sequence, ending in restoration of health. Infections, provoked by outside pathogens, and vaccinations may also provoke Systemic JA or Still's disease, but the crucial aspect is that the child's own body is perceived to be foreign, attacked, and triggers inflammation. The fire of the pyrexia leaves behind a residue of progressive, often severe, joint deformation. *The human I organization's activity, vital for healthy immune regulation, is powerless in the face of dominant one-sided destructive astral body activity* – a basic aspect of rheumatic inflammation.

The first case (▸Chap. 10.9.3.1.1) shows how increased I and astral body activity after the 9th year can aggravate the signs and symptoms of the disease if suppression rather than regulation occurs.

The second case (▸Chap. 10.9.3.1.2) illustrates the problems that may arise with puberty, when the astral body becomes fully present physiologically, and the guiding powers of the individual are limited by awakening needs, and hurts, and consciousness.

10.9.3.1.1 11-year-old boy with Still's disease (Systemic Juvenile Arthritis)

When first seen this 11-year-old boy had been suffering from treatment-resistant Still's disease for nine years. Both parents are dedicated secondary school teachers. The boy's sister is four years older and was born by Caesarian section. The boy's birth, by repeat Caesarian, was a "terrible" experience for the mother, who still recalled her "terrible pain." These exact words will typically be used by nearly all the mothers, which is striking when many histories are reviewed.

When at age 21 months the boy first fell ill, the parents were preoccupied with building a house, especially since their current apartment was damp and there were so-called underground water veins. Their son's illness meant that the building project had to stop, and the family had to continue to live in the unsuitable apartment.

Initially he had fever and polyarticular onset, most severely in the cervical spine. Homoeopathic treatment by several therapists was ineffective, so he was hospitalized at the German Paediatric Rheumatism Centre in Garmisch-Partenkirchen. The most effective treatment was corticosteroids, as usual with Still's disease, but interferon, MTX and cystostatics were ineffective, and cyclosporine only slightly beneficial. Several years later, the experienced hospital medical director regretted that the treatment had failed almost completely. For several months from age 9 to 10, he had a severe episode, with daily fever, exanthematous rash, splenomegaly, and massive polyarticular inflammatory changes. The boy was then no longer able to walk, and needed either to use a wheelchair or to be carried. On that first visit at 11 years of age, knees were in an almost 90°flexion contraction, wrist joints largely destroyed and stiff, and elbows also in severe flexion contraction. He had secondary growth retardation, weighing only 22 kg with a height of 116 cm. Mentally, he had a positive attitude. His face had a very delicate lower jaw and prominent forehead, indicating a shift in balance between head and limbs. Over time the boy impressed us with his balance, remarkably positive optimism, and resilience.

His mother, working as a teacher, was cooperative where treatment was concerned, but inwardly preoccupied by her profession. This inner distraction of a mother or both parents may present in different ways to the physician: intense commitment, especially in caring professions, severe conflict with in-laws or a partner, ambivalence due to personal job compromises, and above all to lingering hurts that arose in connection with the child's arrival. This distraction may lead to the child's sense of inadequate care and attention – a basic theme with rheumatic children and perhaps also a key to the intense jealousy of siblings that is often observed.

The boy was on chronic cortisone treatment and had a positive RF and moderately elevated CRP. He was first treated with

Magnesium carbonicum LM6–8 to stabilize the situation for an extended period. The prescription was based on the following:

- onset in the first seven years of life
- poor growth in conjunction with regulatory failure of the immune system, which Magnesium carbonicum stabilizes [see Soldner, Wilkens und Sommer 2006],
- prior damage to the organism due to numerous toxic drugs – Magnesium carbonicum strengthens coherence in the child's life organization especially if damage was sustained in the first seven-year period,
- refusal to eat green vegetables and appropriate foods; probable hyperacidity.

His refusal to eat greens was a cardinal symptom although green was his favourite colour. The activity of the life organization culminates in the green leaf, where magnesium is the crucial element, making it possible for the leaf to absorb sun forces. The medicament was given alone, also at the mother's request, and resulted in a satisfactory stabilization, allowing discontinuation of the steroids.

After a year and a half, when the patient, living 110 km away, was seen only every three months, there was a dramatic flare in early spring. CRP elevated to 15 times normal, ferritin 10, 800 ng/mL, RF IgG elevated to three times the upper normal, and IgM to five times normal. Fever daily from 4 p. m., with classic Still's rash on the trunk, and severe joint pain. Based on the previous flares, mother predicted a three month episode. Inspite of the distance, the family came on the third day of the episode. Examination showed macular exanthema and definite splenomegaly.

Guiding symptoms for the prescription were

- recurrent, long-term destructive daily fever,
- marked splenomegaly,
- strong and optimistic personality, marked destruction, as if destiny was strking a mighty blow, leaving the I powerless in the body.

Prescription was

- **Chininum sulfuricum D30**, later **C30**, 3 pillules 3 times/day.

This is a medicament used to treat malaria, allopathically as quinine sulfate and homoeopathically as Chininum sulfuricum. Malaria leads to the I's powerlessness in relation to the other levels of existence, ineffective fevers leading to destruction but no healing [see Steiner 1949, 129]. The boy had to go through similar experiences in this episode. Chininum is derived from the alkaloid-rich bark of the cinchona tree, with a bitter taste (relating to the I organization), and remarkable resistance to its environment, the primeval forests of the eastern Andes. It is highly unusual for trees or shrubs to deposit alkaloids in their bark, but an example in our region is Berberis. The prescriber's aim with this bark, a mineralized plant, was to strengthen and link I activity to the astral

body. The balancing action of the I is further promoted by combining the cinchona bark with sulphuric acid.
The goal for this patient was to better link the I organization with the metabolism and limbs. This process occurs physiologically at age nine (see above), exactly the boy's age when the severe flare had impaired walking, standing, and limb growth, all dramatically separating him from his own body. China specifically acts in digestion and metabolism when the I is unable to intervene, resulting in diarrhoea and malabsorption. Similarly, in malaria the I is unable to intervene in the blood itself, which the patient abruptly experiences as extreme weakness and which manifests as hemolysis. Here, too, splenomegaly is a key symptom (▸Chap. 6.3.3.4 on the function of the spleen). The present case demonstrates that China and Chininum sulfuricum are medicaments of the first rank also when there is need for the I's anti-inflammatory power in the joints and the the limbs. The anthroposophic concept of the metabolic-limb system illuminates these pathologic processes.
The treatment took immediate effect, with defervescence in two days; twice in the following 36 months, repeated treatment was necessary and equally effective for acute fever, once with splenomegaly. The boy's Still's disease is no longer evident or progressive. Happily, the family has been able to build their new house and escape the damp environment. Most interestingly, eighteen months later the boy developed an acute right frozen shoulder due to overuse from writing because of severe damage to his elbow and wrist joints.

- **Crotalus terrificus D30 injection** Weleda gave prompt and full improvement;
- **Crotalus horridus D12 pillules** stabilized recovery within a month. In longterm followup, an additional severe flare happened at age 18½, "1st moon", (see Roder 2005.) Triggers were likely school graduation, independence from parents, initiation of vocational training, and starting to drive his specially adapted car. The author, in collaboration with the German Centre of Paediatric and Juvenile Rheumatology, initiated successful treatment with Anakinra (Kineret®) [Skrabl-Baumgartner 2008, 177]. Neither Chininum sulfuricum nor any other homoeopathic medicine was effective acutely. This shows that potential treatment must always be assessed with reference to the patient's age. Urtica Ferro culta D2 Weleda, a"vegetabilized" iron preparation, proved helpful in stabilization. The patient also reported that it supported him in gaining self-confidence and personal initiative.

10.9.3.1.2 17-year-old-girl with Still's disease

For comparison we present the case study of a female patient with Still's disease.

The patient was first seen at the age of seven. The pregnancy was a surprise, to parents who'd recently met and then moved in together. The flat was burglarized during the pregnancy, which came as a shock to the mother who then had cervical insufficiency, treated with cerclage. She had 25 kg pregnancy weight gain. Because of worsening pre-eclampsia and hypertension – as far as the mother remembers, which is all that matters – the birth was induced with oxytocin without release of the cerclage. She experienced horrific pain, then a Caesarian "like an assault", complicated by suture dehiscence, wound infection, and a prolonged stay in intensive care. The premature infant never breastfed. The father, who had medical training, said that his child had been classified as small for 8th month gestational age weighing 2, 200 g. The infant was in neonatal intensive care for three weeks, while his wife recovered from severe pre-eclampsia with hardly any contact with the infant. He said he visited the child daily, but this had"nevertheless been too little attention."

The child vomited frequently, ate irregularly, and crawled late at 10 months. An influenza-like infection occurred before her first birthday, causing knee swelling, and she gradually evolved classic Still's disease. During a lengthy inpatient stay, cortisone was effective, but chronic high doses resulted in growth failure. Classic homoeopathic treatment reduced the dosage of cortisone. At age six, her brother was born in the 30th week of pregnancy. He was fidgety and fussy, had rickets, and obstructive upper respiratory tract infection. One need hardly say how the mother and father experienced these events. Shortly after the birth of her brother, the girl had a flare which was treated unsuccessfully with Methotrexate.

When the girl was seen for initial consultation while on corticosteroids and MTX, her wrists were so painful that she cried on light touch, her left hip had limited abduction, and her knees and ankles were moderately affected. She craved salt and milk, only recognizing after elimination that it aggravated the pain although she'd been on it from birth. She always resisted bedtime and could not fall asleep before 10 pm. She was afraid of nightmares and thunderstorms. She was empathetic and highly observant. At 2 years old she had whooping cough, but otherwise practically no other infections. She was sensitive to cold and wet. The left side was more affected, especially her left hip, which had only 25°of abduction and frequently was severely painful. Later this joint improved temporarily, much to the amazement of the orthopaedic surgeon, until a severe flare at age 15 resulted in complete loss of abduction and extensive loss of range of movement in both hips. This required hip replacement at age 16. Many other joints were involved, especially the right wrist and the ankles. Initially, she responded best to

- **Ledum palustre LM6 dil.**, first 5 drops 3 times/day for many months, later gradually a reduced dosage.
- The main reason for choosing this medicament was the marked dependence of symptoms on cold and wet. The medicinal powers of *Ledum palustre*, Labrador tea, are all the greater the further north and cooler the habitat (edges of moors) [see Simon 2005a]. The LM potency was particularly effective, allowing discontinuation of corticosteroids, MTX and nonsteroidal Anti-Inflammatories for two years.
- The second most important medicament proved to be Bryonia/bryony, the most important potentized medicine for acute inflammatory changes in the hip joint. With its help, acute aggravations with severe pain in the hip joint rapidly resolved.
- **Bryonia D12** and **Bryonia/Stannum pillules.** Wala for acute pain in the hip; 7 (D12) pillules 3 times or 7 pillules 5 times/day, partly on their own, partly with Ledum.

As the patient grew older, injections of

- **Solum Inject amp.** Wala,
  (2 ml s.c. or 10 ml i.v.)

were very helpful for aggravation at onset of cold, wet, or changeable weather. The girl remained inflammation-free (CRP, ESR normalized) with this until her 13th year.

From her 9th year, she had a tendency to adiposity. Mentally, it is notable that although she seems bright, happy, and enthusiastic about school, she was hypersensitive. An episode with severe pain developed at age 13, concurrent with acute depression, and was treated on an inpatient basis with NSAID (naproxen 500 mg twice daily), psychotherapy, intensified physiotherapy, and movement baths when it became impossible to get the girl to do adequate remedial gymnastics as an outpatient, and the family's patience had become exhausted. Solum proved adequate after this on an outpatient basis and acupuncture was started as a new element. Later on, an herbal medicine

Harpagophytum procumbens and

- **Rheuma-Hek®**

in high dosage proved effective in support, limiting the need for NSARs.

Several professionals noticed an unusual mother-daughter interaction especially when her mother did not visit during the first week of her hospitalization at age fifteen. Most appointments involved the father, while the mother complained about the problems her daughter's illness caused at home, the time needed to drive her to a physiotherapist, and so on. Once when the 15 year old girl had to be sent home from school in severe pain and rang up to say she was ill, a midday emergency home visit had to be made by her busy physician. The daughter was alone at home in tears and severe pain, while the mother remained at work.

She had a boyfriend at 15, initiated hormonal contraception, and had her first severe recurrence since starting treatment in our practice, with a sedimentation rate of 100 and CRP four times normal. Another episode of depression accompanied this flare, so she was admitted to the hospital, where she was treated with cortisone and etanercept (Enbrel). During her three month stay, she also received complementary medical treatment. While reviewing all our paediatric rheumatology cases, this patient's forgotten details, including pregnancy and birth history, could be placed in a new perspective as similarities in all the early histories were recognized. When we again discussed the mother's shock at the onset of pregnancy, the attack of obstetrical interventions and all the other events, she felt recognized and accepted, and from that time was a different and happier person. It was only because of this review of the history, eight years after the first appointment, when damage to the joints had already been severe, that it became possible to find a constitutional medicine which improved the severe flare and, more importantly, healed the accompanying depression.

- **Natrium muriaticum C200 pillules**, 3 pillules upto 5 times/day for a total of twelve weeks (the dose being established in close consultation with the patient at a time when she was on steroids and etanercept).

It must be stressed that steroids and etanercept had been given for weeks when this prescription was begun, and inflammation parameters improving, but with unrelenting depression. On the other hand, the patient felt that her rheumatic symptoms also improved further with this medicament. Eight weeks after starting on Natrium muriaticum, the hospital doctors completely discontinued the steroids and etanercept; the inflammation did not recur in the twelve months that followed.

Very definite indications for Natrium muriactium in this case were:

- the long lasting separation from her mother after birth, especially after premature birth,
- difficulty between mother and daughter, ambivalence in an ordinarily nuturing bond that started prenatally and probably contributed to the mother's postpartum depression, which would have benefitted from appropriate treatment,

- clinical signs such as craving for salt, and
- eating disorder, since Natrium muriaticum may be indicated for both anorexia and adiposity due to depression, especially

recurrent depressive episodes in adolescence. Natrium muriaticum is one of the most important single homoeopathic medicines for rheumatic conditions and mirrors their pathogenesis. Looking back unconsciously, feeling trapped, and turning into a column of salt-like Lot's wife-rather than being resilient, presents a therapeutic image for potentized table salt (▸Chap. 6.4.3.6). It may be indicated for children with either early childhood depression or current depression in the closest parent.
The patient has had no recurrences. After bilateral hip replacements, she has enjoyed movement and good quality of life.

10.9.3.2 ANA-positive oligoarthritis and extended oligoarthritis

10.9.3.2.1 2-year-old girl with oligoarthritis

A now 2-year-old term girl, had a birth weight of 2.5 kg (SGA < 3 percentile.) The mother stated that midwife-assisted delivery had been stressful and the child's arrival traumatic. Newborn weight drop of more than 10 % with breast-feeding. "I was not able to breast-feed her completely", voicing a dreadful maternal grief that her child could not be satisfied with the breast, and perhaps an early consequence of the birthing experience.
The child was easy, and even slept through the night from an early age. The mother returned to work when the girl was nine months old. She seemed stressed at appointments, demanding a lot of herself. Her husband was a bank worker. Although the girl pulled up to stand by nine months, she was not walking by her second birthday. At this age she also had a hepatitis B vaccination, immediately followed by an airline trip to the Far East. Looking back, the disease evolved gradually after this long journey and hepatitis vaccination. Extensive oligoarthritis affecting both knee and ankle joints and the right wrist was established at 2¼ years with a knee extension deficit of 20 degrees. ANA 1:1280, CRP only slightly elevated to 3 times normal, no uveitis, rare fevers, only a few infections, but antibiotics twice. She had both a fear and a love-hate relationship with large animals. She was reluctant in new or unforeseen situations; her mother was pregnant again.
Initially

- **Ledum D4** with **Moorextrakt D4 Ledum-Solum D4 dil.**, 5 drops 3 times/day by mouth, was effective.

This is a basic medicament for chronic rheumatoid arthritis in anthroposophic medicine. It was chosen on account of marked aggravation of symptoms in cool, wet weather (see detailed discussion of this medicine by Simon [2005a, 3–15]). The clinical picture showed adequate improvement with this, but not a cure. A brother was born when the girl was three and she had an ambivalent, jealous attitude towards him. Characteristically, apart from joint inflammation with warm, swollen joints, the girl also had a certain hysterical trait. Even with just moderate inflammation, the child would develop complete paralysis in the legs which would be gone once the situation, such as a medical

10

appointment or a playdate was over. These hysterical attacks developed only after her brother was born.

The condition of the joints gradually worsened inspite of various other potentized medicines; on the advice of the family physician, the parents gave NSAIDs in low doses when she was 4½. She had no iridocyclitis. After suffering for two years, with an ANA 1: 1280 and a moderately elevated CRP, a steroid injection was proposed. In this situation – four weeks before the triamcinolone injection – a potentized organ preparation of the most involved joint was given for the first time:

- **Articulatio genus Gl D30 amp.** Wala 1 ml by mouth.

The consequence was an enormous outburst of rage. Treatment continued every five days, later once weekly. Every time she had an outburst, it grew less and less intense. Within just two days she could tiptoe for the first time in months, within five days knee symptoms markedly regressed, and NSAIDs could be discontinued.

Nevertheless, the proposed injection into the right knee was given four weeks later. The ANA had dropped to 1:160 within six months and CRP remained negative. Mentally, the child's response to the organ preparation was so positive that it was as if the jealousy were departing from the knee.

At 30 month follow-up, the child was completely symptom-free. For over a year she was treated with only the organ preparation and supplemented with

- **Articulatio radiocarpea Gl D30 amp.** Wala because the right wrist, which from onset had been moderately affected, was still abnormal after the inflammation in the knee joint had improved.

10.9.3.2.2 4-yearold boy with Polyarthritis

The boy's parents seemed down-to-earth, usually coming together to the appointments. Their passion was off-the-beaten-path adventure travel to distant countries. There was a history of vaginal thrush in 25th week of pregnancy, normal pregnancy, and precipitous birth at 38weeks resulting in an episiotomy and vaginal tear. The boy was the couple's second child. The first child was a scheduled Caesarean, but arrived too quickly, causing considerable injury to the mother. This information puts the birth of this boy in a different light. Was the pregnancy really unremarkable? The parents reported that when mother was in the sixth month of pregnancy, their older toddler son was bitten in the head by the paternal uncle's dog right in front of the parents. All contact with the father's brother, who lived nearby, came to an abrupt halt. The father said that his brother was "very domineering and that things only went right if I behave like a tame and obedient dog." Even after his new nephew's birth, the uncle and parents had not reconciliated.

He was exclusively breast-fed for 5 months. Routine vaccinations were administered, including Hepatitis A and Yellow Fever vaccines at 15 months prior to a six week trip to Mauretania. He started crawling at 7 months and was independently walking at 18 months.

At 20 months of age, although he was asymptomatic, he had empiric antibiotics because his brother had scarlet fever and documented strep. The boy was"never ill" in early childhood. His mother was now pregnant again, which was "too much-brother by the

hand, the boy on my arm, sister in my belly-hoping he'll walk soon." All this only on being questioned, the third pregnancy not mentioned in written history.
The mother reminded the physician of the Natrium muriaticum drug picture. Her family had been refugees. She was blonde, tall, and slender. Her gestures showed distancing from the children; she said she'd started psychotherapy. When her son became ill, all she could think was, "you've got to get through this." Both parents seemed rather cool and aloft showing little emotion, but as a pair they seemed dependable. As the child's treatment continued, they grew friendlier and more open. A nappy (diaper) rash appeared when the boy was 20 months old on a spring holiday to Corsica, which was treated with Nystatin and a sugar-free diet. Several months later, he limped and had his initial episode of left ankle swelling. A month later, his sister was born and the limp disappeared for awhile, or perhaps wasn't noticed. At 24 months he received MMR vaccine and a month later the limp recurred, so an NSAID was given. Following this his parents felt that his angry attitude was impossible to deal with. When the left ankle swelling did not subside, tests were ordered demonstrating ANA-positive JRA. A month later the right knee also swelled, so he was evaluated at a paediatric rheumatology clinic and the diagnosis was confirmed. After naproxen was unsuccessful, he started on MTX and had a steroid injection in the left ankle.
After MTX he was ill and deteriorated."For the first 5 days after MTX, he would refer to himself by his first name, and only then did he use "I" again. His behaviour changed distinctly, and he was sensitive, weepy, impatient, explosive, angry. At 28 months, naproxen was discontinued because of gastric problems and he had a steroid injection in his right knee. He was symptom-free two months later, so by 33 months the MTX could be tapered.
In October, as the weather grew cold, his left ankle swelled again. MTX was discontinued because of intolerance and Ibuprofen was briefly given, then discontinued because of vomiting. Now both ankles were involved, both again were injected with steroids; cervical spine also was now affected. Indomethacin, ice below, and heat above were administered. A few months later off medication, during a trip to Mauretania, both ankles were moderately swollen, worsening with walking. When he returned to the clinic again both ankles, inflamed, knee, wrist, fingers and cervical spine were involved.
At 42 months azathioprine and a steroid injection in his left lower ankle were ineffective. Giardia lamblia infection was diagnosed and metronidazole dispensed. Definite improvement occurred after a diet change to low arachidonic acid, high Omega 3 fatty acids. That summer, on only azathioprine, he was stable with ANA 1:320, CRP 0.2 mg/dL, normal electrophoresis, IgG 11 g/L, Ferritin 20 ng/mL.
Although his hands were less often swollen, when he ate prepared or fast foods they would swell within four hours! Concerned about his appetite, his parents reduced the azathioprine to 25 mg/day, but then he flared with limp and pain in his left ankle and right knee as well as tenosynovitis in his radiocarpal joints. After a gastrointestinal infection, Azathioprine was discontinued. This was his condition when he was first brought to see us.
The boy entered the room like a clown, an imp, initially limping, but then became a frenzy of undisciplined activity. He screamed wildly and his father had to wrestle to hold him. Mother remained very withdrawn and both parents appeared resigned.

He slept well, with his older brother. Originally a warm child, with a warm head and dry feet, he had grown cooler. A year later, when he was five, his mother said, "He makes me angry and exhausted, never listens, patience gets you nowhere." His father was reluctant to pick him up, and just held his hand; his mother found it difficult to touch him at all. His father observed, "things go better if we let him finish things, and don't interrupt, and he is always talking to us." To this his mother responded, "I don't want that – I need time for myself."

When the boy was five, his father had psychotherapy because of panic attacks. For many years he suffered nightmares and ws treated with barbiturates. His own father, the boy's paternal grandfather, had alcoholism and had been severely abused as a child. His mother, the paternal grandmother, had emigrated from East Germany, only connecting with her biologic parents (Stasi background) 15 years before, after reunification.

The boy's mother did not feel that there were problems in her own family's background.

Treatment started by keeping a food diary for 5 days and further improving his diet. Medication prescribed was:

- **Articulatio talocruralis D30 amp** Wala,
  Wednesday morning 0.5 ml by mouth,
- **Articulatio subtalaris D30 amp.** Wala,
  Friday morning 0.5 ml by mouth.
- **Articulatio genus D30 amp.** Wala,
  Monday morning 0.5 ml by mouth.
- **Argentum met. praep. D30 amp.** Weleda mixed with
- **Thymus D30 amp.** Wala and
  Amnion D30 amp. Wala
  aa, 0.5 ml of mixture 4 times/wk in the morning on the remaining days of the week by mouth.

Later Amnion was replaced by **Antimonit D20 amp.** Weleda, as a constitutional medicine to treat the sulphuric, hyperkinetic symptoms. Antimonite (Antimonium crudum) is often helpful with rheumatic diseases, mainly if the originally warm constitution is hysterical, with excess metabolism.

Rhus toxicodendron D30 amp. Wala replaced Thymus, being a deep-acting vegetable medicament and specific for a sense of homelessness, inner restlessness, with typical aggravation in winter, and longing for warmer climes. The plant comes from a southern, equatorial family, making it a 'border crosser' in northern, cooler regions. Rhus tox. is also important in treating periarticular inflammation and tenosynovitis.

Azathioprine and immunosuppressants were not prescribed.

One month after starting treatment the boy improved. He initiated social interaction more often and was painfree off NSAIDs, able to romp and run. Three months later, both ankles felt a bit warm, but otherwise there were no findings. Six months later, after return from a month in warm Morocco, he had a medial malleolar effusion, but recovered quickly. Eight months later, with all joint symptoms resolved but his squeaky, infantile speech was noted, so we gave Aurum/Stibium/Hyoscyamus (▸Chap. 7.5.3). A few months later, after intense swimming, he had pain for two weeks and localized ankle irritation, enthesitis. An important central medicament for inflammation of tendon insertions on ankle and tendovaginitis was prescribed, **Tendo/Allium Cepa comp. amp.** Wala [*Vademecum* 2010, 797]. Fourteen months after his initial consultation, he was a rambunctious kindergartner who still occasionally used his fists, but overall had better self-control and normal speech. His only sequelae were seasonal weather sensitivity and a need for arch supports, so his outcome was assessed as "marvellous" at 24 month followup. In the four years since discontinuation of treatment, he has remained asymptomatic. The boy said, "Mum, I don't have rheumatism any more!" Time will tell, but based on our experience, his prognosis is a complete cure.

10.9.3.2.3 2-year-old girl with oligoarthritis and iridocyclits

Presenting history: In May, at 22 months of age, the girl "twisted her right ankle" and had pain, swelling, and inability to bear weight persist two weeks later.

Her labs showed a CRP 10.6 mg/dL (reference range up to 6), ANA 1:320, negative Borrelia, reduced serum iron, and iridocyclitis on ophthalmolgical exam. She was diagnosed with ANA-positive JRA with iridocyclitis and treated initially with a NSAID and steroid eye drops. When initially seen by the author additional history revealed that 4 weeks after onset, a sister was born. As discussed previously, onset of oligoarthritis correlates often with sibling rivalry. When six weeks of treatment brought normalized eye findings, but no joint improvement, Ibuprofen was prescribed.

The parents are sympathetic, modest people who said "nothing unusual" had happened during their daughter's pregnancy, birth, or infancy. Guided history revealed they had moved. Why? The girl's father had worked in his family's business, which had "always been a struggle", so he had "cut the cord" and quit five months before onset. All contact with his parents and two siblings had been severed, which was very disappointing to the father, his wife, and children. He began a new job just one month before onset. Additional conversation revealed that the mother had suffered during the pregnancy. The family lived together with the paternal grandparents and her interfering mother-in-law had "pounced" on the pregnancy as if"she wanted to have the child." In the 4th week of pregnancy, she'd told the mother, "If you don't eat, we'll send you to the hospital", which shocked the mother speechless. In that moment, she was unable to cry. Two days after the birth, the mother-in-law had taken the 2-day-old infant from her, fed him, and refused to give the wailing infant back. The mother could not say anything and wept when alone later.

Once the father left the grandfather's firm, the mother had begun a new partime job, but went on maternity leave ten days before her daughter "twisted her ankle."

The planned pregnancy had been easy and the baby breastfed for six months. Development had been normal with first words at nine months and walking by 15 months. She had mild bronchitis at 9 months, but otherwise just usual colds and Roseola; she received routine vaccinations. Sleep deteriorated after JRA onset, and she awoke crying from 1–3 a.m. The girl was blonde, quiet, had a large head, and played"like an angel" during the consultation.

Examination showedinflammation, effusion, and heat in the right ankle, accompanied by guarding and limp.

1st prescription:

- **Lac caninum C200**
  3 pillules 3 times.
  Rationale: Competition between "two mothers" (see details ▸Chap. 7.3.2) A week later, child was cheerful in the mornings, but weepy briefly at 11 a.m. Her limping decreased slightly, but the ankle was unchanged.

2nd prescription:

- **Articulatio subtalaris D30 amp.** Wala
- **Articulatio talocruralis D30 amp.** Wala
- **Tendo D30 amp.** Wala
  aa mixed 0.8 mL daily in the mornings.

2 weeks after starting this treatment, the right ankle was a little better. Mild left iridocyclitis 1 drop dexamethasone 5 times daily. She could now walk for 20 minutes without limp.

3rd prescription:

- **+ Iris bovis D30 amp.** Wala,
  0.5 ml by mouth twice/week.
- **Chrysolith D6 trit.** Weleda a good pinch daily at midday [*Vademecum* 2010, 311]

This treatment continued unchanged for the next 18 (!) months. One month after starting treatment, walking improved, but left ankle remained slightly larger than the right, which never regressed completely. Two months after starting treatment she had practically no limping and Ibuprofen dose could be reduced. After three months, ibuprofen gradually discontinued. Curiously, four months after starting treatment, the paternal grandmother *developed systemic lupus erythematosus.* A year after treatment, all eye findings resolved and she had mild tendonitis, just after jumping on a trampoline:

- **Tendo/Allium Cepa comp. pillules** Wala,
  5 globules twice/day.

Right ankle and function normalized. About two years after starting treatment, she continued doing very well although she had subtle connective tissue weaknessand knee joint laxity.

- **Fluorit D6 trit.** Weleda added to the prescription.

Aside from separation anxiety in kindergarten, all was unremarkable.

10.9.3.2.4 3-year-old girl with extended oligoarthritis

A 3-year-old girl from Milan came with severe knee involvement, frequently interfering with walking as well as hot effusions, predominately right-sided of the right hand and digits and right jaw. Aggravation occurred autumn and winter and was so bad that she wanted to stay in bed. She had a notable absence of febrile illnesses. Laboratory tests show ANA > 1:640, CRP elevated to 20 times normal, ESR 50 mm, low ferritin reduced, but no iridocyclitis.

Months later the mother told us that in the 6th month of the pregnancy she and her mother-in-law, who often visited, had a heated argument in front of all four of the children while her husband was gone. The friendly and sensitive mother described her

mother-in-law as powerful and domineering. The fight was such a shock that she could not discuss it further without weeping. Herhusband, also kind and pleasant, seemed helpless at this moment. She had inwardly withdrawn, but remained outwardly pleasant with her mother-in-law, which repeatedly resulted in difficulties. Her own mother lived next door.
Hyperemesis had complicated the pregnancy.
The girl, her fifth child, was creative and radiant, like the sun. She was breastfed for 12 months. She was extremely jealous of her next oldest brother. While on a family camping trip at 15 months old, the girl had febrile bronchitis, which was treated with antibiotics. The toddler sunburned, which someone else brought to the parents' attention, and the return journey had been stressful. The day after their return, she had right knee swelling for the first time.
The girl was at first successfully treated by Italian anthroposophic colleagues, and laboratory values improved. In addition to NSAIDs, she was given potentized metal preparations, Formica, Bryonia and some other medicines. Externally, Solum oil Wala and Phosphorus oil Weleda were applied.
No stabilization was achieved, so many different alternative methods were tried, including a restricted diet.
The author initially geared his treatment to the liver, assuming prior damage from antibiotics, stress and NSAIDs. Lycopodium, Natrium sulfuricum, Bryonia D30 were all ineffective. The Milan hospital recommended treatment with MTX, which the parents declined. After four months of our care, she had neither joint nor pain improvement, so a completely new approach was taken utilizing potentized organ preparations which act directly on the life organization and are particularly important at this age:

- **Articulatio radiocarpea Gl D30 amp.** Wala, **Articulatio genus Gl D30 amp.** Wala, **Thymus Gl D30 amp.** Wala to deal with the autoimmune attack on the joints and the failure of the thymus to regulate immune function. aa ad 3.0 ml, 0.5 ml by mouth in the mornings 6 days/week.
- **Arandisit D15 amp.** Weleda, **Equisetum/Formica amp.** Wala, aa ad 2.0 ml, 0.5 ml at midday, a composition often helpful with rheumatic conditions of potentized horsetail, wood ant and Arandisit, a silicate-type tin mineral [see Simon 2005b, 134f.], which reduces swelling, supports elimination, and regulates astral body function that has grown one-sided.
- **Lac caninum C30 pillules,** 3 pillules at night.

The rationale for Lac caninum is the dysfunctional family, with "several mothers" competing over the child; an indication of proven value established by J. Gnaiger. A lingering hurt in the relationship between these women is particularly characteristic (▸Chap. 10.9.3.8)
Distinct improvement was immediate with this treatment, with decrease of inflammation and effusions, walking without pain, and a radiant child once again. A mistletoe preparation specifically useful in treating rheumatic conditions [see Simon 2005a, 3–10] was added:

- **Iscucin Salicis amp.** Wala, strength A: 0.5 ml once by mouth.

The indications were aggravation of the rheumatic inflammation in cold and wet weather, since potentized willow-grown mistletoe directly stimulates and stabilizes the child's warmth organization and the tendency to joint inflammation and swelling, which willow-grown mistletoe reduces. The warmth organization, directly connected with

immune regulation, was immature, as demonstrated by the lack of febrile illness in early life, and then was acutely stressed and weakened on the holiday before symptom onset. Iscucin Salicis serves very well here to stimulate late maturation. It is given sublingually to young children; older children are given subcutaneous injections. The preparation is not suitable as a first step in acute treatment and may also cause aggravation if given when inflammation is severe, with high IgG, CRP, or ESR. The higher the gamma globulin level on electrophoresis, the more careful must one be in determining the mistletoe dosage. Above all, use it to consolidate treatment.
Lac caninum was gradually reduced and discontinued as mistletoe treatment started. Within four months of the new approach, laboratory values became normal (ESR only 8 mm, hgb 13.1, CRP normal). At 18 months followup, she currently has no symptoms of pain, effusions, or immobility; transient arthralgia, with changes in the weather especially in spring or with infections, responds well now to Bryonia. Treatment and followup continue.

10.9.3.3 9-year-old girl with seronegative polyarthritis

A 9-year-old girl was brought to see us who, at age six years, had developed a rheumatoid factor negative polyarthritis. She had negative ANA and HLA-B27 and was on NSAIDs and MTX when our treatment started.
The mother, a piano teacher, was tentative and, apologized constantly. She squinted due to constant strabismus convergens. The pregnancy's first four months were complicated, but the birth itself had been rapid. The early years were notable for excessive crying, night terrors, Roseola, and chicken pox, with a long "terrible two"phase. Two more siblings followed this first daughter, but she had marked aggressiveness. In contrast to her brother, who was 3 years younger, she was physically mean and hateful to him. The relationship to her youngest brother, who was 4½ years younger, was normal. But, the girl always preferred to be on her own.
The mother described her eldest daughter's character as dominant, highly aggressive, obstinate, always wanting to be first, easily distracted, very creative, gifted in the arts and music, tending to be hysterical, shouting, using coarse expressions, volatile with striking out and biting, not even sparing her mother. Her language development was precocious, but she was afraid at night, in bed, on train journeys. Ambivalence was the main quality of her relationship with her mother, since she craved closeness, but could be highly aggressive, even biting her mother in a rage. She was highly sensitive to touch and pain. Play therapy was discontinued at age five.
At age six, following a fall off her snow sled, the RF-negative polyarthritis emerged. The parents, both musicians, were starting to separate and the girl who was the source of much of the martial strife, wanted to split them apart and have one all to herself. Both parents worked with psychologists.
This is a syndrome definitely belonging to the second seven-year period. The child's polarizing dominated family life, overpowering her mother's weak I organization and bullying her siblings as well as traumatizing her mother physically. The onset of her disease precipitated the marriage crisis with both the child adding to their stress and diminishing real support to the girl.

This was a clear indication for:
Lachesis D12 dil. Weleda, 5 drops twice/day.
After a short primary aggravation, the syndrome cleared completely within six months and has not recurred in three year followup. MTX could be weaned rapidly. Her aggressiveness markedly improved and she was able to acknowledge and apologize for her wrongdoing. The parents have separated; the mother has been helped by painting therapy. The daughter is doing well at school and is also a musician.
A brief update 4 years later:
The parents reunited and recognized in hindsight that the patient's aggressiveness and lability was probably a major element in the marital crisis. Three years ago, this young pianist had an acute recurrence in the hands following tick-borne encephalitis (TBE) vaccination. The family physician had "insisted" on this before a visit to Bavaria, but apparently had not reviewed her history or given information on potential risks. The inflammatory episode came the week after the vaccination. Using **Lachesis** (by mouth) up to the **C200** (*repeated doses required*) it proved possible to resolve by Christmas. Since then no further flares, but repeated signs of irritation affecting the tendons stressed by piano playing.

The exaggerated, premature dynamics of the child's soul organization clearly indicated Lachesis (▸Chap. 6.5.5.4) Bushmaster venom is a prime remedy for aggressive *jealousy*, for *children who seek to break up their parents' relationship, making every calm and harmonious moment an opportunity for aggressive, impulsive disruption*. On the other hand, these children unconsciously sense and suffer because of weakness and dishonesty in their parents' relationship. They have powerful inner potential that may grow into great artistic or social commitment later in life. The psychosomatic genesis of polyarthritis is impressively evident in this case.

10.9.3.4 10-year-old girl with seropositive polyarthritis

The history as given by the mother of a 10-year-old girl with seropositive polyarthritis: "Her birth was traumatic for me. I could have done with help, I did not know what to do with her, not even how to hold her." She had previous painful gynaecological interventions as well as trauma in her relationships to her own parents. After the birth of another child, a son who turned out to have extreme ADHD, the mother developed a chronic degenerative condition, radically changing her ability to care for the children.
The girl's polyarthritis developed shortly after her brother's birth and her mother's illness. Initially she had relatively symmetrical, polyarticular involvement, flared by cold and wet weather. After a severe attack at age nine, rheumatoid factor was positive. She had a history of left hip dysplasia requiring surgical correction. When first seen, this emaciated child was only on high dose NSAID and had acute dramatic inflammation, mainly of her knee joints, which made basic examination painful. She had severe anemia with hemaglobin of 6.7 g/dL and was chilly, with feet so icy cold that she slept in dad's bed to stay warm. She had frequent nightmares, a fear of thunderstorms, and tended to have headaches, sometimes awakening her. She disliked eggs and milk, and had little thirst. Her parents felt that if she had been less miserable, cried less from pain, and was able to walk comfortably, she'd be sanguine. She was clingy with her mother,

who was ill herself and stressed by both her sick daughter and son. She had no real, lasting improvement with Apis mellifica, Bryonia, Dulcamara, or potentized iron preparations, although there was some reduction in pain. After several months,

- **Pulsatilla D200 pillules:** 5 pillules dissolved in 50 mL of water, taken in sips over 3 days

was given for the first time. All symptoms thoroughly improved and labs normalized. The medicament had to be repeated 14 times in the next four years; the indication was always a mild aggravation lasting for more than three days. There were no further episodes of inflammation and, eighteen months after starting treatment, her rheumatoid factor was negative. In the fourteen years since Pulsatilla, she has not had a single recurrence.

10.9.3.5 16-year-old girl with juvenile polyarthritis[1]

From age twelve, the patient had had juvenile polyarthritis with symmetrical polyarticular involvement and had received MTX 10 mg injections for 1 ½ years. The family physician, a homoeopath, had prescribed Nat. mur. C30 daily, among other things, without success. Both parents were accomplished special-needs teachers. The mother was talkative, seemed harsh, and slightly emaciated. The pregnancy was uneventful, but the birth weight was 4.5 kg, and mother felt she was "like a barrel." As a preschooler, the girl was very shy and reticient, clingy, obedient, and cautious around other children, never defending herself, yet also stubborn. Well into puberty by twelve, she was tall, blond, and thin with a strong temperament, frequent headaches, nonspecific abdominal pain, eczema, colds, and worsening polyarthritis. She had warm, swollen elbows and wrists, and was not able to squat on her heels; labs showed mild anaemia, a negative rheumatic factor while on MTX, and a significantly elevated IgG.
The biographical history directed the treatment. When she was 3½, the girl had seen her younger brother fall into a shallow pond and stop breathing. The shock so stunned her that she "froze." Her brother was rescued too late, suffered severe asphyxia, and has been severely disabled, lovingly cared for by the girl and her parents, who already had demanding responsibilities. So the sibling became a trauma for the patient herself; the shock literally shot into her limbs. Psychological trauma is an important biographical motif for patients with polyarthritis. In paediatrics, the maternal experiences always play a role, so the younger the child, the more important this will be. We did not explicitly ask how the mother had felt seeing her lifeless son in the pond and her daughter standing there as if frozen, a daughter who she described in alien terms: "like a barrel" and "like an autistic", which the girl most certainly was not.
It was a great relief to the family to be able just to talk about the event and its consequences.

1 This case goes back over more than 15 years. Not all documents are available any longer. The report is included to inform readers of the impressive medical history.

The prescription was

- **Causticum D30**, followed by **D200:**
  3 pillules 3 times daily for three days for each dose (▸Chap. 6.5.5.3)

Causticum is produced from vegetable ash and a special form of calcium carbonate, which has "gone through hell", recrystallized to marble by applying heat and pressure. The girl's constitution in infancy mirrors this picture.

The central indication in this case was the experience of being paralysed in compassion, the overpowering feeling of being responsible for the suffering of another, an overly close attachment to her mother, and the tendency to direct aggression towards herself.

With this treatment, the girl first became more aggressive and violent, but soon could squat on her heels again; MTX could be discontinued relatively quickly, as well as the NSAIDs. Treatment concluded after two years, when she was well. She has been lost to followup.

10.9.3.6 6-year-old girl with Polymyositis

In late winter, over six weeks, this previously well 5½-year-old girl developed fevers, headaches, limited movement, and abnormal inflammatory markers. That summer she had a tick bite. Six weeks later, she had nightime fevers spiking above 40 °C, migratory arthralgias, no hepatosplenomegaly; CRP elevated to 20 times normal, leucocytes 15 000/µl, ESR 88, and elevated titres for EBV IgM, Mycoplasma, and Anti-streptolysin O. Neither muscle biopsy nor polymyositis-specific antibody testing were done, but a presumptive rheumatic diagnosis was made. Steroids and immunosuppressive treatment proposed were refused by her mother. On the advice of her hospital specialists, she was referred to our practice, now five weeks into another episode. At this first appointment, the child was very stiff, emaciated, pale, suffering impressive pain in the neck flexors (not mentioned in the hospital record) and proximal musculature, as well as daily bouts of fever. She seemed very sensitive and plaintive.

Expanded pertinent history revealed that her maternal grandmother had developed recurrent polymyositis five years earlier. When the child had fever, her intractable neck pain caused a constant right head tilt. Social history revealed intense parental strife with the paternal grandparents. The child was close to her paternal grandmother and was trying to mediate the conflict. Her mother was dark-haired, dull, late for appointments, and made no eye contact. Other professionals had said that the mother had rages and had on one occasion taken up a knife to stab herself in front of her family. Eighteen months before, she had returned to work managing a workshop for people with disabilities, leaving the girl with her grandmother who was suffering from polymyositis. But due to the girl's illness, her mother had been unable to continue to work. The patient had become jealous of her sister, just 18 months younger, and was very attached to her parents, disliking separation from them. She avoided being outside in the sun. Pulsatilla, Ledum, and Causticum scarcely helped at all. Only then was a full family history given, especially the situation concerning the two grandmothers. This led to the prescription of

- **Lac caninum C60**
  3 pillules 3 times/day for 5 days.

The drug proving of Lac caninum actually includes all the muscle symptoms described, especially the neck flexors. But the decisive aspect was the stress caused by her grandmother's illness, which again fits the common picture of the rheumatic child who suffers because of the illness or depression of a close grandmother, who at times takes her mother's place. Additional Lac caninum features were the threat of losing her paternal grandparents and her mother's ambivalence and depression.
The sedimentation rate was still elevated at 56 when Lac caninum treatment began. Complete success came, even in the first week, with defervescence and with return to kindergarten by three weeks. After six weeks ESR normalized at 8. The mother agreed to provide all care for the girl, and not the grandmother. The child remained in good health at nine year followup.

10.9.3.7 Case reports in brief

This history was provided by the **mother of a 6-year-old boy** with oligoarthritis, atopic dermatitis and recurrent bronchitis:
The birth had been"really bad" with vacuum extraction and shoulder dystocia, which the mother described as "catastrophic, a complete surprise." The 3.52 kg postterm boy required an incubator due to hypothermia and hypoxia.
The atopic dermatitis developed in the first six months. She breastfed him for seven months. "Everything revolved just around him." "I was disappointed." "The skin was not perfect." "There would always be one thing or another."
The boy cried when alone, yet rejected cuddles and tenderness. He had received vaccination twice against hepatitis B, since his father suffered from chronic hepatitis B. At age four, he had ANA-positive oligoarthritis, starting in left knee, which was treated conventionally with improved oligoarthritis, but resulted in a massive exacerbation of the atopic dermatitis.

- **Natrium muriaticum LM6 dil.** Arcana
  5 drops in the mornings, and
- **Articulatio genus Gl D30 amp.** Wala
  1 ampoule by mouth once/week

led to almost complete cure of both the atopic dermatitis and joint symptoms, so conventional treatment could be slowly weaned.
A 3-year-old boy with circumscribed scleroderma. He was born to a woman who was homeless, and for the first eight months lived on the street with her. Social services then placed him in a foster family. Scleroderma developed at 2½ years, mainly on the left thigh, lower leg, and the left lower abdomen. He had only erratic contact with his biological mother. Circumscribed scleroderma did not progress while on anthroposophic medical treatment. The child presented with decreasing frequency to the practice. When he was six, the disease returned with rapidly progressive left-sided hemiparesis, abducens paresis, and multiple vascular brainstem lesions on brain imaging studies. High dose steroid pulse therapy partially stabilized the crisis.

It was only when additional history was taken, that the foster mother confided that his biological mother had not contacted the child at all since Christmas, six months before onset; all this time, he had been waiting to hear from her.

A 9-year old girl with Lupus erythematosus, had been adopted from India. Her adoptive mother was a teacher. After the adoption, the adoptive father became increasingly depressed, and the couple separated. At seven years of age the child developed systemic lupus erythematosus, which stabilized initially with conventional treatment. Anthroposophic treatment brought further improvement, although a pubertal flare was again treated conventionally. The patient was apathetic about her origins. Her course seemed to improve when at age sixteen she found a 31-year-old boyfriend. Contact with the patient ended when she was 21, until then developments had continued to be unstable.

10.9.4 Extended therapies for children with rheumatic diseases

On the basis of more than 20 years' experience, C. Tautz has published details of the anthroposophic medicines he has found effective [2005]. The detailed chapter on the anthroposophic treatment of polyarthritis in adults by L. Simon [2005a] also provides a sound foundation. We would refer readers to these works and the *Vademecum of Anthroposophic Medicines* [2010] for the characterization and indication of anthroposophic medicines for rheumatoid arthritis. The authors consider the following particularly important in this context:

- **Quark compresses** during the day for acutely inflamed joints with effusions.

An alternative to be considered is

- **Retterspitz compresses**, depending on age and extent of inflammation from undiluted to 1:10 dilution.

These compresses may be applied cool and also have an effect on the inflammation due to the principle of sour application (▸Chap. 6.5.5.1.2). Sour applications to the skin guide one-sidedly catabolic activity originating from the astral body, to the outside. However, caution is indicated with regard to the generally accepted application of ice.

- **Stannum met. 0.4 % ointment** Weleda (for marked effusion **5 % ointment** Weleda) as an ointment dressing at night supports the forces of the organism in the joint sphere. L. Simon has stressed the relationship which Stannum has to joint cartilage, protection of which is a prime aim of treatment.

For internal use, the following is often effective as metal therapy for rheumatic inflammation using potentized tin (see case studies),

- **Arandisit D6 trit.** Weleda, **D15 amp.** Weleda [see Simon 2005b, 134].

This silicate-type ore from southern Africa reduces swelling and gives structure to both the inflammation of the joint and associated tendons and tendon insertions, which are also commonly involved. It is used both by mouth and s.c. Arandisite is supported above all by

- **Equisetum/Formica pillules/amp.** Wala (see case study ▸Chap. 10.9.3.4) [*Vademecum* 2010, 416]

Both the anthroposophic ophthalmologist, Susanne Vogel [2004] and, in an impressive case study, Tatjana Grah [2002] have written about

- **Uvea comp. amp.** Weleda/**Retina et Chorioidea Gl D30 amp.** Wala, **Quarz D30 amp.** Wala/Weleda injected s.c.
- treating iridocyclitis due to rheumatic disorders. As a bitter principle to encourage the higher levels of existence to penetrate the organization of metabolism and limbs, Grah successfully used the following after this indication, as did other anthroposophic colleagues.
- **Absinthium D3/Resina laricis D1 dil.** Weleda (▶Chap. 6.6) The authors found
- **Iris bovis D30 amp.** Wala

  ½–1 ampoule once/day by mouth in the mornings, later 2 or 3 times/week

effective in several (see case study 10.9.3.2.3) cases, some of which were severe.

Oil dispersion baths, e.g. with

- **Betula e fol. Oleum** Wala (scleroderma) or
- **Ledum oil** (polyarthritis) or
- **Solum oil** Wala (great sensitivity to weather changes and cold)

are particularly valuable in treating

- *circumscribed scleroderma* and *systemic scleroderma,*
- forms of *polyarthritis causing early stiffness* in neurasthenic patients, who tend to be cool. For more on bath therapy, see Simon [2005a].

Professional physiotherapy done regularly, water gymnastics, and provision of splints and aids are all important. In reality these are time-consuming for patients and families, so enthusiastic encouragement is required. In-patient treatment at a paediatric rheumatology or rehabilitation centre can be a most valuable help. Although this aspect of treatment may be considered separate from medical treatment, all patients receiving complementary treatment will also benefit from professional physiotherapy.

Eurythmy therapy enables sick children to copy healthy movements and make them their own, which has a *constructive effect.* Our work has made the authors much more aware of the degree to which *eurythmy therapy directly influences the sphere where pathogenesis has its roots* – in the child's body imitating the movements of the adult. In eurythmy therapy, the acquired disorders of the child's movement become visible. These movements are not only the consequence of pain, but also of the dissonance between child and mother in early childhood. The way the child's soul comes to expression in movement reveals itself. Eurythmy therapy can help the child to overcome ambivalent movement experiences and develop a new, original connection to his or her own movement. This distinguishes eurythmy therapy from physiotherapy, but it does not make physiotherapy superfluous. At the same time important impulses are created for overcoming the autoimmune disease process.

Anthroposophic art therapy makes it possible, especially in the school age child, to work through inner experiences and traumas in a non-verbal and creative way. One important aim is to reorient and transform astral body activity, and its autoimmune destruction, into constructive and nurturing forces. Art therapy is today widely accepted and practised as part of trauma therapy. In the authors' experience, this approach to the treatment of children with rheumatic diseases, who are in either the first or second 7-year period of life, is gaining importance.

Due to the time patients need with outpatient treatment, it may be ideal to start eurythmy and/or art therapy on an inpatient basis in an anthroposophic paediatric unit. In Germany, the Filderklinik Stuttgart or Herdecke Community Hospital both offer these services.

10.9.5 Summary

Our recent work documents the crucial importance of sympathetically searching for expanded biographical connections. The two new case studies in this chapter (▸Chap. 10.9.3.2.2 and ▸Chap. 3) are not extreme cases, but are typicalof the last four years in our practice. Other colleagues have corroborated the value of these connections and treatment principles *for the first 7-year period*. Our patients have taught us that one must ask specifically about background and events, which are typically not viewed as essential for accurate diagnosis. Intense and active listening is essential, since these details are almost never given spontaneously as part of the presenting history.

Our own records show that all the mothers experienced profound disappointment, trauma, or depression in connection with the child's pregnancy, birth, or postpartum period. The striking fact is that when these situations were discussed, all the mothers spontaneously said they had found them stressful, but the physician often did not understand their significance and emotional burden for the mother. Two cases (▸Chap. 10.9.3.2.2 and ▸Chap. 3) also now show the need to listen carefully to father's connections as well.

Hopefully, this growing holistic understanding of parenthood, in all its nuances, will lead to amelioration and prevention of childhood rheumatic conditions. We must truly perceive these mothers, fathers, and families, and then provide effective support for them.

As far as the children are concerned, it holds true that in many cases:

- They often experienced or shared early *trauma* suffered by their mothers in the pregnancy, birth, or breast-feeding period, but do not consciously remember.
- They are *often overly attached to their family*, easily hurt, and often hurtful to others, too.
- *Jealousy* of particular siblings is striking as is the need to have exclusive rights to the parents' attention.
- Conflict between parents and grandparents or serious illness in the grandparents, especially depression and immobilizing diseases, stresses the children. There is often notable difficulty and discord at the parent-grandparent level. This also applies to a child, for instance, with PFAPA(Periodic Fever, Aphthous stomatitis, Pharyngitis, Adenitis) syndrome, a condition on the spectrum of rheumatic diseases.

The efficacy of complementary anthroposophic and homoeopathic treatment will be enhanced by more accurate background history, focused treatment on individual aetiology, age, and the type of disease. Again and again, the process of taking a personal biographic history becomes therapeutic. It offers the patient the experience of being truly perceived by another individual, so profound for each of us that it opens the way to cure, to accepting our own destiny, and to recognizing our self. Every practioner with experience in rheumatology knows that the standard treatment also does not always prove satisfactory and that much is still unknown about long-term consequences. "A critical review of the scientific basis of anti-inflammatory and immunosuppressive therapy reveals the limitations of our knowledge. Yet, despite this ambiguity, these medications must be considered since there is no better alternative." [Horneff and Wahn 2005, 64.6]. These profound words remain true despite increased knowledge of biological medicines. Inspite of their risks, their use can be liberating, offering mobility and freedom from pain that was previously unimaginable. Responsible physicians must be open to all treatment options and seek even more complete communication with the child, parents, and young adults.

10.10 Postoperative treatment

The authors have found the following helpful in post-operative treatment of surgical interventions, including dental extractions:

- **Traumeel Tablets,** Heel®: 1 tablet 5 times/day – *start* only *after* the operation.

This effectively supports wound healing, the resorption of haematomas, and prevention of secondary wound infections.

It is important for patients to avoid all sugar, especially puddings and sweetened drinks, in the recovery stage. Careful attention must be paid to any immobilization required.

To support the circulation and stabilize patients mentally, preoperatively in case of anxieties and sleep disorders, use

- **Aurum/Valeriana comp. pillules.** Wala
  5–10 pillules 5 times/day.

Immediately on emerging from the anaesthetic and to encourage rapid detoxication:

- **Gentiana Magenglobuli** (stomach pillules) Wala
  3–7 pillules 1–3 times/day, depending on duration and depth of anaesthesia, up to 1 week postoperatively is useful.

For operations on the urethra, symptoms after cystoscopy or catheterization, and for all incisions that may have cosmetic consequences, it is helpful to prescribe:

- **Staphisagria D12** (various manuf.)
  5 pillules twice/day for 10–14 days.

Following abdominal procedures and appendectomy especially after perforation, as well as after surgeries in the thorax:

- **Bryonia e rad. D4–6 pillules** Wala
  depending on age and pain, 5–7 pillules, hourly to start.

To care for and treat surgical scars, the helpful combination of:

- **Narbengel** (scar gel; Keloid gel Wala alternating with
- **Echinacea/Viscum comp. Gel** Wala

For marked induration and keloids:

- **Polygonatum 5 % ointment** Weleda has proved effective as an external application.

Wound healing necessitates improved diet, immobilization, and:

- **Calendula D3 amp.** Wala,
  1 ampoule once/day by mouth,

And initially, irrigation with

- **Arnica or Calendula essence** Wala/Weleda diluted 1:10. Calendula is preferred if granulation is inadequate; Arnica if haematoma formation.

Later, or anytime there is excessive dryness:

- **Wecesin Puder (Powder)** Weleda, thinly applied externally several times/day.

References for Chapter 10

(every reference marked with a ■ Bullet point indicates the English translation of the reference above it)

Adebamowo C. A. et al.: High school dietary intake and acne. J Am Acad Dermatol **52,** 207–211. 2005.

Bernuth, G. von: Fetaler und neonataler Kreislauf. In: Pädiatrie. 2. Aufl., 1115–1117. Lentze, M. J., J. Schaub, F. J. Schulte, J. Spranger (Hrsg.). Springer, Berlin, New York 2003.

Deutsche Gesellschaft für Kinderheilkunde und Jugendmedizin: Leitlinien Kinderheilkunde und Jugendmedizin. Urban & Fischer, München 2010.

Fersch, B.: Der Sanddorn. In: Der Merkurstab **57**, 374–375 (2004)

Gasperi, S.: Das Geheimnis der Quelle von Levico-Vetriolo. Der Merkurstab **61,** 228–233 (2008).

Gerlach, L.: Arsen als Heilmittel. In: Rundbrief **29** (1998) der Medizinischen Sektion am Goetheanum, Dornach, 134–139

Girke, M.: Innere Medizin. Salumed Verlag, Berlin 2010.

■ English translation in progress at this time – Ed.

Grah, T.: Therapie einer primär chronischen Polyarthritis mit begleitender Iridocyclitis. Der Merkurstab **55,** 466–467 (2002).

Grandgeorge, D.: Homöopathische Arzneimittelbilder in der Kinderheilkunde. 2. Aufl. Sonntag Verlag, Stuttgart 2004.

Hove JC, Köster, RW, Foronhar, AS, Aurdeo-Bolton G, Fraser SE, Gharib, M: Intracardial fluid forces are an essential epigenetic factor for embryonic cardiogenesis. Nature **421** (2003); www.nature.com/nature (nach einem Hinweis von A. Husemann).

Hildebrandt, G.: Die Zeitgestalt des Herz-Kreislauf-Systems. In: Das Herz des Menschen. 149–188. Bavastro, P., H. C. Kümmell (Hrsg.). Verlag Freies Geistesleben, Stuttgart 1999.

Horneff, G., V. Wahn: Juvenile idiopathische Arthritis. In: Pädiatrische Allergologie und Immunologie. 4. Aufl. Wahn, Seger, Wahn, Holländer (Hrsg.). Urban & Fischer, München 2005.

Husemann, A.: Der Zahnwechsel des Kindes. Verlag Freies Geistesleben, Stuttgart 1996.

Jachens, L.: Die Behandlung von Hautkrankheiten über die Leber. Der Merkurstab **57**, 248–259 (2004).

Joseph A. et al.: Immunologic rheumatic disorders. American Academy of Allergy, Asthma & Immunology,Published online: 10.1016/j.jaci.2009.10.067 (2010).

Kilner, P. J. et al.: Helical and Retrograde Secondary Flow Patterns in the Aortic Arch Studied by the Three-Directional Magnetic Resonance Velouty Mapiry. Circulation **88**, 2235–2247 (1993). Die MR-Aufnahmen von Kilner (Royal-Bromptom-Hospit in London) können via Internet heruntergeladen werden.

Kühne, T., P. Imbach: Idiopathische thrombozytopenische Purpura im Kindesalter. Mschr. f. Kinderheilkunde **154**, 533–539 (2006).

Kümmell, H. C., H.Bettermann: Ergebnisse rhythmologischer Untersuchungen von Cardiodoron am Gesunden. In: Der Merkurstab **49**, 361–371 (1996).

Lauböck, H.: Die Neubewertung der Physiologie von Herz- und Blutbewegung. In: Das Herz des Menschen. 104–130. Bavastro, P., H. C. Kümmell (Hrsg.). Verlag Freies Geistesleben, Stuttgart 1999.

Laue, B. von: Das Blut als Organ des Menschen II. Der Merkurstab **2**, 135 (1995).

Maerker-Stromer, J., P. Höger: Häufige dermatologische Probleme im Kindesalter. Consilium infectiorum **15**, 3, 23–26 (2005).

Melnik, B.: Acne vulgaris. Die Rolle der Diät. Hautarzt **61**, 115–125 (2010).

Müller-Mohnsen, H.: Kontroversen zur Toxizität von Pyrethrum und Pyrethroiden. Internistische Praxis **32**, 2231–2232 (1994).

Roder, F.: Die Mondknoten im Lebenslauf. Verlag Freies Geistesleben, Stuttgart 2005.

Rohen, J. W.: Morphologie des menschlichen Organismus. Verlag Freies Geistesleben, Stuttgart 2000.

- Rohen, J. W.: Functional morphology : the dynamic wholeness of the human organism. Adonis Press, Hillsdale, N. Y. 2007.

Schwarz, R.: Kongenitaler AV-Block II. und III. Grades bei einem 20 Tage alten Neugeborenen. Behandlung mit Cardiodoron mite. Der Merkurstab **58,** 293–296 (2005).

Simon, L: Arzneimittelfindung am Beispiel chronische Polyarthritis. In: Anthroposophische Arzneitherapie. Bd. 1. M. Glöckler (Hrsg.). Wissenschaftliche Verlagsgesellschaft, Stuttgart (2005a).

Simon, L.: "Unerkannte Perlen"im anthroposophischen Arzneimittelschatz. Der Merkurstab **58**, 133–139 (2005b).

Skrabl-Baumgartner, A., Hauer, A.: Biologika in der pädiatrischen Rheumatologie und Gastroenterologie. pädpraxis **72,** 171–186 (2008).

Soldner, G.: Polygonatum officinale 5 % alsExternum bei Phimose. Der Merkurstab **58**, 51 (2005).

Soldner, G., J. Wilkens, M. Sommer: Magnesium chloratum. Der Merkurstab **59,** 112–122 (2006).

Sommer, M.: Kopflausbehandlung – nur mit dem Risiko neurologischer Schäden? Der Merkurstab **47**, 484–486 (1994).

Sommer, M.: Möglichkeiten der Kopflausbehandlung. Der Merkurstab **55**, 470–472 (2002).

Steiner, R., I. Wegman: Grundlegendes zu einer Erweiterung der Heilkunst. Gesamtausgabe Bd. 27. 7. Aufl. Rudolf Steiner Verlag, Dornach 1991.

- Steiner, R., I. Wegman: Fundamentals of therapy : an extension of the art of healing through spiritual-scientific knowledge. GA (complete works) 027. Mercury Press, Spring Valley, N. Y. 1999. Also available as: Extending practical medicine: fundamental principles based on the science of the spirit. Rudolf Steiner Press, London 1996.

Steiner, R.: Geisteswissenschaftliche Gesichtspunkte zur Therapie. Gesamtausgabe Bd. 313. 4. Aufl. Rudolf Steiner Verlag, Dornach 1984.

- Steiner, R.: Anthroposophical spiritual science and medical therapy: second medical course, nine lectures to physicians and medical students, Dornach, April 11–18, 1921. GA (complete works) 313. Mercury Press, Spring Valley, N. Y. 1991.

Steiner, R.: Die Offenbarungen des Karma. Gesamtausgabe Bd. 120. Philosophisch-anthroposophischer Verlag, Dornach 1949. R.Steiner Verlag, Dornach, 8. Aufl.1992.

- Steiner, R. Manifestations of karma: eleven lectures given in Hamburg between 16 and 28 May 1910. Rudolf Steiner Press, London 2010.

Steiner, R.: Eine okkulte Physiologie.Gesamtausgabe Bd. 128. Rudolf Steiner Verlag, Dornach 4. Aufl.1978,5.Aufl. 1991.

- Steiner, R.: An occult physiology: eight lectures given in Prague, 20th to 28th March, 1911. GA (complete works) 128. Rudolf Steiner Press, London 1983.

Steiner, R.: Das Initiatenbewusstsein. Gesamtausgabe Bd. 243 Rudolf Steiner Verlag, Dornach 5. Aufl.1993.

- Steiner, R.: True and false paths in spiritual investigation. GA (complete works) 243. Rudolf Steiner Press/Anthroposophic Press, London/New York 1985.

Steiner, R.: Heilpädagogischer Kurs. Gesamtausgabe Bd. 317. R.Steiner Verlag, Dornach, 8. Aufl.1995.

- Steiner, R.: Education for special needs: the curative education course; twelve lectures for doctors and teachers given at Dornach between 25 June and 7 July 1924. GA (complete works) 317. Rudolf Steiner Press, London 1998.

Steiner, R.: Mediative Betrachtungen und Anleitungen zur Vertiefung der Heilkunst. Gesamtausgabe Bd. 316. Rudolf Steiner Verlag, Dornach, 3. Aufl. 1987.

Stiegele, A.: Zur homöopathischen Behandlung des Lungenabszesses und der fötiden Bronchitis mit Sulfur iodatum. In: Klinische Homöopathie. 5. Aufl. 175–180. Stiegele, A. (Hrsg.). Hippokrates Verlag, Stuttgart 1955.

Tautz, C.: Juvenile idiopathische Arthritis, Komplementäre Therapie. In: Pädiatrie integrativ. Kap.35.1. Schönau, Naumann, Längler, Beuth (Hrsg.). Urban & Fischer, München 2005.

Vademecum Anthroposophische Arzneimittel. 2. Aufl. Der Merkurstab **63**, Supplement (2010).

- Vademecum of anthroposophic medicines, CD format. Medical Section of the School of Spiritual Science, Dornach, Switzerland 2009.

Verhulst, J.: Der Erstgeborene. Verlag Freies Geistesleben, Stuttgart 1999.

Vogel, S.: erkranken – heilen – gesunden: Neue Wege in der Augenheilkunde. L. Staackmann Verlag, München 2. Aufl. 2004.

Wagner, N., Dannecker, G.: Pädiatrische Rheumatologie. Springer, Berlin 2007.

Wahn, V.: Juvenile rheumatoide Arthritis. In: Pädiatrische Allergologie und Immunologie. 3. Aufl. Wahn, Seger, Wahn (Hrsg.). Urban & Fischer, München 1999.

Watanabe: Henoch-Schönlein purpura folllowing influenza vaccinations during the pandemic of influenza A (H1N1). Pediatr. Nephrol published online DOI 10.1007/s00467-010-1722-8.

Weckenmann, M.: Normalisierung neurovegetativ gesteuerter Funktionen durch medikamentöse Langzeittherapie. Therapie über dasNervensystem. Bd. 11. Groß, D. (Hrsg.). Hippokrates, Stuttgart 1973.

Weckenmann, M.: Die Anwendung von Cardiodoron in der Praxis und die dabei beobachteten Wirkungen – Ergebnisse einer Umfrage. Beitr. z. Erw. d. Heilkunst **39**, 245–253 (1986).

Weiß, R. F., V. Fintelmann: Lehrbuch der Phytotherapie. 9. Aufl. Hippokrates, Stuttgart 1999.

Weller, F. et al.: Purpura Schoenlein-Henoch. pädiatrische praxis **70**, 77–92.

11 Eurythmy therapy: principles of effectiveness, areas of application

"At the Waldorf School we had children with such deficits almost from the beginning ... it was not possible for them to follow lessons. A special class was established for these children (...) Observations showed that eurythmy provided something which would get through to them more than anything else, something which they were able to take up directly.
Close involvement with the 'difficult cases', as they were called, led to the most intensive desire to understand the more 'specific' healing elements of eurythmy"
E. Baumann [1952, 7–9]

This is how Elisabeth Baumann, the first eurythmy teacher at the newly established Waldorf School in Stuttgart, described the historic starting point that led to the development of eurythmy therapy. R. Steiner's eurythmy course for physicians and eurythmists was given at a medical conference for anthroposophic medicine in 1921. Paediatrics and education had provided the occasion for this.

Eurythmy therapy is a movement therapy in tune with the modern state of consciousness. Like speech, it covers all levels of human individuality and in this differs from forms of movement that relate only to specific physical problems, e. g. physiotherapy. With eurythmy therapy, the interaction of the human being's powers of soul and spirit as well as the body are taken up and put to therapeutic use.

Eurythmy therapy evolved from the eurythmy which Rudolf Steiner had created as an art form. In eurythmy, the rhythms and sounds of speech – vowels and consonants – are represented in corresponding movements, speech sound forms and rhythms. In eurythmy therapy, these movements and their moods are in effect "reflected" back into the organism of the moving individual instead of being performed for an audience on stage. With eurythmy therapy, the focus is on the interaction which can be achieved by doing certain movements relating to diseased areas of the organism. This is done in a fully awake and attentive state of mind. The patient's individual soul and spirit is thus directed towards certain vital processes, stimulating, modifying and regulating their physiological activities. The vital processes can thus in turn be given impulses, new strength and form. As a result, living powers of growth and healing flow more intensively in the physical body.

The condition R. Steiner [1981, 118] gave when establishing this therapy was "that it should not be used without consulting the physician." The basis is a diagnosis where it is possible to distinguish the physical condition, the dynamics of the life organization, the activity of the soul sphere and the spiritual individuality of the patient and to describe these aspects in a more or less differentiated way. The nature and sequence of the sound movements and rhythms seeks to respond directly to disorders within the above aspects and the way they work together. Eurythmy therapy may be used in treatment and prevention.

Important areas of indication in paediatrics are [see also Kirchner-Bockholdt 1997]:

- allergic conditions, above all asthma (▸Chap. 6.5.5.3) and allergic rhinitis (▸Chap. 6.6.3.3), and also neurodermatitis from the 5th to 7th year of life,
- disorders of pneumatization and resistance to infection, e. g. recurrent sinusitis, adenoids and problems with middle ear ventilaton, bronchitis etc., but not in stages of acute inflammation (▸Chap. 5.1.2.6),
- psychosomatic disorders – anxieties, sleep disorders at school age, enuresis nocturna, migraine, adiposity and anorexia,
- problems at school – attention and concentration problems (ADHS, ▸Chap. 7.5.3.3), lateralization and coordination problems, legasthenia,
- disorders of motor development, motor coordination,
- delayed speech development, stammer,
- visual disorders, with eye movements (special eurythmy therapy for eyes),
- postural and skeletal problems, e. g. scoliosis (▸Chap. 9.3.3), malformation of jaws, osteogenesis imperfecta,
- rheumatic diseases (▸Chap. 10.9.5),
- chronic intestinal diseases,
- the field of special needs education.

In eurythmy therapy children acquire a special, new capacity for movement which addresses their sense and capacity for movement, their sentience and conscious awareness to an equal degree. The aim is to have the child make a consciously done and ensouled movement that will evoke a therapeutic effect in the body. This can at the same time create a counterbalance to mainly mechanical movements directed towards goals devoid of meaning such as competitive sports, for instance. It is to be expected that the need for ensouled, meaningful movement of this kind will grow in future. Recently the therapeutic effect of eurythmy therapy has also be the subject of more broad-based empirical research [see e. g. Langerhorst und Petersen 1999]; a representative cohort study under practice conditions has demonstrated the lasting efficacy of eurythmy therapy [Hamre 2004]. H. B. and E. von Laue have provided eurythmy therapy systematics and a comprehensive literature review [2007]. We would recommend a study of this to anyone who is interested. The comprehensive bibliography for eurythmy therapy published in 2007 [Hachtel, Gaech 2007] contains a full study of sources and the published scientific literature on eurythmy therapy with systematic references (list of indications, list of speech sound sequences, list of all case studies, and literature summaries). The authors are most grateful for this comprehensive bibliography which can again and again provide guidance.

References for Chapter 11

(every reference marked with a ▪ Bullet point indicates the English translation of the reference above it)

Baumann, E.: Einleitung zum Heileurythmiekurs R. Steiners. Rudolf Steiner Verlag, Dornach 1952.

Hachtel, B, Gäch, A.: Bibliographie Heileurythmie. 3. Aufl. Natur-Mensch-Medizin Verlag, Bad Boll 2007.

Hamre, J. H. et al.: Anthroposophic Therapies in Chronic Disease: The Anthroposophic Medicine Outcomes Study (AMOS). Eur. J. Med. Res. **9,** 351–360 (2004).

Kirchner-Bockholdt, M.: Grundelemente der Heil-Eurythmie. Philosophisch-Anthroposophischer Verlag, Dornach 1962, 4. Aufl. 1997.

- Kirchner-Bockholt, M.: Fundamental principles of curative eurythmy. Rudolf Steiner Press, London 1977.

Langerhorst, U., P. Petersen: Heileurythmie – ihre Wirkung und ihre wissenschaftliche Bewertung. Urachhaus, Stuttgart 1999.

Laue, H. B. v., E. von Laue: Zur Physiologie der Heileurythmie. Lautgesetze und Therapieordnungen. Verlag am Goetheanum, Dornach/Schweiz 2007.

- Laue, H. B. v., E. Von Laue: The physiology of eurythmy therapy. Floris Books, Forest Row, England 2010.

Steiner, R.: Heileurythmie. Rudolf Steiner Verlag, Dornach 4. Aufl. 1981.

- Steiner, R.: Eurythmy therapy : 8 lectures given in Dornach, Switzerland, 12–18 Apr 1921, and in Stuttgart, Germany on 28 Oct 1922. GA (complete works) 315. Rudolf Steiner Press, Forest Row, England 2009.

12 Epilogue

The authors' intention with this book is to offer food for thought and concrete help to as many colleagues as possible in their daily striving to do their best for their patients. A complete coverage of paediatrics was not intended. In order to serve the individualization of paediatrics it was necessary to go beyond generally available knowledge and to include our own insights as well as the fruit of collegial conversations and therapeutic experience. Important areas of paediatrics are not covered in this book: for lack of time, experience or competency. The authors regret this, particularly regarding therapeutic education and child and adolescent psychiatry.

f anthroposophic and
edition in its first-ever
tics, vaccinations,
w and further elaborated
, atopic dermatitis,
ts of individual history
ed.

ntegrative medicine is
nd adolescents and
t is an individual
nstitution, psychological
tal circumstances,
hild develops a particular
w to the future and
port of their potential.

logical data
s
medicine

s

nd spiritual aspects

.com

0000

Individual Paediatrics

Soldner / Stellmann

MedPharm

CRC

Soldner / St

Indiv
Paed

Physical, em
of diagnosis
Anthroposop